Manual of
Cardiology

Manual of Cardiology

Kanu Chatterjee
MBBS FRCP (London) FRCP (Edin) FCCP FACC MACP

Clinical Professor of Medicine
Division of Cardiology
The Carver College of Medicine
University of Iowa
Iowa City, Iowa, USA

Emeritus Professor of Medicine
University of California, San Francisco
California, USA

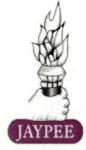

JAYPEE BROTHERS MEDICAL PUBLISHERS
The Health Sciences Publisher
New Delhi | London

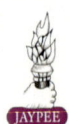

Jaypee Brothers Medical Publishers (P) Ltd

Headquarters
EMCA House
23/23-B, Ansari Road, Daryaganj
New Delhi 110 002, India
Landline: +91-11-23272143, +91-11-23272703
+91-11-23282021, +91-11-23245672
E-mail: jaypee@jaypeebrothers.com

Corporate Office
Jaypee Brothers Medical Publishers (P) Ltd.
4838/24, Ansari Road, Daryaganj
New Delhi 110 002, India
Phone: +91-11-43574357
Fax: +91-11-43574314
E-mail: jaypee@jaypeebrothers.com

Overseas Office
JP Medical Ltd.
83, Victoria Street, London
SW1H 0HW (UK)
Phone: +44-20 3170 8910
E-mail: info@jpmedpub.com

EU GPSR Authorised Representative
Logos Europe, 9 rue Nicolas Poussin
17000, La Rochelle, France
Phone: +33 (0) 6 67 93 73 78
E-mail: Contact@logoseurope.eu

Website: www.jaypeebrothers.com
Website: www.jaypeedigital.com

© 2014, Jaypee Brothers Medical Publishers

The views and opinions expressed in this bo those of the original contributor(s)/author(s) and do not necessarily represent those of editor(s) of the book.

All rights reserved. No part of this publication may be reproduced, stored or transmitted in any form or by any means, electronic, mechanical, photocopying, recording or otherwise, without the prior permission in writing of the publishers.

All brand names and product names used in this book are trade names, service marks, trademarks or registered trademarks of their respective owners. The publisher is not associated with any product or vendor mentioned in this book.

Medical knowledge and practice change constantly. This book is designed to provide accurate, authoritative information about the subject matter in question. However, readers are advised to check the most current information available on procedures included and check information from the manufacturer of each product to be administered, to verify the recommended dose, formula, method and duration of administration, adverse effects and contraindications. It is the responsibility of the practitioner to take all appropriate safety precautions. Neither the publisher nor the author(s)/editor(s) assume any liability for any injury and/or damage to persons or property arising from or related to use of material in this book.

This book is sold on the understanding that the publisher is not engaged in providing professional medical services. If such advice or services are required, the services of a competent medical professional should be sought.

Every effort has been made where necessary to contact holders of copyright to obtain permission to reproduce copyright material. If any have been inadvertently overlooked, the publisher will be pleased to make the necessary arrangements at the irst opportunity.

Inquiries for bulk sales may be solicited at: jaypee@jaypeebrothers.com

Manual of Cardiology

First Edition: 2014, Reprint: **2025**

ISBN 978-93-5152-175-4

Printed in India

Preface

Our knowledge of and ability to treat all kinds of cardiovascular diseases have expanded exponentially in the past few decades. *Manual of Cardiology* provides an up-to-date, practical, and concise text on the evaluation, diagnosis, management, and prevention of a wide spectrum of cardiovascular disease.

The advances in cardiovascular pharmacology have also been considerable. The advantages and disadvantages of diuretic therapy, vasodilators, neurohormone modulators, positive inotropic agents, antilipid, and antithrombotic and antiplatelet agents have been discussed. The clinical pharmacology of these agents in the management of various cardiovascular disorders has been emphasized. During the last two decades, we have witnessed enormous advances in the understanding of the genesis of atrial and ventricular arrhythmias, in the techniques of electrophysiologic and the pharmacologic and nonpharmacologic treatment of arrhythmias, which have been discussed in detail. The new therapeutic modalities for the management of chronic coronary artery diseases have been discovered and devoted to discussion. The diagnosis and management of valvular heart disease and heart failure are discussed in detail as well as chemotherapy and radiation-induced cardiovascular disorders. I have also added modified guidelines for the management of angina, arrhythmias, heart failure, valvular heart diseases, and perioperative cardiac evaluations.

The Manual can serve as a quick reference or a stand-alone source with a focus on hands-on therapeutic guidance for the clinicians. With numerous tables, figures, and algorithms, this book provides the reader with easily accessible information in the most appropriate manner.

Kanu Chatterjee

Contents

1. Cardiovascular Pharmacology　　　1

1.1　Diuretics　1
Introduction　1
Classification of the diuretic compounds　1
Clinical pharmacology of the diuretic compounds　2
Adaptive responses to diuretic administration　4
Individual diuretic classes　5
Clinical use of diuretics in cardiovascular diseases　11
Adverse effects of diuretics　15

1.2　Vasodilators and Neurohormone Modulators　18
Introduction　18
Vasodilator drugs and low blood pressure　19
Arteriolar vasodilators　19
Renin–angiotensin–aldosterone system (RAAS) blockers　22
Mineralocorticoid (aldosterone) receptor blockers　26
Phosphodiesterase type 5 inhibitors　28
Intravenous vasodilators　28
Oral β-adrenergic blocking drugs　29

1.3　Positive Inotropic Drugs　32
Introduction　32
*Intravenously administered, short-term
　positive inotropic therapy　32*

1.4　Antilipid Agents　41
Introduction　41
Appropriate uses　42
Statins　43
Add-on to statin therapy　50
Bile acid sequestrants　50
Ezetimibe　51
Niacin　51
Triglyceride-lowering therapy　52
Fibrates　52
Omega-3 fatty acids　53
Drugs in development　54

1.5　Antithrombotic and Antiplatelet Agents　54
Introduction　54
Clotting, A primer　55
Antithrombotic agents　55
Vitamin K antagonists (VKA)　58
Direct factor Xa inhibitors　59
Direct thrombin inhibitors　60
Antiplatelet agents　63

2. Diagnosis 70

2.1 History and Physical Examination 70
History 70
Physical examination 75

2.2 Plain Film Imaging of Adult Cardiovascular Disease 90
Introduction 90
Chest film technique 90
Cardiac anatomy on chest radiographs 91
Cardiac chamber enlargement 92
Radiographic manifestations of congestive heart failure 96
Cardiac calcifications 98
Acquired valvular heart disease 98
Pericardial disorders 100

2.3 Electrocardiogram 101
Introduction 101
Basis of electrocardiography 101
Component parts of the electrocardiogram 102
Lead systems used to record the electrocardiogram 102
A systematic way of looking at the interpretation of the electrocardiogram 103
Characterization of QRS complex 108
ST–T wave abnormalities 112
"U" wave 113
QT interval 113

2.4 ECG Exercise Testing 115
Introduction 115
Before the test 115
Methodology of exercise testing 117
During the test 119
After the test 126
Screening 128

2.5 Left Ventricle 132
Introduction 132
Systolic function 132
Contrast-enhanced echocardiography 134
Other echo-derived indices of left ventricular systolic function 134
Strain-derived indices 135
Recognizing the etiology of cardiac dysfunction 135
Visual qualitative indicators of systolic dysfunction 135
Diastolic function 136

2.6 Transthoracic Echocardiography 139
Introduction 139
Chamber quantitation 141
Doppler ECHO 143
Diastolic function 143
Pulmonary hypertension 144
Pericardial disease 144

Valvular heart disease　145
　　　Infective endocarditis　148
　　　Intracardiac masses　148
　　　Contrast echocardiography　149
　　　Cardiac resynchronization therapy　149

2.7　Stress Echocardiography　150
　　　Introduction　150
　　　Using stress echocardiography in clinical decisions　150
　　　Future of stress ECHO　155

2.8　Transesophageal Echocardiography　156
　　　Introduction　156
　　　Performance　156
　　　Safety　156
　　　Views　156
　　　Major clinical applications　158
　　　Structural valve assessment　161
　　　Acute aortic dissection　164
　　　Procedural adjunct or intraoperative transesophageal
　　　　echocardiography　165

**2.9　Cardiovascular Nuclear Medicine—
　　　Nuclear Cardiology　167**
　　　Introduction　167
　　　Myocardial perfusion imaging　167
　　　Positron emission tomography perfusion and metabolism　169
　　　Imaging myocardial viability　169
　　　Imaging perfusion　171
　　　Radiation concerns　172

2.10　Cardiac Computed Tomography　173
　　　Introduction　173
　　　Coronary artery disease　173
　　　Myocardium and chambers　176
　　　Pulmonary veins　176
　　　Cardiac veins　177
　　　Valvular disease　177
　　　Pericardium　177
　　　Future　177

2.11　Cardiovascular Magnetic Resonance Imaging　178
　　　Introduction　178
　　　Diagnosis of epicardial coronary artery stenosis　178
　　　Assessment of global and regional left ventricular function
　　　　at rest and during inotropic stress　179
　　　Myocardial perfusion imaging　179
　　　Cardiovascular magnetic resonance coronary angiography　180
　　　Dilated cardiomyopathy　181
　　　Hypertrophic cardiomyopathy　181
　　　Restrictive cardiomyopathy　181
　　　Cardiovascular magnetic resonance-guided therapy　182
　　　Valvular heart disease　182
　　　Diseases with right ventricular predominance　182
　　　Miscellaneous conditions　183

2.12 Molecular Imaging of Vascular Disease 184
Introduction 184
Molecular imaging modalities 184
Molecular imaging of vascular disease processes 186

2.13 Cardiac Hemodynamics and Coronary Physiology 190
Introduction 190
Cardiac catheterization—the basics 190
Cardiac cycle pressure waveforms 192
Hemodynamics in valvular heart disease 193
Hemodynamics in cardiomyopathy 197
Hemodynamics in pericardial disease 198
Coronary hemodynamics 200

2.14 Cardiac Biopsy 201
Introduction 201
Techniques 201
Safety and complications 202
Analysis of EMB tissue 203
Indications 204

2.15 Coronary Angiography and Catheter-based Coronary Intervention 207
Introduction 207
Indications for coronary angiography 207
Contraindications for coronary angiography 207
Patient preparation 209
Sites and techniques of vascular access 209
Catheters for coronary angiography 211
Arterial nomenclature and extent of disease 211
Angiographic projections 212
Congenital anomalies of the coronary circulation 213
General principles for coronary and/or graft cannulation 214
Fluoroscopic imaging system 214
Characteristics of contrast media 214
Access site hemostasis 215
Complications of cardiac catheterization 216
Percutaneous coronary intervention 217
Pharmacotherapy for PCI 221
Parenteral anticoagulant therapy 222
Percutaneous transluminal coronary angioplasty 222
Coronary stents 223
Types of stents 223
Procedural success and complications related to coronary intervention 223

3. Electrophysiology 226

3.1 Arrhythmia Mechanisms 226
Introduction 226
Arrhythmia initiation 226

3.2 Antiarrhythmic Drugs 234
Introduction 234

Arrhythmia mechanisms and antiarrhythmic drugs 234
Indications for antiarrhythmic drug therapy 234
Classification scheme 235
Vaughan–Williams classification 235
Antiarrhythmic drug selection in atrial fibrillation 239
Outpatient versus in-hospital initiation for antiarrhythmic drug therapy 240
Antiarrhythmic drugs in pregnancy and lactation 241
Comparing antiarrhythmic drugs to implantable cardioverter defibrillators in patients at risk of arrhythmic death 242
Antiarrhythmic drug–device interactions 242

3.3 Syncope 243
Introduction 243
Diagnostic tests 245
Approach to the evaluation of syncope 250

3.4 Atrial Fibrillation 253
Introduction 253
Definition and Classification 253
Etiology and Pathogenesis 254
Diagnosis 256
Management 257

3.5 Supraventricular Tachycardia 261
Introduction 261
Classification 261
Diagnosis 265
Treatments 266

3.6 Clinical Spectrum of Ventricular Tachycardia 271
Introduction 271
Monomorphic ventricular tachycardia 272

3.7 Bradycardia and Heart Block 280
Introduction 280
Bradycardia syndromes/diseases 280
Clinical presentation 281
Measurement/diagnosis 281
Sinus node disease 282
AV node disease 282
Hemiblock 283
Bundle branch block 284
Treatment 284

3.8 Arrhythmogenic Right Ventricular Dysplasia/ Cardiomyopathy 285
Introduction 285
Molecular and genetic background 285
Clinical presentation 287
Clinical diagnosis 288
Nonclassical ARVD/C subtypes 289
Molecular genetic analysis 289
Prognosis and therapy 290

3.9 Long QT, Short QT, and Brugada Syndromes 291
Introduction 291
LQT syndrome 291
Brugada syndrome 294

3.10 Cardiac Resynchronization Therapy 296
Introduction 296
CRT: rationale for use 296
CRT in practice 296
Summary of CRT benefit 296
Prediction of response to CRT therapy 299
Role of dyssynchrony imaging 300
Dyssynchrony summary 300
CRT complications 300
Emerging CRT indications 300

3.11 Ambulatory Electrocardiographic Monitoring 305
Introduction 305
Holter monitoring 305
Event recorders 307
Mobile cardiac outpatient telemetry 308
Implantable loop recorders 308

3.12 Cardiac Arrest and Resuscitation 311
Introduction 311
Basic life support 312
Advanced cardiac life support 315
Risks 316
Cessation of resuscitation 318
Postresuscitation care 318

3.13 Risk Stratification for Sudden Cardiac Death 319
Introduction 319
Healthy athletes 319
Brugada syndrome 320
Long QT interval syndrome 320
Early repolarization 320
Short QT syndrome 320
Catecholamine polymorphic ventricular tachycardia 320
Wolff–Parkinson–White syndrome 321
Marfan's syndrome 321
Congenital heart disease 321
Nonischemic cardiomyopathy 322
Coronary artery disease 322

4. Coronary Heart Diseases 324

4.1 Coronary Heart Disease: Risk Factors 324
Introduction 324
CHD screening and prevention 325
Clustering and multiplicative effects of risk factors 325
CHD risk estimation 325
Traditional CHD risk factors 328
Emerging risk factors 332
Subclinical atherosclerosis 332

Translating risk factor screening into event reduction 332

4.2 Acute Coronary Syndrome (Unstable Angina and Non-ST-Segment Elevation Myocardial Infarction): Diagnosis and Early Treatment 333

Introduction 333
Unstable angina and non-ST-segment 333
Clinical features 333
Risk stratification—putting it all together to determine the optimal treatment strategy 336
Early medical therapy 336
Early invasive or initial conservative strategy 340
Revascularization 341

4.3 Acute Coronary Syndrome II (ST-Elevation, Myocardial Infarction, and Post-Myocardial Infarction): Complications and Care 343

Introduction 343
Clinical presentation 343
Reperfusion 345
Early medical therapy 347
Postmyocardial infarction care 348
Complications 350
Special considerations 351
Continued medical therapy for patients with a myocardial infarction 351

4.4 Management of Patients with Coronary Artery Disease and Stable Angina 354

Introduction 354
Current therapeutic approaches for stable angina 354
Antianginal drug therapy 354
Newer antianginal drugs 356
Combination therapy 357
Other drugs in patients with stable angina and chronic CAD 357
Role of myocardial revascularization 357
Comparison of revascularization with pharmacological antianginal therapy 358

4.5 Cardiogenic Shock in Acute Coronary Syndromes 360

Introduction 360
Pathophysiology 360
Other cardiac causes of cardiogenic shock 361
Diagnostic evaluation 363
Medical management 363
Mechanical support 363
Revascularization 363

4.6 Acute Right Ventricular Infarction 364

Introduction 364
Patterns of coronary compromise resulting in RVI 364
Effects of ischemia on RV systolic and diastolic function 365
Effects of reperfusion on ischemic RV dysfunction 365
Rhythm disorders and reflexes associated with RVI 366

Clinical Presentations and Evaluation 366
Noninvasive and hemodynamic evaluation 367
Differential diagnosis of RVI 367
Therapy 367

5. Valvular Heart Diseases   369

5.1 Aortic Valve Disease 369
Aortic stenosis 369
Aortic regurgitation 374

5.2 Mitral Valve Disease 380
Introduction 380
Rheumatic heart disease 380
Mitral stenosis 381
Mitral regurgitation 388

5.3 Tricuspid Valve Disease: Evaluation and Management 397
Introduction 397
Etiology of tricuspid valve disease 397
Clinical presentation 398
Laboratory diagnosis 399
Treatment 400

5.4 Congenital Pulmonic Stenosis 403
Introduction 403
Valvar pulmonic stenosis 403
Isolated infundibular stenosis 408
Supravalvar stenosis 409

5.5 Catheter-based Treatment of Valvular Heart Disease 410
Introduction 410
Catheter-based treatment of mitral valve disease 410
Catheter-based treatment of pulmonary valve disease 413
Catheter-based therapies for aortic stenosis 414

5.6 Infective Endocarditis 417
Introduction 417
Pathogenesis 418
Presentation and diagnosis 422
Management 425

5.7 Prosthetic Heart Valves 433
Risk of valve replacement 433
Types of prosthetic valves 434
Selecting the optimal prosthesis 434
Prosthesis-patient mismatch 437
Long-term management 441
Long-term complications 444

5.8 Antithrombotic Therapy in Valvular Heart Disease 451
Introduction 451
Prophylactic antithrombic therapy 452
Rheumatic valvular heart disease 453
Mitral valve prolapse 453
Calcified or degenerative valvular disease 453

Prosthetic valves 454
Bioprosthetic valves 454
Valvuloplasty and valve repair 455
Management issues 455

6. Vascular Diseases 458

6.1 Evaluation and Management of the Patient with Essential Hypertension 458
Evaluation of the patient with hypertension 458
Antihypertensive therapy 462
Hemodynamic concepts 463
Clinical pharmacologic concepts 463
Treatment algorithms advocated over the years 468

6.2 Peripheral Vascular and Cerebrovascular Disease 469
Introduction 469
Peripheral arterial disease 470
Carotid artery disease 477
Renal artery stenosis 479
Subclavian artery stenosis 480
Mesenteric ischemia 481

6.3 Aortic Dissection and Aneurysm 483
Aortic Dissection *483*
Introduction 483
Classification 483
Clinical examination 484
Diagnosis 485
Treatment 487
Aortic Aneurysm *489*
Introduction 489
Treatment 489
Anatomic substrate for endovascular aneurysm repair 490
Adjunctive devices and techniques 490
Endoleak 490
Late-occurring complications of endovascular aneurysm repair 491
Follow-up imaging 492

6.4 Autonomic Dysfunction and the Cardiovascular System 493
Introduction 493
Autonomic regulation of the cardiovascular system 493
Autonomic testing 495
Primary chronic autonomic failure 497
Secondary and congenital autonomic failure 498
Chronic orthostatic intolerance 498

7. Heart Failure 500

7.1 Diagnosis 500
Analysis of symptoms 500
Physical examination 501

Electrocardiogram 503
Chest radiograph 505
Echocardiography 505
Cardiac magnetic resonance and cardiac tomography 506
Biomarkers 507
Exercise tests and six-minute walk test 510
Myocardial ischemia 511
Genetic studies 512

7.2 Systolic Heart Failure (Heart Failure with Reduced Ejection Fraction) 513

Introduction 513
Ventricular remodeling 514
Functional derangements and hemodynamic consequences 519
Initial treatment of systolic heart failure 520
Symptomatic systolic heart failure 521
Nonpharmacologic treatments 524
Follow-up evaluation 525

7.3 Diastolic Heart Failure (Heart Failure with Preserved Ejection Fraction) 526

Definition 526
Epidemiology and risk factors 526
Pathophysiology 526
Future directions 532

7.4 Cardiorenal Syndrome: The Interplay between Cardiac and Renal Function in Patients with Congestive Heart Failure 534

Definition of the cardiorenal syndrome 534
Role of evidence-based therapies in patients with heart failure and the cardiorenal syndrome 536
Role of ultrafiltration on diuretic resistance and the cardiorenal syndrome 541
Treatment of the cardiorenal syndrome: an approach to the individual patient 541

7.5 Acute Heart Failure Syndromes 545

Introduction 545
Pathophysiology 546
Acute heart failure syndromes management 548
Clinical trials in acute heart failure syndromes 556

7.6 Cardiopulmonary Exercise Testing and Training in Heart Failure 558

Introduction 558
Exercise response in heart failure 559
Cardiopulmonary exercise testing 560
Indications for CPX testing in heart failure 565
Exercise training in heart failure 566

7.7 Advanced Cardiac Therapies for End-stage Heart Failure: Cardiac Transplantation and Mechanical Circulatory Support 568

Introduction 568

Identifying candidates for advanced cardiac therapies 569
Heart transplantation 571
Mechanical circulatory support 581
Future directions 587

8. Myocardial and Pericardial Diseases 591

8.1 Hypertrophic Cardiomyopathy 591
Introduction 591
Pathology 592
Clinical presentation 594
Diagnosis 595
Natural history 598
Management 599
Dual-chamber pacemaker 602

8.2 Dilated Cardiomyopathy 604
Introduction 604
Definition 604
Pathology 604
Etiology 605
Prognosis 608

8.3 Restrictive and Obliterative Cardiomyopathies 610
Introduction 610
Restrictive cardiomyopathies 610
Tropical endomyocardial fibrosis (Davie's disease) 612
Right ventricular endomyocardial fibrosis 612
Left ventricular endomyocardial fibrosis 613
Loeffler's endocarditis 614
Idiopathic restrictive cardiomyopathy 615

8.4 Specific Cardiomyopathies 616
Amyloid Heart Disease *616*
Introduction 616
Overview of cardiac amyloidosis 616
Classification of amyloidosis 617
Cardiac amyloidosis 617
Treatment 621
Peripartum Cardiomyopathy *623*
Introduction 623
Diagnosis 623
Prognosis 623
Treatment 624
Labor and delivery 624
Chemotherapy-induced Cardiomyopathy *625*
Introduction 625
Pathophysiology of anthracycline-induced cardiomyopathy 625
Mechanism of chemotherapy-induced cardiac dysfunction 626
Diagnosis 627
Monitoring 628
Preventive strategies 629
Treatment 629

8.5 Pericardial Disease 631
Introduction 631
Acute pericarditis 631
Chronic relapsing pericarditis 633
Pericardial effusion and pericardial tamponade 634
Constrictive pericarditis 635

8.6 Radiation-induced Heart Disease 641
Introduction 641
Radiation-induced pericardial disease 641
Radiation-induced myocardial disease 642
Radiation-induced coronary artery disease 643
Radiation-induced valvular heart disease 643
Conduction system disease 644
Prevention 644

9. Pulmonary Vascular Disease and Adult Congenital Heart Disease 646

9.1 Pulmonary Arterial Hypertension 646
Definitions and classifications 646
Pathophysiology of pulmonary arterial hypertension 649
Diagnostic evaluation 651
Therapeutic options for the treatment of pulmonary arterial hypertension 657
Treatment algorithm and evaluating response to therapy 661
Therapy of decompensated right heart failure in pulmonary arterial hypertension 662

9.2 Congenital Heart Disease in the Adult Patient 665
Acyanotic Heart Disease 665
Congenital valvar aortic stenosis 665
Coarctation of the aorta 667
Valvar pulmonic stenosis 670
Atrial septal defects 672
Ventricular septal defects 674
Patent ductus arteriosus 677
Other Acyanotic Lesions 680
Ebstein's Anomaly 680
Cyanotic Congenital Heart Disease 682
Palliative shunts 683
Tetralogy of Fallot 683
Truncus arteriosus 690
Total anomalous pulmonary venous return 691

10. Secondary Disorders of the Heart 695

10.1 Alcohol and Arrhythmia 695
Direct effects of ethanol exposure on heart cells and tissues 695
Ethanol ingestion and the normal cardiac conduction system 695

  *Binge drinking and transient clinical arrhythmias—
   holiday heart 695*
  *Alcohol consumption, chronic atrial fibrillation, and
   atrial flutter 696*
  Alcohol consumption and sudden cardiac death 696
  Summary and clinical guidelines 697

10.2 Insulin Resistance and Cardiomyopathy 698
  Introduction 698
  Diastolic heart failure and insulin resistance 698
  Myocardial energy metabolism 699
  Metabolic effects of insulin resistance 700
  Structural effects of insulin resistance 701
  Treatment 702

10.3 Cardiac Complications of Substance Abuse 705
  Introduction 705
  Substances of abuse 705
  Marijuana, tetrahydrocannabinol, hashish 710
  Club drugs: MDMA, GHB, ketamine, rohypnol 710
  Body image drugs 712
  Narcotics 712

10.4 HIV/AIDS and Cardiovascular Disease 713
  Introduction 713
  HIV and coronary heart disease 714
  Surrogate measures of atherosclerosis 716
  HIV-related left ventricular dysfunction and myocarditis 717
  Cerebrovascular disease 718
  Miscellaneous 718

10.5 Systemic Autoimmune Diseases and the Heart 719
  Rheumatoid arthritis 719
  Spondyloarthropathies 721
  Polymyositis—dermatomyositis 723
  Systemic lupus erythematosus 724

10.6 Neurogenic and Stress Cardiomyopathy 726
  Introduction 726
  Neurogenic cardiomyopathy 726
  Stress cardiomyopathy 729

10.7 Kidney and the Heart 732
  Introduction 732
  Pathophysiology 732
  Cardiovascular risk factors in chronic kidney disease 733
  *Spectrum of cardiovascular disease in
   chronic kidney disease 734*
  Diagnostic tests 736
  Principles of treatment of cardiovascular disease 738
  Kidney transplant recipients 738

10.8 Endocrine Heart Disease 740
  Introduction 740
  Diabetes mellitus 740
  Thyroid disease 742

Pituitary disorders 744
Adrenal disorders 745
Parathyroid disorders 747
Carcinoid syndrome 747

10.9 Venous Thromboembolism and Cor Pulmonale 749
Venous thromboembolism 749
Cor pulmonale 758

11. Relevant Issues in Clinical Cardiology 761

11.1 Noncardiac Surgery in Cardiac Patients 761
Introduction 761
Preoperative cardiac risk assessment 761
Preoperative diagnostic testing 764
Preoperative risk mitigation strategies 766
Intraoperative management 768
Management of patients with implanted electronic devices 768
Postoperative management 768

11.2 Gender and Cardiovascular Disease 770
Introduction 770
Prevalence of IHD in women 770
Identification of IHD risk factors in women 770
Assessment of symptoms and myocardial ischemia in women symptom assessment 771
Management of IHD in women 774
Heart failure in women 777
Gender and cardiac arrhythmias 777

11.3 Overview of the Athlete's Heart 779
Introduction 779
Exercise physiology and the athlete's heart: overview 779
Issues relevant to the cardiovascular care of athletes 780

11.4 Cardiovascular Aging 783
Introduction 783
Age-related changes 784
Clinical syndromes 785
Special issues 788

12. Preventive Strategies for Other Cardiovascular Diseases 790

12.1 Prevention of Heart Failure 790
Introduction 790
Staging of heart failure 790
Future perspectives 794

12.2 Stroke: Prevention and Treatment 795
Introduction 795
Definitions 795
Stroke as a symptom 796
Prevention 804

General acute treatment 804
Treatment of acute ischemic stroke 805
Treatment of acute hemorrhagic stroke 807
General in-hospital care and rehabilitation 808

12.3 Rheumatic Fever 810
Introduction 810
Pathogenesis 810
Diagnosis of rheumatic fever 811
Clinical features 812
Treatment 814

13. Evolving Concepts 818

13.1 Preventing Errors in Cardiovascular Medicine 818
Introduction 818
Modern approach to patient safety 818
How to improve patient safety? 819
Communication and culture 820
Learning from mistakes 821
Creating a safe workforce 821
Preventing diagnostic errors 821
What can patients do to keep themselves safe? 822
Changing policy context for patient safety 822

13.2 Integrative Cardiology: The Use of Complementary Therapies and Beyond 823
Nonconventional therapies and cardiology 823
What is integrative medicine? 823
What is integrative cardiology? 823
Dyslipidemia 824
Hypertension 826
Coronary artery disease 828
Heart failure 830

Index 835

Chapter 1

Cardiovascular Pharmacology

1.1 Diuretics

❏ INTRODUCTION

The era of modern diuretic therapy in cardiovascular disease emerged in the late 1950s with the development of effective oral agents with improved tolerability. Until then, the only diuretics available had been intravenous or intramuscular mercurial derivatives, limited by difficulty in use and an unfavorable toxicity profile. Today, the diuretic compounds are recognized as powerful tools that impair sodium reabsorption in the renal tubules. In doing so, they increase the fractional excretion of sodium, affect the rate of urine formation and alter long-term sodium balance. After more than 50 years in clinical use, diuretics remain of considerable importance in the management of cardiovascular diseases. Diuretics have uses other than in hypertension and edematous disorders, such as in the treatment of hypercalcemia, diabetes insipidus, glaucoma, and cerebral edema.

❏ CLASSIFICATION OF THE DIURETIC COMPOUNDS

Modern diuretic compounds are now viewed as a heterogeneous class of drugs that differ remarkably in several aspects, including their chemical derivation, mechanism, and therapeutic efficacy. The most common and clinically useful classification of diuretics is to group them into one of several categories on the basis of the primary site of their interference with sodium reabsorption (Fig. 1):

- Carbonic anhydrase inhibitors (e.g. acetazolamide), acting in the proximal tubule
- High-ceiling or "loop" diuretics (e.g. furosemide, bumetanide, torsemide), acting in thick ascending limb of the loop of Henle
- Thiazide and thiazide-like diuretics (e.g. hydrochlorothiazide, chlorthalidone, metolazone, indapamide) acting in the early portion of the distal convoluted tubule
- A fourth category, which are primarily utilized for their potassium-sparing capabilities, can further be subclassified into the sodium channel blockers (e.g. amiloride, triamterene) and the mineralocorticoid antagonists (e.g. spironolactone, eplerenone). These agents act in the late distal tubule and collecting duct
- A final category of diuretics, the osmotic agents (e.g. mannitol), interfere with sodium reabsorption throughout all segments of the nephron by creating an osmotic force throughout the length of the renal tubule. Distinguishing the diuretic compounds according to their primary site of action is important, as their therapeutic efficacy and primary clinical indications are not completely interchangeable (Table 1).

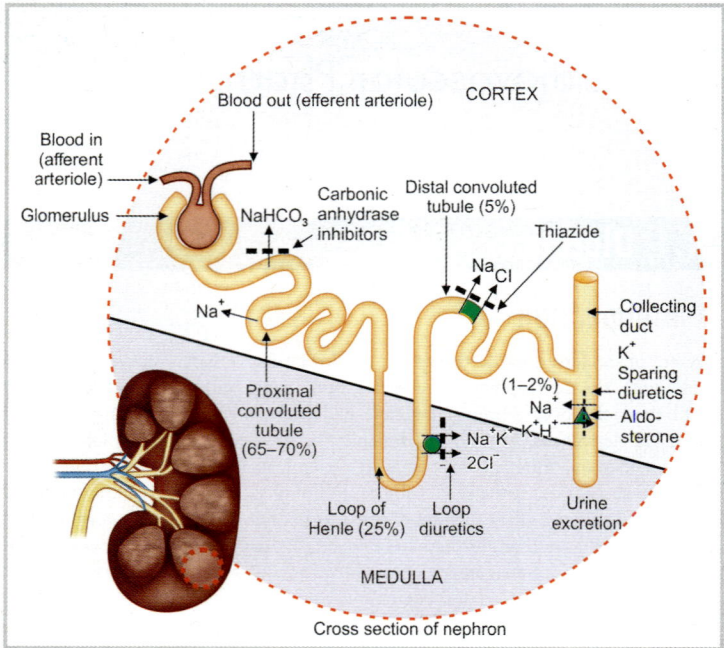

FIGURE 1: Diuretic sites of action in the nephron (Na^+: Sodium; Cl^-: Chloride; K: Potassium; $NaHCO_3$: Sodium bicarbonate; numbers in parentheses reflect the relative percentage of the sodium load reabsorbed in that segment)

Recognizing their sites of action also provides an avenue for additive effects that can be obtained when the different classes of diuretics are used in combination (i.e. "sequential nephron blockade") in certain types of patients.

❏ CLINICAL PHARMACOLOGY OF THE DIURETIC COMPOUNDS

General Pharmacokinetic and Pharmacodynamic Principles

Some generalizations can be made about the pharmacology of the diuretics, despite heterogeneity by class and agent.
- At physiologic pH, diuretics are either organic anions (loops and thiazides) or cations (amiloride and triamterene)
- All diuretics, except mannitol, are highly protein bound, which limits filtration at the glomerulus and traps the diuretic in the vascular space; therefore, they must be actively secreted into the proximal tubule lumen to exert their effect.
- Active transport into the lumen occurs via an organic acid secretory pathway for the carbonic anhydrase inhibitors, loops and thiazides, and a parallel pathway for organic bases
- Mannitol and spironolactone are exceptions; mannitol is freely filtered at the glomerulus and passes through the nephron, acting as a nonreabsorbable solute drawing water along with it, while spironolactone (although protein-bound) enters the renal tubules from plasma by competitively inhibiting the binding of aldosterone to the mineralocorticoid receptor at the basolateral surface

Cardiovascular Pharmacology

Table 1: Characteristics of diuretics: classification, site and mechanism of action, clinical uses

Diuretic classification	Major site of action	Enzyme/channel inhibited	Maximum effect (% of filtered sodium load)	Clinical uses
Carbonic anhydrase inhibitors	Proximal tubule	Carbonic anhydrase	3–5	Glaucoma, metabolic alkalosis, high altitude sickness
High-ceiling or loops	Thick ascending limb of loop of Henle	$Na^+/K^+/2Cl^-$ symporter	20–25	Edematous disorders (congestive heart failure, cirrhosis, nephrotic syndrome), renal insufficiency, hypertension in kidney disease
Thiazide and thiazide-like*	Early distal convoluted tubule	Na^+/Cl^- symporter	5–8	Hypertension, hypercalciuria, diabetes insipidus, pseudohypoaldosteronism type 2 (Gordon's syndrome)
Potassium-sparing	Cortical collecting duct		2–3	
Pteridine derivatives		Epithelial sodium channel		Pseudoaldosteronism (Liddle syndrome), thiazide or loop diuretic-induced hypokalemia or hypomagnesemia
Aldosterone receptor antagonists		Aldosterone receptor		Primary and secondary aldosteronism, congestive heart failure, hyperandrogen states, thiazide or loop diuretic-induced hypokalemia or hypomagnesemia, resistant hypertension (independent of primary aldosteronism), Bartter syndrome
Osmotic agents	Multiple segments	Sugar acts as non-absorbable solute		Cerebral edema, intracranial hypertension

*The terms thiazide and thiazide-like are used to group thiazides based on the presence of a benzothiadiazine molecular structure. Thiazide-like diuretics lack the benzothiadiazine structure but share a similar mechanism of action.

- For the most part, diuretics have direct actions that are site-specific, acting on one or another of the tubular segments but not all of them
- A few agents maintain a degree of secondary activity at another segment (e.g. some thiazides also inhibit carbonic anhydrase), but it is generally considered an irrelevant contribution to their overall therapeutic effect. This is because diuretic action at one site induces important adaptive changes in other segments of the kidney that attempt to preserve sodium, thereby, minimizing the contribution of any secondary site of action to the overall natriuretic effect.

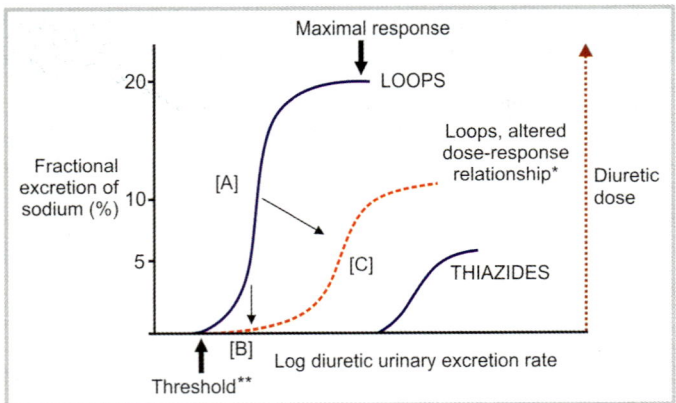

FIGURE 2: Pharmacodynamic illustration of the relationship between diuretic dose and response
* Nephrotic syndrome, congestive heart failure, cirrhosis
** Determinants of diuretic threshold and efficacy include: dose, bioavailability; tubular secretory capacity rate of absorption and time course of delivery. After identifying the threshold dose to achieve effect, a higher diuretic concentration [A] leads to significant natriuresis. When severe sodium retention occurs or sodium intake is reduced, the curve shifts to the right and the previous diuretic serum concentration achieved by the dose in [A] is no longer effective [B]. The dose of the diuretic must be increased to achieve clinically effective natriuresis [C]. Increasing the frequency of doses has no effect on sodium excretion as long as each dose is below the threshold

In general, the desired response is to obtain some meaningful level of natriuresis, which can either correspond to a significant diuresis and reduction in extracellular volume as in the case of loop diuretics to relieve edematous states or a more prolonged low-level diuresis, which reduces systemic vascular resistance and lowers blood pressure, as in the use of thiazides for hypertension. When administered intravenously, bioavailability issues are not present; however, when given orally, diuretic response will be influenced by the rate and extent of absorption, which can be highly variable among diuretic compounds and individual patients. The best index approximating diuretic drug delivery to the intraluminal site of action is its urinary excretion rate, as this corresponds to the observed natriuretic response. This relationship exists for both loops and thiazides (although shallower for thiazides) and can be illustrated using a typical sigmoidal curve (Fig. 2) where the critical determinants are basal response, dose causing 50% response, upper asymptote (maximal response) and slope.

The plasma half-life of a diuretic governs both its expected duration of action and dosing frequency. Loop diuretics have very short half-lives and must be dosed multiple times per day, while thiazides and other distally acting diuretics have half-lives that are sufficient for them to be dosed once or twice daily.

❏ ADAPTIVE RESPONSES TO DIURETIC ADMINISTRATION

The "braking" phenomenon is a term, commonly used to refer to the short-term and long-term adaptive changes observed in the nephron as a result of diuretic administration. These changes are natural compensations intended to protect intravascular volume. Their net result is to stabilize volume losses that lead to the tolerance of the diuretic effect. Diuretic tolerance should be distinguished clinically from diuretic resistance states, the latter describing a phenomenon occurring in conjunction with pathophysiologic conditions, such as renal failure, nephrotic syndrome, congestive heart failure, and cirrhosis. The mechanism of resistance in the setting of these comorbidities is more aptly explained by altered pharmacokinetics and pharmacodynamics rather than physiologic adaptations.

❏ INDIVIDUAL DIURETIC CLASSES

Carbonic Anhydrase Inhibitors

Carbonic anhydrase catalyzes the hydration of bicarbonate in the proximal tubule, thereby, facilitating its reabsorption. Normally, sodium reabsorption accompanies bicarbonate in this process. Inhibitors of carbonic anhydrase (Table 1) interfere with this enzyme activity in the brush border and inside the epithelial cells of the proximal tubule, resulting in impaired sodium, bicarbonate and water reabsorption, as well as a brisk alkaline diuresis. As the majority of the filtered sodium load is reabsorbed in the proximal tubule, one would ordinarily expect a proximally acting agent to produce a substantial diuretic response. However, the net diuretic effect of carbonic anhydrase inhibitors is limited because sodium that is reabsorbed distal to the proximal tubule (mainly in the thick ascending limb of the loop of Henle) offsets these losses. Additionally, the kidney compensates in several ways, which serve to diminish the overall carbonic anhydrase-dependent component of sodium reabsorption. Sodium rejected proximally increases its delivery to the macula densa, which activates the tubuloglomerular feedback mechanism, suppressing the glomerular filtration rate and amount of solutes filtered. Furthermore, the alkaline diuresis caused by the carbonic anhydrase inhibitor reduces bicarbonate levels in the serum, which results in overall less bicarbonate filtration. Acetazolamide (Table 2) demonstrates the most favorable diuretic features among several chemical derivatives of sulfanilamide that were synthesized while searching for more potent carbonic anhydrase inhibitors.

The primary uses of acetazolamide are not directly related to its diuretic action, but rather in the systemic metabolic acidosis induced as a byproduct. This can be helpful in remedying iatrogenic metabolic alkalosis occasionally caused by high doses of loop diuretics (typically in patients with cardiogenic pulmonary edema). Correcting alkalosis in these situations may improve oxygenation.

Additionally, other clinical applications of acetazolamide involve carbonic anhydrase-dependent bicarbonate transport occurring outside the kidney. As carbonic anhydrase is involved in intraocular fluid formation, acetazolamide and its derivatives can be used to decrease intraocular pressure in patients with glaucoma. Acetazolamide has also proven effective in treatment and prophylaxis of acute mountain sickness.

Loop or High-ceiling Diuretics

Loop diuretics (Table 1), so named for their site of action in the thick ascending limb of the loop of Henle. Two agents, furosemide and ethacrynic acid, were developed independently around the same time. Among this group, furosemide was introduced first, followed later by bumetanide and torsemide. The identification and development of these compounds were heralded as major advances in diuretic therapy, as their sizeable effect proved useful in renal insufficiency and heart failure patients unresponsive to other agents. Loop diuretics are often referred to as "high-ceiling" agents due to the substantial diuresis they can cause; maximally effective doses can lead to excretion of 20–25% of filtered sodium, blocking nearly all of

Table 2: Approximate pharmacokinetic parameters of the commonly available diuretics

Diuretic class	Oral bio-availability (%)	Vd (L/kg)	Protein binding (%)	Fate	T½ (hour) (normal)	Duration of action (hour)* (normal)	Additional notes
Carbonic Anhydrase Inhibitors							
Acetazolamide	100	0.2	70–90	R (100%)	6–9	8–12	Metabolic acidosis with prolonged use
Thiazide-type							
Chlorothiazide	15–30	1	70	R (100%)	1.5–2.5	6–12	Rarely used anymore
Hydrochlorothiazide	60–70	2.5	40	R (100%)	3–10	6–12	Increased absorption with food
Bendroflumethiazide	90	1–1.5	94	R (30%), M (70%)	2–5	18–24	Primarily used outside the US
Thiazide-like							
Chlorthalidone	65	3–13	99	R (65%)	50–60	24–72	Binds to carbonic anhydrase in erythrocytes
Metolazone	65	113 (total)	95	R (80%)	8–14	12–24	Retains efficacy in renal insufficiency
Indapamide	71–79	25 (total)	75	M (70%), R (5%)	14	24–36	Possible vasodilatory properties
High-ceiling or loops							
Furosemide	10–100	0.15	91–99	R (50%), 50% conjugated in kidneys	1.5	6	Slightly prolonged T½ in renal insufficiency
Bumetanide	80–100	0.15	90–99	R (60%), M (40%)	1.5	3–6	Slightly prolonged T½ in renal insufficiency

Contd...

Contd...

Table 2: Approximate pharmacokinetic parameters of the commonly available diuretics

Diuretic class	Oral bio-availability (%)	Vd (L/kg)	Protein binding (%)	Fate	T½ (hour) (normal)	Duration of action (hour)* (normal)	Additional notes
Torsemide	80–100	0.2	99	R (20%), M (80%)	3–4	8–12	Slightly prolonged T½ in renal insufficiency
Ethacrynic acid	100	—	90	R (67%), M (33%)	1	4–8	Higher risk of ototoxicity; reserve for patients with documented allergy to other loops
Distal/Collecting duct							
Amiloride	15–25	350 (total)	0	R (50%), 50% fecal	17–26	24	T½ = 100 hours in end stage renal disease
Triamterene	50	—	55–67	M (80%), R (10)	3	7–9	T½ of active metabolite = 3 hours
Spironolactone	65	—	90	M (extent unknown)	1.5	16–24	T½ of active metabolite = 15 hours
Eplerenone	69	43–90 (total)	50	M (extent unknown)	5	24	Less affinity for androgen receptors
Osmotic							
Mannitol	17–20	0.5	0	R (100%)	1	2–8	T½ = 36 hours in end stage renal disease

*refers to natriuretic effect; — indicates insufficient data; R = renal excretion as intact drug; M = hepatically metabolized; Vd = volume of distribution; T½ = elimination half-life.

the reabsorption occurring in this segment. Located within the apical membrane of epithelial cells of the thick ascending limb is the electroneutral $Na^+/K^+/2Cl^-$ cotransporter, which passively carries sodium, potassium, and chloride ions into the cell based on the electrochemical Na^+ gradient generated by the Na^+/K^{+-}ATPase pump of the basolateral membrane. Some potassium is returned to the lumen via K^+ channels of the luminal membrane, such that the net effect of this pathway is Na^+Cl^- reabsorption and a voltage across the tubular wall oriented with the lumen positive in relation to the interstitium. Mechanistically, loop diuretics bind to $Na^+/K^+/2Cl^-$ cotransporter at the chloride site, causing a diuresis of Na^+Cl^- and K^+Cl^-. In addition to prevent its reabsorption, potassium secretion from distal tubular sites is also promoted by loop diuretics by virtue of the increased delivery of sodium to these sites.

All are extensively bound to serum albumin (>95%) and must gain access to the tubular lumen by active secretion through probenecid-sensitive organic anion transporters located in the proximal tubule. This process may be slowed by elevated levels of endogenous organic acids, such as in chronic kidney disease as well as drugs that share the same transporter, including salicylates and nonsteroidal anti-inflammatory drugs.

Thiazide and the Thiazide-like Diuretics

Thiazide diuretics (Table 1) were serendipitously discovered while chemically modifying the sulfa nucleus of acetazolamide in an attempt to develop more potent inhibitors of carbonic anhydrase. The finding that it produced increased chloride rather than bicarbonate accompanying sodium in the urine was an unanticipated consequence, but a major advancement that paved the way for further advances in diuretic therapy. Chlorothiazide, the prototype of the class, became available in 1957, effectively beginning the modern era of diuretic therapy and rendering obsolete the organometallic compounds previously available. Thiazide diuretics inhibit sodium reabsorption from the luminal side in the early segments of the distal tubule, by interfering with the electroneutral Na^+Cl^- symporter located in the apical membrane. The increased delivery of sodium to the collecting duct also increases the exchange with potassium, leading to potassium depletion. Magnesium excretion is also increased with thiazide administration. With few exceptions, the pharmacokinetic parameters of thiazides are not uniformly characterized (Table 2). Generally, all are orally absorbed, have volumes of distribution equal to or greater than equivalent body weight and are extensively bound to plasma proteins.[1] Thiazides must actively be secreted into the proximal tubule, as they are highly protein bound and subject to limited glomerular filtration. Thiazides compete with uric acid for secretion into the proximal tubule by the organic acid secretory system; this leads to reduced uric acid excretion and can precipitate gout in predisposed individuals. Despite heterogeneity in their structure–activity relationships, which has given rise to designations of the analogues as either being thiazide-type or thiazide-like, the general designation of thiazide diuretic is inclusive of all diuretics sharing primary action in the distal tubule. An exception is indapamide, which has less direct evidence for activity at the Na^+Cl^- symporter and has been suggested to possess vasodilatory effects. All thiazides have demonstrated parallel dose-response curves and comparable maximal chloruretic effects. In general, their dose-response curve is much shallower than that of loops (Fig. 2), such that there is a little difference in efficacy between the lowest and maximally effective doses.

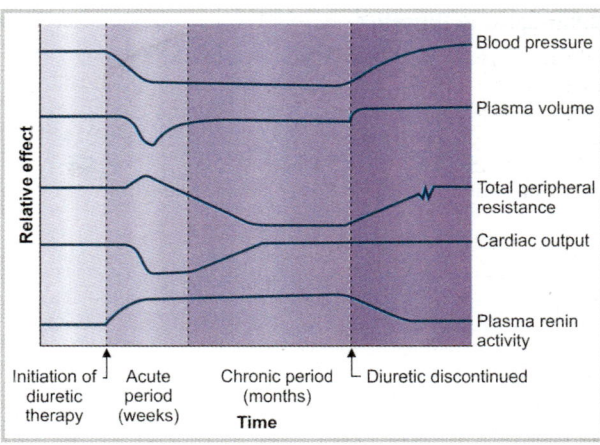

FIGURE 3: Time course of hemodynamic responses to thiazides

There is a significant variation in the metabolism, bioavailability and plasma half-lives of the thiazides (Table 2). The latter two pharmacokinetic features are the most clinically relevant parameters, as they influence the dose and frequency of administration. Chlorothiazide is relatively lipid insoluble and requires large doses to achieve concentrations, which are high enough for the drug to arrive at its site of action. Hydrochlorothiazide, the most widely used thiazide in the United States, has improved bioavailability with approximately 60–70% absorbed orally. Chlorthalidone and metolazone are subjected to a mixed pathway of primarily renal (50–80%) with minor biliary excretion (10%). Other than the 50% reduction in hydrochlorothiazide absorption, noted in patients with heart failure, almost no information exists regarding the influence of disease on the pharmacokinetics of thiazides. As the distal tubule only reabsorbs about 5% of the filtered sodium load, the overt diuretic efficacy of thiazides for volume removal in edematous disorders is limited. However, relative to the loop and other diuretics, an advantage of the thiazides is their long duration of action. This property is a major determinant allowing them to distinguish themselves primarily for their use as antihypertensive agents.

The duration of antihypertensive effect for thiazides exceeds that of their diuretic effect, mainly due to the important hemodynamic changes induced by the prolonged low-level diuresis. These hemodynamic effects can be separated into acute (1–2 weeks) and chronic (several months) periods (Fig. 3).

After commencing regular dosing of a thiazide, blood pressure-lowering is initially attributed to extracellular fluid contraction and reduction in plasma volume. The accompanying decrease in venous return depresses cardiac preload and output, thereby, reducing blood pressure. However, there is a clear dissociation between the degree of initial diuresis and antihypertensive effect, as the eventual chronic response to thiazides cannot be reliably predicted by the degree of initial fall in plasma volume. Other significant changes occurring acutely include a transient rise in peripheral vascular resistance, likely the result of counterregulatory activation of sympathetic nervous and RAAS systems.

Potassium-sparing Diuretics

In the distal tubule and collecting ducts, sodium is reabsorbed through an aldosterone-sensitive sodium channel and by activation of an ATP-dependent sodium–potassium pump. With the help of both mechanisms, potassium and hydrogen are secreted into the lumen to preserve electroneutrality.[1] Potassium-sparing diuretics are divided into two distinct classes:
- Those acting as direct antagonists of cytoplasmic mineralocorticoid receptors and
- Those acting independent of mineralocorticoids.

All potassium-sparing diuretics act primarily at the cortical part of the collecting duct and to a lesser extent in the final segment of the distal convoluted tubule and connecting tubule. As only a small amount of sodium is reabsorbed here, these agents are capable of limited natriuresis (excluding states of mineralocorticoid excess) in most patients. Their primary clinical utility resides in their potassium-sparing capabilities and to a lesser extent, their ability to correct magnesium deficiencies. Spironolactone and eplerenone (Table 2) are competitive antagonists of aldosterone, the most potent of the naturally occurring mineralocorticoids and thereby interfere with the aldosterone mediated exchange of sodium for potassium and hydrogen. Both drugs are rarely used alone, but rather in combination with other diuretics to avoid potassium deficiency. Their aldosterone-blocking capabilities also make them a primary therapy in patients with essential hypertension due to mineralocorticoid excess, such as in primary aldosteronism due to bilateral adrenal hyperplasia or in patients with aldosterone producing adrenal adenomas awaiting surgical resection, or those who are nonsurgical candidates.

The major adverse effects of spironolactone are antiandrogenic and stem from the fact that it is a steroid that competitively inhibits testosterone and progesterone at the cellular level. In particular, gynecomastia can become a concern, especially with high doses. In the dose range of 12.5–50 mg/day, it is rarely a problem. Eplerenone appears to have more selectivity for aldosterone receptors and less affinity for androgen and progestin receptors than spironolactone. Cost differences have traditionally favored spironolactone and it remains to be determined whether eplerenone's safety and efficacy constitute significant advancements over spironolactone. The actions of amiloride and triamterene (Table 2) are quite different than spironolactone and eplerenone. Triamterene has a short half-life (3–6 hours) and duration of effect. Ideally, it should be dosed multiple times per day; however, because it is most commonly used in a fixed-dose combination with hydrochlorothiazide, it is rarely dosed more frequently than once daily. Triamterene is a potential nephrotoxin associated with formation of crystals, nephrolithiasis, interstitial nephritis and acute renal failure. It must be used carefully when other potentially nephrotoxic drugs are coadministered. Amiloride has a much longer half-life (17–26 hours) and can be dosed once or twice daily, achieving steady state in approximately two days. It is preferred in patients with liver disease, as there is no required metabolic activation. However, it is extensively renally cleared and accumulates rapidly when administered in patients with chronic kidney disease.

Osmotic Diuretics

The osmotic diuretic, mannitol (Table 2), is freely filtered through the glomerulus and poorly absorbed. As it is not reabsorbed in the nephron, mannitol does not interfere with specific tubular electrolyte transport systems. Rather, it increases osmolality, as it remains in the tubule lumen and thus impairs the tubular water reabsorption normally driven by the osmotic gradient. As the medullary solute gradient is lost, the urinary concentrating ability of the kidney is greatly reduced and tubular fluid is diluted. The osmotic diuresis that prevails is similar to the glucose-mediated osmotic polyuria and diuresis observed in patients with uncontrolled diabetes. Although some excretion of bicarbonate occurs in the proximal tubule, mannitol's effect is largely in promoting sodium and chloride wasting in the loop of Henle.

Mannitol has been used as a preventive measure against acute renal failure in patients receiving cisplatin, radiocontrast exposure or other high-risk situations; however, there is no evidence that it is any more effective than insuring adequate volume status with parenteral fluids, a more appropriate strategy. In the same manner, mannitol has been investigated for use in oliguric acute renal failure to promote diuresis; again, limited data support this strategy and insuring adequate volume status is a more appropriate approach. Given its significant limitations, mannitol should be only rarely used as a diuretic.

❏ CLINICAL USE OF DIURETICS IN CARDIOVASCULAR DISEASES

Aside from their chemical and mechanistic classifications, diuretics can be categorized functionally into one of three primary uses:
- Treatment of essential hypertension
- Volume removal in edematous disorders
- Correction of potassium and magnesium deficiencies.

Different classes of diuretics are used for a variety of indications, and certain diuretics are more effective on managing a particular condition:
- Thiazide diuretics appear to be the most effective diuretics over the long-term in lowering blood pressure in patients with hypertension
- Loop diuretics are the most powerful diuretics to evoke a substantial diuresis; therefore, they are agents of choice for symptomatic relief in patients with edematous disorders such as congestive heart failure, cirrhosis, and nephrotic syndrome
- Potassium-sparing agents are largely reserved for correcting potassium and magnesium deficiencies associated with thiazide diuretic administration.

While only one type of diuretic is generally used at a time, there are several conditions where diuretic tolerance is encountered. In these situations, combinations of two different types of diuretics are often employed to improve response.

Diuretic Use in Hypertension

General Considerations

Thiazides have been a mainstay in the treatment of hypertension for many years and are preferred agents for chronic therapy in most hypertensive patients where a diuretic is indicated. Thiazide administration typically results in a 10–15/5–10 mm Hg reduction in blood pressure compared to placebo. Thiazide responders are often referred to as having low-renin or salt-sensitive hypertension, in deference to the large contribution volume and sodium play in the maintenance of their blood pressure. These patients typically include the elderly, blacks and high cardiac output states, such as obesity. Although the aforementioned groups are often considered more likely to respond to thiazides, an advantage of thiazides is that they can be effectively combined with nearly any antihypertensive, producing a blood pressure-lowering effect that is additive of the two individual components in almost all cases.

Given their ability to augment efficacy of nearly all other types of antihypertensives, thiazides are powerful tools, which improve the capability of achieving blood pressure goals. In patients considered to have resistant hypertension, lack of appropriate diuretic use has been identified as the primary drug-related cause. Thiazide dosing has evolved in parallel to our progressive understanding of their mechanism of action and dose-response relationships. The dose-response curve for thiazides is much shallower than originally believed. Thiazides are now utilized in significantly lower doses and the term low-dose thiazide has become synonymous with 12.5–25 mg/day of hydrochlorothiazide or its equivalent.

Comparative Efficacy

The ability of thiazides to effectively lower blood pressure translates into reductions in cardiovascular events. Beginning with the completion of the landmark Veteran's Affairs Cooperative Group study in 1967 and continuing through the early 1990s, a series of randomized placebo-controlled trials involving more than 47,000 hypertensive patients convincingly demonstrated these effects. Combined meta-analyses and systematic review show that thiazide-based regimens reduce relative rates of heart failure by 41–49%, stroke by approximately 29–38%, coronary heart disease by 14–21% and overall mortality by 10–11% compared to placebo. Effect sizes are homogeneous throughout major subgroups of patients, including by gender, age and presence of diabetes. The results of these studies have collectively formed the basis for the recommendations contained in the first seven guideline reports of the Joint National Committee, all advocating thiazides as initial therapy for most patients.

Special Considerations

An important clinical issue with thiazides is that they are generally considered less effective in renal insufficiency, particularly when GFR falls below 40 mL/min/1.73 m^2. Larger doses of thiazides have been shown to induce diuresis in patients with chronic kidney disease, but the efficacy of thiazides in this setting has a specific ceiling, which is controlled by several factors, including the reduced delivery of filtered solute and drug to the distal tubule site of action and the fact that the distal tubule is responsible for only a small amount of sodium reabsorption even under normal circumstances. Additionally, increasing the doses of thiazides is impractical given the risk of metabolic and electrolyte side effects.

In the absence of states of mineralocorticoid excess or certain rare genetic conditions, the primary role of potassium-sparing diuretics in the treatment of hypertension is that of an ancillary to help offset the potassium and magnesium wasting induced by thiazides. Spironolactone is advantageous not only in that it can correct thiazide-induced potassium and magnesium wasting, but low doses of 12.5–50 mg daily show significant additive hypotensive effects in patients resistant to treatment regardless of ethnicity or baseline aldosterone level.

Diuretic Use in Edematous Disorders

General Considerations

Loop diuretics are the most potent diuretics available, making them agents of choice in patients with edematous disorders, such as renal insufficiency, hepatic cirrhosis, congestive heart failure and nephrotic syndrome. Loop diuretics are preferred for hypertension or volume control in patients with chronic kidney disease.

Table 3: Ceiling doses and therapeutic regimens for loop diuretics in normal patients and in conditions with reduced diuretic response

Clinical scenario	Furosemide IV	Furosemide PO	Bumetanide IV and PO	Torsemide IV and PO
Continuous infusion rates (mg/hour)	40 mg loading dose		1 mg loading dose	20 mg loading dose
CrCl <25	20, then 40		1, then 2	10, then 20
CrCl 25–75	10, then 20		0.5, then 1	5, then 10
CrCl >75	10		0.5	5
Single-dose ceilings (mg)				
Renal insufficiency* Moderate (CrCl 20–50)	80–160	160	2–3	20–50
Severe (CrCl < 20)	160–200	400	8–10	50–100
Congestive heart failure** (preserved renal function)	40–80	80–160	1–2	20–40
Cirrhosis** (preserved renal function)	40	80	1	10–20
Nephrotic syndrome** (preserved renal function)	80–120	240	2–3	40–60

*Mechanism of reduced effect is impaired delivery to the site of action. The therapeutic strategy is to use sufficiently high enough doses to attain effective amounts at the site of action, and increase frequency of administration of the effective dose.
**Mechanism of reduced effect is diminished nephron response (and binding of diuretic to urinary albumin in nephrotic syndrome). The therapeutic strategy is to increase the frequency of the effective dose.

As previously discussed, the pharmacodynamics of diuretics is altered in most edematous conditions; namely, such that maximal response is lower (Fig. 2). The mechanisms underlying this decreased responsiveness are uncertain, but may relate to increased proximal or distal reabsorption of sodium or an upregulation of the $Na^+/K^+/2Cl^-$ transporter. From a clinical perspective, this means that administering larger single doses will not improve the diuretic response. As in normal patients, it is best to first start with small doses and then titrates upward according to response. This can be achieved practically by sequentially doubling the dose until response is observed or a ceiling dose is reached (Table 3). Escalating doses above these ceiling doses will result in no additional benefit but an increase in side effects. If response is suboptimal, other strategies, such as continuous infusion or using combinations of diuretics as outlined below, may be tried.

Renal Insufficiency

In the absence of heart failure, cirrhosis or nephrotic syndrome, dysregulation of volume homeostasis is usually a late manifestation of renal insufficiency, often not developing until GFR falls to less than 10 mL/min. As renal function declines, the ability to maintain sodium balance diminishes and the fraction of filtered sodium that must be excreted to maintain sodium balance rises progressively. In the setting of constant sodium intake, fractional excretion of sodium must increase fivefold when GFR falls to 20% of normal and tenfold when GFR is 10% of normal.

Normal kidneys are able to accommodate this over a wide range of sodium intake, but patients with renal insufficiency have limited ability to raise the fractional excretion of sodium above 50%. Assuming sodium intake exceeds this reduced maximal excretion, extracellular fluid volume expands, and edema develops. Large doses of thiazides can induce a modest diuresis in patients with renal disease, but loop diuretics are preferred, because they produce a more vigorous and reliable response. Renal clearance of loops falls in parallel with GFR because of decreased renal mass and accumulation of organic acids that compete for proximal secretion. Only 10–20% as much drug may be secreted into the tubular lumen in a patient with a creatinine clearance of 15 mL/min, compared to one with normal renal function. That said, response to the diuretic expressed as fractional excretion of sodium is similar for patients with renal insufficiency to that of healthy patients; thus, residual nephrons seem to respond normally, but the problem is in getting enough drug to the site of action to achieve the diuretic threshold.

Of the thiazides, metolazone is frequently selected for use in combination with a loop because of its long half-life and preserved activity in renal insufficiency. Rarely acetazolamide and collecting duct agents, such as spironolactone and amiloride, are used, but their response is less dramatic than that of a thiazide.

Cirrhosis

Secondary hyperaldosteronism plays an important role in the pathogenesis of sodium retention in patients with cirrhotic edema. Spironolactone is the mainstay of therapy in such patients. Not only it increases patient comfort, but it can also eliminate the need or reduce the interval between paracenteses, an advantage is that protein normally removed during paracenteses can also be spared. The usual dosing range of spironolactone is 50–400 mg/day, but doses above 200 mg/day are often not well tolerated due to painful gynecomastia. An advantage of spironolactone is the once-daily dosing made possible by the sufficiently long half-lives of its active metabolites.

Cirrhotic patients with edema receiving diuretics are prone to complications such as intravascular volume depletion and prerenal azotemia, in up to 20% of patients. Once euvolemia is achieved, maximal diuresis should be limited to 500 mL/day. As in other conditions in which combinations of diuretics are used, close monitoring of electrolytes is necessary. Diuretic therapy should be reduced or discontinued if azotemia develops.

Congestive Heart Failure

Patients with mild heart failure may not have appreciable edema and diuretic therapy is not an absolute necessity, particularly if patients can restrict sodium intake. If hypertension coexists, it is sensible to employ a thiazide diuretic, which may be sufficient to control mild edema, if present. However, most patients with congestive heart failure will eventually develop edema to the extent that requires the use of a loop diuretic. Responsiveness to oral loop diuretics in patients with heart failure is dependent on several factors, including gastrointestinal absorption and tubular secretion. As long as renal function remains preserved, delivery of diuretic into the tubular fluid remains normal in heart failure. However, renal responsiveness to loops as measured by the natriuretic response to maximally effective doses can be one-third to one-fourth than that of healthy individuals. Larger doses will therefore not overcome this diminished response, unless renal insufficiency is present. Rather, the natriuretic response may be increased by giving moderate doses more frequently. In this manner, intravenous therapy is often appropriate in patients with severe heart failure or acute pulmonary edema. A thiazide diuretic can be added in combination to a loop diuretic in situations where the loop diuretic and sodium restriction are not adequate to control the edema. The synergy provided by such combinations can result in profound diuresis and patients must be followed closely to prevent severe hypokalemia and volume depletion to the extent that could induce circulatory collapse.

Nephrotic Syndrome

Diuretic resistance is often encountered in the nephrotic syndrome; a constellation of findings characterized by proteinuria, hypoalbuminemia, and generalized edema. As serum albumin concentrations are low, there is an increase in the permeability of the glomerular basement membrane to plasma proteins. The resulting decrease in plasma oncotic pressure alters Starling forces in the peripheral capillary beds, favoring fluid transudation into the interstitial compartment. Since diuretics are primarily bound to albumin, hypoalbuminemia also causes more diffusion of diuretic into the extracellular fluid, leading to reduction in delivery to the secretory sites and ultimately, the diuretic site of action. In severely hypoalbuminemic patients (<2 g/dL), coadministration of albumin with the loop diuretic (30 mg furosemide mixed with 25 g albumin) may increase the diuretic response. Doses of the loop diuretic must be sufficient not only to overcome urinary binding, but they must also be administered more frequently. Metolazone or another thiazide diuretic may be combined with the loop diuretic as an additional strategy in nephrotic patients.

❑ ADVERSE EFFECTS OF DIURETICS

A number of important and predictable adverse effects can occur with diuretics. Flowchart 1 illustrates some of the more commonly noted effects and the pathways by which they can occur. Both thiazide and loop diuretics increase potassium and magnesium excretion. On an average, potassium will fall by 0.3–0.4 mEq/L with typical dosing. The incidence of clinically relevant hypokalemia with thiazides is reduced when they are combined with ACE inhibitors or ARBs. Diuretic-induced hypokalemia can be managed by coadministering a potassium-sparing diuretic or oral potassium supplements. Potassium-sparing diuretics are generally more effective since they correct the underlying etiology and have the additional effect of reducing magnesium excretion. Maintenance of potassium homeostasis is important, since epidemiologic evidence implicates hypokalemia in the pathogenesis of diuretic dysglycemia and new-onset diabetes. It is important to recognize that new-onset diabetes will occur over time in many hypertensive patients regardless of type of antihypertensive used. Hyponatremia is often caused by diuretics. Several risk factors predispose patients to diuretic-induced hyponatremia, these include:
- Older age
- Female gender
- Psychogenic polydipsia and concurrent antidepressant use (in particular, selective serotonin reuptake inhibitors).

In the presence of these conditions, hyponatremia can occur at any time. Most patients are asymptomatic, but careful monitoring of serum sodium should occur as well as counseling patients to avoid excessive free-water intake in order to minimize risks of its occurrence. Diuretics can increase serum lipid levels, primarily total cholesterol and low-density lipoproteins, approximately 5–7% in the first year of therapy. However, these increases are short lived and the high

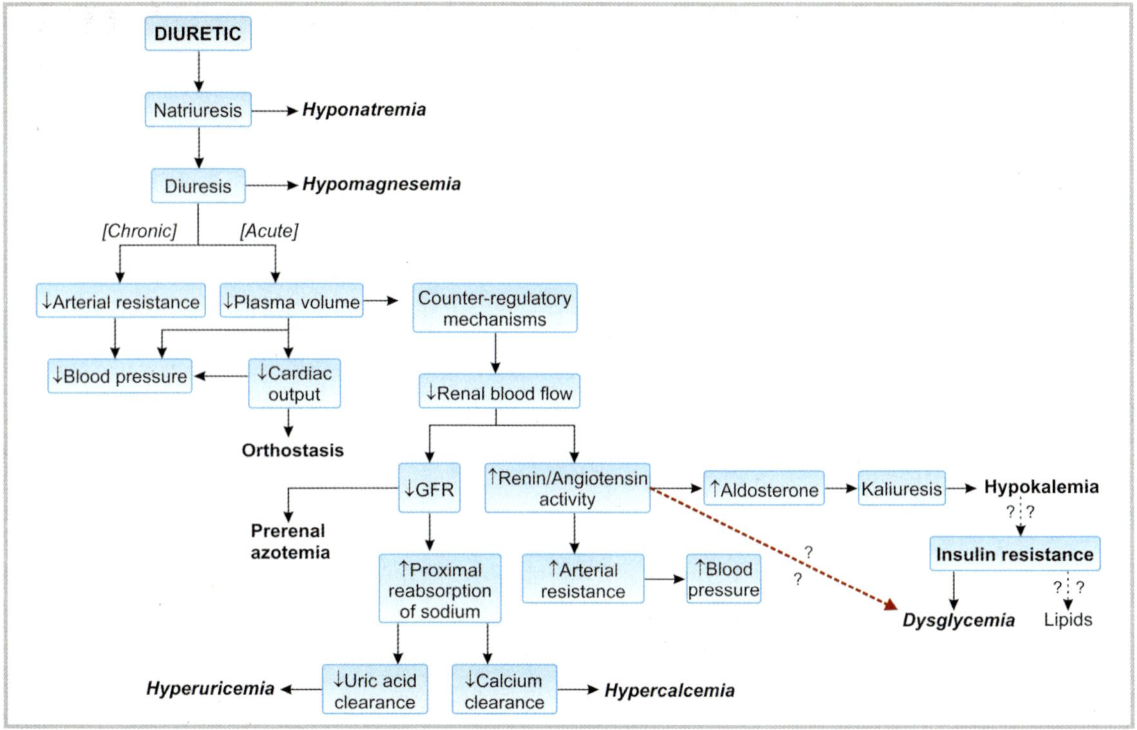

FLOWCHART 1: Proposed mechanisms leading to diuretic complications

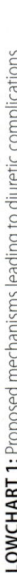

conduction problems or are simply not very powerful vasodilators. They do not play any role in the treatment of heart failure.

Oral Nitrates

Nitrates have been widely used to treat angina by physicians for well over 100 years. It is only in the past 25 years that they have been used to treat systolic heart failure. Their favorable effects on angina, systolic heart failure, mitral regurgitation and coronary spasm are now well known. Nitrates primarily cause venodilation, which typically increases capacitance and reduces preload, thus, lowering end-diastolic volume, reducing cardiac wall tension and diminishing PCWP. Dyspnea is relieved. Larger doses lead to arteriolar dilation, further reducing afterload and improving forward flow. LV cavity size diminishes, reducing mitral regurgitation. It is not surprising that oral nitrate therapy has emerged as an important treatment for systolic heart failure. Nitrates are among the few vasodilators that are able to increase exercise tolerance in patients with systolic heart failure. However, nitrate tolerance occurs in many patients (Fig. 6), thus casting suspicion on long-term efficiency. This can be offset to some extent by hydralazine.

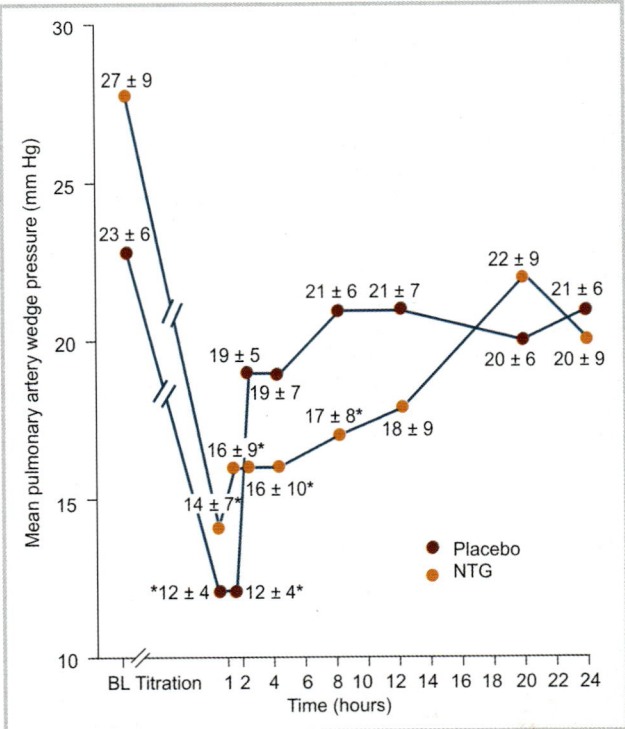

FIGURE 6: The data indicate that tolerance can develop to intravenous nitroglycerin (NTG) over 24 hours. There is a brisk initial response to IV NTG manifested by a fall in pulmonary capillary wedge pressure (PCWP) during titration; but during 24 hours of infusion, PCWP increases back toward control in both the NTG and the placebo arms of the study. (*Source:* Modified from Elkayam U, Kulick D, McIntosh N, et al. Incidence of early tolerance to hemodynamic effects of continuous infusion of NTG in patients with coronary artery disease and heart failure. Circulation. 1987;76:577-84, with permission)

❏ RENIN–ANGIOTENSIN–ALDOSTERONE SYSTEM (RAAS) BLOCKERS

Angiotensin-converting Enzyme Inhibitors (ACE Inhibitors)

ACE inhibitors were introduced into clinical practice in the 1980s for the treatment of hypertension and heart failure. This class of drug therapy has revolutionized therapy for these two conditions and has been demonstrated to improve survival in patients with systolic heart failure. The development of this class of drugs for the treatment of heart failure was predicated on the observation that the RAAS is activated in chronic heart failure and contributes importantly to heightened afterload and to the LV remodeling process.

Angiotensinogen is produced in the liver and is converted in the blood by renin to form a small peptide, angiotensin I (Flowchart 2). Angiotensin I is then further cleaved to form angiotensin II, a very small peptide but potent arteriole constrictor. Angiotensin II subserves a host of other biological activities primarily through the angiotensin II receptor, including promotion of volume retention, activation of and sensitization to the sympathetic nervous system (SNS), thirst, regulation of salt and water balance, modulation of potassium balance, cardiac myocyte, and vascular smooth muscle growth, to name a few. Its actions are central to the development of acute and chronic systolic heart failure.

We now recognize that neurohormonal activation plays a key role in the initiation and progression of heart failure. The RAAS is central to this neurohormonal cascade, as patients with systolic heart failure and high renin levels seemingly derive the most acute benefit from blocking the RAAS. It is now well established that ACE inhibitors slow the progression of heart failure and improve survival in patients with a reduced ejection fraction and congestive heart failure. Much of this improvement is believed to be due to "reverse remodeling".

It is now considered that systolic heart failure is at least in part driven by excessive neurohormonal activation, setting up a vicious cycle of worsening heart failure and death (Flowchart 3). Even though these neurohormonal systems are likely adaptive in an evolutionary sense, and are not simple biomarkers or epiphenomena, they are known to directly contribute to LV remodeling and even patient mortality. The strong notion emerged that pharmacological inhibition of the RAAS (and the SNS) might reduce the progression of LV remodeling, and therefore such drugs should improve patient survival.

ACE inhibitors have now become a standard of care for patients with:
- Hypertension
- Systolic heart failure
- Acute myocardial infarction
- Advanced cardiovascular disease.

Their role in the treatment of patients with systolic heart failure is now undoubted. The drugs acts through a variety of mechanisms:
- They reduce SVR, presumably by inhibiting angiotensin II arteriolar constriction reducing sympathetic tone There is also marked venodilation with a fall in PCWP, presumably due to reduction in sympathetic activity to veins and desensitization of venous capacitance vessels to norepinephrine
- Venous capacitance vessels dilate in response to ACE inhibitors due to reduced sympathetic activity at the neuroeffector level
- These drugs produce a modest improvement in cardiac index and the heart rate may be slightly slow.

Cardiovascular Pharmacology

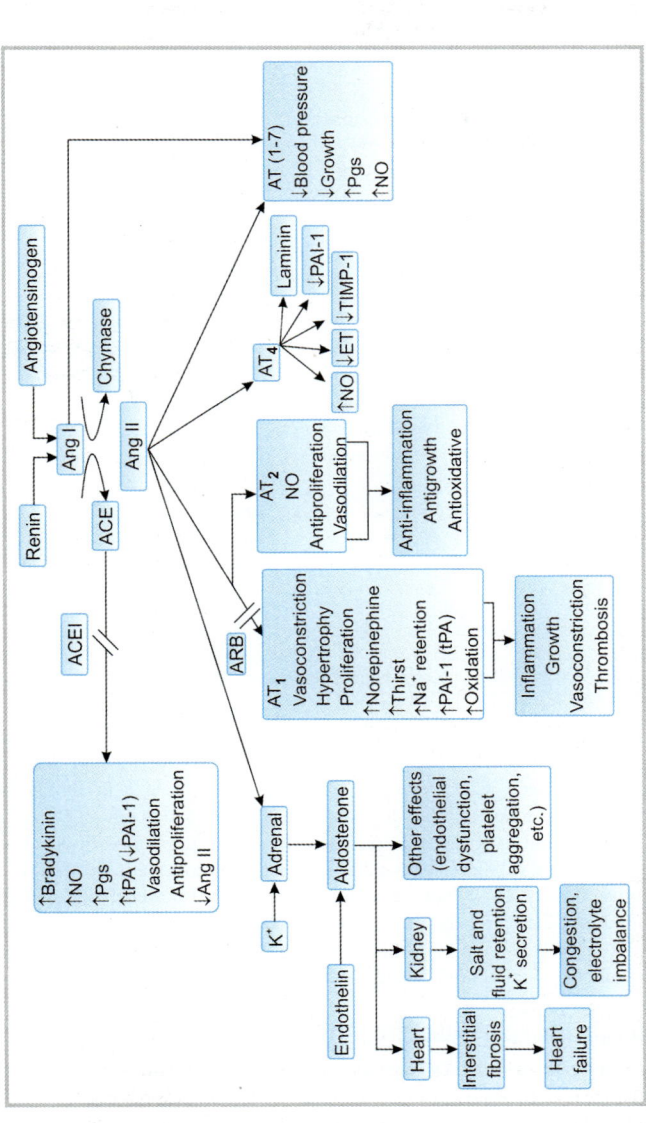

FLOWCHART 2: The renin–angiotensin–aldosterone system

(Abbreviations: ACE: Angiotensin-converting enzyme; ACEI: Angiotensin-converting enzyme inhibitor; ang I: Angiotensin I; ang II: Angiotensin II; AT: Angiotensin receptor; ET: Endothelin; NO: Nitric oxide; PAI: Plasminogen activator inhibitor; PGs: Prostaglandins; TIMP: Tissue inhibitor of metalloproteinase; tPA: Tissue plasminogen activator). (*Source:* Modified from Kalidindi SR, Tang WH, Francis GS. Drug insight: Aldosterone-receptor antagonists in heart failure—The journey continues. Nat Clin Pract Cardiovasc Med. 2007;4(7):368-78, with permission)

FLOWCHART 3: Heart failure is a complex clinical syndrome characterized by extensive neuroendocrine activation. The release of neurohormones appears to be in response to reduced cardiac function and a perceived reduction in effective circulatory volume. It is as if neuroendocrine activity is attempting to protect the blood pressure and maintain circulatory homeostasis. Although this may be adaptive early on, chronic neuroendocrine activation leads to peripheral vasoconstriction, left ventricular remodeling and worsening left ventricular performance, and thus becomes an attractive therapeutic target. Drugs designed to block the exuberant neuroendocrine response, such as ACE inhibitors, have now become the cornerstone of treatment for heart failure

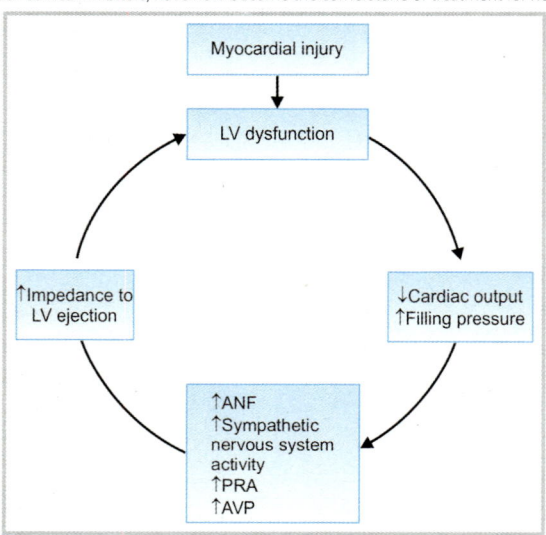

(Abbreviations: LV: Left ventricle; AVP: Arginine vasopressin; ANF: Atrial natriuretic factor; PRA: Plasma renin activity). (*Source:* Francis GS, Tang WH. In: JD Hosenpud, BH Greenberg (Eds). Congestive Heart Failure, 3rd edition. Philadelphia: Lippincott Williams and Wilkins; 2007. pp. 602-19)

There is now a long list of ACE inhibitors to choose from Table 5. They have somewhat dissimilar pharmacodynamics, pharmacokinetics and rates of elimination. In general, it is best to start with small doses of ACE inhibitors and slowly titrate up over days to weeks to a target dose established as safe and effective by use in large clinical trials. It is expected that many patients with advanced systolic heart failure will have about a 20% increase in serum creatinine with ACE inhibitor use. This is usually not a reason to discontinue or lower the dose of the ACE inhibitor. Careful, regular follow-up with a check on electrolytes, blood urea nitrogen (BUN) and serum creatinine is important in the care of these patients when making decisions about altering the dose of ACE inhibitors.

Angiotensin Receptor Blockers (ARBs)

Angiotensin receptors of the AT1 subtype bind angiotensin II with a high structural specificity but limited binding capacity. The remarkable success of ACE inhibitors in the treatment of hypertension, arterial disease, myocardial hypertrophy, heart failure, and diabetic renal disease encouraged the development of alternative drugs to block the RAAS. It was eventually recognized that ACE inhibitor drugs blocked only one of several pathways that reduces angiotensin II activity, and that angiotensin II could "escape" from chronic ACE inhibition. ARBs do not demonstrate this "escape" phenomenon. ARBs do not cause cough. They can be

Cardiovascular Pharmacology

Table 5: Common drugs used in managing chronic heart failure in the United States

Drug	Trade name	Heart failure indication	Post-myocardial infarction indication	Dosing
Angiotensin-converting enzyme (ACE inhibitors)				
Benazepril	*Lotensin*	No	No	5–40 mg QD
Captopril	Capoten	Yes	No	6.25–150 mg TID
Enalapril	Vasotec	Yes	No	2.5–20 mg BID
Fosinopril	Monopril	Yes	No	10–80 mg QD
Lisinopril	Prinivil, Zestril	Yes	No	5–20 mg QD
Moexipril	*Univasc*	No	No	7.5–60 mg QD
Perindopril	*Aceon*	No	No	2–16 mg QD
Quinapril	Accupril	Yes	No	5–20 mg BID
Ramipril	Altace	Yes	Yes	2.5–20 mg QD
Trandolapril	*Mavik*	No	Yes	1–4 mg QD
Zofenopril	*Bifril*	NA	NA	7.5–60 mg QD
Angiotensin II receptor blockers (ARBs)				
Candesartan	Atacand	Yes	No	8–32 mg QD/BID
Eprosartan	*Teveten*	No	No	400–800 mg QD
Irbesartan	*Avapro*	No	No	150–300 QD
Losartan	Cozaar	No	No	50–100 mg QD/BID
Telmisartan	*Telma*	No	No	40–80 QD
Olmesartan	*Benicar*	No	No	20–40 mg QD
Valsartan	Diovan	Yes	No	80–320 mg QD
β-Adrenergic receptor antagonists				
Carvedilol	Coreg	Yes	Yes	3.125–25 mg BID
Metoprolol succinate	Toprol XL	Yes	No	25–200 mg QD
Bisoprolol	*Zebeta*	No	No	1.25–10 mg QD
Nebivolol	*Nabilet*	No	No	1.25–10 mg QD
Aldosterone receptor antagonists				
Spironolactone	Aldactone	Yes	No	25–50 mg QD
Eplerenone	Inspra	No	Yes	25–50 mg QD
Others				
Amlodipine	*Norvasc*	No	No	2.5–10 mg QD
Hydralazine-isosorbide dinitrate	BiDil (37.5/20)	Yes	No	1–2 tablets TID
Digoxin	Digitek	Yes	No	0.125–0.25 mg QD

(Abbreviations: BID: Twice daily; QD: Once daily; TID: Three times daily. Italics indicate a drug that is currently not indicated by the US Food and Drug Administration for treating patients with heart failure). (*Source:* Tang WH, Young JB. Chronic heart failure management. In: EJ Topol (Ed). Textbook of Cardiovascular Medicine, 3rd edition. Philadelphia: Lippincott Williams and Wilkins; 2007. pp. 1373-405) used safely in patients who develop angioedema during treatment with an ACE inhibitor. The incidence of renal dysfunction and hyperkalemia is comparable with ARBs and ACE inhibitors. It is now reasonably clear that ACE inhibitors and ARBs should not be used together, as the likelihood of hyperkalemia, hypotension, and worsening renal function is greater.

Several important points have emerged from many large trials:
- ARBs and ACE inhibitors appear to have very similar efficacy in these patient groups
- If the patient does not tolerate an ACE inhibitor, an ARB is a suitable substitution
- Although generally more expensive, ARBs are better tolerated than ACE inhibitors
- The combination of an ACE inhibitor and an ARB (dual RAAS blocking effect) does not lead to more efficiency and is associated with more hypotension, worsening renal function and hyperkalemia. Despite earlier favorable reports, ARBs do not appear to prevent recurrent atrial fibrillation.

The dose of ARBs has generally been determined by pharmaceutical-generated data and subsequent verification of these doses in large clinical trials (Table 5).

❏ MINERALOCORTICOID (ALDOSTERONE) RECEPTOR BLOCKERS

Aldosterone and Systolic Heart Failure

Aldosterone was structurally identified more than 50 years ago and was soon after designated as mineralocorticoid due to its salt-retaining properties. It also releases potassium from the kidney, gastrointestinal tract, sweat, and salivary glands. It has long been known to play a pathophysiologic role in cardiovascular disease, including congestive heart failure (Flowchart 4). In addition to its mineralocorticoid properties, which can cause hypokalemia and hypomagnesemia, aldosterone contributes in many ways to the development of heart failure.

Inhibition of aldosterone is believed to be favorable due to:
- Reduced collagen deposition and possibly antiremodeling effects
- Reduction in BP
- Prevention of hypokalemia and associated arrhythmias
- Modulation of nitric oxide synthesis (Flowchart 4).

The major mineralocorticoid in heart failure is cortisol and not aldosterone. Serum aldosterone levels are not consistently elevated in patients with heart failure in the absence of diuretics. Accordingly, it is not aldosterone blockade *per se*, but mineralocorticoid receptor blockade that is important. Spironolactone and eplerenone are thus mineralocorticoid receptor blockers more than simply aldosterone receptor blockers.

There is now much greater interest in studying aldosterone receptor blockers. Two landmark studies, the randomized aldosterone evaluation study (RALES) and the myocardial infarction heart failure efficacy and survival study (EPHESUS) have remarkably increased the role of aldosterone mineralocorticoid antagonists for the everyday treatment of systolic heart failure. The drugs spironolactone and eplerenone are now widely used to treat chronic systolic heart failure and post-myocardial infarction heart failure.

Spironolactone and Eplerenone in Chronic Heart Failure

The mechanism of action of spironolactone is complex, as aldosterone mineralo-corticoid modulates many features of the heart failure syndrome. Patients taking

FLOWCHART 4: Aldosterone is a mineralocorticoid that has a central role in a host of biological activities. Many of these activities can be excessive due to dysregulation of aldosterone activity, thus contributing to cardiovascular disease

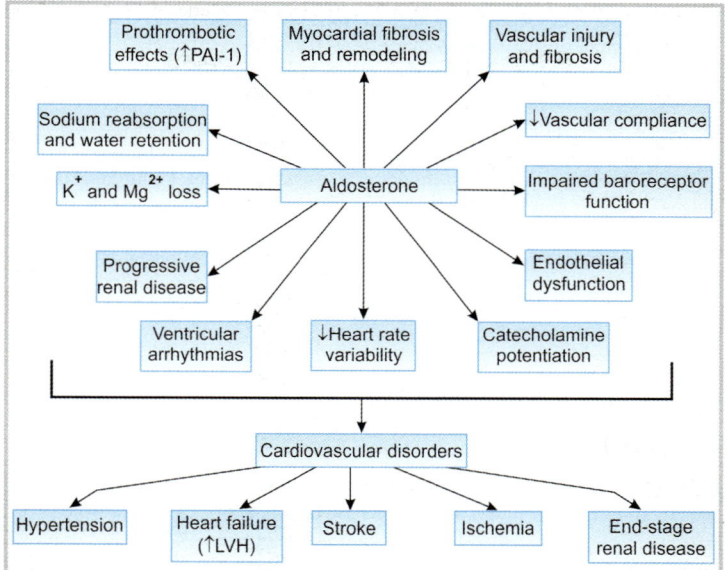

(Abbreviations: LVH: Left ventricular hypertrophy; PAI-1: Plasminogen activator inhibitor-1). (*Source:* Modified from Struthers AD, MacDonald TM. Review of aldosterone and angiotensin-II-induced target organ damage and prevention. Cardiovasc Res. 2004;61:663-70, with permission)

spironolactone need to be frequently and carefully monitored, as hyperkalemia and azotemia can occur with spironolactone, particularly if nonsteroidal anti-inflammatory drugs are used concomitantly.

With the results of RALES trial in 1999, it was clearly demonstrated that spironolactone (25–50 mg per day) added to standard therapy (β-blockers were not yet in widespread use) was safe and reduced mortality by 30%. Death from progressive heart failure and sudden death were both reduced by spironolactone. The patients who participated in RALES were primarily NYHA class III (70%) and IV (30%).

Eplerenone, a newer, more selective aldosterone mineralocorticoid receptor blocker, causes less gynecomastia and breast tenderness than spironolactone. It is more mineralocorticoid specific than spironolactone. EPHESUS was conducted in patients who experienced a recent acute myocardial infarction with an EF of 40% or less who had heart failure, or had a history of diabetes mellitus. Eplerenone (average dose 42.6 mg per day) reduced all-cause mortality by 15%, cardiovascular mortality by 17% and significantly lowered the need for subsequent hospitalization.

The EMPHASIS-HF trial (Effect of Eplerenone versus Placebo on Cardiovascular Mortality and Heart Failure Hospitalization in Subjects with NYHA Class II Chronic Systolic Heart Failure) which employed eplerenone in a large double-blinded trial of patients with more mild (NYHA class II) heart failure was recently stopped prematurely when a favorable response was noted.

❏ PHOSPHODIESTERASE TYPE 5 INHIBITORS

Sildenafil and Tadalafil

Phosphodiesterases are enzymes that hydrolyze the cyclic nucleotides—c-GMP and cyclic adenosine monophosphate (cAMP). Phosphodiesterase 5 (PDE 5) degrades c-GMP via hydrolysis, thus influencing c-GMP's ability to modulate smooth muscle tone, particularly in the venous system of the penile corpus cavernosum and in the pulmonary vasculature.

Sildenafil and tadalafil are useful in patients with pulmonary arterial hypertension who have mild-to-moderately severe symptoms. Preliminary data on sildenafil suggest that its use may also be safe and even beneficial in patients with disproportionate pulmonary hypertension and LV dysfunction. Sildenafil citrate is prescribed in doses of 20 mg TID and tadalafil is much longer acting and is prescribed in doses of 5 mg per day as needed to control pulmonary hypertension. Hypotension can occur with PDE 5 inhibitors, especially when they are used with nitrates.

❏ INTRAVENOUS VASODILATORS

Nitroprusside

Sodium nitroprusside can be dramatic in reversing the deleterious hemodynamics of acute systolic heart failure. Those who have had experience using the drug in this setting are often astonished how quickly the drug lowers PCWP and improves cardiac output, leading to prompt and often striking clinic improvement. The drug is usually started as doses of 10 mcg/min, and gradually titrated up to not more than 400 mcg/min, as needed to control hemodynamic abnormalities and symptoms.

Metabolism and Toxicity of Nitroprusside

Nitroprusside has been used to treat severe heart failure for many years, although the Food and Drug Administration (FDA) has approved it only for severe hypertension and hypotensive surgery. Thiocyanate toxicity can occur, and thiocyanate levels should be checked as needed. Measurement of thiocyanate is a simple, inexpensive colorimetric test, normal levels being less than 10 mg/mL. Metabolic acidosis, anuria, and a prolonged high dose of nitroprusside (>400 mcg/min) can predispose to thiocyanate toxicity, prompting the measurement of thiocyanate levels.

Nitroprusside and Severe Heart Failure

Nitroprusside quickly improves hemodynamics and symptoms in patients with severe heart failure. Even patients with hypotension and shock may improve with nitroprusside, as BP may stabilize or even improve with a large increase in cardiac output. Patients with severe mitral regurgitations or aortic regurgitation may also demonstrate dramatic reversal of serious hemodynamic perturbations with nitroprusside. Patients with severe aortic stenosis and worsening heart failure can be improved with nitroprusside used prior to aortic value replacement, provided they are not hypotensive. It can also be used to stabilize acute heart failure in patients who demonstrate a ruptured interventricular septum following acute myocardial infarction. Recent data indicate that in patients hospitalized with advanced, low-output heart failure, those stabilized in the hospital with nitroprusside may have a more favorable long-term clinical outcome.

Intravenous Nitroglycerin

Similar to nitroprusside, intravenous nitroglycerin has an immediate onset and offset of action. The infusion rate is usually initiated at 10–20 mcg/min and titrated slowly to 200–500 mcg/min as needed to control symptoms and improve hemodynamic parameters. It is not approved by the FDA for the treatment of heart failure but has been widely used for this indication over the past 20 years. Intravenous nitroglycerin is endothelium dependent, and unlike nitroprusside, it has more effect on the venous circulation than on the arterial circulation. However, higher doses of intravenous nitroglycerin decrease SVR, as well as increase venous capacity. Therefore, cardiac output increases and BP can be maintained. PCWP is reduced. Mitral regurgitation improves. There are few data available on the effects of intravenous nitroglycerin on coronary circulation in patients with heart failure. Coronary blood flow appears to improve. This suggests that both the epicardial conductance vessels and the coronary arteriolar resistance vessels are favorably influenced by intravenous nitroglycerin.

Nesiritide

Nesiritide is pure human brain natriuretic peptide (BNP), synthesized using recombinant DNA techniques. It has the same 32-amino acid sequence as endogenous BNP released from the heart. When infused intravenously into the circulation of patients with heart failure, the mean terminal elimination half-life of nesiritide is about 18 minutes. Plasma BNP levels increase about threefold to sixfold with nesiritide infusion.

The largest clinical trial of nesiritide, Vasodilation in the Management of Acute CHF (VMAC), was a comparison study with intravenous nitroglycerin. It demonstrated that nesiritide improved hemodynamic function and self-reported symptoms are more effective than intravenous nitroglycerin or placebo (Figs 7A and B). On this basis, nesiritide was approved by the FDA for heart failure and became widely used for the treatment of acute heart failure. Nesiritide has venous, arterial, and coronary vasodilator properties. Cardiac output improves and PCWP reduces. Hypotension occurs in about 4% of patients, and unlike intravenous nitroglycerin, it can be prolonged (~20 min) because of nesiritide's relatively longer half-life. The effects of nesiritide on renal function are variable, but generally only a modest or neutral renal effect is observed, though worsening renal function has been reported.

❏ ORAL β-ADRENERGIC BLOCKING DRUGS

There is a fundamental belief that the biologically powerful adrenergic nervous system compensates the failing heart by increasing myocyte size (hypertrophy), heart rate and force of contraction (inotropy). The SNS also activates the RAAS, thus conserving intravascular volume and redirecting blood flow to vital organs. However, an overly active SNS has repeatedly been shown to be essentially toxic to myocardial cells in both animals and humans. There have been numerous large randomized trials supporting the concept that blocking the SNS with β-adrenergic blocking drugs in patients with systolic heart failure slows the progression of systolic heart failure and improves patient survival.

It is well known that β-adrenergic receptors downregulate in response to excessive sympathetic drive, presumably in an attempt to protect the cardiac myocyte from overstimulation. Such biological behavior suggests that blocking the receptors pharmacologically may also protect the heart.

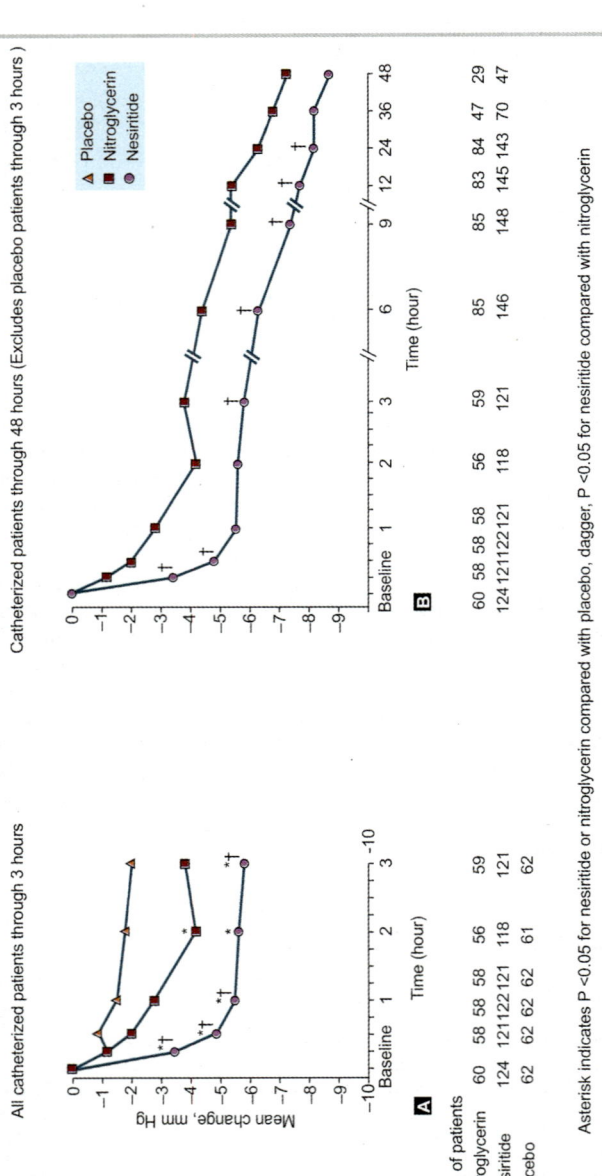

FIGURES 7A AND B: Changes in pulmonary capillary wedge pressure from baseline in response to intravenous nitroglycerin, nesiritide and placebo in patients with heart failure (*Source:* Modified from Publication Committee for the VMAC Investigators (Vasodilatation in the management of Acute CHF). Intravenous nesiritide vs nitroglycerin for treatment of decompensated congestive heart failure: A randomized controlled trial. JAMA.2002;287:1531-40, with permission)

β-adrenergic blocking drugs are now widely used to treat all stages of heart failure. Some patients admitted to the hospital with NYHA class III or IV systolic heart failure may not tolerate β-blockers, because of symptomatic hypotension or low cardiac output. The continuation of β-blocker therapy in patients hospitalized with acute decompensated systolic heart failure is associated with lower postdischarge mortality risk and improved treatment rates.

Although it is unusual nowadays to see patients with heart failure who are naive to either RAAS blockers or β-blockers, occasionally the issue of which class of drug to start first arises. We now have three major heart failure therapeutic strategies aimed at producing reverse remodeling:
- RAAS blocking drugs
- Cardiac resynchronization therapy (CRT)
- β-adrenergic blocking drugs.

Of course, coronary revascularization can also improve LV size and performance in selected patients. These therapies have proven to be the powerful drivers of improved patient survival.

❏ CONCLUSION

Neurohumoral modulating drugs now have a central role in the treatment of patients with systolic heart failure. This was not the case 35 years ago when only digitalis and diuretics were used. Annualized mortality has fallen from ~20% to less than 10% per year commensurate with the use of RAAS and SNS blocking drugs. Of course, ICDs and CRT have also importantly contributed to this mortality reduction. The total cardiovascular death rate burden has fallen substantially in accordance with the widespread use of these therapies. Although, the incidence of ST segment elevation myocardial infarction (STEMI) has also fallen dramatically, incident heart failure continues to increase. There is now much better treatment for hypertension and hyperlipidemia. Paradoxically, as people live longer, we are now seeing a wave of heart failure in the elderly, the fastest growing segment of our population. The scourge of heart failure has not gone away but has rather been shifted to people in their 70s, 80s and 90s. In the end, prevention of heart failure by lifelong control of known risk factors and mechanistic enlightenment, although additional genomic studies may reduce the burden of heart failures even more, as systolic heart failure is likely a largely preventable disorder.

❏ SUGGESTED READINGS

Anand IS, Tam SW, Rector TS, et al. Influence of blood pressure on the effectiveness of a fixed-dose combination of isosorbide dinitrate and hydralazine in the African-American Heart Failure Trial. J Am Coll Cardiol. 2007;49:32-9.

Burnier M, Brunner HR. Angiotensin II receptor antagonists. Lancet. 2000;355:637-45.

CIBIS Investigators and Committees. A randomized trial of ??blockade in heart failure. The Cardiac Insufficiency Bisoprolol Study (CIBIS). Circulation. 1994;90:1765-73.

CIBIS-II Investigators and Committees. The Cardiac Insufficiency Bisoprolol Study II (CIBIS-II): a randomized trial. Lancet. 1999;353:9-13.

Cohn JN. Structural basis for heart failure. Ventricular remodelling and its pharmacological inhibition.

GISSI-AF Investigators. Valsartan for prevention of recurrent atrial fibrillation. N Engl J Med. 2009;360:1606-17.

Guiha NH, Cohn JN, Mikulic E, et al. Treatment of refractory heart failure with infusion of nitroprusside. N Engl J Med. 1974; 291:587-92.

Mullens W, Abrahams Z, Francis GS, et al. Sodium nitroprusside for advanced low-output heart failure. J Am Coll Cardiol. 2008;52:200-7.

ONTARGET Investigators. Telmisartan, ramipril, or both in patients at high risk for vascular events. N Engl J Med. 2008;358:1547-59.

Packer M, Fowler MB, Roecker EB, et al. Effect of carvedilol on the morbidity of patients with severe chronic heart failure: results of the carvedilol prospective randomized cumulative survival (COPERNICUS) study. Circulation. 2002;106:2194-9.

The SOLVD Investigators. Effect of enalapril on survival in patients with reduced left ventricular ejection fraction and congestive heart failure. N Engl J Med. 1991;325:293-302.

VMAC. Intravenous nesiritide vs nitroglycerin for treatment ofdecompensated congestive heart failure. JAMA. 2002;287:1531-40.

Young JB, Dunlap ME, Pfeffer MA, et al. Mortality and morbidity reduction with Candesartan in patients with chronic heart failure and left ventricular systolic dysfunction: results of the CHARM low-left ventricular ejection trials. Circulation. 2004;110:2618-26.

1.3 Positive Inotropic Drugs

❏ INTRODUCTION

Positive inotropic drugs (also know as positive inotropes) are agents that increase the velocity and strength of contraction of the cardiac myocyte and as a consequence, the myocardium and the heart as an organ unit; a few of the measurements of contractility or inotropy include Δ LV systolic upstroke pressure/Δ time, peak slope of LV developed pressure and end-systolic elastance. Positive inotropic drugs are, therefore, generally directed at patients whose overall cardiovascular function is compromised by loss of cardiac contractility resulting in symptoms and signs of depressed stroke volume, cardiac output, hypoperfusion of vital organs and systems and often, hypotension. In general, positive inotropes enhance cardiac contractility via modulation of calcium handling by the cardiomyocyte. The cellular mechanisms of action of the major inotropic drugs are illustrated in Figure 8.

❏ INTRAVENOUSLY ADMINISTERED, SHORT-TERM POSITIVE INOTROPIC THERAPY

The agents under this heading represent a spectrum of pharmacologic properties in addition to their positive inotropic effects. The predominant distinguishing feature among these agents is their effect on vasculature, which can range from vasodilatation to balanced vascular tone to vasoconstriction (Fig. 9 and Table 6). The pharmacologic mechanisms for their positive inotropy on increasing intracellular cyclic adenosine monophosphate (cAMP) by either adrenergic receptor stimulation or inhibition of cAMP degradation (Fig. 8).

Adrenergic Receptor Agonists

Although the adrenergic agonists can evoke tachycardia and dysrhythmias, they do have short elimination half-lives, an ideal pharmacologic property in the monitored critical care setting where a quick "turn on" and "turn off" of cardiovascular effects allow immediate and tightly controlled hemodynamic support.

The catechols (3,4-hydroxyphenyl ring) are the major drug group in the adrenergic family used for positive inotropic therapy. The cardiovascular effects of adrenergic agents used clinically for inotropic and hemodynamic support are individually presented under the heading of each and summarized in Table 6.

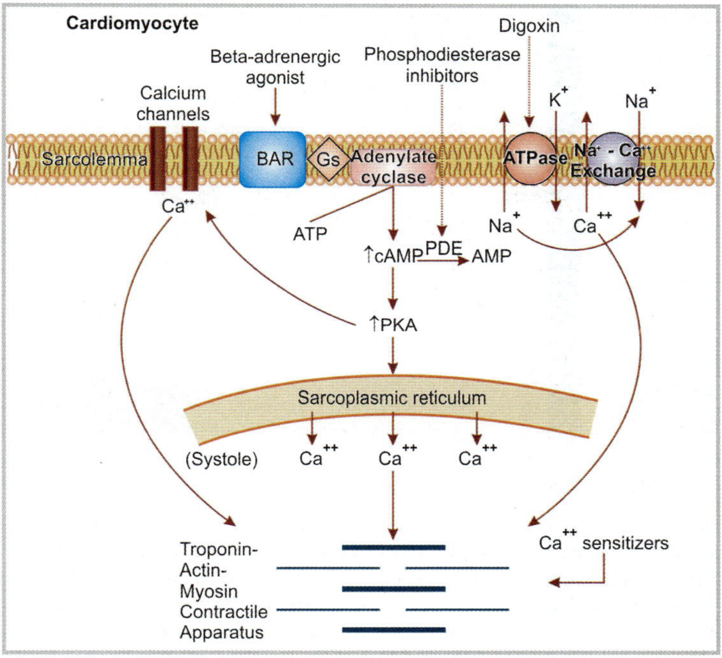

FIGURE 8: The major positive inotropic groups generally act through mechanisms that increase the concentration and availability of intracellular calcium for the actin–myosin contractile apparatus. Beta-adrenergic agonists attach to the beta-adrenergic receptor, activating the Gs protein adenylate cyclase complex to convert ATP to cAMP. cAMP activates protein kinase A, which phosphorylates several intracellular sites resulting in an influx and release of Ca^{++} for systole. Phosphodiesterase inhibitors retard the breakdown of cAMP. Calcium sensitizers act by making the troponin–actin–myosin complex more responsive to available Ca^{++}. By blocking the Na/K ATPase pump, digoxin increases intracellular Na^+ loading of the Na^+-Ca^{++} exchanger, resulting in less extrusion of Ca^{++} from the myocyte. Dashed arrow indicates inhibition. While this illustration depicts the major pharmacologic actions of these positive inotropic groups, their comprehensive mechanisms are considerably more numerous and complex. (Abbreviations: ATP: Adenosine triphosphate; cAMP: Cyclic adenosine monophosphate; AMP: Adenosine monophosphate; PDE: Phosphodiesterase; BAR: Beta-adrenergic receptor; PKA: Protein kinase A)

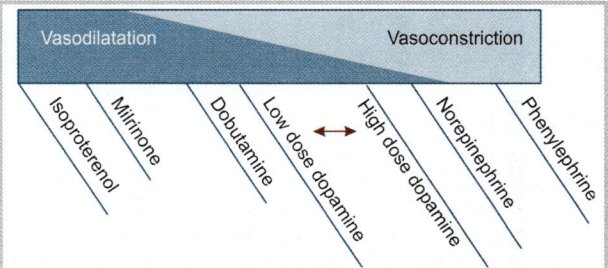

FIGURE 9: The spectrum of net vascular properties of the agents currently available for short-term positive inotropy and cardiovascular support. The vascular effects and responses are a major determinant for selection in individual patients

Table 6: Hemodynamic profiles of the agents currently employed to deliver short-term inotropic and vasoactive support

	Phosphodiesterase inhibitor		Dopamine		Adrenergic agonists	
	Milrinone	Dobutamine	Low dose	Higher dose	Norepinephrine	Phenylephrine
Contractility (inotropy)	↑	↑↑↑	↑	↑↑	↑	↗
Cardiac output	↑↑	↑↑↑	↑	↑	↑	↗
Heart rate (chronotropy)	→↗	→↑	→↑	↑↑	↑	→↑
LV filling pressure	↓↓	↓↓	→	→↑	→↑	→↑
Systemic blood pressure	→↓	→↑	↑	↑↑	↑↑↑	↑↑↑
Systemic vascular resistance	↓↓	↓	↑	↑↑	↑↑↑	↑↑↑
Pulmonary vascular resistance	↓↓	→	↑	→↑	↑	↑

↓ decrease; → minimal to no change; ↗ mild increase; ↑ increase

Dobutamine

Dobutamine is the agent most commonly used for short-term intravenous inotropic support, and its net cardiovascular effects in the setting of left ventricular systolic failure result predominantly from positive inotropic enhancement of depressed cardiac contractility. Dobutamine was developed from methodical manipulation and substitutions on the basic catechol-phenylethylamine molecule.

The major clinical indication for dobutamine administration is short-term inotropic support in patients compromised by ventricular systolic dysfunction, which has resulted in a problematic reduction in blood pressure and systemic perfusion (Table 7).

In the appropriate patient, namely the patient with ventricular systolic dysfunction resulting in a fall in stroke volume and cardiac output, an elevation in left ventricular end-diastolic filling pressure, systemic hypoperfusion and mild-to-moderate reduction in systemic blood pressure, dobutamine increases stroke volume, cardiac output, systemic systolic blood pressure and pulse pressure, and

Table 7: The clinical applications of dobutamine administration

Major indication:

Short-term (hours to days) inotropic and hemodynamic support for patients with ventricular systolic dysfunction resulting in a depressed stroke volume and cardiac output, systemic hypoperfusion, mild-to-moderate systemic hypotension (systolic blood pressures of 70–100 mm Hg) and an elevated left ventricular diastolic filling pressure (>18 mm Hg). This support is maintained until the patient recovers or is directed into more advanced cardiovascular support (e.g. intra-aortic balloon counterpulsation, ventricular assist device) and/or remedial intervention (e.g. coronary artery intervention, valvular repair or replacement, cardiac transplantation).

Additional considerations:

A	Pharmacologic support as needed for patients with severe heart failure undergoing major diagnostic or surgical procedures
B	Cardiovascular hemodynamic support for the heart failure patient through the course of a major illness
C	Pharmacologic bridge in severe heart failure to standard therapies (e.g. angiotensin-converting enzyme inhibitor, beta-adrenergic blocker)
D	As a continuous infusion via indwelling central venous catheter to provide the only means of stabilizing an unstable or decompensated heart failure patient to allow discharge from the hospital (to extended care, home or hospice)
E	For hemodynamic support during weaning from cardiopulmonary bypass and during recovery from cardiac surgery
F	To facilitate recovery of myocardial stunning in the setting of low output cardiac failure
G	As a means of improving renal function and urine output in patients hospitalized for low output, systemic hypoperfusion and volume-overloaded congestive heart failure when renal responsiveness to standard therapy and diuretics is impaired
H	For hemodynamic support during management of cardiac transplant rejection complicated by hemodynamic decompensation
I	To augment systolic function of problematic systolic failure of the right ventricle
J	To assess ventricular (right or left) contractile reserve
K	To evaluate the severity of low-flow, low-gradient aortic valvular stenosis
L	As pharmacologic stress for myocardial perfusion imaging

systemic perfusion, while decreasing pulmonary and systemic vascular resistance and left ventricular filling pressure. While there appears to be a dose-related separation of positive inotropy and beneficial hemodynamic effects from positive chronotropy, higher dosing will evoke a faster heart rate and can provoke ectopic beats and tachydysrhythmias.

Dobutamine can be safely administered to heart failure patients with occlusive coronary disease to attain and maintain a stable clinical and hemodynamic short-term course until the patient is directed to more advanced management (e.g. intra-aortic balloon counterpulsation, coronary angiography and intervention, coronary bypass surgery). Dobutamine may have a favorable effect on myocardial stunning beyond the simple increase in coronary blood flow and myocardial perfusion of the affected region or whole heart.

The most common clinical scenarios for appropriate dobutamine administration (to improve and stabilize hemodynamic and clinical status) include patients managed for:

- Decompensated, hypoperfused, often hypotensive chronic systolic heart failure
- Acute systolic heart failure (e.g. acute myocardial infarction, acute myocarditis)
- Immediately following cardiac surgery + cardiopulmonary bypass.

The various considerations for the administration of dobutamine are presented in Table 7.

Although the usual dose range for dobutamine is 2.0–15.0 mcg/kg/min, many patients can experience clinical and hemodynamic benefit at a lower starting dose of 0.5–1.0 mcg/kg/min and do so with minimal to no increase in heart rate or dysrhythmias. Dosing can be advanced by 1.0–2.0 mcg/kg/min increments every 12–15 or more minutes until the desired clinical and hemodynamic effects are attained. When discontinuing, maintenance doses of less than or equal to 2.0 mcg/kg/min can usually be stopped without difficulty. Higher infusion rates over an extended period generally require weaning over 12–72 hours to avert clinical and hemodynamic deterioration with more abrupt discontinuation.

The pharmacokinetic and pharmacodynamic properties of dobutamine endorse its application as a short-term positive inotropic agent. Most of the drug is eliminated within 12–13 minutes upon discontinuation of the infusion, allowing a rapid dissipation of adverse effects if encountered during the infusion. In human heart failure, there is a direct near-linear relationship between the infusion dose of dobutamine, its plasma levels, and hemodynamic responses.

Adverse effects are largely attributable to its administration in a more ill and compromised patient or due to improper patient and/or dose selection. The most common adverse effects of dobutamine are tachycardia and dysrhythmias. Other side effects, also generally dose related, include headache, tremor, anxiety, palpitations, and nausea. A hypertensive response (elevated systemic systolic blood pressure) can be observed when dobutamine is administered to patients with a history of systemic hypertension or peripheral vascular disease. Patients with high-grade occlusive coronary artery disease can experience angina, myocardial ischemia and infarction, particularly in patients who do not meet the primary indication for use (Table 7) and/or receive excessive initial dosing or excessively rapid advancement of dose. Dobutamine infusions can lower plasma potassium concentrations.

Dopamine

While dopamine, an endogenous precursor of epinephrine and norepinephrine, is the simplest molecule of the adrenergic agents, it has the most complex pharmacology (Fig. 9 and Table 6). In general, dopamine elicits its pharmacodynamic effects through stimulation of dopaminergic receptors (D1 and D2) and adrenergic receptors (β1, β2 and α) and through the neuronal release and reduced neuronal uptake of endogenous norepinephrine. At lower infusion rates (<4.0 mcg/kg/min) in human heart failure, dopamine behaves as a mild vasodilator (dopaminergic), particularly of visceral and renal arterial–arteriolar vascular beds. With increased dosing, this effect is overtaken by dopamine's agonism of adrenergic receptors directly and through its release of norepinephrine from nerve endings; vasodilatation gives way to a net-balanced vascular effect and some positive inotropy at moderate dosing (4.0–8.0 mcg/kg/min) and to considerable vasoconstriction and some retained inotropy at higher doses (>8.0 mcg/kg/min).

In states of low cardiac output, systemic hypoperfusion, and adequate or elevated left ventricular filling pressures, dopamine at less than 4.0 mcg/kg/min can augment ventricular contractility, stroke volume and cardiac output, and reduce systemic and pulmonary vascular resistance; all to a modest degree without a substantial change in systemic blood pressure. As infusion rates move to more than 4.0 mcg/kg/min, vascular resistance, stroke volume and cardiac output plateau and there occurs a substantial dose-related rise in systemic blood pressure. Positive chronotropy and provocation of dysrhythmias are also dose related and can become an undesirable effect at more than or equal to 6.0 mcg/kg/min. Indices of ventricular contractility (positive inotropy) are blunted at higher dosing and during continuous infusion, presumably secondary to the rise in blood pressure, vascular resistance and ventricular afterload and depletion of myocardial norepinephrine stores from dopamine-induced release (and reduced uptake) at nerve endings during high-dose or prolonged infusions.

The most common adverse effects of dopamine administration are similar to those of dobutamine, namely positive chronotropy and dysrhythmias, both dose related. Dopamine crosses the blood–brain barrier to provoke nausea and vomiting in some patients. Intense vasoconstriction by dopamine can lead to ischemia of digits and various organ systems. Subcutaneous infiltration at the infusion site can provoke pain and ischemic changes, potentially reversible with local instillation of phentolamine. Dopamine has been reported to depress minute ventilation in heart failure.

Other Adrenergic Agents

These agents are used in various clinical settings for various indications. Due to overriding vascular effects, they are not employed as primary positive inotropic drugs.

Isoproterenol: This drug is perhaps the purest beta-adrenergic receptor agonist (β1 and β2) available for clinical use. However, its positive inotropic properties are largely overshadowed by strong vasodilatory and positive chronotropic effects (Table 6). Its principal clinical application is rather narrow, namely to increase heart rate in the short-term (until recovery or definitive intervention) in patients with problematic bradycardia or inadequate heart rate response; particularly in clinical situations where intravenous atropine is contraindicated, inadequate, or ineffective. In view of other available, generally safer vasodilating agents (e.g. milrinone, nesiritide, nitrates), isoproterenol is rarely used as a primary vasodilating agent. Adverse effects include flushing, tremor, anxiety, tachycardia, dysrhythmias, and hypotension.

Epinephrine: This endogenous catecholamine stimulates β1, β2 and α1 adrenergic receptors. Epinephrine differs from dobutamine in that its administration is modulated by neuronal uptake and its β2 and α1 effects are more intense than those of dobutamine. In cardiovascular medicine, epinephrine is most often employed during cardiopulmonary resuscitation or as a global hemodynamic support drug during withdrawal for cardiopulmonary bypass and recovery from cardiac surgery. Adverse effects include those described above for dobutamine, dopamine, and isoproterenol.

Norepinephrine and phenylephrine: These agents are predominant α1-adrenergic agonists with mild beta-receptor agonism, and thus, they are viewed as vasopressors (Fig. 9 and Table 6). As such, these compounds are used for vasoconstriction to increase and stabilize systemic blood pressure in states of marked hypotension and shock (vasodilatory and cardiogenic).

Norepinephrine dosing in hypotension and shock generally ranges 0.02–0.40 mcg/kg/min. In addition to the adverse effects described for dopamine, norepinephrine can evoke dose-related systemic hypertension and bradycardia. More intense vasoconstriction with minimal positive inotropy is rendered by phenylephrine.

Phosphodiesterase Inhibitors

Drugs under this grouping are often referred to as "inodilators" because vasodilation is a major component of their pharmacology. In fact, amrinone, studied early in this category, is principally a vasodilator with little to no ability to augment ventricular contraction beyond its unloading effects on the ventricle. Thrombocytopenia during prolonged administration tempered its clinical application. As a therapeutic modality, amrinone has largely been replaced by milrinone.

Milrinone

While milrinone can elicit some positive inotropy through other cellular mechanisms (e.g. activation of the calcium release channel), its cardiovascular effects are principally rendered through inhibition of phosphodiesterase III (PDE III) with consequent impairment of the breakdown metabolism of cAMP (Fig. 8).

In contrast to dobutamine, a positive inotrope with mild vasodilating properties, milrinone is a vasodilator with mild positive inotropic properties. Therefore, for any matched degree of enhanced contractility, milrinone evokes a greater reduction in pulmonary and systemic vascular resistance, systemic blood pressure, and ventricular filling pressures.

In patients with severe low output congestive heart failure, milrinone augments the hemodynamic effects of dobutamine and vice versa. It is not unusual to employ this combination in patients with markedly compromised hemodynamics, generally in the setting of advanced, end-stage heart failure, as a pharmacologic bridge to placement of a ventricular assist device and/or cardiac transplantation.

Milrinone is generally started at 0.20–0.30 mcg/kg/min and gradually advanced as needed to achieve the intended hemodynamic and clinical endpoints and short of evoking tachycardia, dysrhythmias or hypotension. Milrinone has a half-life of 1–3 hours, and thus, the onset of action and equilibration is not as prompt as that seen with the catechol inotropes. The lengthy elimination half-life (1–3 hours) results in a more prolonged recovery from adverse effects, once milrinone is discontinued.

Other Intravenously Administered Positive Inotropic Interventions

A number of additional pharmacologic interventions are known to enhance myocardial contractility.

Calcium Sensitizers

Calcium sensitizers (e.g. levosimendan) augment cardiac contractility by modulating intracellular mechanisms of contraction at the same concentrations of intracellular calcium (Fig. 8).

Levosimendan: Although some of its positive inotropic effect is probably rendered through phosphodiesterase inhibition, levosimendan is reported to enhance myocardial contractility through sensitization of the contractile apparatus to available calcium by increasing or stabilizing calcium binding to troponin C.

Levosimendan behaves as an inodilator in human heart failure; it reduces vascular resistance and ventricular filling pressures, and augments stroke volume and cardiac output. Due to its prominent vasodilating properties, levosimendan should not be considered a first-line drug for low output hypotension or shock. Levosimendan itself has an elimination half-life of 1–2 hours, but a primary active metabolite (OR-1896) has a half-life of more than 75 hours.

Orally Administered Positive Inotropic Agents

Oral inotropes have not fared well over the past two decades as intervention to improve myocardial contractility and performance. While digitalis (currently digoxin) has been used for over 200 years to treat cardiac failure and "dropsy", this coveted role has been reined in by the Digitalis Investigation Group (DIG) trial published in 1997. Many orally administered, non-digitalis agents have been formulated over the past four decades to replace digoxin in the therapeutics of human heart failure; examples include amrinone, milrinone, vesnarinone, pimobendan and butopamine; all were found to be ineffective, to provoke undesirable effects or to adversely affect outcomes.

Digitalis–Digoxin

Most of the enhancement of myocardial contractility by digoxin appears to be generated by inhibiting the Na^+/K^+ ATPase pump of the cardiomyocyte sarcolemma (Fig. 8). This inhibition results in elevation of intracellular sodium, which increases (via blunting of the sodium–calcium exchanger) the intracellular calcium available for contraction. Digitalis may also direct calcium into the myocyte via modulation of the voltage-sensitive sodium channels.

Some of the clinical benefits of digitalis therapy in heart failure likely occur through alteration of sympathetic tone. Heart failure increases sympathetic nervous system tone and reduces parasympathetic tone, resulting in a number of undesirable effects, including increased vascular resistance, tachycardia, renin release and diminished baroreceptor sensitivity; many of these undesirable responses are favorably suppressed or reversed by chronic digitalis administration.

Intravenously administered digoxin in heart failure evokes a modest increase in mean stroke volume, cardiac output and systemic blood pressure, a modest decrease in heart rate and ventricular filling pressures, and little change in vascular resistance; although individual responses can vary widely with better hemodynamic effects noted in the more hemodynamically compromised patients.

The DIG trial has overshadowed all prior studies regarding the use of digitalis chronically in patients with heart failure and sinus rhythm, and has now provided the framework for current digoxin use. Patients were randomized 1:1 to digoxin (median dose 0.25 mg/day) or placebo. Chronic digoxin therapy in the DIG Trial had no effect on total mortality but tended to reduce mortality attributable to heart failure and statistically reduced the combined endpoints of heart failure mortality or hospitalization for heart failure. While this benefit was greatest in patients with lower ejection fractions and worse clinical status, modest improvement was also noted for patients with an LV ejection fraction more than 0.45.

For the overall heart failure population, long-term digoxin administration has a Class IIa indication (level of evidence: B) from the 2009 ACC/AHA Task Force, which stated, "Digitalis can be beneficial in patients with current or prior symptoms of heart failure and reduced left ventricular ejection fraction to decrease hospitalizations in heart failure". Chronic digoxin therapy remains an option to control ventricular rate in the heart failure patient with atrial fibrillation, although this consideration has been challenged. The initial and maintenance oral dose is 0.0625–0.25 mg/day. The 0.125 mg/day dose has largely replaced 0.25 mg/day as the standard maintenance dose because at the lower dose, serum digoxin levels (drawn >8 hours after dosing) typically remain less than or equal to 1.0 ng/mL in patients with normal renal function and clearance. Dose reduction or discontinuation becomes important in patients with renal dysfunction and/or during concomitant administration of medications known to elevate digoxin concentrations (Table 8).

Digoxin's direct effect on sinoatrial and atrioventricular nodal cells and its autonomic properties (reducing sympathetic tone and enhancing parasympathetic tone) leads to many of the manifestations of digoxin toxicity, generally at serum levels more than 2.0 ng/mL, including sinus bradycardia and AV nodal blockade.

Other Orally Administered Positive Inotropic Agents

Hydralazine has positive inotropic properties in human heart failure in addition to its well-established vasodilating, ventricular unloading effects. These inotropic

Table 8: A partial list of agents known to affect, through a number of different mechanisms, serum digoxin concentrations

A	*Decrease levels*
	• Cholestyramine • Salbutamol
	• Sucralfate • Rifampin
	• Kaolin-pectin • Thyroxine
	• Antacids
B	*Increase levels*
	• Antiarrhythmic agents • Antimicrobials
	▪ Amiodarone ▪ Macrolides (-mycin)
	▪ Propafenone ▪ Tetracycline
	▪ Quinidine ▪ Itraconazole
	• Calcium channel blocking agents • Other
	▪ Verapamil ▪ Captopril
	▪ Diltiazem ▪ Carvedilol
	▪ Dihydropyridines (e.g. nifedipine) ▪ Cyclosporine
	• Potassium-sparing diuretics ▪ Indomethacin
	▪ Spironolactone ▪ Omeprazole
	▪ Triamterene ▪ St. John's wort
	▪ Amiloride

and hemodynamic effects can be employed to wean dobutamine (and perhaps, milrinone and low-dose dopamine) from heart failure patients who appear hemodynamically dependent on the intravenous inotrope.

Absolute and relative hypothyroidism can play a major role in the clinical course and outcomes in heart failure. Thyroid hormone replacement enhances myocardial contractility through a number of mechanisms and is of particular clinical importance in these specific patient groups. Whether thyroid hormone intervention merits consideration as a means of augmenting cardiac performance and clinical outcomes in patients with heart failure beyond these groups remains unanswered.

❑ SUGGESTED READINGS

Abraham WT, Adams KF, Fonarow GC, et al. In hospital mortality in patients with acute decompensated heart failure requiring intravenous vasoactive medications: an analysis from the acute decompensated heart failure national registry (ADHERE). J Am Coll Cardiol. 2005;46:57-64.

Bristow MR, Ginsburg R, Umans V, et al. B1- and B2-adrenergic–receptor subpopulations in nonfailing and failing human ventricular myocardium: coupling of both receptor subtypes to muscle contraction and selective B1-receptor downregulation in heart failure. Circ Res. 1986;59:297-309.

Burger AJ, Horton DP, LeJemtel TH, et al. Effect of nesiritide (B-type natriuretic peptide) and dobutamine on ventricular arrhythmias in the treatment of patients with acutely decompensated congestive heart failure: the PRECEDENT study. Am Heart J. 2002;144:1102-8.

Gheorghiade M, Stough WG, Adams K, et al. The pilot randomized study of nesiritide versus dobutamine in heart failure (PRESERVDHF). Am J Cardiol. 2005;96(6A):18G-25G.

Jessup M, Abraham WT, Casey DE, et al. 2009 Focused Update: ACCF/AHA Guidelines for the diagnosis and management of heart failure in adults. Circulation. 2009;119:1977-2016.

Leier CV, Heban PF, Huss P, et al. Comparative systemic and regional hemodynamic effects of dopamine and dobutamine in patients with cardiomyopathic heart failure. Circulation. 1978;58:466-75.

Packer M, Gheorghiade M, Young JB, et al. Withdrawal of digoxin from patients with chronic heart failure treated with angiotensin-converting- enzyme inhibitors. RADIANCE study. N Engl J Med. 1993;329:1-7.

The Digitalis Investigation Group. The effect of digoxin on mortality and morbidity in patients with heart failure. N Engl J Med. 1997;336:525-33.

Tuttle RR, Mills J. Dobutamine: development of a new catecholamine to selectively increase cardiac contractility. Circ Res. 1975;36:185- 96.

1.4 Antilipid Agents

❑ INTRODUCTION

Over 150 years ago, Virchow and his colleagues described the accumulation of lipid as the hallmark of the atherosclerotic plaque. Since then, an extensive body of evidence has shown a direct relationship between blood cholesterol levels and atherosclerotic cardiovascular diseases. The large majority of clinical data come from statin trials. Other lipid modifying drugs have demonstrated more modest cardiovascular benefits.

❑ APPROPRIATE USES

The National Cholesterol Education Program Adult Treatment Panel (NCEP ATP III) has identified two lipid targets for the prevention of cardiovascular diseases, LDL-C and non-high density lipoprotein cholesterol (non-HDL-C) (Table 9). The first target of therapy is *LDL-C,* with treatment goals based on the risk of a coronary heart disease event in the next 10 years. The second target of therapy is non-*HDL-C.* Non-HDL-C is calculated by subtracting HDL-C from total cholesterol and reflects circulating levels of atherogenic apolipoprotein-B containing lipoproteins. The non-HDL-C goal is 30 mg/dL higher than the

Table 9: Overview of lipid treatment goals and strategies			
		Triglycerides (mg/dL)	
	1st target **LDL-C**	**<500** **2nd target** **Non-HDL-C**	**>500**
Objective	**Prevent CVD**	**Prevent CVD**	**Prevent pancreatitis**
Treatment goals	LDL-C goal *High risk:* CHD/CHD risk equivalents* <100 (optional <70) mg/dL *Moderately high risk:* >2 risk factors** with 10-20% 10-year CHD risk† <130 mg/dL (optional < 100 mg/dL) *Moderate risk:* >2 risk factors** with <10% 10-year CHD risk <130 mg/dL *Lower risk:* 0–1 risk factor <160 mg/dL (consider drug therapy LDL >190 mg/dL/optional LDL >160 mg/dL)	Non-HDL-C goal 30 mg/dL higher than LDL goal	Triglycerides < 500 mg/dL
Lifestyle	Therapeutic lifestyle changes	Therapeutic lifestyle changes	• Therapeutic lifestyle changes • Very low-fat (<15%) diet
Drug 1st choice	Statins	Statins	Fibrates
Drug add-on or 2nd choice	Niacin bile-acid sequestrant Ezetimibe	Niacin Ezetimibe Fibrate	Omega-3 fish oil Niacin Statins (high dose)

*Coronary heart disease (CHD) includes a history of myocardial infarction, stable or unstable angina, coronary artery revascularization, or clinically significant myocardial ischemia; CHD risk equivalents include other cardiovascular disease, including peripheral arterial disease, abdominal aortic aneurysm, carotid artery disease (stroke of carotid or intracerebral origin, transient ischemic attack, or >50% carotid artery stenosis), diabetes, and >2 risk factors with >20% 10-year CHD risk

**Risk factors include age (men >45 years, women >55 years), cigarette smoking, hypertension (blood pressure > 140/90 mm Hg or antihypertensive therapy), low HDL-C (<40 mg/dL) and family history of premature CHD (onset in male first degree relative <55 years; first degree female relative <65 years)

†10-year risk of nonfatal myocardial infarction and CHD death estimated by Framingham Scoring

LDL-C goal. Although the NCEP ATP III guidelines recommended using non-HDL-C when triglycerides are 150–500 mg/dL, recent evidence suggests that this recommendation can be simplified to using the non-HDL-C goal when triglycerides are less than 500 mg/dL.

In those with triglyceride levels more than 500 mg/dL, prevention of pancreatitis is the initial objective. Once triglycerides are less than 500 mg/dL, attention can then turn to addressing LDL-C and non-HDL-C levels for cardiovascular prevention. Although low levels of HDL-C and high levels of triglycerides are markers of increased cardiovascular risk, specific treatment targets have not been identified due to the lack of evidence that pharmacologically altering the levels of these two factors per se reduces cardiovascular risk. Cardiovascular prevention efforts in patients with low HDL-C should focus on lifestyle and drug therapy to achieve LDL-C and non-HDL-C goals. In the NCEP ATP III 2004 update, statins were recommended as first line therapy for cardiovascular prevention.

Similar treatment strategies are used to lower LDL-C and non-HDL-C. All patients should be advised to undertake therapeutic lifestyle changes. *Statins* are the drugs of choice based on an extensive record of safely reducing cardiovascular events and overall mortality. Bile acid sequestrants and niacin also reduce cardiovascular risk, although they are less effective and have more adverse effects than statins. Ezetimibe is a well tolerated drug that lowers LDL-C and non-HDL-C but has yet to be established whether ezetimibe reduces cardiovascular risk.

Fibrates are generally the first choice for triglyceride-lowering to prevent pancreatitis. However, fibrates reduce cardiovascular risk less than statins and have safety concerns when used in combination with statins. High doses of omega-3 fish oil, niacin or statins also effectively lower elevated triglycerides. The mechanisms of action, efficacy and safety for each class of drug will now be reviewed.

❑ STATINS

Statins are the foundation of cardiovascular risk reduction. Consistent evidence from more than 100,000 clinical trial participants has shown statins reduce the risk of coronary heart disease and stroke in direct proportion to the magnitude of LDLC lowering. Statins inhibit 3-hydroxy-3-methylglutarul coenzyme A (HMG CoA) reductase, the rate-limiting step in cholesterol synthesis (Fig. 10).

A dose of statin should be used that will lower LDL-C by at least 30–40%. Starting doses of statins generally achieve this degree of LDL-C lowering (pitavastatin 2 mg, atorvastatin 10 mg, lovastatin or pravastatin 40 mg, rosuvastatin 10 mg, simvastatin 40 mg and fluvastatin 80 mg) (Table 10). Reducing LDL-C by more than or equal to 50% or more may be desirable, but usually requires the highest doses of atorvastatin (40–80 mg), rosuvastatin (20–40 mg), or a statin used in combination with another LDL-C lowering agent.

The majority of patients tolerate statins without difficulty. Although commonly reported, muscle complaints are usually not related to statin use. Rhabdomyolysis occurs very rarely and generally in patients with multiple factors predisposing to decreased clearance, such as advanced age, diminished renal function, and medications interfering with statin metabolism. Notably, currently marketed statins are much safer than low-dose aspirin, which has more than 200-fold higher rate of major bleeding than statins have of inducing rhabdomyolysis.

Risk of myopathy and rhabdomyolysis is related to circulating drug levels. Three statins are metabolized by hepatic cytochrome P450 enzyme (CYP) 3A4 and have the most potential for drug interactions—atorvastatin, lovastatin, and

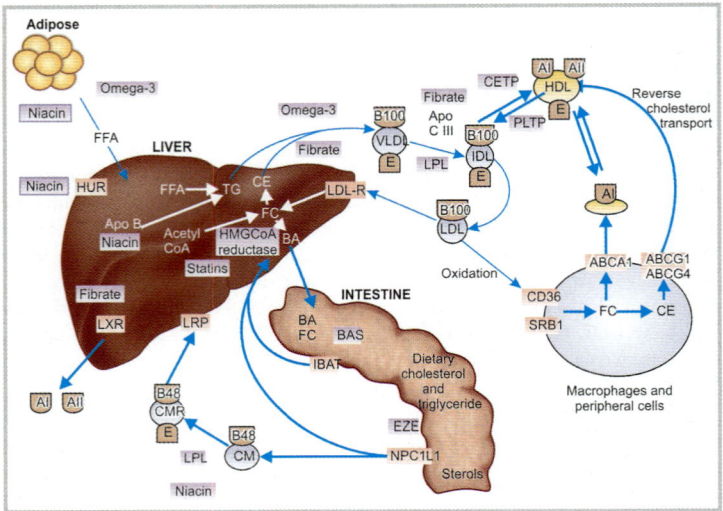

FIGURE 10: Overview of lipid-modifying drug mechanisms.

Statins inhibit the rate-limiting step in cholesterol synthesis, 3-hydroxy-3-methylglutaryl coenzyme A reductase (HMGCoA reductase), which binds acetyl CoA to free cholesterol to create cholesterol esters. Reduction in intrahepatic free cholesterol (FC) increases the number of LDL-receptors (LDL-R) on the cell membrane, facilitating removal of LDL-C from plasma. Bile-acid sequestering agents (BAS) and ezetimibe (EZE) lower plasma LDL-C by lowering intracellular free cholesterol levels. BAS bind bile acids via the intestinal bile acid transporter (IBAT), interrupting the enterohepatic circulation of bile acid FC. EZE acts on the Niemann-Pick C1-Like 1 (NPC1L1) transporter in at the intestinal wall to prevent absorption of dietary and biliary cholesterol. EZE also blocks uptake of plant sterols. Dietary sterol/stanols competitively inhibit the uptake of cholesterol in the intestine. The efficacy of all three intestinally active agents is limited since there is a compensatory increase in hepatic cholesterol synthesis. Niacin acts through a unknown and known mechanisms, including partially inhibiting the release of free fatty acids (FFA) from adipose; increasing lipoprotein lipase (LPL) activity thereby enhancing removal of chylomicron (CM) triglyceride from plasma; decreasing apolipoprotein B (apo B) synthesis, which lowers very low density lipoprotein cholesterol (VLDL-C) and intermediate density lipoprotein cholesterol (IDL-C), and thus plasma triglcyerides; and increasing high density lipoprotein cholesterol (HDL-C) levels through decreased hepatic uptake, likely through the holouptake receptor (HUR) and catabolism. Increased levels of HDL-C may increase reverse cholesterol transport from peripheral cells to the liver. Fibrates lower triglyceride levels by decreasing VLDL secretion and increasing catabolism of triglyceride-rich particles via several mechanisms, including reduced apolipoprotein C (apo C) production which upregulates lipoprotein-lipase-mediated lipolysis and increased cellular FFA uptake as well as increasing FFA catabolism. Fibrates increase HDL-C, induce apolipoprotein A-I and A-II (AI & AII) synthesis via the liver X receptor/retinoid X receptor heterodimer (LXR), Omega-3 fatty acids (O-3) reduce the rate of VLDL synthesis through a number of putative mechanisms inhibiting release of FFA from adipose, inhibiting FFA synthesis, and increasing apo B degradation (Abbreviations: ABC: ATP-binding cassette; B48 or B100: Apolipoprotein B48 or B100; CETP: Cholesterol ester transfer protein; CMR: CM remnant; E: Apolipoprotein E; LRP: LDL receptor-related protein 1; PLTP: Phospholipid transport protein; SRB-1: Steroid receptor binding protein)

simvastatin (remember as "A, L, S") (Table 11). Avoid concomitant use of these three statins with potent inhibitors of CYP3A4, including:

- Azole antifungals (ketoconazole and itraconazole; alternative— fluconazole)
- Macrolide antibiotics (erythromycin and clarithromycin; alternative— azithromycin)
- Rifampicin and protease inhibitors (alternative—indinavir) (Table 12)

Table 10: Percent change in lipids and lipoproteins from baseline for various doses of statins, and statins coadministered with ezetimibe, niacin or fenofibric acid. Doses achieving a 30% to less than 50% reduction in LDL-C are highlighted in light gray and doses achieving more than or equal to 50% reductions are highlighted in dark gray

Statin dose	Fluvastatin	Pitavastatin	Pravastatin	Simvastatin	Atorvastatin	Rosuvastatin	Simvastatin + Ezetimibe 10 mg	Rosuvastatin + Fenofibric acid 135 mg	Lovastatin + ER Niacin 2 g
LDL-C									
2 mg		−36							
4 mg		−43							
10 mg	NR		−20	−28	−37	−46	−46	−37	NR
20 mg	−22		−24	−35	−43	52	−50	−39	NR
40 mg	−25		−30	−39	−48	−55	−56	NR	−42
80 mg	−35		−37	−46	−51	NA	−59	NA	NA
Non-HDL-C									
2 mg		−33							
4 mg		−36							
10 mg	NR		−19	−26	−34	−42	−42	−45	NR
20 mg	NR		−22	−33	−40	−48	−47	−45	NR
40 mg	NR		−27	−36	−45	−51	−51	NR	NR
80 mg	NR		NR	−42	−48	NA	−55	NA	NR

Contd...

Contd...

Table 10: Percent change in lipids and lipoproteins from baseline for various doses of statins, and statins coadministered with ezetimibe, niacin or fenofibric acid. Doses achieving a 30% to less than 50% reduction in LDL-C are highlighted in light gray and doses achieving more than or equal to 50% reductions are highlighted in dark gray

Statin dose	Fluvastatin	Pitavastatin	Pravastatin	Simvastatin	Atorvastatin	Rosuvastatin	Simvastatin + Ezetimibe 10 mg	Rosuvastatin + Fenofibric acid 135 mg	Lovastatin + ER Niacin 2 g
Triglycerides									
2 mg		–19							
4 mg		–18							
10 mg	NR		–8	–12	–20	–20	–24	–47	NR
20 mg	–12		–8	–18	–23	–24	–26	–43	NR
40 mg	–14		–13	–15	–27	–26	–29	NR	–44
80 mg	–19		–19	–18	–28	—	–26	NA	NR
HDL-C									
2 mg		+7							
4 mg		+5							
10 mg	NR		+3	+5	+6	+8	+8	+20	NR
20 mg	+3		+4	+6	+5	+10	+9	+19	NR
40 mg	+4		+6	+5	+4	+10	+9	NR	+30
80 mg	+11		+3	+7	+2		+7	NA	NR

(Abbreviations: ER: Extended release; NA: Dose not approved; NR: Not reported).

Table 11: Summary of comparative pharmacokinetics of statins in healthy volunteers

	Atorvastatin	Fluvastatin	Lovastatin	Pitavastatin	Pravastatin	Rosuvastatin	Simvastatin
Major metabolic enzyme	CYP3A4	CYP2C9	CYP3A4 Glucuronidation	Minimal CYP450 Glucuronidation	No CYP450 Glucuronidation	Some CYP 2C8 Glucuronidation	CYP3A4 Glucuronidation
Renal excretion (%)	≤2	<6	≥10	15	20	10	13
Absorption (%)	30	98	30–31	51	34	40–60	60–80
Prodrug	No	No	Yes	No	No	No	Yes
t_{max} (hour)	1.0–2.0	0.5–1.0	2.0–4.0	1.0	1.0–1.5	3.0–5.0	1.3–3.0
$T_{1/2}$ (hour)	14–15	3.0	2.0	12	2.0	20	1.4–3.0
Lipophilicity (logP)	4.06	3.24	4.30	—	−0.23	—/33	4.68
Protein binding (%)	>98	>98	>95	99	43–54	88	95
Affinity for Pgp transporter	Yes	No	Yes	—	Yes	No	Yes
Hepatic first-pass metabolism (%)	20–30	40–70	40–70	—	50–70	50–70	50–80
Systemic active metabolites (no.)	Yes (2)	No	Yes (3)	No	No	Minimal	Yes (3)
Bioavailability (%)	12–14	29	<5	51	18	20	<5

Table 12: Selected clinically relevant statin drug interactions

Drug interactions	Atorvastatin	Fluvastatin	Lovastatin	Pitavastatin	Pravastatin	Rosuvastatin	Simvastatin
Gemfibrozil Alternative: Fenofibrate	+	+	++	+	++	+	++
Cyclosporine	++		++	++	++	++	++
HIV protease inhibitors Alternative: Indinavir	+		+	+		+	+
Ketoconazole, itraconazole Alternative: Fluconazole	+		+				+
Erythromycin, clarithromycin, telithromycin Alternative: Azithromycin	+	+	++				+
Rifampicin	+		+	+			+
Diltiazem, verapamil Alternatives: Amlodipine, nifedipine			+				+, ++
Amiodarone			+				+
Digoxin	+						+
Fluoxetine, fluvoxamine, sertraline, nefazodone Alternative: paroxetine, venlataxine	+		+				+

Cardiovascular Pharmacology

FLOWCHART 5: An approach to managing muscle and other symptoms in statin-treated patients

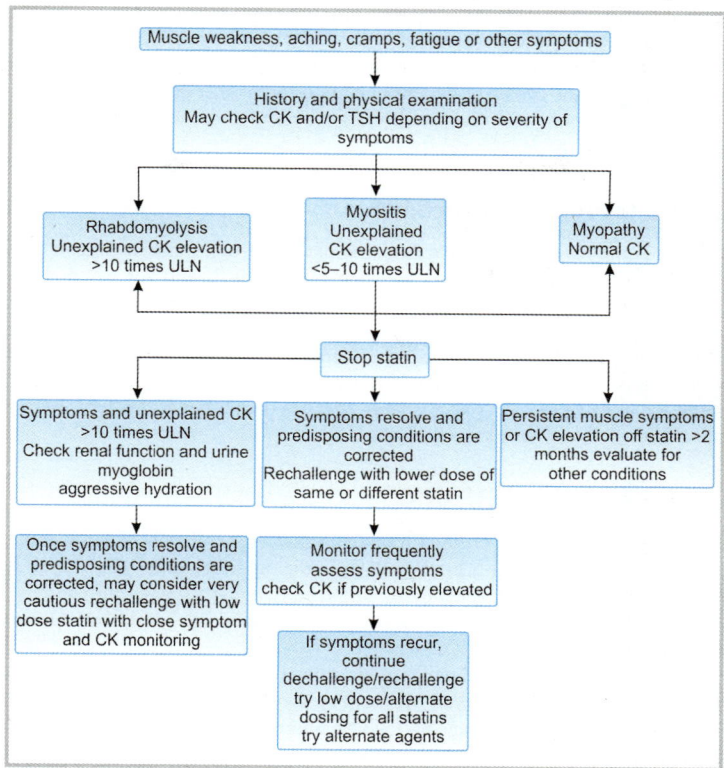

- Lower doses of simvastatin and lovastatin are recommended for patients receiving weaker CYP3A4 inhibitors amiodarone, calcium channel blockers diltiazem and verapamil (alternatives— amlodipine and nifedipine) Interactions with some antidepressants (alternatives—paroxetine and venlafaxine) have also been reported.

Although statins are primarily metabolized by the liver, some statins have relatively greater renal excretion—lovastatin, pitavastatin, pravastatin, rosuvastatin, and simvastatin. Dose adjustment may be considered in those with markedly impaired renal excretion. All statins should be used with caution in patients with a glomerular filtration rate less than 30 since substantially impaired renal excretion is also a marker for other patient characteristics that may increase the potential for adverse muscle effects, including advanced age, frailty, and polypharmacy.

An approach to the management of muscle and other symptoms in statin-treated patients is provided in Flowchart 5. Persistent muscle pain or weakness affecting the proximal muscles is the most common manifestation of statin intolerance. The general approach is to discontinue the statin until symptoms resolve, and then rechallenge with a low dose of the same or another statin.

Abnormal liver function tests are also common among patients receiving statins but are not usually related to statin use. Persistent elevations in hepatic alanine transaminase (ALT; which is the most specific test for drug-related hepatotoxicity) in long-term clinical trials are uncommon and related to increasing statin dose. As long as a stable pattern of ALT elevation has been established, statins can still be used in these patients for cardiovascular prevention with regular ALT monitoring. In patients with unexplained ALT elevations greater than 3 times the upper limit of normal, the statin should be discontinued along with other potential hepatotoxic agents. The patient monitored until levels return to baseline or an etiology is established.

❏ ADD-ON TO STATIN THERAPY

Consideration may be given to adding a second agent to a statin in patients who have not achieved their LDL-C and non-HDLC goals and for whom more aggressive therapy is deemed appropriate. It should be noted, however, at this time there is insufficient clinical trial evidence that adding a second agent to statin therapy will result in additional cardiovascular event reduction. Ezetimibe, bile acid sequestrants and niacin 2 g will lower LDL-C, an additional 15% when added to statin therapy (Table 13). Niacin is more effective than other agents for lowering non-HDL-C due to greater increases in HDL-C.

❏ BILE ACID SEQUESTRANTS

Bile acid sequestrants interrupt the enterohepatic recirculation of cholesterol-rich bile acids by irreversibly binding them in the intestinal lumen (Fig. 10). Bile acid sequestrants are not systemically absorbed. Cholestyramine and colestipol modestly decrease CHD risk in long-term clinical trials, as would be expected from their modest effect on LDL-C.

As monotherapy, bile acid sequestrants at the recommended dosage will lower LDL-C by about 15% and non-HDL-C by about 10%. Bile acid sequestrants increase triglycerides on average by 15–30%, and the largest triglyceride increases occur in patients with more severe hypertriglyceridemia. Bile acid sequestrants

Table 13: Lipid lowering options for patients who have not achieved LDL-C and non-HDL-C goals on statin therapy

Drug	Percent changes from baseline			
	LDL-C	Non-HDL-C	Triglyceride	HDL-C
Double statin dose	–6%	–6%	–2 to –12%	–2 to +2%
Ezetimibe 10 mg	–15 to –20%	–12%	–9%	NS
Niacin 2 g	–1 to –8%	–15 to –31%*	–24%	+18 to +21%
Bile acid binding agent Colestipol 2 scoops (6 g) Cholestyramine 2 scoops (8 g) Coleselvalam 6 tabs or suspension (3.75 g)	–6 to –16%	–5 to –8%	0 to +23%	+1 to +7%
Fenofibrate 145 mg Fenofibric acid 135 mg	–6 to +4%	–3 to –23%*	–15 to –27%	+10 to +13%
Gemfibrozil 600 mg BID	+7%	+2%	–18%	0%
Marine omega-3 fatty acids	–6 to +10%	–7 to –9%	0 to –27%	+2 to +4%

*Calculated by subtracting mean HDL-C from mean total cholesterol

are contraindicated in those with triglyceride levels more than 400 mg/dL and should be used with caution when triglycerides are 200–400 mg/dL. Colesevelam has been shown to reduce hemoglobin A1C levels by about 0.5% in diabetics with inadequate glycemic control, with greater benefit in those with hemoglobin A1C levels more than 8.0%. Notably, average triglyceride levels were less than 200 mg/dL in these studies.

Adverse intestinal effects, such as bloating, constipation and bowel obstruction, limit their use, although these effects are less common with colesevelam. Colestipol and cholestyramine decrease the absorption of anionic drugs and vitamins (vitamins A, D and K, and folic acid) and should be administered 1 hour after or 4 hours before estrogen, progestin, warfarin, digoxin, thyroxine, phenobarbitol, propranolol, thiazide diuretics, tetracycline, vancomycin, penicillin G, niacin, or ezetimibe.

❏ EZETIMIBE

Ezetimibe also acts in the intestine where it selectively inhibits uptake of cholesterol by blocking Niemann-Pick C1-Like 1 receptor, a critical mediator of cholesterol absorption, at the brush border of the small intestine (Fig. 10). By reducing cholesterol absorption from bile acids and diet, ezetimibe reduces intracellular cholesterol levels, which in turn, upregulates LDL receptors to lower plasma cholesterol levels. Statins and bile acid sequestrants act similarly through this final cholesterol-lowering pathway. Ezetimibe and its active metabolites undergo extensive enterohepatic recirculation limiting systemic exposure.

As monotherapy, ezetimibe lowers LDL-C and non-HDL-C by about 20%. When used with a statin, ezetimibe lowers LDL-C by 15–20% with a lesser effect on non-HDL-C (Table 4). A combination of tablet of ezetimibe 10 mg and simvastatin 80 mg lowers LDL-C by about 60%, similar to the highest doses of atorvastatin and rosuvastatin.

Ezetimibe has minimal adverse effects and does not appear to increase the risk of myopathy when used in conjunction with a statin. No dose adjustments are needed in patients with renal or hepatic insufficiency. Statin-ezetimibe combinations cause persistent hepatic ALT elevations greater than 3 times the upper limit of normal at a rate similar to atorvastatin 80 mg. The value of ezetimibe when added to statin therapy for cardiovascular prevention is unclear.

❏ NIACIN

Niacin can improve all lipid parameters, although effects are highly variable between patients. Therefore, niacin should only be continued in those experiencing a significant therapeutic response in the targeted lipid parameter(s) until clinical trial data are available regarding its cardiovascular risk reduction benefits added to a statin. Not all of niacin's mechanisms of action have been elucidated. Niacin lowers LDL-C and VLDLC by decreasing apolipoprotein B synthesis. Triglyceride reductions result from partial inhibition of fatty acid release from adipose tissue, leading to decreased hepatic triglyceride synthesis, as well as through increased lipoprotein lipase activity which increases the rate of chylomicron triglyceride removal from plasma (Fig. 10). Niacin-induced increases in HDL-C levels are likely related to decreased triglyceride levels, and may result from decreased hepatic uptake and catabolism of HDL-C. Niacin undergoes extensive first pass metabolism in the liver, through enzymatic pathways separate from those metabolizing statins, and is rapidly excreted in urine. Niacin has few important drug interactions although it is extensively bound to cholestyramine.

One gram of niacin will raise HDL-C by 15% and lower triglycerides by 25%, but has little effect on LDL-C or non- HDL-C levels. At the 2 g dose, niacin will lower LDL-C by about 15%, and further increase HDL-C (+ 25%) and lower triglycerides (- 30%). Niacin 2 g will also lower lipoprotein by about 20%, although it is not known whether this will further reduce cardiovascular risk. When added to a statin, niacin retains the HDL-C raising and non-HDL-C and triglyceride lowering properties for niacin monotherapy, although some attenuation of LDL-C lowering may occur.

Immediate-release, or crystalline, niacin may have substantial cutaneous effects, such as flushing and itching, that are reduced with extended-release niacin formulations. A higher dose of aspirin (325 mg), ibuprofen 200 mg, or another nonsteroidal anti-inflammatory drug (NSAID) taken 30–60 minutes prior to niacin administration can alleviate flushing, redness, itching, rash, and dryness.

Niacin adherence may be improved titrating the dose gradually over a period of weeks to months. Flushing rates usually substantially diminish after 4 weeks of extended-release niacin use, and rarely occur after 1 year of use. Ingestion with a snack or meal slows absorption.

Doses of extended-release niacin greater than 2 g/day are contraindicated due to a very high rate of serious hepatotoxicity, including liver failure. Sustained-release niacin, which is available over the counter, should be avoided, especially in doses of more than 1.5 g daily. Serum ALT should be monitored every 6–12 weeks during the first 6–12 months of niacin treatment, and every 6 months thereafter. Niacin should be discontinued if:

- Hepatic transaminase levels are persistently more than 3 times the upper limit of normal
- Bilirubin is more than 3 mg/dL
- Prothrombin time is elevated
- Symptoms of nausea, vomiting, or malaise are present.

❏ TRIGLYCERIDE-LOWERING THERAPY

Triglycerides are not a target of therapy for cardiovascular risk reduction. Although those with triglyceride levels more than 150 mg/dL are at increased cardiovascular risk, adjustment for low HDL-C levels and insulin resistance eliminates the majority of the risk associated with elevated triglycerides. Nor are triglyceride changes from drug therapy associated with reduced cardiovascular risk. In those with severe hypertriglyceridemia (>500 mg/dL), triglycerides are the target of therapy to prevent pancreatitis.

❏ FIBRATES

Fibrates are nuclear peroxisome proliferator-activated (PPAR) receptor-α agonists that upregulate the gene for lipoprotein lipase and downregulate the gene for apolipoprotein C-III, an inhibitor of lipoprotein lipase. Lipoprotein lipase increases triglyceride hydrolysis (which decreases VLDL-C secretion) and increases catabolism of triglyceride-rich particles (Fig. 10).

Gemfibrozil undergoes glucuronidation in the liver and is 70% renally excreted. Gemfibrozil potently inhibits glucuronidation of other drugs, including all statins. Fenofibrate is also metabolized via glucuronidation and is primarily renally excreted. However, fenofibrate and fenofibric acid, its active metabolite, are much less potent inhibitors of glucuronidation than gemfibrozil, and have little effect on statin levels. Fibrates may substantially increase prothrombin time and international normalized ratios in patients receiving warfarin. Warfarin dose may need to be decreased by 25–35%.

Fenofibrate very modestly reduces cardiovascular risk to the degree expected from the magnitude of its modest LDL-C and non-HDL-C changes. Conversely, gemfibrozil reduces cardiovascular risk more than expected from the minimal changes observed in LDL-C and non-HDL-C. The risk reduction with gemfibrozil is independent of triglyceride changes and has been largely attributable to the use of gemfibrozil itself.

As monotherapy, fenofibrate is slightly more effective than gemfibrozil for lowering LDL-C (11% vs 1%, respectively) and non-HDL-C (18% vs 13%), although both may increase LDL-C levels in hypertriglyceridemic patients. Both drugs lower triglycerides by about 45% and raise HDL-C by about 10%.

Fibrates increase the risk of myopathy, abnormal transaminase levels, and creatinine elevations. Fibrate monotherapy increases the risk of myopathy. The risk for gemfibrozil is twofold higher than for fenofibrate. When used with a statin, gemfibrozil has a 33-fold higher risk of myopathy than fenofibrate, in part due to greater inhibition of glucuronidation. Fenofibrate appears to have little impact on statin blood levels, and so is the drug of choice for combination with low-to-moderate dose statins.

Rises in creatinine levels can occur in patients taking fenofibrate, although the clinical significance of this is unclear. The dose of fenofibrate should be reduced if creatinine rises above the normal range, and the patient carefully monitoring for adverse effects. Fenofibrate dose should be reduced in patients with glomerular filtration rates less than 60 mL/min/1.73 m^2, and fenofibrate completely avoided when it is less than 15 mL/min/1.73 m^2. Fenofibrate is nondialyzable and must be avoided in dialysis and renal transplant patients. A reduced dose of gemfibrozil can be used in these patients. Gemfibrozil also has significant renal excretion and concomitant use with statins with renal clearance should be avoided.

❏ OMEGA-3 FATTY ACIDS

The omega-3 fatty acids eicosopentanoic acid (EPA) and docohexanoic acid (DHA) in doses more than 3 g daily can lower triglyceride levels about as much as a fibrate. EPA and DHA come from marine sources (fish and seaweed) and are the only omega-3 fatty acids that lower triglycerides. Alpha-linolenic acid is an omega-3 fatty acid derived from land-based plant sources is minimally converted to EPA and DHA and has minimal lipid effects.

EPA and DHA, including intake from fatty fish once or twice a week, have been shown to reduce the risk of coronary death, although the mechanisms through which this occur is unclear. Triglyceride-lowering *per se* does not appear to reduce cardiovascular risk in studies to date. EPA and DHA are rapidly absorbed with a long half-life due to extensive incorporation into cell membranes.

A 3–4 g dose of EPA/DHA is needed to lower triglycerides by 30–45%. Very concentrated fish oil is available over-the-counter or by prescription.

The most common adverse effects of omega-3 fish oil are fishy eructation, nausea and intestinal complaints. Pharmaceutical grade fish oil is highly refined and has fewer adverse gastrointestinal effects. Doses of omega-3 fatty acids less than 6 g daily do not increase glucose levels or the risk of bleeding with aspirin or anticoagulants.

❑ DRUGS IN DEVELOPMENT

Several drugs with novel mechanisms influencing the metabolism of LDL-C, VLDL-C, and HDL-C are in development. Several at-risk populations may benefit from LDL-C and non-HDL-C lowering agents, including those who are intolerant of statins, those with familial hypercholesterolemia or other forms of severe hyperlipidemia, and those needing additional lipid modification to reach their treatment targets.

❑ SUGGESTED READINGS

Grundy SM, Cleeman JI, Merz CNB, et al. Implications of recent clinical trials for the National Cholesterol Education Program Adult Treatment Panel III guidelines. Circulation. 2004;110:227-39.

National Cholesterol Education Panel. Third Report of the National Cholesterol Education Program (NCEP) Expert Panel on Detection, valuation, and Treatment of High Blood Cholesterol in Adults (Adult Treatment Panel III) Final Report. Circulation. 2002;106:3143-421.

Robinson JG, Smith B, Maheshwari N, et al. Pleiotropic effects of statins: benefit beyond cholesterol reduction? A meta-regression analysis J Am Coll Cardiol. 2005;46:1855-62.

Robinson JG. Pharmacologic treatment of dyslipidemia and cardiovascular disease. In: Kwiterovich P (Ed). The Johns Hopkins Textbook of Dyslipidemia. Phildelphia: Wolters Kluwer;2010. pp.266-76.

The Accord Study Group. Effects of Combination Lipid Therapy in Type 2 Diabetes Mellitus. N Engl J Med. 2010: NEJMoa1001282.

The FIELD study investigators. Effects of long-term fenofibrate therapy on cardiovascular events in 9795 people with type 2 diabetes mellitus (the FIELD study): randomised controlled trial. Lancet. 2005;366:1849-61.

US Food and Drug Administration. FDA Drug Safety Communication: ongoing safety review of high-dose Zocor (simvastatin) and increased risk of muscle injury. March 19, 2010; http://www.fda.gov/ Drugs/DrugSafety/PostmarketDrugSafety Informationfor Patientsand Providers/ucm204882.htm Accessed June 2010.

Vandenberg B, Robinson J. Management of the patient with statin intolerance. Curr Atheroscler Rep. 2010;12:48-57.

1.5 Antithrombotic and Antiplatelet Agents

❑ INTRODUCTION

Arterial and venous thromboses are a major cause of death and disability worldwide. A majority of myocardial infarctions (MI) and cerebrovascular accidents (CVA) are caused by unregulated arterial thrombosis after rupture of an atherosclerotic plaque. Venous thromboembolism (VTE)—deep vein thrombosis (DVT) and pulmonary embolism (PE)—and embolic stroke secondary to atrial fibrillation (AF) are the result of pathologic venous clot. As prevention and treatment of these entities is fundamental to the discipline, anticoagulants are an elemental component of the cardiologist's armamentarium. Warfarin, heparin, and aspirin have been the standards of antithrombotic and antiplatelet therapeutics, but in the past 15 years low molecular weight heparins (LMWH) and the platelet ADP receptor antagonist clopidogrel have markedly altered the standards of treatment.

❑ CLOTTING, A PRIMER

Prior to discussing individual agents, a brief update on thrombosis: the classic, waterfall cascade, as described by Davie and Ratnoff in 1964, served as a useful basis for understanding the mechanisms underlying clotting (Fig. 11). The addition of an "extrinsic" pathway, triggered by tissue factor (TF) activation of factor VII after endothelial injury, and recognition of factors V and VIII as cofactors transformed the linear cascade into a Y. This new schema placed factor Xa (fXa) in a central position as the first, integrative step of a common pathway. Conveniently, the activated partial thromboplastin time (aPTT) and prothrombin time (PT) are well suited to interrogate for gross abnormalities in the enzymes constituting the intrinsic and extrinsic portions of the cascade.

Subsequent research has revealed additional components of the clotting system and highlighted the importance of feedback and inhibition (Fig. 12). Understanding of the central role played by thrombin has lead to the development of new direct thrombin inhibitors (DTI) that show promise in treating venous and arterial thrombi. The second development is discovery of multiple platelet signaling pathways. The recognition of additional activating pathways—unaffected by aspirin—has lead to the development of new antiplatelet agents that are essential for treatment of arterial thrombi.

❑ ANTITHROMBOTIC AGENTS

Heparins and Indirect Xa Inhibitors

Unfractionated heparin (UFH) is the prototype intravenous anticoagulant. Derived from porcine intestinal mucosa, UFH is a polysaccharide with average molecular weight of 15 kDa. A specific pentasaccharide sequence within this polymer binds to antithrombin III (AT), inducing a conformational change that allows direct and potent fXa inhibition. The AT-heparin complex also inhibits thrombin. The UFH

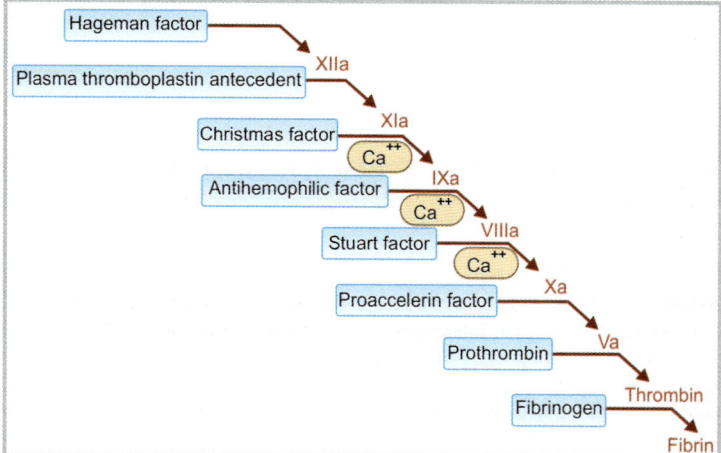

FIGURE 11: Classic waterfall cascade: initially conceived as a linear series of reactions in which each enzyme activated the next to produce fibrin. Original enzyme names are denoted in black with conversion to active enzyme in red using current nomenclature. Although TF and factor VII were not recognized as part of the original clotting cascade, it depicted the sequence of reactions of the intrinsic pathway quite accurately

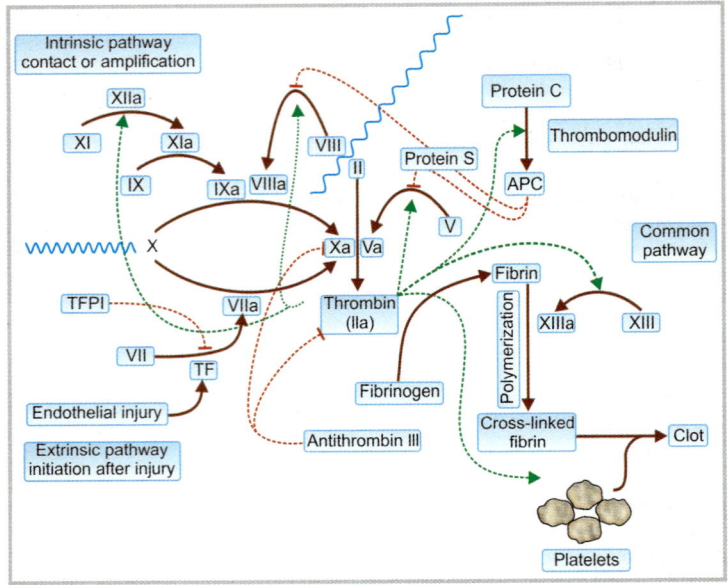

FIGURE 12: Clotting cascade as currently understood: the intrinsic pathway (upper left) proceeds through factors XI, IX and VIII to activation of fX. Activation of fXI can occur through fXIIa, as occurs after addition of a negatively charged trigger in the aPTT, or through thrombin feedback. After endothelial injury, exposed tissue factor complexes with and activates fVII via the extrinsic pathway, which activates fX in turn. The common pathway integrates procoagulant signal and leads to conversion of fibrinogen to fibrin by thrombin. Thrombin and fXa, the two principal anticoagulant targets, are components of the common pathway. *Legend:* Inactive proenzymes are gray. Active enzymes are black and denoted by an a. Black arrows signify activation reactions. Molecules astride the arrows are activating proteases. Enzymes depicted in smaller type act as cofactors for coagulation proteases. Green, dotted arrows signify action by thrombin as an activating enzyme. Antithrombotic molecules are written in red and their sites of action are denoted by red dotted lines

does not enhance AT inhibition of thrombin, but rather serves as a physical bridge, approximating the two molecules. A heparin must have 18 or more saccharide units (MW ~ 5.4 kDa) to facilitate AT-thrombin interaction. Given the average size of a UFH molecule, the vast majority can inhibit thrombin and fXa (an inhibition ratio of 1:1).

Unfractionated heparin can be used in any situation in which parenteral anticoagulation is required. UFH is well suited to short-term or high-risk anticoagulation due to its short half-life (1–2 hours) and potential for reversal with protamine. There are a small number of indications in which heparin is the current standard of care (bivalirudin, discussed below, may replace UFH for indication 4):

1. Patients with a high bleeding risk with indication for short-term anticoagulation.
2. Patients with renal impairment; as LMWH is cleared by the kidneys, it is contraindicated in patients with CrCl <30 mL/min. UFH is not dependent on renal excretion.
3. Massive PE or extensive DVT; LMWH was not studied in these populations.
4. PCI; short half-life, ease of point-of-care monitoring with aPTT or activated clotting time (ACT).

5. Cardiopulmonary bypass (CPB) and other extracorporeal circuits due to experience and full reversibility.

The UFH is extensively bound to plasma proteins (including platelet factor 4 (PF4) and high molecular weight vWF multimers) whose concentrations vary from patient to patient. The effect on individual patients is variable and UFH must be monitored to achieve appropriate anticoagulation. The aPTT should be tested 4–6 hours after the initiation of therapy. Once the therapeutic aPTT is reached, usually 1.5–2 times reference, UFH can be safely monitored on a daily basis so long as dosing remains constant. The UFH also requires regular monitoring of platelet count due to the risk of heparin-induced thrombocytopenia (HIT, also known as HTTS).

Low Molecular Weight Heparins

Low molecular weight heparins (LMWH) including enoxaparin, Dalteparin, and nadroparin. LMWH exerts majority of its effect through indirect inhibition of fXa with an anti-Xa/anti-IIa ratio of ~3.8. In contrast to heparin, exclusively renal excretion occurs in a dose-dependent fashion.

The LMWH has high (90%) bioavailability, which translates to predictable plasma levels after SQ administration. The half-life of most LMWH is approximately 4 hours, which allows daily or BID administration. These properties allow weight-based administration without a daily monitoring requirement, a significant convenience and cost advantage. The LMWH is also better suited for long-term therapy, as patients can self-administer SQ injections. The appropriate use of LMWH in the catheterization lab remains unsettled, due to potential increased bleeding risk, and falls outside the scope of this chapter. LMWH have the following FDA indications:
- Prophylaxis of DVT in patients undergoing abdominal surgery (40 mg SQ daily), total knee replacement or total hip replacement (30 mg SQ BID) and medically ill patients (40 mg SQ daily) with limited mobility
- Inpatient treatment of acute DVT with or without PE
- Outpatient treatment of acute DVT without PE
- Prophylaxis of recurrent ischemia in patients with unstable angina and NSTEMI in conjunction with aspirin
- Treatment of acute STEMI with thrombolysis in conjunction with aspirin; whether managed medically or subsequent PCI
- Extended treatment of VTE in patients with cancer (dalteparin).

Fondaparinux

Fondaparinux is a synthetic analogue of the ATIII binding pentasaccharide sequence found in heparins, producing equivalent fXa inhibition to LMWH. Administered in IV form only, it is 100% bioavailable.

Although theoretic advantages of fondaparinux exist, including more predictable dosing, evidence is lacking that fondaparinux is superior to LMWH. The drug is broadly approved for treatment of:
- Acute DVT
- PE
- DVT prophylaxis in a manner similar to LMWH.

Fondaparinux has been found to be non-inferior at 9 days with respect to patient outcomes with fewer bleeding episodes and improved 30 days mortality in the OASIS-5 study. Based on these findings, fondaparinux receives a class 1 indication as alternative therapy to either UFH or LMWH in the recent ACCF/

AHA Focused Update of the Guidelines for the Management of Patients with Unstable Angina/Non-ST Elevation Myocardial Infarction. However, guiding catheter thrombosis and other intraprocedural thrombotic effects were increased in patients treated solely with fondaparinux who underwent subsequent PCI. This finding greatly tempered enthusiasm for the drug as a potential UFH replacement in ACS.

Overall, similar to LMWH, fondaparinux is principally cleared by the kidneys, and is contraindicated in patients with CrCl less than 30. Unlike LMWH, it is contraindicated in patients less than 50 kg, which may exclude a large number of elderly patients and women.

Idrabiotaparinux

Idrabiotaparinux is a hypermethylated fondaparinux derivative with half-life of 130 hours, designed as a once weekly drug. Like fondaparinux, it is primarily excreted via the kidney. Originally developed as idraparinux, the drug was tested as extended therapy for prevention of VTE in patients with acute DVT or PE. In this study, idraparinux 2.5 mg SQ weekly was equivalent to standard therapy (LMWH and warfarin) with less observed bleeding in patients with DVT, but inferior to standard therapy after PE. The development of idraparinux was halted due to the increased risk of bleeding, long half-life and irreversibility.

Renamed idrabiotaparinux after addition of a biotin moiety, the compound was now reversible by IV administration of avidin, a protein derived from eggs. Like protamine, avidin binds tightly to idrabiotaparinux, leading to rapid clearance.

❏ VITAMIN K ANTAGONISTS (VKA)

Warfarin

Warfarin is the oral anticoagulant against which all newer anticoagulants are measured. Despite its many drawbacks (see below), it has been successfully used to treat a wide range of thrombotic conditions.

Warfarin sodium is a dicurmarol derivative that blocks addition of γ-carboxyglutamic acid (Gla) to factors II, VII, IX, X, protein C and protein S by the vitamin K epoxide reductase (VKOR) enzyme complex. Inhibition of this reaction impairs the final, activating step in hepatic synthesis of these vitamin K-dependent clotting factors (Fig. 13).

The VKA are currently indicated for the treatment of the following conditions:
- Antiphospholipid antibody syndrome (APLAS)
- Primary prevention of stroke or systemic embolism in patients with atrial fibrillation
- Secondary prevention of recurrent CVA
- Secondary CAD prophylaxis after ACS or MI
- Heparin-induced thrombocytopenia (HIT)
- Impaired LV function
- Peripheral arterial occlusive disease
- Prosthetic cardiac valve
- Endocarditis without intracerebral abscess
- Protein C deficiency
- Protein S deficiency
- Pulmonary embolism—acute treatment and secondary prophylaxis
- Venous thromboembolism (VTE, including DVT)—acute treatment and secondary prophylaxis.

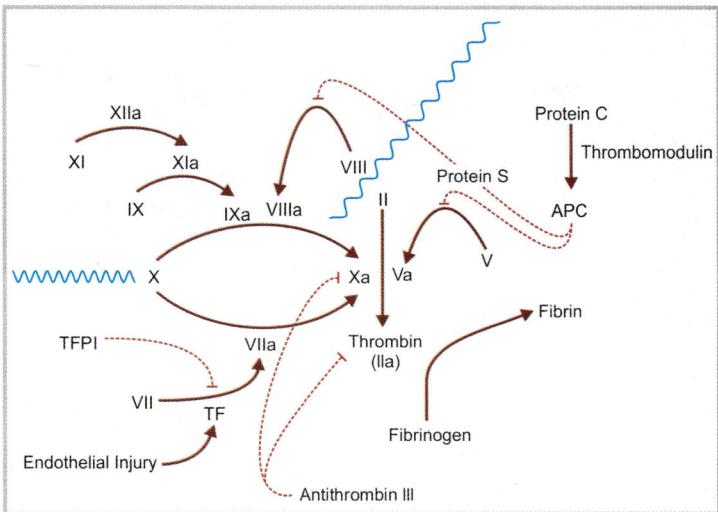

FIGURE 13: Sites of warfarin effect: vitamin K is a cofactor of γ-glutamyl carboxylase, which adds a carboxyl moiety to several proteases of the clotting cascade. Proteases requiring carboxylation are II (prothrombin), VII, IX, X and anticoagulant proteins C and S. Without addition of the carboxyl group, these enzymes are inactive. Warfarin is an inhibitor of vitamin K epoxide reductase (VKOR). If vitamin K remains oxidized through inhibition of VKOR, it cannot function as a cofactor and hepatic carboxylation of these enzymes is decreased. The names of affected enzymes are blurred in the figure

Given the extensive number of indications, a dosing discussion for each is beyond the scope of this chapter and best obtained from disease specific resources, such as AHA/ACC guidelines (e.g. AF, heart failure, valvular heart disease, etc.), ACCP evidence-based clinical practice guidelines (e.g. PE, VTE, etc.) and Micromedex.

The significant cost and burden of monitoring, numerous drug interactions and a narrow therapeutic window make warfarin therapy challenging for patients and providers. Recent studies have shown that, on average, the typical patient on long-term anticoagulation for AF is within the therapeutic range just over 50% of the time. In specialized anticoagulation clinics, this percentage increases to 63%. Conversely, elevated INR (especially >4.0) places patients at risk for bleeding complications. Patient adherence is an additional barrier to successful therapy with VKAs.

❑ DIRECT FACTOR XA INHIBITORS

The direct fXa inhibitors are a new class of (primarily) orally formulated anticoagulants that have pharmacologic profiles similar to that of LMWH. The promise of this class lies in its potential to replace warfarin for long-term indications without need for routine monitoring or "bridging" during the perioperative period. Early studies indicate that the direct fXa inhibitors may also replace LMWH in some settings such as postoperative DVT prophylaxis. It remains to be seen whether the therapeutic index of these drugs is wide enough to permit use of in a broad range of clinical settings.

Rivaroxaban

Rivaroxaban, an oral agent, is the prototype drug in this class and was approved by the FDA in late 2011 for prevention of stroke and systemic embolism in persons with atrial fibrillation. This new class of inhibitors directly inhibits fXa without involvement of AT III. Direct inhibitors can bind to the prothrombinase complex, not accessible to AT III-mediated indirect inhibitors, with resultant reduction in thrombin generation.

Rivaroxaban prolongs PT to a greater extent than aPTT, but due to variable interaction with assay reagents these values cannot be used reliably for monitoring. The compound has high oral bioavailability (>80%), reaches maximum concentration in 2–4 hours with a 7–11 hours terminal half-life. These properties permit daily, weight-based dosing, obviating the need for monitoring in many patients.

Apixaban

Apixaban is a second direct fXa inhibitor in advanced stages of testing. Like rivaroxaban, the molecule is a selective, reversible fXa inhibitor that reaches maximum plasma concentrations quickly (~3 hours) after administration, and has a prolonged half-life (8–14 hours). About 50% of absorption occurs after oral administration. The drug is metabolized, predominantly, through nonhepatic pathways with renal excretion a major (~30%) route of elimination. Uses of potent inhibitors (azole antifungals, macrolide antibiotics and PI) are contraindicated in conjunction with apixaban.

Dose ranging studies for DVT prophylaxis after orthopedic surgery, DVT and demonstrated prevention of thrombosis efficacy and acceptable safety profile. An initial comparison of apixaban (2.5 mg PO BID) to enoxaparin (30 mg SQ BID) after TKA did not demonstrate non-inferiority due to an unexpectedly low event rate. Less bleeding was observed in the apixaban group and the drugs' safety profiles were comparable.

❏ DIRECT THROMBIN INHIBITORS

Thrombin is a key point of propagation in thrombosis and hemostasis. Not only does active thrombin convert fibrinogen to fibrin but also creates a positive feedback loop by activating factors V, VIII and XI. It also acts as a potent activator of platelets. Given this central location in the clotting cascade, it is an attractive anticoagulant target. UFH indirectly inhibits thrombin, mediated by AT III, but this complex has limited activity against fibrin-bound thrombin. The inability to inhibit fibrin-bound thrombin, the site of clot propagation, is a potentially significant limitation. The direct thrombin inhibitors (DTI) are designed to overcome this limitation. Thrombin's activity can be inhibited at three separate locations on the molecule: (i) the active, catalytic site; (ii) exosite 1, the dock for substrates, such as fibrin, and (iii) exosite 2, the heparin binding domain. Two classes of DTI are distinguished by their mechanism of inhibition. The bivalent DTI are derived from hirudin, a naturally occurring compound that was isolated from the leech in 1905—the first anticoagulant. The bivalent DTI, as the name suggests, exert their inhibitory effect through binding to exosite 1 and the catalytic site. Univalent DTI, in contrast, are small synthetic molecules that bind only to the active site.

Hirudin

Hirudin, isolated from *Hirudo medicinalis* is not used as a commercial anticoagulant. The 2 recombinant hirudins (r-hirudin or lepirudin and desulfato-hirudin or desirudin) differ at a single amino acid and are used in clinical practice. Referred to generically as hirudin, the 3 molecules are pharmacologically interchangeable.

Hirudin forms an irreversible 1:1 complex with thrombin and interacts minimally with plasma proteins. Hirudin has a short half-life in patients with normal renal function. Excretion is predominantly renal. Functional half-life is extended in patients with renal dysfunction and can reach 5 days in patients with absent kidney function. The aPTT is the test for choice of monitoring hirudin anticoagulation, but the response is linear only to 60–70 seconds. Beyond that point, the aPTT will underestimate the level of coagulation.

Hirudins have two specific indications. Based on the HAT trials, lepirudin is approved for treatment of HIT complicated by thrombosis. In these studies, the incidence of new thrombosis was significantly lowered, by 93%, in the hirudin groups as compared to historical controls. The risks for limb amputation or death were equivalent in the two groups. Current standards advocate immediate heparin withdrawal, regardless of thrombosis at the time of diagnosis; followed by immediate parenteral anticoagulation until a therapeutic INR has been reached with a VKA. Given its ability to inhibit clot-bound thrombin, lepirudin was also studied as an alterative to heparin during PCI. In these studies, hirudin was more effective in prevention of ischemic end-points but not significantly better than heparin in prevention of cardiovascular death or MI at 1 week. Higher rates of bleeding and increased transfusion requirements observed in the studies negated the potential beneficial effects.

The two primary limitations of hirudins are mutually reinforcing. The extreme dependence on normal renal function to maintain predictable anticoagulation can make avoiding over anticoagulation difficult. Given the increased rate of bleeding, treatment of elderly or critically ill patients is challenging and requires close monitoring. Besides these, There is no antidote to hirudin. When bleeding is life-threatening , only specific HD filters are effective for removal.

Bivalirudin

Bivalirudin is a synthetic, bivalent DTI and hirudin analogue. Unlike hirudin, the molecule is cleaved after binding, producing transient inhibition of thrombin. Bivalirudin has a lower affinity for thrombin than hirudin by 1000-fold and does not spur antibody formation. The drug is degraded by proteolytic and hepatic mechanisms. Dose adjustment is required in patients with renal impairment.

Due to short half-life and IV formulation, bivalirudin is administered as a continuous infusion after an initial bolus. The principal indication is as an alternative anticoagulant during PCI. Bivalirudin can also be used for treatment of HIT/HTTS, but its mode of administration makes use impractical in noncritical care settings. Current FDA indications are:

- Use as an anticoagulant in patients with unstable angina undergoing percutaneous transluminal coronary angioplasty (PTCA)
- Use as an anticoagulant in patients undergoing percutaneous coronary intervention (PCI) with provisional use of glycoprotein IIb/IIIa inhibitor (GPI) is indicated
- Bivalirudin is indicated for patients with or at risk of HIT/HITTS undergoing PCI.

The two main limitations of bivalirudin are its exclusively parenteral formulation and its route of excretion, requiring dose adjustment patients with renal dysfunction. Assuming normal renal function, the half-life of bivalirudin is approximately 25 minutes. Coagulation parameters return to normal 1 hour after cessation of IV infusion. As with all anticoagulants, it confers an increased risk of bleeding, but the lower rates of bleeding in the aforementioned trials make it an appropriate alternative during PCI, PTCA or CABG. The aPTT can be used for monitoring at lower levels of anticoagulation; up to 3 times the upper limit of normal. Above this limit, the test is no longer sensitive.

Argatroban

Argatroban is a synthetic, small molecule derived from L-arginine. This univalent DTI, as a prototype of the class, reversibly inhibits only the active site of thrombin. Argatroban otherwise behaves similarly to bivalirudin, inhibiting both free and clot-bound thrombin. The molecule is metabolized in the liver and excreted, principally, in the feces without significant renal involvement. Argatroban is administered intravenously. The plasma half-life is 45 minutes and steady state anticoagulation is reached in 1–3 hours.

Argatroban has two FDA indications and is used principally in patients with HIT and significant renal dysfunction:
- Prophylaxis or treatment of thrombosis in patients with HIT
- Use during PCI in patients with documented or at risk for HIT.

Efficacy data from studies has shown that prompt treatment with intravenous argatroban (to an INR of 1.5–3 for 5–7 days) which resulted in a significant decrease in new thrombosis (28% vs 38.8%) when compared to historical HIT controls treated with placebo. The principal advantage of argatroban is ease of use in patients with impaired renal function. In treatment of HIT and during PCI, no dose-adjustment of argatroban for renal dysfunction is required. In patients with HIT, the level of anticoagulation can be safely monitored using the aPTT so long as the desired therapeutic range in less than 3 times the upper limit of normal.

Allergic reactions after argatroban administration have manifested in a variety of clinical settings. Greater than 95% of these reactions occurred in patients who were concomitantly treated with thrombolytic therapy (e.g. streptokinase) or iodine-based contrast media. Coadministration with other antithrombotic or antiplatelet agents is associated with an increased risk of bleeding.

Ximelagatran

Ximelagatran was the first oral, univalent direct thrombin inhibitor to reach advanced stages of preclinical testing. Phase III trials of ximelagatran have demonstrated efficacy in several clinical settings: postoperative DVT prophylaxis, acute DVT treatment, secondary prevention of ACS, and stroke prevention in patients with AF. A British meta-analysis comparing ximelagatran to standard dose enoxaparin showed improved VTE prophylaxis, but increased serious bleeding.

Dabigatran

Dabigatran is a univalent, oral DTI that potently inhibits thrombin, similar to ximelagatran. It is approved in the EU and Canada for perioperative DVT prophylaxis in orthopedic patients. The structure of dabigatran etexilate, the orally formulated prodrug, is distinct from ximelagatran. Metabolism proceeds through plasma esterases, rather than hepatic enzymes, and it has been found to be non-hepatotoxic. It is theorized that rapid plasma metabolism quickly lowers inactive precursor concentrations, preventing a ximelagatran-like toxicity. The drug reaches peak plasma concentrations in 1.5 hours and exhibits a 14–17 hours half-life. Twice-daily dosing is standard.

The FDA has unanimously recommended approval the 150 mg PO BID dose of dabigatran for stroke prevention in AF. Additional recommendations include:
- A 75 mg tablet for daily use in renal impairment
- Use of 110 mg PO BID dose for patients with elevated bleeding risk
- Phase IV testing of higher dose dabigatran in the above clinical setting

A dose of 150 mg orally BID has demonstrated equivalence to standard therapy (SQ enoxaparin followed by dose adjusted warfarin) in 6-month treatment of acute VTE, both DVT and PE in the RE-COVER study. Other studies may determine whether dabigatran replaces warfarin as the drug of choice for treatment and long-term prevention of VTE. Dabigatran should immediately fill a need for patients with inadequate access to an anticoagulation clinic or for whom increased bleeding risk makes warfarin therapy unacceptable.

❑ ANTIPLATELET AGENTS

Platelets instigate and catalyze arterial thrombosis in a stepwise process (Fig. 14). Each step presents a potential therapeutic target for inhibition of thrombosis. At injury outset, platelets adhere to sub-endothelial matrix components, minimizing the breach in the endothelial wall. Although few therapeutics that interrupt adherence have been studied, development potential will be discussed briefly. Also

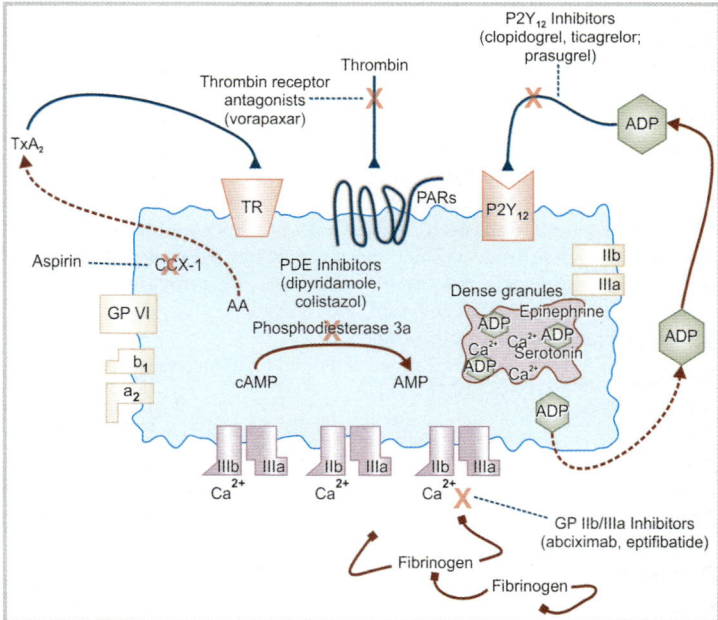

FIGURE 14: Antiplatelet agents: Depicted at right are the major sites of action of the five extant classes of antiplatelet drugs. Aspirin is the major inhibitor of the TxA_2 pathway. Clopidogrel and ticagrelor inhibit $P2Y_{12}$ activation by ADP. GP IIb/IIIa inhibitors inhibit fibrinogen binding and platelet aggregation

exposed by endothelial injury, TF binds factor VII, initiates the clotting cascade and generates thrombin, which is a potent activator of platelets. ADP and TxA_2 are also crucial signals that lead to platelet activation and recruitment. The most established antiplatelet therapies, aspirin (an inhibitor of TXA_2 synthesis) and clopidogrel (an ADP/$P2Y_{12}$ antagonist), aim to disrupt this second step. Once activated, intracellular signaling produces a conformational change in the GP IIb/IIIa (aIIbb3) receptor that favors fibrinogen binding (as well as vWF and fibronectin). *Aggregation* is the result of avid platelet binding, via the abundant aIIbb3, to many fibrinogen molecules. The two aIIbb3 binding regions of fibrinogen produce extensive platelet cross-linking. This final step is inhibited by the parenteral glycoprotein IIb/IIIa inhibitors (GPI), which will be discussed only briefly in this section, due to their limited use outside the catheterization lab.

Inhibitors of Platelet Adhesion

At present, there are no clinically available inhibitors of platelet adhesion. *In vitro* and animal models have demonstrated that inhibition of multiple receptors can reduce platelet adhesion to the subendothelial matrix. Animal models have demonstrated protection from arterial thrombosis when adhesion is inhibited. A monoclonal antibody directed against the murine GPVI receptor led to a long-term prevention from thrombosis. Together, these findings make inhibitors of adhesion an attractive target for drug development.

Aegyptin, a mosquito derived molecule has been shown to prevents *in vivo* platelet aggregation and thrombosis after laser-induced carotid injury in rats without excess bleeding. Saratin, a leech derived compound, prevents platelet and vWF binding to collagen under high-shear conditions.

Inhibitors of Platelet Activation

TXA_2 Pathway Inhibitors

Aspirin or acetylsalicylic acid (ASA) is the prototype TXA_2 pathway inhibitor. NSAIDs, ibuprofen and naproxen, which reversibly inhibit cyclooxygenase (COX), and selective COX-2 inhibitors, such as celecoxib, are members of the class, as are ridogrel and terbogrel, which combine a TxA_2 synthase inhibitor and TxA_2/prostaglandin endoperoxide receptor antagonist. While these combination drugs have theoretic advantages over aspirin, they have not proven clinically more efficacious and have produced untoward side effects.

Current indications for ASA use include:
- A dose of 325 mg daily for 1 month followed by 81 mg daily for life—ACS, including STEMI, NSTEMI and UA
- A dose of 325 mg daily for 1 month followed by 81 mg daily for life—following PCI
- A dose of 81 mg daily for life—for secondary prevention of MI in patients with CAD, PAOD or documented pulmonary artery disease
- A dose of 81 mg daily for life—after CABG, carotid endarterectomy or peripheral vascular bypass
- A dose of 1300 mg daily—for symptomatic intracranial arterial stenosis
- A dose of 81–325 mg daily—prevention of embolic stroke in patients with AF and CHADS2 score of 1 or contraindications to warfarin use
- A dose of 50–325 mg daily, preferably in combination with dipyridamole 200 mg twice daily—secondary prevention of CVA after stoke or TIA

- A dose of 325 mg once—administered 24–48 hours after acute stroke (of note, ASA is not recommended within 24 hours of thrombolytic therapy)
- A dose of 81–162 mg daily—for patients with heart failure and reduced ejection fraction
- A dose of 100 mg daily—for patients with polycythema vera and no contraindication to ASA use.

Of note, ASA is not formally indicated for primary prevention. In 2009, the US Preventative Services Task Force recommended encouragement of daily, low-dose ASA use for primary prevention of cardiovascular disease (CVD) in men aged between 45 and 79 years and women between 55 and 79 years without mention of risk factors or diabetes (DM). Recently published meta-analyses and RCT have questioned the benefit of ASA for primary prevention due to a poor risk–benefit ratio. A 2010 position statement of the American Diabetes Association (ADA) and American Heart Association was released that included the provision that recommendation of low-dose (75–162 mg) ASA in patients with DM and an elevated 10-year risk for CVD is "reasonable". It continued that ASA should *not* be recommended for primary prevention in men with age less than 50 years and women less than 60 years with DM without additional CVD risk factors.

The main adverse effect of ASA is bleeding, most commonly GI, although rates are low. The yearly risk of major GI bleed is 0.05–0.1% among patients treated with low-dose ASA, twice the baseline rate. Factors that increase the risk of bleeding are:
- Increasing age
- Previous GI bleeding (GIB) or peptic ulcer disease
- Concomitant use of warfarin, NSAIDs, or steroids.

The most recent AHA/American College of Gastroenterology guidelines advocate GI prophylaxis for any patient prescribed long-term antiplatelet therapy. For patients on dual antiplatelet therapy, such as ASA and clopidogrel, a PPI is the recommended agent to prevent GI bleeding. For patients on single antiplatelet therapy, PPI is recommended when gastroesophageal reflux disease or the above risk factors are present.

Increased postoperative bleeding, but not death, has also been reported after CABG in patients with preoperative ASA use. This effect was observed only in conjunction with doses greater than or equal to 325 mg daily. This finding would indicate that continuation of low-dose ASA, rather than cessation 5 days prior, would be appropriate therapy for patients undergoing CABG. Cessation of antiplatelet therapy after MI or stent placement, especially within the recommended treatment windows, is associated with elevated risk of thrombosis.

Inhibitors of ADP/P2Y$_{12}$ Signaling

Clopidogrel: Clopidogrel (Plavix) is the prototype P2Y$_{12}$ inhibitor, a second-generation thienopyridine. The first generation drug of this class, ticlopidine, is discussed subsequently. Thienopyridines selectively and irreversibly inhibit the P2Y$_{12}$ receptor, reducing ADP-dependent platelet aggregation. After ingestion, 15% of clopidogrel is converted to an active metabolite by the hepatic CYP system. Within 2 hours of a 300 mg oral dose, the active metabolite produces 40% inhibition of ADP-induced platelet aggregation. Due to irreversible P2Y$_{12}$ inhibition, platelet inhibition is maintained for 48 hours, despite the 8-hour half-life of the active metabolite.

After loading, daily administration of 75 mg increases platelet inhibition to approximately 60%, the maximum achievable. A larger loading dose; 600 mg, achieves maximum platelet inhibition in 2 hours. Clinically, loading with 600 mg prior to PCI improves 30-day clinical outcome without increasing rates of bleeding. Clopidogrel was approved on the basis of a single large trial, in which it (75 mg daily) was compared directly with ASA 325 mg daily for secondary prevention of CVD in patients with symptomatic peripheral arterial disease (PAD), recent MI or recent ischemic stroke (both <35 days). Current indications for clopidogrel include:

- ACS
  - For patients with NSTEMI or unstable angina, a 300 mg loading dose followed by 75 mg daily in combination with daily ASA
  - For patients with STEMI; 75 mg daily in combination with ASA, with or without thrombolytics. Loading dose is optional in this setting, but 600 mg appears appropriate for patients proceeding to PCI
- Secondary prevention of CVD with documented MI, stroke, or PAD.

Dual antiplatelet therapy may improve secondary prevention in the highest risk patients, but increased bleeding has limited wide use. Current indications do not specify duration of dual antiplatelet therapy, but the recommended minimum length of therapy for patients implanted with bare metal stents is 1 month. Optimal duration of dual antiplatelet therapy after DES remains uncertain due to reports of stent thrombosis beyond 1 year.

Incidence of bleeding increases when clopidogrel is added to ASA as part of dual antiplatelet therapy. As discussed above, PPI is currently indicated for all patients receiving dual antiplatelet therapy. Concern has arisen that concomitant use of PPI and clopidogrel attenuates the effect of the latter.

A black box warning was recently added to clopidogrel, warning of adverse events among patients with genetic polymorphisms of 2C19 that impair metabolism. An ACCF/AHA response did not advise routine CYP testing or alteration of clinical practice, citing a paucity of prospective outcome data or predictive value of routine genetic testing.

Prasugrel

Prasugrel is a third generation thienopyridine. Like clopidogrel, an active metabolite irreversibly inhibits the $P2Y_{12}$ receptor. The liver converts prasugrel more efficiently to its active metabolite compared to clopidogrel. Prasugrel produces complete inhibition of platelet aggregation by 1 hour. Despite structural similarities, prasugrel is unaffected by common polymorphisms of 2C19 and 2C9, another CYP450 enzyme implicated in reduced clopidogrel metabolism. These pharmacologic distinctions have correlated with increased *in vivo* platelet inhibition when compared to clopidogrel.

Prasugrel was approved for clinical use in 2009. Prasugrel is currently indicated for:
- Patients with unstable angina or NSTEMI
- Patients with STEMI when managed with immediate or delayed PCI.

A class III recommendation (indicating harm) regarding prasugrel has been included in the most recent STEMI and UA/SNTEMI guidelines.160,281 It should not be used in patients with *"history of stroke and transient ischemic attack for whom primary PCI is planned, prasugrel is not recommended as part of a dual-antiplatelet therapy regimen."* Prasugrel received an extensive black box warning based on the increased risks for bleeding. Prasugrel is contraindicated in patients with age more than 75 years, except for those at highest risk, due to increased risk of fatal and ICH. The drug is contraindicated if urgent CABG is 'likely' and should be discontinued 7 days prior to any surgery.

Phosphodiesterase (PDE) Inhibitors
Dipyridamole
The prototype drug in the class, acts by increasing intracellular levels of cyclic adenosine monophosphate (cAMP). Increased cAMP levels, in turn, reduce platelet activation by inhibiting calcium mobilization. Several *in vitro* mechanisms of action have been demonstrated; inhibition of platelet PDE, reduction of adenosine uptake by platelets and stimulation of prostacyclin (PGI2) release by endothelial cells.

Indications and efficacy: Dipyridamole was introduced for treatment of angina. The antiplatelet properties of the drug were discovered later, leading to its repurposing as an antithrombotic agent. It has proven ineffective as a lone anticoagulant. The current indications for dipyridamole are:
- 100 mg four times daily in conjunction with warfarin to reduce thrombotic complications after implantation of a mechanical heart valve
- Extended-release dipyridamole (ERDP) 200 mg in conjunction with ASA 25 mg used twice daily for secondary prevention of stroke after TIA or completed ischemic stroke due to thrombosis.

Headache is the principal adverse effect of dipyridamole treatment, affecting one-third of treated patients and a leading cause of drug discontinuation. Increased rates of diarrhea and other GI complaints have also been reported. The combination is contraindicated in patients with severe hepatic impairment or severe renal impairment (GFR <10 mL/min).

Cilostazol: Cilostazol is an inhibitor of platelet PDE3A, which like dipyridamole, also acts as a vasodilator. Thrombin activates PDE3A (via PAR-1, below), reducing the intracellular cAMP concentration and promoting platelet activation. Given the antagonism of thrombin signaling in platelets, it is not surprising that cilostazol exerts antiplatelet effects. The principal route of drug metabolism is hepatic (CYP3A4 and 3A5) and fecal excretion predominates.

Cilostazol was granted FDA only for approval for the treatment of symptomatic claudication in a dose of 50–100 mg twice daily. Cilostazol treatment has been shown to significant increases in pain-free walking distance for patients with disabling disease (but without limb ischemia or pain at rest). More recently, cilostazol has been tested as an adjunctive antiplatelet therapy after PCI. The addition of cilostazol to dual antiplatelet therapy after bare metal stent placement was associated with decreased angiographic stenosis at 6 months. No reduction in MI or mortality was reported in the association with the reduction in stenosis. The effect was most pronounced in diabetic subjects, long lesions and small-diameter vessels, situations in which DES would be preferentially used.

The principal adverse effects of cilostazol are headache and diarrhea, as with dipyridamole. Palpitations are the unique side effect associated with cilostazol. Caution should be exercised when cilostazol is used in concert with inhibitors of CYP3A4/5 such as macrolide antibiotics, selective serotonin reuptake inhibitors, azole antifungals and warfarin. Additionally, grapefruit juice was associated with purpura in a patient using cilostazol.

Thrombin Receptor Antagonists
Thrombin signaling via PARs appears to be the most potent of the three parallel platelet activation pathways.

Vorapaxar: Vorapaxar is an oral inhibitor of PAR1 and prototype thrombin receptor antagonists (TRA). Vorapaxar was derived from himbacine, a compound isolated from the bark of the Australian magnolia. Vorapaxar dose-dependently inhibited platelet aggregation in vitro and does not affect traditional measures of coagulation. The drug is rapidly absorbed but slowly eliminated with a half-life of 165–311 hours. Return of platelet function occurs, on average, 1 month after drug cessation. The drug is excreted in the feces and dose adjustment for renal function in not required.

Inhibitors of Platelet Aggregation

Three glycoprotein IIb/IIIa inhibitors (GPI) have received FDA approval for use in ACS or adjunctive therapy during PCI. In aggregate, these agents significantly reduce death and MI through 6 months. Oral GPI have shown no clinical benefit and are associated with increased mortality. The clinical indications for GPI use have become more limited with time. A complete discussion of GPI indications and use is located in sections discussing catheterization and PCI.

The first approved agent, *abciximab*, is a chimeric protein composed of Fab (fragment, antigen binding) regions from the murine 7E3 antibody and the Fc of human immunoglobulin. Abciximab in conjunction with coronary stenting has shown to lead to a marked improvement in clinical outcome at both 30 days and 6 months. Abciximab has demonstrated benefit over placebo in patients with elevated troponin at the time of PCI. Abciximab is not cleared by the kidneys and is safe in patients with CKD or ESRD.

Eptifibatide: Eptifibatide is small molecule GPI modeled after a component of pigmy rattlesnake (*Sistrurus miliarius barbouri*) venom. A peptide-based compound, eptifibatide binds tightly to aIIbb3, producing dose-dependent reversible inhibition. Significantly lower rates of MI and death occurred in patients with ACS treated with eptifibatide, in addition to heparin and ASA, with or without subsequent PCI. The ESPRIT trial demonstrated reduced rates of MI and death at 1 year when used in conjunction with standard therapy during PCI. Subsequently no benefit was reported with scheduled eptifibatide prior to PCI as compared to provisional use after procedural thrombotic complication.

Tirofiban: Tirofiban is a second small molecule, nonpeptide GPI. Although never compared directly with eptifibatide, it is used interchangeably due to similar mechanisms of action and clearance. When compared directly to abciximab, tirofiban use was associated with increased rates of MI.

❑ SUGGESTED READINGS

Antman EM, Morrow DA, McCabe CH, et al. ExTRACT-TIMI 25 investigators. Enoxaparin versus unfractionated heparin with fibrinolysis for ST-elevation myocardial infarction. N Engl J Med. 2006;354:1477-88.

Bhatt DL, Scheiman J, Abraham NS, et al. ACCF/ACG/AHA 2008 expert consensus document on reducing the gastrointestinal risks of antiplatelet therapy and NSAID use: a report of the American College of Cardiology Foundation Task Force on Clinical Expert Consensus Documents. J Am Coll Cardiol. 2008;52:1502-17.

Briefing Information for the September 20, 2010 Meeting of the Cardiovascular and Renal Drugs Advisory Committee. http:// www.fda.gov/AdvisoryCommittees/Committees MeetingMaterials/Drugs/CardiovascularandRenal DrugsAdvisoryCommittee/ucm226008.htm.

Clagett GP, Sobel M, Jackson MR, et al. Antithrombotic therapy in peripheral arterial occlusive disease: the Seventh ACCP Conference on Antithrombotic and Thrombolytic Therapy. Chest, 2004;126:609S- 26S.

Davie, EW, Ratnoff OD. Waterfall sequence for intrinsic blood clotting. Science. 1965;145:1310-2.

Gailani D, Renne´ T. The intrinsic pathway of coagulation: a target for treating thromboembolic disease? J Thromb Haemost. 2007; 5:1106-12.

Holmes DR Jr, Dehmer GJ, Kaul S, et al. ACCF/AHA clopidogrel clinical alert: approaches to the FDA "Boxed Warning": a report of the American College of Cardiology Foundation Task Force on Clinical Expert Consensus Documents and the American Heart Association. Circulation. 2010;122:537-57.

Pignone M, Alberts MJ, Colwell JA, et al. Aspirin for primary prevention of cardiovascular events in people with diabetes: a position statement of the American Diabetes Association, a scientific statement of the American Heart Association, and an expert consensus document of the American College of Cardiology Foundation. Circulation. 2010;121:2694-701.

The Fifth Organization to Assess Strategies in Acute Ischemic Syndromes Investigators. Comparison of fondaparinux and enoxaparin in acute coronary syndromes. N Engl J Med. 2006;354: 1464-76.

The Platelet Receptor Inhibition in Ischemic Syndrome Management in Patients Limited by Unstable Signs and Symptoms (PRISM-PLUS) Study Investigators. Inhibition of the platelet glycoprotein IIb/IIIa receptor with tirofiban in unstable angina and non-Q-wave myocardial infarction. N Engl J Med. 1998;338:1488-97.

Wright RS, Anderson JL, Adams CD, et al. 2011 ACCF/AHA focused update of the guidelines for the management of patients with unstable angina/non–ST-elevation myocardial infarction (updating the 2007 guideline): a report of the American College of Cardiology Foundation/American Heart Association Task Force on Practice Guidelines. Circulation. 2011;123:2022-60.

Chapter 2

Diagnosis

2.1 History and Physical Examination

The history and physical examination are essential, not only for the diagnosis of cardiovascular disorders but also to assess severity, to establish a plan of management and to assess the prognosis. Appropriate history and physical examination are also essential to decide what tests are necessary for a patient, as presently a plethora of tests is available for the diagnosis and management of the same cardiac disorder. It should also be appreciated that "history and physical examination" are cost-effective. During examination of the patient, the physician can also gain the confidence of the patient and of the family and can establish a good rapport that is necessary for the appropriate management of the problem of the patient.

❏ HISTORY

General Approach

During history taking, it is desirable to allow the patient to present the symptoms without interruption. Frequent interruptions give the impression that the physician is in hurry and impatient and disinterested. After the patient describes the symptoms, it is appropriate to discuss with the patient and the family to ascertain the chronology of symptoms and their severity. It is pertinent to enquire about each symptom. The major symptoms associated with cardiovascular disorders are chest pain or discomfort, dyspnea, palpitations, dizziness, and syncope.

Analysis of Symptoms

Chest Pain or Discomfort

Chest pain is one of the very common presenting symptoms that patients present to the cardiologists. The chest pain or discomfort can be caused by various cardiac and noncardiac causes, which are summarized in Tables 1 to 4.

Angina pectoris is a symptom of both of chronic coronary artery disease and of acute coronary syndromes. For the diagnosis of angina pectoris, it is imperative to enquire about the character, location, site of radiation, duration, and precipitating and relieving factors of the chest discomfort. While elucidating the history, the following thing should be noted:

Table 1: Cardiac chest pain	
• Coronary artery disease	• Noncoronary artery disease
• Acute coronary syndromes	• Aortic dissection
• Stable angina	• Acute pulmonary embolism
• Ischemic cardiomyopathy	

Table 2: Noncardiac chest pain

- Pulmonary
  - Pleuritis
  - Pneumonia
  - Tracheobronchitis
  - Pneumothorax
  - Mediastinitis
  - Tumor

Table 3: Cardiac causes of chest discomfort

- Aortic stenosis
- Aortic regurgitations
- Hypertrophic cardiomyopathy
- Restrictive cardiomyopathy
- Pulmonary hypertension

Table 4: Noncardiac chest pain

- Musculoskeletal
  - Costochondritis
  - Intercostal muscle cramps
  - Cervical disk disease
- Other causes
  - Herpes zoster
  - Emotional
  - Chest wall tumor
  - Disorders of breast

Character: Frequently, it is described as "heaviness", "pressure", "tightness", "squeezing" or "band across the chest". The character of angina pectoris is usually "dull and deep" and not "sharp and superficial".

Location: The location of the chest discomfort can be retrosternal, epigastric or left pectoral. When chest pain is much localized and can be indicated by one or two finger tips, it is unlikely to be angina pectoris.

Radiation: The radiation of angina pain may be to one or both shoulders, one or both arms and hands, one or both sides of the neck, lower jaw and interscapular area. The radiation can also occur to armpits, epigastrium and subcostal areas. The pain radiates from the center to the periphery (centripetal) and rarely centrifugal.

Intensity: The intensity of angina increases slowly and reaches its peak in minutes, not instantaneously. Similarly, it is relieved gradually, not abruptly. Analysis of the duration of chest discomfort is also helpful to decide whether it is ischemic or nonischemic pain.

Gestures: Patient's gestures during describing the chest discomfort have been thought to be useful in the diagnosis of its etiology.

Precipitating and relieving factors: The precipitating and relieving factors of the chest discomfort should be analyzed to determine its etiology. Classic angina (Heberden's angina) is precipitated by exercise or by emotional stress and is relieved when the exercise is discontinued. It tends to occur often after meals.

Exposure to cold weather precipitates angina more easily in patients with classic angina. Similarly, carrying heavy objects and heavy meals are also frequent precipitating factors. The character, location, and radiation of chest discomfort are similar in the different clinical subsets of angina. However, some distinctive features can be recognized in various subsets.

The atypical presentations frequently called "angina equivalents" are dyspnea, indigestion and belching, and dizziness and syncope without chest pain. The atypical presentations are more common in diabetics, women, and the elderly. A few clinical features of angina are summarized in Tables 5 and 6.

Table 5: Clinical features of stable angina

- Location
  - Usually retrosternal, can be epigastric, interscapular
- Localization
  - Usually diffuse, difficult to localize
  - When is very localized (point sign)—unlikely to be angina
- Quality
  - Pressure, heaviness, squeezing, indigestion
- Radiation
  - One or both arms, upper back, neck, epigastrium, shoulder
  - Lower jaw (upper jaw, head, lower back, lower abdomen, or lower extremities radiation is not feature of angina)
- Duration
  - Usually 1–10 minutes (not a few seconds or hours)
- Precipitating factors
  - Physical activity, emotional stress, sexual intercourse
- Aggravating factors
  - Cold weather, heavy meals
- Relieving factors
  - Cessation of activity, nitroglycerin (if relief is instantaneous it is unlikely to be angina)
- Associated symptoms
  - Usually none, occasionally dyspnea

Table 6: Clinical features of chest pain in acute coronary syndromes

- Location
  - Same as stable angina
- Quality
  - Same as stable angina
- Duration
  - Usually longer than stable angina
- Relieving factors
  - Usually unrelieved by rest or nitroglycerin
- Associated symptoms
  - Dyspnea, sweating, weakness, nausea, vomiting presyncope, or syncope

Chest pain resulting from acute aortic dissection is usually severe. The location can be anterior chest. Radiation to the back is common. The downward radiation along the spine is very suggestive of aortic dissection. The onset of pain is frequently instantaneous and the maximal severity may occur at the onset. A few clinical features of pain of acute pericarditis, pulmonary embolism and acute aortic dissection are summarized in Table 7.

The severity of angina is assessed by the Canadian Cardiovascular Society (CCS) functional classification (Table 8) or specific activity scale (Table 9). CCS is most frequently used to assess the severity of angina.

In suspected patients inquiries should be made about the risk factors. The modifiable and nonmodifiable risk factors for atherosclerotic coronary artery diseases are summarized in Table 10.

Dyspnea

Dyspnea is an uncomfortable sensation of breathing. It is also defined as "labored" breathing. Dyspnea can occur during exertion (exertional), during recumbency

Table 7: Clinical features of chest pain due to acute pericarditis, acute pulmonary embolism, and acute aortic dissection

Acute pericarditis	Acute pulmonary embolism	Acute aortic dissection

- Location
  - Anterior chest, superficial
- Character
  - Sharp, can be pleuritic
- Radiation
  - Supraspinatus areas, shoulders, back
- Relieving factors
  - Worse in supine position, less severe in sitting and leaning forward position, relieved by analgesics, nonsteroidals and steroids
	- Location
	  - Usually retrosternal
	- Quality
	  - Deep, may be similar to acute coronary syndromes
	- Associated symptoms
	  - Tachypnea and dyspnea
		- Location
		  - Chest, back
		- Quality
		  - Shearing, tearing
		- Onset
		  - Instantaneous
		- Radiation
		  - Downwards along the spine

Table 8: Canadian Cardiovascular Society (CCS) functional classification

Class I
- Ordinary physical activity, such as walking and climbing stairs, does not cause angina
- Angina with strenuous or rapid or prolonged exertion at work or recreation

Class II
- Slight limitation of ordinary activity. Walking or climbing stairs rapidly, walking uphill, walking or stair climbing after meals, in cold, in wind or when under emotional stress, or only during the few hours after awakening
- Walking more than two blocks on the level, and climbing more than one flight of ordinary stairs at a normal pace and in normal conditions

Class III
- Marked limitation of ordinary physical activity
- Walking 1–2 blocks on the level and climbing more than one flight in normal conditions

Class IV
- Inability to carry on any physical activity without discomfort—anginal syndrome may be present at rest

Table 9: Specific activity scale

Class I
- Patients can perform to completion any activity requiring ≤7 metabolic equivalents [e.g. can carry 24 lbs up eight steps; carry objects that weigh 80 lbs, do outdoor work (shovel snow, spade soil); do recreational activities (skiing, basketball, squash, handball, jog/walk 5 mph)]

Class II
- Patients can perform to completion any activity requiring ≤5 metabolic equivalents (e.g. have sexual intercourse without stopping, garden, rake, weed, roller skate, dance fox trot, walk 4 mph on level ground), but cannot and do not perform to completion activities requiring ≥7 metabolic equivalents

Class III
- Patients can perform to completion any activity requiring ≥2 metabolic equivalents (e.g. shower without stopping, strip and make bed, clean windows, walk 2.5 mph, bowl, play golf, dress without stopping), but cannot and do not perform to completion any activities requiring ≥ 5 metabolic equivalents

Class IV
- Patients cannot or do not perform to completion activities requiring ≥2 metabolic equivalents. Cannot carry out activities listed above (Specific Activity Scale Class III)

Table 10: Cardiac and pulmonary causes of dyspnea

Differential diagnosis of dyspnea

Cardiac
- CHF
- CAD
- Cardiomyopathy
- Valvular dysfunction
- LVH
- Pericardial diseases
- Arrhythmias
- Congenital HD

Pulmonary
- COPD
- Asthma
- Restrictive lung diseases
- Hereditary lung diseases
- Pneumothorax

(Abbreviations: CHF: Congestive heart disease; HD: Heart disease; CAD: Coronary heart disease; LVH: Left ventricular hypertrophy)

Table 11: Cardiac cause of dyspnea

Dyspnea

Cardiac or noncardiac dyspnea

Physical examination:
- Signs of heart failure—diagnostic of cardiac cause, e.g. S3, elevated JVP, positive HJR

Presence of cardiac pathology:
- Very suggestive of cardiac cause

Chest X-ray:
- Very helpful when findings of pulmonary venous congestion or pulmonary hypertension are present

ECG:
- Normal electrocardiogram
- A negative predictive value has over 90%

(Abbreviations: JVP: Jugular venous pressure; HJR: Hepatojugular reflux)

(orthopnea) or even with standing (platypnea). There are both cardiac and noncardiac (Table 10) causes of dyspnea. Many patients have both cardiac and pulmonary disease. To distinguish between cardiac and noncardiac dyspnea, the measurements of serum B-type natriuretic peptide (BNP) or N-terminal ProBNP (NTBNP) is helpful. In noncardiac dyspnea, the natriuretic peptide levels are normal, and in patients with heart failure, they are substantially elevated.

Exertional dyspnea can be caused by both cardiac and noncardiac causes. Exertional dyspnea is an important symptom of chronic heart failure. Orthopnea is defined when patients develop dyspnea lying flat and feel better when the upper part of the torso is elevated.

There are many cardiac conditions, which can be associated with episodic severe dyspnea. In between the episodes of dyspnea, these patients are relatively asymptomatic and may have good exercise tolerance. Careful cardiovascular examination may also reveal the etiology of dyspnea. For example, evidence of valvular and myocardial heart diseases suggests cardiac cause of dyspnea (Table 11).

Palpitation

Palpitation is perceived as an uncomfortable sensation in the chest associated with heartbeats. The most frequent cause of palpitation is premature atrial or ventricular contractions. The premature beat itself is not felt; the normal beat following the compensatory pause is felt as a strong beat. The patients usually describe this uncomfortable sensation as "a thump", "skipped beat", "the heart is coming out of chest", "heart stops" and "heart stops beating". The frequent premature beats may also be associated with other symptoms, such as dizziness, sinking feeling, shortness of breath and chest pain.

Syncope

Syncope is defined as transient loss of consciousness. Patients with presyncope complain of dizziness and near fainting, although they do not loose consciousness completely. The mechanism of cardiac syncope is reduced cerebral perfusion resulting from decreased cardiac output and hypotension.

A careful history is helpful for the diagnosis of the cause of syncope. Enquiry should be made about the circumstances in which syncope occurred, whether it was accompanied or preceded by palpitation, whether it occurs during exertion or it can also occur at rest, and whether it occurs only during upright position or it is unrelated to body position.

Edema

Patients with edema present with the symptom of "swelling", usually of the lower extremities. Both cardiac and noncardiac conditions may be associated with edema. Enquiries should be made regarding the initial location and progression of edema. Right heart failure with systemic venous hypertension causes dependent edema, such as in the ankles, feet, and legs. In bedridden patients, edema can be predominantly in the back. Generalized edema is uncommon in heart failure and usually suggests permeability edema, such as in patients with hypoalbuminemia.

Cough

Paroxysms of cough may be the presenting symptoms in cardiac and noncardiac patients. Patients with left heart failure may complain of nocturnal cough with or without dyspnea. Paroxysms of nonproductive cough are bothersome complications of angiotensin-converting enzyme inhibitor therapy.

Hemoptysis

Hemoptysis is an uncommon presenting symptom of cardiac patients. Patients with hemodynamic pulmonary edema may present with history of frothy pink, blood-tinged sputum. These patients also have dyspnea.

Recurrent hemoptysis may be a presenting symptom in patients with precapillary pulmonary arterial hypertension and Eisenmenger's syndrome. Hemoptysis associated with pleuritic chest pain should raise the suspicion of pulmonary embolism. Patients on anticoagulation therapy may present with hemoptysis.

It should be appreciated, however, that frank hemoptysis is an uncommon presenting symptom of cardiac patients, and primary bronchopulmonary disease, such as malignancy, should always be suspected.

❏ PHYSICAL EXAMINATION

Physical examination like history taking, is an integral part of evaluation of a patient with suspected or established cardiovascular disorders.

General Appearance

The physical examination starts with the inspection. During inspection, the physician has the opportunity to observe the patient's expression, skin color, posture, and general health status. During inspection, the nutritional status of the patient can be determined. Obesity or cachexia can easily be recognized. Obesity is a risk factor for metabolic syndrome, coronary artery disease, and heart failure.

Examination of the Skin

Examination of the color of the skin can reveal presence of cyanosis, jaundice and slaty, and bronze discoloration. Cyanosis is characterized by bluish discoloration of the skin and mucous membrane. Most frequently cyanosis is due to presence of abnormal amount of reduced hemoglobin. Cyanosis can be central, peripheral or mixed. Central cyanosis is due to intracardiac or intrapulmonary right-to-left shunt. The amount of desaturated hemoglobin is increased in central cyanosis and best recognized inspecting the buccal mucous membrane, tongue, and oropharyngeal mucous membrane.

Jaundice due to hyperbilirubinemia is occasionally seen in patients with severe right heart failure associated with congestive hepatopathy. Patients with portopulmonary hypertension may also have jaundice. A few abnormalities of skin, which can be associated with cardiovascular disorders are summarized in Table 12.

Examination of the Musculoskeletal System

The majority of congenital heart disease with musculoskeletal abnormalities is encountered in the pediatric population. In adult cardiology practices a few conditions, although distinctly uncommon, may be seen (Table 13).

Table 12: Skin abnormalities and cardiovascular disorders

- Cyanosis
  - Central—intracardiac and intrapulmonary right-to-left shunt
  - Peripheral—low cardiac output, increased peripheral oxygen extraction
- Methemoglobinemia—bluish discoloration of the skin
  - Hereditary (rare) and acquired (nitrate and nitrite toxicity)
- Jaundice—yellow discoloration
  - Prosthetic valve malfunction—hemolysis
  - Portopulmonary hypertension
  - Severe congestive hepatopathy
- Bronze discoloration—slaty color of the skin
  - Primary or secondary hemochromatosis
  - Atrial or ventricular arrhythmias
  - Restrictive cardiomyopathy, dilated cardiomyopathy
- Amiodarone skin toxicity—benign
- Butterfly rash of the face—lupus erythematosus
  - Valvular disease (Libman–Sack endocarditis)
  - Pulmonary arterial hypertension
- Malar flush of the face—
  - Severe mitral stenosis
  - Severe precapillary pulmonary hypertension
- Plantar and palmar keratosis and wooly hair—naxos disease
  - Arrhythmogenic right ventricular dysplasia

Contd...

Contd...

Table 12: Skin abnormalities and cardiovascular disorders

- Telangiectasia of lips, tongue and buccal mucous membrane—
  - Osler–Weber–Rendu syndrome
  - Arteriovenous malformations
- Xanthomatosis—tendon xanthoma, xanthoma in the palmar crease, with or without xanthelasma—familial hyperlipidemia
  - Premature coronary artery disease
- Cutaneous lentiginosis—LEOPARD syndrome
  - Conduction defects, congenital pulmonary stenosis
- Petechiae and purpuric skin rash—bacterial endocarditis
  - Valvular heart disease
- Blotchy cyanosis—carcinoid heart disease
  - Right-sided valvular heart disease
- Livid reticularis—reticular purplish skin rash
  - Lupus erythematosus
  - Valvular heart disease, pulmonary hypertension
  - Blue toes syndrome
  - Cholesterol emboli
- Atrophic skin lesions—necrobiosis diabeticorum
  - Increased risks of cardiovascular disease
- Annular skin rash with clear center—Lyme disease
  - Heart block, myocarditis
- Tightening of the skin, flexion contractures of the fingers, telangiectasia-scleroderma, CREST syndrome
  - Pulmonary arterial hypertension

Table 13: Musculoskeletal abnormalities associated with cardiovascular disorders

- Marfan's syndrome
  - Aortic regurgitation, mitral regurgitation, aortic disease
- Ehler–Danlos syndrome
  - Mitral regurgitation, aortic disease
- Turner's syndrome
  - Coarctation of aorta
- Holt–Oram syndrome
  - Atrial septal defect
- Down syndrome
  - Ventricular septal defect, atrioventricular cushion defects
- Rheumatoid arthritis
  - Aortic regurgitation, heart block
- Ankylosing spondylosis
  - Aortic and mitral valve disease, heart block
- Clubbing of the fingers and toes
  - Congenital cyanotic heart disease, bacterial endocarditis
- Straight back syndrome
  - Mitral valve prolapse
- Clubbing of fingers and toes
  - Congenital cyanotic heart disease, bacterial endocarditis

Finger and toes should be examined for clubbing. The drumstick type of clubbing is seen in cardiovascular diseases, such as congenital cyanotic heart disease and bacterial endocarditis. Bacterial endocarditis can be also associated with splinter hemorrhage, Janeway and Osler nodes and valvular regurgitations. Heberden's nodes, which are usually seen in the fingers, result from osteoarthritis and are not associated with cardiovascular disorder.

Measurement of Arterial Pressure

At present, in most institutions, automated techniques are used for the measurement of blood pressure. The various techniques of measuring blood pressure, their advantages and disadvantages, and pitfalls are discussed in the section on clinical hypertension.

Examination of the Jugular Venous Pulse

Careful examination of the jugular venous pulse and pressure provides information regarding the hemodynamic changes in the right side of the heart. It has been suggested that for estimation of jugular venous pressure, it is easier and preferable to examine the external jugular vein. However, it has also been suggested that if pulsation is present and visible, the examination of the internal jugular veins is preferable to that of the external jugular veins, as the internal jugular veins are in a direct line with the superior vena cava.

Estimation of Jugular Venous Pressure

The jugular venous pressure can be estimated by examining either external or internal jugular veins (Fig. 1). Conventionally, the upper torso is elevated to 30–40 degrees and the top of the venous pulsation is determined and 5 cm is added to the height assuming that right atrium is located 5 cm below the sternal angle (angle of Louis). However, it has been suggested that 10 cm should be added rather than 5 cm, if the torso is elevated to 45 degrees or greater. It should be appreciated that the external jugular venous pulse may not be recognized in patients with a fat and short neck. Kinking and thrombotic obstruction of the external jugular veins may also cause a spuriously higher central venous pressure.

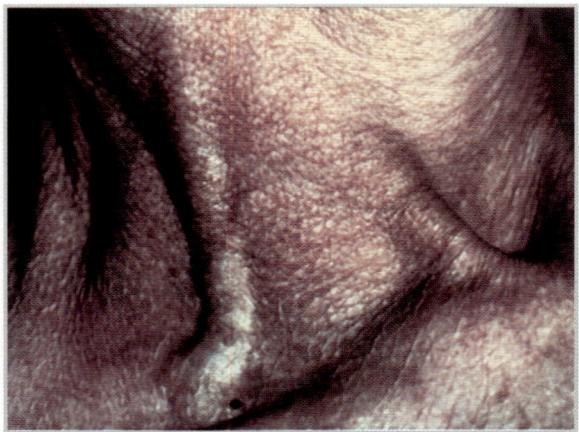

FIGURE 1: Courses of the external and internal jugular veins. The external jugular vein runs from lateral to the medial side of the neck across the sternocleidomastoid muscle. The internal jugular vein starts at the root of the neck in between the two heads of the sternocleidomastoid muscle and runs superiorly toward the angle of the jaw

Table 14: Causes of increased central venous and right atrial pressures

- Tricuspid valve obstruction—
  - Rheumatic tricuspid valve stenosis (usually associated with mitral and/or aortic valve disease)
  - Right atrial myxoma
  - Carcinoid heart disease
  - Neoplastic disease
- Right ventricular failure—
  - Systolic—
    Primary-RV infarction
    Secondary-pulmonary hypertension
  - Diastolic—
    Right ventricular hypertrophy
  - Pericardial disease
  - Pericardial effusion
  - Constrictive pericarditis
- Primary tricuspid regurgitation—
  - Traumatic
  - Ruptured chordae
  - Ebstein's anomaly
  - Carcinoid heart disease
  - Rheumatic heart disease
  - Neoplastic disease
- Generalized volume overload—
  - Glomerulonephritis
  - Anemia
  - Large atrioventous communications
  - Isolated right ventricular volume overload
  - Atrial septal defects

Elevated central venous pressure suggests that the right atrial pressure is elevated. The upper limit of normal right atrial pressure in the supine position is about 7 mm Hg. Some of the causes of increased central venous and right atrial pressures are summarized in Table 14.

Jugular Venous Pulsations

The jugular venous pulse characters are best analyzed by examining the internal jugular veins. When the right atrial pressure waveforms are recorded during cardiac catheterization, three positive waves (a, c and v) and two negative waves (x and y descents) are recognized. The "a" wave occurs during atrial systole with increased right atrial pressure due to atrial contraction (Fig. 2). The "c" wave is related to bulging of the closed tricuspid valve into the right atrium at the beginning of the right ventricular systole. The "x" descent is primarily due to atrial relaxation with a fall in right atrial pressure. The downward descent of the tricuspid valve apparatus also contributes to the genesis of the "x" descent.

After complete relaxation of the right atrium and the nadir of "x" descent, the right atrial pressure rises as the systemic venous return to the right atrium continues. With the onset of right ventricular systole when the tricuspid valve closes, the right atrial pressure rises and the "v" wave begins. The right atrial pressure continues to rise as the systemic venous return to the right atrium continues.

The peak of the "v" wave coincides with the end of the right ventricular systole and can be recognized by timing with the down slope of the carotid pulse. The "y" descent begins with the opening of the tricuspid valve and continues during the rapid filling phase of the right ventricle with a concurrent pressure decline in the right atrium.

The hepatojugular reflux, also called abdominojugular reflux, is assessed during sustained abdominal compression by applying firm pressure over the abdomen for 10–15 seconds. Normally, during abdominal compression, the jugular venous pressure increases transiently by 1–3 cm.

Arterial Pulse

The contour, character and amplitude of the arterial pulses are related to left ventricular stroke volume, left ventricular velocity of ejection, aortic dP/dT,

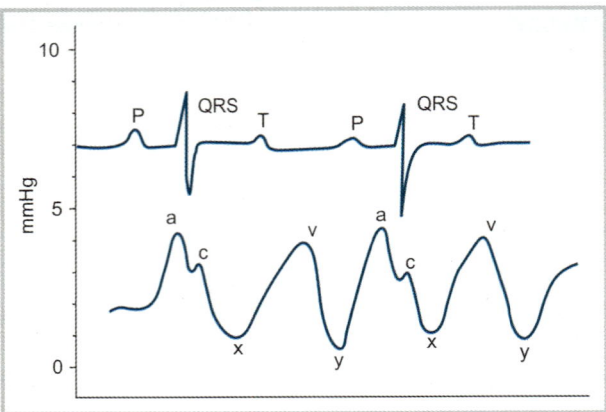

FIGURE 2: The schematic illustrations of right atrial pressure waveforms, which reveal three positive "a", "c" and "v" waves and two negative waves "x" and "y" descent. The "a" wave occurs during atrial systole following P wave of the electrocardiogram. The "c" wave occurs at the onset of right ventricular systole when the closed tricuspid valve bulges into the right atrium. It occurs just after the QRS complex of the electrocardiogram. The "x" descent is related to atrial relaxation. The peak of the "v" wave coincides with the end of right ventricular systole. It coincides with the end of the T-wave of the electrocardiogram. The "y" descent is caused by the opening of the tricuspid valve and during the rapid filling phase (P: P wave; QRS: QRS complex; T: T wave. Normally the magnitude of "a" wave is greater than "v" wave and is less than 7 mm Hg)

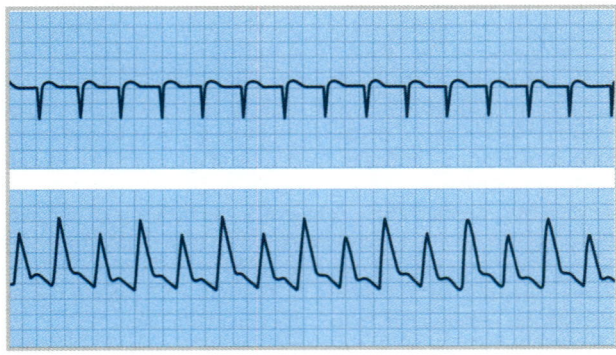

FIGURE 3: The characteristic "strong and weak alternating sequences of arterial pulses" in a patient with systolic heart failure are illustrated. The upper panel is an electrocardiogram showing normal sinus rhythm. The lower panel is directly recorded arterial pressure, showing alternating higher and lower arterial pressure

systemic vascular resistance, and the capacity and compliance of the arterial vascular system.

Examination of the volume and contours of arterial pulses provides important diagnostic clues regarding the underlying etiology of the pathophysiologic condition. Decreased amplitude may reflect reduced stroke volume irrespective of its etiology. Pulsus alternans in presence of regular rhythm indicates reduced left ventricular ejection fraction (Fig. 3).

Table 15: Cardiovascular physical examination
Palpable precordial impulses
• Prominent systolic left parasternal impulse
▪ RV failure
• Sustained LV apical impulse
▪ Reduced LVEF
▪ Increased LV mass
• Palpable PA impulse
▪ Left-to-right shunt
▪ Pulmonary hypertension
▪ Pulmonary stenosis

(Abbreviations: LV: Left ventricle; RV: Right ventricle; LVEF: Left ventricle ejection fraction; PA: Pulmonary artery)

It should be appreciated that the absence of pulsus alternans does not exclude systolic heart failure. However, the presence of pulsus alternans is almost diagnostic of reduced left ventricular ejection fraction, although it is present in only about 10% of patients with chronic systolic heart failure. In patients with acute coronary syndrome, in approximately 25% of patients pulsus alternans can be appreciated.

The pulsus paradoxus is characterized by a fall in arterial pressure during inspiration more than 10 mm Hg. Normally systolic arterial pressure falls during inspiration by an average of 8–12 mm Hg. In cardiac tamponade there is a substantially greater decrease in the arterial pressure during inspiration. The magnitude of the pulsus paradoxus can be better appreciated if the blood pressure is recorded by the sphygmomanometer. The cuff pressure should be decreased slowly. The systolic pressure at expiration is noted. With a further reduction of cuff pressure, the systolic pressure during inspiration is noted and the difference between these two systolic blood pressures provides an estimate of pulsus paradoxus. More severe the tamponade, a greater fall in arterial pressure occurs during inspiration.

Examination of the Precordial Pulsation

Precordial cardiovascular pulsations are best appreciated with the patient in supine position with the upper torso elevated not more than 45 degree. During inspection, the left ventricular apical impulse is usually visible over the left fifth intercostal space medial to the anterior axillary line. In patients with severe volume overload of the left ventricle, such as due to severe mitral or aortic regurgitation, an accentuated left ventricular apical impulse along with pulsation of the entire precordium may be visible. The left ventricular apical impulse, also called apex beat, is examined with the patient in a partial left lateral decubitus position. A few clinical conditions and mechanisms of precordial impulses are summarized in Table 15.

Auscultation

The heart sounds are schematically illustrated in Figure 4. The analysis of the heart sounds should precede analysis of the heart murmurs. The high-frequency heart sounds, such as first (S1) and second (S2) and murmurs due to aortic and mitral regurgitation are better appreciated with the use of the diaphragm of the stethoscope. The lower frequency heart sounds, such as third (S3) and fourth (S4) and mid-diastolic rumbles are better heard with the bell of the stethoscope.

The S1 occurs just before the upstroke of the carotid pulse at the beginning of the isovolumic systole. At the bedside, S1 and S2 are best recognized by timing with carotid pulse upstroke and down stroke, respectively.

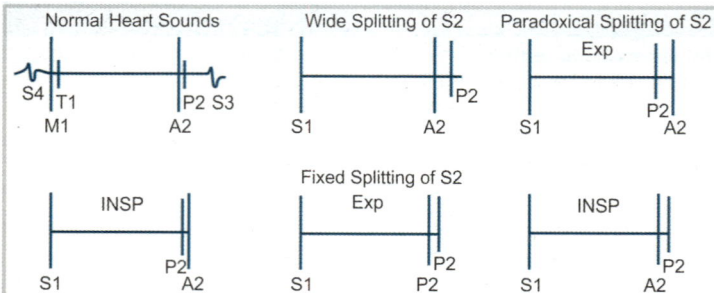

FIGURE 4: Schematic illustration of the heart sounds. S4 is the presystolic low pitch atrial sound. The S1 consists of higher pitch mitral (M1) and tricuspid valve (T1) closure sounds. The S2 consists of higher pitch closure sounds of aortic (A2) and pulmonary (P2) valves. The S3 is a lower pitch early diastolic filling sound. The wide splitting of S2 is defined when the interval between A2 and P2 is longer than normal. The A2 precedes P2 and during inspiration the interval between A2 and P2 widens. The paradoxical splitting is defined when P2 precedes A2 during the expiratory phase of the respiratory cycle and during inspiration the P2-A2 interval shortens. The "fixed splitting" is defined when the A2-P2 interval remains relatively unchanged during expiration and inspiration. (Abbreviations: S4: Fourth heart sound; M1: Mitral valve closure sound; T1: The tricuspid valve closure sound; A2: The aortic valve closure sound; P2: The pulmonary valve closure sound; S3: The third heart sound)

Table 16: Clinical conditions that can be associated with altered intensity and splitting of the first heart sound

- Increased intensity—
  - Mitral valve obstruction
  - Short PR interval
  - Enhanced left ventricular contractile function
  - Holosystolic mitral valve prolapse
- Decreased intensity—
  - Long PR interval
  - Decreased left ventricular contractile function
  - Increased left ventricular diastolic pressure
  - Premature closure of the mitral valve (severe acute aortic regurgitation)
  - Immobile mitral valve
  - Large pericardial effusion
- Changing intensity—
  - AV dissociation
  - Atrial fibrillation
- Wide splitting—
  - Right bundle branch block
  - Premature ventricular contractions
  - Ventricular tachycardia
  - Atrial septal defect
- Reversed splitting—
  - Severe mitral stenosis
  - Auscultatory alternans
  - Tamponade
  - Electrical alternans

The maximal intensity of S1 is appreciated over the cardiac apex. A variety of clinical conditions can cause alterations in the first and second heart sounds, and these are listed in Tables 16 and 17.

The S3 and S4 are low pitch sounds and originate in the ventricles. They are often termed ventricular filling sounds and are associated with ventricular filling and an increase in ventricular dimensions. The S3 occurs with the beginning of passive ventricular filling after the relaxation is completed. It coincides with end of the rapid filling phase of the apexcardiogram. The S4 occurs during atrial systole. Both S3 and S4 are better appreciated with the bell of the stethoscope.

The ejection sounds are related to the opening of the semilunar valves at the beginning of the ventricular ejection. The aortic ejection sound is related to the

Table 17: Clinical conditions that may be associated with changes in intensity and splitting of the second heart sound	
Increased intensity of A2	• Systemic hypertension • Coarctation of the aorta • Ascending aortic aneurysm
Decreased intensity of A2	• Calcific aortic stenosis • Severe aortic regurgitation
Increased intensity of P2	• Pulmonary arterial hypertension • Peripheral pulmonary artery branch stenosis • Idiopathic dilatation of the pulmonary artery
Decreased intensity of P2	• Pulmonary valve stenosis • Congenital absence of pulmonary valve
Wide splitting of S2	• Right bundle branch block • Left ventricular pacing • Accessory pathway with left ventricular preexcitation • Premature beats of left ventricular origin • Fascicular tachycardia • Right ventricular outflow obstruction • Pulmonary arterial hypertension
Wide and "fixed" splitting of S2	• Atrial septal defects • Common atrium • Right ventricular failure
Reversed (paradoxic) splitting of S2	• Left bundle branch block • Right ventricular pacing • Accessory pathway with right ventricular preexcitation • Premature beats of right ventricular origin • Right ventricular tachycardia • Severe aortic regurgitation • Large patent ductus arteriosus • Left ventricular outflow obstruction • Systemic hypertension • Severe tricuspid regurgitation (rare)
Single S2	• Eisenmenger syndrome with ventricular septal defect • Single ventricle

(Abbreviations: A2: Aortic component of the second heart sound; P2: Pulmonic component of the second heart sound; S2: Second heart sound)

opening of the aortic valve and the pulmonary ejection sound is that of opening of the pulmonary valve.

The prolapse of the mitral valve is the most common cause of midsystolic clicks (MSC). The S1–MSC interval is longer than the S4–S1 or M1–T1 intervals. In mitral valve prolapse, in a given patient the click diameter of the left ventricle is fixed. The S1–MSC intervals vary with changes in left ventricular volumes. During the supine position the S1–MSC interval is longer because the left ventricular end-diastolic volume is larger and the click diameter is reached later.

The high-pitch sounds associated with the opening of the mitral or tricuspid valves are called opening snaps and occur in early diastole. These sounds coincide with their rapid opening to the maximal open position and are appreciated in patients with mitral or tricuspid valve stenosis. The opening snaps are best heard with the diaphragm of the stethoscope.

> **Table 18: The timing and characters of the various types of murmurs**
>
> **Systolic murmurs**
> - Ejection systolic starts after S1 and does not extend to S2
> - Pansystolic starts with S1 and extends to S2 (mitral, tricuspid regurgitation, VSD)
> - Early systolic starts with S1 and does not extend to S2 (mitral, tricuspid regurgitation, VSD)
> - Late systolic starts after S1 and extends to S2 (mild MR or TR)
>
> **Diastolic murmurs**
> - Early diastolic starts with S2 (AI, PI)
> - Mid-diastolic starts after S2 (MS, TS, AFM)
> - Presystolic starts after S2 and extends to S1 (MS, AFM)
> - Continuous murmurs—encompass both systole and diastole (arteriovenous communication—PDA, AV fistula, mammary shuffle)
>
> (Abbreviations: PDA: Patent ductus arteriosus; AV: Atrioventricuar; AFM: Austin Flint murmur; TS: Tricuspid stenosis; MS: Mitral stenosis; AI: Aortic insufficiency; PI: Pulmonary insufficiency; MR: Mitral regurgitation; TR: Tricuspid regurgitation; VSD: Ventricular septal defect; AS: Aortic stenosis; PS: Pulmonary stenosis)

Auscultation of Heart Murmurs

The various types of cardiac murmurs and some of their causes are summarized in Table 18. In clinical practice, significant valvular heart disease is first diagnosed by detecting a murmur. Detection of murmur by auscultation has a sensitivity of 70% and a specificity of 98%. The guidelines recommend that all patients with suspected valvular heart disease should have echocardiography for establishing the cause of the murmur.

The murmurs can be systolic, diastolic, or continuous. The systolic murmurs are further classified as midsystolic (ejection) murmurs or regurgitant murmurs. The ejection systolic murmurs are related to left or right ventricular ejection to aorta or pulmonary artery, respectively. By definition, ejection systolic murmur begins after S1 and at the end of isovolumic systole. The interval between S1 and the onset of the murmur is related to the duration of the isovolumic systole. It ends at the end of ejection and before the closure of the semilunar valves, i.e. before A2 and P2. The interval between the end of the murmur and A2 or P2 is related to the duration of aortic or pulmonary hang out times. The intensity of the ejection systolic murmur increases (crescendo) during acceleration of blood flow in early systole, and the intensity decreases (decrescendo) with deceleration of flow in late systole (the crescendo-decrescendo murmurs).

The regurgitant systolic murmurs are classified into:
- Holosystolic or pansystolic—the murmur starts with S1 and terminates at or after S2
- Early systolic—the early systolic murmur starts with S1 and ends before S2
- Late systolic—the late systolic murmur starts after S1 and terminates at S2.

The diastolic murmurs are classified into:
- Early diastolic—early diastolic murmur which begins with S2 and terminates before S1
- Mid-diastolic—mid-diastolic murmur which starts after S2 and ends at or before 1
- Late-diastolic—late diastolic or presystolic murmur which starts in late diastole after S2 and terminates at S1.

The continuous murmurs begin in systole and continue into diastole.

Ejection Systolic Murmurs

The ejection systolic murmurs may result from fixed or dynamic obstruction of the left ventricular outflow tract. The murmurs are of harsh quality. The fixed obstruction may be at the level of aortic valve, or it can be supravalvular or subvalvular. The characters and duration of the murmur may be similar in valvular, supravalvular, and subvalvular aortic stenosis. However, there are other distinctive features of valvular, supravalvular, and subvalvular aortic stenosis. Aortic valve stenosis is frequently associated with an anacrotic carotid pulse, delayed upstroke and delayed peak (Fig. 5). The murmur radiates to both carotids. The supravalvular, valvular, and subvalvular aortic stenosis may all be associated with murmurs of aortic regurgitation.

Aortic valve sclerosis is associated with a short ejection systolic murmur. The murmur is best heard over the right second intercostal space and generally is not loud. In patients with bicuspid aortic valve without aortic stenosis, a short ejection systolic murmur preceded by an ejection sound is frequently heard and an early diastolic murmur of trivial aortic regurgitation may also be present. The carotid pulse and S2 are normal. A transthoracic echocardiogram is recommended in both the situations to confirm the diagnosis. In dynamic left ventricular outflow tract obstruction due to hypertrophic obstructive cardiomyopathy (HOCM), an ejection systolic murmur is always present.

Innocent Murmurs

The innocent murmurs are typical ejection systolic murmurs and are not associated with any other abnormal findings. The duration and intensity of innocent murmurs are variable. The innocent murmurs are related to increased flow across semilunar valves. The high cardiac output, such as with anemia, thyrotoxicosis and pregnancy, may be associated with flow murmurs. In over 80% of normal pregnant women, a pulmonary ejection systolic murmur can be heard.

Pulmonary Outflow Obstruction

An ejection systolic murmur is present in pulmonary valve, supravalvular or subvalvular stenosis. The pulmonary valve stenosis is associated with a harsh

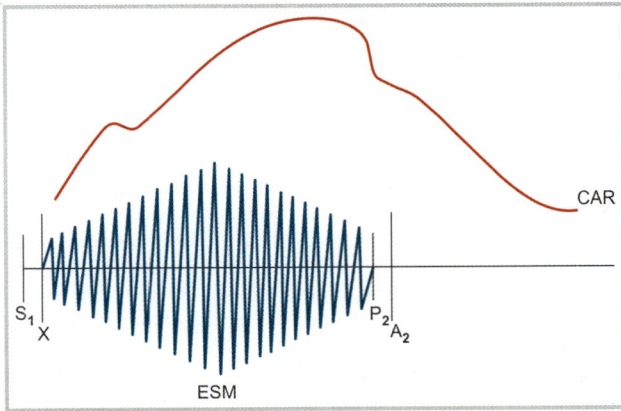

FIGURE 5: Schematic illustrations of the characters of the ejection systolic murmur and changes in carotid pulse in aortic valve stenosis. (Abbreviations: S1: First heart sound; A2: Aortic valve closure sound; P2: Pulmonary valve closure sound; ESM: Ejection systolic murmur; X: Aortic ejection sound; CAR: Carotid pulse)

ejection systolic murmur, which is best heard over the left second interspace. It is usually preceded by the pulmonary ejection sound. The intensity of the murmur increases during inspiration but that of the ejection sound decreases. The duration of the murmur correlates with the severity of stenosis. The interval between A2 and P2 also correlates directly with the severity.

The idiopathic dilatation of the pulmonary artery is associated with a relatively short ejection systolic murmur, an ejection sound and a widely split S2 with normal intensity of P2. The auscultatory findings are similar in pulmonary hypertension; however, in pulmonary arterial hypertension the intensity of P2 is increased and the splitting of S2 is narrower.

Regurgitant Murmurs

The systolic regurgitant murmurs start with S1 and may or may not extend to S2. When the murmur extends to S2 or beyond, it is called pansystolic. It is caused when blood flows from a chamber whose pressure throughout the systole is higher than the pressure in the chamber receiving the flow. Mitral or tricuspid valve regurgitation and unrestricted ventricular septal defect are the major causes of holosystolic murmurs. When the murmur does not extend to S2, it is termed early systolic regurgitant murmur. When the murmur starts after S1 and extends to S2, it is termed late systolic murmur.

Mitral regurgitation: The murmurs of mitral regurgitation are high pitched and best appreciated with the diaphragm of the stethoscope over cardiac apex with the patient in partial left lateral decubitus position. The intensity of the murmur in part determines radiation. The direction of radiation is along the direction of regurgitation jet from left ventricle to left atrium.

The physical findings of acute severe mitral regurgitation are different than those of chronic severe mitral regurgitation. Acute severe mitral regurgitation, e.g. due to ruptured chordae, is associated with sudden onset of dyspnea due to pulmonary edema. The physical findings are characterized by an early systolic regurgitant murmur, evidence for pulmonary hypertension, and a hyperdynamic left ventricular apical impulse and normal left ventricular ejection fraction. The murmur terminates in mid-systole or late systole when the left atrial pressure equalizes with left ventricular systolic pressure.

The physical findings of chronic severe mitral regurgitation are characterized by a holosystolic murmur, a widely split S2 and an S3. The murmur frequently extends beyond A2 as the left ventricular pressure still remains higher than the left atrial pressure even after the closure of the aortic valve. The cardiac enlargement is also appreciated. The left ventricular apical impulse is hyperdynamic indicating normal ejection fraction.

Tricuspid regurgitation: The tricuspid regurgitation murmur can be holosystolic, early systolic, or late systolic. The early and late systolic murmurs indicate mild tricuspid regurgitation. The holosystolic murmur is usually associated with more severe tricuspid regurgitation. The murmurs of tricuspid regurgitation are best heard over the lower left parasternal area and the intensity increases during inspiration (Carvallo's sign, sometimes spelled Carvello's). During inspiration there is increased systemic venous return, which is associated with more severe tricuspid regurgitation. Presence of a right ventricular S3 and a mid-diastolic flow murmur, which also increase in intensity during inspiration, indicates more severe tricuspid regurgitation. These auscultatory findings are frequently detected in patients with atrial septal defect and a large left-to-right shunt.

Diastolic Murmurs

Early Diastolic Murmurs

Early diastolic murmurs result most frequently, either from aortic or pulmonary regurgitation. The aortic and pulmonary regurgitation murmurs start with or shortly after A2 or P2, respectively. These murmurs are of relatively higher pitched and best heard with the use of the diaphragm of the stethoscope.

Aortic regurgitation: Auscultation is essential for the diagnosis of aortic regurgitation. The detection of an early diastolic murmur during auscultation has a positive likelihood ratio of 8.8 for the presence of aortic regurgitation and indicates that when an early diastolic murmur is heard, the likelihood of presence of aortic regurgitation is very high.

The murmur is best heard when a firm pressure is applied with the diaphragm of the stethoscope and the patient leaning forward and during held expiration. Auscultation should be performed over the right second interspace, along left sternal border and over the cardiac apex for the detection of the murmur. The radiation of aortic regurgitation murmur is toward cardiac apex. The murmur has a decrescendo configuration and a "blowing" quality. Occasionally, the murmur can have a musical quality (diastolic whoop), which appears to be due to flail everted aortic cusp.

The physical findings of chronic hemodynamically significant aortic regurgitation are illustrated in Figure 6 and Table 19. The early diastolic murmur is longer in duration and can be pandiastolic. A low-pitched mid-diastolic murmur, called "Austin Flint" murmur, may be heard. The intensity of A2 is usually decreased, but it does not necessarily indicate severe aortic regurgitation.

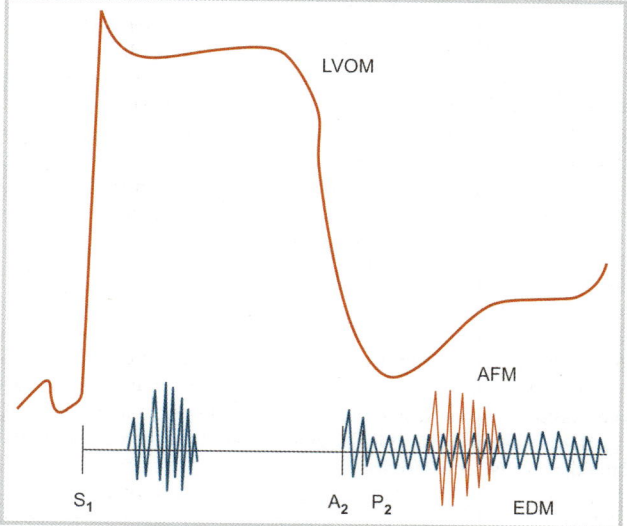

FIGURE 6: Schematic illustrations of physical findings in chronic severe aortic regurgitation showing a long early diastolic murmur, Austin Flint murmur (AFM), reversed splitting of S2 and hyperdynamic left ventricular impulse. (Abbreviations: EDM: Early diastolic murmur; A2: Aortic component of second heart sound; P2: Pulmonic component of second heart sound; S1: First heart sound; LVOM: Left ventricular outward murmur)

Table 19: Differences in the physical findings in acute and chronic severe aortic regurgitation		
	Acute	**Chronic**
Carotid pulse small volume	small volume	bisferiens quality, large volume, sharp upstroke
S1	decreased intensity or absent	decreased intensity or normal
S2	normal or decreased	normal or decreased
P2	increased	normal or increased
Apical impulse	normal and nondisplaced	displaced, normal or sustained
S4	absent	present
EDM	short	long or short
AFM	absent	present

(Abbreviations: S1: First heart sound; S2: Second heart sound; P2: Pulmonic component of second heart sound; S4: Fourth heart sound; EDM: Early diastolic murmur; AFM: Austin Flint murmur)

Presence of the physical findings of pulmonary hypertension and right heart failure indirectly suggest severe aortic regurgitation. The carotid pulse upstroke is sharp and may have a bisferiens character. The apical impulse is usually displaced laterally and downward due to dilatation of the left ventricle.

Pulmonic regurgitation: Very mild or trivial pulmonary valve regurgitation is detected in many normal subjects by echo-Doppler studies and do not have any clinical significance. In the adult patients, the most common cause of pulmonic regurgitation is pulmonary hypertension (Graham–Steel murmur). It is high pitched and starts with a loud P2 and has a "blowing" quality. The duration is variable. The murmur may increase in intensity during inspiration. An echocardiographic study is essential to exclude aortic regurgitation.

Mid-diastolic Murmurs

The mid-diastolic murmurs are low- or medium-pitched murmurs and have rumbling quality and thus these murmurs are frequently called "rumbles". An anatomic or functional obstruction of the atrioventricular valves is associated with mid-diastolic murmurs.

Mitral stenosis: The characteristic auscultatory findings of mitral stenosis are a loud S1, a mid-diastolic murmur with or without presystolic accentuation. It is best heard with the bell of the stethoscope over the cardiac apex with the patient in the left lateral decubitus. The murmur originates in the left ventricular cavity explaining why it is best heard over the cardiac apex. The presystolic component of the mid-diastolic murmur can be present even in presence of atrial fibrillation. The mid-diastolic murmur due to mitral stenosis is preceded by the opening snap until the mitral valve is heavily calcified and immobile. The duration of the murmur correlates directly with the severity of mitral stenosis.

Tricuspid stenosis: The auscultatory findings of tricuspid stenosis are very similar to those of mitral stenosis (Fig. 7). However, in tricuspid stenosis, the intensity of the murmur increases during inspiration because of increased gradient across the tricuspid valve (Carvallo' sign). The mid-diastolic murmur can be associated with an opening snap. The physical findings of tricuspid valve stenosis are summarized in Table 20.

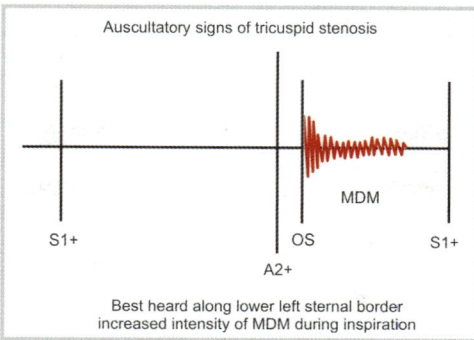

FIGURE 7: Schematic illustrations of auscultatory signs of tricuspid stenosis. Right sided opening snap (OS), mid-diastolic murmur (MDM) and increased intensity of the first heart sound (S1+). (Abbreviation: A2+: Aortic component of the second heart sound)

Table 20: Tricuspid stenosis—physical findings

- Elevated jugular venous pressure with prominent "a" wave and slow "y" descent
- Mid diastolic rumble, which increases in intensity during inspiration
- Right-sided opening snap
- Right-sided presystolic murmur
- Presystolic hepatic pulsation

When isolated tricuspid stenosis is present, right atrial myxoma or carcinoid heart disease should be suspected. An echocardiographic study is mandatory. Left and right atrial myxomas can be associated with auscultatory findings that are similar to those of mitral and tricuspid valve stenosis. The "tumor plop" sounds can be similar to opening snaps.

Austin Flint murmur: It is a low-pitched rumbling murmur associated with aortic regurgitation. Controversy exists about the genesis of the murmur. Fluttering of the mitral valve and relative mitral stenosis due to movement of the mitral valve leaflets to the semi-closed position has been proposed as the potential mechanisms. It is however present most frequently in patients with hemodynamically significant aortic regurgitation.

Continuous Murmurs

The continuous murmurs begin in systole and extend to diastole. These murmurs result from blood flow from a higher pressure chamber or vessel to a lower pressure chamber or vessel. In the adult patient, a patent ductus arteriosus and a venous hum are the usual causes of continuous murmurs. The venous hum can be easily diagnosed at the bedside. The venous hum is not heard in supine position. Pressure at the root of the neck also causes disappearance of the venous hum. The "mammary soufflé" associated with pregnancy is another cause of benign continuous murmur. Fistulous communication between an internal mammary artery graft to the vein accompanying the left anterior descending coronary artery is another rare cause of continuous murmur.

❏ SUGGESTED READINGS

Bonow RO, Carabello BA, Chatterjee K, et al. 2008 Focused update incorporated into the ACC/AHA 2006 guidelines for the management of patients with valvular heart disease: a report of the American College of Cardiology/American Heart Association Task Force on Practice Guidelines (Writing Committee to Revise the 1998 Guidelines for the Management of Patients with Valvular Heart Disease): endorsed by the Society of Cardiovascular Anesthesiologists, Society for Cardiovascular Angiography and Interventions, and Society of Thoracic Surgeons. Circulation. 2008;118:e523.

Devine PJ, Sullenberger LE, Bellin DA, et al. Jugular venous pulse: window into the right heart. South Med J. 2007;100:1022-7.

Goldman L, Hashimoto B, Cook EF, et al. Comparative reproducibility and validity of systems for assessing cardiovascular functional class: advantages of a new specific activity scale. Circulation. 1981;64:1227-34.

Lee CH, Xiao HB, Gibson DG. Jugular venous "a" wave in dilated cardiomyopathy: sign of abbreviated right ventricular filling time. Br Heart J. 1991;65:342-5.

Marcus GM, Cohen J, Varosy P, et al. The utility of gestures in patients with chest discomfort. Am J Med. 2007;120:83-9.

Perloff JK. Auscultatory and phonocardiographic manifestations of pulmonary hypertension. Prog Cardiovasc Dis. 1967;9:303-40.

Rutishauser W, Wirz P, Gander M, et al. Atriogenic diastolic reflux in patients with atrioventricular block. Circulation. 1966;34:807-17.

The Criteria Committee of the New York Association. Nomenclature and Criteria for Diagnosis, 9th edition. Boston: Little Brown;1994. pp. 253-6.

Willems J, Roelandt J, Kesteloot H. The jugular venous pulse tracing. Proc Vth European Cong Cardiol. 1968. p. 433.

2.2 Plain Film Imaging of Adult Cardiovascular Disease

❏ INTRODUCTION

Plain film radiography of the chest offers valuable information about the cardiovascular system, and appropriately, should serve as the initial investigative test in patients suspected of having cardiovascular disease, especially those with presenting with chest pain. Furthermore, by analysis of cardiac morphology, pulmonary vasculature and the vascular pedicle, chest films can provide additional semiquantitative information about heart function, pulmonary blood flow, and circulating blood volume.

❏ CHEST FILM TECHNIQUE

Radiographic assessment of the thoracic cardiovascular structures ideally requires the acquisition of two projections of the chest. This is primarily due to the oblique position of the heart within the chest. Frontal chest radiographs can be obtained either with the ventral chest closest to the film (PA projection) or reversed (AP film). Conventionally, frontal radiographs of the chest obtained within the department are usually obtained in the PA projection while all portable films use an AP technique. Selection between these two options, however, is not entirely academic, as there are significant changes relating to heart size between these two examination. Since the heart is located ventrally within the chest cavity, the

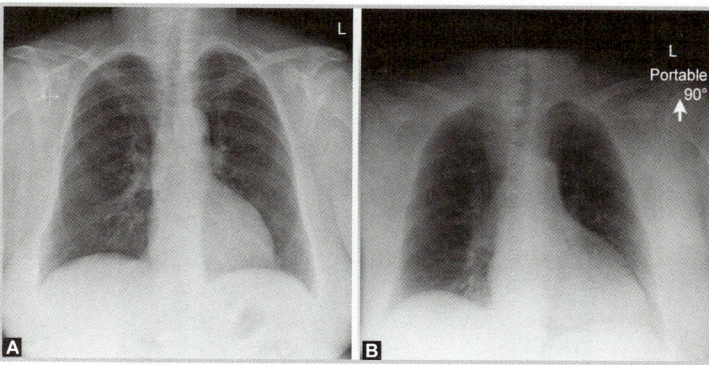

FIGURES 8A AND B: PA vs AP films: (A) PA film and (B) AP film on the same patient days apart. Note the significant increase in the size of the cardiac silhouette on the AP film due to magnification

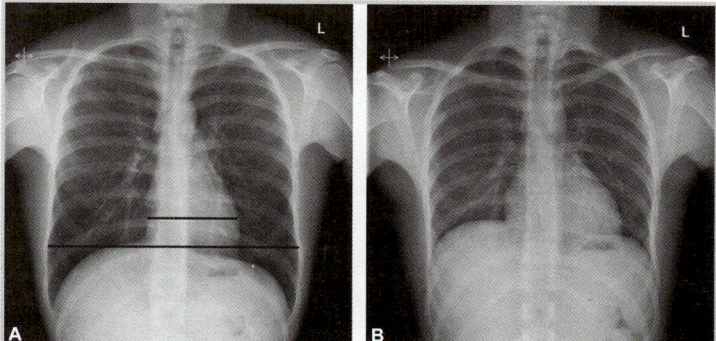

FIGURES 9A AND B: (A) Inspiratory vs (B) expiratory PA chest films. Horizontal lines reflect points of measurements for the cardiothoracic ratio (TR). Note the apparent increase in the size of the heart with expiration (B)

divergence of the X-ray beam which occurs with AP films results in an undesirable artifactual magnification of the cardiac silhouette (Figs 8A and B).

Qualitative assessment of cardiac enlargement can be quickly established radiographically by measuring the cardiothoracic ratio (CTR). This ratio, as measured on upright PA chest radiographs, refers to the ratio of the transverse diameter of the cardiac silhouette (measured horizontally) compared to the transverse chest diameter (as measured horizontally from inner margins of the ribs at the level of the right diaphragm). A normal CTR measured by this method should be 0.5 or smaller, provided there is good inspiratory effort. Decreases in lung volumes will produce an artificial increase in the systolic time ratio (STR), due the more horizontal axis of the heart along the left diaphragm (Figs 9A and B).

❏ CARDIAC ANATOMY ON CHEST RADIOGRAPHS

On the frontal radiograph (Fig. 10), the heart is normally orientated slight to the left of midline with the interventricular septum normally orientated 30 degrees left anterior oblique (LAO). This orientation results in superimpositioning of the right

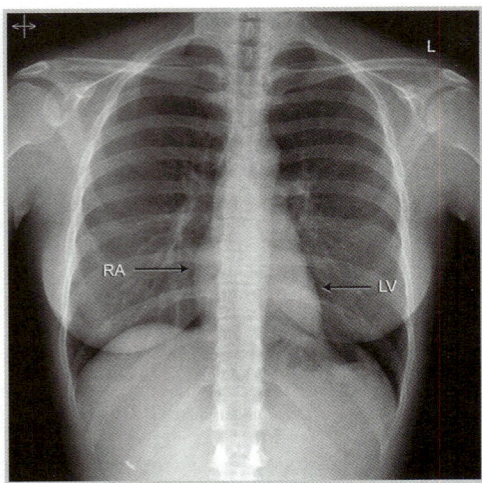

FIGURE 10: Normal PA chest film. The left ventricle (LV) forms the left heart border while the right heart border is composed of the lateral margin of the right atrium (RA)

ventricle in front of the left ventricle. As such, the left heart border is composed entirely of the left ventricle. On the right side, the right atrium composes the right heart shadow (Fig. 10B). The shadow of the superior vena cava (SVC) comprises the vertical right paramedian shadow coursing inferiorly from the upper mediastinum to the right atrium. In the middle of the SVC, directly superior to the proximal right mainstem bronchus lies the azygous vein, which appears as a teardrop vascular shadow reflecting the anterior course of this vein as it empties into the SVC.

On frontal radiographs, the concept of the three cardiac mogul shadows comprising the left cardiomediastinal silhouette needs to addressed. The superior most mogul reflects the aortic knob. Inferiorly, the left hilum (pulmonary artery) comprises the second mogul. While not normally present, the third mogul arises when there is enlargement of the left atrial appendage.

On the lateral radiograph (Fig. 11), the cardiac silhouette occupies the retrosternal region with the apex directly inferiorly toward the xiphoid process. Anteriorly, the right ventricle creates the anterior cardiac border. The left atrium forms the superior portion of the posterior aspect of the cardiac silhouette, with the mainstem bronchi immediately superiorly. The left ventricle forms the lower portion of the posterior margin of the heart shadow, with the diaphragm immediately below it.

❑ CARDIAC CHAMBER ENLARGEMENT

Left Ventricular Enlargement

Enlargement of the left ventricle will result in an enlarged cardiac silhouette, producing a bulbous left cardiac apex, which is displaced down and out on the frontal radiograph (Fig. 12). On the lateral projection (Fig. 13), the left ventricular shadow will extend toward the thoracic spine away from the posterior border of the IVC. Normally, the posterior edge of the left ventricular shadow should reside within two centimeters of the posterior edge of the IVC at a point two centimeters

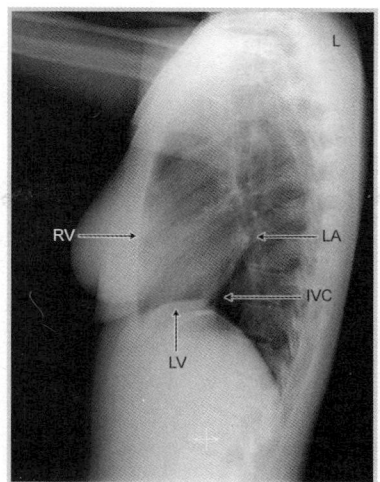

FIGURE 11: Normal cardiac anatomy on lateral radiograph. The right ventricle (RV) forms the ventral border of the cardiac silhouette while the inferoposterior border is composed of the left ventricle (LV). The left atrium (LA) composes the posterior-most border of the cardiac silhouette. The posterior border of the inferior vena cava (IVC) is also demonstrated to good advantage

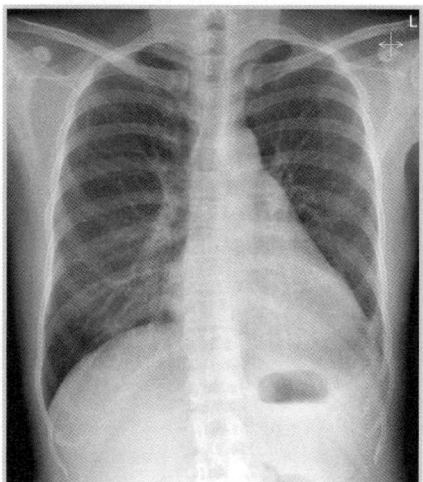

FIGURE 12: Left ventricular enlargement. PA chest film showing classic down and out configuration of the cardiac silhouette

above the diaphragm (Rigler's rule). With left ventricular hypertrophy, cardiac morphology is generally preserved with no apparent increase in size or change in left ventriclular configuration.

Right Ventricular Enlargement

Right ventricular enlargement, although uncommon, is manifested by uplifting of the ventricular apex on frontal projections producing the "boot-shaped" heart

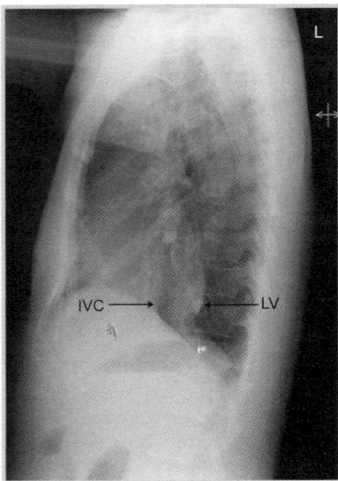

FIGURE 13: Left ventricular enlargement. Lateral film shows posterior displacement of the left ventricular shadow relative to the inferior vena cava (arrows)

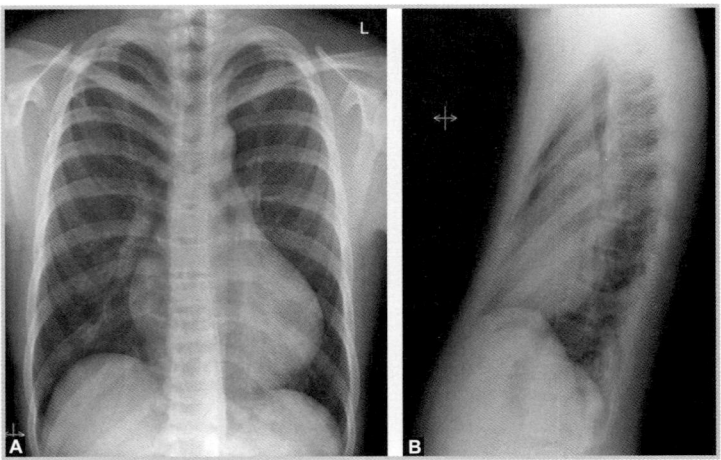

FIGURES 14A AND B: Right ventricular enlargement. PA and lateral films in patient with tetralogy of Fallot. (A) The PA film shows the upturned ventricular shadow producing the *"coer en sabot"* or boot shaped heart. (B) The lateral film shows filling in of the retrosternal region by the enlarged right ventricle

or *coer en sabot* configuration. On the lateral film there should be corresponding encroachment toward the sternum with "filling in" the retrosternal clear space (Figs 14A and B).

Left Atrial Enlargement

Left atrial/appendage enlargement will result in the formation of the third mogul as described above (Figs 15A and B).

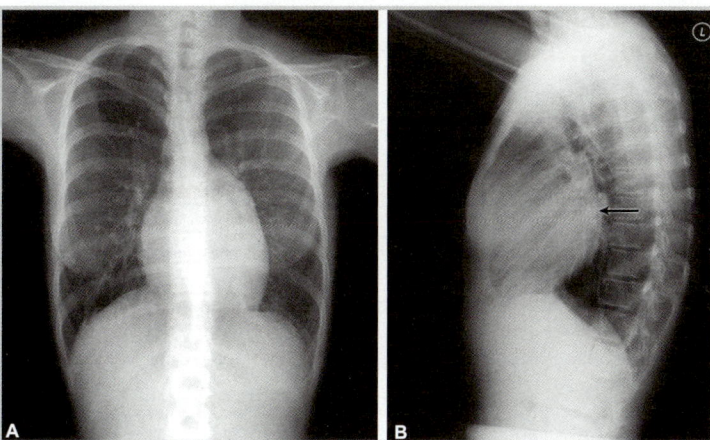

FIGURES 15A AND B: Left atrial enlargement. (A) PA and (B) lateral chest films showing classic cardiac silhouette of left atrial dilatation. On the PA film, there is bulging of the left cardiac border (third mogul). On the lateral film, note the conspicuous posterior displacement of the left atrial shadow (arrow).

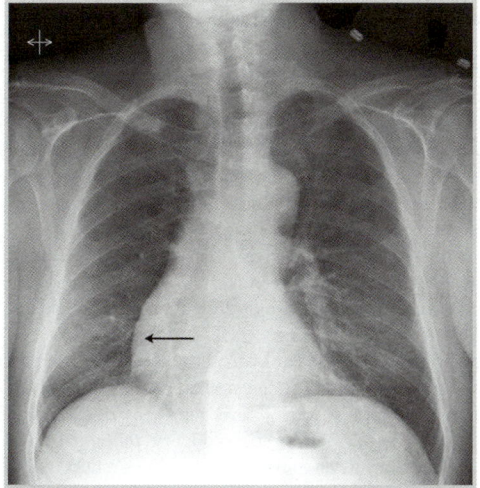

FIGURE 16: Right atrial enlargement. PA chest film showing lateral prominence of the right heart border (arrow) in patient with tricuspid insufficiency

Right Atrial Enlargement

Right atrial enlargement often goes relatively unnoticed but will result in lateral displacement of the right cardiac border on the frontal radiograph (Fig. 16). A sausage-shaped density may become more evident as the atrial appendage enlarges.

❏ RADIOGRAPHIC MANIFESTATIONS OF CONGESTIVE HEART FAILURE

Plain film radiography of the chest is an excellent modality to diagnose and measure the effectiveness of therapy in patients with congestive heart failure. In fact, it has been established that the characteristic stages of radiographic features of congestive heart failure on chest films correlate very well with hemodynamic measurements obtained with left atrial wedge pressures as determined with Swan Ganz catheterization.

The radiographic stages relate to the physiologic changes and hemodynamic perturbations occurring along the capillary and venous regions of the pulmonary circulation. The physiologic factors that determine the quantity of extravascular fluid depend on several factors:
- Intravascular hydrostatic pressure (promoting fluid escape from the intravascular space)
- Plasma oncotic pressure and interstitial hydrostatic pressures (which acts to keep intravascular fluid within vessels)
- Interstitial oncotic forces (acting to pull fluid out of the intravascular spaces).

Normally, these opposing forces result in a net positive fluid escape from the intravascular spaces into the interstitum, which is in turn, returned to the central venous circulation via the lymphatics. In heart failure, as hydrostatic forces within the pulmonary arterial circulation increase, there are corresponding and predictable radiographic changes, which reflect the increase of both increased pulmonary blood flow and eventual transudation of fluid out around the arterioles and capillaries into the perivascular interstitum and lymphatic spaces.

In the earliest stages of cardiac decompensation where there is only a modest increase in left atrial wedge pressures above normal (16–18 mm Hg), chest radiographs will demonstrate an increase in the size of the pulmonary vessels in the upper lobes reflecting shunting of blood flow to the upper lobes. This recruitment phenomenon, known as cephalad redistribution, results in disruption of normal A:B ratio whereby the caliber of the vessel becomes larger than the adjacent bronchus. Despite this redistribution, the pulmonary vessels should remain sharply defined as should the associated bronchus.

In the second stage of congestive heart failure, corresponding to wedge pressures around 18 mm Hg, there is enough intravascular hydrostatic force at the venule side of the capillary to increase or drive fluid out into the interstitial spaces surrounding the artery and bronchus.

With further increases in vascular hydrostatic pressures, more fluid accumulates in the interstium of the lungs. Fine linear shadows develop, which are known as Kerley lines. Radiographically, Kerley lines represent thickening (edema) of the intralobular septae that surround the secondary pulmonary lobule. Normally invisible on chest films, the development of septal lines reflect both interstitial fluid and augmentation of lymphatic flow, and become radiographically visible as either long linear shadows emanating out into the middle paracentral regions of both lungs (Kerley A lines) (Fig. 17) or as parallel shorter subpleural lines (Kerley B lines) running perpendicular to the pleural surface (usually in the middle and lower lung zones regions). Kerley C lines, which are believed to represent summation of Kerley B lines, typically are found in the lower lung zone regions but are more central, slightly longer and much less common than B lines.

In cases of significant elevations of hydrostatic pressures (wedge pressures greater than 25 mm Hg), after the interstitial space is saturated and no longer capable of accommodating additional fluid, migration of fluid occurs into the

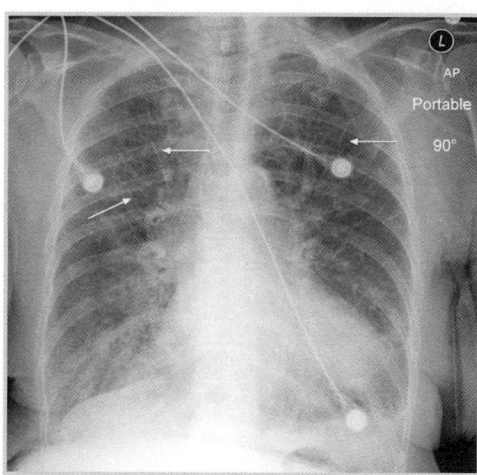

FIGURE 17: Interstitial edema. PA radiograph of patient in moderate congestive heart failure showing Kerley A (arrows) and parallel Kerley B lines in the lung bases reflecting interstitial edema

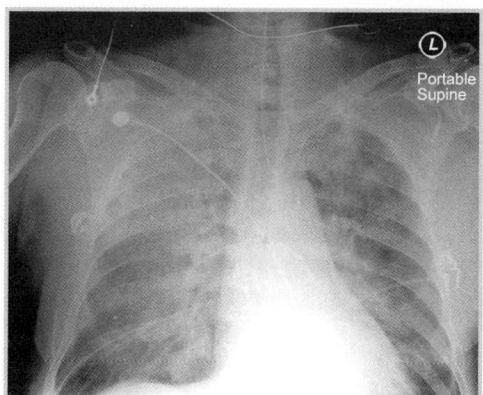

FIGURE 18: Pulmonary edema in patient with severe congestive heart failure due to acute myocardial infarction

lower pressure environment of the alveoli and airways. Chest radiographs will exhibit the classic perihilar haze or batwing airspace changes of pulmonary edema. Again, radiographically this phenomenon should be bilateral, and characteristically symmetric in distribution. In cases of severe heart failure, the edema may become generalized resulting in uniformly opaque lung tissue (Fig. 18).

The concept of the vascular pedicle needs to be addressed when evaluating radiographs for heart failure. The vascular pedicle refers to the conglomerate radiographic shadows encompassing both the venous and arterial circulation within the mediastinum. The vascular pedicle width is determined on frontal radiographs by drawing a line across the mid portion of the mediastinum extending from where the right mainstem bronchus crosses the SVC, to a point intersecting a vertical line drawn the origin of the left brachiocephalic artery (Fig. 19).

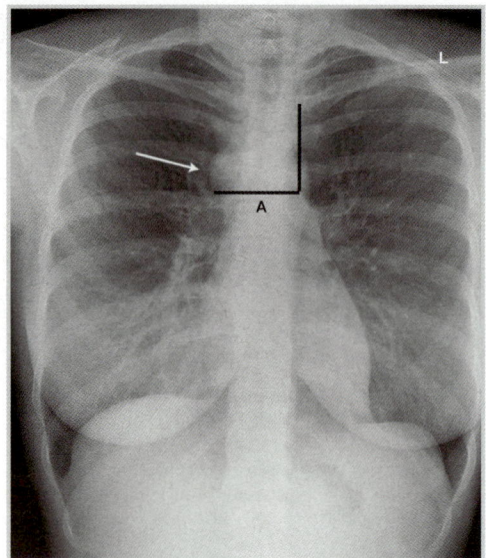

FIGURE 19: Vascular pedicle. Assessment of the vascular pedicle can easily be determined on PA chest radiographs by drawing a horizontal line from the junction of the SVC and right mainstem bronchus to a point drawn perpendicular from the left innominate artery. The horizontal line (A) represents the vascular pedicle, which should be normally around 5 cm in length

❑ CARDIAC CALCIFICATIONS

Evaluation of unusual of calcifications overlying the cardiac silhouette may provide important clues about specific disease processes, which may not be clinically suspected. The identification of coronary calcium indicates severe, advance atherosclerosis. Identification of coronary calcium implies significant disease with an higher likelihood of significant stenosis and is even more significant in patients with acute chest pain syndromes. Linear myocardial calcifications may be encountered in patients with a history of prior myocardial infarction, and if protuberant, may indicate associated formation of ventricular aneurysm. Valvular calcifications when identified on chest films generally are also associated with significant valvular stenosis.

❑ ACQUIRED VALVULAR HEART DISEASE

Aortic and mitral valve disorders are the most commonly encountered forms of valvular heart disease in adults and both have characteristic radiographic manifestations. Characteristically, most of these disorders stem from either congenital structural valvular abnormalities or rheumatic heart disease.

Aortic Stenosis

The most common form of congenital heart disease is the biscuspid aortic valve with a prevalence of 1–2% in the general population. The typical radiographic feature of aortic stenosis, which is related to the severity of stenosis is poststenotic

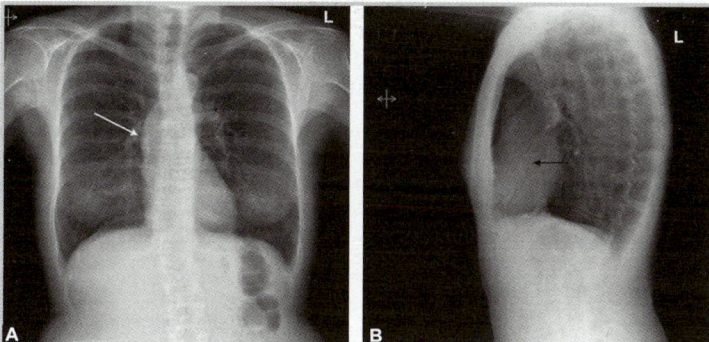

FIGURES 20A AND B: Aortic stenosis. (A) PA film shows dilatation of the ascending thoracic aorta (arrow) without associated left ventricular dilatation. (B) Lateral film shows calcification of the aortic valve (arrow)

dilatation of the ascending thoracic aorta due to the jet effect of blood exiting the stenotic valve (Figs 20A and B).

Aortic Insufficiency

Aortic insufficiency in adults can be attributed to either aortic valve disease or disorders of the aortic root, such as aneurysm or dissection. The radiographic manifestations of aortic insufficiency like aortic stenosis are related to both the severity and duration of the disease. Features of aortic insufficiency on chest films include both dilatation of the ascending thoracic aorta with associated left ventricular enlargement. Enlargement of the left atrium rarely occurs providing competency of the mitral valve.

Mitral Stenosis

Most cases of mitral stenosis are a sequela of rheumatic fever. The radiographic manifestations of mitral stenosis coincide with the degree of the severity of the stenosis. Characteristically, radiographs will usually are diagnostic for this disease and demonstrate left atrial enlargement, which can be marked in severe. Severe stenosis at the mitral valve resulting in significant left heart obstruction and may also produce radiographic changes of congestive heart failure as well as pulmonary arterial hypertension.

Mitral Regurgitation

While associated with rheumatic heart disease, mitral valve insufficiency in adults is more commonly seen in mitral valve prolapse. Chest films demonstrate marked left atrial enlargement with pulmonary venous hypertension. Frequently, there is a component of associated dilatation of the left ventricle as well, especially in long-standing cases. Occasionally, in cases of severe mitral regurgitation, passive venous congestion with or without pulmonary edema may be encountered. Unilateral right upper lobe edema/hemorrhage secondary to the jet effect of regurgitant blood entering the right upper lobe pulmonary vein may also occasionally be encountered.

Pulmonary Valve Stenosis

Pulmonary valve stenosis is generally a component of congenital heart disease and is an uncommon acquired valvular disorder in adult, resulting from fusion on the commissures. In any case, the typical radiographic feature of pulmonary stenosis is unilateral dilatation of the left pulmonary artery arising from the poststenotic jet effect of blood exiting the pulmonary valve. Long-standing cases may show associated enlargement of the right ventricular shadow.

Pulmonary Valve Insufficiency

Distinctly uncommon in adults, insufficiency of the pulmonary valve often is not associated with any specific morphologic changes of the cardiovascular structures on chest films other than occasional right heart enlargement.

Tricuspid Insufficiency

In most cases of triscuspid insufficiency, there are no discernible radiographic changes suggestive of this disease. When severe, prominence of the right heart border reflecting right atrial enlargement occurs (Fig. 16). Associated widening of the vascular pedicle (especially SVC shadow) and dilatation of the azygous vein may also present indicating an increase in right atrial pressure.

❏ PERICARDIAL DISORDERS

Pericardial Effusion

It is important to realize that the heart shadow as demonstrated on plain films is composed of both the heart and the surrounding pericardial sac. As such, an apparent increase in the heart shadow may be due to either intrinsic cardiac chamber(s) dilatation or alternatively reflect accumulation of fluid in the pericardial space. While small pericardial effusions usually will go undetected by chest films, large amounts will alter the overall shape of the heart shadow resulting in a globular relatively featureless cardiac silhouette (aka water bottle configuration) (Fig. 21). The lateral film may show an opaque line (fat pad sign) along the ventral surface of the heart reflecting separation of visceral and parietal pericardial fat by the effusion.

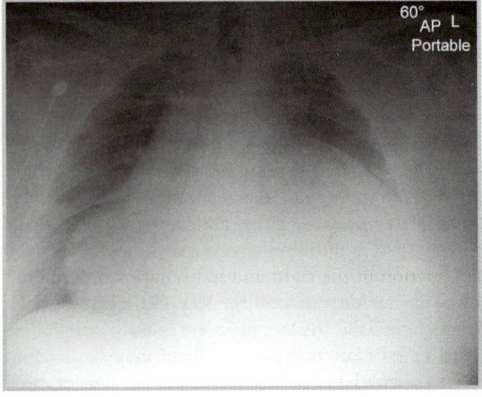

FIGURE 21: Pericardial effusion. PA chest films shows marked global enlargement (water bottle configuration) of the cardiac silhouette secondary to a large pericardial effusion

2.3 Electrocardiogram

❏ INTRODUCTION

The electrocardiogram remains one of the most valuable, most readily available, and relatively least expensive laboratory tools. Its accurate interpretation is absolutely critical to patient care. While computer-assisted interpretation of the 12 lead electrocardiogram is almost universally available, the computer-based interpretation should never be assumed accurate.

❏ BASIS OF ELECTROCARDIOGRAPHY

The electrocardiogram in its most basic sense represents the recording of electrical potentials from the heart projected on to the body surface and fed into a galvanometer set-up as a voltmeter. The electrical potentials are produced by depolarization and repolarization of the atrial and ventricular myocardial cells of the heart.

The heart's activation normally begins with the discharge of the sinoatrial node located in the right atrium beginning just below the superior vena cava. This discharge is of such a tiny magnitude that the electrocardiogram cannot record it. Nevertheless, this leads to the depolarization of the atrial musculature from the high right atrium, over the right atrium, and over to the left atrium creating what has been designated as a p wave. Under normal circumstances, this depolarizing wave then moves from the atrial chambers and passes on to the discrete conduction pathways connecting the atrium to the ventricular musculature, specifically through the atrioventricular (AV) node, then through the common bundle or bundle of His, and then out simultaneously through the right and left bundle branches to activate the ventricular musculature. The depolarization then proceeds through the AV bundle (common bundle or bundle of His) that penetrates the dense connective tissue of the central fibrous body and runs down along the right ventricular side of the membranous interventricular septum. The common bundle then bifurcates into the right and left bundles. The right bundle runs as a quite discrete bundle along a particularly prominent trabecular band known as the moderator band across to the base of the anterior papillary muscle of the right ventricle. The left bundle passes beneath the membranous part of the interventricular septum to reach the left side of the septum where it eventually divides into two broad bands. The anterior division is relatively more discrete and activates the anterior superior portion of the left ventricle. The much broader band is the posterior division that activates the posterior inferior portion of the left ventricle. All three bundles fan out as the Purkinje fibers of the interior of the ventricles activating the ventricular musculature from the endocardial to epicardial surface. The septal depolarization under normal circumstances accounts for a dominate portion of the initial portion of the depolarization of the ventricles recorded by the electrocardiogram and designated the QRS complex. Continued conduction in the right and left bundles is occurring simultaneously while this septal activation is occurring. The right and left bundles carry their impulse on to the interior of the free walls of the two ventricles as they spread out as cells identical to themselves known as Purkinje cells coating the endocardial surface of the two ventricles. This leads to depolarization of the entire ventricular muscles masses from endocardium to epicardium.

❑ COMPONENT PARTS OF THE ELECTROCARDIOGRAM

The depolarization of the atrial chambers produces waves called p waves. The repolarization of the atrial chambers is usually not evident on the surface ECG tracing. The summation of all the depolarizations of the ventricular chambers (a summation of phase 0 of all the action potentials of the ventricular myocardial cell depolarizations) is expressed as the QRS complex. By custom, a Q wave must be an initial deflection of a QRS complex and must be a negative or downward deflection. All upward or positive deflections are called R waves and negative deflections that are not the initial deflection of the QRS complex are called S waves. If there is more than one R or S wave in the complex, the second deflection is labeled R prime (R') or S prime (S'). Descriptively sometimes R or S waves may be represented by capital or lower case letters depending on the size of the deflection. The summation of the repolarization of the ventricular chambers (primarily the phase 3 of the action potentials of the ventricular myocardial cells) is represented on the ECG by the T wave. The deflection or direction of the T wave is generally in the same direction as the major direction of the QRS complex for most leads since the left ventricle, which by its mass dominates the formation of the QRS complex, depolarizes from the endocardium out to the epicardium but repolarizes from the epicardium inward to the endocardium. The T wave may be followed by a low voltage wave, named the U wave. The origin of this wave remains in dispute.

❑ LEAD SYSTEMS USED TO RECORD THE ELECTROCARDIOGRAM

The original system devised by Einthoven consists of the leads from the left arm, the right arm and left leg set up to compare the recordings from one extremity to a second extremity by feeding the recordings into the either side of the voltmeter. The three potential combinations have been designated as bipolar leads. As designed by Einthoven, lead I is the comparison of the left arm potentials versus the right arm potentials connected to the voltmeter so that an upright wave is recorded in lead I when the left arm's potential is positive relative to the right arm's electrical potential. Einthoven's second lead, lead II, consists of the comparison of the potentials on the left leg versus the right arm connected so that an upright deflection in lead II occurs when the left leg's potential is positive compared to the right arm's potential. Lead III is a comparison of the potentials from the left leg versus the left arm connected to the voltmeter so that this lead registers an upright deflection when the left leg's potential is positive relative to the left arm's potential. Thus the three leads create a triangle with three points of view separated by 60 degrees. Kirchhoff's second law based on the conservation of energy states that the algebraic sum of the potentials around a closed path must be zero. This means that the electrical potential recorded in lead II is equal to the sum of the potentials recorded in leads I and III.

Frank Wilson et al. developed a system of recording electrical potentials from a single extremity compared to an "indifferent electrode" whose recorded potentials are minimal. The purpose was to record just the potentials from a given extremity representing each of the apices of Einthoven's triangle. Electrocardiographic leads using this system are indicated by the letter V, hence VR, VL, and VF. The connections to the voltmeter are such that an upright wave is recorded in VR when its potentials are positive. Emanuel Goldberger modified this V lead system, as it pertains to the extremity leads in such a way as to increase the amplitude of the potentials recorded. This augmentation of the potential recorded from a given extremity is indicated by the "a" preceding the name of that lead, i.e. aVR, aVL and aVF. From the standpoint of vectors for each lead, the potential recorded in any given lead is already described by any two leads equidistant from that leads point of view. For instance, lead aVF is completely described by the sum of lead II and lead III divided by 2. The formulae usually presented then are as follows:

II = I + III;
aVF = (II + III)/2.

All other comparisons can be given by algebraic rearrangement of these two equations.

Later, the precordial leads were developed using Wilson's central terminal versus the exploring electrode placed at various positions on the chest wall. For accuracy of electrocardiographic interpretations and especially in comparing serial recordings, the correct placement of the precordial leads is absolutely essential. Lead V1 must be placed in the 4th intercostal space just to the right of the sternal border; lead V2 in the 4th intercostal space just to the left of the sternal border; lead V4 at the left midclavicular line in the 5th intercostal space; lead V3 at the midpoint of a diagonal line connecting leads lead V2 and lead V4. Lead V5 is placed at the anterior axillary line at the anterior axillary line's intersection with a line extending out perpendicular to the rostral–caudal line of the body from the position of V4. Lead V6 is placed at the midaxillary line along the same line as V4 and V5. The midaxillary line is best defined in terms of lead placement as the mid or central plane of the thorax. There is a common misconception that V5 and V6 stay in the same interspace as V4. If the anterior axillary line is not well defined, lead V5 should be placed midway between V4 and V6.

❏ A SYSTEMATIC WAY OF LOOKING AT THE INTERPRETATION OF THE ELECTROCARDIOGRAM

Identification of Atrial Activity

Proceeding in a systematic fashion helps to prevent omissions and leads to better conclusions. It is recommended that analysis should start with identification of the atrial activity. In identifying the name of the atrial activity, the first question should be is the atrial activity "sinus activity". This is based on the rate (for adults perhaps as low as 40 per minute and up to 180 when at rest and faced with high output stresses such as fever, infection, etc. and up to about 200 with maximal exercise). The maximal heart rate for the adult with exercise can be roughly estimated by subtracting the person's age from 220. If the activity fits within these ranges, then sinus activity is a potential diagnosis. The next criterion is the morphology of the p waves, especially in lead II. At the slower rates, the p of sinus activity should be upright or flat but not inverted in lead II and at faster rates definitely upright in lead II. The p morphology generally remains constant in appearance, although at the slower rates associated with sinus arrhythmia the p wave in lead II may be more upright when the p to p interval is shorter and more flat when the p to p interval is longer. The third criterion on the electrocardiogram is that the p intervals are reasonably regular. With high vagal tone producing slower rates, such as in athletes, the p to p interval may expand and shorten in synchrony with inspiration and exhalation, a normal variant called sinus arrhythmia.

If the conclusion is that the atrial activity is not sinus, the observed atrial activity should be categorized into one of three groups:

1. "Organized": specifically that the atrial wave morphology in any given lead maintains a constant morphology and a constant atrial wave to atrial wave interval. If the conclusion is that the atrial activity is organized but not sinus, then the proper diagnosis can usually be based on the rate of the atrial waves and their morphology. Based on these considerations, usually the conclusion will be that the atrial activity represents atrial flutter (Fig. 22), an ectopic atrial tachycardia (re-entrant or focal ectopic) (Fig. 23) or retrograde p waves.
2. "Chaotic": specifically that the atrial morphology in any given lead is constantly varying in morphology and wave to wave interval. If the atrial activity is not organized but instead is chaotic, i.e. constantly varying in morphology and wave to wave interval, the two most likely rhythms are atrial fibrillation and multifocal atrial tachycardia. An atrial wave with consistent p wave morphology but an irregular p to p interval is retrograde activation of the atria from conduction from a source distal to the AV node, e.g. a ventricular tachycardia, but conducting retrograde back up through the AV node with a ventriculoatrial second degree block, e.g. with Mobitz I (Wenckebach) characteristics.
3. The atrial activity cannot be found consistently or is only detected for only one or two beats during the rhythm strip. Under these circumstances, characterizing the dominant QRS complexes into one of three general observational groups is helpful. The first such group would be regular R-to-R intervals with "narrow" QRS complexes. This breaks down into a slow variety and a fast variety. The slow variety would in general consist of a heart rate of 60 BPM or less with plenty of room between QRS complexes to allow for detection of atrial waves. If no such waves can be observed in any of the 12 leads, it is likely that this represents atrial asystole with the expected emergence of a junctional escape rhythm. The more common situation is the "fast" variety in which there is rapid QRS rates of about 100–220 BPM. The likely candidates explaining this finding include sinus tachycardia where the sinus p waves have become difficult to identify, atrial flutter with 2 to 1 AV conduction and "paroxysmal supraventricular tachycardia" (usually AV nodal using reentrant supraventricular tachycardia) (Fig. 24).

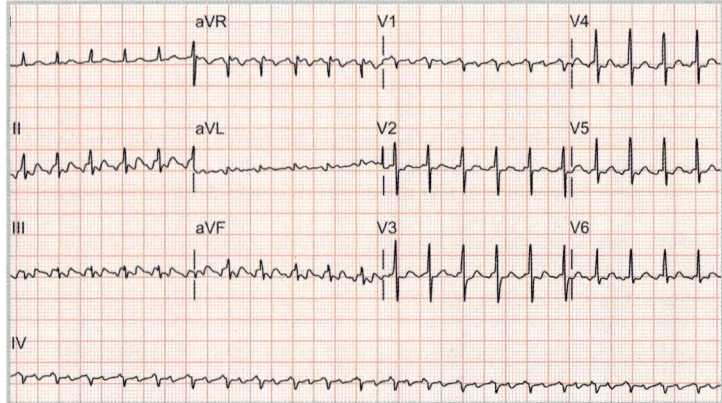

FIGURE 22: An example of atrial flutter with 2:1 conduction

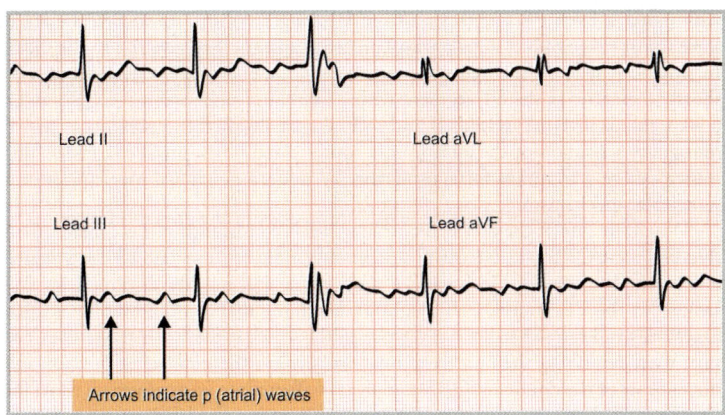

FIGURE 23: An example of focal ectopic atrial tachycardia with 2:1 atrioventricular block

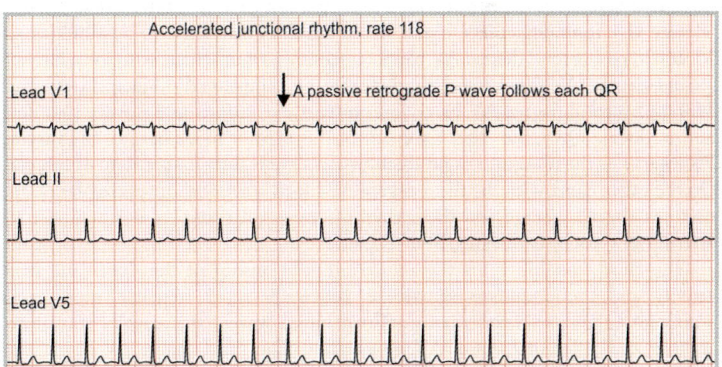

FIGURE 24: An example of atrioventricular reentrant tachycardia (AVNRT)

The next possibility under the "cannot find the atrial activity section", is that the dominant QRS intervals are varying in an irregularly irregular way, i.e. a completely unpredictable and unpatterned R-to-R variation. A reasonable assumption under the circumstance when no atrial activity can be discerned is that the rhythm is "fine" (very low amplitude) atrial fibrillation.

The final observational is that the above two steps did not lead to a reasonable diagnosis or, more commonly, that there are regular but wide (>120 msec) regular QRSs. Under this circumstance, moving to the ventricular analysis to be described subsequently is useful in choosing whether the QRSs reflect a ventricular rhythm versus a rhythm that is not of ventricular origin and is not from an atrial source.

Given that an atrial activity has been identified, the next step is to identify in a general way what the numerical relationship is between the dominant atrial waves and the dominant QRSs. Simplistically, the first possibility is that the dominant atrial activity and the dominant QRSs exist in a one to one relationship. Thus one atrial wave would need to be observed for each dominant QRS complexes with either a fixed PR length or a fixed RP length. With a fixed PR, the atrial wave (most commonly a sinus p wave) proceeds antegrade to give rise to the QRS. In situations where the atrial wave is found at the end of the QRS complex or shortly thereafter in the ST segment with a fixed interval between the QRS and a p wave that is inverted in leads II and aVF, almost always this represents a passive retrograde activation of the atria from a source distal to the atrial chambers. This source can be a reentrant focus using the AV node, a junctional mechanism or a ventricular mechanism.

When the rate of the dominant atrial waves is consistently always greater than the dominant QRS rate, almost invariably this indicates a second or third degree AV block. The type of block can be most easily and quickly discerned by first looking at the PR intervals, although not assuming that a p followed by a QRS necessarily indicates that the p gives rise to the QRS. If the PR interval does not vary, then describing the numerical relation between the number of p waves and the number of the dominant QRS complexes will produce an appropriate name for the block. If there are two waves for each QRS with a fixed PR, the appropriate name is 2 to 1 second degree AV block. If there is a fixed ratio of 3 or more p waves per QRS with a fixed PR, the appropriate name would be advanced second degree AV block. All others fitting the description of more dominant p waves than dominant QRS complexes but with a fixed PR can be appropriately diagnosed as Mobitz II second degree AV block. If the PR does vary, the two possibilities are Mobitz type I second degree AV block (essentially synonymous with Wenckebach second degree AV block) and third degree or complete AV block. Given that Mobitz I second degree AV block intermittently manifests as a p wave that does not produce a QRS, the other hallmark of this type of block besides the varying PR interval is the intermittent production of a significantly longer R-to-R interval. On the other hand, with the third degree AV block junctional or ventricular escape rhythms should emerge and these rhythms are regular and do not demonstrate intermittent, patently obvious, R-to-R pauses.

The third possibility for the numerical relationship of the dominant atrial activity and the dominant ventricular activity is more frequent, more rapid dominant QRS complexes than dominant atrial waves. This usually constitutes another and different form of AV dissociation than third degree AV block. This usually represents interference AV dissociation created by a slowing of the sinus rate below the rate of normal physiologic escape pacemakers, usually junctional escape pacemakers, and/or development of a pathological ectopic tachycardia, from a source distal to the AV node, regardless if that is junctional or ventricular (Fig. 25).

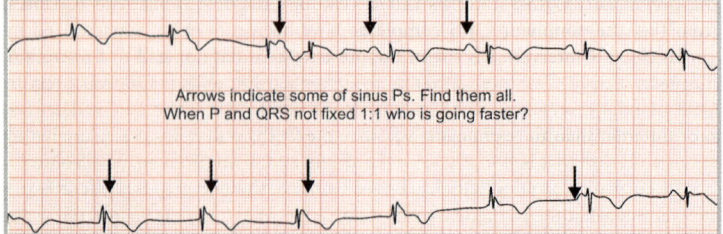

FIGURE 25: An example of sinus bradycardia with junctional escape rhythm creating interference atrioventricular dissociation

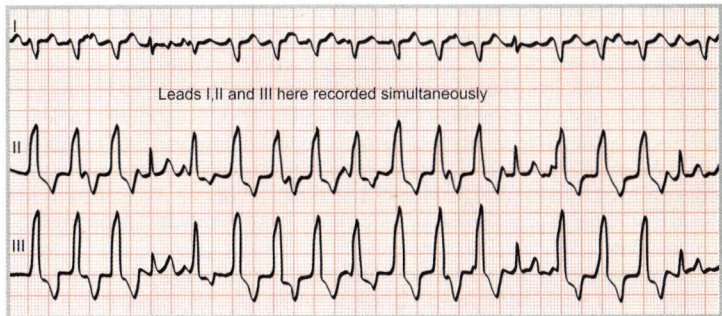

FIGURE 26: An example of accelerated idioventricular rhythm

Given that as stated above, the QRS complexes are likely the result of a ventricular rhythm or a nonventricular rhythm that is not of atrial origin. The next step in sorting out the possibilities is to note if the dominant QRS complexes are unusually wide, specifically 120 msecs or greater. In making this determination, the measurement should take into account the inscription of the QRS in all 12 leads, using the widest inscription found for the dominant QRS. If the QRS is less than 120 msecs, it is quite likely that the rhythm producing the QRS complexes is not of ventricular origin. Thus the likely possibilities become a junctional escape rhythm recognized by its rate of about 60 BPM or less, an accelerated junctional rhythm recognized by its rate of greater than 70 BPM but less than 130 BPM, or the paroxysmal (usually AV nodal using reentrant) supraventricular tachycardia recognized by its rate of about 140 BPM or more. If the QRS duration is 120 msecs or greater, knowledge of the morphology of the QRS complexes prior to the onset of the rhythm disturbance can be critical. If the QRS prior to the onset of a pathological tachycardia happened to be a left bundle branch block and the patient then developed a paroxysmal supraventricular tachycardia, it would be likely that the QRS complexes under this circumstance would be identical to those prior to the tachycardia and thus would simulate a ventricular tachycardia. If the QRS complexes are wide and not identical to those prior to the onset of the rhythm disturbance, the correct diagnosis can usually be made by noting the QRS rate. If the rate is less than 40 BPM, the diagnosis is ventricular escape rhythm. If the rate is about 55–110, the diagnosis is accelerated idioventricular rhythm (Fig. 26). If the rate is above 120 BPM, the diagnosis is ventricular tachycardia.

Having completed the analysis to this point, the next step is to look for unexpected early QRS complexes and to look for unexpected long R-to-R pauses, given that the dominant QRS complexes have been otherwise characterized by regular R-to-R intervals. Except in the presence of interference AV dissociation, unexpected early QRS complexes would represent ectopic premature beats of atrial, junctional or ventricular origin. If the premature complex (whether identical to or different than the dominant QRS complexes in morphology) is preceded by a premature p wave, then it is reasonably to presume that the premature beat is an atrial premature beat, usually associated with a noncompensatory pause (the R-to-R interval encompassing the premature beat being less than the R-to-R interval preceding or following the premature beat). If the premature beat is distinctly different than the prior QRSs and does not have a premature p in front of it, then it is reasonable to presume that the beat is a ventricular premature beat, which will usually produce a fully compensatory pause (the R-to-R interval encompassing the premature beat being essentially twice the R-to-R interval preceding or following the premature beat).

Attention should then turn to identifying any long R-to-R intervals (unexpected pauses) interrupting otherwise regular R-to-R intervals. To define the reason for an unexpectedly long pause, observe what has occurred during the pause. An early p represents a nonconducted atrial premature beat; an on time p represents the appearance of Mobitz I or II second degree AV block and the absence of either a premature p or an on time p represents sinoatrial arrest or sinoatrial block.

One final commentary is necessary with regard to rhythm analysis. This involves the presence of atrial and/or ventricular electronic pacing. Pacing spikes are vertical slashes occurring during the rhythm. What they are pacing is given by the wave that follows them, i.e. an atrial wave for atrial pacing, a QRS for ventricular pacing, or neither if the pacing fails to capture.

❏ CHARACTERIZATION OF QRS COMPLEX

Having characterized the rhythm fully, the next step is to characterize the QRS complexes. However, if the dominant QRS complexes represent a ventricular rhythm (ventricular escape, accelerated idioventricular rhythm or ventricular tachycardia), such an analysis is not reasonable since that QRS has already been deformed by the rhythm and the QRS diagnoses to follow cannot be made with accuracy. Given that the QRS complexes concerned do not represent a ventricular rhythm, e.g. a ventricular escape rhythm, then the clinician can reasonably proceed with the QRS analysis.

Having determined that the QRSs in question are unusually wide, attention should shift to determine if the PR interval is unusually short, usually less than 120 msecs. The absence of any PR segment associated with the wide QRS complexes almost always indicates the diagnosis of the Wolff-Parkinson-White anomaly (preexcitation sydrome) due to the presence of an anomalous or accessory conducting pathway from atrium to ventricle (Fig. 27).

If the QRS is wide, a very practical next step is to look in lead V1. The reason is that this will almost always allow the interpreter to determine if there is a right bundle branch block. This conduction disturbance produces a delayed and prolonged depolarization of the right ventricle causing R waves to be found as the

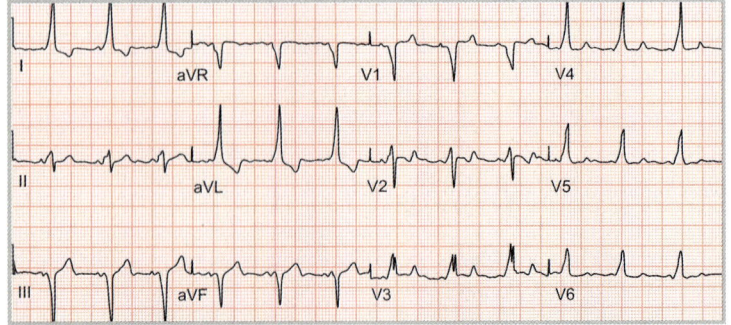

FIGURE 27: An example of accessory pathway

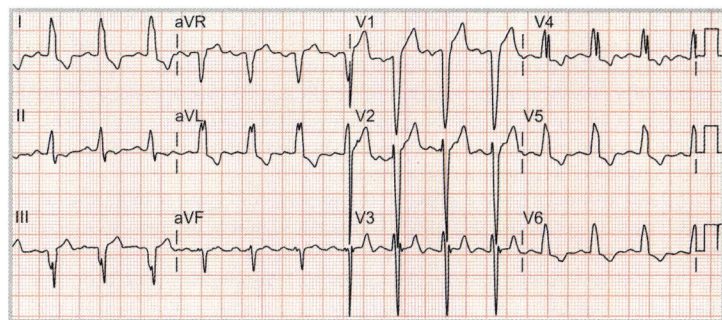

FIGURE 28: An example of left bundle branch block

terminal portion of the QRS with these depolarizing forces directed anteriorly and rightward toward lead V1. It does not matter in this circumstance if the pattern is the traditional rSR' pattern or a qR pattern or even just a tall, although fractured R wave. Having made the diagnosis of right bundle branch block, the interpreter can proceed on to the next two steps, specifically determination of the QRS axis and the search for pathological Q waves indicative of the presence of a myocardial infarction.

If inspection of the EKG does not confirm the presence of a right bundle branch block, but rather shows a tiny r-large S wave or a QS pattern in lead V1, left bundle branch block then needs consideration. Classic left bundle branch block is best confirmed by finding notching or fracturing in the middle of the QRS complex with a QRS duration of at least 120 msecs (Fig. 28). This notching is usually best seen in the leads with tall R waves, although it may be observed in those with deep S waves. Since a left bundle branch block implies a completely distorted activation of the left ventricle, attempting to make other diagnoses, such as left ventricular hypertrophy or myocardial infarction, cannot be done with a great deal of accuracy.

The QRS axis, to be discussed next, is almost always either a normal axis or a left axis. While those with normal versus left axis differ generally in their clinical presentation, the axis itself does not seem to have relevance to the conduction disturbance itself. In very rare instances a left bundle branch block will demonstrate a right axis deviation. The range of the normal mean frontal plane QRS axis is dependent on the age group of the individuals, shifting leftward with increasing age. For adults the normal axis is from about positive 90 degrees up and leftward to minus 30 degrees. Arbitrarily moderate left axis deviation is between minus 30 and minus 45 degrees and marked left axis deviation is from minus 45 to minus 90 degrees. When marked left axis deviation is present (i.e. an axis of minus 45 degrees to minus 90 degrees), a diagnosis of left anterior hemiblock is appropriate. Right axis deviation in adults has been divided into moderated right axis deviation when the axis is from plus 90 to plus 120 degrees and marked right axis deviation when the axis is between plus 120 and plus 180 degrees. When right axis deviation is present, three general considerations should come to mind: (i) right ventricular hypertrophy and/or emphysema, (ii) high lateral myocardial infarction, and (iii) left posterior hemiblock. Often other electrocardiographic features and other clinical information will need to be assessed in order to choose among these three. Technically, the determination of the axis by the electrocardiographer uses the area inscribed the Q, R, and S waves. This is the manner in which the axis is determined by most computer-assisted electrocardiographic interpretations. This works well when the individual deflections in a given lead are of about the same width. However, in the presence of a right bundle branch block, it would be advisable to ignore the contribution of the wide terminal deflection to the QRS when estimating the axis, especially when trying to suggest the additional presence of left anterior or left posterior hemiblock.

Attention should now be given to the presence of Q waves indicative of the presence of a myocardial infarction. Currently, Q waves of equal to or greater than 0.3 s width and equal to or greater than 0.1 mV depth (1 mm depth on the usual electrocardiographic recording) when found in leads I or II or aVF or one of the precordial leads V2 through V6 correlate well with the diagnosis of myocardial infarction. In addition smaller q waves in V2 of 0.02 s duration should be considered abnormal and suggestive of a prior myocardial infarction.

Having completed analysis for the presence of pathological Q waves, attention can turn to the relative amplitudes of the negative and positive QRS deflections in the precordial leads. This starts with an analysis of the relative amplitudes of R waves in lead V1. Reasonable screening criteria for unusually prominent R waves in lead V1 would include an R or R prime that is greater than 0.5 mV (5 mm height) and also is greater than the amplitude of any negative deflection in lead V1. This would reflect unusually prominent anteriorly directed forces which could be explained by addition of electromotive forces anteriorly, i.e. right ventricular hypertrophy or destruction of equivalent forces posteriorly, i.e. a posterior myocardial infarction (in truth probably a posterolateral infarction). The choice between the two possibilities is based on accompanying electrocardiographic features.

If the R or R prime is bigger than 5 mm tall or taller than the depth of any negative wave in V1 but not both the possibilities would be: (i) possibly still a normal variant, (ii) right ventricular hypertrophy, (iii) a posterior infarction, and (iv) a right bundle branch block that is not quite as wide as usual, an "incomplete" right bundle branch block (Flowchart 1). If right axis deviation is present, this would favour either incomplete right bundle branch block or right ventricular hypertrophy. If other evidence of conduction disturbance exists, e.g. Mobitz type 2 second degree AV block, then the former would be favored. If not, right ventricular hypertrophy would be favored.

Observation then proceeds to assessment of unusually deep negative waves in the right precordial leads and unusually tall R waves in lateral leads. Using the voltages recorded in these leads has been used to suggest the presence of left ventricular hypertrophy (Fig. 29). The problem with the electrocardiographic diagnosis of left ventricular hypertrophy based solely on voltage criteria is that the sensitivity of such criteria using precordial leads is only about 50% and about 10–15% of normal people will be labeled as having left ventricular hypertrophy when they do not have it. Using voltage criteria from the limb leads, such as lead I or lead aVL, eliminates much of the inaccuracy related to people without left ventricular hypertrophy but only identifies about 15% of those who do have left ventricular hypertrophy. The presence of the typical ST and T abnormality accompanying left ventricular hypertrophy (called by some a "strain pattern") and found in the tall R wave leads as so beautifully demonstrated by Romhilt and Estes only reduces the false-positives but still leaves the sensitivity at about 50%. Finally, newer imaging modalities, such as magnetic resonance imaging, are now beginning to help sort out the relative values of various voltage criteria. For the time being, using a combined sum of the largest negative wave in V1 or V2 plus

Diagnosis

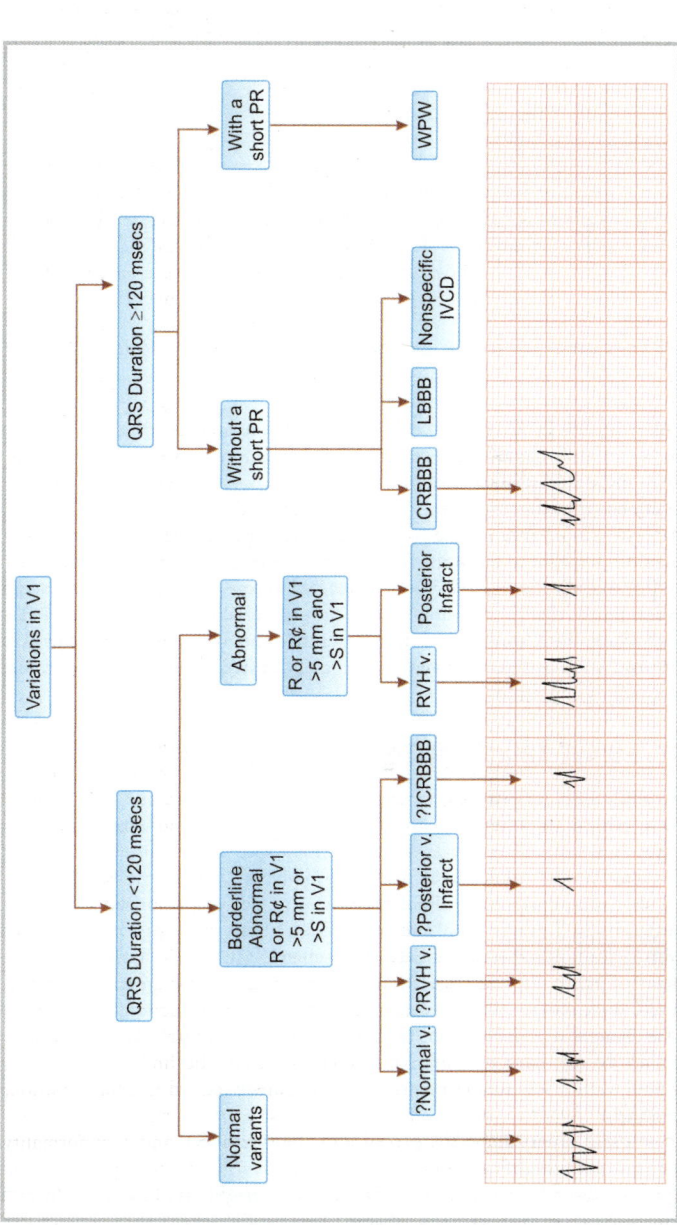

FLOWCHART 1: Variations in V1

(Abbreviations: +: Consider possible; RVH: Right ventricular hypertrophy; ICRBBB: Incomplete right bundle branch block; CRBBB: Complete right bundle branch block; LBBB: Left bundle branch block; IVCD: Intraventricular conduction defect; WPW: Wolff–Parkinson–White anomaly)

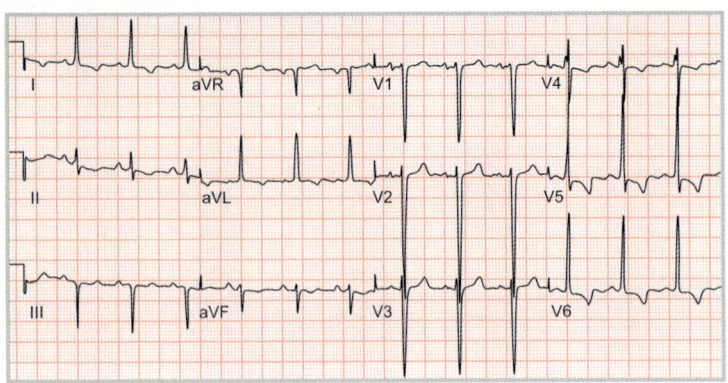

FIGURE 29: An example of left ventricular hypertrophy with secondary repolarization abnormality

the tallest R wave in V5 or V6 of more than 35 mm in an individual over 35 years of age as an electrocardiographic screening to suggest possible left ventricular hypertrophy would seem reasonable.

Completion of the inspection of the precordial leads involves looking for "poor r wave progression" and/or "late precordial transition". Descriptively "poor r wave progression" is meant to mean that there is an unusually small initial r wave in lead V2 and/or that the r wave in V3 is not larger than the r wave in V2. Late precordial transition means that the transition across the precordial leads from right to left to the lead where the R wave has become larger than the S wave has not occurred by at least lead V5. Transition before that in the right precordial leads, including lead V2 is usually a normal finding.

❏ ST–T WAVE ABNORMALITIES

In the adult with no prior electrocardiogram for comparison, the leads that are the most critical are the same leads as suggested for identification of pathological Q waves indicative of a myocardial infarction. Specifically this would exclude leads aVR, III, aVL and V1. Consistently in the adult the T waves in leads I and II should be upright and should be isoelectric or upright in lead aVF. In the precordial leads, T waves should be isoelectric or upright in lead V2 and always upright in leads V3 through V6. In the pediatric age group, inverted T waves extending further leftward than lead V2 are often present. Having identified definite T wave abnormalities always requires clinical correlation without assuming that the changes represent serious cardiac abnormality. Certainly they could reflect a relatively benign condition, such as hyperventilation, following meals in young, conditions such as low serum potassium or the presence of a drug affecting cardiac ion channels.

In general observable ST depressions other than in lead aVR should be considered abnormalities. While many of these ST depressions are quite nonspecific, the ST segments manifesting as a straight line that is horizontal or downsloping in two spatially adjacent leads should suggest serious cardiac ischemia as a highly likely possibility. Standards have been published that state that ST elevations with a J point elevation of equal to or greater than 0.2 mV (2 mm) in men and equal to or greater than 0.15 mV in women in leads V2–

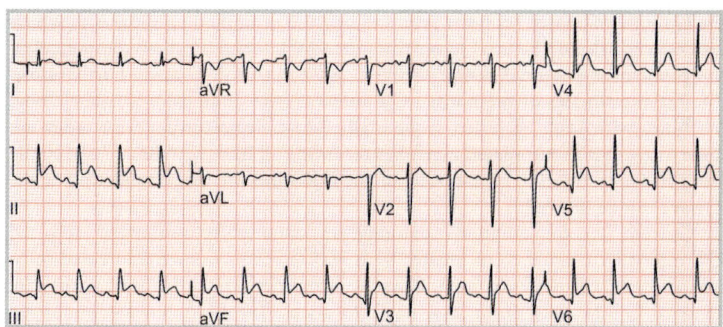

FIGURE 30: An example of acute pericarditis

V3 and equal to or greater than 0.1 in any other two contiguous leads should be considered as indicative of acute myocardial ischemia in the absence of left bundle branch block or left ventricular hypertrophy. Diffuse ST elevations may be defined as ST elevation in leads I, II, aVF, and usually III plus leads V2 through V6. The finding of this diffuse ST elevation should strongly suggest the presence of acute pericarditis (Fig. 30). Nevertheless, for both localized ST elevations and diffuse ST elevations, the overlap with ST elevations representing such normal variants as "early repolarization" is quite real. Prior electrocardiograms are most helpful in making this discrimination. In addition ST elevations that are greater with faster heart rates than those elevations recorded on prior electrocardiograms with slower heart rates favors epicardial injury from pericarditis over early repolarization.

❏ "U" WAVE

U wave is a low amplitude wave of about 0.3 mV (0.3 mm) following the T wave. It is most likely to be observed in leads V2 and V3. Under normal circumstances, it most commonly observed at heart rates of 65 or less and uncommonly with heart rates above. Under these circumstances, it is a normal finding. Its physiologic explanation is still debated. Exaggeration of the amplitude of the U wave may exist by itself without accompanying ST or T wave abnormality. More commonly exaggerated amplitude of the U wave may be associated with ST depression and/or diminished T wave amplitude. In some instances the U wave may fuse with the T wave. Under these circumstances, search for causative factors is critical, including hypokalemia as well as cardioactive and other medications that lead to a prolonged QT interval as well congenital varieties of the long QT syndrome.

❏ QT INTERVAL

QT interval is derived by the measurement from the onset of the QRS complex representing the onset of ventricular depolarization to the end of the T wave representing the latest indication of ventricular repolarization. There are major problems with defining the normal QT interval because of variations on a gender and age basis, because of difficulties in determining the end of the T wave, because of lack of consensus as the best way to correct for the normal variation in the QT interval based on heart rate, and because of unified opinion as to which lead or leads should be used to measure the QT interval. Further compounding the problem is potential fusion of the U wave with the T wave. Furthermore, the initial estimates of the normal QT interval were done using single channel machines with leads recorded sequentially. Most electrocardiograms today are done using digital automated machines recording all leads simultaneously. In the latter instance, the true initial onset of the QRS and the true completion of the T wave can be derived.

Current recommendations defining an abnormally prolonged adjusted QT interval are equal to or greater than 460 msecs in women and equal to or greater than 450 msecs in men. Current recommendation defines a short rate adjusted QT as equal to or less than 390 msecs. The FDA has recommended that rate corrected QT intervals should be subdivided into three severities when considering QT prolonging properties of drugs: greater than 450 msecs, greater than 480 msecs and greater than 500 msecs. Adjustment of the QT interval in situations where the QRS duration is prolonged can be done by using the QT interval minus the QRS duration and applying established standards for this JT interval.

Finally, all QT prolongations generated by computer-assisted automated electrocardiographic machines should be confirmed by visual inspection by the interpreter.

❏ SUGGESTED READINGS

Hancock WE, Deal BJ, Mirvis DM, et al. AHA/ACCF/HRS recommendation and interpretation of the electrocardiogram: Part V: electrocardiogram changes associated with cardiac chamber hypertrophy: a scientific statement from the American Heart Association Electrocardiography and Arrhythmias Committee, Council on Clinical Cardiology; the American College of Cardiology Foundation; and the Heart Rhythm Society: Endorsed by the International Society for Computerized Electrcardiology. Circulation. 2009;119:e251-61.

Rautaharju PM, Surawicz B, Gettes LS. AHA/ACCF/HRS recommendations for the standardization and interpretation of the electrocardiogram: Part IV: the ST segment, T and U waves, and the QT interval: a scientific statement from the American Heart Association Electrocardiography and Arrythmias Committee, Council on Clinical cardiology; the American College of Cardiology Foundation; and the Heart Rhythm Society: Endorsed by the International Society for Computerized Electrocardiology. Circulation. 2009;119:e241-50.

Wagner GS, Macfarlane P, Wellens, et al. AHA/ACCF/HRS recommendations for the standardization and interpretation of the electrocardiogram: Part VI: Acute Ischemia/Infarction: a scientific statement from the American Heart Association Electrcardiography and Arrhythmias Committee, Council on Clinical cardiology; the American College of Cardiology Foundation; and the Heart Rhythm Society: Endorsed by the International Society for Computerized Electrocardiology. Circulation. 2009;119:e262-70.

2.4 ECG Exercise Testing

❑ INTRODUCTION

Exercise testing is a noninvasive tool to evaluate the cardiovascular system's response to exercise under carefully controlled conditions. Exercise is the body's most common physiologic stress, and it places major demands on the cardiopulmonary system. Thus, exercise can be considered the most practical test of cardiac perfusion and function. The exercise test, alone and in combination with other noninvasive modalities, remains an important testing method due to its high yield of diagnostic, prognostic, and functional information.

❑ BEFORE THE TEST

Indications for Exercise Testing (Patient Selection)

The indications for an exercise test according to the guidelines are now presented and will be discussed later.

Exercise Testing for Diagnosis

The ACC/AHA guidelines for the diagnostic use of the standard exercise test have stated that it is appropriate for testing of adult male or female patients (including those with complete right bundle-branch block or with less than one millimeter of resting ST depression) with an *intermediate pretest probability* of coronary artery disease (CAD) based on gender, age, and symptoms (Table 21).

Exercise Testing for Prognosis

Indications for exercise testing to assess risk and prognosis in patients with symptoms or with a prior history of CAD:

Table 21: Pretest probability of coronary artery disease by symptoms, gender, and age					
Age[a]	Gender	Typical/ anginaa[b]	Atypical/ probable angina	Nonanginal chest pain	Asymptomatic
30–39	Men	Intermediate	Intermediate	Low	Very low
	Women	Intermediate	Very low	Very low	Very low
40–49	Men	High	Intermediate	Intermediate	Low
	Women	Intermediate	Low	Very low	Very low
50–59	Men	High	Intermediate	Intermediate	Low
	Women	Intermediate	Intermediate	Low	Very low
60–69	Men	High	Intermediate	Intermediate	Low
	Women	High	Intermediate	Intermediate	Low

[a]There are no data for patients younger than 30 or older than 69, but it can be assumed that the prevalence of CAD is low for those less than 30 years of age and higher for those over 69 years of age.
[b]High = >90%, intermediate = 10–90%, low = <10%, very low = <5%.

Class I (Definitely Appropriate)

Conditions for which there is evidence and/or general agreement that the standard exercise test is useful and helpful to assess risk and prognosis in patients with symptoms or a prior history of CAD who:
- Are undergoing initial evaluation with suspected or known CAD. Specific exceptions are noted below in Class IIb
- Have suspected or known CAD previously evaluated with significant change in clinical status.

Class IIb (May Be Appropriate)

Conditions for which there is conflicting evidence and/or a divergence of opinion that the standard exercise test is useful and helpful to assess risk and prognosis in patients with symptoms or a prior history of CAD but the usefulness/efficacy is less well established.
- Patients who demonstrate the following ECG abnormalities:
    - Preexcitation (Wolff–Parkinson–White) syndrome
    - Electronically paced ventricular rhythm
    - More than one millimeter of resting ST depression
    - Complete left bundle branch block
- Patients with a stable clinical course who undergo periodic monitoring to guide management.

Exercise Testing Patients Presenting with Acute Coronary Syndromes

The CNR Cardiology Research Group in Italy has found that a large body of evidence still supports the use of the exercise ECG as the most cost-effective tool for prognostic purposes as well as for quality of life assessment following ACS. This is consistent with the ACC/AHA guidelines, which state that patients who are pain free, have either a normal or nondiagnostic ECG or one that is unchanged from previous tracings, and have a normal set of initial cardiac enzymes are appropriate candidates for further evaluation with exercise ECG stress testing. If the patient is low risk and does not experience any further ischemic discomfort has a low risk follow-up 12-lead ECG after 6–8 hours of observation, the patient may be considered for an early exercise test. Ideally, this test is performed before discharge and is supervised by an experienced physician.

Exercise Testing Patients with Heart Failure

Traditionally, exercise tests were thought to only be a tool to diagnose coronary disease; however, it is now recognized to have major applications for assessing functional capabilities, therapeutic interventions, and estimating prognosis in heart failure. Numerous hemodynamic abnormalities underlie the reduced exercise capacity commonly observed in chronic heart failure, including:
- Impaired heart rate responses
- Inability to distribute cardiac output normally
- Abnormal arterial vasodilatory capacity
- Abnormal cellular metabolism in skeletal muscle
- Higher than normal systemic vascular resistance
- Higher than normal pulmonary pressures
- Ventilatory abnormalities that increase the work of breathing and cause exertional dyspnea.

Table 22: Benefits of exercise testing post-MI

Predischarge submaximal test
- Optimizing discharge
- Altering medical therapy
- Triaging for intensity of follow-up
- First step in rehabilitation—assurance, encouragement
- Reassuring spouse
- Recognizing exercise-induced ischemia and dysrhythmias

Maximal test for return to normal activities
- Determining limitations
- Prognostication
- Reassuring employers
- Determining level of disability
- Triaging for invasive studies
- Deciding on medications
- Exercise prescription
- Continued rehabilitation

Exercise Testing Patients after Myocardial Infarction

The benefits of performing an exercise test in post-MI patients are listed in Table 22. Evaluation of patients with exercise testing can expedite and optimize their discharge from the hospital. An exercise test prior to discharge is helpful in providing patients with guidelines for exercise at home, reassuring them of their physical status, advising them to resume or increase their activity level, advising them on timing of return to work and in determining the risk of complications.

Exercise testing is also an important tool in exercise training as part of comprehensive cardiac rehabilitation. It can be used to develop and modify an exercise prescription, assist in providing activity counseling and assess the patient's progress by comparing physiologic response at the initiation of the exercise training program to response after weeks or months of training.

Contraindications to Exercise Testing

Table 23 lists some of the absolute and relative contraindications to exercise testing that must be considered prior to prescribing a test for a patient.

❏ METHODOLOGY OF EXERCISE TESTING

Use of proper methodology is critical for patient safety and accurate results. Updated guidelines are available from the AHA/ACC that are based on a multitude of research studies over the last 20 years and have led to greater uniformity in methods.

Safety Precautions and Equipment

The safety precautions outlined in the guidelines are explicit with regard to the requirements for exercise testing. Besides emergency equipment, the safety and accuracy of the testing equipment must be considered. The treadmill should have front and side rails to help subjects steady themselves and should be calibrated monthly.

> **Table 23: Contraindications to exercise testing**
>
> **Absolute**
> - High-risk unstable angina
> - Uncontrolled cardiac arrhythmias causing symptoms or hemodynamic compromise
> - Symptomatic severe aortic stenosis
> - Uncontrolled symptomatic heart failure
> - Acute pulmonary embolus or pulmonary infarction
> - Acute myocarditis or pericarditis
> - Acute aortic dissection
>
> **Relative[a]**
> - Left main coronary stenosis
> - Moderate stenotic valvular heart disease
> - Electrolyte abnormalities
> - Severe arterial hypertension[b]
> - Tachyarrhythmias or bradyarrhythmias
> - Hypertrophic cardiomyopathy and other forms of outflow tract obstruction
> - Mental or physical impairment leading to inability to exercise adequately
> - High-degree atrioventricular block
>
> [a]Relative contraindications can be superseded if the benefits of exercise outweigh the risks.
> [b]In the absence of definitive evidence, the committee suggested systolic blood pressure (SBP) of greater than 200 mm Hg and/or diastolic blood pressure of greater than 110 mm Hg.
> (*Source:* Gibbons, Balady, Bricker, et al.)

Pretest Preparations

When the test is scheduled, the patient should be instructed not to eat, drink or smoke at least 2 hours prior to the test and to come dressed for exercise, including proper footwear. During the pretest evaluation, the patient's usual level of exercise activity should be established to help determine a baseline and an appropriate target workload for testing. The physician should also review the patient's medical history, considering any conditions that can increase the risk of testing. Table 23 lists the absolute and relative contraindications to exercise testing.

The next important methodological issue is when to terminate for safety reasons and these indications are summarized in Table 24.

Exercise Test Modalities

Three types of exercise can be used to stress the cardiovascular system:
- **Isometric:** Isometric exercise, defined as constant muscular contraction without movement (such as handgrip), imposes a disproportionate pressure load on the left ventricle relative to the body's ability to supply oxygen. Isometric exercise is not recommended for routine exercise testing
- **Dynamic:** Dynamic exercise is defined as rhythmic muscular activity resulting in movement, and it initiates a more appropriate increase in cardiac output and oxygen exchange. This chapter considers only dynamic exercise testing, because a delivered workload can be calibrated accurately and the physiologic response measured easily.
- **Combination approach**.

Bicycle Ergometer versus Treadmill

The bicycle ergometer usually costs less, takes up less space, and makes less noise than a treadmill. Although bicycling is a dynamic exercise, most individuals

> **Table 24: Indications for terminating exercise testing**
>
> **Absolute indications**
> - Moderate-to-severe angina
> - Increasing nervous system symptoms (e.g. ataxia, dizziness or near-syncope)
> - Signs of poor perfusion (cyanosis or pallor)
> - Technical difficulties in monitoring ECG or SBP
> - Subject's desire to stop
> - Sustained ventricular tachycardia
> - ST-segment elevation (≥1.0 mm) in leads without diagnostic Q waves (other than V1 or aVR)
>
> **Relative indications**
> - Drop in SBP of ≥10 mm Hg from baseline blood pressure despite an increase in workload in the absence of other evidence of ischemia
> - ST or QRS changes such as excessive ST-segment depression (>2 mm of horizontal or down-sloping ST-segment depression) or marked axis shift
> - Arrhythmias other than sustained ventricular tachycardia, including multifocal PVCs, triplets of PVCs, supraventricular tachycardia, heart block, or bradyarrhythmias
> - Fatigue, shortness of breath, wheezing, leg cramps, or claudication
> - Development of bundle-branch block or intraventricular conduction delay, which cannot be distinguished from ventricular tachycardia
> - Increasing chest pain
> - Hypertensive response[a]
>
> (Abbreviation: PVCs: Premature ventricular contractions)
>
> [a]In the absence of definitive evidence, the committee suggests SBP of >250 mm Hg and/or a diastolic blood pressure of >115 mm Hg.
>
> (*Source:* Gibbons, Balady, Bricker, et al.)

perform more work on a treadmill because a greater muscle mass is involved. These factors create considerable variability in test results, which is reflected in most studies comparing exercise on an upright cycle ergometer versus a treadmill exercise. Specifically, while maximal heart rate values have been demonstrated to be roughly similar, maximal oxygen uptake has been shown to be up to 25% greater during treadmill exercise.

Exercise Protocols

The most common protocols, their stages and the predicted oxygen cost of each stage are illustrated in Figure 31. The exercise protocol should be progressive with even increments in speed and grade whenever possible. Recent guidelines suggest that protocols should be individualized for each subject such that test duration is approximately 8–12 minutes. Because ramp testing uses small and even increments, it permits a more accurate estimation of exercise capacity and can be individualized to yield targeted test duration.

❑ DURING THE TEST

Physiology Review

This would be a good time to do a quick review of some of the basic principles of physiology that are pertinent to understanding the mechanisms behind the body's response to exercise. For brief overviews of the major central and peripheral adaptations that occur from rest to maximal exercise (Figs 32A and B).

Functional class	Clinical status	O_2 cost mL/kg/min	METs	Bicycle ergometer	Treadmill protocols: Bruce (mph)	Bruce (% GR)	Bulke-wate	Ellestad (mph)	Ellestad (%GR)	McHonry (mph)	McHonry (%GR)	Naughton	METs
				1 watt-6 kpds; For 70 kg body weight, kpds	3 min stages		% GT at 3.3 mph 1-min stages	3/2/3 min stagess				2-min stages 3.0 mph %GR	
					5.5	2.0							
Normal and I	Healthy dependent on age, activity	56.0	16		5.0	18	26, 25	6	15			32.5	16
		52.5	15				24, 23					30.0	15
		49.0	14	1500			22, 21	5	15	mph	%GR	27.5	14
		45.5	13		4.2	16	20, 19			3.3	21	25.0	13
		42.0	12	1350			18			3.3	18	22.5	12
		38.5	11	1200			17, 16	5	10	3.3	15	20.0	11
	Sedentary healthy	35.0	10	1050	3.4	14	15					17.5	10
		31.5	9	900			14, 13					15.0	9
		28.0	8				12, 11	4	10	3.3	12	12.5	8
	Limited	24.5	7	750	2.5	12	10	3	10			10.0	7
II	Symptomatic	21.0	6	600			9, 8			3.3	9	7.5	6
		17.5	5	450	1.7	10	7, 6	1.7	10	3.3	6	5.0	5
III		14.0	4	300	1.7	5	5, 4					2.5	4
		10.5	3				3			2.0	3	0.0	3
IV		7.0	2	150	1.7	0	2						2
		3.5	1				1						1

FIGURE 31: The most common protocols, their stages, and the predicted oxygen cost of each stage (Abbreviations: GR: Grade; METs: Metabolic equivalents)

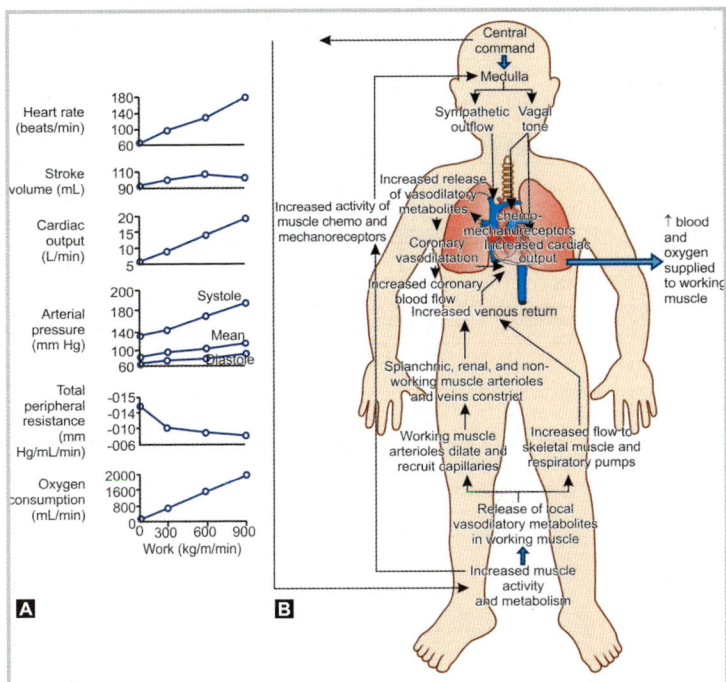

FIGURES 32A AND B: (A) Graphs of the hemodynamic responses to dynamic exercise. (B) Sequence of physiological responses to dynamic exercise (*Source:* Modified from Cardiovascular Physiology at a Glance, Blackwell Publishers, 2004)

Table 25: Two basic principles of exercise physiology	
Myocardial oxygen consumption =	Heart rate × SBP (determinants include wall tension = left ventricular pressure × volume; contractility; and heart rate)
Ventilatory oxygen consumption (VO$_2$) =	External work performed, or cardiac output[a] × A-VO$_2$ difference

(Abbreviations: A-VO$_2$: Arteriovenous oxygen difference; VO$_2$: Volume oxygen consumption; vol%: Volume percent).
[a]The arteriovenous O$_2$ difference is approximately 15–17 vol% at maximal exercise in most individuals; therefore, VO$_{2max}$ generally reflects the extent to which cardiac output increases.

Oxygen Consumption

Two basic principles of exercise physiology are important to understand in regard to exercise testing. The first is a *physiologic* principle: total body oxygen uptake and myocardial oxygen uptake are distinct in their determinants, and in the way, they are measured or estimated (Table 25).

Total body or ventilatory oxygen uptake [volume oxygen consumption (VO$_2$)] is the amount of oxygen extracted from inspired air (Flowcharts 2 and 3). The determinants of VO$_2$ are cardiac output and the peripheral arteriovenous oxygen difference. Maximal arteriovenous difference is physiologically limited to roughly 15–17 mL/dL. Thus maximal arteriovenous difference behaves more or less as a

FLOWCHART 2: Central determinants of maximal oxygen uptake

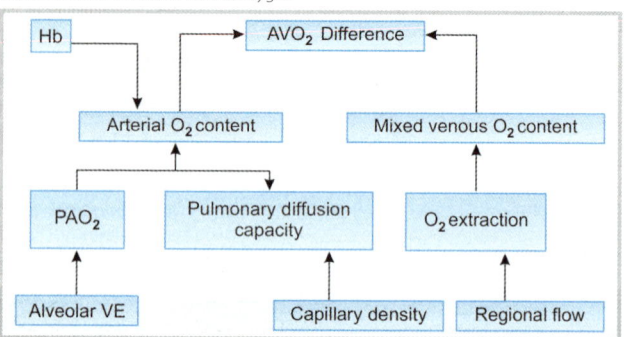

(*Source:* Myers J, Froelicher VF. Hemodynamic determinants of exercise capacity in chronic heart failure. Ann Intern Med. 1991;115:377-86)

FLOWCHART 3: Peripheral determinants of maximal oxygen uptake. The A-VO$_2$ difference is the difference between arterial and venous oxygen

(*Abbreviations:* A-VO$_2$: Arteriovenous oxygen difference; Hb: Hemoglobin; PAO$_2$: Partial pressure of alveolar oxygen; VE: Minute ventilation). (*Source:* Myers J, Froelicher VF. Hemodynamic determinants of exercise capacity in chronic heart failure. Ann Intern Med. 1991;115:377-86)

constant, making maximal oxygen uptake an indirect estimate of maximal cardiac output.

Myocardial oxygen uptake is the amount of oxygen consumed by the heart muscle. The determinants of myocardial oxygen uptake include intramyocardial wall tension (left ventricular pressure and end-diastolic volume), contractility, and heart rate. It has been shown that myocardial oxygen uptake can be estimated by the product of heart rate and SBP, or double product.

Acute Cardiopulmonary Response to Exercise

The intact cardiovascular system responds to acute exercise with a series of adjustments that assure the following (Fig. 32). This response requires a major redistribution of cardiac output along with a number of local metabolic changes. The usual measure of the capacity of the body to deliver and use oxygen is the maximal oxygen consumption (VO$_{2max}$).

The cardiopulmonary limits (VO$_{2max}$) are defined by the following:

- A central component (cardiac output) describes the capacity of the heart to function as a pump
- Peripheral factors (arteriovenous oxygen difference) describe the capacity of the lung to oxygenate the blood delivered to it as well as the capacity of the working muscle to extract this oxygen from the blood.

Central Factors

Heart rate: Sympathetic and parasympathetic nervous system influences are responsible for the cardiovascular system's first response to exercise, which is an increase in heart rate. Vagal withdrawal is responsible for the initial 10–30 beats per minute change, whereas the remainder is thought to be largely caused by increased sympathetic outflow. Of the two major components of cardiac output, heart rate and stroke volume, heart rate is responsible for most of the increase in cardiac output during exercise, particularly at higher levels. Heart rate increases linearly with workload and oxygen uptake.

The heart rate response to exercise is influenced by several factors, and of these, age is the most important factor as a significant decline in maximal heart rate occurs with increasing age.

Stroke volume: It is equal to the difference between end-diastolic and end-systolic volume. Thus, a greater diastolic filling (preload) will increase stroke volume, or factors that increase arterial blood pressure will resist ventricular outflow (afterload) and result in a reduced stroke volume. During exercise, stroke volume increases up to approximately 50–60% of maximal capacity, after which increases in cardiac output are caused by further increases in heart rate. Evidence suggests that this adaptation is caused more by increases in preload, and possibly local adaptations that reduce peripheral vascular resistance, rather than by increases in myocardial contractility. The end-diastolic and end-systolic responses to acute exercise are certainly dependent on presence and type of disease, exercise intensity, and exercise position.

End-systolic volume: It depends on two factors:
- Contractility: It describes the forcefulness of the heart's contraction. Increasing contractility results in a greater stroke volume and thus greater cardiac output. Contractility is commonly quantified by the ejection fraction
- *Afterload:* It is a measure of the force resisting the ejection of blood by the heart. Increased afterload (or aortic pressure, as is observed with chronic hypertension) results in a reduced ejection fraction and increased end-diastolic and end-systolic volumes. During dynamic exercise, the total peripheral resistance is reduced by vasodilation and thus, despite even a fivefold increase in cardiac output among normal subjects during exercise, mean arterial pressure increases only moderately.

Peripheral Factors (Arteriovenous Oxygen Difference)

Oxygen extraction by the tissues during exercise reflects the difference between the oxygen content of the arteries and the veins, yielding a typical arteriovenous oxygen difference (A-VO_2) at rest of 4–6 mL O_2/100 mL. During exercise, this difference widens as the working tissues extract greater amounts of oxygen; venous oxygen content reaches very low levels and A-VO_2 can be as high as 16–18 mL O_2/100 mL with exhaustive exercise. Some oxygenated blood always returns to the heart; however, as smaller amounts of blood continue to flow through, metabolically less active tissues do not fully extract oxygen. The A-VO_2 is generally considered to widen by a relatively *fixed* amount during exercise, and differences in VO_{2max} are predominantly explained by differences in cardiac output.

Determinants of arterial oxygen content: Arterial oxygen content is related to the partial pressure of arterial oxygen, which is determined in the lung by alveolar ventilation and pulmonary diffusion capacity, as well as hemoglobin content of the blood. In the absence of pulmonary disease, arterial oxygen content and saturation are usually normal throughout exercise. Patients with symptomatic pulmonary disease often neither ventilate the alveoli adequately nor diffuse oxygen from the lung into the bloodstream normally, resulting in a decrease in arterial oxygen saturation during exercise.

Determinants of venous oxygen content: Venous oxygen content reflects the capacity to extract oxygen from the blood. Muscle blood flow increases in proportion to increased oxygen requirement, which is determined by increased work rate. The increase in blood flow is brought about not only by the increase in cardiac output but also by a preferential redistribution of the cardiac output to the exercising muscle. Locally produced vasodilatory mechanisms along with possible neurogenic dilatation resulting from higher sympathetic activity reduce local vascular resistance and mediate the greater skeletal muscle blood flow. A marked increase in the number of open capillaries reduces diffusion distances, increases capillary blood volume and increases mean transit time, facilitating oxygen delivery to the muscle.

Autonomic Control

Neural Control Mechanisms

The neural control mechanisms responsible for the cardiovascular response to exercise occur through two processes that initiate and maintain this response:

1. *Central command*: Neural impulses, arising from the central nervous system, recruit motor units, excite medullary and spinal neuronal circuits and cause the cardiovascular changes during exercise.
2. *Muscle afferents*: Muscle contraction stimulates afferent endings within the skeletal muscle, which in turn, reflexively evoke the cardiovascular changes.

Pharmacologic blockade studies have helped elucidate the differential contributions of the two autonomic branches during exercise. Blockade of parasympathetic control with atropine reveals that most of the initial response to exercise, up to a heart rate of 100–120 beats per minute (bpm), is attributable to the withdrawal of tonic vagal activity. Vagal withdrawal induces a rapid increase in heart rate and cardiac output. Conversely, blockade of sympathetic control with propranolol reveals the importance of augmented sympathetic activity during moderate and heavy exercise.

Autonomic Modulation During Immediate Recovery from Exercise

Autonomic physiology during recovery from acute bouts of exercise involves reactivation of the parasympathetic system and deactivation of sympathetic activity. A delay in heart rate recovery has been used as a marker of autonomic dysfunction and/or failure of the cardiovascular system to respond to the normal autonomic responses to exercise. The change in heart rate from peak exercise to minute 1 or 2 of recovery appears to distinguish and prognosticate survival. Early recovery after acute bouts of exercise appears to be dominated by parasympathetic reactivation, with sympathetic withdrawal becoming more important later in recovery.

Hemodynamics

The increased demand for myocardial oxygen required by dynamic exercise is the key to the use of exercise testing as a diagnostic tool for CAD. Myocardial oxygen consumption cannot be directly measured in a practical manner, but its relative demand can be estimated from its determinants, such as heart rate, wall tension (left ventricular pressure and diastolic volume), contractility, and cardiac work.

Heart Rate

Age-predicted maximal heart rate targets are relatively useless for clinical purposes, and they should not be used for exercise testing end-points. It is surprising how much steeper the age-related decline in maximal heart rate is in clinically referred populations as compared with age-matched normal subjects or volunteers.

Exercise Capacity

Exercise capacity is influenced by many factors other than age and gender, including health, activity level, body composition and the exercise mode and protocol used. Exercise capacity should not be reported in total time, rather as the oxygen uptake or MET equivalent of the workload achieved. This method permits the comparison of the results of many different exercise testing protocols.

Blood pressure: The SBP should rise with increasing treadmill workload, whereas diastolic blood pressure usually remains approximately the same or drops.

Possible complications: Most complications can be avoided by measuring blood pressure, monitoring the ECG, questioning the patient about symptoms and levels of fatigue and assessing appearance during the test.

Subjects should be reminded not to grasp the front or side rails because this decreases the work performed and creates noise in the ECG.

To ensure the safety of exercise testing, the following list of the most dangerous circumstances in the exercise testing laboratory should be recognized:

- An ST-segment elevation (without baseline diagnostic Q waves) can be associated with dangerous arrhythmias and infarction and usually occurs in V_2 or aVF rather than V_5
- When a patient with an ischemic cardiomyopathy exhibits severe chest pain due to ischemia (angina pectoris), a cool down walk is advisable
- When a patient develops exertional hypotension accompanied by ischemia (angina or ST-segment depression) or when it occurs in a patient with a history of congestive heart failure (CHF), cardiomyopathy or recent myocardial infarction (MI), safety is a serious issue

Recovery after Exercise

For maximal sensitivity, patients should return to a supine as soon as possible during the post-exercise period. It is advisable to record approximately 10 seconds of ECG data while the patient is standing motionless but still at near-maximal heart rate and then have the patient lie down. Having the patient perform a cool-down walk after the test can delay or eliminate the appearance of ST-segment.

Monitoring should continue for at least 5 minutes after exercise or until changes stabilize. An abnormal response occurring only in the recovery period is neither unusual nor necessarily suggestive of a false-positive result. The third minute is critical for ST analysis. Noise should not be a problem, and ST depression at that time has important implications regarding the presence and severity of CAD.

Diagnostic Scores

Studies considering non-ECG data consistently demonstrate that the multivariable equations outperform simple ST diagnostic criteria. These equations generally provide a predictive accuracy of 80% (ROC area of 0.80). To obtain the best diagnostic characteristics with the exercise test, clinical and non-ECG test responses should be considered. We have validated simple scores for both men and women.

❏ AFTER THE TEST

ECG Interpretation: Factors Determining Prognosis

ST-segment Analysis

ST-segment depression represents global subendocardial ischemia, with a direction determined largely by the placement of the heart in the chest. ST depression does not localize coronary artery lesions. ST depression in the inferior leads is most often caused by the atrial repolarization wave, which begins in the PR segment and can often extend into the beginning of the ST-segment. Severe transmural ischemia, resulting in wall motion abnormalities, causes a shift of the vector in the direction of the wall motion abnormality. Preexisting areas of wall motion abnormality (i.e. scar), however, usually indicated by a Q wave are also capable of causing such shifts resulting in ST elevation without the presence of ischemia. While the resting ECG exhibits Q waves from an old MI, ST elevations are caused by ischemia, wall-motion abnormalities, or both, whereas accompanying ST depression can be caused by a second area of ischemia or reciprocal changes. When the resting ECG is normal, however, ST elevation is a result of severe ischemia (spasm or a critical lesion), although accompanying ST depression is reciprocal. Exercise-induced ST depression loses its diagnostic power in patients with left bundle-branch block, Wolff–Parkinson–White (WPW) syndrome, electronic pacemakers, intraventricular conduction defects (IVCDs) with inverted T waves and in patients with more than 1 mm of resting ST depression. ST-segment changes isolated to the inferior leads are more likely to be false-positive responses unless profound (i.e. >1 mm). The various patterns of ST-segment changes are illustrated in Figures 33A and B.

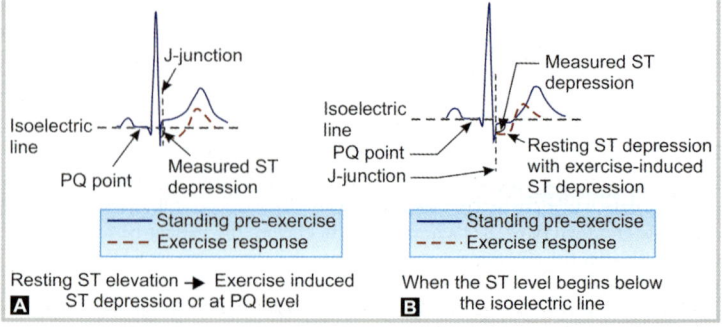

FIGURES 33A AND B: The various patterns of ST-segment shift. The standard criterion for abnormal is 1 mm of horizontal or downsloping ST-segment depression below the PR isoelectric line or 1 mm further depression, if there is baseline depression

Precordial lead V_5 alone consistently outperforms the inferior leads or the combination of leads V_5 with II, because lead II has been shown to have a high false-positive rate. Exercise-induced ST-segment depression in inferior limb leads is a poor marker for CAD in and of itself. In patients without prior MI and normal resting electrocardiograms, ST depression in precordial lead V_5 along with V_4 and V_6 are reliable markers for CAD, and the monitoring of inferior limb leads adds little additional diagnostic information. This said, however, elevation inferiorly should not be ignored.

Exercise-induced Arrhythmias

As with resting ventricular arrhythmias, exercise-induced ventricular arrhythmias have an independent association with death in most patients with coronary disease and in asymptomatic individuals. The risk can be more delayed (> 6 years) than that associated with ST depression. Nonsustained ventricular tachycardia is uncommon during routine clinical treadmill testing but is usually well-tolerated if exhibited. When healthy individuals exhibit premature ventricular contractions (PVCs) during testing, there is no need for immediate concern.

Prognostic Utilization of Exercise Testing

The two principal reasons for estimating prognosis are to:
- Provide accurate answers to patients' questions regarding the probable outcome of their illnesses
- Identify those patients in whom interventions might improve outcome and which measures to take to achieve such benefits.

Exercise capacity is the primary predictor of prognosis in all categories of patients. With each decrease in the MET value achieved there is a 10–20% increase in overall mortality. Exercise capacity interacts with age such that even after accounting for age and gender, exercise capacity is a weaker predictor of death in elderly individuals than younger individuals undergoing exercise stress testing.

There are ample data supporting the use of exercise testing as the first noninvasive step after the history, physical examination and resting ECG in the prognostic evaluation of CAD patients. It accomplishes both the purposes of prognostic testing to provide information regarding the patient's status and to help make recommendations for optimal management. This assessment should always include calculation of a properly designed score such as the Duke Treadmill Score or the VA Treadmill Score (Table 26). Recently, we have added to the Duke nomogram to improve its prognostic value (Fig. 34).

In summary, VO_{2max} or other related measures should not be used as the only prognostic markers in heart failure. The combination of cardiopulmonary exercise data and other clinical and hemodynamic responses in multivariate scores has been shown to more powerfully stratify risk.

Table 26: Prognostic scores: the Duke Treadmill Score and the VA Treadmill score
Duke score = METs – 5 × (mm E-I ST depression) – 4 × (TMAP index)
VA score = 5 × (CHF/Dig) + mm E-I ST depression + change in SBP score – METs
(Abbreviations: CHF: Congestive heart failure; METs: Metabolic equivalents; SBP: Systolic blood pressure; TMAP: Treadmill angina pectoris).
TMAP score: 0 if no angina, 1 if angina occurred during test, 2 if angina was the reason for stopping.
Change in SBP score: from 0 for rise greater than 40 mm Hg to 5 for drop below rest.

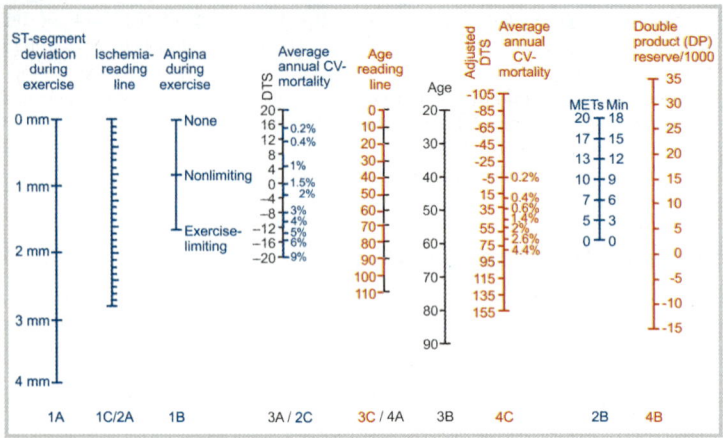

FIGURE 34: Age and double product (DP) adjusted Duke Treadmill Score (DTS) nomogram. Determination of average annual CV mortality adjusted for age and DP reserve proceeds as follows: at first, DTS will be obtained as described before; briefly, the marks for the observed amount of exercise-induced ST-segment deviation (1A) and degree of angina (1B) on their respective lines are connected with a straight edge. The point where this line intersects the ischemia-reading line (1C) is noted. Then, the mark for ischemia (2A) is connected with that for exercise duration in minutes or the equivalent in METs (2B). The point at which this line intersects the DTS line indicates the amount of DTS and the average annual CV mortality (2C). Subsequently, the point at which the drawing line from the marks for DTS (3A) to the corresponding value for age (3B) intersects age—DTS line indicates average annual CV mortality adjusted for age (3C). Finally, the point where the modified DTS line intersects the line drawn from the age—DTS line (4A) to the corresponding value for DP reserve/1,000 (4B) indicates average annual CV mortality adjusted for age and DP reserve (4C) (*Source:* Modified from Sadrzadeh Rafie AH, et al. Age and double product (SBP x heart rate) reserve-adjusted modification of the Duke Treadmill Score nomogram in men. Am J Cardiol. 2008;102:1407-12

❏ SCREENING

Screening for asymptomatic CAD has become a topic of increased interest as some recent data suggest efficacy of the statins in reducing the risk of cardiac events even in asymptomatic individuals. Global risk factor equations, such as the Framingham score, should be the first step in screening asymptomatic individuals for preclinical coronary. These are available as nomograms that can easily applied by healthcare professionals, or be calculated as part of a computerized patient record. Several additional testing procedures that have promise for screening include the simple ankle-brachial index (particularly in the elderly), C-reactive protein and other emerging biomarkers, carotid ultrasound measurements of intimal medial thickness, and the resting ECG (particularly spatial QRS-T wave angle).

❏ CONCLUSION

The exercise test complements the medical history and the physical examination, and it remains the second most commonly performed cardiologic procedure next to the routine ECG. The addition of echocardiography or myocardial perfusion imaging does not negate the importance of the ECG or clinical and hemodynamic responses to exercise. The renewed efforts to control costs undoubtedly will support

Table 27: Exercise testing rules to maximize information obtained

- The exercise protocol should be progressive, with even increments in speed and grade whenever possible
- The treadmill protocol should be adjusted to the patient, and one protocol is not appropriate for all patients; consider using a manual or automated ramp protocol
- Report exercise capacity in METs, not minutes of exercise
- Hyperventilation prior to testing is not indicated
- ST-segment measurements should be made at ST0 (J-junction), and ST-segment depression should be considered abnormal only if horizontal or downsloping
- Raw ECG waveforms should be considered first and then supplemented by computer-enhanced (filtered and averaged) waveforms when the raw data are acceptable
- In testing for diagnostic purposes, patients should be placed supine as soon as possible after exercise, with a cool-down walk avoided
- The 3-minutes recovery period is critical to include in analysis of the ST-segment response
- Measurement of SBP during exercise is extremely important and exertional hypotension is ominous; manual blood pressure measurement techniques are preferred
- Age-predicted heart rate targets are largely useless due to the wide scatter for any age; exercise tests should be symptom limited
- A treadmill score should be calculated for every patient; use of multiple scores or a computerized consensus score should be considered as part of the treadmill report

(Abbreviaition: METs: Metabolic equivalents).

the role of the exercise test. Convincing evidence that treadmill scores enhance the diagnostic and prognostic power of the exercise test certainly has cost-efficacy implications. Use of proper methodology is paramount for safety and obtaining accurate and comparable results. The use of specific criteria for exclusion and termination, interaction with the subject and appropriate emergency equipment is essential. Table 27 lists important rules to follow for getting the most information from the standard exercise test.

The ACC/AHA guidelines for exercise testing clearly indicate the correct uses of exercise testing. Since the last guidelines, exercise testing has been extended as the first diagnostic test in women and in individuals with right bundle-branch block and resting ST-segment depression. The use of diagnostic scores and prognostic scores, such as the Duke Treadmill score, increases the value of the exercise test. In fact, the use of scores results in test characteristics that approach the nuclear and echocardiographic add-ons to the exercise test.

MODIFIED SUMMARY OF GUIDELINES
AAA/AHA 2002 Guideline Update for Exercise Testing: Summary Article:
A Report of the American College of Cardiology/American Heart Association Task Force on Practice Guidelines
(Committee to Update the 1997 Exercise Testing Guidelines)
Circulation 2002;106:1883–92

Modified by Kanu Chatterjee

Class I: Conditions for which there is evidence and/or general agreement that a given procedure/therapy is useful and effective.

Class II: Conditions for which there is conflicting evidence and/or a divergence of opinion about the usefulness/efficacy of performing the procedure/therapy.

Class IIa: Weight of evidence/opinion is in favor of usefulness/efficacy.

Class IIb: Usefulness/efficacy is less well established by evidence/opinion.

Class III: Conditions for which there is evidence and/or general agreement that a procedure/therapy is not useful/effective and in some cases may be harmful.

Level A (highest): Derived from multiple randomized clinical trials.

Level B (intermediate): Data are on the basis of a limited number of randomized trials, nonrandomized studies or observational registries.

Level C (lowest): Primary basis for the recommendation was expert opinion.

Exercise Testing Guideline Recommendation

Class I:
1. Patients undergoing initial evaluation with suspected or known CAD including patients with complete right bundle-branch block or less that 1 mm ST depression (Level of Evidence B).
2. Patients with known or suspected CAD previously evaluated presenting with new or changing symptoms (Level of Evidence B).
3. Low-risk unstable angina patients (Level of Evidence B).
4. Intermediate-risk unstable angina patients 2–3 days after presentation and without evidence active ischemia or heart failure (Level of Evidence B).

Class IIa: Intermediate-risk unstable angina patients with negative cardiac markers and without significant change in ECG (Level of Evidence B).

Class IIb:
1. Patients with ECG abnormalities of preexcitation, electronically paced ventricular rhythm, 1 mm or more resting ST depression, patients with LBBB or QRS duration of >120 ms.
2. Patients with a stable clinical course who undergo periodic monitoring to guide treatment (Level of Evidence B).

Class III:
1. Patients with severe comorbidity likely to limit the expectancy and/or candidacy for revascularization.
2. High-risk unstable angina patients (Level of Evidence C).

Patients with Acute Coronary Syndrome

Class I:
1. Submaximal exercise at about 4–6 days before discharge for assessment of prognosis, activity prescription or for evaluation of medical therapy.
2. Symptom limited exercise test about 14–21 days after discharge for assessment of prognosis, activity prescription, or evaluation medical therapy if predischarge exercise test has not been done.
3. Symptom limited exercise test at 3–6 weeks after discharge to assess prognosis, activity prescription or evaluation of medical therapy if early exercise test was submaximal.

Class IIa: After discharge for activity counseling and/or exercise training as part of cardiac rehabilitation in patients who have undergone reavascularization.

Class IIb:
1. In patients with ECG abnormalities of LBBB, preexcitation syndrome, left ventricular hypertrophy, digoxin therapy, greater than 1 mm resting ST depression electronically paced ventricular rhythm.
2. Periodic monitoring in patients who continue to participate in exercise training or cardiac rehabilitation.

Class III:
1. Severe comorbidity likely to limit life expectancy and/or candidacy for revascularization.
2. To evaluate patients with acute myocardial infarction with uncompensated heart failure, cardiac arrythmia or noncardiac conditions that limit the ability to exercise (Level of Evidence C).
3. Predischarge exercise test in patients who had already cardiac catheterization (Level of Evidence C).

Asymptomatic Diabetic Patients

Class IIa: Evaluation of asymptomatic patients with diabetes who plan to do vigorous exercise.
(Level of Evidence C)

Class IIb:
1. Evaluation of patients with multiple risk factors as guide to risk-reduction therapy
2. Evaluation of asymptomatic men older than 45 years or women older than 55 years who plan to do vigorous exercise or who are involved in an occupation in which exercise impairment may impact public safety or who are at high risk for CAD.

Class III: Routine screening of asymptomatic men or women.

Patients with Valvular Heart Disease

Class I: In patients with chronic aortic regurgitation for assessment of symptoms and functional capacity in whom it is difficult assess symptoms.

Class IIa:
1. In patients with chronic aortic regurgitation for evaluation of symptoms and functional capacity before participation in athletic activity.
2. In patients with chronic aortic regurgitation for assessment of prognosis before aortic valve replacement in asymptomatic or minimally symptomatic patients with left ventricular dysfunction.

Class IIb: Evaluation of patients with valvular heart disease (see guidelines in valvular heart disease).

Class III: For diagnosis of CAD in patients with moderate to severe valvular heart disease or with LBBB, electronically paced rhythm, preexcitation syndrome or greater than 1 mm ST depression in the rest ECG.

Patients with Rhythm Disorders

Class I:
1. For identification of appropriate settings in patients with rate-adaptive pacemakers
2. For evaluation of congenital complete heart block in patients considering increased physical activity or participation in competitive sports (Level of Evidence C).

Class IIa:
1. Evaluation of patients with known or suspected exercise-induced arrhythmias
2. Evaluation medical, surgical or ablation therapy in patients with exercise-induced arrhythmias (including atrial fibrillation).

Class IIb:
1. Investigation of isolated ventricular ectopic beats in middle aged patients without other evidence of CAD.
2. For investigation of prolonged first degree atrioventricular block or type I second degree Wenckebach, left bundle-branch block, right bundle-branch block or isolated ectopic beats in young persons considering participation in competitive sports (Level of Evidence C).

Class III: Routine investigations of isolated ectopic beats in young patients.

❏ SUGGESTED READINGS

American College of Sports Medicine. Guidelines for Exercise Testing and Prescription, 6th edition. Baltimore: Lippincott, Williams and Wilkins; 2000.

COCATS Guidelines. Guidelines for Training in Adult Cardiovascular Medicine, Core Cardiology Training Symposium. June 27- 28, 1994. American College of Cardiology. J Am Coll Cardiol. 1995;25:1-34.

Fletcher GF, et al. Exercise standards for testing and training: A statement for healthcare professionals from the American Heart Association. Circulation. 2001;104:1694-740.

Gibbons RJ, et al. ACC/AHA 2002 guideline update for exercise testing: summary article: a report of the American College of Cardiology/American Heart Association Task Force on Practice Guidelines (Committee to Update the 1997 Exercise Testing Guidelines). Circulation. 2002;106:1883-92.

Rafie AH, et al. Age-adjusted modification of the Duke Treadmill Score nomogram. Am Heart J. 2008;155:1033-8.

Schlant RC, Friesinger GC 2nd, Leonard JJ. Clinical competence in exercise testing. A statement for physicians from the ACP/ACC/AHA Task Force on Clinical Privileges in Cardiology. J Am Coll Cardiol. 1990;16:1061-5.

2.5 Left Ventricle

❏ INTRODUCTION

Echocardiography is the most commonly used clinical diagnostic tool for the evaluation of left ventricular (LV) systolic and diastolic function. In addition to measuring LV ejection fraction (EF), echocardiography provides clinically useful information about various aspects of LV structure and function. For instance, the anatomy of the LV may be altered in several pathologically significant ways and can be accurately measured and expressed by measuring cross-sectional segments of the LV from sets of echocardiographic images.

❏ SYSTOLIC FUNCTION

The reliable, precise, cost-effective and expeditious characterization of regional and global systolic LV function is best accomplished by echocardiography. Quantitative expressions of global LV function may be obtained directly by calculation of left ventricular ejection fraction (LVEF) from its components, end-systolic volume (ESV) and end-diastolic volume (EDV), by determination of rate of pressure rise in the left ventricle from spectral Doppler flow signals, by low velocity tissue Doppler signals from annular and myocardial motion and by determination of global strain and strain rate using either tissue Doppler or speckle tracking. An initial impression of LV systolic function may be accomplished by visual evaluation of LV contraction. The standard views from the apical and parasternal windows are sufficient for this purpose. One usually starts with parasternal long- and short-axis views of the LV. From the apical window, the LV should be examined in standard 4-chamber, 2-chamber and long axis views. The LV may also be evaluated from the subcostal window in both short- and long-axis views.

Left Ventricular Ejection Fraction

The most commonly applied measure of the global LV systolic function in the clinical setting is the EF of the left ventricle (LVEF), or the fraction of the LV diastolic volume ejected with each contraction. There are a number of reasons for the universality of LVEF: it expresses the complex motion of a three-dimensional (3D) structure with a simple number; it is easy to measure or estimate; it is interchangeable when determined by different methods; it parallels LV contractility; its prognostic significance and clinical utility for treatment stratification are considered established. to the point where they will be automated.

It is recommended calculation of LV volumes should be dome in all patients both for their own inherent value and as the sole means of calculating EF. There are several reasons for this recommendation:

- When performed properly from technically adequate images, quantitatively acquired volume and EF are more accurate than the visual estimation and the gap in accuracy continues to widen with improvement of imaging techniques
- Quantitation provides additional valuable informations—LV volume and mass—which are superior in outcome prediction to linear dimensions
- Continuous feedback to the echocardiographer allows maintenance of skill in visual estimation of LV global function; the ability of the physician to perform accurate visual estimation further increases the reliability of calculations, allowing the reader to identify those studies, in which calculations were performed poorly, and repeat or correct those measurements. In the final analysis, visual estimation, however skillful the observer, is less reliable than quantification by a skilled sonographer.

Linear Measurements in the Assessment of LV Function

Linear dimensions (so-called m-mode) should be performed under 2D guidance, and only if the beam can be directed perpendicular to the transected LV walls and cavity long axis. The use of linear dimensions may lead to two types of errors: the first is from the incorrect positioning of the ultrasound beam that may be corrected by meticulous use of 2D echo guidance. The second is that linear dimensions sample only a limited area near the LV base; assumptions regarding the geometric shape and symmetry of the left ventricle must be made to derive indices of global LV function.

The derived functional indices from single dimensional measurements include: fractional shortening of the left ventricle, E-point to septal separation (EPSS), and the amplitude of the aortic root motion.

Components of Ejection Fraction

End-systolic Volume

Left ventricular end-systolic volume indexed (ESVI) to BSA is a simple yet powerful stand-alone marker of ventricular remodeling that can and should be measured routinely in the clinical practice of echocardiography. The authors recommend first considering ESVI when judging systolic function.

Left Ventricular End-systolic Volume and Clinical Outcomes

A decrease in ESV with angiotensin-converting enzyme inhibitor therapy has been associated with a reduction in cardiac events in patients with moderately decreased LV systolic function. Using LV contrast ventriculography, end-systolic volume has been shown to be an important predictor of both postoperative ventricular function and survival after coronary artery bypass grafting in patients with decreased LV function. The aforementioned studies have consistently shown that large increases in ESV predict adverse cardiovascular outcomes in participants with LV systolic dysfunction.

End-diastolic Volume

End-diastole is the moment in the cardiac cycle when the left ventricle completes filling and reaches its largest volume. A healthy heart has the property of increasing diastolic volume in response to a spectrum of preloads without altering its elliptical shape and with only small increases in filling pressure. In normality, ESV changes are small so that changes in stroke volume are mainly mediated by increases in EDV. Due to relative preload dependence, EDV changes and degrees of enlargement are less reliable indicators of myocardial contractility.

❑ CONTRAST-ENHANCED ECHOCARDIOGRAPHY

Suboptimal endocardial border definition limits the accurate measurement of LV volumes by echocardiography. Endocardial border definition is particularly challenging in the setting of obesity, chronic lung disease, ventilator support and chest wall deformities. Contrast echocardiography, by increasing the mismatch between the acoustic impedance of blood and that of myocardium enhances the discrimination between myocardial tissue and the blood pool and improves the accuracy of echocardiography to quantitate LV volumes. These advantages are particularly apparent in large spherical hearts in which the lateral and anterior walls are situated in the portion of the image with the poorest resolution. In the authors' experience, sonographers are likely to foreshorten the image of a spherically dilated ventricle in order to image the lateral wall and confuse trabeculations along the lateral wall with the true endocardium. The 2008 ASE consensus statement recommends the use of contrast agents in difficult-to-image patients with reduced image quality, where greater than or equal to 2 contiguous segments are not seen on unenhanced images and in patients requiring accurate quantification of LVEF regardless of image quality, with the intention of increasing the confidence of the interpreting physician in assessing LV volumes and systolic function.

❑ OTHER ECHO-DERIVED INDICES OF LEFT VENTRICULAR SYSTOLIC FUNCTION

Left ventricular stroke volume is routinely calculated by multiplication of the velocity-time integral (VTI) of the pulsed wave Doppler flow signal from the LVOT, by the crosssectional area of the LVOT calculated from its radius [Area = pi × (radius)2]. VTI of forward blood flow is the length of the column of blood in centimeter, passing through the LVOT during systole. Multiplication of this value by the crosssectional area, through which this column is moving, provides an expression of stroke volume. The product of stroke volume and heart rate is cardiac output in l/min. Since the size of the LVOT is usually a function of BSA, in our practice, the authors prefer to use VTI and minute distance (VTI × heart rate) as analogs of stroke volume. Normal VTI from LVOT pulsed wave Doppler is between 18 cm and 23 cm and normal minute distance between 10 m/min and 20 m/min. Another index of global LV systolic function is the velocity of pressure increase in the left ventricle at the initial part of ejection period (dP/dt).

❏ STRAIN-DERIVED INDICES

In echocardiography parlance, strain is defined as myocardial deformation relative to its baseline dimension due to a stress. The rate of deformation over time is termed strain rate. Both strain and strain rates can be measured using tissue pulsed Doppler and speckle tracking. The former technique uses gated tissue Doppler to compare the myocardial motion of two points, usually 1 cm apart, along a single beam of interrogation; this method is angle dependent. The newer strain measurement technique that uses the grayscale speckle pattern of myocardial images is angle-independent. Strain and strain rate can be used to evaluate both regional and global LV systolic and diastolic function. Moreover, these deformation indices can quantify myocardial function in various planes, including longitudinal, circumferential and radial. These measures may be useful in determining early systolic dysfunction (regional and global) in the setting of normal EF.

❏ RECOGNIZING THE ETIOLOGY OF CARDIAC DYSFUNCTION

According to the report of the World Health Organization/International Society and Federation of Cardiology Task Force on the definition and classification of cardiomyopathies, there are five major types of cardiomyopathy (i.e. diseases of the myocardium associated with cardiac dysfunction) that can be appreciated by echocardiography. These conditions can affect either ventricle, but are most often recognized when they involve the left chamber.
1. Dilated cardiomyopathy arising as primary myocardial disease of unknown etiology or as disorders of ischemic, toxic, familial or infective origin.
2. Hypertrophic cardiomyopathy, arising as a primary condition or secondary process to conditions, such as aortic stenosis or hypertension.
3. Restrictive or infiltrative cardiomyopathies, such as cardiacamyloidosis.
4. Arrhythmogenic right ventricular dysplasia or cardiomyopathy (not discussed here).
5. Unclassified cardiomyopathy including endomyocardial fibroelastosis and ventricular noncompaction.

❏ VISUAL QUALITATIVE INDICATORS OF SYSTOLIC DYSFUNCTION

Earlier in this chapter the authors discussed their recommendations concerning the visual estimation of EF. Foremost among these was that visual estimation be used as confirmatory evidence of quantitation rather than for primary evaluation. The authors believe that among the more useful qualitative findings associated with all stages of systolic dysfunction are *sphericity* and *descent of the cardiac base*.

The shape of the healthy left ventricle is elliptical and the ratio of its long axis to its short axis is approximately 2:1. In decompensated states, particularly those with volume overload, its shape becomes spherical with the ratio of the axes approaching unity (1:1). Although this ratio has been correlated with EF, the concept of sphericity is most useful when appreciated visually.

Left Ventricular Mass

Left ventricular hypertrophy is universal as an early compensatory change in LV disease and is commonly encountered in patients with ischemic heart disease, congestive HF and advanced age. Concentric LVH, in which LV mass is increased with preserved size and function, may occur in response to chronically increased afterload. Eccentric LVH is seen with ventricular remodeling and chamber enlargement in response to acute or progressive decline in systolic function and typically accompanies a dilated cardiomyopathy.

The wall thickness of the LV has long been an informative m-mode echocardiographic measurement. Taken by itself, the linear thickness of the septum or of the posterior wall, or both, has been used as an index of LVH (>1.1 cm). The ratio of posterior wall thickness to septal thickness is used as an index of asymmetric hypertrophy (>1.3:1). As in the case of LV cavitary dimension, many laboratories use the simple linear measurement of wall thickness to assess LV mass indirectly and some extrapolate LV mass indirectly by an algorithm that extrapolates wall thickness from linear dimensions of opposing walls and subtended cavity.

❏ DIASTOLIC FUNCTION

Echocardiography allows detailed investigation and integration of the complex array of flow related events that occur during LV filling. Whereas systolic function or the process of ejection is known as *inotropy*, diastolic function or the process of filling is termed *lusitropy*.

Echocardiographic analysis of the diastolic function of the left ventricle is based on multiple parameters, including pulsed wave Doppler of the transmitral flow, flow patterns in the pulmonary veins, flow propagation velocity by color m-mode of the LV inflow tract and tissue Doppler studies of motion of the LV base in diastole. In addition, left atrial volume provides a measure of the chronicity of abnormal LV filling conditions.

Types of Diastolic Dysfunction

Abnormalities of diastolic function exist along a continuum, which, based on echocardiographic parameters, may be categorized into four relatively distinct types: (i) impaired relaxation of the left ventricle (type 1 diastolic dysfunction), (ii) pseudonormal filling (type 2 diastolic dysfunction), (iii) restrictive filling (type 3 diastolic dysfunction) that is reversible with Valsalva maneuver, and (iv) type 4 diastolic dysfunctionrestrictive pattern that is irreversible with Valsalva maneuver. Figure 35 shows the mitral inflow at rest and its response to Valsalva in the subgroups of diastolic dysfunction. Pulmonary vein and DTI patterns are also depicted for each of the subgroups.

Impaired Relaxation of the Left Ventricle

The initial stage of LV diastolic dysfunction is manifest by impaired or slowed relaxation of the left ventricle (type 1 diastolic dysfunction). It is characterized by slowing of the energy-consuming process governing ventricular relaxation; the filling pressures usually remain normal, with brief elevation at the end of diastole at the time of atrial contraction. Because the elevation of the presystolic a wave at end diastole is brief, the mean diastolic pressure remains low. However, when tachycardia intervenes, diastole shortens and the contribution of the A wave to mean diastolic pressure increases; in many patients, exercise intolerance results. Furthermore, patients with type 1 dysfunction may be intolerant to atrial fibrillation because the loss of atrial contraction causes left atrial pressure to rise in compensation for the loss of 60% of filling volume by active transport and refilling atrium with an equal amount through the suction of active relaxation. Delayed relaxation can be recognized by examination of mitral inflow where the ratio of the E and A waves

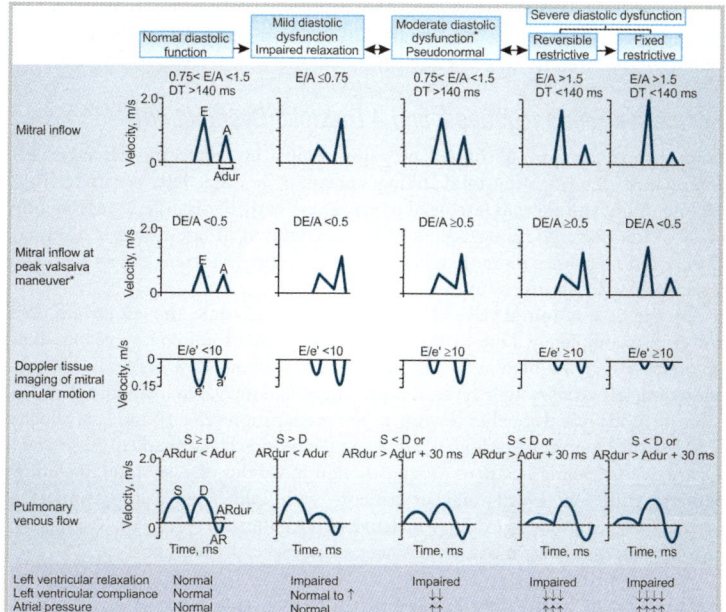

FIGURE 35: Types of transmitral flow (upper row) and corresponding types of tissue Doppler interrogation of the mitral annular motion (lower row). Sample volume is placed on the interventricular septal part of the mitral annulus from the apical 4-chamber view. Tissue Doppler recording allows discrimination of normal and pseudonormal flow. (Abbreviations: A: Transmitral flow during atrial systole; Am: Mitral annular motion during atrial systole; E: Early diastolic transmitral flow; Em: Early diastolic motion of the mitral annulus)

is less than 1, IVRT is prolonged and deceleration time (pre-A wave deceleration of inflow) (DT) lengthened. Pulmonary venous flow demonstrates pronounced systolic dominance associated with augmented atrial relaxation and decreased VTI of the diastolic wave, and slowed propagation velocity (Vp). The Em velocity on the tissue Doppler recording of mitral annular motion is also reduced. This filling pattern is consistent with essentially normal mean LV and LA diastolic pressures and does not impart a worsened prognosis in coronary disease.

Pseudonormal Filling

The next stage, stage 2, in the decline in diastolic function that follows impaired LV diastolic function (stage 1) is associated with elevation of the LV and left atrial diastolic pressure. Although LV relaxation remains slowed, higher left atrial pressure leads to an increase in early transmitral filling (E wave) velocity and impaired LV compliance leads to rapid termination of filling when ventricular capacity is prematurely achieved. The abrupt termination of filling shortens the deceleration time toward normal. The increase in left atrial pressure also causes mitral valve to open sooner with consequent shortening of the IVRT. The elevation of LV filling pressures is a direct consequence of decreased chamber compliance, which sees the pressure in the left ventricle rise more rapidly during filling. These changes "pseudonormalize" transmitral flow, and make it difficult to distinguish from normal. However, with the Valsalva maneuver, preload decreases, left atrial pressure drops and the "pseudonormal" pattern may temporarily revert back to the pattern of impaired LV relaxation (stage 1).

Restrictive Filling (Grades 3 and 4 Diastolic Dysfunction)

Further increase in LV filling pressure results in worsening effective LV compliance. During diastolic filling, pressure in the left ventricle rises exponentially, and exceeds left atrial pressure very early in diastole. Consequently, most of the diastolic filling occurs early, contribution of late filling is minimal, E to A ratio becomes more than 2:1, deceleration time shortens to less than 140 msec and IVRT shortens further.

By the time of mitral valve closure at the end of diastole, the left atrium does not empty completely. Due to this, the systolic wave of pulmonary venous flow becomes severely blunted and most of pulmonary venous flow occurs in diastole. Moreover, left atrial systolic reversal is prolonged and increased in amplitude. Also, color m-mode reveals further slowing of the propagation velocity and Em velocity on the tissue Doppler recording of mitral annular motion is also markedly decreased. Restrictive LV filling is a poor prognostic sign in various disease states, including patients with low LVEF and in patients with infiltrative cardiomyopathies. Patients who continue to exhibit restrictive filling pattern despite Valsalva (stage 4) or following aggressive medical treatment are at especially high risk.

Evaluation of Left Ventricular Filling Pressures

The ultimate significance of diastolic parameters is due to their ability to noninvasively evaluate LV filling pressure. Identification of the diastolic filling pattern provides an approximate understanding of the level of LV filling pressure. Typically, delayed relaxation pattern is associated with normal filling pressures, pseudonormal pattern with mild-to-moderate elevation of pressures and restrictive pattern with markedly elevated filling pressures. In addition, deceleration time of early diastolic filling may be an accurate indicator of LV filling pressure in patients with low LVEF, in whom a deceleration time less than 150 msec nearly always indicates mean left atrial pressure above 25 mm Hg.

However patterns of mitral inflow as predictors of filling pressure are vulnerable to confounding. Heart rate, preload, afterload, contractility, valvular regurgitation, and the position of the sample volume may influence transmitral flow independently of diastolic function.

❏ CONCLUSION

Left ventricular systolic and diastolic parameters can be comprehensively measured by echocardiography/Doppler and provide a wealth of information about ejection and filling functions and have strong prognostic significance. However, they are best utilized when interpreted together in an expertly performed comprehensive echocardiographic study in the light of the pertinent clinical questions and context.

❏ SUGGESTED READINGS

Byrd BF 3rd, Wahr D, Wang YS, et al. Left ventricular mass and volume/mass ratio determined by two-dimensional echocardiography in normal adults. J Am Coll Cardiol. 1985;6:1021-5.

Lang RM, Bierig M, Devereux RB, et al. Recommendations for chamber quantification: a report from the American Society of Echocardiography's Guidelines and Standards Committee and the Chamber Quantification Writing Group, developed in conjunction with the European Association of Echocardiography, a branch of the European Society of Cardiology. J Am Soc Echocardiogr. 2005;18: 1440-63.

Mulvagh SL, Rakowski H, Vannan MA, et al. American Society of Echocardiography Consensus Statement on the clinical applications of ultrasonic contrast agents in echocardiography. J Am Soc Echocardiogr. 2008;21:1179-201.

Richardson P, McKenna W, Bristow M, et al. Report of the 1995 World Health Organization/International Society and Federation of Cardiology Task Force on the definition and classification of cardiomyopathies. Circulation. 1996;93:841-2.

Schiller NB, Shah PM, Crawford M, et al. Recommendations for quantitation of the left ventricle by two-dimensional echocardiography. American Society of Echocardiography Committee on Standards, Subcommittee on Quantitation of Two-Dimensional Echocardiograms. J Am Soc Echocardiogr. 1989;2:358-67.

2.6 Transthoracic Echocardiography

❑ INTRODUCTION

Echocardiography is the examination of the heart using reflected sound waves. The early clinically applied technology was mmode (i.e. motion-based mode). This provided a one dimensional view of the heart with motion recorded at a high frame rate of 1,000–2,000 frames per second. A variety of two-dimensional (2D) methods have become available for cross-sectional display of cardiac structures, but at a lower frame rate of 30–100 frames per second. Doppler techniques provide the recording of intracardiac blood flow, and with color Doppler, the Doppler signal is displayed as 2D imaging using color to denote the direction and character of flow. Echocardiography is widely recognized as an appropriate imaging modality in evaluating patients with a variety of symptoms and signs of heart disease (Table 28).

Table 28: Appropriate indications for echocardiography

Symptoms
- Dyspnea
- Chest pain with suspected myocardial ischemia in patients with nondiagnostic laboratory markers and ECG and in whom a resting echocardiogram can be performed during pain
- Light-headedness or syncope
- TIA or cerebrovascular event

Prior testing that is concerning for heart disease (e.g. abnormal chest X-ray or electrocardiogram, elevated BNP)

Native valve disease
- Murmur
- Suspected mitral valve prolapse
- Initial evaluation of known or suspected native valve stenosis or regurgitation
- Routine (yearly) re-evaluation of asymptomatic patient with severe native valvular stenosis or regurgitation
- Re-evaluation of patient with native valve stenosis or regurgitation with a change in clinical status

Contd...

Contd...

Table 28: Appropriate indications for echocardiography

Prosthetic valve
- Initial evaluation of prosthetic valve for establishment of baseline after placement
- Re-evaluation due to suspected dysfunction or thrombosis or a change in clinical status

Infective endocarditis
- Initial evaluation of suspected infective endocarditis with positive blood culture or new murmur
- Re-evaluation of infective endocarditis in patients with virulent organism, severe hemodynamic lesion, aortic involvement, persistent bacteremia, a change in clinical status or symptomatic deterioration.

Known or suspected adult congenital heart disease

Sustained or nonsustained ventricular tachycardia

Evaluation of intracardiac and extracardiac structures and chambers
- Cardiovascular source of embolus
- Evaluation for cardiac mass due to suspected tumor or thrombus
- Evaluation of pericardial conditions such as effusion, constrictive pericarditis and tamponade

Known or suspected Marfan disease for evaluation of proximal aortic root and/or mitral valve

Heart failure
- Initial evaluation of known or suspected heart failure (systolic or diastolic)
- Re-evaluation to guide therapy in a patient with a change in clinical status

Pacing device evaluation
- Evaluation for dyssynchrony in patient being considered for cardiac resynchronization therapy
- Known implanted pacing device with symptoms possibly due to suboptimal pacing device settings to re-evaluate for dyssynchrony and/or revision of pacing device setting

Hypertrophic cardiomyopathy
- Initial evaluation of known or suspected hypertrophic cardiomyopathy
- Re-evaluation of known hypertrophic cardiomyopathy in a patient with a change in clinical status to guide or evaluate therapy

Cardiomyopathy
- Evaluation of suspected restrictive, infiltrative, or genetic cardiomyopathy
- Screening for structure and function in first-degree relatives of patients with inherited cardiomyopathy

Cardiotoxic agents
- Baseline and serial re-evaluation in patients undergoing therapy with cardiotoxic agents

Myocardial infarction
- Initial evaluation of LV function after acute MI
- Re-evaluation of LV function following MI during recovery when results will guide therapy
- Evaluation of suspected complication of myocardial ischemia/infarction such as acute mitral regurgitation, ventricular septal defect, heart failure, thrombus and RV involvement

Pulmonary
- Respiratory failure with suspected cardiac etiology
- Known or suspected pulmonary embolism to guide therapy (i.e. thrombectomy and thrombolytics)
- Evaluation of known or suspected pulmonary hypertension including evaluation of RV function and estimated pulmonary artery pressure

Hemodynamic instability of uncertain or suspected cardiac etiology

❑ CHAMBER QUANTITATION

Left ventricular linear dimensions are important measurements in the management of patients with heart disease, especially in patients with volume overload due to valvular heart disease. LV internal dimensions at end-diastole (LVIDd) and at endsystole (LVIDs) are usually made from parasternal long axis images at the level of the minor axis (i.e. perpendicular to the long axis of the left ventricle), at the level of the mitral leaflet tips or chords with measurements obtained at the tissueblood interface (Fig. 36). The normal reference range for LV end diastolic diameter varies with gender: women, less than or equal to 5.3 cm [<3.2 cm/m^2 when indexed for body surface area (BSA)] and men, less than or equal to 5.9 cm (<3.1 cm/m^2 when indexed for BSA).

The development of LV hypertrophy predicts increased risk of stroke, systolic heart failure and mortality; however, reduction in LV mass corresponds with improved outcomes. Wall thickness is measured at end-diastole with normal thickness less than or equal to 0.9 cm. Left ventricular ejection fraction (LVEF) predicts mortality and is proportional to survival (i.e. the lower the LVEF, the lower the individual patient's survival). In addition, LVEF guides therapeutic decision-making, helping to identify patients for drug therapy initiation (e.g. angiotensin converting enzyme inhibitors and beta-blockers in patients with LVEF <40%) and for implantation of internal cardiac defibrillators. Regional wall motion of the left ventricle can be assessed with 2D echocardiography. A standard model of analysis involves dividing the left ventricle into 17 segments (Fig. 37). The identification of segments is useful for the identification of coronary perfusion territories.

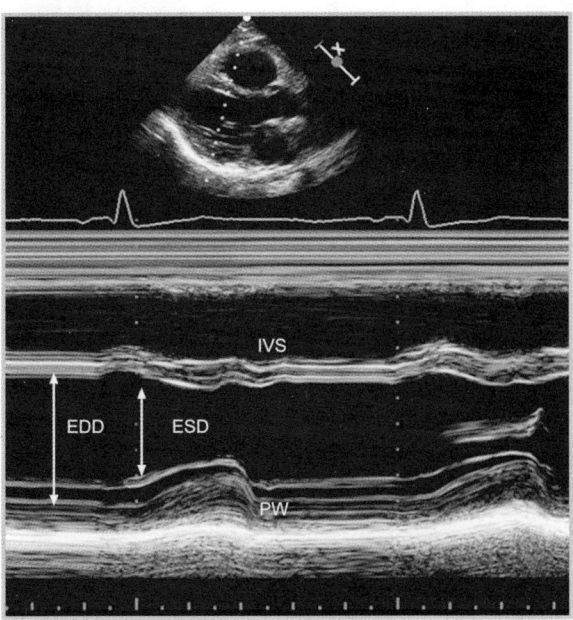

FIGURE 36: Measurement of left ventricular end-diastolic dimensions (EDD) and end-systolic dimensions (ESD) from m-mode of the LV using the parasternal long axis view (inset) for landmark identification. (Abbreviations: IVS: Interventricular septum; PW: Posterior wall)

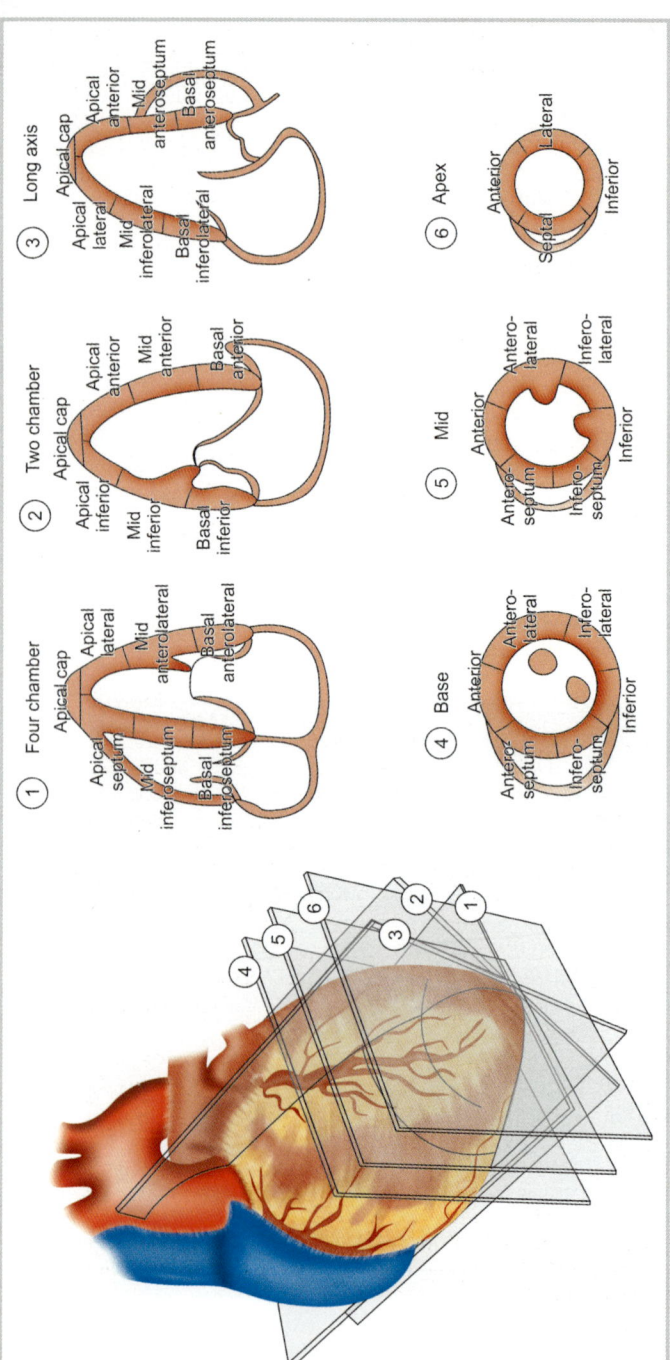

FIGURE 37: Seventeen segment model of left ventricular regional wall analysis based on apical and parasternal short axis views. (*Source:* Modified from Lang RM, Bierig M, Devereux RB, et al. Recommendations for chamber quantification: a report from the American Society of Echocardiography's guidelines and standards committee and the chamber quantification writing group, developed in conjunction with the European Association of Echocardiography, a branch of the European Society of Cardiology. J Am Soc Echo. 2005:18:1440-63, with permission)

Right ventricular (RV) size is influenced by afterload and pressure changes as well as diseases, such as myocardial infarction and RV dysplasia. In the apical 4-chamber view, the RV area or midcavity diameter should be smaller that the LV, otherwise RV dilation is present. Right ventricular (RV) diameter is measure at end diastole and dilation is present with basal minor diameter greater than 4.2 cm, mid level diameter greater than 3.5 cm or major length greater than 8.6 cm. Left atrial (LA) enlargement as determined by echocardiography is a predictor of cardiovascular outcomes. Left artrial (LA) size is measured at ventricular end systole, when the LA chamber is at its largest dimension. Right atrial (RA) enlargement has adverse prognostic implications in patients with pulmonary hypertension.

❏ DOPPLER ECHO

There are three modalities: (i) pulsed wave; (ii) continuous wave, and (iii) color Doppler. Pulsed wave Doppler measures flow velocity within a specific site (i.e. range gate) but is limited in the measurement of high velocities. Continuous wave Doppler can record high velocities but cannot localize the site of origin of the velocity. Color Doppler estimates flow velocities within regions of interest with the 2D image. Color Doppler provides a rapid assessment of flow with a spatial and directional (colorcoded) display of velocities on a 2D echo. Pulsed and continuous wave Doppler provides quantitation of flow velocity and pressure gradient.

❏ DIASTOLIC FUNCTION

Approximately one half of patients with a new diagnosis of heart failure have normal or near normal LV systolic function and these patients frequently have abnormalities of diastolic function. Morphologic abnormalities include LV hypertrophy. Wall thickness and LV mass can be assessed and with increased filling pressures, LA volume increases which can also be assessed with 2D echocardiography. Doppler measurement of mitral inflow velocities, pulmonary vein velocities and LV myocardial tissue velocities are used to provide additional assessment of LV diastolic dysfunction (Figs 38A to C). These are obtained from the apical 4-chamber view which allows proper alignment of the Doppler beam. The major mitral inflow velocity parameters are: peak early filling (E) and late diastolic filling (A) velocities, the E/A ratio and deceleration time (DT) of early filling velocity. In addition, the isovolumic relaxation period can be determined by placing continuous wave Doppler beam in the LVOT to simultaneously display the end of aortic ejection and the onset of mitral inflow.

The four mitral inflow patterns are (i) normal (i.e. the mitral E velocity is dominant), (ii) impaired LV relaxation (i.e. the mitral A velocity is dominant), (iii) restrictive filling (i.e. elevated mitral E velocity with shortened DT) and (iv) pseudonormal (i.e. normal mitral E velocity dominance).

A Doppler beam placed into a pulmonary vein will provide a recording of the systolic (S) and diastolic (D) velocities. The S velocity is influenced by changes in LA pressure, contraction and relaxation. The D velocity is influenced by changes in LV filling and compliance. With an increase in LA pressure, the S velocity is expected to decrease and the D velocity increases (similar to the E velocity increase on mitral inflow Doppler).

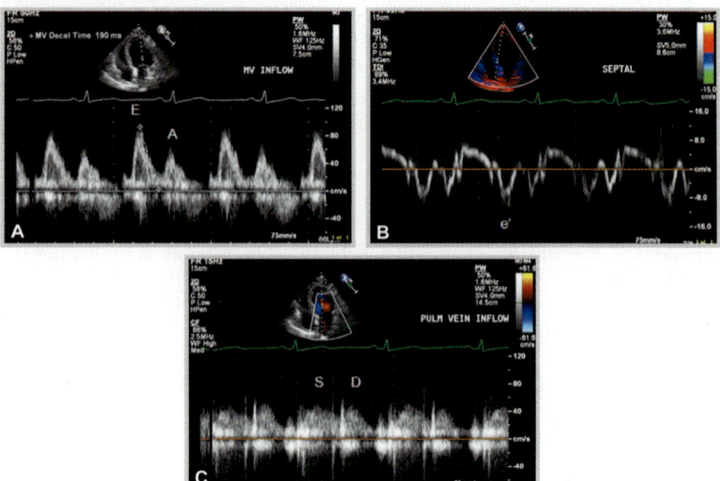

FIGURES 38A TO C: Diastolic function assessment with Doppler echocardiography. (A) Mitral inflow Doppler velocity profiles of early (E) and late atrial (A) filling. (B) Septal wall tissue Doppler imaging for assessment of e'. (C) Pulmonary vein Doppler velocity profiles for measurement of systolic (S) and diastolic (D) velocities

❑ PULMONARY HYPERTENSION

Pulmonary arterial (PA) hypertension results from restricted flow through the PA circulation, increased pulmonary vascular resistance and ultimately in right heart failure. Pulmonary arterial hypertension is defined as mean PA pressure greater than 25 mm Hg at rest, PA wedge pressure less than 15 mm Hg and pulmonary vascular resistance greater than 3 Wood Units. Pulmonary hypertension can also result from disorders associated with elevated LV filling pressures, such as LV dysfunction (either systolic or diastolic) and valvular heart disease. Transthoracic echocardiography (TTE) may identify conditions that predispose to PH or suggest a specific disease entity. A complete 2D and Doppler echo study can provide an estimate of RV systolic pressure or cardiac sequelae of PH. Right ventricular (RV) systolic pressure greater than 40 mm Hg generally warrants further evaluation in the patient with unexplained dyspnea. Other findings of PH are RA or RV enlargement or interventricular septal flattening. The presence of any degree of pericardial effusion, RA enlargement and RV enlargement or dysfunction is predictor of poor prognosis.

The RA pressure can be estimated by the inferior vena cava appearance. A normal RA pressure of 0–5 mm Hg is predicted by an inferior vena cava diameter of less than 2.1 cm with collapse greater than 50% with a sniff. An elevated RA pressure of 10–20 mm Hg is suggested by inferior vena cava diameter greater than 2.1 cm with collapse less than 50% with a sniff.

❑ PERICARDIAL DISEASE

Echocardiography can be useful in detecting a variety of conditions that affect the pericardium including (i) effusion, (ii) tamponade, (iii) constriction, (iv) partial or complete absence of the pericardium, and (v) pericardial cysts or tumors. Pericardial effusion is recognized as an echo-free space between the visceral and the parietal pericardium surrounding the heart. Small effusions are generally limited to the posterior atrioventricular groove. As the effusion increases, fluid extends laterally and with large effusion, fluid surrounds the heart.

When the ability of the pericardium to stretch is exceeded by fluid accumulation, pericardial sac pressure increases and may exceed intracardiac pressures during the cycle, resulting in tamponade physiology. The signs of tamponade include RA wall inversion and diastolic compression of the RV free wall. Plethora of the inferior vena cava is a useful indicator of elevated RA pressure. Tamponade produces reciprocal respiration-related changes in diastolic filling of the LV and the RV, and exaggerated respiratory changes in mitral and tricuspid inflow velocities can be demonstrated by pulsed Doppler.

❑ VALVULAR HEART DISEASE

Aortic Stenosis

The most common cause of aortic stenosis in adults is calcification of a normal trileaflet or a congenital bicuspid valve. Anatomic evaluation of the AV with 2D echo is based on a combination of short and long axis images to identify the number of leaflets, and to describe leaflet mobility, thickness and calcification. Unfortunately, the accuracy of direct planimetry of the valve area is limited by artefacts from calcification. Doppler echocardiography allows the determination of the level of obstruction and the quantitation of the pressure gradient. The primary hemodynamic parameters for the clinical evaluation of aortic stenosis severity are jet velocity, mean transaortic gradient and valve area by the continuity equation. Jet velocity is measured across the narrowed AV using continuous wave Doppler ultrasound. Multiple acoustic windows are interrogated and the highest velocity is used.

When low LV systolic function accompanies severe aortic stenosis, the transvalvular velocity and gradient may be low due to the low-flow state. Low-flow, low-gradient aortic steosis generally refers to the presence of: (i) valve area less than 1.0 cm^2, (ii) LVEF less than 40%, and (iii) mean pressure gradient less than 30–40 mm Hg. Obstruction to LV ejection can occur at several levels: subaortic (LVOT), aortic (valvular) and supravalvular. Hypertrophic cardiomyopathy is characterized by inappropriate hypertrophy, interstitial fibrosis, myocardial disarray and impaired LV performance. Asymmetric LV hypertrophy typically involves the septum, but almost any myocardial segment can be involved.

Aortic Regurgitation

Chronic aortic regurgitation is a condition of combined volume and pressure overload. While the LV may compensate for the increased load, eventually depressed contractility may occur, sometimes while the patient remains asymptomatic. Color Doppler evaluation of aortic regurgitation includes the measurement of the regurgitant jet size, the vena contracta through the orifice, and the flow convergence toward the regurgitant orifice area.

Continuous and pulsed wave Doppler methods for quantitation of aortic regurgitation are based on velocity measurements from systolic and diastolic velocity profiles. The rate of deceleration of the diastolic regurgitant jet (i.e. deceleration slope) reflects the equalization of pressures between the aorta and

Table 29: Classification of mitral stenosis severity			
	Mild	Moderate	Severe
Valve area (cm^2)	>1.5	1.0–1.5	<1.0
Mean gradient (mm Hg)	<5	5–10	>10
Pulmonary artery systolic pressure (mm Hg)	<30	30–50	>50

the left ventricle. As aortic regurgitation severity increases, the deceleration slope increases.

Mitral Stenosis

The principal cause of mitral stenosis is rheumatic heart disease, and despite a decrease in the prevalence of rheumatic fever, mitral stenosis remains a significant problem, particularly due to immigration from developing countries. Direct measurement of the valve area is possible by tracing the valve orifice area from the parasternal short axis view. However, careful attention to gain settings is needed since excessive setting may lead to underestimation of area. In addition, scanning should be performed from the apex to base of the LV to assure that the area is measured at the level of the leaflet tips (i.e. the smallest measurable orifice).

Recommendations for classification of mitral stenosis severity (Table 29) are based on Doppler assessment of the mitral stenosis as well as secondary findings of pulmonary hypertension severity.

The estimation of the diastolic pressure gradient across the mitral valve in mitral stenosis uses the modified Bernoulli equation ($\Delta P = 4v2$). For accurate measurement, the Doppler ultrasound beam must be oriented parallel to flow, so the apical 4-chamber view is preferred for imaging. Doppler ultrasound provides an alternative method to direct planimetry for assessing valve area. The decline in velocity of diastolic transmitral blood flow is inversely proportional to valve area according to the formula:

$$\text{Mitral valve area} = 220/T_{1/2}$$

where $T_{1/2}$ is the time (in msec) between the maximum mitral gradient in early diastole and the point at which the gradient is half the maximum initial value. In the valve area equation, 220 is an empirically derived constant (Fig. 39).

Mitral Regurgitation

An initial comprehensive TTE in a patient with suspected MR provides a baseline assessment left-sided chamber size and LVEF. In addition, TTE provides an approximation of MR severity, anatomic information regarding mechanism and PA pressure. Changes from baseline values are useful in guiding the timing of mitral valve surgery.

The echocardiographic examination of the mitral valve begins with a 2D echo evaluation since the etiology of regurgitation may be visualized. Examples include underlying mitral valve prolapse and annular dilatation due to LV enlargement. Color flow Doppler evaluation includes visualization of the origin of the regurgitant jet and its width (i.e. the vena contracta), as well as spatial orientation in the left atrium. The vena contracta is the narrowest portion of a jet that occurs at or just downstream from the orifice and represents a measure of the effective regurgitant orifice area. The size of the vena contracta is independent of flow rate and driving force.

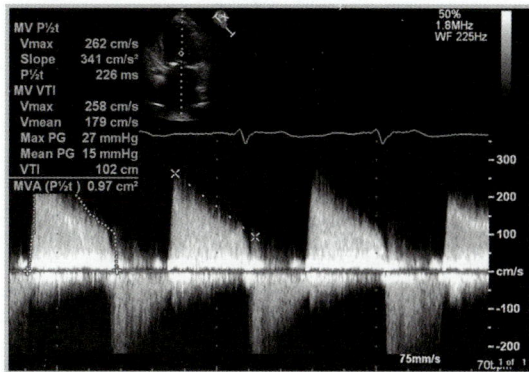

FIGURE 39: Continuous wave Doppler demonstrating severe mitral stenosis. The pressure half-time (P1/2t) is 226 ms, predicting a valve area of 0.97 cm^2

Continuous wave Doppler signal of the regurgitant jet measures maximum velocity which does not provide quantitation of jet severity. However, the contour of the profile and its density are useful. Pulsed Doppler evaluation of the mitral inflow velocity at the mitral leaflet tips provides measurement of the early and late filling velocities. As regurgitation severity increases, there is loss of relative contribution of atrial filling and an increase in early filling.

Tricuspid Stenosis

Isolated tricuspid stenosis is uncommon and the same principles as for mitral stenosis apply. However, an empiric constant of 190 has been proposed and the mean gradient in significant tricuspid stenosis is lower than for mitral stenosis. Hemodynamically significant stenosis is defined as a mean pressure gradient greater than 5 mm Hg, and $T_{1/2}$ greater than 190 msec (corresponding to a valve area less than 1.0 cm^2 and assuming an empiric constant of 190). Additional supportive findings on 2D echocardiography include enlargement of the RA and dilatation of the inferior vena cava.

Tricuspid Regurgitation

Similar to MR, tricuspid regurgitation is assessed by integrating information on right-sided chamber size, septal motion and Doppler parameters. Significant tricuspid regurgitation is often associated with RA and RV enlargement and in the presence of significant volume overload of the RV, there may be paradoxical septal motion. Right atrial (RA) pressure estimation can be appreciated by the size and respiratory variation of the inferior vena cava.

Color Doppler methods for assessing severity include measuring jet area, the vena contracta, and the effective regurgitant orifice area using methods described above for MR. Pulsed Doppler can measure the RV filling velocities and with severe tricuspid regurgitation, early filling velocities are elevated and can be greater than 1.0 m/sec.

Pulmonic Stenosis

Isolated pulmonic stenosis is usually congenital in origin. The severity of stenosis is determined by the pressure gradient as calculated from the modified Bernoulli equation. The grading of severity based on peak pressure gradient is mild [<36 mm Hg (corresponding to peak velocity <3 m/sec)], moderate [36–64 mm Hg (or a peak velocity of 3–4 m/sec)], and severe [>64 mm Hg (or a peak velocity of >4 m/sec)]. Evaluation of the valve's anatomy with 2D echo may provide additional information.

Pulmonic Regurgitation

Mild pulmonic regurgitation may be present in normal subjects; however, significant regurgitation suggests the presence of underlying structural heart disease. Color Doppler flow mapping is the most widely used method for detection and regurgitation. The jet or vena contracta widths are common measurements in the assessment of regurgitation severity. As severity of regurgitation increases, continuous wave Doppler demonstrates a rapid deceleration of diastolic flow as diastolic pressure in PA and RV equalize.

❏ INFECTIVE ENDOCARDITIS

Echocardiography is central to the diagnosis and management of patients with infective endocarditis. Transesophageal echocardiography (TTE) is an appropriate test for the detection of valvular vegetation, with or without positive blood cultures for the diagnosis of infective endocarditis, although TEE is considered more sensitive than TTE in detecting vegetations. In addition, TTE can characterize the hemodynamic severity of valvular lesions and potential complications of endocarditis (e.g. abscess, valve perforation, shunt). Transesophageal echocardiography is also recommended for reassessment of high-risk patients (e.g. those with a virulent organism, clinical deterioration, persistent or recurrent fever, new murmur or persistent bacteremia).

Positive echocardiographic evidence of infective endocarditis is defined as an "oscillating intracardiac mass on valve or supporting structures, in the path of regurgitant jets, or on implanted material in the absence of an alternative anatomic explanation; or abscess; or new partial dehiscence of prosthetic valve; or new valvular regurgitation". Transesophageal echocardiography has a sensitivity of 60–65% and specificity of 94–96% in the detection of vegetations. In contrast, improved sensitivity of 85–98% is reported for TEE. False negative TTE studies are more frequent with small vegetations, presence of prosthetic material or technically deficient studies.

Current recommendations for the use of TEE in patients with endocarditis include: (i) symptomatic patients with infective endocarditis if TTE is nondiagnostic (to assess hemodynamic severity of a valve lesion), (ii) patients with valvular heart disease and positive blood culture if TTE is nondiagnostic, (iii) patients with possible complications of infective endocarditis, and (iv) patients with suspected prosthetic valve endocarditis.

❏ INTRACARDIAC MASSES

Abnormal intracardiac masses are typically echodensities that represent thrombus or tumor. However, there are normal variants that can be confused with mass lesions. Primary tumors are uncommon and about 75% are benign, usually representing myxoma in the adult and rhabdomyoma in children under 15 years. About 75–90% of myxomas are found in the LA, pedunculated and attached to the interatrial septum, in or adjacent to the fossa ovalis. Angiosarcoma is the most common sarcoma and has a propensity to occur on the right side of the heart, especially in the RA. Rhabdomyosarcoma can occur in any cardiac chamber, grow rapidly and have usually invaded the pericardium by the time of diagnosis. Metastatic tumors are up to 40 times more common than primary tumors, and are typically encountered in patients with widespread systemic tumor dissemination.

❏ CONTRAST ECHOCARDIOGRAPHY

Echo contrast agents used in contrast echocardiography include agitated saline for the assessment of right-to-left intracardiac shunts and manufactured microbubbles with shell composition of lipid, human albumin or phospholipid and gas (e.g. air, perfluoropropane, sulfur hexafluoride, etc.). Manufactured contrast agents may be useful in improving the accuracy and reproducibility of the assessment of LV structure and function at rest and during stress. Suboptimal echocardiograms can be converted to diagnostic examinations in 75–90% of patients due to improved endocardial definition.

❏ CARDIAC RESYNCHRONIZATION THERAPY

Echocardiography has been used to improve patient selection for chronic resynchronization therapy (CRT), also referred to as biventricular pacing, and to optimize device settings after implantation. Unfortunately, approximately 25–35% of patients undergoing CRT do not have an appropriate response. While a number of explanations have been proposed for the suboptimal response, the absence of dyssynchrony (i.e. regions of early and late contraction within the left ventricle) is a likely factor and can potentially be identified by echocardiography. M-mode echo provides excellent temporal resolution due to a sampling rate 1,000/sec. A delay from septal wall peak inward motion to posterior wall peak inward motion of greater than or equal to 130 msec has been proposed as a marker of dyssynchrony.

❏ SUGGESTED READINGS

Baumgartner H, Hung J, Bermejo J, et al. Echocardiographic assessment of valve stenosis: EAE/ASE recommendations for clinical practice. J Am Soc Echocardiogr. 2009;22:1-23.

Bonow RO, Carabello BA, Chatterjee K, et al. ACC/AHA 2006 guidelines for the management of patients with valvular heart disease. Executive Summary. Circulation. 2006;114:450-527.

Douglas PS, Khandheria B, Stainback RF, et al. ACCF/ASE/ACEP/ASNC/SCAI/SCCT/SCMR 2007 appropriateness criteria for transthoracic and transesophageal echocardiography. J Am Coll Cardiol. 2007;50:187-204.

Gorcsan J 3rd, Abraham T, Agler DA, et al. Echocardiography for cardiac resynchronization therapy: recommendations for performance and reporting—a report from the American Society of Echocardiography dyssynchrony writing group. J Am Soc Echocardiogr. 2008;21:191-213.

Lang RM, Bierig M, Devereux RB, et al. Recommendations for chamber quantification: a report from the American Society of Echocardiography's guidelines and standards committee and the chamber quantification writing group, developed in conjunction with the European Association of Echocardiography, a branch of the European Society of Cardiology. J Am Soc Echo. 2005;18:1440-63.

Quinones MA, Otto CM, Stoddard M, et al. Recommendations for quantification of Doppler echocardiography: a report from the Doppler Quantification Task Force of the Nomenclature and Standards Committee of the American Society of Echocardiography. J Am Soc Echocardiogr. 2002;15:167-84.

Zoghbi WA, Enriquez-Sarano M, Foster E, et al. Recommendations for evaluation of the severity of native valvular regurgitation with two-dimensional and Doppler echocardiography. J Am Soc Echocardiogr. 2003;16:777-802.

2.7 Stress Echocardiography

❏ INTRODUCTION

Coronary artery disease (CAD) has been the number one killer in Western society since the turn of the century. Identifying those at risk and preventing the sequelae of ischemic disease is thus a major goal of current-day practice. Stress echocardiography (SE) has been used in this regard for over a quarter of a century. Given the rapid escalation in use and the associated costs associated with SE, it is necessary for both cardiologists and noncardiologists alike to have an in-depth understanding of all clinical uses.

❏ USING STRESS ECHOCARDIOGRAPHY IN CLINICAL DECISIONS

Pathophysiology Involved in Stress Echo

The major uses of SE have been in (i) diagnosing and (ii) estimating risk in patients with suspected or known ischemic disease. In order to establish a diagnosis of ischemic disease, SE must show a functional mismatch between myocardial oxygen supply and demand. The "gold standard", however, is not a functional test, rather an anatomic measurement of coronary stenosis. In addition, the reduction in blood flow necessary to produce ischemia, and hence, a wall motion abnormality has been variably defined in the literature. Both 50% and 70% stenoses of a major epicardial artery (as defined by coronary angiography) have been used to derive sensitivity or specificity of SE.

The increase in myocardial oxygen demand achieved by stress testing can occur by various mechanisms. Three general modalities are commonly used: (i) an exercise stress which produces a dynamic increase in myocardial oxygen demand, (ii) a pharmacologic stress (dobutamine), which increases in myocardial oxygen demand, and (iii) a vasodilator stress, which produces a coronary "steal".

Stress Echocardiography and the Diagnosis of Coronary Artery Disease

Exercise Stress Echo (ESE)

Assessment prior to an exercise stress echo: All stress testing begins with a review of the indication(s) for the stress test in particular, and contraindications for stress testing in general (Table 30).

Indications for SE have been outlined by several groups with the most recent being the appropriateness criteria endorsed by the major cardiac societies. In the area of diagnosis of ischemic disease, the most common appropriate indications include the following: (i) diagnosis of chest pain syndromes in patients with intermediate probability of disease, (ii) diagnosis of chest pain syndrome in patients with abnormal baseline EKG, and (iii) diagnosis in patients with prior equivocal stress testing.

Contraindications to exercise stress echocardiography (ESE) are similar to those outlined for exercise testing in general. They are listed in Table 31.

The final clinical decision to be made before starting an exercise test is to review the medication list for medications which may interfere with testing or with test interpretation. Concomitant use of beta blockers may result in an inability to

Table 30: Checklist for patient assessment prior to exercise stress echocardiography

Appropriate clinical indications
No contraindications to exercise
Ability to exercise—DASI score
- Exercise limitations
- Musculoskeletal limitations

Clinical symptom review
- Pretest probability
- Pretest score (Morise)

Baseline EKG review
- Normal
- Baseline abnormalities

Current medications
- Beta blocker (held for 48 hours)
- Diltiazem or verapamil
- Long acting nitrates
- Digoxin

Table 31: Contraindications to exercise testing

- Acute myocardial infarction, recent
- Unstable angina (not stabilized by medical therapy or recent pain at rest)
- Uncontrolled heart failure
- Uncontrolled symptomatic arrhythmias
- Symptomatic severe aortic stenosis
- Acute pulmonary embolus or pulmonary infarction
- Deep vein thrombosis
- Acute myocarditis or pericarditis
- Acute aortic dissection (or recent aortic surgery)
- Uncontrolled hypertension (>220/120 mm Hg)
- Significant left main coronary stenosis
- Significant electrolyte abnormalities (particularly hyper or hypokalemia)
- Severe hypertrophic cardiomyopathy
- High-degree atrioventricular block
- Inability to exercise adequately due to physical or mental limitation

achieve 85% of maximum predicted HR, and as a result, has been reported to lower the sensitivity of testing. Therefore, if beta blockers can be discontinued safely prior to testing, then it is recommended that they be discontinued for approximately 4–5 half-lives or 48 hours prior to testing. Similarly, other drugs which slow HR response (diltiazem and verapamil) or alter the ischemic response (nitrates) should be reviewed and discontinued if clinically appropriate.

Choosing an exercise protocol: The choice of the type of exercise is often made by what is available at one's own institution. In the United States, exercise treadmill is the most common form of stress exercise. Outside of the United States, exercise using a bicycle ergometer is performed more frequently. There are advantages and disadvantages to both. Exercise treadmill has the advantage in that walking is familiar to all, whereas patients may not be as familiar with use of a bike. From an SE standpoint, however, imaging must be performed after the completion of treadmill exercise and carries the risk that ischemic wall motion abnormalities will have resolved before imaging can be completed. In contrast, imaging is performed continuously during bicycle exercise, although image degradation due to motion

Table 32: Endpoints for stress echocardiography

- Achievement of target heart rate
- Symptom limitation
- Protocol completion (i.e. maximal dobutamine or dipyridamole dose)
- Significant wall motion abnormality (see text)
- Ischemic EKG response (i.e. ≥2 mm ST depression or ST elevation >1 mm in non-Q wave lead)
- Severe ischemic symptoms (i.e. chest discomfort or exertional dyspnea)
- Severe hypertension (systolic BP >220 mm Hg or diastolic BP >120 mm Hg)
- Hypotension or fall in BP >20 mm Hg with exercise
- Arrhythmias (SVT, VT, heart block, BBB)
- CNS symptoms

artifact can be troublesome. The most common protocol used in exercise treadmill testing is the Bruce protocol. This protocol has the advantage of widespread use and literature validation.

Conducting the exercise stress echo: A detailed account of the technique required to conduct treadmill exercise testing is beyond the scope of this chapter. Comments about the protocol will be limited to the additional considerations associated with echo imaging.

Baseline echo images should be reviewed prior to the start of exercise. Segments within all coronary distributions should be visualized prior to starting exercise. If two or more segments cannot be visualized, then use of a contrast agent should be considered. Given the US food and drug administration (FDA) black box warning associated with the use of contrast agents, use of perflutren contrast agents cannot be used in many situations. In the majority of cases, a symptom limited exercise study is recommended unless a study endpoint is reached. Exercise end-points have been outlined by the ACC and AHA in guidelines published in 2002. Exercise endpoints are listed in Table 32.

Interpretation of exercise stress echo: Final interpretation of the ESE should consider all components of the study: symptoms, EKG changes, blood pressure (BP) response, echo imaging and exercise tolerance. Reports should contain all of the information that is standard in exercise treadmill studies. The most widely used method of echo interpretation is visual. Function in each myocardial segment is evaluated at rest and then compared at peak exercise. Contraction in each segment is graded as normal or hyperdynamic, hypokinetic, akinetic or dyskinetic. Both the timing of wall motion and thickening should be considered as ischemia results in both delayed contraction and relaxation.

Pharmacologic Stress Echo

Assessing the patient prior to pharmacologic stress testing: Similar to the ESE, pharmacologic SE starts with a review of the indication(s) for the stress test and contraindications for stress agent to be used (Table 33). As with ESE, the reader is referred to the appropriateness criteria for SE for a review of the indications. Appropriate indications for use of dobutamine stress echocardiography (DSE) for diagnosis are similar to those listed for use of ESE (Table 30).

Contraindications to DSE differ considerably from ESE. Contraindications for both dobutamine use and atropine use should be reviewed. A detailed list can be found in Table 34.

When performed in the setting of acute chest pain, serial cardiac enzymes should also be documented to be normal before proceeding with the test. The final

Table 33: Checklist for patient assessment prior to pharmacologic stress testing/echocardiography

- Appropriate clinical indications
- No Contraindications to:
  - Dobutamine:
    - Contraindications
    - Precautions due to known side effects of dobutamine
    - Other considerations
  - Atropine:
    - Contraindications
    - Precautions due to known side effects of atropine
    - Beta blockers (if needed to reverse ischemic response)
    - Dipyridamole
- Clinical symptoms:
  - Pretest probability
  - Clinically stable
- Baseline EKG
  - Baseline abnormalities
  - Previous EKG available for comparison
- Current medication use:
  - Beta blocker held?
  - Diltiazem or verapamil held? (particularly if high dose)
  - Xanthine containing medications or caffeine (if using dipyridamole)

Table 34: Contraindications and precautions with use of dobutamine and atropine

Contraindications to dobutamine
- Symptomatic severe aortic stenosis
- Acute aortic dissection
- Recent or unstable coronary syndrome
- Obstructive hypertrophic cardiomyopathy
- Hypersensitivity

Conditions which may worsen due to dobutamine side effects
- Uncontrolled atrial fibrillation or PSVT
- Uncontrolled hypertension
- Known ventricular arrhythmias

Precautions with other conditions
- Electrolyte abnormalities (particularly hypokalemia)
- Intraventricular thrombus
- Arterial aneurysms
- High degree AV block
- Significant asthma and high risk patients (higher need for use of beta blockers as reversal agent)

Contraindications to atropine
- Narrow angle glaucoma
- Obstructive GI disease
- Myasthenia gravis
- Hypersensitivity to atropine or anticholinergics
- Significant BPH or obstructive uropathy

Conditions which may worsen because of atropine side effects
- Uncontrolled atrial fibrillation or PSVT
- Uncontrolled hypertension
- Known ventricular arrhythmias

clinical decision before starting a DSE is a review of the medications. Beta blockers are routinely stopped 48 hours (4–5 half-lives) before the study if the question is one of diagnosis. If dipyridamole stress is being considered, all xanthine containing medications should be stopped for 72 hours or caffeine containing substances should be stopped 24 hours prior to testing.

Pharmacologic stress echo protocols: (i) Dobutamine stress protocol: The protocols begin at 10 /g/kg per minute and now increase to a maximum dose of 50 mcg/kg per minute. Atropine is added at the doses listed above. Use of atropine at the end of the protocol also allows additional time for dobutamine to reach steady state. If there is a vagal response to dobutamine with manifest bradycardia and relative hypotension, atropine may be added prior to the end of the dobutamine protocol. This is not uncommonly seen at dobutamine doses of 40 mcg/kg per minute or greater. In settings where atropine will not be used or is contraindicated, an additional 3 minutes may be added to protocol to ensure that dobutamine reaches steady state.

Dipyridamole stress protocol: Protocols vary but generally can be divided into two types. The first standard, longer protocol consists of dipyridamole intravenously at a total dose of 0.84 mg/kg over 10 minutes. The initial infusion rate is 0.56 mg/kg for 4 minutes, followed by a 4 minute period of no infusion. A second infusion follows at a lower dose of 0.28 mg/kg. If no endpoint is reached, atropine can be added in doses of 0.25 mg up to a maximal dose of 1 mg. The second, shorter protocol consists of dipyridamole infusion at the 0.84 mg/kg over 6 minutes.

Interpretating the pharmacologic stress echo: The most widely used method of echo imaging interpretation is visual. Like ESE, function in each myocardial segment is evaluated at baseline, and then compared at peak dobutamine or dipyridamole dose. With use of dobutamine, however, comparison with low dose must be considered. An ischemic biphasic response may occur in which an increase in contractility is seen at low dose, followed by no further change or a decrease at peak dose. As with ESE, contraction in each segment is graded as normal or hyperdynamic, hypokinetic, akinetic, or dyskinetic. Both the timing of wall motion and thickening are evaluated. A wall motion scoring system, such as the ASE 16 segment model or the 17 segment model, can be used in a semiquantitative way to report the findings. The overall change in ventricular cavity size in systole should also be reviewed.

In summary, diagnosis of ischemic disease can be assessed with either exercise or pharmacologic SE. The choice of the testing modality should be based on the ability of the patient to exercise, the presence or absence of baseline EKG abnormalities, and the experience of the echocardiography lab. When used in patients with appropriate indications, both study types have been shown to identify patients at risk of ischemic disease with a high degree of accuracy.

Stress Echo and Myocardial Viability

In addition to use in diagnosis and prognosis of ischemic disease, SE has also been used to determine myocardial viability. In patients with resting wall motion abnormalities, viable myocardium is felt to be present when an increase in contractility or increase in endocardial motion can be demonstrated in response to stress. Given that revascularization may benefit up to 50% of patients with chronic "hibernating" myocardial (myocardium that is chronically ischemic and, therefore, dysfunctional), determination of viability may have a significant impact on management decisions.

DSE is the preferred testing modality and has been reported to be the most specific test. The assessment prior to the start of the procedure is similar to that described under diagnostic testing. The protocol, however, varies slightly and is much less aggressive. Dobutamine infusion starts at 5 μg/kg per minute for 3 minutes and increases to 10 μg/kg per minute for an additional 3 minutes. In patients with critical coronary disease, some have advocated starting at an even lower dose— 2.5 μg/kg per minute. The endpoints include the following: (i) a lack of increase in baseline contractility suggesting myocardial necrosis, (ii) an increase in myocardial contractility suggesting myocardial stunning or hibernation, or (iii) a biphasic response in which an increase in contractility is seen at the lower dose, but regional wall motion worsens at the higher dose as ischemia is induced.

Stress Echo and the Assessment of Hemodynamics of Valvular Disease

Because both cardiac structure and valvular hemodynamics can be assessed, SE is increasingly being used to assess valvular heart disease. The most common uses of SE have included assessment of patients with valvular stenosis. ACC/AHA guidelines support use of SE in the assessment of asymptomatic patients with severe aortic stenosis (AS) (class IIb), patients with AS and LV dysfunction, and in patients with mitral stenosis who are either asymptomatic with severe mitral stenosis, or who are symptomatic with mild to moderate mitral stenosis at rest (class I recommendation, level of evidence C). The role of SE in patients with mitral regurgitation or aortic regurgitation is less clear.

❏ FUTURE OF STRESS ECHO

In summary, SE has been proven to be vital resource in evaluation of CAD. Future advances with a focus on 3-dimensional SE, tissue Doppler and contrast perfusion scoring will likely further enhance its usefulness. Given the lack of radiation exposure and cost effectiveness, it will likely to be used for many years to come. Future studies of comparative effectiveness research will likely help to refine its use as a diagnostic and prognostic tool in cardiovascular disease.

❏ SUGGESTED READINGS

Douglas PS, Khandheria B, Stainback RF, et al. ACCF/ASE/ACEP/ AHA/ASNC/SCAI/SCCT/SCMR 2008 appropriateness criteria for stress echocardiography: a report of the American College of Cardiology Foundation Appropriateness Criteria Task Force, American Society of Echocardiography, American College of Emergency Physicians, American Heart Association, American Society of Nuclear Cardiology, Society for Cardiovascular Angiography and Interventions, Society of Cardiovascular Computed Tomography, and Society for Cardiovascular Magnetic Resonance endorsed by the Heart Rhythm Society and the Society of Critical Care Medicine. J Am Coll Cardiol. 2008;51:1127-47.

Gibbons RJ, Balady GJ, Beasley JW, et al. ACC/AHA Guidelines for Exercise Testing. A report of the American College of Cardiology/ American Heart Association Task Force on Practice Guidelines (Committee on Exercise Testing). J Am Coll Cardiol. 1997;30:260-311.

Gibbons RJ, Balady GJ, Bricker JT, et al. ACC/AHA 2002 guideline update for exercise testing: summary article. A report of the American College of Cardiology/American Heart Association Task Force on Practice Guidelines. J Am Coll Cardiol. 2002;40:1531-40.

Hill J, Timmis A. Exercise tolerance testing. BMJ. 2002;324:1084-7.

Sicari R, Nihoyannopoulos P, Evangelista A, et al. Stress echocardiography expert consensus statement: European Association of Echocardiography (EAE) (a registered branch of the ESC). Eur J Echocardiogr. 2008;9:415-37.

Smith SC, Feldman TE, Hirshfeld JW, et al. ACC/AHA/SCAI 2005 Guideline Update for Percutaneous Coronary Intervention—summary article: a report of the American College of Cardiology/American Heart Association Task Force on Practice Guidelines (ACC/AHA/SCAI Writing Committee to Update the 2001 Guidelines for Percutaneous Coronary Intervention). Circulation. 2006;113:156-75.

2.8 Transesophageal Echocardiography

❏ INTRODUCTION

Over the past few decades, transesophageal echocardiography (TEE) has become a commonly performed imaging modality that is complementary to transthoracic echocardiography (TTE). It is widely available, portable, provides real-time imaging, and may be performed in a variety of clinical settings. The use of the esophagus as an acoustic window has permitted the use of higher frequency transducers than those used in TTE studies.

❏ PERFORMANCE

Transesophageal echocardiography should be performed in a laboratory equipped with appropriate tools as well as trained personnel. In addition to the ultrasound machine and multiplane imaging probe, the laboratory must possess the necessary sanitizing equipment to disinfect the TEE probes and transducers. Since performing TEE requires conscious sedation, it necessitates the assistance of a nurse or another qualified assistant who monitors the patient's vital signs, arterial saturation and level of consciousness throughout the procedure. The patient's airway is also monitored with suctioning of oral secretions as necessary to reduce the risk of aspiration. Prior to esophageal intubation, a careful history is obtained from the patient to exclude significant laryngeal or gastroesophageal pathology. The patient is kept fasting for at least 6 hours, and peripheral IV access is obtained to provide moderate conscious sedation with low doses of an IV benzodiazepine and a narcotic. The oropharynx is anesthetized. The patient is then placed in the left lateral decubitus position with the neck flexed. The TEE probe is positioned in the posterior oropharynx. The esophagus is then intubated as the patient initiates a swallow.

❏ SAFETY

The procedural risks of TEE are relatively small but may include transient throat pain, laryngospasm, aspiration, hypoxemia, hypotension, dysrhythmia, bleeding, esophageal rupture, or even death. In general, bleeding complications are rare and usually mild in the face of therapeutic levels of anticoagulation. The risk of bacteremia with TEE is very low and most operators do not routinely treat with prophylactic antibiotics. Methemoglobinemia is a potentially life-threatening complication of topical benzocaine use. Contraindications to TEE include esophageal stricture, diverticulum, tumor and recent esophageal or gastric surgery. Relative contraindications include prior mediastinal irradiation, esophageal varices and coagulopathy. Patients should always be questioned about a history of dysphagia, esophageal varices, and/or liver disease before attempting intubation.

❏ VIEWS

Using a multiplane transesophageal echoscope, standard echocardiographic views of the heart may be obtained. The American Society of Echocardiography (ASE) recommends 20 cross-sectional views composing a comprehensive TEE examination (Fig. 40). The probe is initially advanced into the proximal esophagus, and images are taken from four general positions: (i) the basal esophagus, (ii) mid esophagus or 4-chamber view, (iii) transgastric, and (iv) aortic positions. In addition, the plane of the scan may be rotated through an arc of 180°. At 0°, the plane of interrogation is horizontal or transverse to the heart. More vertical orientation of the crystal provides longitudinal sectioning of the heart. The probe may also be manipulated anteriorly or posteriorly by flexing or extending the probe respectively in the coronal plane.

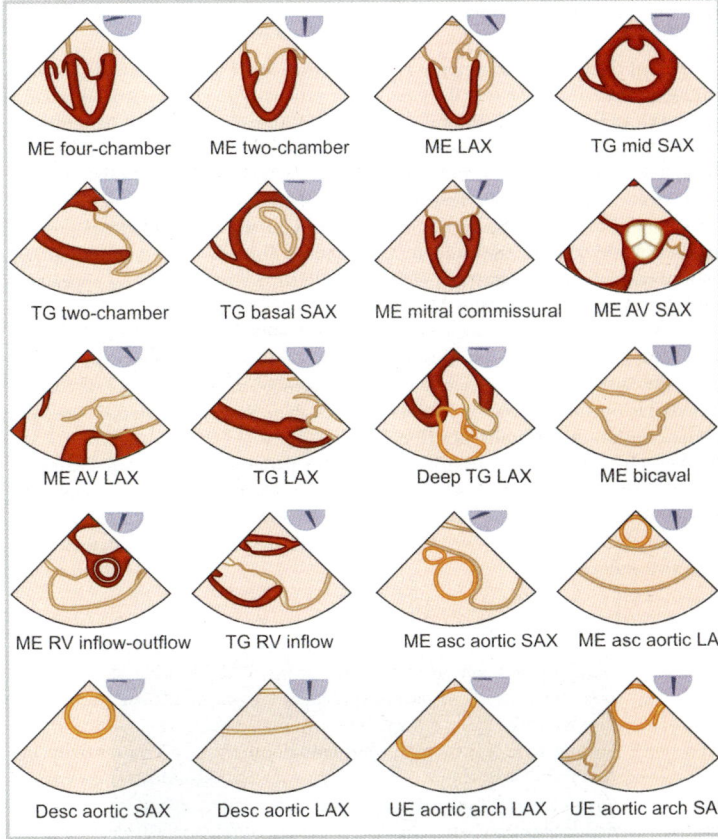

FIGURE 40: Twenty cross-sectional views composing the recommended comprehensive TEE examination. Approximate multiplane angle is indicated by the icon adjacent to each view. (Abbreviations: ME: Mid esophageal; LAX: Long axis; TG: Transgastric; SAX: Short axis; AV: Aortic valve; RV: Right ventricle; Asc: Ascending; Desc: Descending; UE: Upper esophageal). (*Source:* Reproduced with permission from Shanewise JS et al. ASE/SCA guidelines for performing a comprehensive intraoperative multiplane TEE. J Am Soc Echocardiogr. 1999;12:884-900)

❏ MAJOR CLINICAL APPLICATIONS

Source of Embolism

According to the 2011 ASE appropriateness criteria, TEE evaluation for cardiovascular source of embolic event in a stroke patient with no identified noncardiac source is considered highly appropriate (score 7/9). Up to 15–20% of ischemic strokes may be on the basis of an intracardiac source. Transesophageal echocardiography (TEE) has been found to be superior to TTE in detecting cardiac sources of embolism and may also be a more cost-effective approach in their detection. The yield of TEE is higher in patients with clinical cardiac disease.

Masses

Left atrial thrombus is commonly associated with atrial fibrillation and rheumatic mitral stenosis. It may be seen in up to 27% of patients with chronic atrial fibrillation (Fig. 41). Left ventricular thrombus occurs in approximately 5% of patients with acute myocardial infarction, particularly when the infarct is anterior in location. It is also seen in about 4% of patients with dilated cardiomyopathy; these patients also have an even greater risk of developing left atrial thrombus. Prosthetic valves may develop thrombus, especially mechanical valves in the atrioventricular position, in the setting of subtherapeutic anticoagulation. Thrombi may display high-risk characteristics for embolization, which include large size, protruding appearance, high mobility, and central echolucency.

Aortic atherosclerotic plaques are associated with hypertension and are more common in elderly patients. Plaques may be categorized as simple or complex with the latter being more prone to thromboembolization. Features of complex atheromas include a wall thickness greater than 4 mm, ulceration, mobility, pedunculation, and echolucency (Fig. 42).

Vegetative lesions are readily identified in patients with clinical features of infective endocarditis (Fig. 43). Vegetation size greater than 1 cm, vegetation mobility and mitral location are all risk factors for systemic embolization. Additionally, TEE permits visualization of perivalvular abscess in patients with infective endocarditis.

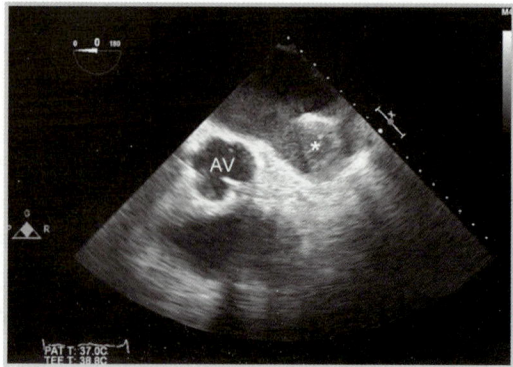

FIGURE 41: Transesophageal echocardiography (TEE) showing a left atrial appendage thrombus (depicted by the asterisk) in a patient with chronic atrial fibrillation. Note the presence of smoke in the left atrium. (Abbreviations: LA: Left atrium; AV: Aortic valve)

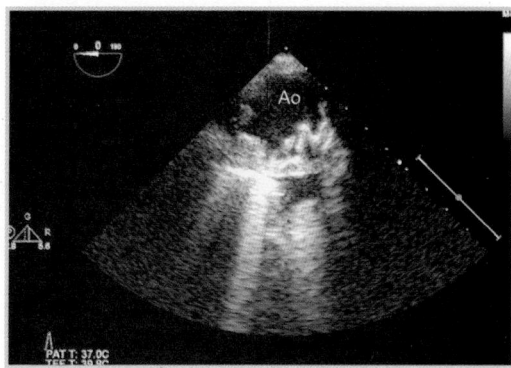

FIGURE 42: Transesophageal echocardiography (TEE) showing an example of atheroma in the descending aorta. Note the complex appearance of the atheroma with echodense and echolucent areas. (Abbreviation: Ao: Aorta)

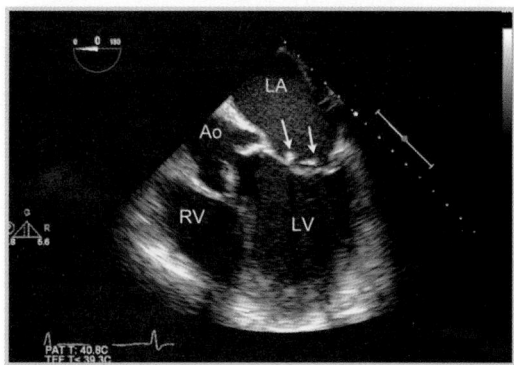

FIGURE 43: An example of vegetations (indicated by the arrows) involving the mitral valve in a patient with infective endocarditis. (Abbreviations: LA: Left atrium; Ao: Aorta; RV: Right ventricle; LV: Left ventricle)

Primary cardiac tumors commonly include myxomas and papillary fibroelastomas. Myxomas are usually benign tumors found in the left atrium attached to the interatrial septum in the region of the fossa ovale (Fig. 44). They may present with embolization greater than 50% of the time.

Passageways for Paradoxic Embolization

Interatrial septal abnormalities are associated with thromboembolic events. Patients with an interatrial shunt may have intermittent right-to-left shunting, particularly if there is a transient increase in right-sided pressure as occurs with coughing or performing a Valsalva maneuver. In this setting, venous thrombi may potentially enter the systemic circulation resulting in paradoxical embolism. Right-to-left shunting may be demonstrated by the administration of intravenous agitated saline contrast. An atrial septal aneurysm is a congenital variant with redundant, mobile, interatrial septal tissue in the region of the fossa with a base measuring 15 mm and an excursion of at least 10 mm during the cardiorespiratory cycle. Atrial septal aneurysms are associated with patent foramen ovale (Fig. 45).

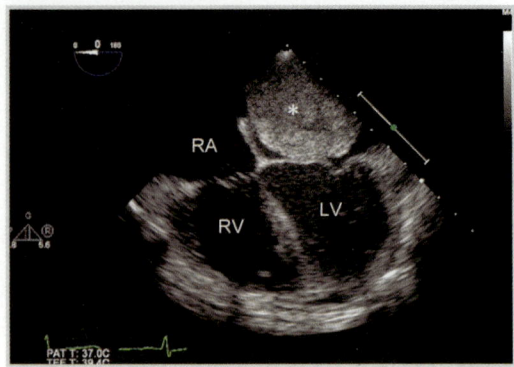

FIGURE 44: An example of a myxoma (depicted by the asterisk) in the left atrium. Myxomas vary in size and sometimes may occupy most of the left atrium. In this case, the tumor impedes the blood flow to the left ventricle during diastole which may lead to hemodynamic instability. (Abbreviations: RA: Right atrium; RV: Right ventricle; LV: Left ventricle)

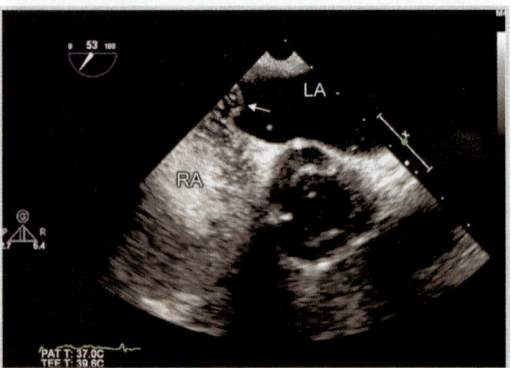

FIGURE 45: Interatrial septal aneurysm (denoted by the arrow) is often associated with a patent foramen ovale demonstrated by a positive bubble study in this patient. (Abbreviations: LA: Left atrium; RA: Right atrium)

Atrial Fibrillation

Atrial fibrillation is associated with a 4–6-fold increased risk of thromboembolism presumably from left atrial appendage thrombi. The conversion of atrial fibrillation to sinus rhythm involves a small risk of clots that may form in the left atrial appendage during or shortly after sinus rhythm restoration. With the advent of TEE, the left atrial appendage can be assessed for the presence of thrombus. This is the basis of a TEE-guided strategy for cardioversion.

Endocarditis

Transesophageal echocardiography has geatly facilitated the diagnosis of endocarditis. It permits improved detection of small vegetations and the identification of coexisting paravalvular abnormalities. Although the procedure is minimally invasive and entails added expense, it has been shown to have higher sensitivity and specificity than TTE and is also better able to assess complications

❏ STRUCTURAL VALVE ASSESSMENT

Transesophageal echocardiography is an ideal technique for visualization of the mitral valve apparatus owing to the proximity of the TEE probe to the left atrium. Mitral valve prolapse (Fig. 46) and flail mitral valve (Fig. 47) are readily assessed by TEE. Another use of TEE is to identify the mechanism and severity of mitral valve regurgitation (Figs 48 and 49). In patients with mitral stenosis in whom a high quality transthoracic echo can be obtained, TEE may not necessarily provide additional information. However TEE is capable of demonstrating high-resolution images of mitral stenosis (Fig. 50).

Transesophageal echocardiography is also a valuable tool for assessment of aortic stenosis (Figs 51 and 52) and aortic regurgitation (Fig. 53).

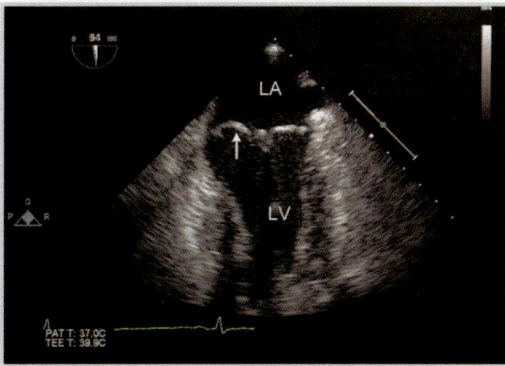

FIGURE 46: A 2-chamber view shows prolapse of the mitral valve posterior leaflet (arrow). (Abbreviations: LA: Left atrium; LV: Left ventricle)

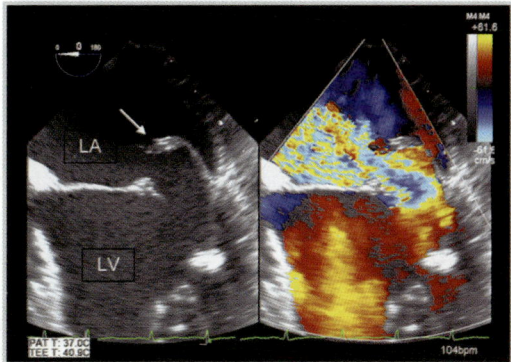

FIGURE 47: Close-up view of mitral valve showing flail posterior leaflet (arrow). The right-sided image demonstrates a regurgitant jet directed anteriorly. (Abbreviations: LA: Left atrium; LV: Left ventricle)

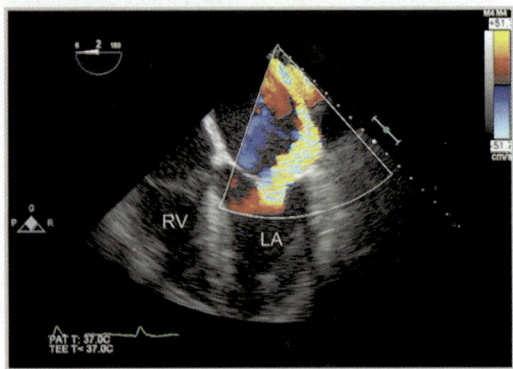

FIGURE 48: A 4-chamber view showing mitral regurgitation. Note the eccentric posteriorly directed MR jet indicating anterior MV pathology

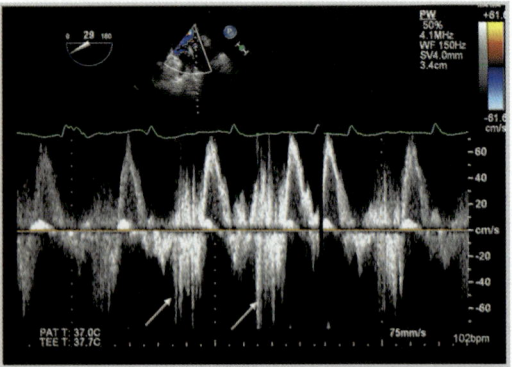

FIGURE 49: Pulmonary vein pulse Doppler imaging recorded from transesophageal echocardiography (TEE) in a patient with mitral regurgitation. Note the systolic flow reversal through the pulmonary vein indicating severe mitral regurgitation

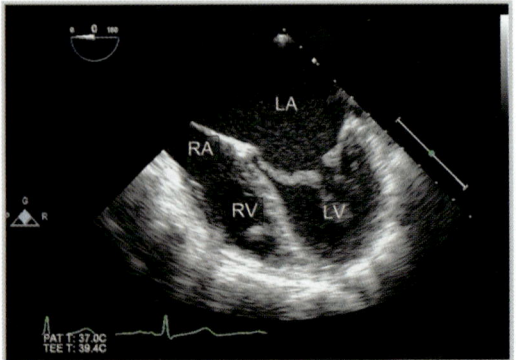

FIGURE 50: A 4-chamber view transesophageal echocardiography (TEE) showing rheumatic mitral stenosis. Note the thickened mitral valve leaflets with restricted mobility. (Abbreviations: LA: Left atrium; RA: Right atrium; RV: Right ventricle; LV: Left ventricle)

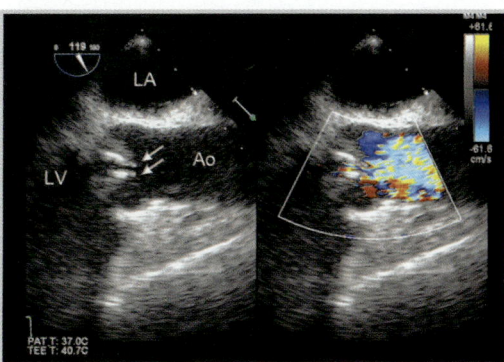

FIGURE 51: A long axis view transesophageal echocardiography (TEE) through the aortic valve from a patient with aortic stenosis. Note the severely restricted aortic valve leaflet mobility (arrows) causing turbulent flow (depicted by color Doppler on the right-sided image). (Abbreviations: LA: Left atrium; LV: Left ventricle; Ao: Aorta)

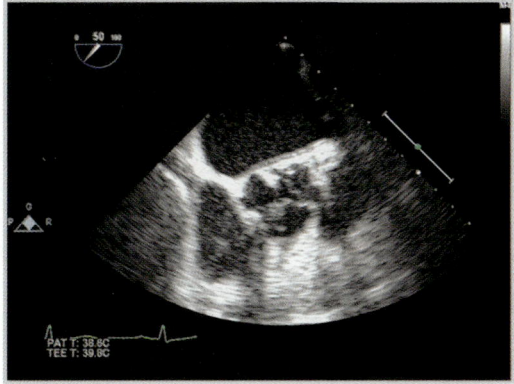

FIGURE 52: A short axis view of aortic valve in a patient with aortic stenosis showing restricted aortic valve leaflet mobility

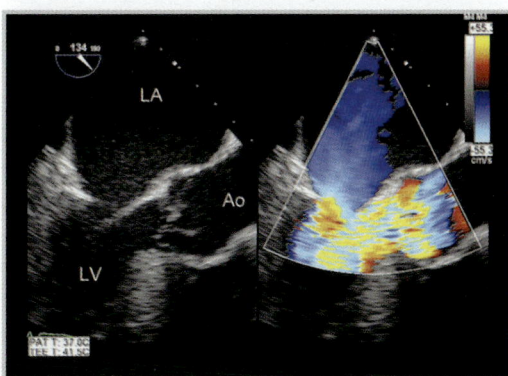

FIGURE 53: A 3-chamber view transesophageal echocardiography (TEE) showing long axis of the aortic valve with severe aortic insufficiency. (Abbreviations: LA: Left atrium; LV: Left ventricle; Ao: Aorta)

The valvular structures on the right side of the heart being positioned anteriorly (in the far field of view from the TEE probe) are less conducive to assessment by TEE. However, the tricuspid valve in most cases can be assessed fairly accurately in transgastric view. Four-chamber view is suitable for diagnosis of tricuspid regurgitation (Fig. 54). Pulmonary valvular abnormalities are relatively rare and not necessarily easier evaluated by transesophageal echocardiography.

❏ ACUTE AORTIC DISSECTION

Transesophageal echocardiography has significant advantages over magnetic resonance imaging (MRI) or computed tomography (CT) in the assessment of acute aortic dissection. It may be rapidly performed at the bedside of patients who are unstable for transport to MRI or CT suites. The characteristic finding in patients with an aortic dissection is the identification of an intimal flap (Figs 55 and 56). Furthermore, the location and extent of the flap as well as

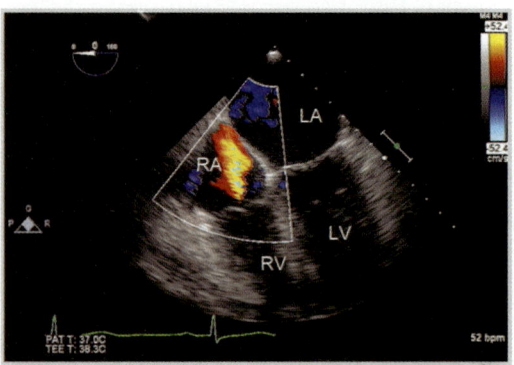

FIGURE 54: A 4-chamber view TEE showing tricuspid regurgitation. (Abbreviations: LA: Left atrium; RA: Right atrium; RV: Right ventricle; LV: Left ventricle)

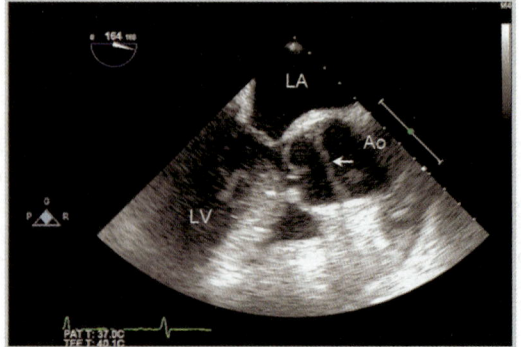

FIGURE 55: A 3-chamber view transesophageal echocardiography (TEE) demonstrating type A aortic dissection. The arrow denotes the dissection flap. (Abbreviations: LA: Left atrium; Ao: Aorta; LV: Left ventricle)

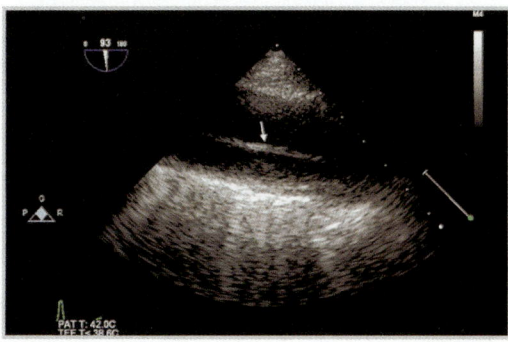

FIGURE 56: Longitudinal view of the descending aorta demonstrating type B aortic dissection. The arrow indicates the dissection flap

entry and exit points may be well delineated by TEE. Additional pertinent findings on TEE would include the aortic diameter, presence of thrombus in the false lumen, presence of a pericardial effusion, presence of aortic regurgitation, or involvement of branch vessels or coronary arteries. An aortic intramural hematoma is characterized by thickening of the aortic wall greater than 7 mm and may be either crescentic or circular in nature with evidence of an intramural accumulation of blood. A penetrating atherosclerotic ulcer may be identified as an ulcerlike projection into an aortic intramural hematoma, usually in the descending aorta. These entities may coexist with an aortic dissection, and they are managed in a similar fashion.

❏ PROCEDURAL ADJUNCT OR INTRAOPERATIVE TRANSESOPHAGEAL ECHOCARDIOGRAPHY

Transesophageal echocardiography is commonly used as an adjunct to fluoroscopic imaging during interventional procedures in the cardiac catheterization laboratory. In patients with significant right-to-left shunting, percutaneous closure of an atrial septal defect or patent foramen ovale is an attractive alternative to open surgical repair. Transesophageal echocardiography offers the advantage of real time imaging of the interatrial septum as well as the surrounding structures, the closure device and catheters. The atrial septal defect size may be measured by TEE for selection of the appropriate closure device (Fig. 57). The position and deployment of the device is also guided by TEE. Further, the adequacy of closure of the defect and the detection of potential complications may be determined with TEE. Transesophageal echocardiography is also used to guide many aspects of mitral balloon valvuloplasty. It may be used for patient selection, guidance of transseptal puncture, exclusion of left atrial appendage thrombus, and wire and balloon positioning. It is also used to assess for potential complications of the procedure, including atrial septal defect, worsening mitral regurgitation, or cardiac tamponade and may shorten procedural and fluoroscopic times. Intraoperative TEE is increasingly performed for the evaluation of the mitral valve during surgical repair. A comprehensive examination of the mitral valve can accurately guide the surgeon.

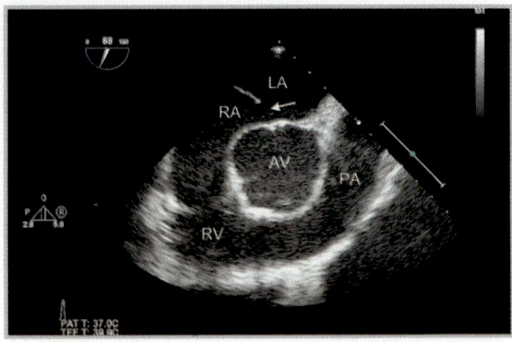

FIGURE 57: Short-axis view through aortic valve demonstrating a defect in interatrial septum (depicted by the arrow), which represents an example of secundum atrial septal defect. (Abbreviations: LA: Left atrium; RA: Right atrium; RV: Right ventricle; PA: Pulmonary artery; AV: Aortic valve)

❏ CONCLUSION

Transesophageal echocardiography provides significant complementary information to TTE. Although semiinvasive in nature, it is generally safe when performed by appropriately trained operators. It may be rapidly performed at the bedside of critically ill patients. In some clinical applications, it is superior to TTE, such as the detection of left atrial appendage thrombus, vegetations, aortic dissection and prosthetic mitral valve function. Transesophageal echocardiography will likely continue to expand in its application with future technologic advancements including 3D echocardiography.

❏ SUGGESTED READINGS

Bayer AS, Bolger AF, Taubert KA, et al. Diagnosis and management of infective endocarditis and its complications. Circulation. 1998;98:2936-48.

Frazin L, Talano JV, Stephanides L, et al. Esophageal echocardiography. Circulation. 1976;54: 102-8.

Hisinaga KHA, Nagata K, Yoshida S. A new transesophageal real time two-dimensional echocardiographic system using a flexible tube and its clinical application. Pro Jpn Soc Ultrasonics Med. 1977;32:43-4.

Keren A, Kim CB, Hu BS, et al. Accuracy of biplane and multiplane tranesophageal echocardiography in diagnosis of typical acute aortic dissection and intramural hematoma. J Am Coll Cardiol. 1996;28:627-36.

Peterson GE, Brickner E, Reimold SC. Transesophageal echocardiography. Clinical indications and applications. Circulation. 2003;107:2398-402.

Sengupta PP, Khandheria BK. Transesophageal echocardiography. Heart. 2005;91(4):541-7.

Side CD, Gosling RG. Non-surgical assessment of cardiac function. Nature. 1971;232:335-6.

2.9 Cardiovascular Nuclear Medicine— Nuclear Cardiology

❏ INTRODUCTION

The primary advantage of nuclear medicine methods is their ability to image physiology. Nowhere is this more apparent and valued than in their cardiac applications. Stress single photon emission computed tomography (SPECT) perfusion studies are performed for the diagnosis, localization, and risk stratification of coronary artery disease (CAD). With its growing availability of positron emission tomography (PET) myocardial perfusion studies are increasingly applied. The field is invigorated by new instrumentation, new acquisition, processing, and display hardware and software, new stress testing (ST) and imaging agents, and the integration of computed tomographic methods.

❏ MYOCARDIAL PERFUSION IMAGING

Image Acquisition Protocols

Protocols for ST with exercise, regadenoson, adenosine, dipyridamole and dobutamine have been established. The imaging protocols, whether one or two day, applying ^{99m}Tc-based sestamibi or tetrofosmin or combined radiotracers, performed in the sequence of rest versus stress or the reverse, are varied and may be individualized to the patient and. Adding low level exercise to vasodilator stress appears to reduce background image activity but adds nothing to diagnostic accuracy. Each protocol has its advantages and disadvantages.

Image Display

The perfusion image display divides the left ventricular (LV) myocardium into 17 or 20 segments, which may be grouped to represent the distribution of the three coronary arteries on a polar map of regional LV activity. An objective 5-point semi-quantitative scoring system is applied in each segment to grade the severity and together, the extent, of regional and global myocardial perfusion defects.

Gated Myocardial Perfusion Imaging

^{99m}Tc-based perfusion tracers permit a high injected dose and allow acquisition of gated studies with adequate count statistics in each of 8 or 16 frames. Gated studies and their assessment of LV systolic function add to the ability of the perfusion method to risk stratify CAD where decremental left ventricular ejection fraction (LVEF) with stress, raises dramatically the prognostic risk related to any image perfusion defect. The "partial volume effect" produces intensity changes linearly related to myocardial wall thickening, the basis for accuracy in the measurement of percent wall thickening on gated perfusion images (Figs 58).

Interpretation

Myocardial perfusion imaging presents a map of regional myocardial perfusion. Normal images are rarely the result of artefacts, but abnormal images are not uncommonly based in artefact. The polar map objectively identifies and compares areas of reduced activity to a normal gender matched normal control set. However,

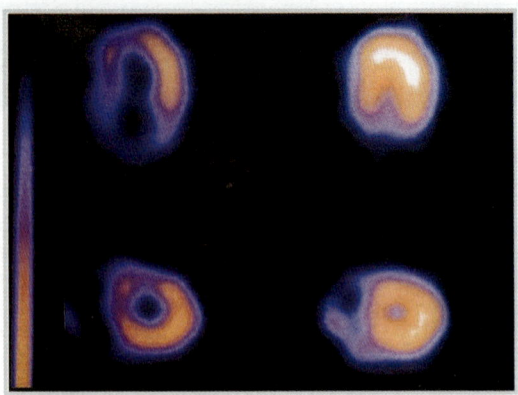

FIGURE 58: Gated sestamibi imaging. Shown are end-diastolic (left) and end-systolic (right) gated ^{99m}Tc-sestamibi perfusion images in a normal heart in selected short (above) and horizontal long axis (below) SPECT slices. Inward systolic motion is evident as well as brightening, or increased intensity during systole. The latter, a result of partial volume effect, is well correlated with myocardial thickening (*Source:* Modified from Botvinick EH, Dae M, O'Connell JW, et al. The scintigraphic evaluation of the cardiovascular system. In: Parmley WW, Chatterjee K (Eds). Cardiology. Philadelphia: JB Lippincott; 1991)

areas of reduced activity unrelated to perfusion may relate to patient motion, attenuation by the breast, chest wall or diaphragm and must be clarified. SPECT attenuation correction (AC) and prone imaging have been used to distinguish such effects and improve diagnostic accuracy. AC methods aid viability evaluation, help overcome ambiguities related to high background activity, aid security in the evaluation of stress only studies, and improve the accuracy of quantitative image parameters. AC is optional for SPECT image acquisition but is mandatory for PET which requires AC to fix the errors introduced by the gross loss of data intrinsic to its 360° acquisition.

Clinical Applications of Myocardial Perfusion Imaging in the Emergency Department—With Acute Chest Pain Syndromes

^{99m}Tc-based myocardial perfusion imaging (MPI) is a useful tool in the triage and evaluation of patients in the acute ED setting. Rest MPI has been shown to be as accurate as serum enzyme analysis for MI diagnosis and has the advantage of speed, where two troponin determinations over 6 hours after chest pain (CP) onset are required to exclude an event. Rest MPI has a high negative predictive value, 99–100%, for the exclusion of acute MI or subsequent cardiac events. Acute rest MPI is especially useful in patients with acute CP and normal or nonspecific rest ECGs. Of course, the full extent of myocardium at ischemic risk is most certainly determined with subsequent stress MPI. The study may remain diagnostic with radionuclide injection as long as 6 hours after cessation of symptoms.

Unstable Angina/Non-ST Elevation Myocardial Infarction

The presence and extent of reversible perfusion defects on MPI is a useful tool in predicting future cardiac events. If no recurrent ischemia or signs of congestive heart failure (CHF) are evident, vasodilator pharmacological stress MPI may be recommended in those patients with unstable angina/non-ST elevation myocardial infarction (UA/NSTEMI) to assess inducible ischemia and help decide whether an early invasive strategy is warranted. For ACS (UA/NSTEMI, STEMI or CP syndrome) with coronary angiogram and stenosis of uncertain significance, MPI can again be helpful in determining the significance of the lesion.

Follow-up after Initial ACS Evaluation Strategy

The initial goal of evaluating patients with suspected ACS and nonischemic ECG results in the ED, through use of either resting MPI or serial cardiac serum markers, is to determine the likelihood of ACS and to stratify patient risk. Subsequent assessment of symptoms and risk usually requires some form of ST. Decisions about the type of stress used (treadmill exercise or pharmacologic stress) and the type of analysis performed (ECG testing alone or ECG testing in conjunction with gated-MPI) can be made based on well-established clinical protocols, such as those outlined in the American College of Cardiology (ACC)/American Heart Association (AHA) Stable Angina Guidelines. It is recommended either that such ST is performed in the ED before the patient is discharged or that the patient is discharged with an appointment for an outpatient stress test within 1 week. A thorough review of this subject was written by Kontos et al.

❏ POSITRON EMISSION TOMOGRAPHY PERFUSION AND METABOLISM

PET and Spect Technology

Compared with SPECT, PET has superior image resolution. A number of factors make it most accurate for CAD diagnosis and prognosis and the index imaging method for assessment of myocardial viability. Major advances in PET technology add to its intrinsic physical advantages over SPECT and have contributed to its rapid growth and current application. Combined PET/CT instruments have proliferated widely for use in oncology making the instrumentation more available and the application of PET MPI possible. Reimbursement makes it practical. PET MPI combined with calcium scoring and CTCA add to its interest among practitioners. PET quantitation of flow reserve adds advantages beyond other methods and raises excitement for the future.

PET tracers are plentiful but suffer from their generally short half-life and their generation in cyclotrons rather than generators. Among PET perfusion agents, only ^{82}Rb is generator produced and available to institutions without a cyclotron. 13N ammonia is cyclotron produced and well applied for flow quantitation. Each has physical, kinetic and flow related advantages beyond ^{99m}Tc-based radiotracers. Single photon emission computed tomography (SPECT) technology is moving rapidly, seeking to equal or surpass the advantages of PET. New instruments, imaging methods and computer software provide new solid state detectors with rapid camera rotation and list mode acquisition.

❏ IMAGING MYOCARDIAL VIABILITY

Principles

When myocardium demonstrates systolic dysfunction, the question of myocardial viability arises. Dysfunctional myocardium may be scarred and beyond salvage, or it may be viable in one of several forms. Viable but dysfunctional myocardium may be ischemic, even in the absence of overt ischemic symptoms or signs, or "stunned" or "hibernating". Dysfunctional but viable myocardium is salvageable and may be restored to function with revascularization; a non inconsequential consideration in patients with systolic dysfunction and severe CHF (Tables 35 to 37). Here, with failure of medical treatment, reversal of dysfunction in extensive "hibernating" areas could be lifesaving and present an important and preferred choice to heart transplantation, which too often is not an available option.

Nonscintigraphic Imaging Options

The improvement of wall motion with low dose dobutamine stress echocardiography is a more subjective noninvasive alternate manner of determining myocardial viability. MRI and delayed (gadolinium) contrast enhancement, indicating scar on MRI, are another alternative methods for viability assessment. However, SPECT and PET methods remain the most frequently applied, best documented, and most trusted methods for determination of myocardial viability. They stand as the comparative gold standard for all other methods and the one to which they aspire.

Table 35: Spectrum of myocardial pathophysiology and viability

Myocardial state	Rest wall motion	Rest/stress perfusion	Metabolism
Normal	Normal	Normal	Normal
Scar	Abnormal	Abnormal—fixed defect	Abnormal
Ischemia	Normal	Abnormal—reversible defect	Normal
Stunned (Transient, post-ischemic dysfunction)	Abnormal	Normal	Normal
Hibernating (dysfunction due to marginal blood supply, serial stunning)	Abnormal	Reversible or fixed defects	Preserved

Table 36: The basis for imaging myocardial viability

Viatility method	Principles
^{201}Tl perfusion imaging/MR contrast enhancement	Membrane integrity
MIBI/Tetrafosmin perfusion imaging	Mitochondrial integrity
Low dose dobutamine/MR imaging	Inotropic contractile response
PET	Preserved metabolism

Table 37: Scintigraphic evidence of myocardial viability and functional reversibility (in the presence of rest wall motion abnormalities and related coronary disease)

- Evidence of preserved perfusion in a dysfunctional segment
- Extensive reversible perfusion abnormalities in a region of abnormal wall motion
- Delayed redistribution of ^{201}Tl in a region with abnormal wall motion
- Post-reinjection ^{201}Tl uptake
- Modest fixed defect in a region with extensive wall motion abnormalities
- PET perfusion-metabolism mismatch
- Evidence of fatty acid uptake (metabolism)

Scintigraphic Imaging Options— Perfusion Related

Most prominent among scintigraphic indicators of viability is the maintenance of regional perfusion. The presence of ^{201}Tl or ^{82}Rb, potassium analogues which enter the cell by energy requiring active transport, or any of the ^{99m}Tc perfusion tracers, which enter viable cells by diffusion, indicates viability. Here, the level of radiotracer uptake is directly proportional to the likelihood of viability and restoration of function after revascularization. ^{201}Tl is initially distributed to the myocardium in proportion to regional flow. With time the intracellular ^{201}Tl distribution parallels intracellular space or viability. These distributions are generally the same, but if viable cells are ischemic at rest, an initial rest related perfusion defect may "fill in" or normalize with time. Delayed ^{201}Tl imaging at 4 and 24 hours or the delayed "reinjection" of a small dose of the radionuclide may normalize perfusion, an indicator of viability. The time to redistribution is directly proportional to the severity of the stenosis and related flow abnormality. Reinjection and related viability detection appear to be augmented with nitroglycerin. Administration of nitrates has been advocated to increase radiotracer uptake and optimize the evaluation of viability with single photon perfusion agents.

Scintigraphic Imaging Options—Metabolism-based

With fasting or with ischemia, myocardial metabolism shifts from its primary metabolite, fatty acids, to glucose. Imaging a radiolabeled analogue of glucose, 18F-deoxyglucose (FDG), which is trapped in the myocyte but not metabolized, remains the noninvasive imaging standard for myocardial viability. Scintigraphically, the density of a perfusion defect at rest has been found proportional to the likelihood of viability. However, even severe PET perfusion defects are roughly divided between those which are and those which are not, viable. Here, viability is determined by evidence of 18F-FDG uptake, revealing a perfusion-metabolism mismatch and indicating active metabolism in the area of underperfusion. Guidelines have been published for application of cardiac PET studies as well as for qualifications to practice cardiac PET.

❏ IMAGING PERFUSION

Rubidium (^{82}Rb) Chloride

Strontium generator produced ^{82}Rb (T 1/2 = 75 sec) is being applied with increasing frequency for pharmacologic stress MPI. Compared with current ^{99m}Tc-based agents it has improved imaging characteristics and better spatial resolution, superior flow linearity, shorter acquisition time with imaging begun at the time of radionuclide administration and completed within 1 hour, more rigorous AC and ready availability. The review of ^{82}Rb PET MPI presented in the PET guidelines notes an overall diagnostic sensitivity of 89% and specificity of 86% for CAD, superior to SPECT MPI. The method is clearly advantageous for use in heavy patients and women where issues of attenuation often cloud interpretation.

Nitrogen (^{13}N) Ammonia

With cyclotron produced ^{13}N ($T_{1/2}$ = 75 sec) ammonia, the longer agent half-life permits the performance of gated exercise MPI. Guidelines have been developed for patient preparation for data acquisition, interpretation and reporting of both 18F-FDG cardiac PET for myocardial viability and for PET perfusion imaging performed with generator produced ^{82}Rb as well as with cyclotron produced ^{13}N ammonia. Future applications with PET/CT scanners could find PET perfusion and CT coronary anatomy fused noninvasively into an image with optimal information content.

❏ RADIATION CONCERNS

When taken in the context of natural background radiation, manmade radiation represents 18% of that delivered. Yet, this is primarily medical in origin and, of course, may be controlled by design and application of diagnostic and therapeutic methods. The seventh report of the National Research Council's Committee on the Biological Effects of Ionizing Radiation (BIER) on the medical effects of low dose ionizing radiation was released in 2005. It assumes a linear dose response relationship between exposure to ionizing radiation and the development of solid and hematologic cancers in humans.

While the public attitudes toward nuclear power as a method of energy generation had recently been mellowed with realization of its benefits, an increased and almost certainly exaggerated concern has emerged with the recent events related to the natural disaster in Japan. Unfair and biased use of this public fear and prejudice by other physicians for their own benefit must not be permitted. The public must be made aware that radiation is a fact of life to which they are exposed constantly with increased exposure at altitude and even when sleeping with their partner. While all accept these as reasonable and even necessary exposures with an acceptable risk, so too are appropriately applied diagnostic nuclear imaging and radiographic methods.

❏ SUGGESTED READINGS

Galvin JM, Brown KA. The site of acute myocardial infarction is related to the coronary territory of transient defects on prior myocardial perfusion imaging. J Nucl Cardiol. 1996;3:382-8.

Hendel RC, Berman DS, Di Carli MF, et al. ACCF/ASNC/ACR/AHA/ASE/SCCT/SCMR/SNM 2009 appropriate use criteria for cardiac radionuclide imaging: a report of the American College of Cardiology Foundation appropriate use criteria Task Force, the American Society of Nuclear Cardiology, the American College of Radiology, the American Heart Association, the American Society of Echocardiography, the Society of Cardiovascular Computed Tomography, the Society for Cardiovascular Magnetic Resonance, and the Society of Nuclear Medicine. J Am Coll Cardiol. 2009;53:2201-29.

Hendel RC, Berman DS, Di Carli MF, et al. Cardiac radionuclide imaging: a report of the American College of Cardiology Foundation Appropriate Use Criteria Task Force, the American Society of Nuclear Cardiology, the American College of Radiology, the American Heart Association, the American Society of Echocardiography, the Society of Cardiovascular Computed Tomography, the Society for Cardiovascular Magnetic Resonance, and the Society of Nuclear Medicine Endorsed by the American College of Emergency Physicians published online May 18, 2009.

Henzlova MJ, Cerqueira MD, Hansen CL, et al. ASNC imaging guidelines for nuclear cardiology procedures, stress protocols and tracers. J Nucl Cardiol [online]. Available from www. onlinejnc. Com .

Little WC, Constantinescu M, Applegate RJ, et al. Can coronary angiography predict the site of a subsequent myocardial infarction in patients with mild to moderate coronary artery disease? Circulation. 1988;78:1157-66.

2.10 Cardiac Computed Tomography

❏ INTRODUCTION

Soon after Sir Godfrey Hounsfield first developed his prototype computed tomography (CT) scanner in the early 1970s, there was interest in imaging the heart. The first scientific report of CT of the heart was in 1976. Reports of EKG-gated image acquisition and the concept of "stop-action" heart imaging occurred in 1977. The first scanners acquired data over several minutes, and image analysis was done overnight by assistance of primitive computer technology. Improvements in technology over the years lead to progressive improvements in image acquisition protocols and dramatic reduction in radiation. Current top of the line scanners can acquire a single phase image of the whole heart within a fraction of a second with radiation dose that is 60–80% less than a standard abdominal or chest CT. Due to progressive improvement in CT technology, both hardware and software, the image acquisition can be done in a few seconds and computerized processing of raw data takes a few minutes resulting in thousands of images covering the whole heart from different parts of the cardiac cycle.

Basic Principles of Computed Tomography

Image acquisition during CT relies on catching X-ray beams as they travel through the body. This requires an X-ray generator and X-ray detector. To produce an axial image or a "slice" of the body, with minimal artifacts, the X-ray beam has to travel through the body at multiple angles, and images are produced from the attenuation pattern of X-rays as they reach the detectors.

X-ray beams are generated identically to X-rays during standard chest X-ray. X-ray generator will produce X-ray beams of differing *energy* [kilovoltage (kV)] profiles and *current* [milliamperes (mA)]. Most commonly used energy profile is 100 or 120 kV based on patient size. Imaging acquisition done simultaneously with multiple energy profiles (ranging 80–140 kV) can allow for better tissue discrimination (e.g. dual energy imaging). The X-ray detectors generate images by the assistance of complex mathematical models calculated by computer, hence the prior nomenclature of computer-assisted tomography or "CAT" scanning. Current high-end CT detectors have multiple rows of detectors that can capture 64–320 slices or images during partial rotation.

In combination with standard reconstruction algorithm using 50% overlapping, the *spatial resolution* can be as low as 0.4 mm. The X-ray detectors generate images by the assistance of complex mathematical models calculated by computer; hence, the prior nomenclature of computer-assisted tomography or "CAT" scanning.

Due to cardiac motion, it is essential to have EKG gating during image acquisition and reconstruction. As images are always acquired with EKG data present and reconstruction of raw data is always done based on the corresponding EKG, it could be stated that all cardiac CT is done with retrospective gating (Table 38). But in general, when referring to prospective or retrospective EKG gating a reference is made to how the X-ray generation is controlled.

❏ CORONARY ARTERY DISEASE

The coronary arteries can be evaluated by CT both with and without contrast. Noncontrast CT is best suited for assessment of coronary calcifications in primary

Table 38: CT protocol terms

General protocol terms	Scan mode	Pitch	Prospective EKG gated X-ray generation	EKG editing	Image reconstruction	When used	Radiation
Retrospective	Helical mode	0.2–0.5	No	Yes	Retrospective	Irregular heart rhythm, e.g. atrial fibrillation	Highest
Dose modulated	Helical mode	0.2–0.5	Yes—Prospective modulation of current (mA)	Yes	Retrospective	Coronary and ventricular function analysis	Intermediate
FLASH or high pitch	Helical mode	3.4	Yes—Prospective during diastole only	No	Retrospective	Coronary analysis when heart rate is below 65 bpm	Lowest
Prospective or step and shoot	Axial mode	1	Yes—Prospective interrupted mode (on and off)	If padding (window) is increased	Retrospective	Coronary analysis when heart rate is below 65 bpm	Lowest
Sequential adaptive	Axial mode	1	Yes—Mix of modulation and interrupted mode	Limited	Retrospective	Coronary analysis when heart rate is below 65 bpm	Low—Intermediate

prevention. Contrast CT angiography is reserved for symptomatic patients primarily to exclude presence of obstructive disease. Patients with previously known coronary disease have less benefit from contrast CT due to blooming artifacts from coronary calcifications.

Noncontrast CT and Coronary Calcifications

Noncontrast CT can estimate atherosclerotic burden but has limited value in predicting coronary stenosis. The magnitude of coronary calcifications correlates well with atherosclerotic burden in histologic studies but not as well with stenosis analysis. Assessment of coronary calcium by CT was first done in the late 1980s and proposal for a quantification method was presented by Agatston et al. in 1990. The Agatston score is generally referred to as "calcium scoring". Other methods to quantify the coronary calcifications are based on volume and but these are not used in clinical practice. In general, Agatston score less than 100 is considered to convey low risk and greater than 300–400 high risk.

Contrast CT and Coronary Angiography

EKG gated contrast enhanced CT is primarily used to exclude the presence of obstructive coronary disease in patients with chest discomfort. Patients with known coronary disease are generally not considered good candidates for CT due to blooming artifacts from coronary calcium that can limit stenosis analysis. Contrast enhanced CT differs from invasive angiography since it not only determines stenosis but also assesses the presence of atherosclerotic plaque and type of plaque similar to intravascular ultrasound (IVUS).

Careful selection of patients for coronary CT is very important to minimize risk to the patient and optimize appropriate use. Due to high sensitivity and high negative predictive value, CT is best suited for symptomatic patients with intermediate or low risk for obstructive coronary disease.

In general, CT is highly sensitive for detection of coronary disease and has the ability to detect disease before a vessel has hemodynamically significant stenosis. CT is able to characterize coronary plaque into—calcified, noncalcified and mixed plaque (mixture of calcified and noncalcified plaque elements). The greatest strength of CT is the low event rate of 0.17–0.37% in patients with a normal coronary CT.

Coronary Stent

Coronary stent evaluation by CT is limited by blooming artifacts. The stent size, design and metal type will have varying effect on artifacts. Stents with diameter greater than 3–3.5 mm are better suited than smaller stents. Asymptomatic patients with stents are not appropriate for cardiac CT.

Coronary Bypass Grafts

Coronary bypass grafts can be evaluated by contrast CT with good results due to large diameter of the grafts and lack of motion. Metal clip artifacts and severe native coronary disease with diffuse coronary calcifications have limited the clinical applicability. As such cardiac CT has limited clinical use in routine evaluation of bypass graft patency.

Anomalous Coronary Arteries

Screening for anomalous coronary vessels with EKG gated contrast CT is considered Class I indication. CT allows for more accurate evaluation of the course of the vessels where exclusion of interarterial course is paramount. The anomalous vessels are of great variety and the course of the proximal portion of each vessel determines the clinical significance.

❏ MYOCARDIUM AND CHAMBERS

There has been progressive improvement in spatial and temporal resolution that allows for accurate assessment of ventricular ejection fraction plus regional systolic wall thickening over time. Due to radiation involved with CT, other techniques, such as echocardiography and magnetic resonance imaging (MRI) are considered first line imaging techniques for assessing the myocardium and chambers. *Dual source* CT scanners have been able to show excellent image quality irrespective of heart rate and during phantom imaging able to assess global function with greater accuracy than MRI. Right ventricular systolic function can also be assessed by CT with equal or better interobserver and intraobserver variability than MRI. Left ventricular ejection fraction measured by CT has prognostic value that can supplement clinical history and coronary findings

Qualitative and quantitative myocardial perfusion analysis can be performed by CT. Combining coronary analysis with myocardial contrast enhancement and wall motion analysis improves accuracy of coronary analysis and is expected to be a cost-effective way of analyzing ischemic heart disease in the future. For image evaluation of myocardial perfusion defects the image settings are different than during coronary evaluation. Additionally increased images thickness (5–10 mm) with average or MinIP has superior contrast to noise ratio compared to MIP and thin slices images.

Current clinical use for detection of myocardial scar by CT is aimed at patients who are not able to undergo MRI due to presence of an ICD. These are typically patients with reoccurring ventricular tachycardia awaiting catheter ablation therapy. In these cases, CT can possibly detect the location of scar by hypoenhancement during the first pass imaging, wall thinning, delayed enhancement and exclude mural thrombus. Additionally the CT images can be used for anatomic mapping for the ablation procedure, similar to common practice of mapping left atrium during ablation of atrial fibrillation. Left ventricular thrombus can be easily accessed by CT and apical thrombus is frequently detected on nongated contrast enhanced CT of the chest.

❏ PULMONARY VEINS

With the advent of radiofrequency ablation for atrial fibrillation, there is an increased need for visualization of the left atrium, left atrial appendage and pulmonary veins. Other imaging modalities, such as transesophageal echocardiography, intracardiac echocardiography and MRI can also delineate these structures. CT is frequently the test of choice due to its widespread availability and the ease of performance. The excellent contrast to noise ratio of CT images makes them well-suited for developing a 3D map of the highly variable anatomy of the left atrium, appendage and pulmonary veins prior to the ablation procedure. Integration of the 3D map with electroanatomic mapping and real-time location of ablation catheters is thought to increase safety and efficacy of the procedure in addition to facilitating shorter periprocedural fluoroscopic time.

❏ CARDIAC VEINS

Cardiac venous anatomy is readily assessed by CT. This requires slight delay of image acquisition time to allow adequate levophase maturation. Cardiac venous anatomy is highly variable and theoretically it could be assessed prior to placement of the left ventricular pacemaker lead.

❏ VALVULAR DISEASE

Evaluation of valves by CT is, in general, done as a byproduct of coronary analysis. Echocardiography remains the gold standard for valvular assessment due to safety, lack of radiation, higher temporal resolution and ability to assess the functional significance of valvular lesions. CT is considered appropriate when the significant valvular dysfunction is suspected and other noninvasive methods are inadequate. Assessment of valves by CT is primarily done by morphologic evaluation, and functional assessment is limited. Estimations of flow by combination of volume and area measurements over time are still investigational and expected to be limited by temporal resolution and assumption of intact integrity of other valves.

❏ PERICARDIUM

Superior spatial resolution of CT allows for excellent visualization and characterization of pericardial pathology. Initial imaging modality for pericardial disease is echocardiography but CT offers advantages over echocardiography in regards to superior spatial resolution, detection of calcification and characterization of adjacent intrathoracic structures. High spatial resolution and separation of myocardium from pericardium by epicardial fat allows for accurate measurements of pericardial thickness.

Malignant Cardiac Neoplasm

Angiosarcomas are malignant and usually arise from the right atrium with associated pericardial or pleural effusions, metastatic lung lesions and right-sided heart failure. On CT, it is often broad-based with heterogeneous enhancement or a low-attenuated mass, which might be nodular or irregular. Myxosarcomas are a rare form of a primary malignant cardiac tumor and very difficult to differentiate from a myxomas on CT. Metastatic cardiac tumors make up the bulk of malignant cardiac tumors. Most of the tumors originate through direct or transvenous invasion from the lungs, breasts, esophagus or other mediastinal tumors. CT findings of metastatic malignant tumors are usually nonspecific.

❏ FUTURE

The future of cardiac CT is very promising. The fast pace of technology has allowed a progressive improvement in CT scanning methods. At current time, we are able to acquire an image of the whole heart within a third of a second and with considerably less radiation than is used by other standard tests, such as SPECT, CT chest, CT abdomen and CT of the head. With progression of technology, we can expect to see better spatial resolution, lower radiation, and better tissue characterization.

❏ SUGGESTED READINGS

Beckmann EC. CT scanning the early days. Br J Radiol. 2006;79:5-8.

Garcia MJ, Lessick J, Hoffmann MH, et al. Accuracy of 16-row multidetector computed tomography for the assessment of coronary artery stenosis. JAMA. 2006;296:403-11.

Gerber TC, Carr JJ, Arai AE, et al. Ionizing radiation in cardiac imaging: a science advisory from the American Heart Association Committee on Cardiac Imaging of the Council on Clinical Cardiology and Committee on Cardiovascular Imaging and Intervention of the Council on Cardiovascular Radiology and Intervention. Circulation. 2009;119:1056-65.

Greenland P, Bonow RO, Brundage BH, et al. American College of Cardiology Foundation Clinical Expert Consensus Task Force (ACCF/AHA Writing Committee to Update the 2000 Expert Consensus Document on Electron Beam Computed Tomography); Society of Atherosclerosis Imaging and Prevention; Society of Cardiovascular Computed Tomography. ACCF/AHA 2007 clinical expert consensus document on coronary artery calcium scoring by computed tomography in global cardiovascular risk assessment and in evaluation of patients with chest pain: a report of the American College of Cardiology Foundation Clinical Expert Consensus Task Force (ACCF/AHA Writing Committee to Update the 2000 Expert Consensus Document on Electron Beam Computed Tomography) developed in collaboration with the Society of Atherosclerosis Imaging and Prevention and the Society of Cardiovascular Computed Tomography. J Am Coll Cardiol. 2007;49:378-402.

Greenland P, Alpert JS, Beller GA, et al. American College of Cardiology Foundation/American Heart Association Task Force on Practice Guidelines. 2010 ACCF/AHA guideline for assessment of cardiovascular risk in asymptomatic adults: a report of the American College of Cardiology Foundation/American Heart Association Task Force on Practice Guidelines. Circulation. 2010;122:e584-636.

2.11 Cardiovascular Magnetic Resonance Imaging

❏ INTRODUCTION

History of magnetic resonance imaging (MRI) for characterization of cardiovascular morphology and function has been one of continuous innovations and refinements for over 25 years. Advancements in device design, image acquisition methodology, and image analysis are rapidly translated into standardized methods for broad application in clinical cardiovascular medicine and cardiovascular research.

Information Provided by Cardiovascular Magnetic Resonance

Morphology, kinematics, and tissue characterization together form the crux of cardiovascular assessment with CMR. Assessments of left and right ventricular volumes and mass are highly reproducible and, when indexed for body habitus, are able to report relatively narrow reference ranges (Table 39). It is important to note, however, that reference ranges depend somewhat upon the specific CMR image acquisition method, and vary by sex and ethnic lineage.

❏ DIAGNOSIS OF EPICARDIAL CORONARY ARTERY STENOSIS

Myocardial infarction caused by flow limitation in epicardial coronary arteries [coronary artery stenosis (CAS)] is responsible for about one-sixth of all deaths in

Table 39: Normal values for CMR using true-FISP acquisition		
	Males*	**Females***
LVEDV (mL)	168.5 ± 33.4	134.9 ± 19.3
LVESV (mL)	60.8 ± 16.0	48.9 ± 10.7
LVSV (mL)	107.7 ± 20.7	86.0 ± 12.3
LVEF (%)	64.2 ± 4.6	64.0 ± 4.9
LV Mass (g)	133.2 ± 23.9	90.2 ± 12.0
LV EDV/BSA (mL/m^2)	82.3 ± 14.7	77.7 ± 10.8
LV Mass/BSA (g/m^2)	64.7 ± 9.3	52.0 ± 7.4
LV EDV/HT (mL/m)	95.0 ± 17.3	82.6 ± 10.9
LV Mass/HT (g/m)	75.1 ± 12.3	55.3 ± 7.0
RVEDV (mL)	176.5 ± 33.0	130.6 ± 23.7
RVESV (mL)	79.3 ± 16.2	52.3 ± 9.9
RVSV (mL)	97.8 ± 18.7	78.3 ± 16.9
RVEF (%)	55.1 ± 3.7	59.8 ± 5.0
RV EDV/BSA (mL/m^2)	86.2 ± 14.1	75.2 ± 13.8
RV EDV/HT (mL/m)	99.5 ± 16.9	80.0 ± 14.2

*mean ± SD
(Abbreviations: LV: Left ventricle; RV: Right ventricle; EDV: End-diastolic volume; ESV: End-systolic volume; SV: Stroke volume; EF: Ejection fraction; BSA: Body surface area; HT: Height; true-FISP: True fast imaging with steady-state precession)
(*Source:* Alfakih, Plein S, Thiele H, et al. Normal human left and right ventricular dimensions for MRI as assessed by turbo gradient echo and steady-state free precession imaging sequences. J Magn Reson Imaging. 2003;17:329-9, with permission)

the United States. Since myocardial infarction and sudden cardiac death (SCD) are often not preceded by intractable symptoms, a diagnostic armamentarium has been developed for the purpose of detecting disease in the epicardial coronary arteries.

❏ ASSESSMENT OF GLOBAL AND REGIONAL LEFT VENTRICULAR FUNCTION AT REST AND DURING INOTROPIC STRESS

Ischemia is detected when the increased myocardial oxygen demand induced by inotrope infusion exceeds its supply, resulting in a wall motion abnormality. Assessment of global and regional left ventricular systolic function during stepped infusion of the inotrope dobutamine has emerged as the CMR method most widely employed for detection of CAS. Optimal diagnostic sensitivity is achieved when heart rate is raised to greater than or equal to 85% of predicted maximum, which often requires coadministration of the muscarinic blocker atropine.

❏ MYOCARDIAL PERFUSION IMAGING

Adenosinergic drugs cause vasodilation in coronary resistance vessels. In the presence of flow-limiting epicardial coronary stenosis, resistance arteries will be at least partially dilated at rest in order to maintain normal myocardial perfusion. During vasodilator stress, then, the incremental increase in tissue perfusion will be diminished in regions subserved by a stenotic epicardial vessel, compared to regions subserved by nonstenotic epicardial vessels, forming the basis for recognition of CAS. A comprehensive CMR evaluation, which includes perfusion assessment during adenosine stress provides incremental prognostic information, over and above consideration of routine clinical variables.

❏ CARDIOVASCULAR MAGNETIC RESONANCE CORONARY ANGIOGRAPHY

The CMR is useful to identify the origin and proximal course of the coronary arteries for the purpose of confirming or rejecting the presence of anomalies (Figs 59A and B). The CMR has been employed to identify the presence of coronary aneurysms in patients with Kawasaki disease. Coronary artery bypass graft patency can be ascertained with high diagnostic accuracy.

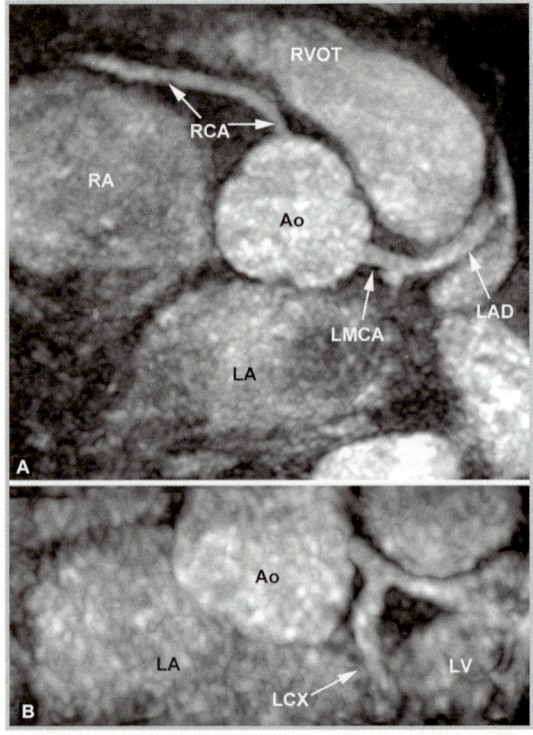

FIGURES 59A AND B: Free-breathing True-FISP 3-D coronary angiogram from a young man with chest pain, dyspnea, abnormal ECG, and elevated serum cardiac troponin-T. The origins and courses of the proximal coronary arteries are normal, effectively ruling out coronary anomaly as the etiology of the patient's clinical findings (Abbreviations: Ao: Aorta; RA: Right atrium; LA: Left atrium; RVOT: Right ventricular outflow tract; LV: Left ventricle; LMCA: Left main coronary artery; LAD: Left anterior descending coronary artery; LCX: Left circumflex coronary artery; RCA: Right coronary artery) (*Source:* Alan H. Stolpen, MD, PhD, Department of Radiology, University of Iowa Carver College of Medicine)

❑ DILATED CARDIOMYOPATHY

Dilated cardiomyopathy (DCM) is the most common cause of heart failure, and the most frequent reason for referral for heart transplantation or mechanical cardiac assist device implantation. Applications of established CMR methods can be useful in decision-making in selected patients with DCM.

Coronary Artery Stenoses

In patients presenting with systolic heart failure due to DCM, it is incumbent upon the clinician to ascertain the presence or absence of flow-limiting coronary artery stenoses (CAS). As noted above, CMR can be useful for identifying patients with DCM due to CAS. The unique ability of CMR to depict the transmural extent of ischemic scar allows accurate prediction of functional recovery after successful revascularization, and directly influences prognosis in patients with ischemic DCM.

The CMR is emerging as the diagnostic procedure of choice for identification of myocarditis in patients presenting with incident left ventricular dysfunction. The CMR localization of myocardial inflammation has been found to improve the diagnostic yield of endomyocardial biopsy in some, but not all, studies.

❑ HYPERTROPHIC CARDIOMYOPATHY

Hypertrophic cardiomyopathy (HCM) is a leading cause of sudden death in young people and in competitive athletes. Cellular hypertrophy with myocyte disarray and increased interstitial collagen are histopathologic hallmarks of the disease. Clinical manifestations include diastolic heart failure, arrhythmic and neurogenic syncope and SCD. Since sudden death commonly occurs in the absence of intractable symptoms, risk stratification algorithms have been proposed and are in continuous evolution.

The CMR can offer higher diagnostic sensitivity for HCM than echocardiography. This is more often the case when the left ventricular region of hypertrophy occurs in a location other than the basal interventricular septum, or when visualization of the heart with echocardiography is suboptimal. The CMR can provide diagnostic certainty in such cases, where the clinical suspicion of apical HCM is high. In some cases, CMR can be useful to definitively discriminate between apical HCM and left ventricular noncompaction (LVNC). In patients with HCM, there is frequently involvement of the RV, a finding of uncertain clinical significance.

The CMR can be helpful in elucidating the risk profile in individual patients. In addition to higher diagnostic sensitivity for the disease itself, Rickers et al. reported that CMR identified patients with wall thickness greater than 3 cm in 10% of cases where echocardiography did not.

HCM is associated with functional abnormalities of the microcirculation, which may correlate with its clinical course. Abnormalities of myocardial energetics can be ascertained in patients with HCM, and often precede onset of symptoms.

❑ RESTRICTIVE CARDIOMYOPATHY

Restrictive cardiomyopathy (RCM) comprises a diverse set of conditions, which often entail a long period of clinical latency, followed by progressive cardiac dysfunction and death due to refractory heart failure or SCD. The CMR can be useful for discriminating between the two conditions. Constrictive pericarditis is readily identified using methods described below. In a patient with a clinical diagnosis of heart failure, CMR provides quantitative corroboration of the salient features of restrictive cardiomyopathy early in the course of disease—normal or decreased left ventricular end-diastolic volume, normal or increased left ventricular mass, preserved or only mildly decreased left ventricular ejection fraction.

In addition to morphologic and functional data, CMR can identify expansion of the extracellular space—a common finding in restrictive cardiomyopathy caused by amyloidosis, Fabry's disease, sarcoidosis, and hypereosinophilic syndromes. Iron overload states represent a special case for the diagnosis of restrictive cardiomyopathy. Clinically important levels of iron deposited in myocardium can sufficiently alter the local CMR signal so as to be diagnostic.

❏ CARDIOVASCULAR MAGNETIC RESONANCE-GUIDED THERAPY

In some cases, e.g. hypereosinophilia, therapeutic decisions are guided by routine clinical assessments and laboratory testing. In other cases, longitudinal CMR studies can help optimize management of chronic conditions responsible for restrictive cardiomyopathy.

Plasma cell dyscrasias can cause restrictive cardiomyopathy via deposition of immunoglobulin components in myocardium—a form of amyloidosis. The CMR can identify the extent of cardiac amyloidosis in such patients, along with critical cardiac function data, which guide therapy. The CMR is useful for identification of thalassemia major patients at risk of heart failure due to iron overload, and longitudinal CMR studies are useful to determine efficacy of chelation therapy.

❏ VALVULAR HEART DISEASE

Echocardiography, via transthoracic or transesophageal approaches, is most often the procedure of choice for assessment of the morphology of the cardiac valves. The CMR studies usually require compilation of image data over multiple cardiac cycles, in order to achieve sufficient signal-to-noise ratios—a requirement not ideally suited to visualization of thin structures exhibiting complex motion during the cardiac cycle. "real-time" CMR techniques have been applied, but do not generally offer improved valve visualization compared to best-quality echocardiographic images.

The CMR can be useful for assessment of valve morphology and function when echocardiographic images are suboptimal but is more often utilized to characterize the impact of valve disease upon cardiac chamber morphology and function.

❏ DISEASES WITH RIGHT VENTRICULAR PREDOMINANCE

Right ventricular morphology and function are often altered in patients with left ventricular disease. In addition, a number of conditions exert preferential effects on the RV, with relative sparing of the LV. The superior quantitative accuracy of CMR characterizations of right ventricular volumes and mass facilitate evaluation with a high degree of confidence. In addition, techniques capable of quantitating through plane blood velocity (velocity encoding) provide useful information in cases where left and right ventricular stroke volumes are unequal, and where there is significant valvular regurgitation.

Intracardiac Shunt

In adults with intracardiac shunting of blood, clinical decision-making and prognosis depend critically upon right ventricular morphology and function. The shape of the RV defies simple characterization, which creates difficulty in obtaining quantitative assessments with techniques, such as echocardiography, which acquire images on only a few planes.

The CMR provides quantitative evaluation of intracardiac shunting utilizing three complementary and corroborative methods: (i) ventriculographic comparison of left and right ventricular stroke volumes, (ii) calculation of stroke volumes in the main pulmonary artery and ascending aorta by means of velocity encoding techniques, and (iii) calculation of volumetric flow in the shunt itself using velocity encoding techniques.

Pulmonary Artery Hypertension

Primary pulmonary hypertension is a progressive disease of resistance arteries in the lungs, in the absence of a systemic disease known to affect pulmonary artery pressure. Secondary pulmonary hypertension can develop as a complication of diverse disease processes—collagen vascular disorders, pulmonary embolism, congenital malformations of the heart or great vessels, cor pulmonale, or mass effects.

Although advanced 3D echocardiographic techniques are under development to address this need, CMR methods continue to serve as the reference standard for such methods, and CMR yields superior reproducibility with lower interobserver bias.

❏ MISCELLANEOUS CONDITIONS

Cardiac Thrombi

The diagnosis of LV mural thrombus is usually based on clinical suspicion and confirmation of characteristic findings on echocardiography. More recently, CMR has been shown to provide increased diagnostic accuracy in patients at high-risk for mural thrombus and consequent systemic embolization. The CMR has diagnostic accuracy similar to transesophageal echocardiography for detection of left atrial appendage mural thrombi and is less invasive.

Cardiac Masses

The CMR can be useful to discriminate between solid-tissue cardiac masses and mural thrombi. Information regarding tissue character and vascularity augment decisions about treatment and prognosis.

Pericardial Disease

The CMR is a useful adjunct for assessment of pericardial disease and its functional consequences. The CMR can estimate pericardial effusion. However echocardiography is the imaging technique of choice and clinical application of CMR for the diagnosis and management of pericardial effusion is limited. However, CMR can be used to assess pericardial thickness in patients with suspected constrictive pericarditis.

❑ SUGGESTED READINGS

Bonow RO, Carabello BA, Kanu C, et al. ACC/AHA 2006 guidelines for the management of patients with valvular heart disease: a report of the American College of Cardiology/American Heart Association Task Force on Practice Guidelines (writing committee to revise the 1998 Guidelines for the Management of Patients With Valvular Heart Disease): developed in collaboration with the Society of Cardiovascular Anesthesiologists: endorsed by the Society for Cardiovascular Angiography and Interventions and the Society of Thoracic Surgeons. Circulation. 2006;114:e84-231.

Hunt SA, Abraham WT, Chin MH, et al. 2009 focused update incorporated into the ACC/AHA 2005 Guidelines for the Diagnosis and Management of Heart Failure in Adults: a report of the American College of Cardiology Foundation/American Heart Association Task Force on Practice Guidelines: developed in collaboration with the International Society for Heart and Lung Transplantation. Circulation. 2009;119:e391-479.

Malm S, Frigstad S, Sagberg E, et al. Real-time simultaneous triplane contrast echocardiography gives rapid, accurate, and reproducible assessment of left ventricular volumes and ejection fraction: a comparison with magnetic resonance imaging. J Am Soc Echocardiogr. 2006;19:1494-501.

Ridgway JP. Cardiovascular magnetic resonance physics for clinicians. J Cardiovasc Magn Reson. 2010;12:71.

Rodgers GP, Ayanian JZ, Balady G, et al. American College of Cardiology/American Heart Association Clinical Competence Statement on Stress Testing. A Report of the American College of Cardiology/American Heart Association/American College of Physicians-American Society of Internal Medicine Task Force on Clinical Competence. Circulation. 2000;102:1726-38.

Tandri H, Daya SK, Nasir K, et al. Normal reference values for the adult right ventricle by magnetic resonance imaging. Am J Cardiol. 2006;98:1660-4.

2.12 Molecular Imaging of Vascular Disease

❑ INTRODUCTION

With the discovery of new molecular targets and pathways that both expand our knowledge base and refine classical teachings, there is an ongoing role for technological advances to illuminate these areas by offering improved diagnostic and therapeutic clinical tools. Molecular imaging aims to capitalize on these advances by employing small molecules and nanoparticles, which are coupled with imaging agents to visualize cellular and molecular events in living subjects, complementing clinical, anatomical and physiological imaging modalities.

❑ MOLECULAR IMAGING MODALITIES

A wealth of different imaging modalities have been utilized for cardiovascular molecular imaging, each of which offers certain advantages and limitations as outlined in (Table 40). Factors of importance include sensitivity, spatial and temporal resolution, depth penetration, scan time, radiation exposure and cost among others. Compared to other applications, such as cancer detection, cardiovascular molecular imaging also poses significant additional difficulties due to cardiac and respiratory motion artifacts for myocardial imaging, small vessel size for coronary plaque detection, and competing signals from adjacent blood flow.

Of the imaging strategies in current clinical practice, superparamagnetic nanoparticles for magnetic resonance imaging (MRI) and 18F-fluorodeoxyglucose

Table 40: Comparison of small animal molecular imaging modalities

Technique	Resolution	Depth	Sensitivity	Scan time	Multi-channel	Agents	Clinical
Computed tomography (CT)	50 µm	Unlimited	+	Seconds to minutes	Yes	Iodine moieties	Yes
Magnetic resonance imaging (MRI)	10–100 µm	Unlimited	++	Minutes to hours	Yes	Paramagnetic and magnetic particles	Yes
Contrast-enhanced ultrasound (CEU)	50 µm	Centimeters	++	Seconds to minutes	No	Microbubbles	Yes
Single photon emission computed tomography (SPECT)	0.3–1 mm	Unlimited	+++	Minutes	Dual	Radiolabeled compounds (^{99m}Tc, ^{111}In, ^{131}I, ^{67}Ga, ^{201}Tl)	Yes
Positron emission tomography (PET)	1–2 mm	Unlimited	+++	Seconds to minutes	No	Radiolabeled compounds (^{18}F, ^{64}Cu, ^{11}C, ^{68}Ga)	Yes
Bioluminescence imaging (BLI)	3–5 mm	Millimeters	+++	Seconds to minutes	Multiple	Luciferase, luminol	Potential
Fluorescence reflectance imaging (FRI)	1 mm	Millimeters	+++	Seconds to minutes	Multiple	Fluorophores, photoproteins	Yes
Fluorescence mediated tomography (FMT)	1 mm	Centimeters	++	Minutes	Multiple	Near-infrared fluorophores	Developing
Intravital microscopy	1 µm	Micrometers	++	Seconds to hours	Multiple	Fluorophores, photoproteins	Developing

+ millimolar or less; ++ micromolar; +++ nanomolar or greater

(FDG) for positron emission tomography (PET) provide illustrative examples of the technical tradeoffs inherent to all of the different modalities. Imaging strategies, such as 18FDG-PET, offer high sensitivity of detection but relatively poor spatial resolution.

Combinatory use of multiple imaging modalities into hybrid imaging strategies is frequently utilized to overcome the limitations of a single imaging platform. Other molecular imaging modalities include contrast-enhanced ultrasound imaging with ligand-coated microbubbles and optical imaging strategies that utilize fluorescence (intravital microscopy, fluorescence molecular tomography, intravascular catheter-based imaging) and bioluminescence reporter gene imaging.

❏ MOLECULAR IMAGING OF VASCULAR DISEASE PROCESSES

With an ever growing armamentarium of molecular imaging probes available for use and in development, there has been extensive growth of molecular imaging applications in vascular disease. High-priority areas include atherosclerosis, thrombosis, aneurysmal disease and vascular injury. While most molecular imaging probes are in preclinical testing and development phases, and only a few agents that are FDA approved are present, this balance is likely to shift significantly in the coming years with the translation of these new emerging agents into the clinical arena.

Atherosclerosis

Atherosclerotic vascular disease, fueled by lipid deposition, endovascular inflammation and leukocytic infiltration of the vessel wall, is an important and well-studied focus of molecular imaging studies. Atherosclerosis is a top priority within molecular imaging, with the goal of early detection and preventative treatment of lipid-rich "vulnerable" plaques that have the highest likelihood to rupture, resulting in an acute coronary syndrome, peripheral arterial occlusion or cerebrovascular accident.

From a clinical perspective, there are presently two major platforms for atherosclerosis detection, 18FDG-PET imaging and ultrasmall superparamagnetic iron oxide (USPIO) nanoparticle-enhanced MRI, both of which can identify inflammatory foci in larger caliber arteries, such as the carotid, aorta, and femoral beds.

Inflammation

Large arteries (e.g. carotid, aorta, and iliofemoral): Infiltration of the vessel wall with leukocytes in atherosclerosis predominantly composed of the key effector cells monocytes and macrophages, represent tissue sites of active inflammation and vessel remodeling.

Ultrasmall superparamagnetic iron oxide: Clinical ultrasmall superparamagnetic iron oxide (USPIO) are magnetic nanoparticles composed of a 3 nm superparamagnetic iron oxide core that induce MRI tissue contrast by strongly influencing local signals in T2- and T2*-weighted images. To allow sufficient tissue accumulation and blood pool washout of nonspecific circulating signal, MRI is performed 24–36 hours following USPIO injection and the images are collected over 1–2 hours. Due to its T2 relaxation effects, USPIO are detected as dark "negative" reductions in MRI signal.

18F-Fluorodeoxyglucose: The other major clinical atherosclerosis molecular imaging platform features 18FDG-PET. 18FDG is a glucose analogue that becomes concentrated within metabolically active cells where it emits positrons (110 minute half life) for detection by clinical PET scanners. Intracellular concentration of 18FDG occurs following active transport of the agent into the cytosol through normal glucose transport pathways where it becomes trapped upon phosphorylation by the enzyme hexokinase. Compared to USPIO-enhanced MRI, 18FDG-PET is significantly more sensitive but must be coupled with coregistered CT (or other anatomical modality) to provide the high degree of spatial resolution required to enable precise tissue localization, which exposes the patient to additional ionizing radiation.

Coronary arteries: Coronary atherosclerotic plaque imaging is highly challenging due to the small size of the vessels, the motion of surrounding myocardium during systole and diastole, as well as respirophasic variations. To overcome these challenges, imaging modalities must have both high spatial and temporal resolution, as well as high sensitivity, a combination not easily found in a single entity.

18FDG: While 18FDG targeted imaging of coronary arterial plaques is limited by high background signal from the adjacent highly metabolically active myocardium, there is recent evidence that noninvasive coronary molecular imaging may be possible with 18FDG-PET/CT utilizing a specialized myocardial suppression protocol where patients consumed a high fat and low carbohydrate meal, the night before the study, and then drank a vegetable oil formulation on the morning of the study.

Molecular CT imaging: Macrophages can be targeted with N1177, an iodinated nanoparticle CT contrast agent dispersed with surfactant. Given the excellent spatiotemporal resolution of modern multidetector CT imaging systems, already in clinical use for coronary artery imaging and the potential to discriminate atherosclerotic plaque constituents, such as calcium versus fibrous tissue or lipid, the addition of molecular targeted imaging agents, such as N1177 to coronary CT assessment, offers heightened ability to identify high-risk macrophage-laden coronary atherosclerotic plaques that may prove future use in preventing ischemic events.

NIRF imaging: Intravascular molecular imaging technologies are also being advanced, exemplified by the development of a prototype intravascular catheter that allows real time, high resolution *in vivo* NIRF sensing of atherosclerotic plaque through flowing blood. Evaluation in atherosclerosis-laden rabbit iliac arteries, of similar size to human coronary vessels, was performed after intravenous administration of a cysteine protease-activatable NIRF imaging agent (ProSense750) that can detect vascular inflammation.

Macrophages: A lipid-based gadolinium MRI probe shows strong affinity for the macrophage scavenger receptor-B (CD36), to enable noninvasive positive contrast MRI of plaque macrophages.

Proteases: There is also a particular focus on detecting enzymatic activity as a marker of active inflammatory changes and tissue destruction. In addition to cathepsin protease imaging, MMPs are frequently pursued targets on multiple platforms including an NIRF protease activity sensor, a positive-contrast gadolinium chelate p947 for MRI and the radionuclide SPECT tracers ^{111}In-RP782 and ^{99m}Tc-MMP.

Adhesion molecules: Endothelial surface glycoprotein receptors upregulated during inflammation, such as VCAM-1, E-selectin and P-selectin, have also been targeted using phage-display derived VCAM-1 specific nanoparticles, coated microbubbles for contrast-enhanced ultrasound, iodine-containing liposomes conjugated to a receptor binding peptide with CT, microparticles of iron oxide and 18F-labeled small affinity ligand.

Oxidative Stress

The oxidation of phospholipids in atheroma contributes to the activation and recruitment of monocyte/macrophages and the production of enzymes, such as MMP, that degrade local tissue strength thus destabilizing plaque constituents. Detection of proinflammatory oxidative products by noninvasive molecular imaging may provide prospective information on the risk of individual plaques for future events or on the efficacy of therapeutics. Enzymatic detection agents for myeloperoxidase (MPO), a macrophage-derived product, have been evaluated by blue light bioluminescence using a small molecule luminol that activates fluorescence when oxidizing species are present, as well as by MRI with the gadolinium agent bis-5HTDTPA(Gd).

Neovascularization

New vessel formation occurs during states where growth factors, such as vascular endothelial growth factor (VEGF) and others, are released stimulating endothelial and other supporting cells to create new blood channels. Endothelial cells organizing into interconnected vascular tubes and networks are anchored to extracellular matrix proteins in part through expression of the $\alpha_V\beta_3$ integrin surface receptor, a common target for neovascularization molecular imaging studies. A number of promising agents have been preclinically tested, including many agents for integrin $\alpha_V\beta_3$, which can be detected by the peptide sequence RGD or RGD mimetics. Noninvasive plaque angiogenesis imaging was initially shown with paramagnetic integrin $\alpha_V\beta_3$-targeted agents for MRI.

Apoptosis

Programmed cell death or apoptosis contributes to weakening of the fibrous cap via smooth muscle cell loss and facilitates expansion of the unstable lipid-filled necrotic core. Molecular signaling markers can identify cells destined for apoptotic demise, via annexin protein binding to exposed phosphatidylserine residues or via components of the caspase enzyme family that activate and execute the apoptotic cascade. The most widely utilized annexin-based imaging agents for apoptosis detection are high sensitivity SPECT-based tracers, such as ^{99m}Tc-annexin and ^{111}In-annexin, and can be combined with other readouts such as 18FDG-derived inflammation or MMP presence. In a limited number of patients with transient ischemic attacks scheduled for carotid endarterectomy, ^{99m}Tc-annexin A5 SPECT imaging has illuminated the relationship between apoptotic activity and carotid plaque instability

Calcification

Vascular calcification is increasingly linked to chronic vascular inflammation, likely representing the terminal phase of inflammatory lesions. In atherosclerosis, microcalcifications within plaques portend a greater risk for rupture and on a larger scale global coronary calcium scoring correlates with risk of future cardiovascular events. Currently available probes include optical agents, such as fluorescently labeled enzymes substrates that identify the bone mineral component hydroxyapatite.

The mechanism of bone mineral deposition in atherosclerotic calcification has been explored in molecular imaging studies of hypercholesterolemic mice with surgically induced renal failure to accelerate osteogenesis by using multichannel intravital fluorescence molecular imaging with a fluorescent quenched substrate for cathepsin S (CatS) and an optical bone mineral targeting agent (osteosense).

Thrombosis

Molecular imaging of key thrombus-associated molecules and cells has the potential to biologically refine anatomical imaging methods, such as ultrasound or CT. Moreover, molecular imaging strategies may provide additional guidance into optimal therapeutic strategies to treat fibrin-rich or platelet-rich thrombi. Other advantages include the ability to replace invasive thrombosis imaging strategies with noninvasive options. For example, intracardiac thrombus formation, as may occur in the atrial appendage from atrial fibrillation, often requires transesophageal echocardiography for diagnosis. Another clinical arena of importance is arteriolar thrombosis syndromes, where flow-based diagnostic methods may be limited due to spatial resolution and possibly nephrotoxic contrast material and radiation exposure.

Outlook

Molecular imaging studies are yielding unparalleled *in vivo* insight into clinical aspects of vascular disease, including atherosclerosis, thrombosis, aneurysm formation and vascular injury. Clinical development of high-yield molecular imaging agents and the development of coronary-artery targeted imaging systems remain top priorities for the field. Preclinically, the emphasis remains on developing new highly sensitive, multifunctional/multimodal imaging agents with excellent safety and pharmacokinetic profiles. For molecular imaging to integrate into routine clinical practice, clear utility beyond functional and anatomical imaging will need to be established. In the near term, molecular imaging will likely assess the biological effects of new pharmacotherapies aimed to mitigate vascular disease. Thereafter, molecular imaging should improve the risk stratification and the clinical management of many vascular disease states.

❏ SUGGESTED READINGS

Burke AP, Farb A, Malcom GT, et al. Coronary risk factors and plaque morphology in men with coronary disease who died suddenly. N Engl J Med. 1997;336:1276-82.

Graebe M, Pedersen SF, Borgwardt L, et al. Molecular pathology in vulnerable carotid plaques: correlation with [18]-fluorodeoxyglucose positron emission tomography (FDG-PET). Eur J Vasc Endovasc Surg. 2009;37:714-21.

Jaffer FA, Libby P, Weissleder R. Molecular imaging of cardiovascular disease. Circulation. 2007;116:1052-61.

Sanz J, Fayad ZA. Imaging of atherosclerotic cardiovascular disease. Nature. 2008;451:953-7.

2.13 Cardiac Hemodynamics and Coronary Physiology

❑ INTRODUCTION

The first living human cardiac catheterization was performed in 1929 by a German surgical resident physician, Werner Forssmann, when he inserted a urological catheter into his own antecubital vein, passed it to his right atrium, and then walked to the X-ray room to document the position of the catheter in his heart. Forssmann later won the Nobel prize for his contributions to physiology and medicine.

❑ CARDIAC CATHETERIZATION—THE BASICS

Proper cardiac diagnosis and disease management relies on accurate hemodynamic data acquisition. Traditionally, the transducer is placed at the mid-chest level by dividing the patient's anterior-posterior chest diameter by two. To optimize confidence in data, the clinician should be astute to recognize artifacts that affect data integrity. The catheter, loose equipment connections, transducer, or amplifier and gain settings may create artifacts in pressure waveforms. Catheter kink or blood, contrast media, or air in the catheter can result in reduced pressure transmission and overdampening of the pressure waveform (Figs 60A to C).

Cardiac catheterization is a relatively safe procedure, however, knowledge of the relative contraindications and possible complications of cardiac catheterization are important in assessing the risks and benefits of the procedure (Tables 41 and 42). Furthermore, risk assessment must be performed on an individual basis as the risks associated with each procedure will vary based on the patient's comorbidities.

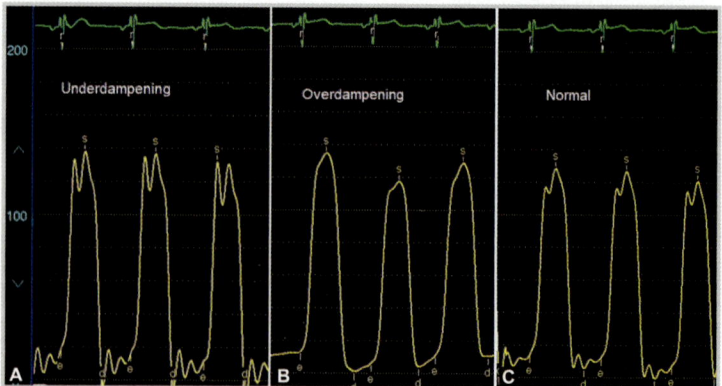

FIGURES 60A TO C: Left ventricle pressure waveform (A) Underdampening of pressure waveforms results when either excessive catheter movement or air bubble oscillations produce artifacts in peaks and dips of the pressure waveform, with falsely elevated systolic pressure and low diastolic pressure; (B) Catheter kink or blood, contrast media, or air in the catheter can result in reduced pressure transmission and overdampening of the pressure waveform, with smooth contour of the waveform; (C) Normal waveform (Abbreviations: s: systolic; d: diastolic; e: end-diastolic pressure)

Table 41: Risks of cardiac catheterization and coronary angiography*

Complication	Risk (%)
Mortality	0.11
Myocardial infarction	0.05
Cerebrovascular accident	0.07
Arrhythmia	0.38
Vascular complications	0.43
Contrast reaction	0.37
Hemodynamic complication	0.26
Perforation of heart chamber	0.03
Other complications	0.28
Total of major complications	1.70

*Number of patients = 59,792

Source: Scanlon PJ, Faxon DP, Audet AM, et al. ACC/AHA guidelines for coronary angiography: A report of the American College of Cardiology/American Heart Association Task Force on Practice Guidelines (Committee on Coronary Angiography). J Am Coll Cardiol. 1999; 33:1760.

Table 42: Relative contraindications to coronary angiography

- Acute renal failure
- Chronic renal failure secondary to diabetes
- Active gastrointestinal bleed
- Unexplained fever that may be due to infection
- Untreated active infection
- Acute stroke
- Severe anemia
- Severe uncontrolled hypertension
- Severe symptomatic electrolyte imbalance
- Severe lack of patient cooperation, due to psychological or severe systemic illness
- Severe concomitant illness that drastically shortens life expectancy or increases risk of therapeutic intervention
- Patient refusal to consider definitive therapy such angioplasty or coronary artery bypass graft or valve surgery
- Digitalis intoxication
- Documented anaphylactoid reaction to angiographic contrast media
- Severe peripheral vascular disease limiting vascular access
- Decompensated congestive heart failure or acute pulmonary edema
- Severe coagulopathy
- Aortic valve endocarditis

Source: Scanlon PJ, Faxon DP, Audet AM, et al. ACC/AHA guidelines for coronary angiography: A report of the American College of Cardiology/American Heart Association Task Force on Practice Guidelines (Committee on Coronary Angiography). J Am Coll Cardiol. 1999; 33:1760-1.

Right Heart Catheterization

Right heart catheterization is performed for assessment of right heart pressures, pulmonary arterial and pulmonary arterial wedge pressure (PAWP), which estimates left atrial pressure and to calculate resistance of systemic and pulmonary vascular beds. This information is useful in studying conditions, such as valvular heart disease, cardiac shunts, heart failure, and pulmonary hypertension and to establish the etiology of shock.

❑ CARDIAC CYCLE PRESSURE WAVEFORMS

Atrial Pressures

The right atrial pressure tracing exhibits "a" and "v" waves that reflect an increase in the atrial pressure with atrial contraction and filling during ventricular systole, respectively. The "a" wave is followed by a "c" deflection that results from closure of the tricuspid valve during isovolumetric ventricular contraction. During the x-descent, the atrium relaxes with a decline in pressure. The y-descent following the "v" wave reflects atrial emptying after opening of the tricuspid valve (Fig. 61).

Ventricular Pressures

In the absence of valve stenosis, systolic pressures of the right and left ventricle pressure equal those of the pulmonary artery and aorta, respectively. Ventricular diastolic pressures are dependent on myocardial compliance, which is inversely proportional to the slope of the pressure-volume curve. Wall thickness, volume, ischemia and medications affect myocardial compliance by altering the pressure-volume curve. Impaired myocardial compliance results in a "stiffer" chamber and elevation of ventricular end-diastolic pressure.

Left ventricle end-diastolic pressure (LVEDP) is approximately equal to left atrial and PAWP. During left heart catheterization, LVEDP is usually measured using a pigtail catheter placed in the left ventricle. However, if more accurate pressure recordings are required, a high-fidelity manometer can be used instead of a fluid-filled catheter.

LVEDP is measured on the left ventricular pressure tracing at a point just prior to isovolumetric contraction and immediately after the "a" wave of the PAWP tracing. LVEDP also corresponds to the "R" wave of the electrocardiogram tracing (Fig. 62).

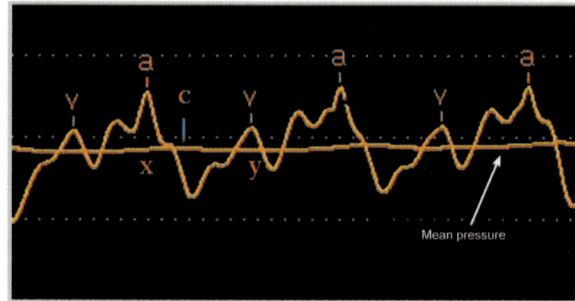

FIGURE 61: Right atrial pressure waveform. The "a" and "v" waves that reflect an increase in the atrial pressure with atrial contraction and filling during ventricular systole, respectively. The "c" deflection results from closure of the tricuspid valve during isovolumetric ventricular contraction. The atrium relaxes with a decline in pressure during the x-descent and the y-descent occurs during atrial emptying. Left atrial pressure waveform is similar to the right atrium but with increased amplitude of the "a" and "v" waves.

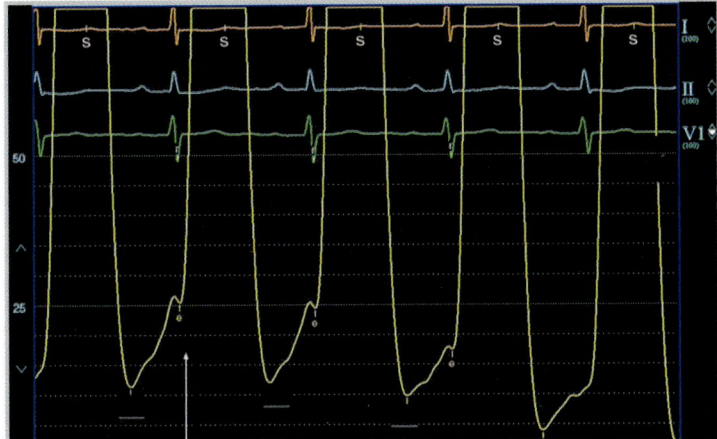

FIGURE 62: Identification of left-ventricle end diastolic pressure. Left ventricle pressure (yellow) and ECG leads tracing. LVEDP corresponds to the "R" wave of the electrocardiogram tracing. LVEDP may also be measured at a point just prior to isovolumetric contraction and immediately after the "a" wave of the PAWP tracing (Abbreviation: e: end-diastolic pressure)

❑ HEMODYNAMICS IN VALVULAR HEART DISEASE

Aortic Stenosis

Valvular AS is most often due to calcific degeneration of the valve seen in the elderly population. Young adults with AS often have a congenital malformation of the valve that contributes to the development of AS. AS may also be supravalvular or subvavular. Current guidelines discourage invasive hemodynamic evaluation of aortic stenosis when noninvasive findings regarding the severity of aortic stenosis by echocardiography are unequivocal. Invasive evaluation is reserved for situations in which there is a discrepancy between echocardiographic findings and patient's symptoms.

Hemodynamic measurements in AS reveal a gradient between the systolic aortic and the left ventricular pressures (Fig. 63).

Aortic Regurgitation

Although characterization of aortic regurgitation (AR) by echocardiography is often adequate, aortic angiography provides further information on aortic root size and qualitative information on regurgitation of blood across the aortic valve in to the left ventricle. Aortic angiography is performed with a multi-side-hole catheter positioned just above the sinus of Valsalva in the left anterior oblique projection and a power injector is used to inject contrast. AR is graded on a scale of 1–4:

Grade 1 (mild) minimal contrast opacifies the left ventricle
Grade 2 (moderate) opacification of entire left ventricular
Grade 3 (moderately severe) dense opacification of left ventricle over sequential cardiac cycles and
Grade 4 (severe) dense opacification of entire left ventricle in one cardiac cycle (Fig. 64).

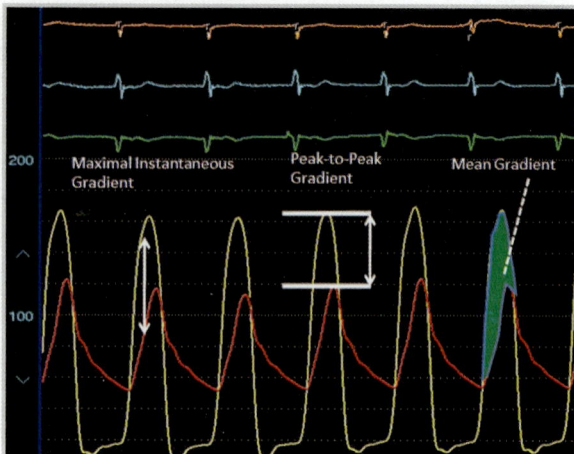

FIGURE 63: Aortic-left ventricular systolic gradient in aortic stenosis. Maximal instantaneous gradient is the maximum pressure gradient between the aorta (red) and left ventricle (yellow) at a single point in time. Peak-to-peak gradient is the absolute difference between peak aortic systolic pressure and peak left ventricular systolic pressure. Mean gradient is defined by the area between the systolic left ventricular and aortic hemodynamic tracings (green shaded area)

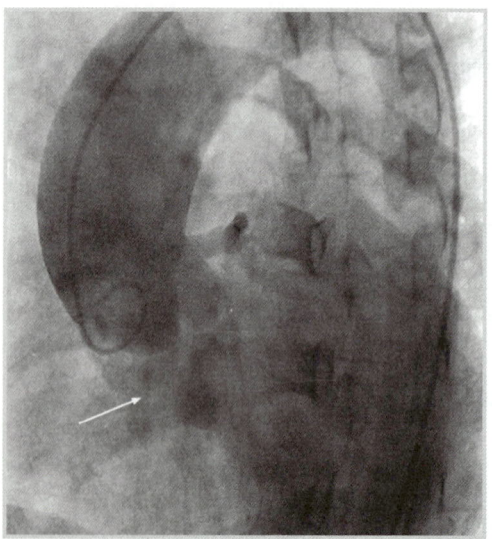

FIGURE 64: Aortic regurgitation on aortic angiography. Aortogram performed with pigtail catheter in the aorta demonstrating grade 2 aortic regurgitation, with moderate opacification of the left ventricle

The pathophysiology and cardiac hemodynamics of acute and chronic AR are different. Recognizing the different patterns in the LVEDP and pulse pressure aid in making this distinction and are described below.

Chronic Aortic Regurgitation

As blood volume regurgitates from the aorta to the left ventricular chamber in diastole, arterial diastolic pressure falls. As the severity of AR worsens, the left ventricular end-diastolic volume also increases. An increased left ventricular ejection volume results in augmented arterial systolic pressure. Therefore, the pulse pressure increases as is evident on the aortic pressure waveform. Hemodynamically significant AR results in a bisferiens pulse, which is a double peak of the aortic systolic contour separated by a mid-systolic dip.

Increased wall stress from a chronically volume overloaded left ventricular chamber results in eccentric hypertrophy. The compliance of the left ventricular eventually begins to deteriorate and results in a modest rise in the LVEDP along with an increased slope of the ventricular diastolic waveform.

Acute Aortic Regurgitation

Acute AR may result from aortic dissection involving the aortic root, trauma, or valve perforation from endocarditis. Unlike chronic AR, an increase in the aortic pulse pressure may not be as impressive acutely due to the absence of both an increased ventricular ejection velocity and decreased systemic vascular resistance. Pulsus alternans may be evident on the aortic pressure waveform with beat-to-beat variation in systolic amplitude due to variations in myocardial contraction strength.

Mitral Stenosis

Hemodynamic assessment of mitral stenosis (MS) requires simultaneous right and left cardiac catheterization. Mean gradients by Doppler methods and valve area by planimetery, may be obtained by echocardiography. During valvuloplasty, resolution of the mitral valve gradient and the undesirable development of mitral regurgitation are monitored by hemodynamics.

Measurement of the mean mitral valve gradient is made by the diastolic area difference between the left atrial and the left ventricular diastolic pressure waveforms (Fig. 65).

PAWP approximates left atrial pressure and may be used as a surrogate to limit the risk associated with transeptal puncture. However, since the PAWP waveform is delayed 40–120 msec with respect to the left atrial pressure waveform, the tracing should be phase shifted so that the peak of the PAWP "v" wave is placed on the downslope of the left ventricular pressure tracing.

Mitral Regurgitation

Disruption of any component of the mitral valve apparatus may result in regurgitation of blood from the left ventricle to the atrium during systole. 2D-echocardiography provides anatomical information on mitral valve structures and Doppler calculations quantify mitral regurgitation (MR). Left ventriculography provides a qualitative assessment of mitral incompetence, which is performed using a pigtail catheter with side-holes in the 30 degrees right anterior oblique projection using 30 mL of contrast at a rate of 10 mL/second. Severity of MR on ventriculography is graded on a scale of 1–4:

Grade 1 (mild) contrast partially opacifies the left atrium
Grade 2 (moderate) complete yet faint opacification of left atrium
Grade 3 (moderately severe) opacification of left atrium and left ventricle are comparable
Grade 4 (severely) dense opacification of complete left atrium in one beat.

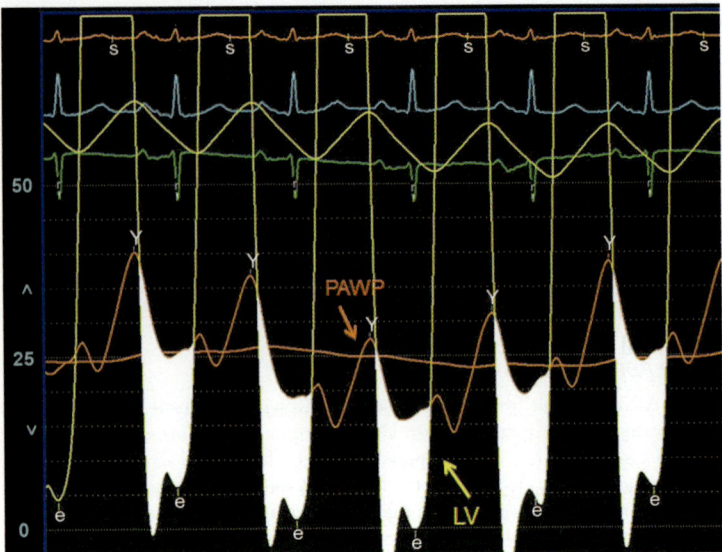

FIGURE 65: Mitral stenosis, diastolic gradient. Mean mitral valve gradient is determined by the diastolic area difference between the pulmonary arterial wedge pressure (PAWP) tracing in orange and left ventricle (LV) pressure tracing in yellow

Pulmonic Stenosis

Pulmonic stenosis (PS) is rare and most often congenital in etiology. PS may be valvular, supra- or subvalvular. Echocardiography can be useful in identifying the location of the stenosis and quantifying the gradient. Right ventriculography to evaluate PS may be performed with a pigtail or Berman catheter.

Catheter pullback from the pulmonary artery to the right ventricle quantifies and locates the obstruction. Quantification of the gradient may also be performed by a double lumen catheter or placement of catheters in the pulmonary artery and right ventricle simultaneously. A gradient across the pulmonic valve of greater than 50 mm Hg indicates severe PS and lesser than 25 mm Hg indicates mild PS. Diastolic pressures provide important diagnostic information to identify the location of the obstruction.

Pulmonic Regurgitation

Minimal pulmonic regurgitation (PR) is present in normal individuals. Significant PR may be due to processes involving the pulmonic valve or secondary to pulmonary hypertension. Significant PR results in a widened pulmonary arterial pulse pressure. A rapid rise in the right ventricular diastolic pressure is evidenced with an elevated RVEDP approaching pulmonary arterial diastolic pressure.

Pulmonary arteriography is of limited value as a catheter across the pulmonic valve causes PR itself. Therefore, echocardiography has greater utility in defining the severity and characteristics of the PR jet.

Tricuspid Stenosis

Tricuspid stenosis (TS) is rare, yet when present, may be congenital in etiology or secondary to rheumatic or carcinoid heart disease. Doppler and 2D echocardiography provide useful information on valve gradient and area, as well as other coexisting valvular heart disease. Hemodynamic tracings reveal elevated right atrial pressure with blunted y-descent due to impairment of right ventricular filling. Simultaneous catheters in the right atrium and right ventricle demonstrate the presence of a discrete diastolic gradient between the right atrium and ventricle. A mean gradient greater than or equal to 5 mm Hg across the tricuspid valve suggests hemodynamically significant TS. Varying degrees of tricuspid regurgitation almost always accompanies TS due to leaflet restriction and incomplete coaptation.

Tricuspid Regurgitation

Trace tricuspid regurgitation (TR) is present in normal patients without consequence due to the complex closure of the tricuspid valve leaflets. Doppler and 2D-echocardiography provide information on jet severity and direction, hepatic vein systolic flow reversal, right ventricular size, valve morphology, and the presence of pulmonary hypertension. A negative jet on right atrial angiography or contrast reflux across the tricuspid valve with right ventriculography provides a qualitative assessment of TR.

Hemodynamic tracing of right atrial pressure demonstrates a large "v" wave. However, it is important to note that the height of the "v" wave is also dependent on right atrial size and compliance. Thus, the absence of a tall "v" wave does not exclude the diagnosis of severe tricuspid regurgitation.

❏ HEMODYNAMICS IN CARDIOMYOPATHY

Cardiomyopathy of any cause is usually associated with changes in cardiac hemodynamics, including elevation of end-diastolic pressures in the affected ventricle(s), reduced cardiac output, reduced mixed venous oxygen saturation, and elevated atrial pressures. In more advanced cardiomyopathy, pulsus alternans may be observed, and it signifies ventricular dysfunction.

Hypertrophic Obstructive Cardiomyopathy

Hemodynamics in left ventricular cavitary obstruction is amongst the most interesting in diagnostic catheterization. Variants of hypertrophic obstructive cardiomyopathy (HOCM) exist and not all patients with hypertrophic cardiomyopathy have an obstructive component. Likewise, not all patients with intracavitary obstruction have HOCM. For example, myocardial infarction or Takosubo's cardiomyopathy may alter myocardial contractility and generate an intracavitary gradient. When present, the intracavitary obstruction can be localized in the apex, mid-cavity or outflow tract of the left ventricle. Ventriculography provides a visual assessment of cavitary obliteration during systole.

Restrictive Cardiomyopathy

Restrictive cardiomyopathy (RCM) results from infiltrative myocardial diseases as well as other rare conditions. Direct myocardial involvement of an infiltrative process results in reduced myocardial compliance and biventricular diastolic dysfunction, often with preserved systolic function.

| Table 43: Sensitivity and specificity of hemodynamic parameters in constrictive pericarditis |

	Constrictive pericarditis	Restrictive cardiomyopathy	Sensitivity (%)	Specificity (%)
LVEDP-RVEDP*	≤5 mm Hg	>5 mm Hg	60	38
Pulmonary artery systolic pressure	<55 mm Hg	>55 mm Hg	93	24
Right ventricular systolic and EDP	>1/3	≤1/3	93	38
Respiratory variation in mean right atrial pressure	Absent	Present	93	48
Left ventricular diastolic rapid filling wave	>7 mm Hg	≤7 mm Hg	93	57
Ventricular interdependence	Present	Absent	100	95

(Abbreviations: *LV: Left ventricle; RV: Right ventricle; EDP: End-diastolic pressure). (*Source:* Hurrell DG, Nishimura RA, Higano ST, et al. Value of dynamic respiratory changes in left and right ventricular pressures for the diagnosis of constrictive pericarditis. Circulation. 1996; 93:2007-13)

Evaluation of hemodynamics in RCM is performed by right heart catheterization to assess right atrial, right ventricular, pulmonary artery, and PAWPs. Simultaneous catheters in the right and left ventricles allow analysis of the change in ventricular pressures during the respiratory cycle and help distinguish RCM from constrictive pericarditis; ventricular interdependence that occurs in constrictive pericarditis is not seen in RCM.

Biventricular diastolic pressures in RCM are elevated and often near equal within 5 mm Hg. However, since left ventricular involvement exceeds that of the right ventricle, LVEDP is greater than RVEDP. The ventricular diastolic tracing has a characteristic "dip-and-plateau" or "square-root sign" configuration due to abrupt cessation of ventricular filling followed by a restriction to further filling from impaired relaxation of the ventricle. Pulmonary artery pressures in RCM are generally high and may exceed 55 mm Hg.

Restrictive cardiomyopathy and constrictive pericarditis share many similar properties. However, distinguishing the two conditions is extremely important, as the treatment for the latter is surgical pericardiectomy. Several hemodynamic parameters to better distinguish these conditions have been evaluated (Table 43). Perhaps the most reliable is respirophasic concordance in RCM; left and right ventricular pressures follow normal physiologic properties with a decrease in systolic pressure during inspiration and increase in expiration.

❑ HEMODYNAMICS IN PERICARDIAL DISEASE

The pericardium consists of visceral and parietal layers separated by a minimal amount of serous fluid, and extends to cover the heart and great vessels, excluding a portion of the left atrium and pulmonary veins. This anatomical relationship is important in understanding the physiology and hemodynamics of constrictive pericarditis.

Constrictive Pericarditis

In constrictive pericarditis, a rigid thickened pericardium uncouples the pericardial and cardiac pressures from intrathoracic pressures; the variations in pressures with the respiratory cycle are no longer transmitted. Thus, producing an inspiratory increase in jugular venous pressure, also known as Kussmaul's sign. The right atrial

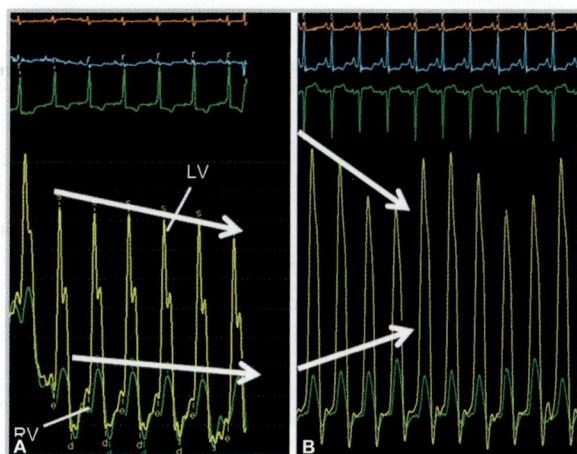

FIGURES 66A AND B: Respirophasic waveforms in (A) restrictive cardiomyopathy with ventricular concordance of right and left ventricle pressures with a parallel change in right ventricle (RV) and left ventricle (LV) pressures (arrows). (B) Constrictive pericarditis demonstrating ventricular discordance of the right and left ventricle pressures

pressure tracing reveals a steep y-descent due to rapid filling in early diastole. A prominent "a" wave during atrial contraction occurs due to elevated pressure, followed by a blunted x-descent secondary to impairment in ventricular filling; resulting in an "M" configuration of the right atrial pressure tracing.

The rigid pericardium impairs the ventricular compliance and diastolic pressures are elevated and near equal. Intrathoracic pressures are transmitted to the pulmonary veins and a portion of the left atrium not encased by the pericardium. However, the pressure of the pericardial bound left ventricle does not vary with intrathoracic pressure as a result of the dissociation from pericardial pressures in constrictive pericarditis. Thus, the effective filling gradient across the mitral valve is decreased in inspiration. With the reduced left ventricular volume and elevated right ventricular diastolic pressure, the interventricular septum shifts to the left. Ventricular interdependence or discordance during the respirophasic cycle is demonstrated by simultaneous catheters in the right and left ventricles (Figs 66A and B).

Cardiac Tamponade

Between the visceral and parietal layers of the pericardium, there is the pericardial space that normally contains less than 35 mL of plasma ultrafiltrate, or pericardial fluid. Normal pericardial pressure is between 5 and 5 mm Hg.

The hemodynamics of cardiac tamponade shares similarities to constrictive pericarditis, with an elevation and near equalization of diastolic pressures. Right atrial pressure is elevated, however, unlike constrictive pericarditis, a blunted y-descent is present on the right atrial pressure waveform in cardiac tamponade. Unlike constrictive pericarditis, the dip-and-plateau configuration of the diastolic ventricular pressure tracing is not seen in cardiac tamponade. This is due to the lack of sudden restriction to filling.

❏ CORONARY HEMODYNAMICS

Coronary angiography provides information on luminal contrast opacification and visual estimation of luminal diameter stenosis often dictates whether coronary intervention is performed. Based on the angiographic views and plaque characteristics, such as eccentricity, angiography may not capture the area of maximal stenosis.

Fractional Flow Reserve

Fractional flow reserve (FFR) is a physiologic coronary study performed percutaneously at the time of coronary angiography to detect ischemia-producing stenoses. FFR is calculated as the ratio of mean coronary artery pressure distal to the coronary lesion of interest at maximal hyperemia to the mean aortic pressure.

A FFR of lesser than 0.75 correlates with ischemia when compared to non-invasive stress testing with a sensitivity of 88% and specificity of 100%. Interestingly, the largest study to date using FFR to guide percutaneous intervention in patients with multivessel disease, found that using FFR lesser than 0.8 to guide decision making reduced the primary endpoint of death, nonfatal myocardial infarction and repeat revascularization.

Coronary Flow Reserve

Similar to FFR, coronary flow reserve (CFR) is a physiologic coronary study performed percutaneously at the time of coronary angiography for the detection of ischemia-producing stenoses. The technique of CFR involves use of a doppler tipped guidewire that transmits ultrasound Doppler waves from which coronary flow can be assessed. CFR is the ratio of coronary flow distal to a stenosis at maximal hyperemia to basal coronary blood flow measured in a coronary artery without stenosis. A CFR of lesser than 2 identifies an ischemia-producing stenosis.

Unlike FFR, CFR is influenced by conditions that affect vascular resistance such as microvascular disease and myocardial hypertrophy. Therefore, it has utility in the assessment of microvascular disease and is an important research tool. Coronary flow is also influenced by hemodynamic variations, such as tachycardia. Since CFR reflects both epicardial and microvascular flow, one must be aware of limitations with this technique in assessing the significance of coronary stenosis.

Index of Microcirculatory Resistance

Assessment of microcirculation is best performed by measuring the index of microvascular resistance (IMR). This may be important in symptomatic patients with risk factors for epicardial coronary artery disease and yet no angiographic evidence of significant epicardial disease. Similar to FFR, IMR is performed by measuring the pressure distal to the coronary stenosis with a pressure sensor wire. A coronary thermodilution curve is generated using a pressor sensory wire with proximal and distal thermistor. The mean transit time is measured from the coronary thermodilution curve and the inverse of mean transit time is a surrogate of absolute flow.

❏ SUGGESTED READINGS

Berry D. History of Cardiology: Werner Forssmann, MD. Circulation. 2006;113:f26-8.
Cohen MV, Gorlin R. Modified orifice equation for the calculation of mitral valve area. Am Heart J. 1972;84:839-40.

Grossman W. Percutaneous approach including trans-septal and apical puncture. In: Baim DS (Ed). Cardiac Catheterization, Angiography, and Intervention, 7th edition. Philadelphia: Lippincott; 2006. pp. 79- 106.

Grossman W. Profiles in valvular heart disease. In: Baim DS (Ed). Cardiac Catheterization, Angiography and Intervention, 7th edition. Philadelphia: Lippincott; 2006. pp. 653-6.

Higano ST, Azrak E, Tahirkheli NK, et al. Constrictive physiology. In: Kern MJ, Lim MJ, Goldstein JA (Eds). Hemodynamic Rounds, 3rd edition. New York: Wiley-Blackwell; 2009. pp. 231-45.

2.14 Cardiac Biopsy

❑ INTRODUCTION

The development and refinement of endomyocardial biopsy (EMB) has significantly advanced our understanding of many cardiac diseases, which once confounded even the most astute clinicians. In fact, for several conditions, EMB is the only modality that provides a definitive diagnosis and, therefore, is the "gold standard" upon which other tests should be compared. The EMB has also helped to change the landscape of certain situations such post heart transplant patients. Despite these benefits, there have been few, large, randomized controlled trials supporting the use of EMB in the clinical arena.

❑ TECHNIQUES

A transvenous approach is taken for right ventricular EMB. Either the femoral vein or the internal jugular vein (either right or left) is cannulated with an introducer sheath via the modified Seldinger technique (Fig. 67). Electrocardiographic rhythm, blood pressure and pulse oximetry should be monitored in all patients undergoing EMB. Ultrasound guidance can facilitate identification of the vein of interest for purposes of cannulation and has been shown to reduce procedure time and complications. In addition, in patients with normal or low right atrial pressure, elevating the patient's legs, using the Trendelenburg (head-down) position, or having the patient perform a Valsalva maneuver all elevate central venous pressure (CVP) which distends the internal jugular vein and allows for easier cannulation. Once the internal jugular vein has been cannulated, a 40 cm J guidewire is advanced into the right atrium. Then a sheath (7–9 French) with a side-arm and back-bleed valve (Cordis Corporation) is advanced over the guidewire. The CVP is then recorded via the side arm before the biopsy.

Next, the bioptome is inserted into the sheath with the tip pointed toward the lateral wall of the right atrium and advanced to the right atrium under either echocardiographic or fluoroscopic guidance. At the level of the mid-right atrium, the bioptome is rotated anteriorly in a clockwise direction approximately 180 degrees and is advanced through the tricuspid valve apparatus toward the right ventricle. The bioptome is then advanced to the interventricular septum. The bioptome position in the right ventricle should be confirmed with fluoroscopy (30-degree right anterior oblique and 60-degree left anterior oblique views). The bioptome should appear to lie across the spine and below the upper margin of the left hemidiaphragm. The goal of this step is to take proper precaution to avoid the thin, right ventricular free wall. Next, the jaws are opened and the bioptome is advanced to the right ventricular muscular septum. Proper localization of the

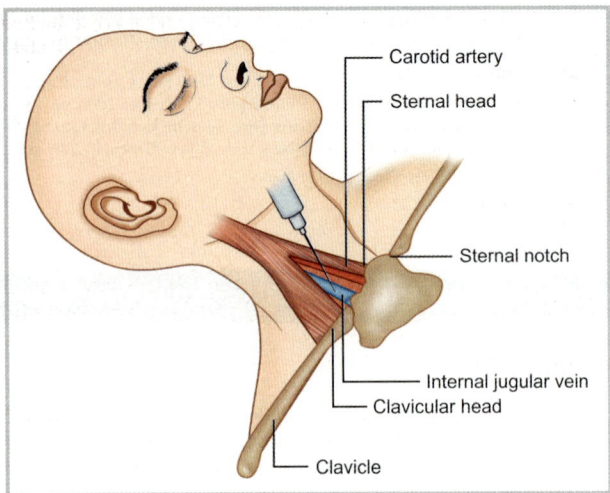

FIGURE 67: Regional anatomy for right internal jugular vein puncture. With the patient's head rotated to the left, the sternal notch, clavicle and the sternal and clavicular heads of the sternocleidomastoid muscle are identified. A skin nick is made between the two heads of the muscle, two fingerbreadths above the top of the clavicle, and the needle is inserted at an angle of 30–40° from vertical, and 20–30° right of sagittal. This approach leads to reliable puncture of the internal jugular vein and aims the needle away from the more medially located carotid artery (Source: Grossman's cardiac catheterization, angiography and intervention by LWW, 2000)

bioptome is evidenced by lack of further advancement, the occurrence of premature ventricular contractions, and the transmission of ventricular impulses to the operator's hand. The jaws are then closed and allowed a brief delay to sever the tissue. The bioptome and enclosed sample are then slowly retracted all the way out of the sheath. Three to five separate biopsies should usually be obtained to account for sampling error. The samples are then placed in specific preservatives depending upon the diagnosis suspected. If a balloon-tipped pulmonary artery catheter was used to perform a right heart catheterization, such as during EMB for transplant rejection, it is our practice to advance the balloon-tipped pulmonary artery catheter to the right atrium for several minutes after completion of the EMB to ensure stable right atrial pressures and to screen for possible myocardial perforation which could lead to tamponade. Alternatively, repeat CVP measurement is obtained at conclusion of the biopsy through the side arm.

Left ventricular biopsy remains limited to individual cases in which the suspected disease is limited to the left ventricle. The femoral artery is often used as the percutaneous access site for left ventricular biopsy. In this approach, a preformed sheath is employed to maintain arterial patency. In addition, to avoid embolic events, the sheath must be maintained under constant pressurized infusion. Given the potential for serious consequences of left-sided embolization, aspirin or other antiplatelet agents are generally combined with heparin for left ventricular biopsy.

❑ SAFETY AND COMPLICATIONS

Despite the invasive nature of the procedure and potential for severe complications, EMB is now considered a very safe technique. The EMB complications can be categorized as to those that occur in the acute setting and those that occur after a delayed period of time. Immediate periprocedural risks include perforation with pericardial tamponade, pneumothorax, pulmonary embolization, ventricular, and supraventricular arrhythmias, heart block, recurrent laryngeal nerve paresis, damage to the tricuspid valve and creation of an arteriovenous fistula within the heart. Like any invasive procedure, degree of risk is heavily dependent upon operator's experience. In addition, baseline clinical features of the patient, access site and type of bioptome are also likely important. Delayed complications include access site bleeding, damage to the tricuspid valve, pericardial tamponade and deep vein thrombosis.

One of the most significant complications with EMB is cardiac perforation leading to tamponade. Several clinical features that have been associated with increased risk of perforation include: increased right ventricular systolic pressures, bleeding diathesis, recent receipt of heparin and right ventricular enlargement. Cardiac perforation should be suspected if the patient complains of chest pain with a biopsy pass, unexpected bradycardia or hypotension is encountered, or if the EMB samples float in 10% formalin (suggesting the presence of cardiac fat). In these circumstances, right atrial pressure, fluoroscopic appearance of the heart border and possibly bedside echocardiography should be used to monitor for hemopericardium. If confirmed, urgent pericardiocentesis should be performed. In most cases, in a patient with normal coagulation parameters, catheter drainage is sufficient to stabilize the patient. However, on occasion, it may be necessary to consult thoracic surgeons to evacuate the pericardial space.

❑ ANALYSIS OF EMB TISSUE

The utility of EMB for diagnosis of suspected cardiac conditions is heavily dependent upon proper sampling technique, careful handling of the EMB sample and initial preparation of the sample in appropriate fixatives. In general, an attempt should be made to obtain samples from greater than 1 region of the right ventricular septum. In addition, between 5 and 10 samples of 1–2 mm^3 in size should be obtained to minimize sampling errors. Biopsy samples should be removed gently from the jaws of the bioptome with a fine needle (not forceps) and placed on moistened filter paper. Next, the samples should be transferred to a container with 10% neutral buffered formalin for light microscopy or 4% glutaraldehyde for transmission electron microscopy. The EMB samples can also be snap frozen in OCT embedding medium and stored at −80°F for molecular studies, immunohistochemistry or immunofluorescence. In general, flash freezing is appropriate for culture, polymerase chain reaction (PCR) or reverse transcriptase PCR (rtPCR) to identify viruses but is not well-suited for standard histological preparations due to the development of ice crystal artefacts.

Light Microscopy and Stains

Once the EMB samples have been fixed and transported from the catheterization laboratory to the pathology laboratory, they are then embedded in paraffin and serial 4/m thick sections are cut and sequentially numbered. The specimens are then stained with hematoxylin and eosin (H&E) as well as Movat or elastic trichrome stain to visualize collagen and elastic tissue. It is a common practice for many laboratories to routinely stain one slide for iron on men and all postmenopausal women to screen for hemochromatosis. In addition, Congo red staining may be performed to screen for amyloidosis.

Cardiotropic Virus Detection

The EMB samples can also be screened for cardiotropic viruses. Identification of viral genomes from EMB samples has recently become more feasible due to the development of rapid, quantitative (qPCR) and qualitative (nested PCR) molecular techniques. Several studies have reported a high incidence of viral genome detection in the myocardium of patients with suspected myocarditis and dilated cardiomyopathy (DCM). The most common viruses detected in the myocardium include enteroviruses, adenoviruses, parvovirus B19, cytomegalovirus (CMV), influenza, respiratory syncytial virus, herpes simplex virus, Epstein-Barr virus, human herpes 6, HIV, and hepatitis C.

❑ INDICATIONS

The utility of EMB for the diagnosis of cardiovascular conditions are limited to case series and cohorts. As a result, one of the most difficult decisions facing the clinician is determining under what circumstances performing an EMB would lead to a clinically meaningful diagnosis or change in therapy while taking into account the risk of harm from the procedure itself. Recognizing the need for a comprehensive review of the literature and a unified set of recommendations, the American Heart Association (AHA), the American College of Cardiology Foundation (ACCF) and the European Society of Cardiology (ESC) convened a multidisciplinary group of experts, and recently released a joint scientific statement. In this statement, the authors review 14 clinical case scenarios where EMB might be considered and provide Class I–III recommendations along with levels of evidence (Levels A–C) to support these recommendations (Table 44).

The two clinical scenarios that received a Class I indication for EMB were:
- In the setting of unexplained, new-onset heart failure of less than 2 weeks' duration associated with a normal-sized or dilated left ventricle in addition to hemodynamic compromise
- In the setting of unexplained, new-onset heart failure of 2 weeks to 3 months duration associated with a dilated left ventricle and new ventricular arrhythmias, Mobitz type II second- or third-degree atrioventricular (AV) heart block, or failure to respond to usual care within 1–2 weeks

The EMB should be performed in these two settings to identify three clinical entities: (i) lymphocytic myocarditis, (ii) giant cell myocarditis (GCM), or (iii) necrotizing eosinophilic myocarditis. Identification of these clinical entities is important both for prognostic as well as therapeutic purposes.

❑ SUMMARY

The EMB has led to a greater understanding of many cardiac diseases and continues to provide useful diagnostic information to the clinician. While recommendations about the utility of EMB are limited by the lack of large, randomized trials, there appears to be consensus regarding the use of EMB in the clinical scenario of the acute onset of decompensated heart failure of less than 3 months duration as well as in monitoring of cardiac allograft rejection. The EMB is also recognized to play an important role in the diagnostic algorithms of many other cardiac disease states, although its practical use should be evaluated in the context of the diseases being considered (i.e. it is important to rule out diseases or identify diseases with specific therapies that influence outcome). With the advent of newer techniques and improved bioptomes, complication rates have declined significantly.

Table 44: The role of endomyocardial biopsy in 14 clinical scenarios

Scenario number	Clinical scenario	Class of recommendation (I, IIa, IIb, III)	Level of evidence (A, B, C)
1.	New-onset heart failure of <2 weeks' duration associated with a normal-sized or dilated left ventricle and hemodynamic compromise	I	B
2.	New-onset heart failure of 2 weeks' to 3 months' duration associated with a dilated left ventricle and new ventricular arrhythmias, second- or third-degree heart block, or failure to respond to usual care within 1–2 weeks	I	B
3.	Heart failure of >3 months' duration associated with a dilated left ventricle and new ventricular arrhythmias, second- or third-degree heart block, or failure to respond to usual care within 1–2 weeks	IIa	C
4.	Heart failure associated with a DCM of any duration associated with suspected allergic reaction and/or eosinophilia	IIa	C
5.	Heart failure associated with suspected anthracycline cardiomyopathy	IIa	C
6.	Heart failure associated with unexplained restrictive cardiomyopathy	IIa	C
7.	Suspected cardiac tumors	IIa	C
8.	Unexplained cardiomyopathy in children	IIa	C
9.	New-onset heart failure of 2 weeks' to 3 months' duration associated with a dilated left ventricle, without new ventricular arrhythmias or second- or third-degree heart block, that responds to usual care within 1–2 weeks	IIb	B
10.	Heart failure of >3 months' duration assoicated with a dilated left ventricle, without new ventricular arrhythmias or second- or third-degree heart block, that responds to usual care within 1–2 weeks	IIb	C
11.	Heart failure associated with unexplained HCM	IIb	C
12.	Suspected ARVD/C	IIb	C
13.	Unexplained ventricular arrhythmias	IIb	C
14.	Unexplained atrial fibrillation	III	C

MODIFIED SUMMARIES OF GUIDELINES AHA/ACC/ESC SCIENTIFIC STATEMENT. THE ROLE OF ENDOMYOCARDIAL BIOPSY IN THE MANAGEMENT OF CARDIOVASCULAR DISEASE. CIRCULATION. 2007;116:2216-33

Kanu Chatterjee

Class I: Conditions for which there is evidence or there is general agreement that a given procedure is beneficial, useful and effective.

Class II: Conditions for which there is conflicting evidence and/or a divergence of opinion about the usefulness/efficacy of a procedure or treatment.

Class IIa: Conditions for which the weight of evidence/opinion is in favor of usefulness/efficacy.

Class IIb: Conditions for which usefulness/efficacy is less well established by evidence/opinion.

Class III: Conditions for which there is evidence and/or general agreement that a procedure/treatment is not useful and in some cases may be harmful.

THE LEVELS OF EVIDENCE

Level A (highest): Multiple randomized clinical trials.

Level B: (intermediate): Limited number of randomized trials, nonrandomized studies and registries.

Level C: Primarily expert consensus.

Class I

1. Unexplained, new-onset heart failure, 2 weeks duration with a normal or dilated left ventricle and hemodynamic compromise (level of evidence B).
2. Unexplained new-onset heart failure of 2 weeks to 3 months' duration with a dilated left ventricle and new ventricular arrhythmias or advanced atrioventricular heart block or failure to respond to usual care in 1–2 weeks (level of evidence B).

Class IIa

1. Unexplained heart failure of greater than 3 months' duration with a dilated left ventricle and new ventricular arrhythmias or advanced atrioventricular heart block or failure to respond to usual care within 1–2 weeks. (level of evidence C).
2. Unexplained heart failure with a dilated cardiomyopathy of any duration and suspected allergic reaction and eosinophilia (level of evidence C).
3. Unexplained heart failure and suspected anthracycline cardiomyopathy (level of evidence C).
4. Heart failure with unexplained restrictive cardiomyopathy (level of evidence C).
5. With suspected (non-myxoma 0 cardiac tumors) (level of evidence C).
6. Unexplained cardiomyopathy in children (level of evidence C).

Class IIb

1. Unexplained new-onset heart failure of 2 weeks to 3 months' duration with a dilated left ventricle but without new ventricular arrhythmias or advanced atrioventricular heart block that responds to usual care within 1–2 weeks (level of evidence B).
2. Unexplained heart failure of greater than 3 months' duration with a dilated left ventricle without new ventricular arrhythmias or advanced atrioventricular heart block that responds to usual care within 1–2 weeks (level of evidence C).
3. Suspected arrhythmogenic right ventricular dysplasia/cardiomyopathy (level of evidence C).
4. Unexplained ventricular arrhythmias (level of evidence C).

Class III

Unexplained atrial fibrillation (level of evidence C).

❏ SUGGESTED READINGS

Brunner-La Rocca HP, Sutsch G, Schneider J, et al. Natural course of moderate cardiac allograft rejection (International Society for Heart Transplantation grade 2) early and late after transplantation. Circulation. 1996;94:1334-8.

Caves PK, Stinson EB, Dong E Jr. New instrument for transvenous cardiac biopsy. Am J Cardiol. 1974;33:264-7.

Chan KL, Veinot J, Leach A, et al. Diagnosis of left atrial sarcoma by transvenous endomyocardial biopsy. Can J Cardiol. 2001;17:206-8.

Cooper LT, Baughman KL, Feldman AM, et al. The role of endomyocardial biopsy in the management of cardiovascular disease. J Am Coll Cardiol. 2007;50:1914-31.

Flipse TR, Tazelaar HD. Diagnosis of malignant cardiac disease by endomyocardial biopsy. Mayo Clin Proc. 1990;65:1415-22.

Sakakibara S, Konno S. Endomyocardial biopsy. Jpn Heart J. 1962;3:537-43.

2.15 Coronary Angiography and Catheter-based Coronary Intervention

❏ INTRODUCTION

The first attempt to image the coronary arteries began in the late 1940s. In 1953, Seldinger first introduced a method of percutaneous arterial catheterization to study the coronary arteries. Coronary angiography has subsequently become one of the most widely used invasive procedures in cardiovascular medicine and remains the gold standard for identifying the presence or absence of atherosclerotic coronary artery disease (CAD). The methods used to perform coronary angiography have continued to improve substantially over time. Smaller (5–6 French) high-flow injection catheters have replaced larger (8 French) thick-walled catheters. The smaller sheath sizes and the introduction and development of radial artery access for coronary catheterization have allowed same-day outpatient coronary angiography, early ambulation and discharge.

❏ INDICATIONS FOR CORONARY ANGIOGRAPHY

The American College of Cardiology/American Heart Association (ACC/AHA) Task Force has established indications for coronary angiography in patients with known or suspected CAD (Table 45).

❏ CONTRAINDICATIONS FOR CORONARY ANGIOGRAPHY

With the exception of patient refusal, there are no absolute contraindications to coronary angiography. Significant relative contraindications include ongoing stroke or cerebrovascular accident (CVA) within a month, recent head trauma, significant active bleeding, anemia with hemoglobin less than 8 mg/dL, uncontrolled systemic hypertension, digitalis toxicity, previous contrast reaction without pretreatment with corticosteroids, severe electrolyte imbalance, unexplained fever, and untreated infection. The risks and benefits of the procedure and alternative evaluation techniques—if potentially indicated— should always be carefully reviewed with the patient and family in all circumstances prior to coronary angiography, but especially in the presence of relative contraindications (Table 46).

Table 45: Indications for coronary angiography

ACC/AHA guideline summary: Coronary angiography for risk stratification in patients with chronic stable angina

Class I: There is evidence and/or general agreement that coronary angiography should be performed to risk stratify patients with chronic stable angina in the following settings:

- Disabling anginal symptoms [Canadian Cardiovascular Society (CCS) classes III and IV] despite medical therapy
- High-risk criteria on noninvasive testing independent of the severity of angina
- Survivors of sudden cardiac death or serious ventricular arrhythmia
- Symptoms and signs of heart failure
- Clinical features suggest that the patient has a high likelihood of severe coronary artery disease

Class IIa: The evidence or opinion is in favor of performing coronary angiography to risk stratify patients with chronic stable angina in the following settings:

- Left ventricular ejection fraction less than 45%, CCS class I or II angina and evidence, on noninvasive testing, of ischemia that does not meet high-risk criteria
- Noninvasive testing does not reveal adequate prognostic information

Class IIb: The evidence or opinion is less well established for performing coronary angiography to risk stratify patients with chronic stable angina in the following settings:

- Left ventricular ejection fraction greater than 45%, CCS class I or II angina and evidence, on noninvasive testing, of ischemia that does not meet high-risk criteria
- CCS class III or IV angina that improves to class I or II with medical therapy
- CCS class I or II angina but unacceptable side effects to adequate medical therapy

Class III: There is evidence and/or general agreement that coronary angiography should not be performed to risk stratify patients with chronic stable angina in the following settings:

- CCS class I or II angina that responds to medical therapy and, on noninvasive testing, shows no evidence of ischemia
- Patient preference to avoid revascularization

(*Source:* Gibbons RJ, Abrams J, Chatterjee K, et al. ACC/AHA 2002 guidelines update for the management of patients with chronic stable angina—summary article: a report of the American College of Cardiology/American Heart Association Task Force on Practice Guidelines (Committee on the Management of Patients with Chronic Stable Angina). Circulation. 2003;107:149)

Table 46: Contraindications to cardiac catheterization

Absolute contraindications
- Inadequate equipment or catheterization facility
- Patient refusal

Relative contraindications
- Acute gastrointestinal bleeding or anemia
- Anticoagulation (or known uncontrolled bleeding diathesis)
- Electrolyte imbalance
- Infection or fever
- Medication intoxication (e.g. digitalis, phenothiazine)
- Pregnancy
- Recent cerebral vascular accident (>1 mon)
- Renal failure
- Uncontrolled congestive heart failure, high blood pressure, arrhythmias
- Uncooperative patient

❏ PATIENT PREPARATION

The procedure should be explained to the patient in simple terms and informed consent to perform the procedure is then obtained. The operator should clearly explain the potential risks and benefits for cardiac catheterization to the patient and family. Patients with diabetes mellitus, renal insufficiency or previous reported hypersensitivity to iodinated contrast media constitute groups who need special consideration. For diabetic patients, insulin dosing should be adjusted to minimize the risk of periprocedural hypoglycemia. Patients with renal insufficiency should have interventions for renal function preservation following contrast administration. These should include volume repletion with intravenous (IV) fluids before contrast administration, consideration of N-acetylcysteine administration and consideration of biplane angiography if available.

❏ SITES AND TECHNIQUES OF VASCULAR ACCESS

The site of vascular access is determined by the anticipated pathologic and anatomic findings relevant to the patient. Prior to the procedure, assessment of all peripheral pulses is mandatory. If a transradial approach is being considered, an Allen's test should also be performed to confirm candidacy for this approach.

Femoral Artery Approach

Percutaneous femoral arterial catheterization remains the most widely used vascular access site for coronary angiography. In order to reduce access site complications, obtaining access to the common femoral artery below the inguinal ligament is strongly recommended. Before the puncture, fluoroscopy of the tip of a metal clamp placed near the medial edge of the middle of the head of the femur is often performed. This step is done to enhance the likelihood of puncturing the common femoral artery, while remaining below the inguinal ligament. This location in the middle of the femoral head is typically the location of the common femoral artery in most patients, although there is certainly anatomic variation (Fig. 68). Adequate local anesthesia should be administered. A skin nick is then placed approximately 1-1/2–2 fingerbreadths (3 cm) below the inguinal ligament and directly over the femoral artery pulsation. Palpation identifies the middle of the artery and the needle is advanced at a 30–45° angle to the vessel, preferably puncturing only the front wall. Once brisk arterial flow through the needle is established, the guidewire is advanced through the needle to the descending aorta. If any resistance to passage of the wire is encountered, the operator should stop immediately and use fluoroscopy to visualize advancement of the wire. Once the wire is successfully placed into the descending aorta to the level of the diaphragm, the needle is then exchanged for a valved sheath, which is usually 4–6 French in size for femoral access diagnostic procedures.

Transradial Approach

The superficial location of the radial artery makes it easily accessible in most patients. There is dual blood supply to the hand via the radial and the ulnar arteries which decreases the potential of any meaningful clinical sequelae in the case of a procedure-related radial artery occlusion. Patient comfort is enhanced as there is no need for flat bedrest after a transradial procedure. Patients with a palpable radial pulse and a normal Allen's test are generally candidates for the transradial approach. The ideal point to access the radial artery is just proximal to the styloid

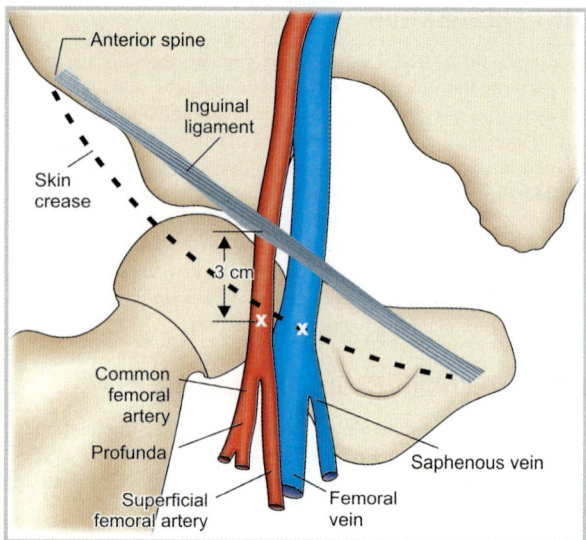

FIGURE 68: Femoral artery access site. Anatomy relevant to percutaneous catheterization of the femoral artery (FA) and vein. The right FA vein passes underneath the inguinal ligament, which connects the anteriorsuperior iliac spine and pubic tubercle. The arterial skin nick (indicated by X) should be placed approximately 1-1/2–2 fingerbreadths (3 cm) below the inguinal ligament and directly over the FA pulsation

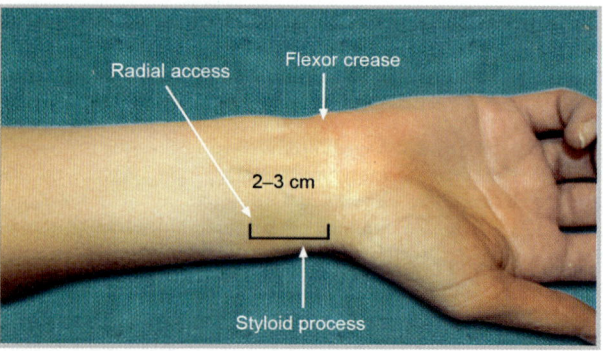

FIGURE 69: Ideal radial artery access site: just proximal to the styloid process (usually 2–3 cm from the flexor crease)

process of the radius. This is usually about 2–3 cm above the flexor crease (Fig. 69). A small amount of local anesthesia is given to the area. The radial artery can be accessed with two different techniques. In the first, the radial pulse is palpated at the site indicated previously. Then, a short (2.5 cm) 21 gauge needle is advanced into the radial artery at a 30–40° angle. Once pulsatile flow is obtained, a 0.021 inch diameter guidewire is advanced in the radial artery. A hydrophilic coated sheath (typically 5 French) is advanced into the radial artery—no skin nick is usually needed. As soon as the sheath is placed, a spasmolytic cocktail containing a calcium channel blocker and nitroglycerin is administered to prevent arterial spasm. Heparin is also always given during transradial catheterization, as this is known to decrease the chance of procedural related radial artery occlusion.

The second technique for obtaining radial arterial access involves the use of an IV catheter to puncture the radial artery instead of a bare needle. Once a backflow of blood is noted in the hub of the IV catheter, the catheter is advanced to also puncture the posterior wall of the vessel. The needle is then removed and the plastic cannula is slowly withdrawn until pulsatile flow is obtained. Then a guidewire (0.021–0.025 inch) is advanced into the radial artery and the IV catheter is then exchanged for the sheath and spasmolytic cocktail and heparin are given.

Brachial Artery Approach

With the recent development and increase in the use of transradial catheterization, the brachial approach for catheterization has become less commonly used. In the past, brachial arterial access for coronary angiography was performed primarily with a cutdown approach. However, this technique has largely fallen out of favor in the performance of coronary angiography. Currently, when brachial access is used for coronary angiography, access is gained percutaneously, often with a 21G needle and 0.021 inch guidewire. The brachial artery is typically accessed 2–3 cm above the antecubital fossa, where the vessel is still relatively superficial. Accessing the vessel more proximal than this typically increases the risk of access difficulty and complications as the vessel is generally deeper in this area. There can be spasm of the brachial artery, but this is much less common and can be treated with spasmolytic medications.

❑ CATHETERS FOR CORONARY ANGIOGRAPHY

Numerous shapes and sizes of catheters are available to the angiographer. Routinely used catheters that are preshaped for normal anatomy are available for both the radial and the femoral approaches. There is an additional array of shapes and sizes to aid the operator with the various coronary artery anatomical variations that are encountered (Figs 70 and 71).

❑ ARTERIAL NOMENCLATURE AND EXTENT OF DISEASE

The major epicardial vessels and their second- and third-order branches can be visualized using coronary angiography. The network of smaller intramyocardial branches is generally not seen secondary to their size, cardiac motion and

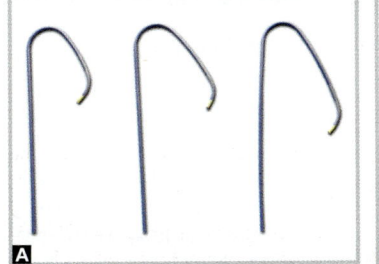
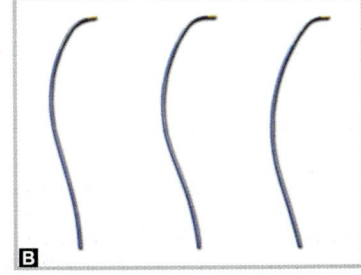

FIGURES 70A AND B: (A) Judkins left 4,5,6 catheters (left to right); (B) Judkins right 3.5,4,5 catheters (left to right). (*Source:* Boston Scientific)

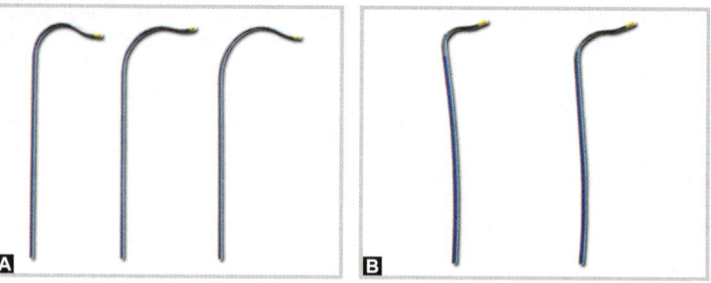

FIGURES 71A AND B: (A) Amplatz left 1,2,3 catheters (left to right); (B) Amplatz right 1,2 catheters (left to right). (*Source:* Boston Scientific.)

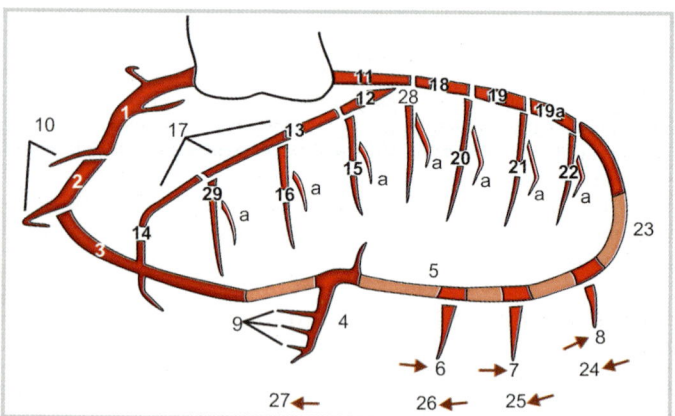

FIGURE 72: The coronary artery map used by the BARI investigators. The map is derived from that used in CASS with the addition of branch segments for the diagonal, marginal, and ramus vessels

limitations in resolution of angiographic systems. These fourth-order and higher "resistance" vessels play a major role in autoregulation of coronary blood flow. Coronary perfusion in these smaller branch vessels can be quantitatively assessed using the myocardial blush score which has important prognostic significance in patients with STEMI and those undergoing percutaneous coronary intervention (PCI). The Coronary Artery Surgery Study (CASS) investigators established the nomenclature most commonly used to describe the coronary anatomy, defining 27 segments in three major coronary arteries (Fig. 72). The Bypass Angioplasty Revascularization Investigators (BARI) study modified these criteria with the addition of two segments for the ramus intermedius and addition of the third diagonal branch.

❏ ANGIOGRAPHIC PROJECTIONS

The major coronary arteries traverse the interventricular and atrioventricular (AV) grooves, aligned with the long and short axes of the heart, respectively. Since the heart is oriented obliquely in the thoracic cavity, the coronary circulation is generally visualized in the right anterior oblique (RAO) and LAO projections to furnish true posteroanterior and lateral views of the heart. However, without sagittal angulations, these views are limited by vessel foreshortening and superimposition of branches. Simultaneous rotation of the X-ray beam in the sagittal plane provides a better view of the major coronary arteries and their branches. It is recommended that the coronary arteries be visualized in both the LAO and RAO projections using both cranial and caudal angulation with all segments of the vessels visualized in at least two preferably orthogonal views.

❏ CONGENITAL ANOMALIES OF THE CORONARY CIRCULATION

Coronary anomalies may occur in 1–5% of patients undergoing coronary angiography, depending on the threshold for defining an anatomical variant (Table 47). The Documentation of precise ischemia risk for some of these anomalies using conventional exercise stress testing or intravascular Doppler flow studies is poorly predictive and may fail to detect significant anatomic abnormalities. Accordingly, coronary artery anomalies are divided into those that cause and those that do not cause myocardial ischemia (Table 48).

Table 47: Incidence of coronary anomalies among 1950 angiograms

Variable	Number	Percent
Coronary anomalies	110	5.64
Split RCA	24	1.23
Ectopic RCA (right cusp)	22	1.13
Ectopic RCA (left cusp)	18	0.92
Fistulas	17	0.87
Absent left main coronary artery	13	0.67
Lcx artery arising from right cusp	13	0.67
LCA arising from right cusp	3	0.15
Low origin of RCA	2	0.1
Other anomalies	3	0.15

(*Source:* Angelini P (Ed). Coronary Artery Anomalies: A Comprehensive Approach. Philadelphia: Lippincott Williams and Wilkins; 1999. p. 42.)

Table 48: Ischemia occurring in coronary anomalies

Type of ischemia	Coronary anomaly
No ischemia	Majority of anomalies (split RCA, ectopic RCA from right cusp, ectopic RCA from left cusp)
Episodic ischemia	Anomalous origin of a coronary artery from the opposite sinus (ACAOS); coronary artery fistulas; myocardial bridge
Obligatory	Anomalous left coronary artery from the pulmonary ischemia artery (ALCAPA); coronary ostial atresia or severe stenosis

(Abbreviations: RCA: Right coronary artery; ACAOS: Anomalous origin of a coronary artery from the opposite sinus; ALCAPA: Anomalous left coronary artery from the pulmonary artery) (*Source:* Angelini P (Ed). Coronary Artery Anomalies: A Comprehensive Approach. Philadelphia; Lippincott Williams and Wilkins: 1999. p. 42)

❏ GENERAL PRINCIPLES FOR CORONARY AND/OR GRAFT CANNULATION

Coronary cannulation is typically performed using an approximate 30° LAO projection. Pressure is constantly transduced from the tip of the catheter throughout the procedure to monitor for pressure damping or ventricularization. Either of these phenomena may indicate a severe stenosis with wedging of the catheter into the stenosis, or that the catheter tip is positioned against the coronary vessel wall. Injection of contrast when there is damping or ventricularization of the pressure waveform should be avoided as the incidence of coronary dissection or ventricular arrhythmia is clearly increased in this situation. Whenever pressure waveform damping is present, the catheter should be repositioned until a normal waveform appears or nonselective injections performed to assess the possibility of an ostial stenosis or other anatomical reason for the pressure damping. Subsequently, a smaller French or different shape catheter may be considered to safely perform the angiogram.

Left Main Coronary Artery Cannulation

As previously noted, the Judkins left 4.0 coronary catheter is used most often to engage the LMCA in femoral access procedures, with a gentle advancement under fluoroscopic guidance. However, if the Judkins left catheter begins to turnout of profile (so that one or both curves of the catheter are no longer visualized en face), it can be rotated clockwise very slightly and advanced slowly to enter the left sinus of Valsalva, permitting the catheter tip to engage the ostium of the LMCA.

Right Coronary Artery Cannulation

As with the LMCA, cannulation of the RCA is also generally performed in the LAO view but requires different maneuvers than those for cannulation of the LMCA. Whereas the Judkins left catheter naturally seeks the ostium of the LMCA, the Judkins right or Amplatz right catheters that are typically used to engage the RCA must be rotated to engage the vessel.

❏ FLUOROSCOPIC IMAGING SYSTEM

The basic principle of radiographic coronary imaging is that radiation produced by the X-ray tube is attenuated as it passes through the body. This attenuation of the X-ray is detected by the image intensifier (Fig. 73). Iodinated contrast medium is injected into the coronary arteries which enhances the absorption of the X-rays and produces a sharp contrast with the surrounding cardiac tissues. The X-ray shadow is then converted into a visible light image by the image intensifier and displayed on fluoroscopic monitors.

❏ CHARACTERISTICS OF CONTRAST MEDIA

All types of contrast media contain three iodine molecules attached to a fully substituted benzene ring. The fourth position in the standard ionic agent is taken up by sodium or methylglucamine as a cation; the remaining two positions of the benzene ring have side chains of diatrizoate, metrizoate, or iothalamate. All contrast media is excreted predominantly (99%) by glomerular filtration with about 1% excreted by the biliary system. The normal half-time of excretion is 20 minutes. To reduce the osmotic effects of contrast medium, the number of dissolved particles must be decreased or the molal concentration of iodine per particle must

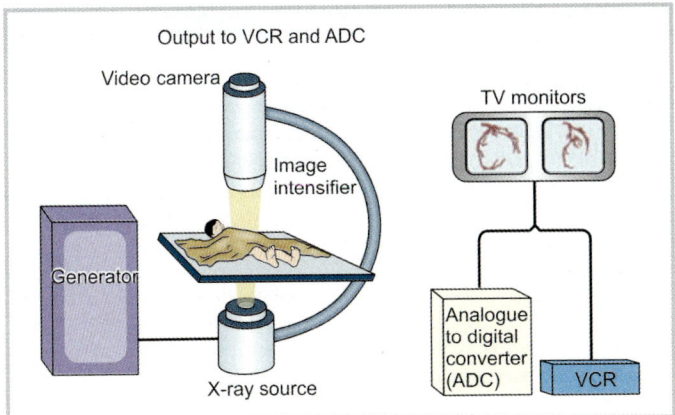

FIGURE 73: Cineangiographic equipment. The major components include: a generator, X-ray tube, image intensifier attached to a positioner, such as a C-arm, optical system, videocamera, videocassette recorder (VCR), analogue to digital converter (ADC), and television monitors

be increased. New-generation, nonionic, monomeric and ionic dimeric contrast agents have approximately the same viscosity and iodine concentration but have only one-half or less of the osmolality of the ionic agents. Currently, nonionic, low-osmolar agents are preferred in all patients, but especially in adults with poor LV function; patients with renal disease, especially those with diabetes; and patients with a history of serious reaction to contrast media or with multiple allergies.

Contrast Media Reactions

There are three types of contrast allergies: (i) minor cutaneous and mucosal manifestations, (ii) smooth muscle and minor anaphylactoid responses, and (iii) major cardiovascular and anaphylactoid responses. Major reactions involving laryngeal or pulmonary edema often are accompanied by minor or less severe reactions. Nonionic contrast media has replaced ionic contrast media for most patients to minimize the chance of allergic or other adverse contrast reactions. Table 49 lists the adverse reactions associated with radiocontrast materials. Patients with diabetes, renal insufficiency or volume depletion from any cause are at risk for contrast-induced nephropathy (CIN). Advanced preparations to limit the chance of CIN include volume repletion (IV fluid administration, holding diuretics) and maintenance of large-volume urine flow (>200 mL/hour).

❏ ACCESS SITE HEMOSTASIS

After the catheterization procedure has been completed and the catheters removed, the sheath is flushed. If heparin has been given, an activated clotting time (ACT) is obtained for femoral or brachial access procedures. The sheath is removed when the ACT is 150–180 seconds. To remove the femoral arterial sheath, gentle pressure is applied proximal to the puncture site while the sheath is removed, taking care not to crush the sheath and/or strip clot into the distal artery. Once the sheath is removed, firm downward pressure is then applied just proximal to the arteriotomy for 15–30 minutes, with gradual reduction in pressure after

Table 49: Reactions associated with contrast media

- Allergic (anaphylactoid) reactions
  - Grade I: Single episode of emesis, nausea, sneezing or vertigo
  - Grade II: Hives; multiple episodes of emesis, fevers or chills
  - Grade III: Clinical shock, bronchospasm, laryngospasm or edema, loss of consciousness, hypotension, hypertension, cardiac arrhythmia, angioedema or pulmonary edema
- Cardiovascular toxicity
- Electrophysiologic
- Bradycardia (asystole, heart block)
- Tachycardia (sinus, ventricular)
- Ventricular fibrillation
- Hemodynamic
- Hypotension (cardiac depression, vasodilation)
- Heart failure (cardiac depression, increased intravascular volume)
- Nephrotoxicity
- Discomfort
- Nausea, vomiting
- Heat and flushing
- Hyperthyroidism

the initial 10–15 minutes. After manual hemostasis is achieved, a small adhesive bandage is used to cover the wound. Additional methods to secure postprocedure arterial hemostasis include external hemostasis pads, mechanical pressure clamps, and vascular closure devices. A variety of vascular closure devices are currently available. These devices do reduce the time to obtain hemostasis and allow earlier ambulation. They may be particularly helpful in anticoagulated patients, patients with back pain or an inability to lie flat. The brachial sheath is removed in relatively the same manner as a femoral sheath. There are, however, no mechanical pressure clamp devices or closure devices for use with brachial access.

❏ COMPLICATIONS OF CARDIAC CATHETERIZATION

The cumulative incidence of the major risks of stroke, death and MI is approximately 0.1%. The minor risks of vascular injury, allergic reaction, bleeding, hematoma and infection range from 0.04% to 5% (Table 50).

Access Site Complications

The most common complication noted with femoral access catheterization is hemorrhage and local hematoma formation. These complications occur more frequently with increasing size of the access sheath, concomitant venous access, increased amounts of anticoagulation, female patients, obesity and also low body weight. Other possible access site complications (in order of decreasing frequency) include retroperitoneal hematoma, pseudoaneurysm, arteriovenous (AV) fistula and arterial thrombosis. The frequency of access site complications is increased in obese patients, during high-risk procedures, in critically ill elderly patients with extensive atheromatous disease.

Other Complications

Embolic stroke is a rare complication of diagnostic coronary angiography but, when it occurs, it can be devastating. Embolic stroke more commonly occurs in patients

Table 50: Complications and risk for cardiac catheterization [SCAI Registry (%)]

Mortality	0.11
Myocardial infarction	0.05
Cerebrovascular accident	0.07
Arrhythmias	0.38
Vascular complications	0.43
Contrast reaction	0.37
Hemodynamic complications	0.26
Perforation of heart chamber	0.03
Other complications	0.28
Total of major complications	1.70

(*Source:* Adapted from Scanlon P, Faxon D, Audet A, et al. ACC/AHA guidelines for coronary angiography. J Am Coll Cardiol.1999;33:1756)

with significant aortic atheroma. Giving heparin for longer duration procedures (such as bypass graft procedures, aortic valve assessment) or in patients at higher risk for stroke should be considered. Catheter induced coronary artery dissection is an infrequent but important complication to be aware about. Nerve pain after diagnostic catheterization is infrequent, but can occur. With the expanded use of complex PCI, patients may now return for multiple procedures over their lifetime which can subject them to the risk of cumulative radiation injury.

❑ PERCUTANEOUS CORONARY INTERVENTION

The term "angina pectoris" was used to describe a syndrome characterized by a sensation of "strangling and anxiety" in the chest. This was attributed to myocardial ischemia arising from increased myocardial oxygen consumption due to obstructive CAD. Treatment of this syndrome was initially done with coronary artery bypass surgery, first introduced in 1968. Due to limitations, percutaneous treatment was considered feasible in only 10% of all patients needing revascularization. Today, PCI encompasses a broad array of procedures, including angioplasty, stenting and various "niche" devices which all together allow the performance of safe and effective percutaneous revascularization in many different clinical situations (Table 51).

Table 51: Indications for PCI

Common indications for percutaneous coronary interventions according to patient presentation:

Patients with asymptomatic ischemia or CCS class I or II angina

Class IIa
PCI is reasonable in patients with 1 or more significant lesions in 1 or 2 coronary arteries suitable for PCI. The vessels intended to be treated must subtend a moderate to large area of viable myocardium or be associated with a moderate-to-severe degree of ischemia on noninvasive testing. It is also indicated in patients with recurrent stenosis after PCI with large area of viable myocardium. PCI can also be offered to patients with significant left main disease (> 50%), who are not eligible for CABG

Contd...

Contd...

Table 51: Indications for PCI

Class IIb

(1) The effectiveness of PCI for patients with asymptomatic ischemia or CCS class I or II angina who have 2- or 3-vessel disease with significant proximal LAD CAD who are otherwise eligible for CABG with 1 arterial conduit and who have treated diabetes or abnormal LV function is not well established. However, it can be considered in patients with nonproximal LAD disease in a vessel that serves a moderate area of viable myocardium with demonstrable ischemia on testing

Class III

PCI is generally not recommended in patients with asymptomatic ischemia or CCS class I or II angina who do not meet the criteria as listed under the class II recommendations or who have 1 or more of the following:

1. Only a small area of viable myocardium at risk.
2. No objective evidence of ischemia.
3. Lesions that have a low likelihood of successful dilatation.
4. Mild symptoms those are unlikely to be due to myocardial ischemia.
5. Factors associated with increased risk of morbidity or mortality.
6. Left main disease and eligibility for CABG.
7. Insignificant disease (< 50% coronary stenosis).

Patients with CCS class III angina

Class IIa

1. It is reasonable that PCI be performed in patients with CCS class III angina and single-vessel or multivessel CAD who are undergoing medical therapy and who have 1 or more significant lesions in 1 or more coronary arteries suitable for PCI with a high likelihood of success and low risk of morbidity or mortality.
2. It is reasonable that PCI be performed in patients with CCS class III angina with single-vessel or multivessel CAD who are undergoing medical therapy with focal saphenous vein graft lesions or multiple stenoses who are poor candidates for reoperative surgery.
3. Use of PCI is reasonable in patients with CCS class III angina with significant left main CAD (> 50% diameter stenosis) who are candidates for revascularization but are not eligible for CABG.

Class IIb

1. PCI may be considered in patients with CCS class III angina with single-vessel or multivessel CAD who are undergoing medical therapy and who have 1 or more lesions to be dilated with a reduced likelihood of success.
2. PCI may be considered in patients with CCS class III angina and no evidence of ischemia on noninvasive testing or who are undergoing medical therapy and have 2- or 3-vessel CAD with significant proximal LAD CAD and treated diabetes or abnormal LV function.

Class III

PCI is not recommended for patients with CCS class III angina with single-vessel or multivessel CAD, no evidence of myocardial injury or ischemia on objective testing, and no trial of medical therapy, or who have 1 of the following:

1. Only a small area of myocardium at risk.
2. All lesions or the culprit lesion to be dilated with morphology that conveys a low likelihood of success.
3. A high risk of procedure-related morbidity or mortality.
4. Insignificant disease (< 50% coronary stenosis).
5. Significant left main CAD and candidacy for CABG.

Patients with UA or NSTEMI

Class I

An early invasive PCI strategy is indicated for patients with UA or NSTEMI who have no serious comorbidity and coronary lesions amenable to PCI. Patients must have any of the following high-risk features:

1. Recurrent ischemia despite intensive antiischemic therapy.

Contd...

Contd...

Table 51: Indications for PCI

2. Elevated troponin level.
3. New ST segment depression.
4. HF symptoms or new or worsening mitral regurgitation.
5. Depressed LV systolic function.
6. Hemodynamic instability.
7. Sustained ventricular tachycardia.
8. PCI within 6 months.
9. Prior CABG.

Class IIa

1. It is reasonable that PCI be performed in patients with UA or NSTEMI and single-vessel or multivessel CAD who are undergoing medical therapy with focal saphenous vein graft lesions or multiple stenoses who are poor candidates for reoperative surgery.
2. In the absence of high-risk features associated with UA or NSTEMI, it is reasonable to perform PCI in patients with amenable lesions and no contraindication for PCI with either an early invasive or early conservative strategy.
3. Use of PCI is reasonable in patients with UA or NSTEMI with significant left main CAD (>50% diameter stenosis) who are candidates for revascularization but are not eligible for CABG.

Class IIb

1. In the absence of high-risk features associated with UA or NSTEMI, PCI may be considered in patients with single-vessel or multivessel CAD who are undergoing medical therapy and who have 1 or more lesions to be dilated with reduced likelihood of success.
2. PCI may be considered in patients with UA or NSTEMI who are undergoing medical therapy who have 2- or 3-vessel disease, significant proximal LAD CAD, and treated diabetes or abnormal LV function.

Class III

In the absence of high-risk features associated with UA or NSTEMI, PCI is not recommended for patients with UA or NSTEMI who have single-vessel or multivessel CAD and no trial of medical therapy, or who have 1 or more of the following:

1. Only a small area of myocardium at risk.
2. All lesions or the culprit lesion to be dilated with morphology that conveys a low likelihood of success.
3. A high risk of procedure-related morbidity or mortality.
4. Insignificant disease (< 50% coronary stenosis).
5. Significant left main CAD and candidacy for CABG.

STEMI

Class I

General considerations:

1. If immediately available, primary PCI should be performed in patients with STEMI who can undergo PCI of the infarct artery within 12 hours of symptom onset, if performed in a timely fashion (balloon inflation goal within 90 minutes of presentation).

Specific considerations:

2. Primary PCI should be performed for patients less than 75 years old with ST elevation or presumably new left bundle-branch block who develop shock within 36 hours of MI and are suitable for revascularization that can be performed within 18 hours of shock, unless further support is futile because of the patient's wishes or contraindications/unsuitability for further invasive care.
3. Primary PCI should be performed in patients with severe congestive heart failure and/or pulmonary edema (Killip class 3) and onset of symptoms within 12 hours.

Class IIa

1. Primary PCI is reasonable for selected patients 75 years or older with ST elevation or left bundle-branch block or who develop shock within 36 hours of MI and are suitable for revascularization that can be performed within 18 hours of shock. Patients with good prior functional status who are suitable for revascularization and agree to invasive care may be selected for such an invasive strategy.

Contd...

Contd...

Table 51: Indications for PCI

2. It is reasonable to perform primary PCI for patients with onset of symptoms within the prior 12–24 hours and 1 or more of the following:
   A. Severe congestive heart failure.
   B. Hemodynamic or electrical instability.
   C. Evidence of persistent ischemia.

Class III

1. Elective PCI should not be performed in a noninfarct related artery at the time of primary PCI of the infarct related artery in patients without hemodynamic compromise.
2. Primary PCI should not be performed in asymptomatic patients more than 12 hours after onset of STEMI who are hemodynamically and electrically stable.

PCI after successful fibrinolysis or for patients not undergoing primary reperfusion.

Class I

1. In patients whose anatomy is suitable, PCI should be performed when there is objective evidence of recurrent MI.
2. In patients whose anatomy is suitable, PCI should be performed for moderate or severe spontaneous or provocable myocardial ischemia during recovery from STEMI.
3. In patients whose anatomy is suitable, PCI should be performed for cardiogenic shock or hemodynamic instability.

Class IIa

1. It is reasonable to perform routine PCI in patients with LV ejection fraction less than or equal to 40%, HF, or serious ventricular arrhythmias.
2. It is reasonable to perform PCI when there is documented clinical heart failure during the acute episode, even though subsequent evaluation shows preserved LV function.

Class IIb

PCI might be considered as part of an invasive strategy after fibrinolytic therapy.

Percutaneous intervention in patients with prior coronary bypass surgery

Class I

1. When technically feasible, PCI should be performed in patients with early ischemia (usually within 30 days) after CABG.
2. It is recommended that embolic protection devices (EPD) be used when technically feasible in patients undergoing PCI to saphenous vein grafts.

Class IIa

1. PCI is reasonable in patients with ischemia that occurs 1–3 years after CABG and who have preserved LV function with discrete lesions in graft conduits.
2. PCI is reasonable in patients with disabling angina secondary to new disease in a native coronary circulation after CABG.
3. PCI is reasonable in patients with diseased vein grafts more than 3 years after CABG.
4. PCI is reasonable when technically feasible in patients with a patent left internal mammary artery graft who have clinically significant obstructions in other vessels.

Class III

1. PCI is not recommended in patients with prior CABG for chronic total vein graft occlusions.
2. PCI is not recommended in patients who have multiple target lesions with prior CABG and who have multivessel disease, failure of multiple SVGs and impaired LV function unless repeat CABG poses excessive risk due to severe comorbid conditions.

(*Source:* Modified from: King SB, Smith SC, Hirshfeld JW, et al. 2007 focused update of the ACC/AHA/SCAI 2005 guideline update for percutaneous coronary intervention. Circulation. 2008;117:261; and Modified from: Kushner FG, Hand M, Smith SC, et al. 2009 focused updates: ACC/AHA guidelines for the management of patients with ST-elevation myocardial infarction. Circulation. 2009;120:2271.)

❏ PHARMACOTHERAPY FOR PCI

Treatment with antiplatelet and anticoagulant medications is a requirement for the safe and successful performance of any PCI. Some of the most commonly used medications during PCI are described below.

Antiplatelet Therapy

Aspirin

Aspirin irreversibly inhibits cyclooxygenase and thus blocks the synthesis of thromboxane A2, a vasoconstricting agent that promotes platelet aggregation. Aspirin substantially reduces periprocedural MI caused by thrombotic occlusions compared with placebo and has been established as a standard for all patients undergoing PCI. Patients taking daily aspirin should receive 75–325 mg aspirin before PCI. Patients not already taking daily long-term aspirin therapy should be given 300–325 mg of aspirin at least 2 hours and preferably 24 hours before PCI is performed.

Thienopyridines

Dual antiplatelet therapy with aspirin and a thienopyridine is required in any PCI that includes stenting. The indicated duration of dual antiplatelet therapy specifically related to stenting varies, depending on if bare metal or drug-eluting stents are used. Dual antiplatelet therapy is needed for at least 1 month with bare metal stent placement and for at least 1 year if a drug-eluting stent is placed. Clopidogrel inhibits platelet activation by irreversibly blocking the ADP (P2Y12) receptor. Along with aspirin, clopidogrel is routinely administered prior to stent implantation. Recent evidence also supports its use in non-stent PCI. An initial clopidogrel dose of 600 mg is needed to produce potent inhibition of ADP-induced platelet aggregation within 2 hours. A 300 mg loading dose can be used when longer pretreatment is possible and has been shown to produce maximal platelet inhibition within 24 hours with substantial inhibition at 15 hours.

Prasugrel is a more potent P2Y12 ADP receptor inhibitor that has a more rapid onset of action and higher levels of platelet inhibition than higher dose clopidogrel. In patients with an acute coronary syndrome undergoing PCI who are at low bleeding risk and have not had a previous stroke, prasugrel 60 mg loading dose should be given as soon as possible after definition of the coronary anatomy and continued for the appropriate course after stent placement, depending on the type of stent used.

Ticagrelor is a reversible oral P2Y12 receptor antagonist which provides faster, greater and more consistent ADP-receptor inhibition than clopidogrel. Current evidence suggests that in the absence of risk factors for bleeding, dual antiplatelet therapy should be continued for at least 1 month after BMS placement and for 1 year after drugeluting stents (DES) placement.

IIb/IIIa Platelet Receptor Inhibitors

Thrombin and collagen are potent platelet agonists that can cause ADP and serotonin release and activate glycoprotein (GP) IIb/ IIIa fibrinogen receptors on the platelet surface. The first such agent approved by the FDA was abciximab, a monoclonal antibody. Abciximab was shown to reduce ischemic complications and late clinical events in high-risk angioplasty. The other IIb/IIIa receptor inhibitors approved by the FDA include eptifibatide, a peptide and tirofiban, a small nonpeptide molecule. These are both competitive inhibitors. Each of these agents reduces a composite end point of death or nonfatal MI in the setting of coronary intervention and in acute coronary syndromes.

❑ PARENTERAL ANTICOAGULANT THERAPY

Intravenous anticoagulation is always given during PCI to prevent thrombosis during the procedure. This practice was historically initiated because of the central role of thrombin in arterial thrombosis. Anticoagulation is used in conjunction with antiplatelet therapy for PCI. There are a few options of different agents to use for anticoagulation during PCI.

Heparin

For PCI, heparin monitoring is usually performed via the ACT, since the partial thromboplastin time (PTT) becomes prolonged at the heparin concentrations used in these procedures. The most recent American College of Cardiology/American Heart Association/Society for Cardiovascular Angiography and Intervention guideline update for PCI also recommends that intravenous, unfractionated heparin (UFH) should be given using a weight-adjusted bolus of 70–100 IU/kg to achieve an ACT between 250 and 350 seconds, in patients who do not receive a GP IIb/IIIa inhibitor. Postprocedural heparin is not recommended in patients with an uncomplicated procedure.

Enoxaparin

Although seemingly safe and as effective as unfractionated heparin, the clinical role of low molecular weight heparin remains uncertain as a routine strategy for PCI. It seems reasonable to continue enoxaparin rather than switching to unfractionated heparin once it has been initiated, but it must be redosed at the time of the PCI in most cases.

Bivalirudin

Bivalirudin is a specific direct thrombin inhibitor. Trials showed that bivalirudin is statistically noninferior to unfractionated heparin for the prevention of ischemic complications in patients undergoing PCI with stenting.

Bivalirudin is one of the alternatives in patients with known or suspected heparin-induced thrombocytopenia who require PCI. One potential disadvantage of bivalirudin is its increased cost compared to unfractionated heparin. Although, reduction of bleeding complications may certainly balance out this initial increased cost. One last thing to keep in mind about bivalirudin is that there is no reversing agent for its anticoagulant effect.

❑ PERCUTANEOUS TRANSLUMINAL CORONARY ANGIOPLASTY

Percutaneous transluminal coronary angioplasty (PTCA) expands the coronary lumen by stretching and tearing the atherosclerotic plaque and vessel wall and, to a lesser extent, by redistributing atherosclerotic plaque along its longitudinal axis. Elastic recoil of the stretched vessel wall generally leaves a 30–35% residual diameter stenosis, and the vessel expansion can result in propagating coronary dissections, leading to abrupt vessel closure in 5–8% of patients. Due to significant technological advances (stent development primarily) and the increased rates of abrupt vessel closure and restenosis with PTCA alone compared to stenting that has been demonstrated, "stand alone" PTCA has a limited role in PCI today.

❏ CORONARY STENTS

PTCA was associated with two major limitations: acute (during the procedure) or subacute (after the procedure and within 30 days) vessel closure and late (4–8 months postprocedure) restenosis. The development and use of intracoronary stents and the enhanced use of various antithrombotic therapies have resulted in significant reductions in both of these complications. Due to these advantages, stenting is now performed in the majority of PCIs. Despite substantial improvements in early and late outcomes with bare metal stenting compared to PTCA, restenosis of these stents can occur in the months to years after bare metal stenting.

❏ TYPES OF STENTS

There are many different types of intracoronary stents. They can generally be considered according to metal composition, open versus closed cell design, and whether or not they are capable of eluting drugs for local delivery. Currently available intracoronary stents are generally composed of either stainless steel or a cobalt–chromium alloy. In general, cobalt–chromium stents tend to be more flexible, while the stainless steel designs may offer greater radial strength for bulky lesions or those involving the more fibromuscular aorto-ostial locations.

Today, intracoronary stents come premounted on a compliant balloon are delivered through a coronary guide catheter over a guidewire to the lesion and deployed by inflation of the balloon. Optimal stenting is performed in a way that reduces the minimal residual luminal stenosis to as small as possible. Given the current availability of low profile stent delivery systems, many stenting procedures are completed with a direct stenting technique where the first intervention to the lesion is the placement of the stent. Lesion should always be dilated with a balloon before stent deployment is attempted if there is any concern that the lesion may not dilate optimally with initial stent deployment. Significant lesion calcification and the fibrotic, sometimes resistant plaque in cases of restenosis are situations where lesion predilation should be strongly considered.

❏ PROCEDURAL SUCCESS AND COMPLICATIONS RELATED TO CORONARY INTERVENTION

Procedural success after PCI is measured both in terms of the angiographic success in treating the diseased vessel as well as in the complication rates related to the performance of the procedure. Complications during coronary interventions can be considered as those that are common to the complications that occur with diagnostic coronary angiography, or those that occur specifically as a result of the coronary intervention. Anatomic (or angiographic) success after PCI is defined as the attainment of a residual diameter stenosis of less than 50% after PTCA or less than 20% after stenting. A number of clinical, angiographic and technical variables predict the risk of procedural failure and complications in patients undergoing PCI. Major complications include death, MI or stroke; minor complications include transient ischemic attacks, vascular access site complications, CIN and a host of angiographic complications (Table 52).

Table 52: Variables associated with early failure and complications after percutaneous coronary intervention

Clinical variables
- Women
- Advanced age
- Diabetes mellitus
- Unstable or Canadian Cardiovascular Society (CCS) Class IV angina
- Congestive heart failure
- Cardiogenic shock
- Renal insufficiency
- Preprocedural instability requiring intra-aortic balloon pump support
- Preprocedural elevation of C-reactive protein
- Multivessel coronary artery disease

Anatomic variables
- Multivessel CAD-
- Left main disease
- Thrombus
- SVG intervention
- ACC/AHA type B2 and C lesion morphology
- Chronic total coronary occlusion
- Large area of myocardium at risk
- PCI of vessel supplying collaterals to a large artery

Procedural factors
- A higher final percentage diameter stenosis
- Smaller minimal lumen diameter
- Presence of a residual dissection or trans-stenotic pressure gradient

❑ SUGGESTED READINGS

Anderson HV, Shaw RE, Brindis RG, et al. A contemporary overview of percutaneous coronary interventions. The American College of Cardiology-National Cardiovascular Data Registry (ACC-NCDR). J Am Coll Cardiol. 2002;39:1096-103.

Angelini P. Coronary artery anomalies—current clinical issues: definitions, classification, incidence, clinical relevance, and treatment guidelines. Tex Heart Inst J. 2002;29:271-8.

Campeau L. Percutaneous radial artery approach for coronary angiography. Cathet Cardiovasc Diagn. 1989;16:3-7.

Chew DP, Bhatt DL, Lincoff AM, et al. Defining the optimal activated clotting time during percutaneous coronary intervention: aggregate results from 6 randomized, controlled trials. Circulation. 2001;103: 961-6.

Douglas JS, King SB. Complications of coronary arteriography: management during and following the procedure. In: King SB, Douglas JS (Eds). Coronary Arteriography. New York: McGraw-Hill; 1984. pp. 302-13.

Gibbons RJ, Abrams J, Chatterjee K, et al. ACC/AHA 2002 guideline update for the management of patients with chronic stable angina— summary article: a report of the American College of Cardiology/ American Heart Association Task Force on Practice Guidelines (Committee on the Management of Patients with Chronic Stable Angina). Circulation. 2003;107:149-58.

Jolly SS, Amlani S, Hamon M, et al. Radial versus femoral access for coronary angiography or intervention and the impact on major bleeding and ischemic events: a systematic review and meta-analysis of randomized trials. Am Heart J. 2009;157:132-40.

Kiemeneij F, Laarman GJ, Odekerken D, et al. A randomized comparison of percutaneous transluminal coronary angioplasty by the radial, brachial and femoral approaches: the access study. J Am Coll Cardiol. 1997;29:1269-75.

Krone RJ, Shaw RE, Klein LW, et al. Evaluation of the ACC/AHA/ SCAI lesion classification system in the current "stent era" of coronary interventions (from the ACC–National Cardiovascular Data Registry). Am J Cardiol. 2003;92:389-94.

Smith S, Feldman TE, Hirshfeld JW, et al. ACC/AHA/SCAI 2005 guideline update for percutaneous coronary intervention: a report of the American College of Cardiology/American Heart Association Task Force on Practice Guidelines (ACC/AHA/SCAI Writing Committee to Update the 2001 Guidelines for Percutaneous Coronary Intervention). J Am Coll Cardiol. 2006;47:e1-121.

Sutton JM, Ellis SG, Roubin GS, et al. Major clinical events after coronary stenting. The multicenter registry of acute and elective Gianturco-Roubin stent placement. The Gianturco-Roubin Intracoronary Stent Investigator Group. Circulation. 1994;89:1126-37.

Chapter 3

Electrophysiology

3.1 Arrhythmia Mechanisms

❏ INTRODUCTION

Arrhythmias require initiating conditions and a hospitable substrate for perpetuation. Triggers and substrates are often considered as unrelated or independent events. However, new findings suggest that triggers and substrates may be connected, particularly in structural heart disease, by hyperactivity of signaling molecules, intracellular Ca^{2+} and reactive oxygen species (ROS). There is now a body of evidence to support a view that the increased ROS and disturbed intracellular Ca^{2+} homeostasis that mark structural heart disease contribute to arrhythmia initiation, while actively promoting a proarrhythmic substrate. Ion channels are the fundamental effectors that determine membrane currents and arrhythmias, but ion channels are regulated by multiple factors in myocardium, including intracellular Ca^{2+}, phosphorylation and ROS. These same factors participate in responses to common forms of myocardial injury, including ischemia and infarction, which lead to proarrhythmic adaptations in myocardium.

❏ ARRHYTHMIA INITIATION

Molecular and Cellular Mechanisms

Ion channels and exchangers are the fundamental units directing physiological and pathological membrane excitability and conduction.

$$E = \frac{RT}{zF} \ln \frac{[\text{ion outside cell}]}{[\text{ion inside cell}]} = 2.303 \frac{RT}{zF} \log_{10} \frac{[\text{ion outside cell}]}{[\text{ion inside cell}]}$$

Nernst Equation E-equilibrium potential or Nernst potential is the cell membrane potential that is necessary to oppose the diffusion of an ion across the cell membrane as motivated by the concentration gradient of each ion (R—universal gas constant; T—temperature in degrees Kelvin; z—valence: F—Faraday's constant). At 25°C, RT/F = 25.693 mV.

Selective membrane permeability coupled with active pumps (ATPases) allow for an electrochemical gradient across cell membranes. The Nernst equation is a powerful, but simplified (i.e. relies exclusively on two ions), description of a half cell that predicts how ionic gradients determine cell membrane potential. The maintenance of Na^+ and K^+ gradients under conditions of selective membrane permeability requires a Na^+ and K^+ 'pump'—the Na^+/K^+ ATPase. The Na^+/K^+ pump transports extracellular Na^+ $[Na^+]o$ and intracellular K^+ $[K^+]i$ against their concentration gradients, a process that requires energy input from ATP hydrolysis. The Na^+/K^+ ATPase is required to maintain physiological $[Na^+]o$ (~145 mM), $[K^+]o$ (~4 mM) and $[Na^+]i$ (~10 mM), $[K^+]i$ (~140 mM) in the face of the tendency of these gradients to dissipate with repetitive opening of Na^+ and K^+ channel proteins.

Under resting conditions myocardial cell membrane potentials approximate the equilibrium potential for K+, ~ −90 mV, where the cytosolic side of the membrane is negative and the extracellular side of the membrane is positive, because the cell membrane permeability is greatest for K+ under resting conditions. The resting membrane permeability to K+ occurs because a particular ion channel, the inward rectifier, opens at the negative potentials present in resting membranes.

$$Eeq, K^+ = \frac{RT}{zF} \ln \frac{[K^+]_0}{[K^+]_i}$$

Nernst Equation for K^+.

The resting membrane potential is highly dependent upon [K+]o and the resting membrane potential determines membrane excitability in part because voltage-gated Na+ channels (mostly NaV1.5) begin to inactivate at membrane potentials more positive than −100 mV. At 37 °C (~310 °K) the equilibrium potential for K+ (Eeq, K+) is −91 mV for [K+]o = 4.5 mM and [K+]i = 140 mM. If the [K+]o is reduced to 2.5 mM the Eeq, K+ is −107.5 mV (and more NaV1.5 channels are available to activate), and if the [K+]o = 6.5 mM, the Eeq, K+ is −82 mV (with reduced NaV1.5 channel availability). Thus, the Nernst equation provides quantitative insight into the importance of K+ homeostasis for normal cardiac electrophysiology.

Ion channels are protein complexes embedded in cell membranes. All ion channels consist of a pore forming a subunit. Some a subunits (e.g. K+ channels) aggregate with identical or similar a subunits to form a cell membrane spanning pore. This pore is the conductance pathway that allows individual ions to cross lipid bilayer membranes with high throughput. Ion channels are configured for relative ion selectivity. The specific amino acids lining the pore create a 'filter' that selects ionic species for conductance based on ionic size and charge. In solution ions are effectively larger due to a sphere of hydration that is a result of charge associated water molecules. Ion channels open and close in response to a blend of various stimuli. In contracting atrial and ventricular myocardium and in specialized pacemaking [sinoatrial node (SAN)] and conduction tissue (atrioventricular node and His-Purkinje system) the most important and best understood ion channels are primarily opened by changes in membrane potential. These so-called 'voltage-gated ion channels' all contain a cell membrane spanning domain enriched in charged amino acids that act as a membrane voltage sensor. The voltage sensor moves in response to changes in the membrane potential, and these movements are allosterically coupled to the pore domain. Voltage-gated ion channels open and close in response to a change in membrane potential, but also inactivate.

Ion channels are not the only source of ionic membrane currents. In myocardium, the Na+/Ca2+ exchanger is the predominant mechanism for removing Ca2+ from the cytoplasm to the extracellular space. The Na+/Ca2+ exchanger transfers a Ca2+ for 3Na+ (forward exchange mode). Because there is a single net positive charge moved to exchange a Ca2+ ion from the cytoplasm to the extracellular space, the Na+/Ca2+ exchanger produces a small inward Na+ current in forward mode. Although the Na+/Ca2+ exchanger does not directly require ATP, the Na+ gradient necessary for forward mode exchange depends upon the ATP-requiring Na+/K+ ATPase. The Na+/K+ ATPase and a sarcolemmal Ca2+ ATPase produce small, but measurable currents. The Na+/Ca2+ exchanger current, although small in magnitude compared to NaV or CaV channel currents, contributes to AP duration. It is essential for the direct myocardial inotropic actions of digitalis glycosides, which inhibit the Na+/K+ ATPase leading to accumulation of [Na+]i and consequent increase in [Ca2+]i, because the gradient for Ca2+ extrusion by Na+/Ca2+ exchanger is less favorable than when [Na+]i is lower.

Action Potentials Require Orchestrated Ion Channel Opening and Inactivation

Action potentials are the fundamental unit of membrane excitability (Fig. 1). In most myocardial cells action potentials are initiated by opening of voltage-gated Na+ channels, NaV1.5. The inward NaV1.5 current (INa) depolarizes atrial and ventricular myocytes in a few milliseconds. The brevity of INa is due to the rapidity of the inactivation process, which competes with activation to modulate the peak current. The membrane potential depolarizes (becomes more positive) from the negative resting potential (~ −80 mV) to approach the reversal potential for Na+, estimated by the Nernst equation (~ +50 mV). Specialized myocytes that are dedicated more to automaticity (i.e. SAN) and conduction (i.e. the atrioventricular node) than contraction rely on ICa for their (phase 0) action potential upstroke. Membrane depolarization activates a combination of voltage-gated ion channels, but the most prominent are depolarizing inward CaV1.2/1.3 currents (ICa) and several distinct, but structurally related repolarizing inward K+ channel (KVx) currents (IK). The interplay between ICa and IK largely determines the duration of the myocardial action potentials, which last hundreds of milliseconds. Atrial and ventricular myocardial action potentials have different shapes and electrophysiological properties. In fact, there are important heterogeneities in action potential configuration within the atrium and ventricle. The ventricular

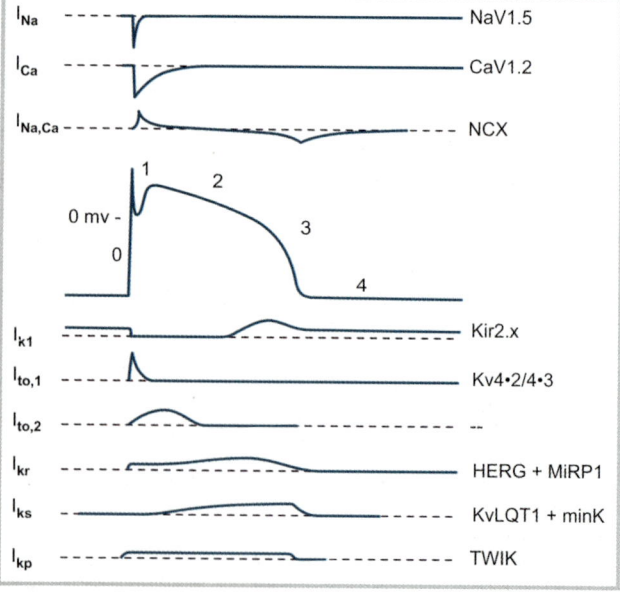

FIGURE 1: The action potential duration and configuration is shaped by the interplay between inward and outward-going ionic currents. The top two tracings represent NaV1.5 and CaV1.2 inward currents that initiate and sustain action potential depolarization. The third tracing from the top is the Na+/Ca2+ exchanger (NCX) that can produce inward (forward mode) and outward (reverse mode) currents at various action potential phases. The ventricular action potential is labeled by phase (0–4). The lower six tracings represent some of the K+ currents that contribute to action potential repolarization

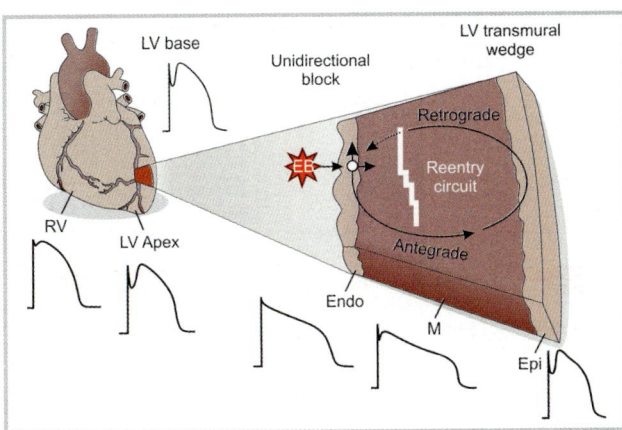

FIGURE 2: Ventricular action potentials are heterogeneous and vary between base and apex and across the myocardium from endocardium to epicardium. M cells in the mid-myocardium have characteristically long action potentials with a reduced phase 1. Structural defects, such as scar tissue, can serve as a structural barrier that supports a reentry circuit for arrhythmias. Exaggeration of action potential heterogeneities, by genetic disease or acquired disease, can also support a reentry circuit, even in the absence of scar

endocardium, midmyocardium and epicardium show prominent differences in action potential configuration, due to variability in expression of repolarizing K^+ currents (Fig. 2).

Action Potential Physiology: A Consequence of Ion Channel and Cellular Properties

Myocardial action potentials are distinguished from action potentials in other excitable tissues by their extreme length, lasting up to hundreds of milliseconds. In contrast, action potentials in most neurons last only a few milliseconds. Cardiac action potentials are often described in phases (Fig. 1). Phase 0 marks the abrupt depolarization from the resting potential and is attributable to NaV1.5 current in most myocardial cells. Cardiac action potentials are long because of their plateau. The action potential plateau occurs because of a fine balance, mostly between depolarizing inward CaV current, a small persistent (slowly inactivating) component of NaV1.5 current, and activation of repolarizing K^+ currents.

Action potentials can be repetitively initiated in atrial and ventricular myocardium within the time constraints of the tissue refractory period (Figs 3A and B). The refractory period is determined in large part by the duration of the cardiac action potential. Action potentials are initiated by positive (inward) current sufficient to depolarize the membrane potential to the threshold for activation of NaV1.5 in contracting myocardium or CaV1 in specialized conduction tissue. During phase 2 of the action potential plateau myocardial cells are absolutely refractory, meaning that no amount of inward current is adequate to elicit an action potential. Later, in the course of action potential repolarization (phase 3), an action potential can be stimulated, but only by a larger inward current than would be necessary after completion of action potential repolarization. Tissue where an action potential can only be stimulated by a supranormal current is said to be

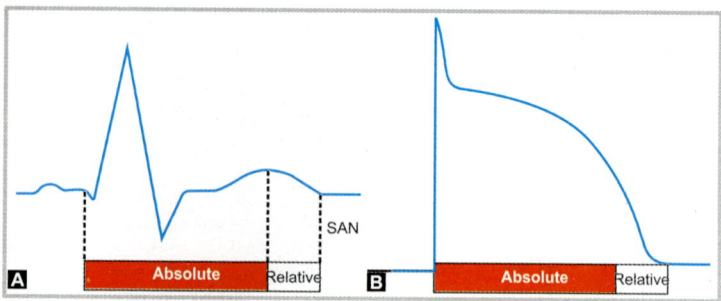

FIGURES 3A AND B: Tissue refractoriness to excitation is determined by action potential repolarization and reflected in the surface ECG. (A) A schematic ECG tracing. (B) The surface ECG is a reflection of many action potentials. Myocardial tissue is absolutely refractory to repeat stimulation (dark bars) until late in repolarization. Tissue is potentially excitable prior to completion of repolarization, but initiation of excitation requires a supranormal depolarizing current, a state of relative refractoriness (light bars).

relatively refractory. Under physiological conditions action potentials shorten in response to shorter stimulation intervals (i.e. faster rates), due to a process called restitution. Action potential restitution occurs, in part, because rapid simulation enhances net outward repolarizing current. Action potential restitution is impaired in genetic long QT syndromes (LQTS), where repolarizing currents are defective, or in common forms of heart failure where reduction in repolarizing currents is a signature event in the proarrhythmic electrical remodeling process. Tissue refractoriness can persist after action potential repolarization under conditions of reduced availability of inward currents responsible for phase 0 depolarization (i.e. NaV1.5 in contracting myocardium and CaV1.2 and CaV1.3 in specialized conduction tissue). Various factors contribute to availability of these channels to open, including cell membrane potential (e.g. fewer NaV and CaV channels are available to open at depolarized potentials because membrane depolarization favors inactivation), oxidation, pH, $[Ca^{2+}]i$, ischemia and autonomic tone. Thus, cell membrane excitability depends on multiple input variables that ultimately converge on ion channels and APs.

Action Potentials: Designed for Automaticity and to Initiate Contraction

Myocardial action potentials are committed to the major tasks of myocardium: rhythmic, repetitive beating and mechanical work that propels blood through the circulatory system. Sinoatrial node (SAN) action potentials have a specialized, late diastolic component or phase 4 where membrane depolarization leads to activation of CaV channel currents to drive phase 0 depolarization. The slope of phase 4 is the membrane potential mechanism for increasing (steeper slope) or decreasing (shallower slope) heart rate (Fig. 4). In healthy hearts, the activity of phase 4 is largely confined to the SAN, where the steady increase in net inward current during late diastolic depolarization is augmented by b adrenergic receptor stimulation and reduced by muscarinic receptor stimulation. Multiple currents likely contribute to physiological phase 4 depolarization in SAN, but recent evidence suggests that two currents play a critical role in physiological pacing. The classical 'pacemaker' current is a Na^+/K^+ selective cation current carried by an *HCN4* gene encoded channel. The *HCN4* current, also called the funny current (If) is enhanced by cyclic AMP, which

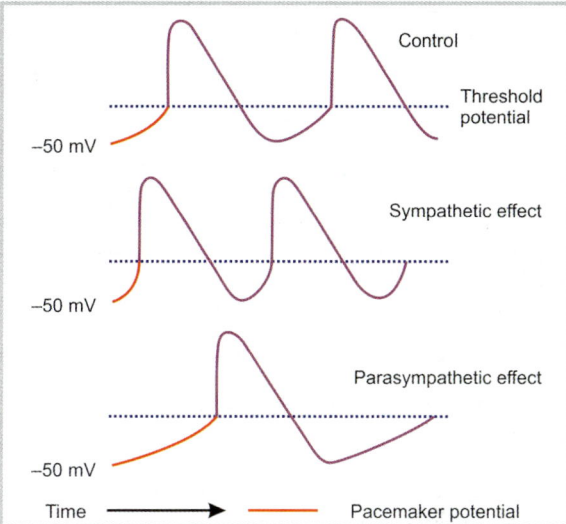

FIGURE 4: The cell membrane potential for determining heart rate in sinoatrial nodal cells is set by the steepness of phase 4 (pacemaker) potential. Steeper phase 4 allows the membrane potential to reach the threshold for action potential initiation more rapidly than shallow phase 4 depolarization

confers increased activity (and steeper phase 4) with a adrenergic receptor agonist stimulation. More recent understanding of physiological automaticity in SAN cells suggests that SR Ca^{2+} release enhances inward Na^+/Ca^{2+} exchanger current. The relationship between spontaneous SAN cell SR Ca^{2+} release and inward Na^+/Ca^{2+} exchanger current that contributes to phase 4 depolarization has been called a 'Ca^{2+} clock mechanism' of pacing. The Ca^{2+} clock is responsive to a adrenergic receptor agonist stimulation because cellular Ca^{2+} entry by CaV1 currents and SR Ca^{2+} release are both increased by catecholamines. While the Ca^{2+} clock appears to contribute to the normal physiology of SAN cells, SR Ca^{2+} leak and increased inward Na^+/Ca^{2+} exchanger current is known to induce DADs and trigger arrhythmias in atrial and ventricular myocardium under conditions of pathological stress. Thus, physiological automaticity resembles pathological triggering, suggesting that so-called 'triggered' arrhythmias are a natural consequence of excitation–contraction coupling.

Action Potential Physiology: Reflected by the Surface Electrocardiogram

The ECG is a surface report on myocardial electrical activity. Although multiple factors influence ECG parameters, the basic intervals (PR, QRS, QT) reflect ion channel-directed AP parameters. The PR interval is the duration required for an electrical impulse to conduct from the point of 'break out' near the SAN to the ventricle. In diseased myocardium, impaired atrial and His–Purkinje conduction may contribute to PR prolongation. The QRS interval reflects the speed of conduction and depolarization through the right and left ventricles. The QRS interval can be prolonged by NaV or Cx gene defects or antagonist drugs, injury or disease in the His–Purkinje system or myocardial injury, including myocardial ischemia, infarction and scar. The QT interval corresponds to ventricular repolarization. Ventricular repolarization is complex, due to the physiological variation in repolarizing ionic currents in endocardium, mid-myocardium and epicardium, as well as between the ventricular apex and base. QT interval prolongation can occur in long QT syndromes that are due to intrinsic defects in repolarizing ionic currents or their cellular localization (LQTS). Ion channel antagonist drugs are the most common reason for QT interval prolongation. Importantly, a wide variety of drugs are antagonists of the hERG (human ether-a-go-go related gene) or *KCNH2* encoded KV11.1 K$^+$ channel a subunit protein that conducts the rapid delayed rectifier current (IKr). Rectifier current antagonist properties are a major obstacle for drug development because of the link between QT prolongation, Torsade de Pointes ventricular arrhythmia and sudden death. Diseases of ion channel encoding genes that alter membrane repolarization can result in AP and QT interval lengthening (Long QT syndromes) or AP and QT interval shortening (Short QT syndromes). Failing myocardium from a variety of causes (e.g. myocardial infarction, valvular disease, genetic disease) undergoes a proarrhythmic electrical remodeling process where repolarizing K$^+$ currents are reduced resulting in AP and QT interval prolongation. Understanding basic electrophysiological principles constitutes the foundation for understanding arrhythmia mechanisms and for interpreting ECGs.

Afterdepolarizations and Triggered Arrhythmias

Afterdepolarizations are arrhythmia-initiating oscillations in cell membrane potential. Early afterdepolarizations (EADs) occur during the plateau phases (2 and 3) of AP repolarization. Delayed afterdepolarizations (DADs) occur after AP repolarization, during phase 4. EADs and DADs can trigger an arrhythmia by propagating to adjacent tissue under favorable source-sink conditions. EADs and DADs of sufficient magnitude depolarize the cell membrane to reach the threshold for activation of NaV and/or CaV channel currents to initiate AP phase 0. Both EADs and DADs can be thought to arise as a consequence of corruption of key components of CICR.

EADs and DADs are hypothesized to initiate life-threatening arrhythmias in long QT syndromes, catecholaminergic polymorphic VT, atrial fibrillation, and ventricular arrhythmias in heart failure. Long QT syndromes are mostly the result of dominant or dominant negative mutations that cause a defect in depolarization that results in AP prolongation, CaMKII is activated in atrial fibrillation and during AP prolongation, due to enhanced Ca^{2+} entry, and is thought to promote arrhythmias by enhancing CaV1 current facilitation, the noninactivating component of NaV1.5 and SR Ca^{2+} leak in animal and cellular models.

Proarrhythmic Substrates

Cardiac arrhythmias are often initiated by afterdepolarizations, but sustained by a mechanism called reentry (Fig. 5). Reentry can occur over a large tissue domain (e.g. typical atrial flutter, bundle branch reentry ventricular tachycardia, the atrioventricular reciprocating tachycardia), or in a small volume of tissue (e.g. atrioventricular nodal tachycardia, fasicular ventricular tachycardia). Processes that lead to myocardial scar formation, such as myocardial infarction, can favor reentry by producing regions of slowed conduction. Physiological electrical heterogeneity is exaggerated by proarrhythmic drugs, and in animal models of mycoardial hypertrophy. Enhanced dispersion of repolarization is thought to support a voltage gradient that constitutes a functional reentrant circuit. Reduced INa, as occurs in the Brugada syndrome, can also induce a functional reentrant circuit by unmasking enhanced transient outward K$^+$ current in AP phase 1.

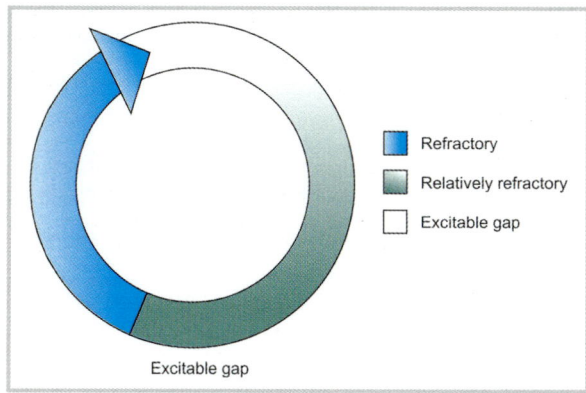

FIGURE 5: A simplified reentrant circuit with core components indicated by color coding

Proarrhythmic Triggers and Substrates: Promoted in Failing Hearts

Although afterdepolarizations and reentry are distinct entities, there is a growing appreciation that common biological factors can promote development of proarrhythmic triggers and substrates in heart failure. CaMKII has emerged as a signal that drives structural and electrical components of myocardial injury, providing a molecular rationale to explain why failing hearts are prone to arrhythmias. Failing myocardium is consistently marked by AP prolongation, loss of normal intracellular Ca^{2+} homeostasis, increased ROS and increased expression of CaMKII. These factors favor EADs because the prolonged AP plateau occurs over a membrane potential window permissive for CaV1.2 opening. After myocardial infarction the border-zone tissue between nonliving scar and normal myocytes serves as a substrate for reentry. Surviving border-zone tissue undergoes electrical remodeling marked by reduced NaV1.5 expression that is due, at least in part, to reduction in ion channel-targeting ankyrin G expression. Loss of NaV1.5 current contributes to conduction slowing. In addition, borderzone tissue is enriched in ROS and ROS activated CaMKII is increased in the MI border-zone. The prosurvival effects of CaMKII inhibition are likely multifactorial, and have been mapped to CaV1.2, SR Ca^{2+}, and mitochondria. CaMKII activation after MI results in activation of inflammatory signaling by increased nuclear factor for κB (NF-κB) transcription. Thus, understanding CaMKII signaling provides insight into how a properly positioned nodal signal can produce the twin phenotypes of heart failure and arrhythmias.

❏ SUGGESTED READINGS

Grant AO. Cardiac ion channels. Circ Arrhythm Electrophysiol. 2009;2:185-94.

Grueter CE, Abiria SA, Dzhura I, et al. L-Type Ca(2+) channel facilitation mediated by phosphorylation of the beta subunit by CaMKII 1. Mol Cell. 2006;23:641-50.

Hodgkin AL, Huxley AF. A quantitative description of membrane current and its application to conduction and excitation in nerve. Journal of Physiology. 1952;117:500-44.

Kurita T, Ohe T, Shimizu W, et al. Early afterdepolarizationlike activity in patients with class IA induced long QT syndrome and torsades de pointes. Pacing and Clinical Electrophysiology. 1997;20:695-705.

Pogwizd SM, McKenzie JP, Cain ME. Mechanisms underlying spontaneous and induced ventricular arrhythmias in patients with idiopathic dilated cardiomyopathy. Circ. 1998;98:2404-14.

Roden DM, Balser JR, George AL Jr., et al. Cardiac ion channels. Annu Rev Physiol. 2002;64:431-75.

Sun XH, Protasi F, Takahashi M, et al. Molecular architecture of membranes involved in excitation-contraction coupling of cardiac muscle. Journal of Cell Biology. 1995;129:659-71.

Tessier S, Karczewski P, Krause EG, et al. Regulation of the transient outward K(+) current by Ca(2+)/calmodulin-dependent protein kinases II in human atrial myocytes. Circulation Research. 1999;85:810-9.

Tomaselli GF, Barth AS. Sudden cardio arrest: oxidative stress irritates the heart. Nat Med. 2010;16:648-9.

Yang Y, Zhu WZ, Joiner ML, et al. Calmodulin kinase II inhibition protects against myocardial cell apoptosis in vivo 3. Am J Physiol Heart Circ Physiol. 2006;291:H3065–H75.

3.2 Antiarrhythmic Drugs

❏ INTRODUCTION

Antiarrhythmic drugs (AADs) were developed to suppress cardiac arrhythmias, and therefore improve survival, symptoms and morbidity. The AAD therapy has undergone constant evolution as new therapies have emerged and the risk benefit profile of these drugs on major clinical endpoints is better understood. Currently, AADs, for the most part, are used as an adjunct to therapies that target and cure the rhythm like catheter ablation or those directed against the underlying structural heart disease.

❏ ARRHYTHMIA MECHANISMS AND ANTIARRHYTHMIC DRUGS

Cardiac tachyarrhythmias are due to several well-understood mechanisms, including various forms of reentry, triggered activity and automaticity. The AADs can affect cardiac ionic channels and receptors to affect properties that alter the chance of initiation, perpetuation and termination of tachyarrhythmias. The AADs can affect cardiac excitability, conduction, and refractoriness.

❏ INDICATIONS FOR ANTIARRHYTHMIC DRUG THERAPY

The AADs are now mainly used to treat atrial tachyarrhythmias, particularly atrial fibrillation (AF). While mortality outcome with regard to rhythm control with an AAD is not superior to rate control, symptom reduction and improvement in quality of life can be superior in select patients who have AF and atrial flutter. The AADs are used to treat other supraventricular tachyarrhythmias, including AV node reentry, sinoatrial reentry, AV reentry tachycardia and atrial tachycardias. Occasionally, AADs are used to suppress ventricular and atrial ectopy including nonsustained and even sustained ventricular tachycardia (VT) but their use is balanced by potential adverse effects. The AADs can be used as primary therapy for patients with idiopathic VT but for patients with underlying structural heart disease and VT, AADs are not generally recommended as primary therapy unless there are specific reasons to do so in lieu of ablation therapy and/or implantable devices. The reason for this is that the proarrhythmic effects of the drugs can exceed the benefits.

Table 1: The Vaughan–Williams classification of antiarrhythmic drugs			
Class	**Drug**	**Ion channel effect**	**Electrophysiological effect**
I		Block inward Na^+ channel and outward K^+ channels	
IA	Quinidine Procainamide Disopyramide		Slow conduction velocity (predominant effect) and increase refractoriness
IB	Lidocaine Mexiletine		Shorten APD, especially in depolarized cells
IC	Flecainide Propafenone		Marked conduction slowing (minimal effect on refractoriness)
II	Beta-blockers	Beta-adrenoceptor blockade	Sympatholytic effect
III	Sotalol	Block Ikr and beta-receptors	Prolong refractoriness and APD
	Amiodarone	Blocks multiple potassium channels, Na^+ channels, Ca^{++} channels, beta-receptors	Prolong refractoriness and APD
	Dronedarone	Blocks multiple potassium channels, Na^+ channels, Ca^{++} channels, beta-receptors	Prolong refractoriness and APD
	Ibutilide	Blocks Ikr and late Na^+ current	Prolong refractoriness and APD
	Dofetilide	Blocks Ikr	Prolong refractoriness and APD
	Azimilide	Blocks Ikr and Iks	Prolong refractoriness and APD
IV	Calcium channel blockers	Blocks Ca^{++} channels	Negative chronotropic and inotropic effects

(Abbreviations: APD: Action potential duration; Ikr: Rapid rectifier current; IKs: Delayed rectifier current)

❑ CLASSIFICATION SCHEME

The Vaughan-Williams classification, the most commonly used and by far the most clinically relevant, classifies the drugs based on their most prominent electrophysiological action (Table 1).

❑ VAUGHAN–WILLIAMS CLASSIFICATION

Class I: Sodium channel blockers

Class IA, e.g. quinidine, procainamide, disopyramide

Class IB, e.g. lidocaine, mexiletine, phenytoin

Class IC, e.g. flecainide, propafenone

Class II: Sympathetic antagonists—beta-blockers

Class III: Prolong repolarization, e.g. sotalol, amiodarone, dofetilide, ibutilide, dronedarone, azimilide

Class IV: Calcium channel antagonists

The dosing, common uses and adverse effects of the orally available AADs are shown in Table 2.

Table 2: Dosing, uses and side effects of orally available antiarrhythmic drugs

Class	Drug	Maintenance oral dosing	Side effects	Uses
IA	Quinidine	300–600 mg every 6 hours	• Nausea, vomiting, diarrhea, anorexia, abdominal pain • Tinnitus, hearing loss, visual disturbance, confusion (cinchonism) • Thrombocytopenia, hemolytic anemia, anaphylaxis • Hypotension, QRS prolongation, syncope, torsades de pointes, QT prolongation	• PVCs • Sustained VT and VF • Short QT syndrome • Brugada syndrome • AF • Atrial flutter
	Procainamide	250–1,000 mg every 4–6 hours (no longer available)	• Rash, myalgia, vasculitis, Raynaud • Fever, agranulocytosis • Hypotension, bradycardia, QT prolongation, torsades de pointes • Drug-induced lupus	• Sustained VT • Unmasking Brugada syndrome • AF in WPW
	Disopyramide	100–200 mg every 6 hours	• Urinary retention, constipation, glaucoma, xerostomia • QT prolongation, torsades de pointes • Reduced ventricular contractility	• PVCs • VT • Hypertrophic CMP • AF
IB	Mexiletine	200–300 mg every 8 hours	• Tremor, dysarthria, dizziness, diplopia, nystagmus, anxiety • Nausea, vomiting, dyspepsia • Hypotension, bradycardia	• VT and VF • Reduction of ICD shocks
IC	Flecainide	100–200 mg two times daily	• Negative inotropy, AV block, bradycardia • Decreases pacing threshold • Confusion, irritability	• Paroxysmal AF • SVTs • VT • PVCs unmasking Brugada syndrome
	Propafenone	150–300 mg every 8 hours	• Dizziness, blurred vision • Bronchospasm • AV block, bradycardia, heart failure exacerbation • Decreases pacing threshold	• Paroxysmal AF • SVTs • VT • PVCs
II	Beta-blocker	Beta-blocker specific	• Hypotension, bradycardia, heart block, heart failure exacerbation • Bronchospasm • Depression • Impairment of sexual function	• Atrial arrhythmias • Rate control in AF • SVTs • PVCs • VT • VF

Contd...

Contd...

Table 2: Dosing, uses and side effects of orally available antiarrhythmic drugs

Class	Drug	Maintenance oral dosing	Side effects	Uses
III	Amiodarone	1,200–1,800 mg daily for the first 7–10 days, then taper gradually to 200–400 mg daily	• Pulmonary fibrosis • Abnormal liver function tests • Hyperthyroidism or hypothyroidism • Bradycardia, heart failure exacerbation • Tremor, paresthesia • Photosensitivity • Corneal deposits	• VT • VF • Reduction of ICD shocks • AF • Atrial flutter • AF in WPW • Other SVTs
	Sotalol	80–160 mg every 12 hours	• Bradycardia, torsades de pointes	• Sustained VT/VF • VT in ARVD • Reduction of ICD shocks • AF • Atrial flutter
	Dofetilide	250–500 mcg twice daily	• Torsade de pointes	• AF
	Dronedarone	400 mg twice daily	• Gastrointestinal side effects	• To reduce the risk of cardiovascular hospitalization in patients with non-permanent AF and associated cardiac risk factors • Rhythm control in AF
IV	Calcium channel blocker (Verapamil)	80–160 mg every 8 hours	• Hypotension, bradycardia, AV block	• Idiopathic VT • PVCs • Rate control in AF • SVTs

(Abbreviations: AF: Atrial fibrillation; CMP: Cardiomyopathy; ICD: Implantable cardioverter defibrillator; PVCs: Premature ventricular contractions; SVTs: Supraventricular tachycardias; VF: Ventricular fibrillation; VT: Ventricular tachycardia; WPW: Wolff-Parkinson-White syndrome)

Class I Antiarrhythmic Drugs: Sodium Channel Blockers

The class I antiarrhythmic drugs primarily act by slowing conductance of sodium (Na+) across the cell membrane. These drugs, therefore, interfere with the depolarization phase of the cardiac action potential ("phase 0") and also decrease responsiveness to excitation (reduction in Vmax). Class I drugs are further classified into IA (quinidine, procainamide, and disopyramide), IB (mexiletine, lidocaine), and IC (flecainide, propafenone). Depending on the type, class I drugs can block sodium channels (class IC drugs) or alter the ability of the sodium channel to conduct; the effect on the channel can be short or prolonged.

Class IA Antiarrhythmic Drugs

Class IA drugs slow conduction in atrial and ventricular myocardium and have a moderate effect on slowing myocardial conduction by moderate effect on phase 0 (Vmax) but they also have other effects. These drugs prolong repolarization by their effects on potassium channels. Disopyramide, in particular, can have an anticholinergic effect. Additionally, these drugs have vasodilatory (intravenous procainamide and quinidine), negative inotropic (disopyramide), and vagolytic (quinidine and disopyramide effects).

Class IB Antiarrhythmic Drugs

As a group, class IB drugs block sodium channels in both activated and inactivated states but do not delay channel recovery. They affect conduction in ventricular myocardium and have little, if any, effect on atrial myocardium or on AV conduction. This results in shortening of action potential duration and refractoriness. Lidocaine may affect ischemic myocardium preferentially. Their efficacy is increased at high heart rates and also in depolarized tissues, which makes them effective in treatment of ventricular arrhythmias in the ischemic myocardium.

Class IC Antiarrhythmic Drugs

The currently available class IC drugs are potent sodium channel blockers and cause marked conduction slowing in cardiac tissues without exerting any effects on refractoriness. Their sodium channel blocking effects are exaggerated at high heart rates (use dependency) and in depolarized tissues. At therapeutic doses, class IC drugs prolong the PR and QRS intervals without having significant effects on the QTc interval. Class IC drugs also exert negative inotropic effects and can worsen heart failure in patients with left ventricular dysfunction. The use of these drugs is not recommended in patients who have ventricular dysfunction, who have marked left ventricular hypertrophy, or who have ischemic heart disease.

Class II Antiarrhythmic Drugs: Beta-adrenoceptor Blockers

Beta-adrenergic blocking drugs are one of the most efficacious drugs used in clinical cardiology for a variety of purposes, including treatment of congestive heart failure and myocardial ischemia. Beta-blockers also have AAD properties and can reduce the risk of sudden cardiac death by a number of mechanisms, can reduce ventricular tachyarrhythmias in select patients, can inhibit AF, can prevent paroxysmal supraventricular tachyarrhythmias of various types and can have additive effects to other AADs. Additionally, beta-blockers can slow AV nodal conduction in patients with rapid atrial tachyarrhythmias, including AF and atrial flutter.

Beta-blockers work by a variety of mechanisms. They can suppress automaticity and the triggers for atrial tachycardias, AF, and ventricular fibrillation. They can also interfere with the reentry circuit in patients with AV node reentry and with AV reentry tachycardia (by facilitating blockade in the AV node). Beta-blockers may facilitate the effects of class I AADs since their efficacy may be blunted under conditions of catecholamine excess.

Class III Antiarrhythmic Drugs: Drugs, which Prolong Repolarization

All clinically available class III drugs block the rapid component of the delayed-rectifier potassium channel (Ikr), resulting in an increase in action potential duration and refractoriness in various cardiac tissues, the hallmark of a class III AAD. With class III AADs, reverse use dependence can also occur. In this situation, the AAD effect is most pronounced during slow heart rates. The class III AADs (d-sotalol and N-acetylprocainamide—a metabolite of procainamide, but not amiodarone) demonstrate reverse use dependence. Quinidine can show reverse use dependence for the potassium channel.

Class IV Antiarrhythmic Drugs: Calcium Channel Antagonists

Verapamil blocks the L-type calcium channel and can be used to slow AV nodal conduction to control the ventricular response rate atrial flutter and AF, but it could also be used to prevent recurrence of AV nodal reentry and AV reentry supraventricular tachycardia. Furthermore, verapamil can prevent triggered activity and inhibit idiopathic right ventricular outflow tract tachycardias by this mechanism. Additionally, verapamil can affect reentrant mechanisms responsible for idiopathic left VT. The dose of verapamil is 120–480 mg a day in single or divided doses. Diltiazem, another calcium channel blocker that can be used to control the ventricular response rate in AF, is available in both intravenous and oral formulations.

Miscellaneous Drugs: Adenosine

Adenosine is an ultrashort acting purinergic agonist; it is vagotonic. It binds to the adenosine A1 receptor. Adenosine activates the IKACH, ADO channels present in the atrium, sinus node and the AV node. This results in increased outward potassium current, which leads to shortening of atrial action potential and membrane hyperpolarization and transient AV nodal block and sinus node, depression. These IKADO channels are not present in the ventricular myocytes and therefore, adenosine has not much of an effect in the ventricular myocardium. Indirectly, adenosine has an antiadrenergic action due to a decrease in cyclic AMP. Adverse effects with adenosine typically include dyspnea, chest tightness, flushing and exacerbation of bronchospasm.

These are typically short-lasting and resolve quickly.

❑ ANTIARRHYTHMIC DRUG SELECTION IN ATRIAL FIBRILLATION

The 2011 ACC/AHA/ESC Guidelines for Management of AF provides recommendations regarding AAD selection if rhythm control is planned for AF (Flowchart 1). The recommendations are primarily based on AAD safety than on drug efficacy. For patients with no evidence of structural heart disease or have hypertension without substantial left ventricular hypertrophy, flecainide, propafenone, sotalol or dronedarone is first-line therapy, followed by amiodarone, dofetilide, or catheter ablation. For patients with hypertension and substantial left ventricular hypertrophy, amiodarone is the first choice drug, with catheter ablation as the second-line choice. In patients with coronary artery disease, dofetilide or sotalol is first-line, followed by amiodarone or catheter ablation. For heart failure

FLOWCHART 1: Antiarrhythmic drug selection, based on underlying structural heart disease, for maintenance of sinus rhythm in atrial fibrillation

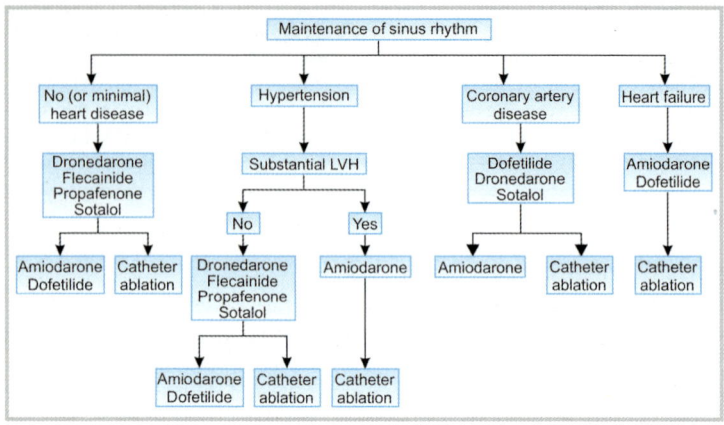

Source: Modified from Wann LS, Curtis AB, January CT, et al. 2011 ACCF/AHA/HRS focused update on the management of patients with atrial fibrillation (updating the 2006 guideline): a report of the American College of Cardiology Foundation/American Heart Association Task Force on Practice Guidelines. Circulation. 2011;123:104-23

patients, amiodarone or dofetilide is first-line therapy, followed by catheter ablation. Most recently, dronedarone has been included in the guidelines and has a role in the treatment of AF as stated in the package insert as "an AAD indicated to reduce the risk of cardiovascular hospitalization in patients with paroxysmal or persistent AF or atrial flutter, with a recent episode of AF or atrial flutter and associated cardiovascular risk factors (i.e. age >70, hypertension, diabetes, prior cerebrovascular accident, left atrial diameter >50 mm or left ventricular ejection fraction <40%), who are in sinus rhythm or who will be cardioverted".

❑ OUTPATIENT VERSUS IN-HOSPITAL INITIATION FOR ANTIARRHYTHMIC DRUG THERAPY

The location of initiation of an AAD depends on the severity of the arrhythmia and the risk of starting the AAD. It is recommended that all class IA AADs be initiated in the hospital due to risk of torsades de pointes, which at times can be idiosyncratic and non-dose dependent. Class IB AADs, specifically mexiletine, can be started and titrated as an outpatient because the risk of proarrhythmia is small, but in most cases, this drug is started in the hospital due to the fact that most patients whom this drug is initiated have unstable ventricular arrhythmias. Class IC AADs can generally be started outside the hospital for AF as the early risk of proarrhythmia is low as long as the patient has no underlying structural heart disease and no evidence for cardiac ischemia. There is a small risk of rapid rates in AF with one-to-one conduction and atrial flutter, but with proper AV nodal blocking drugs, this risk can be offset. Amiodarone can be started as an outpatient for patients who have AF and atrial flutter as the proarrhythmic risk is low. On the other hand, most patients with VT are considered unstable, and therefore, the initiation of amiodarone normally begins in the hospital. A patient may not be fully loaded with amiodarone, but nevertheless, the drug should be started in the hospital. Sotalol and dofetilide should be initiated in the hospital due to the risk of developing QT prolongation and torsades de pointes. Dofetilide must be started in the hospital based on strict guidelines about how the drug should be initiated and titrated. Dronedarone is generally not proarrhythmic and can be started outside the hospital.

❏ ANTIARRHYTHMIC DRUGS IN PREGNANCY AND LACTATION

An overview of the effect of various AADs in pregnancy and lactation is presented in Table 3. Sotalol is the only pregnancy category B drug [either animal-reproduction studies have not demonstrated a fetal risk, but there are no controlled studies in pregnant women, or animal-reproduction studies have shown an adverse effect (other than a decrease in fertility) that was not confirmed in controlled studies in women in the first trimester (and there is no evidence of a risk in later trimesters)], while amiodarone is classified as pregnancy category D drug [there is positive evidence of human fetal risk, but the benefits from use in pregnant women may be acceptable despite the risk (e.g. if the drug is needed in a life-threatening situation or for a serious disease for which safer drugs cannot be used or are ineffective)]. Dronedarone is a pregnancy category X drug (studies in animals or human beings have demonstrated fetal abnormalities, or there is evidence of fetal risk based on human experience or both, and the risk of the use of the drug in pregnant women clearly outweighs any possible benefit. The drug is contraindicated in women who are or may become pregnant) and so is contraindicated in women who are or may become pregnant. The rest of the AADs are considered pregnancy category C drug [either studies in animals have revealed adverse effects on the fetus (teratogenic or embryocidal or other) and there are no controlled studies in women, or studies in women and animals are not available. Drugs should be given only if the potential benefit justifies the potential risk to the fetus]. The use of beta-blockers during pregnancy is relatively safe. The only exception is atenolol, which is a pregnancy category D drug.

Table 3: Antiarrhythmic drugs in pregnancy and lactation

Drug	Pregnancy	Lactation
Quinidine	C	Excreted
Procainamide	C	Excreted
Disopyramide	C	Excreted
Mexiletine	C	Excreted
Flecainide	C	Excreted
Propafenone	C	?
Sotalol	B	Excreted
Dofetilide	C	?
Dronedarone	X	?
Amiodarone	D	Excreted

❑ COMPARING ANTIARRHYTHMIC DRUGS TO IMPLANTABLE CARDIOVERTER DEFIBRILLATORS IN PATIENTS AT RISK OF ARRHYTHMIC DEATH

Several large, randomized, prospective, multicenter, controlled clinical trials compared ICDs versus AADs. The Antiarrhythmics Versus Implantable Defibrillators (AVID) trial randomized patients resuscitated from a cardiac arrest to an ICD, empiric amiodarone (mean dose of 300 mg; 90% of patients) or sotalol. The group runnings ICDs had a significant 39% (one year), 27% (two year) and 31% (three year) mortality reduction when compared to AADs. Only those patients with left ventricular ejection fraction between 20% and 34% showed a survival benefit with ICD (83%) when compared to amiodarone (72%).

ICDs are superior to AADs for both primary and secondary prevention of mortality, presumably due to sudden cardiac death. The AADs should be reserved only for patients who are not candidates for an ICD, who refuse ICD therapy, and for select patients with genetic disorders that respond well to a specific AAD.

❑ ANTIARRHYTHMIC DRUG–DEVICE INTERACTIONS

The ICD has emerged as the primary therapeutic modality for prevention of sudden cardiac death. Concomitant AAD therapy may be required in select ICD patients to suppress recurrent atrial and ventricular arrhythmias and to reduce the incidence and frequency of both appropriate and inappropriate shocks. When used in this setting, AADs can affect device functioning in several ways:
- AADs can increase defibrillation and pacing thresholds
- AADs can slow VT rate to below the programmed ICD detection rate
- AADs can cause sinus and AV node dysfunction, resulting in bradycardia and AV block
- AADs can be proarrhythmic.

It is important to be aware of these potential interactions when selecting an appropriate AAD and also during device programming. Amiodarone and sotalol are the two most common AADs used in an ICD population. Table 4 lists the effect of various AADs on pacing and defibrillation thresholds.

Table 4: Effect of antiarrhythmic drugs on defibrillation and pacing thresholds		
Drug	**Pacing threshold**	**Defibrillation threshold**
Quinidine	Increase	Increase
Procainamide	Increase	No change/increase
Lidocaine	No change	Increase
Flecainide	Increase	Increase
Beta-blockers	Increase	Decreases
Digoxin	Decrease	Decrease/no change
Ibutilide	Not known	Decrease
Sotalol	No effect	Decrease
Amiodarone	No effect	Increase
Dofetilide	No change	Decrease
Verapamil	Increase	Not known

❑ CONCLUSION

Antiarrhythmic drug therapy continues to play a critical role in the management of atrial and ventricular arrhythmias. The role of AADs has evolved in the face of advances in curative therapy for specific arrhythmias, as well as for underlying diseases. It is fair to say that the history of AAD therapy has come full circle. Irrespective of effects on survival, AADs are an integral part of the pharmacological armamentarium to combat AF, to treat ventricular arrhythmias in the structurally normal heart and in those with channelopathies, to suppress sustained ventricular arrhythmias in patients with structural heart disease who either have an ICD or are not candidates for one. The field of AAD therapy continues to evolve as newer drugs that target novel mechanisms are being actively developed and, with currently available drugs finding new indications for their use.

❑ SUGGESTED READINGS

Goldschlager N, Epstein AE, Naccarelli GV, et al. A practical guide for clinicians who treat patients with amiodarone: 2007. Heart Rhythm. 2007;4:1250-9.

Gopinathannair R, Sullivan RM, Olshansky B. Update on medical management of atrial fibrillation in the modern era. Heart Rhythm. 2009;6:S17-22.

Harrison DC. Antiarrhythmic drug classification: new science and practical applications. Am J Cardiol. 1985;56:185-7.

Vaughan Williams EM. A classification of antiarrhythmic actions reassessed after a decade of new drugs. J Clin Pharmacol. 1984;24: 129-47.

Wann LS, Curtis AB, January CT, et al. 2011 ACCF/AHA/HRS focused update on the management of patients with atrial fibrillation (updating the 2006 guideline): a report of the American College of Cardiology Foundation/American Heart Association Task Force on Practice Guidelines. Circulation. 2011;123:104-23.

3.3 Syncope

❑ INTRODUCTION

Syncope is a sudden and transient loss of consciousness associated with loss of postural tone, followed by complete and spontaneous recovery. The mechanism for transient loss of consciousness associated with syncope is cerebral hypoperfusion with reduced blood flow to the reticular activating system. A common phrase used in clinical medicine is presyncope, which is considered to represent a warning or prodrome for frank syncope. In the case of presyncope, symptoms, such as dizziness and graying out are not followed by frank loss of consciousness. Many physicians evaluate and treat presyncope in a similar manner to syncope; although a reasonable approach, there is no strong clinical data to support similar etiologies and outcomes.

It is important to acknowledge that the definition of syncope (and thus etiologic classification) varies even among experts. Using a more general definition of transient loss of consciousness, some experts include neurologic (e.g. seizure and concussion), metabolic (e.g. hypoxia) and psychiatric conditions as forms of syncope, while others who emphasize cerebral hypoperfusion consider syncope as one of the several causes of transient loss of consciousness and classify some neurologic, metabolic and psychiatric mechanisms as separate entities (Flowchart 2). Using this

FLOWCHART 2: Classification of mechanistic causes for transient loss of consciousness and syncope

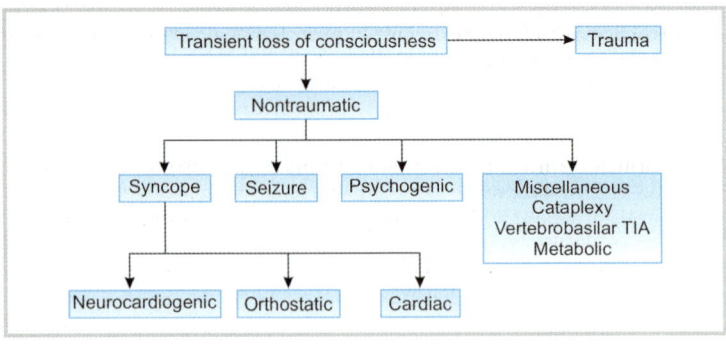

more restrictive definition of syncope, the three most important causes of transient loss of consciousness are: (i) syncope; (ii) seizure and (iii) psychogenic blackouts. Determining the correct cause of syncope is the key to approaching therapy, if the initial working clinical diagnosis is erroneous, subsequent investigations and even the final diagnosis and treatment may also be incorrect. Regardless of definition, syncope may represent a harbinger for sudden death, and often the diagnostic evaluation focuses on identifying or ruling out potential life-threatening causes of syncope, such as ventricular arrhythmias or aortic stenosis. For this reason, the diagnostic workup for the patient with syncope revolves around two different but related issues: (i) identification of the specific mechanism for syncope and (ii) risk stratification to estimate short-term and long-term risk of adverse outcomes.

Causes and Classification of Syncope

As discussed earlier, syncope is but one cause of transient loss of consciousness. Syncope can further be classified into three general causes: (i) reflex or neurally mediated syncope, (ii) syncope due to orthostatic hypotension, and (iii) cardiac syncope (Flowchart 2).

Reflex or neurally mediated syncope is the most common cause of syncope. One form, often called vasovagal syncope or the "common faint", is the single most common cause of syncope. In all forms of reflex syncope, triggering of the afferent limb of a reflex arc leads to hypotension due to vasodilation (vasodepressor effect) and decreased heart rate (vagal effect). In vasovagal syncope the afferent limb can be triggered by a variety of conditions, such as heat, hypovolemia, pain, or fear and anxiety while in conditions often called—situational syncope, triggering occurs from specific actions such as micturition, cough or swallow. Finally, particularly in older patients, the afferent limb can be triggered by carotid sinus stimulation.

A second cause of syncope is orthostatic hypotension. Normally with standing, accumulation of fluid in the legs results in the initiation of a complex neurologic reflex response that maintains systemic blood pressure. In orthostatic hypotension, this response is insufficient, leading to a decrease in systemic blood pressure. Diabetes is the most common cause of autonomic neuropathy in the United States and can be associated with relatively high mortality rates (25–50% mortality at 5–8 years). Another form of autonomic dysfunction, which can be associated with syncope is the postural orthostatic tachycardia syndrome (POTS).

The third cause of syncope is a cardiac abnormality. Etiologies of cardiac syncope can broadly be divided into abnormal heart rhythms and obstruction to flow. Both rapid heart rates and slow heart rates can cause cerebral hypoperfusion and syncope. Obstruction to blood flow can be due aortic stenosis, pulmonary valve stenosis or dynamic left ventricular outflow tract obstruction in some patients with hypertrophic cardiomyopathy (HCM).

❏ DIAGNOSTIC TESTS

The evaluation of syncope is often challenging and in up to 40% of cases no specific cause can be identified; this is especially true in older patients. The history and physical examination play an essential role in evaluating patients with syncope. No test has found to be the "gold standard", underscoring the importance of careful initial evaluation by the history and the physical examination and choosing subsequent tests based on this initial assessment.

History and Physical Examination

The history and physical examination play an important role in establishing cause of transient loss of consciousness and, in particular, for differentiating between syncope and seizure as this distinction can be difficult (Flowchart 2).

Once the clinician has decided that an episode of transient loss of consciousness is most likely due to syncope, the history and physical examination can provide further clues as to its specific cause. Pertinent questions should include a history prior of cardiac disease and diagnosis, if known; family history of arrhythmias, syncope and sudden death, knowledge of an abnormal electrocardiogram, medications, positional changes that occurred prior to the syncopal spell (including headturning), prodromal symptoms, and history of prior syncopal events. Features of the clinical history that are more commonly associated with significant arrhythmias, such as ventricular tachycardia or bradycardia due to advanced or complete heart block include male sex, age older than 50 years, fewer than three episodes of syncope and duration of warning prior to syncope of less than 6 seconds. Conversely, a history of diabetes, prior arrhythmia, no recollection of the episode and palpitations preceding syncope more likely made a cardiac cause. Similarly, a first event over 35 years of age or bystanders describing the patient "turning blue" were also associated with a cardiac cause of syncope.

The physical examination has a central role in evaluation of syncope. A complete cardiac examination should be performed to assess the presence of structural cardiac disease. Orthostatic vital signs are an essential part of the physical examination in a patient. The POTS is defined as an increase in heart rate more than 25–30 beats per minute within 5 minutes of standing with symptoms. Cardiac auscultatory findings, such as murmurs or gallops, are important for identifying the presence and severity of structural cardiac disease, such as aortic stenosis and HCM. On palpation, findings, such as a left ventricular heave or a sustained left ventricular impulse, can alert the clinician to the presence of structural heart disease, such as left ventricular hypertrophy or ventricular dilation, due to cardiomyopathy or past myocardial infarction that will make more likely a cardiac cause of syncope. Finally, performing carotid sinus massage (CSM) is important in patients with syncope over 40 years of age.

Blood Tests

Routine blood tests, including electrolytes, tests for anemia (hematocrit or hemoglobin) and glucose, although commonly performed, generally have a low diagnostic yield in evaluation of syncope. The exception may be the presence of anemia; anemia has been incorporated into several prognostic algorithms used for risk stratification of patients with syncope. It is important to note that the most recent guidelines do not specifically recommend any blood tests for the evaluation of syncope.

Electrocardiogram

A 12 lead ECG is a basic part of the workup in all patients with syncope. Although the diagnostic yield of a baseline ECG is low (5–10%), it is an inexpensive and widely available test that can be used to quickly risk stratify patients, particularly if it is abnormal.

There are some ECG patterns that can be used to identify potential causes for syncope: Wolff–Parkinson–White Syndrome, Long QT syndrome, Brugada syndrome, arrhythmogenic right ventricular cardiomyopathy, and HCM.

Echocardiography

Both the AHA/ACCF and ESC guidelines state that the echocardiogram plays a central role in syncopal patients with suspected cardiac disease. Echocardiography has a low diagnostic yield in patients with a normal physical examination and normal ECG and need not necessarily be obtained in all patients with syncope. A structural abnormality noted during echocardiography does not per se establish a diagnostic cause for syncope.

Exercise Testing

Exercise testing has a low diagnostic yield in the evaluation of syncope (<5%). However, it may particularly be useful in those patients with exertional syncope. Published guidelines are not uniform in their recommendations; however, the AHA/ACCF scientific statement (but not the ESC guidelines) suggest that exercise testing should be more widely applied to any patient with unexplained syncope, particularly those with coronary artery disease or those at risk for coronary artery disease.

Continuous ECG Monitoring

External Devices (24 Hours Ambulatory ECG Recorders, Event Recorders)

Since intermittent bradycardia or tachycardia are the most common cardiac etiologies for syncope, an ECG obtained when the patient is having symptoms is critical for determining whether an arrhythmia is the cause of symptoms. Since most episodes of syncope are usually separated by long periods of time the yield of monitoring less than 48 hours is at best 1–2%.

Implantable Loop Recorders

More recently implantable loop recorders (ILRs) that are placed subcutaneously in the left upper chest and that have larger memories and the ability to continuously monitor the ECG formore than 1 year have been developed by several manufacturers.

Current guidelines recommend an ILR for patients with recurrent but infrequent episodes of syncope in whom there is a high index of suspicion for an arrhythmogenic cause after a negative initial workup. The ILR has gradually supplanted invasive electrophysiology studies and tilt table testing as the diagnostic test of choice for patients with syncope. The ILR is ideal for obtaining a heart rhythm correlation for a patient with intermittent symptoms.

Signal Averaged ECG

In some patients with structural heart disease, low amplitude signals in the terminal portion of the QRS complexes can sometimes be observed using special recording techniques that obtain a number of QRS complexes (allowing random noise to cancel out) and use special filtering algorithms. Late potentials are thought to arise from delayed depolarization of the abnormal myocardium and thus reflect nonhomogeneous depolarization. The signal averaged ECG (SAECG) may be useful in rare circumstances; for example, in some cases the SAECG can help identify patients with arrhythmogenic right ventricular cardiomyopathy.

Upright Tilt Table Testing

Upright tilt table testing is commonly obtained in the diagnostic workup of syncope. The physiology of standing is complex, but when the patient is moved from the supine to the upright position, approximately 300–600 mL of blood pools in the lower extremities and lower portion of the abdomen, which in turn leads to a 25–50% decrease in intravascular volume. In response to the decrease in stroke volume a complex interplay of various cardioregulatory systems normally results in maintenance of blood pressure despite the redistribution of blood.

The ESC has developed detailed guidelines for the methodology, indications and diagnostic criteria for tilt table testing. In general, tilt table testing is recommended when it is important to identify whether the patient is susceptible to vasovagal syncope (e.g. a patient with a structurally normal heart that has a single episode of syncope associated with significant injury) or to help differentiate between reflex syncope from orthostatic hypotension.

Electrophysiology Study

The electrophysiology study (EPS) is an invasive test that may be useful for workup of syncope in selected patients. In EPS, using specialized electrode catheters placed in the heart, the clinician can define cardiac electrophysiologic properties, such as sinus node and AV node function, and evaluate the mechanism for any inducible ventricular tachycardia or supraventricular tachycardia under controlled conditions.

Currently, EPS is reasonable for evaluating patients with syncope and coronary artery disease with prior myocardial infarction that do not meet criteria for an ICD implant or those patients that meet criteria for ICD implant, but where further risk stratification information might change a clinical decision (usually whether or not to implant an ICD). The EPS is also reasonable for the patient with syncope and evidence for abnormal atrioventricular conduction where defining the site of block will impact clinical decision-making.

Cardiac Catheterization

Cardiac catheterization is generally not indicated for the workup of syncope unless accompanied by symptoms suggestive of significant coronary artery disease.

Neurologic Tests

Computed tomography (CT) scans, electroencephalography (EEG) and carotid duplex scans are often obtained for the evaluation of patients with transient loss of

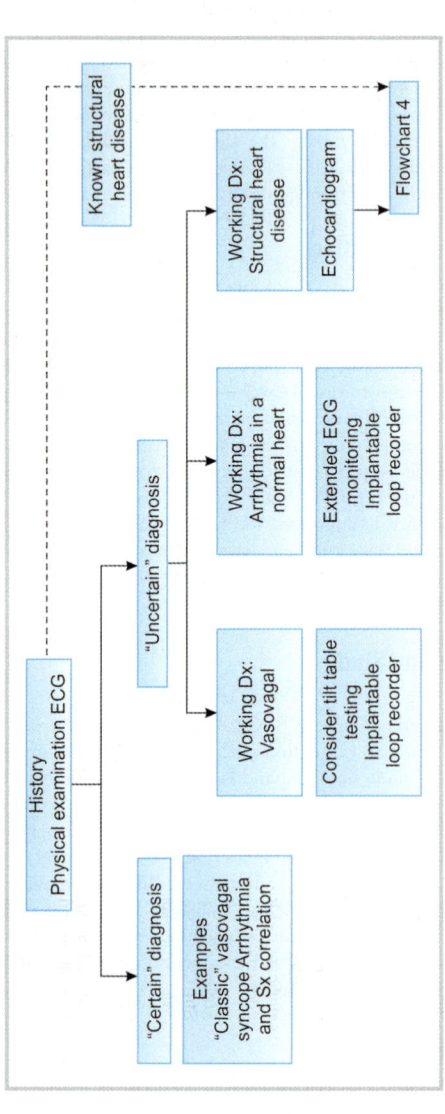

FLOWCHART 3: Diagnostic evaluation of a patient with syncope

Electrophysiology

FLOWCHART 4: Diagnostic and therapeutic considerations in a patient with syncope and structural heart disease

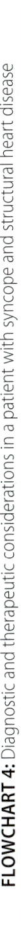

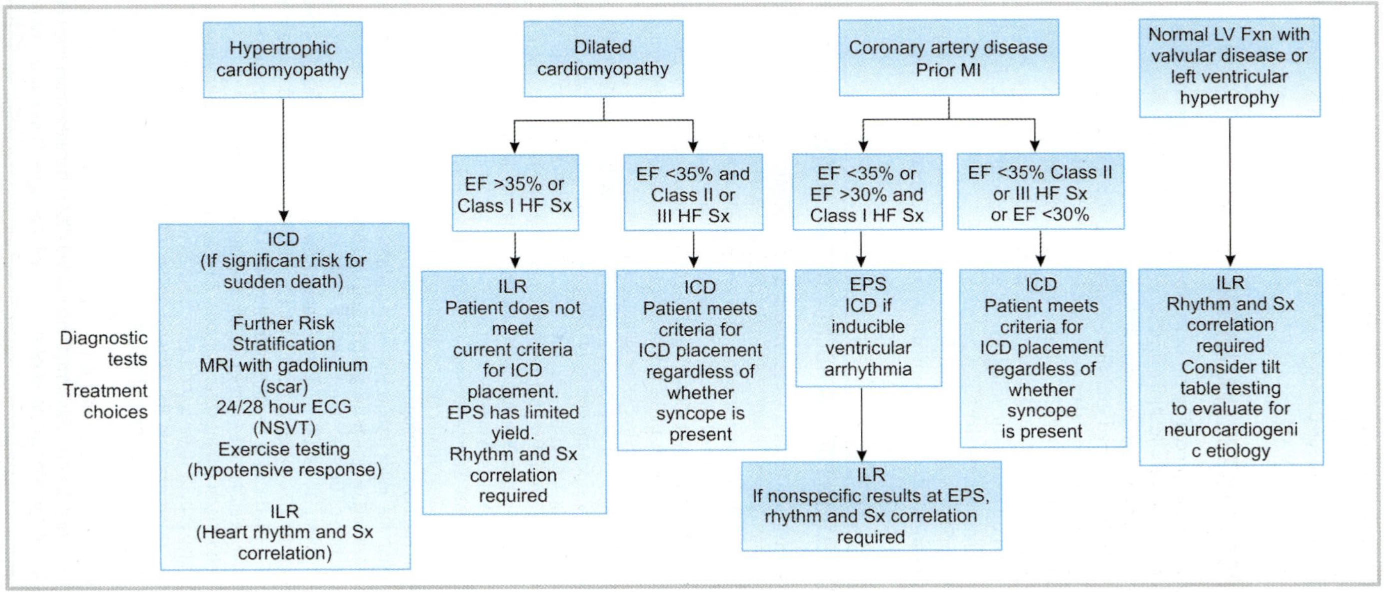

(Abbreviations: ICD: Implantable cardiac defibrillator; ILR: Implantable loop recorder; EF: Ejection fraction)

consciousness. Multiple studies have shown that the diagnostic yield of these tests is extremely low (1–3%) in unselected patient populations. It is recommended that these tests should be ordered only if indicated by clinical findings that specifically suggest a neurologic process.

❑ APPROACH TO THE EVALUATION OF SYNCOPE

As outlined in the preceding sections, there are many tests available for the assessment of syncope and indiscriminate use of diagnostic tests can lead to an expensive evaluation that provides little insight into the management of the patient. Recently published guidelines emphasize the importance of the history and a comprehensive physical examination in the initial evaluation of syncope and also recommend a baseline ECG. Since future risk is largely dependent on whether the patient has a cardiac cause of syncope and whether the patient has structural heart disease most diagnostic and risk-stratification algorithms use this issue as the first decision point (Flowchart 3).

In the patient with structural heart disease identified by history, physical examination and ECG the appropriate workup will depend on the type of disease present (Flowchart 4).

> ### GUIDELINES FOR EMERGENCY DEPARTMENT EVALUATION
>
> One of the most significant sources for high cost in patients with syncope is hospital admission that ranges 26–60%. For this reason a number of investigators have evaluated the utility of algorithms for identifying patients at higher risk for significant events and have developed syncope management units (similar to the concept of chest pain units) that allow expedited and more efficient management of patients with syncope. The components of the risk stratification rules vary and some have debated whether the rules are effective for reducing cost (Table 5).
>
> The Osservatorio Epidemiologico sulla Sincope nel Lazio (OESIL) risk score was derived from a patient cohort of 270 patients that presented with syncope in 6 community hospitals in the Lazio region of Italy. Multivariate analysis identified four independent predictors that predicted risk: History of cardiovascular disease, age more than 65 years, syncope without a prodrome and an abnormal ECG. The 12 month mortality increased linearly from 0% (no risk factors present) to 57% (all four risk factors present). Several subsequent studies have validated the OESIL risk score for predicting one year risk in other patient cohorts.
>
> The San Francisco Syncope Rule was developed to predict short-term outcomes (7 days after the index event).The investigators evaluated multiple variables but simplified their rule to include five elements: (1) abnormal ECG; (2) shortness of breath; (3) hematocrit less than 30%; (4) systolic blood pressure less than 90 mm Hg and (5) a history heart failure. Often the mnemonic chess is used to more easily remember the components: C: Congestive heart failure; H: Hematocrit; E: ECG; S: Systolic blood pressure; S—shortness of breath. Similar to the OESIL risk score subsequent studies have generally validated the utility of the San Francisco Syncope Rule.
>
> In the short-term prognosis of syncope (STePS) study 676 patients with syncope were evaluated at both 10 days and 1 year. Severe outcomes (death, major therapeutic procedures, readmission to the hospital within 10 days) were observed in 6.1% of patients (mainly rehospitalization) at 10 day follow-up. Severe outcomes were observed mainly in patients who were admitted (14.7%) compared to those who were discharged from the emergency department (2.0%). The main mechanistic cause for severe outcomes was arrhythmia-related (25/41 patients, most often due to implantation of a permanent pacemaker), although five patients died had a variety of

causes, none specifically arrhythmia related (disseminated intravascular coagulation, pulmonary edema, aortic dissection, pulmonary embolism and stroke). Predictors of short-term risk included an abnormal ECG, concomitant trauma and absence of preceding symptoms. Interestingly, factors associated with long-term adverse outcomes were different from the short-term risk predictors and included age more than 65 years and history of neoplasm, cerebrovascular disease and heart disease (structural heart disease or ventricular arrhythmias).

Table 5: Comparison of the components and primary outcomes for four different risk stratification schemes

Algorithm				Components:				Endpoint
	Age	Sx and Hx	PE	ECG	Anemia	O_2	BNP	
OESIL	>65 years	Sudden onset CVD		Q waves, ST Δ's, LVH, BBB, Arrhythmia				1 year mortality
SFSR*		SOB, HF Hx	SBP < 90 mm Hg	Δ's, from a prior ECG, Arrhythmia	Hct $\leq 30\%$			7 day mortality and serious outcomes
STePS[†]	>65 years	Trauma, Sudden onset Hx CVA or CVD, Male		Q waves LVH, LBBB, Arrhythmia				10 day and 1 year mortality and serious outcomes
ROSE**		Chest pain		Q waves, LBBB, HR ≤ 50 bpm	Hb ≤ 9 g/dL; fecal blood	$\leq 94\%$	>300 pg/ml	30 day serious outcomes

(Abbreviations: OESIL: Osservatorio Epidemiologico sulla Sincope nel Lazio; SFSR: *San Francisco Syncope Rule. Serious Outcomes: Myocardial infarction, arrhythmia, pulmonary embolism, stroke, subarachnoid hemorrhage, significant hemorrhage or any condition causing or likely to cause a return ED visit and hospitalization for a related event; [†]STePS: Short Term Prognosis of Syncope. Serious Outcomes: Need for major therapeutic procedures and early (within 10 days) readmission to hospital; **ROSE: Risk stratification of Syncope in the Emergency Department. Serious Outcomes: Acute myocardial infarction, serious arrhythmia, hemorrhage, pulmonary embolus; Hx: History; PE: Physical examination; O_2: Oxygen saturation; BNP: Brain natriuretic peptide; Time frame: Time of endpoint evaluation; HR: Heart rate; PVC: Premature ventricular contractions; SOB: Shortness of breath; CVD: Cardiovascular disease; CVA: Cerebrovascular accident; LVH: Left ventricular hypertrophy; LBBB: Left bundle branch block)

In the risk stratification of syncope in the emergency department (ROSE) study a cohort of 550 patients with syncope was evaluated. One-month serious outcome (acute myocardial infarction, life-threatening arrhythmia, requirement for ICD or permanent pacemaker implant, hemorrhage requiring transfusion, pulmonary embolus or significant neurologic event) or allcause death occurred in 40 (7.3%) patients in the derivation cohort. Independent predictors were B-type BNP concentration ≥ 300 pg/mL[odds ratio (OR): 7.3], positive fecal occult blood (OR: 13.2), hemoglobin ≤ 9.0 g/dL (OR: 6.7), oxygen saturation $\leq 94\%$ (OR: 3.0) and Q-wave on the presenting ECG (OR: 2.8). One-month serious outcome or all-cause death occurred in 39 (7.1%) patients in the validation cohort. The ROSE rule (the presence of any of the independent predictors) had a sensitivity and specificity of 87.2% and 65.5%, respectively, and a negative predictive value of 98.5% for a serious outcome or death at one month. An elevated BNP concentration alone was a major predictor of serious cardiovascular outcomes (8 of 22 events, 36%) and all-cause deaths (8 of 9 deaths, 89%).

Another strategy for reducing the cost of syncope is streamlining the process of evaluation using syncope or transient loss of consciousness units. In the Syncope Evaluation in the Emergency Department Study (SEEDS), 103 patients were randomized to standard care or a specialized syncope unit that provided early evaluation and focused diagnostic testing. Patients randomized to the syncope unit were less likely to require hospital admission (syncope unit: 43% vs standard care: 98%) and more likely to have a presumptive diagnosis (syncope unit: 67% vs standard care: 10%) on discharge from the emergency department or from the syncope unit.

Several groups have argued the obvious importance of developing a consistent method for risk stratification of patients with syncope. Although the currently published rules vary some basic points can be made. First it is important to decide whether or not to assign a working diagnosis of a cardiac cause of syncope. All of the risk stratification schemes use two or more criteria for identifying a group of patients with a higher likelihood for cardiac syncope. An abnormal ECG (Q waves, bundle branch block or atrioventricular block) is a component in all of the risk stratification schemes. Criteria, such as age more than 65 (OESIL), history of cardiovascular disease (OESIL) or presence of congestive heart failure (San Francisco Syncope Rule) and elevated BNP (ROSE)are all parameters that increase the likelihood of identifying a patient with a cardiac cause for syncope. Second, criteria that evaluate for noncardiac causes of syncope focus on conditions associated with higher short-term risk, such as pulmonary embolus (O_2 saturation <90% in the San Francisco Syncope Rule or < 94% in ROSE), significant anemia (hematocrit <30% in the San Francisco Syncope Rule and hemoglobin <9.0 g/dL in ROSE), or shock from any cause (SBP <90 mm Hg in the San Francisco Syncope Rule) or gastrointestinal bleeding (fecal occult blood in ROSE).

GUIDELINES/OFFICIAL RECOMMENDATIONS

There have been formal statements on syncope from two cardiology groups. The AHA/ACCF in collaboration with the Heart Rhythm Society published a scientific statement on the evaluation of syncope in 2006. The writing group recommends a history, physical examination and ECG in all patients with syncope. If the cause of syncope remains unexplained (not neurally mediated or orthostatic) they recommend an echocardiogram, an exercise test and ischemia evaluation. If these tests are normal, no additional testing is required for an isolated benign event. However, if recurrent episodes of syncope or if the episode is associated with significant injury, the clinician should use tests that evaluate the cardiac rhythm during symptoms. The choice among 24–48 hours ambulatory ECG monitoring, external event recorder or an ILR will depend on the frequency of the episodes and the severity of symptoms (syncope vs presyncope). The scientific statement provides a concise practical framework on the evaluation of syncope but does not address emergency room evaluation or subsequent treatment.

More recently, the ESC has published a comprehensive guidelines document that discusses both diagnosis and management of syncope. Similar to the scientific statement from the cardiology societies based in the United States, they recommend an initial evaluation that includes history, physical examination (with orthostatic blood pressure measurements) and an ECG. They emphasize that the clinician should attempt to answer three specific questions:
1. Is it a syncopal episode or not?
2. Has an etiologic diagnosis been determined?
3. Is there evidence for a high risk of a cardiovascular event or death?

If these questions cannot be answered with the initial evaluation, additional tests, such as an echocardiography and other types of cardiac imaging, exercise testing, tilt table testing, cardiac rhythm monitoring and other tests, can be chosen depending on the clinical situation.

❏ SUGGESTED READINGS

Benditt DG, Olshansky B, Wieling W. The ACCF/AHA scientific statement on syncope needs rethinking. J Am Coll Cardiol. Ad Hoc Syncope Consortium. 2006;48:2598-9; (author reply) Epub 2006;2599.

Brignole M, Sutton R, Menozzi C, et al. International Study on Syncope of Uncertain Etiology 2 (ISSUE 2) Group. Early application of an implantable loop recorder allows effective specific therapy in patients with recurrent suspected neurally mediated syncope. Eur Heart J. 2006;27:1085-92.

European Heart Rhythm Association (EHRA), Heart Failure Association (H FA), Heart Rhythm Society (HRS), et al. Guidelines for the diagnosis and management of syncope (version 2009): the Task Force for the Diagnosis and Management of Syncope of the European Society of Cardiology (ESC). Eur Heart J. 2009;30:2631-71.

Shen WK, Decker WW, Smars PA, et al. Syncope Evaluation in the Emergency Department Study (SEEDS): a multidisciplinary approach to syncope management. Circulation. 2004;110:3636-45.

Strickberger SA, Benson DW, Biaggioni I, et al. AHA/ACCF scientific statement on the evaluation of syncope: from the American Heart Association Councils on Clinical Cardiology, Cardiovascular Nursing, Cardiovascular Disease in the Young, and Stroke, and the Quality of Care and Outcomes Research Interdisciplinary Working Group; and the American College of Cardiology Foundation In Collaboration With the Heart Rhythm Society. J Am Coll Cardiol. 2006;47:473-84.

3.4 Atrial Fibrillation

❏ INTRODUCTION

Atrial fibrillation (AF) is the most common sustained arrhythmia in adults and is associated with substantial morbidity, mortality, and cost. AF is characterized by disorganized atrial electrical activity and irregular ventricular rates. AF can result in heart failure, thromboembolism, impaired quality of life and may increase mortality. While AF is frequently associated with structural heart disease, it can occur in isolation (lone AF) or in association with noncardiac diseases.

❏ DEFINITION AND CLASSIFICATION

Atrial fibrillation is easily recognized on the surface of ECG as an irregular supraventricular rhythm (irregular QRS complexes), with a loss of clear P-waves and/or the presence of fibrillatory waves (Fig. 6). AF in response to a reversible cause (e.g. hyperthyroidism, pericarditis, hypoxia, pneumonia, surgery, pulmonary embolism) is called "secondary AF". AF can also occur in association with valve disease (typically mitral stenosis or regurgitation), in association with other structural heart disease (congestive heart failure, right ventricular dysfunction) or other known risks (e.g. hypertension, pulmonary disease, sleep apnea). AF that occurs without any overt heart disease, pulmonary disease, or hypertension (HTN) is called "lone AF".

While several classification schemes have been proposed for AF, the most widely used is based on the duration of AF episodes and whether intervention is required to terminate AF. AF is called "paroxysmal" when episodes terminate spontaneously in less than seven days from onset. When two or more such episodes occur, paroxysmal AF is called "recurrent". When AF lasts longer than seven days

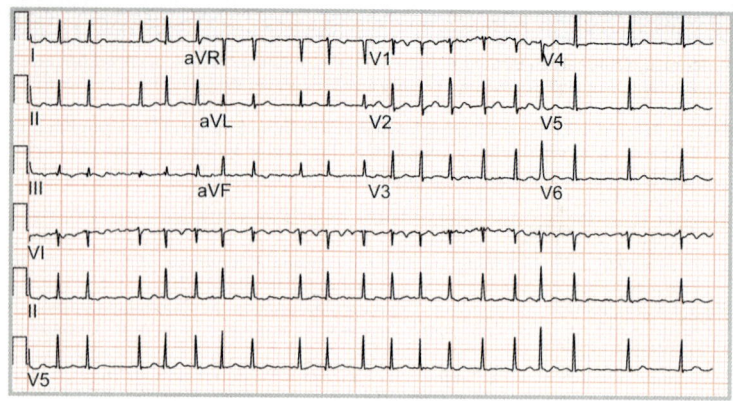

FIGURE 6: Typical ECG of atrial fibrillation showing an absence of P waves, the presence of fibrillatory waves (visible in lead V1), and a rapid, irregular ventricular response

or requires pharmacological or electrical conversion, it is called "persistent". AF that is resistant to drugs or cardioversion is called "permanent". It should be noted that these definitions are not necessarily always clean; for example, some patients with persistent AF may have periods where their AF is paroxysmal.

❏ ETIOLOGY AND PATHOGENESIS

While short episodes of AF lasting a few seconds can be induced in normal atria, longer episodes require a vulnerable atrial substrate. This vulnerable substrate can be due to atrial enlargement, atrial fibrosis or other electrophysiological abnormalities of the atrial myocardium (Table 6). For spontaneous AF to occur, there also needs to be a trigger. This is typically premature atrial depolarizations or short bursts of atrial tachycardia that interact with a vulnerable substrate to spontaneously induce AF. While the triggering activity may arise from anywhere in the atria, evidence to date suggests that majority arise from the pulmonary veins.

Structural Heart Disease

AF is most frequently associated with underlying structural heart disease. In the Framingham Study cohort, the major echocardiographic predictors of the development of AF, apart from valvular disease, were LV systolic dysfunction, LV hypertrophy and atrial enlargement. In addition, a variety of noncardiac conditions can result in AF, and AF can occur in the absence of any other discernible cardiac or non-cardiac disease. The cardiac causes are listed in Table 7.

Electrophysiological Abnormalities

AF is associated with several other electrophysiological disorders of the heart, which in some cases may trigger episodes of AF directly and in other cases may be indicators of a diseased atrial substrate that is prone to developing AF (Table 7).

Noncardiac Causes

Hypertension is the most common noncardiac cause of AF. In population-based series, hypertension confers an adjusted relative risk of 1.5 for the development of

Table 6: Factors predisposing to atrial fibrillation

Electrophysiological abnormalities
Enhanced automaticity (focal AF)
Conduction abnormality (reentry)

Atrial pressure elevation
Mitral or tricuspid valve disease
Myocardial disease (primary or secondary, leading to systolic or diastolic dysfunction)
Semilunar valve abnormalities (causing ventricular hypertrophy)
Systemic or pulmonary hypertension
Intracardiac tumors or thrombi

Atrial ischemia
Coronary artery disease

Inflammatory or infiltrative atrial disease
Pericarditis
Amyloidosis
Myocarditis
Age-induced atrial fibrotic change

Drugs
Alcohol
Caffeine

Endocrine disorders
Hyperthyroidism
Pheochromocytoma

Changes in autonomic tone
Increased parasympathetic activity
Increased sympathetic activity

Primary or metastatic disease in or adjacent to the atrial wall

Postoperative
Cardiac, pulmonary or esophageal surgery

Congenital heart disease

Neurogenic
Subarachnoid hemorrhage
Nonhemorrhagic, major stroke

Idiopathic (lone AF)

Familial AF

Table 7 Cardiac causes of Heart failure

Structural disease
- Valvular heart disease
- Heart failure
- Ischemic heart disease
- Hypertrophic cardiomyopathy

Electrophysiological abnormalities
- Atrial tachycardia and pulmonary venous activity
- Supraventricular tachycardia
- Conduction system disease
- Cardiac nervous system dysfunction

AF. Hyperthyroidism is common cause of AF. One percent of patients with new-onset AF have overt hyperthyroidism, while an additional 5–6% have subclinical hyperthyroidism. Conditions associated with systemic inflammation, metabolic stress or atrial enlargement, such as diabetes, obesity, postsurgical state, and sepsis are all associated with the development of AF.

Chronic obstructive pulmonary disease (COPD) is associated with a relative risk of 1.3–1.8 for the development of AF, depending on the severity of lung disease. Obstructive sleep apnea (OSA) is also associated with AF, and may be an under-recognized cause of the arrhythmia. Heavy alcohol use is strongly associated with AF. In addition, a variety of medications can precipitate episodes of AF, including modulators nervous system function, diuretics and cardiac inotropic agents.

❏ DIAGNOSIS

Presentation

As assessed by remote monitoring, most individual episodes of AF are asymptomatic and many patients are unaware of their arrhythmia. Those who are symptomatic exhibit a broad spectrum of complaints, most commonly palpitations, dyspnea, and symptoms of congestive heart failure. In otherwise healthy patients without accessory pathways, syncope is an unusual presentation for AF. Noncardiac symptoms associated with AF include polyuria and thromboembolic events, most commonly acute embolic stroke.

Physical Examination

The physical examination of patients with AF is also highly variable. Patients in AF can have heart rates ranging from bradycardia to extreme tachycardia depending on the integrity of AV nodal conduction, medications, autonomic tone and the presence of accessory pathways. Due to loss of atrial mechanical function, A-waves are absent from the jugular venous pulsation and a fourth heart sound is not audible in AF. Owing to the variable ventricular filling time in AF, the intensity of heart sounds can change beat to beat.

Electrocardiogram

Although the hallmarks of AF on the surface ECG are loss of P-waves and an irregular ventricular response, AF must still be distinguished from other supraventricular tachycardias associated with an irregular ventricular response, including atrial flutter with variable block and multifocal atrial tachycardia. The latter is typically associated with lung disease, and is characterized by at least three distinct P-wave morphologies on the surface ECG, whereas the fibrillatory waves in AF are more rapid and variable in morphology. In certain patients, however, fibrillatory waves can be "coarse" and at first glance may be difficult to distinguish from flutter waves. Careful examination of the surface ECG in such patients usually unmasks subtle variation in the amplitudes and frequency of apparent flutter waves that reveal the true rhythm to be AF. In the setting of complete AV block with a junctional escape, accelerated junctional rhythms, ventricular tachycardia or ventricular pacing, the ventricular rate in AF can be regular. In such cases, it is important to focus on the nature of the atrial activity to make the diagnosis of AF.

Diagnostic Testing

All patients presenting with new-onset AF should undergo appropriate testing for a reversible cause. All patients with new-onset AF should receive an assessment of thyroid function. Additional laboratory testing should be guided by the history and physical examination. All patients with AF should receive an echocardiogram, since the most common cause of AF is structural heart disease.

❏ MANAGEMENT

New-onset Atrial Fibrillation

Newly diagnosed AF should prompt a diagnostic workup for a reversible cause. In general, when a reversible cause is identified, initial treatment should be directed at the underlying precipitating factor rather than the AF. Patients with new-onset AF presenting to the emergency room can in most cases be managed safely without hospital admission. Hospital admission may be warranted for patients with concurrent medical conditions requiring inpatient treatment, for the elderly, and for patients with significant structural heart disease, ischemia, hemodynamic instability or preexcited AF.

Immediate reversion to sinus rhythm is warranted in patients with hemodynamic instability, active ischemia, severe heart failure symptoms, or AF with ventricular preexcitation. In such cases, while it is ideal to confirm absence of an intracardiac thrombus using a transesophageal echocardiogram, this may not be possible due to the urgency of the situation. At a minimum, systemic anticoagulation should be administered prior to cardioversion unless strongly contraindicated.

When urgent cardioversion is not indicated, it is acceptable to pursue an initial rate control strategy for patients who are mildly or moderately symptomatic. About 70% of patients with new-onset AF of less than 72 hours duration will spontaneously convert to sinus rhythm without intervention. For the remainder, reversion to sinus rhythm with cardioversion, either electrical or chemical, may be reasonable if the risk of short-term AF recurrence is relatively low or unknown. This is the case in younger patients (<65) with structurally normal hearts and in patients with reversible causes for AF once the underlying cause is addressed. Antiarrhythmic drug therapy is generally reserved for patients with recurrent AF and is not routinely administered to patients after cardioversion for new-onset AF.

Rate Control Versus Rhythm Control in Recurrent AF

In approaching the patient with recurrent paroxysmal or persistent AF, the clinician must decide whether to attempt to maintain sinus rhythm. Theoretically, maintaining sinus rhythm would prevent symptoms associated with AF, normalize heart rate, maintain AV synchrony and the atrial contribution to cardiac output, and prevent deleterious atrial remodeling. Moreover, the epidemiological data on outcomes in AF raise hope that patients in whom sinus rhythm can be maintained might have improved quality of life and reduced mortality. On the other hand, the pharmacological tools available to maintain sinus rhythm are limited, and the attempt to maintain AF may be associated with side effects of these medications.

Currently, there is no algorithmic or guideline-driven approach that determines in whom rhythm control should be attempted. Relevant considerations are age, comorbidities, patient preference, risk of antiarrhythmic drugs, the likelihood of maintaining sinus rhythm, and whether the patient has symptoms due to AF even with adequate rate control. Thus, in older patients with structural heart disease and/

or hypertension and no symptoms, rate control may be a reasonable first strategy; while in younger patients or in patients with lone AF with symptoms, rhythm control may be a reasonable initial choice.

Restoration of Sinus Rhythm

Once a rhythm control strategy is selected, the initial step is to restore sinus rhythm. Reversion to sinus rhythm without early recurrence of AF is more likely when the duration of AF is less than one year, the left atrium is not markedly enlarged, and structural heart disease is minimal. It is also safe to cardiovert low-risk patients without a history of rheumatic heart disease or prior thromboembolism when the duration of the AF episode is less than 48 hours without a TEE. In these cases, intravenous heparin or equivalent should be administered before cardioversion. Patients should be therapeutically anticoagulated from the time of cardioversion for at least 1 month. After that, thromboembolic risk should be reassessed and addressed as indicated.

Electrical cardioversion is highly effective for restoration of sinus rhythm in patients with paroxysmal AF. Chemical cardioversion is also effective for reversion to sinus rhythm, but in general it is not as effective as electrical cardioversion. Class III agents, such as amiodarone, ibutilide and dofetilide, are the most effective drugs for cardioversion of long-standing AF, while class 1C agents flecainide and propafenone are also effective when the duration of AF is less than 7 days. When using ibutilide or dofetilide, special attention should be paid to electrolytes and QT interval, as these medications confer a significant short-term risk of torsades de pointes.

Pharmacological Approaches

In general, once a decision to attempt rhythm control has been made, the choice of antiarrhythmic drugs is primarily dictated by risks and side-effect potential, which are largely determined by the presence or absence of structural heart disease. Flowchart 5 shows a scheme recommended in the 2006 ACC/AHA/ESC Guidelines for management of AF. This section presents an overview of the Class 1 and Class 3 medications used to maintain sinus rhythm and the evidence supporting their use in specific populations.

Due to the role of the RAAS system in the pathogenesis of AF, the use of angiotensin receptor blockers (ARB) and angiotensin converting enzyme inhibitors has been explored in AF. Particularly for patients with hypertension, left ventricular dysfunction or diabetes, but possibly even for patients without many comorbidities, RAAS inhibition can be an important adjunctive therapy for AF.

Maintenance of Sinus Rhythm—Invasive Approaches

Nonpharmacological approaches to maintenance of sinus rhythm include catheter ablation, surgical ablation, pacing, and atrial defibrillation. The finding that physiological pacing modes in bradycardic patients with AF can prevent recurrences has led to a variety of pacing strategies to maintain sinus rhythm, including multisite pacing, alternative site pacing, and overdrive suppression of AF. With the exception of small subpopulations these strategies have not been shown to be effective. Patients with AF should therefore not receive permanent pacemakers for the purpose of AF suppression, although selection of physiological pacing modes and minimization of ventricular pacing can prevent AF episodes in patients receiving pacemakers for other reasons.

FLOWCHART 5: 2006 American College of Cardiology (ACC)/American Heart Association (AHA)/European Society of Cardiology (ESC) algorithm for antiarrhythmic drug therapy to maintain sinus rhythm in patients with recurrent paroxysmal or persistent AF. Patients should first be categorized by severity of heart disease (left to right) and treatment selection should proceed from top to bottom. Within boxes, drugs are listed alphabetically and not by order of preference

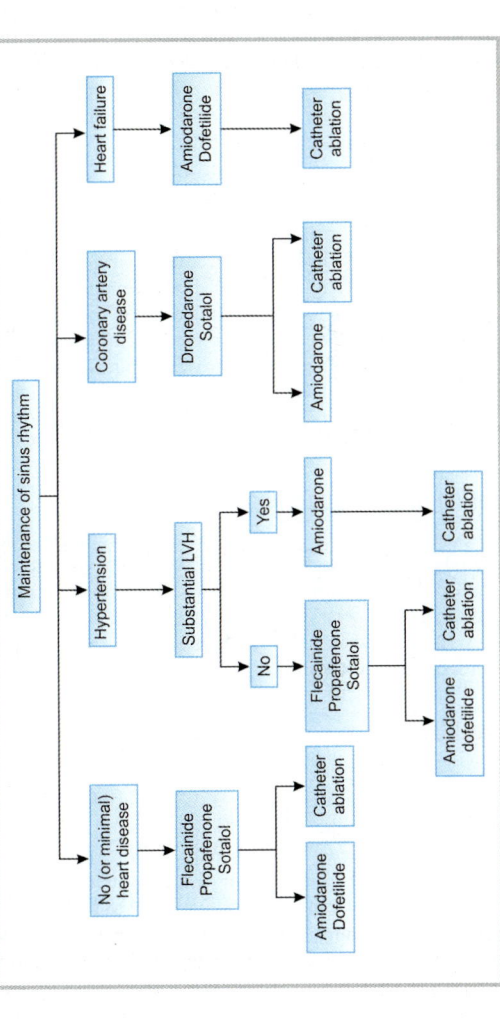

Catheter Ablation

The development of catheter ablation for AF began with the observation that rapid firing originating in the pulmonary veins frequently triggered AF. At present, ablation techniques for AF vary widely among practitioners and the optimal approach has yet to be defined. Most commonly, contiguous or nearly contiguous lesions are created around each of the four pulmonary veins, and electrical isolation is confirmed with a combination of recording and pacing within the pulmonary veins. As ablation causes atrial inflammation in the short run, early recurrence of AF is common after ablation and does not necessarily indicate long-term procedural non-success.

Strategies for Rate Control

The recommended target for rate control in AF is 80 bpm at rest and less than 120 bpm with moderate activity, although these numbers are not based on prospective trials. The mainstays for rate control in AF are beta-adrenergic blockers and the non-dihydropyridine calcium channel blockers diltiazem and verapamil. These medications slow AV nodal conduction and prolong AV nodal refractoriness, thereby reducing the frequency of fibrillatory waves that can be conducted to the ventricles. As oral therapy for ambulatory AF patients, digoxin can be a useful adjunctive agent for rate control, but is less effective as monotherapy for rate control in AF and should not be used in this way. Dronederone is also an effective rate control agent and can be used for this purpose even if not effective at maintaining sinus rhythm.

Prevention of Thromboembolism

It is imperative that all patients with AF undergo risk stratification for thromboembolic events, regardless of AF type and regardless of treatment strategy. Anticoagulation with warfarin lowers the risk of stroke for nearly all patients with AF; however, in the lowest risk patients, the risk of major bleeding due to warfarin therapy exceeds the value of this marginal risk reduction. For such patients, aspirin can be an acceptable alternative.

❏ CONCLUSION

Although major advances in the understanding and treatment of AF have occurred recently—such as the understanding of the role of the pulmonary veins in AF and the development of catheter ablation for AF—we still do not have an understanding of the etiology of the underlying substrate of AF and thus no targeted treatments to prevent or reverse AF exist. Current treatment strategies are aimed at preventing stroke, and either rate control or rhythm control to prevent rapid ventricular rates and symptoms. In general, treatment options for persistent and permanent AF are limited to stroke prevention and rate control. Future research will hopefully define the substrate(s) that predispose to AF and thereby allow directed therapy to prevent or reverse AF.

❏ SUGGESTED READINGS

Benjamin EJ, Wolf PA, D'Agostino RB, et al. Impact of atrial fibrillation on the risk of death: the Framingham heart study. Circulation. 1998;98:946-52.

Fuster V, Rydén LE, Cannom DS, et al. ACC/AHA/ESC 2006 Guidelines for the Management of Patients with Atrial Fibrillation: a report of the American College of Cardiology/

American Heart Association Task Force on Practice Guidelines and the European Society of Cardiology Committee for Practice Guidelines (Writing Committee to Revise the 2001 Guidelines for the Management of Patients With Atrial Fibrillation): developed in collaboration with the European Heart Rhythm Association and the Heart Rhythm Society. Circulation. 2006;114:e257-e354.

Lamassa M, Di Carlo A, Pracucci G, et al. Characteristics, outcome, and care of stroke associated with atrial fibrillation in Europe: data from a multicenter multinational hospital-based registry (The European Community Stroke Project). Stroke. 2001;32:392-8.

Patients with nonvalvular atrial fibrillation at low risk of stroke during treatment with aspirin: stroke Prevention in Atrial Fibrillation III study. The SPAF III Writing Committee for the Stroke Prevention in Atrial Fibrillation Investigators. JAMA. 1998;279:1273-7.

3.5 Supraventricular Tachycardia

❑ INTRODUCTION

Supraventricular tachycardia (SVT) is a heart rhythm disturbance, initiated in the atria or ventricles, with atrial rates exceeding 100 beats per minute (bpm), that requires tissue above the His bundle in order to be perpetuated. SVTs can be symptomatic or asymptomatic, slow or fast, regular or irregular, sustained or nonsustained, paroxysmal, persistent or permanent, and may be due to various mechanisms involving tissue in the atria, AV node, His Purkinje system and/or the ventricles.

❑ CLASSIFICATION

Supraventricular tachycardias are either AV nodal dependent or AV nodal independent (Table 8). AV nodal dependent SVTs require AV nodal conduction in

Table 8: Classification of supraventricular tachycardias

AV nodal dependent
- AV nodal reentry
- AV reentry
    - Orthodromic AV reciprocating tachycardia
    - Antidromic AV reciprocating tachycardia

AV nodal independent
- Atrial tachycardias
    - Sinoatrial reentry
    - Focal (triggered, automatic, microreentry)
    - Macroreentry (scar mediated, congenital heart disease)
- Junctional ectopic tachycardia
- Atria flutter
    - Right atrial flutter
        - Clockwise
        - Counterclockwise
    - Left atrial flutter
        - Mitral reentry
        - Scar mediated
        - Pulmonary vein
- Atrial fibrillation

FLOWCHART 6: Supraventricular tachycardia—AVRT (Panel A), AVNRT (Panel B) and AT (Panel C)

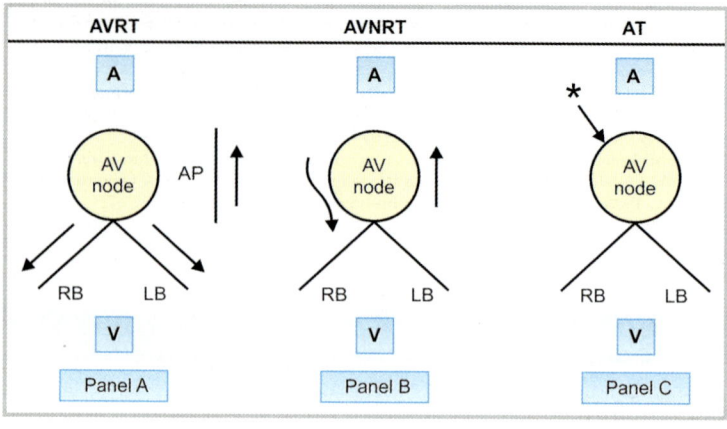

order to perpetuate. These SVTs generally have a regular ventricular rate. The two common forms of SVT are atrioventricular nodal reentry tachycardia (AVNRT) and atrioventricular reciprocating tachycardia (AVRT). AV nodal independent SVTs require only atrial tissue and do not require AV nodal activation for the tachycardia to occur. They can have a regular ventricular response, as seen in sinoatrial reentry, nonparoxysmal junctional ectopic tachycardia (JET), monomorphic atrial tachycardia (AT), and atrial flutter (AFL) with a fixed or variable AV conduction ratio or an irregular ventricular response as seen with AFib, AFL with variable AV conduction and multifocal atrial tachycardia (MAT). Almost all irregular SVTs are AV nodal independent. AV nodal dependent SVTs can occasionally be irregular, especially at the initiation and termination of the tachycardia. AV nodal independent SVTs can be associated with complete AV block such that the ventricular rhythm is a junctional or ventricular escape (Flowchart 6).

Atrial-based AV Nodal Independent SVT

Sinus Tachycardia

Sinus tachycardia is ubiquitous, occurs with sympathetic activation, and may be due to specific triggers, such as infection, heart failure, pulmonary embolus or hyperthyroidism. It is not generally considered to be SVT. Sinus tachycardia tends to start with gradual acceleration and usually stops with an even more gradual deceleration. In some instances, it can be difficult to distinguish sinus tachycardia from SVT. The P wave morphology in sinus tachycardia is similar to that in sinus rhythm, although due to sympathetic stimulation of the sinus node, exit from the sinus node may be more superior and thus the P wave may shift slightly in sinus tachycardia. Rates rarely exceed 200 bpm, except in children or during extreme physical activity. The P wave normally precedes the QRS complex but this depends on AV nodal conduction.

Atrial Flutter

Atrial flutter is a macroreentrant rapid AT, typically involving the right atrium. It tends to coexist with AFib (although most AFib originates from the left atrium) and tends to occur in patients with structural heart disease. The atrial rate,

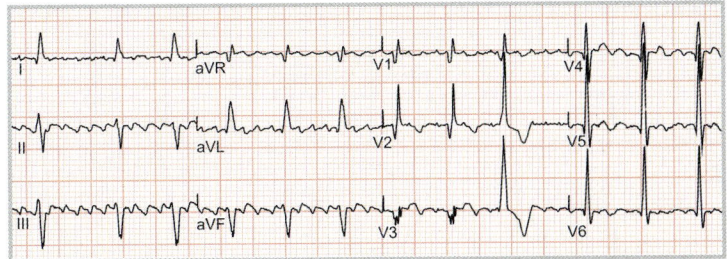

FIGURE 7: "Saw tooth" flutter waves are seen in the inferior leads in "typical" counterclockwise, isthmus-dependent atrial flutter. Usually, this form of atrial flutter demonstrates upright P waves in lead V1. Here, there is variable AV conduction

without drug therapy, exceeds 200 bpm but can be as high as 350 bpm. The most common form of AFL, due to counterclockwise electrical activation in the right atrium around the tricuspid ring utilizing an isthmus of tissue, the cavotricuspid isthmus, has a "saw tooth" appearance in the inferior leads with no isoelectric segment between beats (Fig. 7). Approximately 10% of typical AFL is perpetuated by clockwise activation around the tricuspid ring. Atypical forms of right AFL involve upper loop or lower loop reentry mechanisms. These flutters do not show the "typical" electrocardiographic appearance or rate and may require an alternative approach during ablation procedures. Some AFL due to scar can be associated with congenital heart disease; these often have very unusual reentrant pathways.

Atrial Tachycardia

Atrial tachycardia can originate from the left atrium, right atrium, vena cavae or pulmonary veins [Flowchart 6 (Panel C)]. The tachycardia can be focal or macroreentrant involving large areas of the atria. Focal forms can be microreentrant or due to an automatic or triggered mechanism. Monomorphic AT represents about 5–10% of all regular SVTs. The P wave precedes the QRS complex but generally has a morphology distinct from the sinus P wave. The PR interval may vary. The atrial rates are generally 120–200 bpm. The conduction can be 1:1 but AV block can be present. An "A-A-V" pattern can be seen during AT.

Intra-atrial Reentrant Tachycardia

Macroreentry or microreentry AT often utilizes areas of scar at incisions from prior cardiac surgery or corrected congenital heart disease (such as a Fontan procedure) and represents 5–10% of SVTs. This type of tachycardia is distinguishable from AFL as there are discrete P waves separated by an isoelectric baseline. Adenosine may terminate atrial re-entrant SVTs in 15% of cases.

Sinoatrial Reentry Tachycardia

Sinoatrial reentry tachycardia (SART) is a unique, uncommon form of regular AT due to a reentrant mechanism involving the sinoatrial node. The P wave morphology is often similar to that in sinus rhythm with the exit point in the right atrium slightly below the sinus node (Figs 8A and B) but it can masquerade as other forms of SVT. This tachycardia starts and stops abruptly and tends to be slower and more irregular than other types of SVT. Patients with AVNRT may also have associated SVTs, such as sinoatrial reentry.

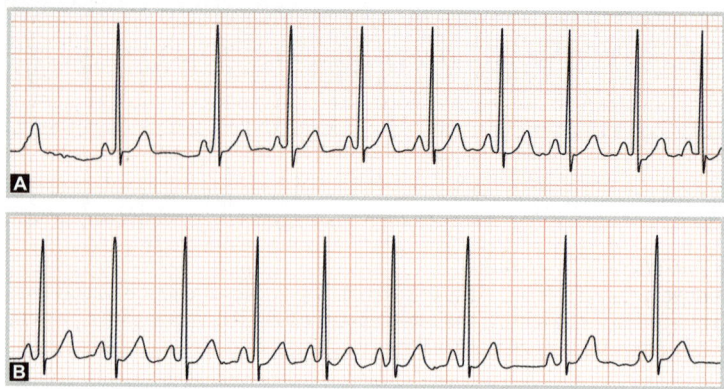

FIGURES 8A AND B: This rhythm strip demonstrates an abrupt change (speeding and slowing) in heart rate with an upright P wave in the inferior leads. The P wave morphology does not change and is similar to that in sinus rhythm. This is expected in typical sinoatrial reentrant supraventricular tachycardia

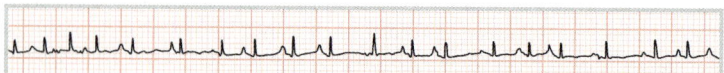

FIGURE 9: This rhythm strip shows multifocal atrial tachycardia, with at least three distinct P wave morphologies present. This type of tachycardia is often related to severe pulmonary disease and treatment of the underlying disease is the best way to eliminate the tachycardia. The prognosis is generally poor but not directly related to the atrial tachycardia itself. While there is no specific antiarrhythmic treatment for this tachycardia, amiodarone or verapamil may be effective

Multifocal Atrial Tachycardia

In MAT, atrial activation occurs from multiple locations leading to at least three different morphologies of P waves (Fig. 9). The atrial rate is between 110 bpm and 170 bpm. In some cases, it can be difficult to distinguish from "coarse" AFib.

AV Nodal Dependent SVT

Atrioventricular Nodal Reentrant Tachycardia

Atrioventricular nodal reentrant tachycardia is due to the presence of two physiological and anatomical ("slow" and "fast") AV nodal pathways. Typically, activation proceeds down the "slow" perinodal pathway and returns via the retrograde "fast" perinodal pathway [Flowchart 6 (Panel B)]. The rates of AVNRT are usually between 150 bpm and 200 bpm, but it can be as fast as 250 bpm. Slow or fast AVNRT usually begins with a premature atrial depolarization followed by a long PR interval. There can be a pseudo R' in lead V1 and a pseudo S wave in the inferior leads, a retrograde P wave seen in other leads or not. AVNRT can be present with a bundle branch block, and this can be tachycardia dependent.

Atrioventricular Reentry Tachycardia

Atrioventricular reciprocating tachycardia is a macroreentrant tachycardia involving activation of the atria and ventricles through anterograde and retrograde conducting AV pathways [the AV node and an accessory pathway. Typically, the antegrade conduction during AVRT is via the AV node with retrograde conduction via an independent accessory pathway. When this occurs, it is known as "orthodromic AV reciprocating tachycardia" [Flowchart 6 (Panel A)], representing approximately 30% of all regular SVTs. It is more common in young males and tends to be faster than AVNRT. During this tachycardia, the P wave is distinctly after the QRS complex, and this tachycardia is often termed "long RP tachycardia".

Preexcitation Syndromes

Manifest antegrade conduction through an accessory pathway can "preexcite" the ventricles and cause a fusion complex or complete conduction via the antegrade accessory pathway. The AV connection can occur by way of the left ventricle, the right ventricle, or the septum at virtually any location between the atria and the ventricles. When this is present in sinus rhythm, the pattern on the ECG is known as the "Wolff–Parkinson–White" (WPW) pattern. When this pattern is associated with palpitations, this is known as WPW syndrome.

❏ DIAGNOSIS

The clinical presentation can be diagnostic of SVT, and it may be possible to proceed with further evaluation and therapy on this basis alone. Classic symptoms include abrupt onset of rapid palpitations with associated dyspnea, chest discomfort, dizziness, and light headedness. These symptoms often abruptly terminate when the patient utilizes vagal maneuvers that are learned over time in an attempt to abate the symptoms.

The physical examination can aid in determining the specific type of SVT. The neck veins may show prominent pulsations with each beat, consistent with cannon A waves, common in typical AVNRT. Alternatively, patients with AFL may have flutter waves seen as pulsations in the neck at a rate faster than the pulse itself. An irregularly irregular pulse or a pulse deficit would be consistent with AFib. Additionally, important information from the physical examination includes blood pressure recordings as well as evidence for hemodynamic compromise or the presence of congestive heart failure.

Bedside maneuvers, such as carotid sinus massage or Valsalva, can terminate tachycardia abruptly. They can also uncover the presence of an AV nodal independent tachycardia, such as AFL. These maneuvers can also slow down the sinus rate and stop sinoatrial reentry as well. Adenosine can stop some ATs.

Electrophysiology Studies

Invasive electrophysiology studies are used either for diagnosis of SVT in patients with classic symptoms or for determination of the mechanism of SVT for those who have recorded episodes or have a wide QRS tachycardia that may be SVT or VT. During the electrophysiology study, 2–5 intravenous catheter sheaths are placed and recording and stimulating catheter electrodes are placed in specific sites of the heart to record electrical activation and to stimulate the heart to initiate tachycardia and understand its mechanism.

After SVT is initiated in the electrophysiology laboratory, the relationships of the atria, ventricles and His bundle during extrastimulus testing and during tachycardia can help to determine the tachycardia mechanism. Transient entrainment may help to understand the location and mechanism of the SVT.

❑ TREATMENTS

The goal of treatment is to terminate tachycardia acutely, maintain normal sinus rhythm, control ventricular response rate, eliminate symptoms, normalize hemodynamics, and prevent worsening of any underlying cardiovascular conditions due to SVT.

Acute Care

Acute management depends on the type and severity of symptoms related to the SVT and the type of SVT (Table 9). Acute interventions are designed to slow the ventricular rate (for AV nodal independent SVTs) and/or terminate the tachycardia. Therapies include drugs to cardiovert and prevent recurrence, drugs used to slow the AV conduction and the ventricular rate, and direct current cardioversion. Acute management requires careful electrocardiographic and hemodynamic monitoring. Patients remaining in SVT and having ventricular rates that cannot be controlled require hospital admission. Other indications for admission include frequent recurrences, resistance to initial drug therapy, initiation of new antiarrhythmic drugs, radiofrequency (RF) catheter ablation (elective or urgent) or adverse consequences from SVT (heart failure exacerbation, hypotension, myocardial ischemia) (Flowchart 7).

AV Nodal-dependent SVT or Regular SVT

The first line treatment for an AV nodal-dependent tachycardia is a vagal maneuver, such as carotid sinus massage, to create transient AV block and terminate the tachycardia. Patients can learn to perform vagal maneuvers and stop tachycardia on their own without the need for medical intervention. Carotid sinus massage is an easy and effective methodology to stop AV nodal dependent SVT but should only be used in the absence of a carotid bruit and/or absence of significant carotid disease. In this procedure, the head should be turned away from the side being compressed (usually the right side) and a firm compression with 2–3 fingers is applied over the bulb of the carotid. Sometimes, carotid massage can be combined with a Valsalva maneuver and even the Trendelenburg position to facilitate conversion. Another vagal reflex, the "diving reflex" in which the face is placed in cold water, may be effective.

Adenosine (Flowchart 8) can differentiate AV nodal independent versus AV nodal dependent SVT and can be used to help to make a diagnosis, but like AVNRT, SART can respond to autonomic maneuvers and adenosine. Adenosine effectively and rapidly terminates AV nodal-dependent SVTs. It is generally effective even if borderline hypotension is present. The advantage of adenosine is its rapid onset and short half-life.

Intravenous calcium channel antagonists, verapamil and diltiazem, can also terminate SVT. Intravenous verapamil at doses of 5–15 mg can be effective; the duration of action is 5–45 minutes. Intravenous diltiazem can be used in doses of 0.15 mg/kg, 0.25 mg/kg and 0.45 mg/kg. Calcium channel blockers have negative inotropic effects and therefore can cause hypotension; use is not recommended when the patient is hypotensive or has ventricular dysfunction. It should be avoided in patients with preexcited AFib (i.e. antegrade activation via an accessory pathway). It should never be used when there is an undiagnosed wide QRS complex tachycardia as the results could be disastrous.

Intravenous beta-adrenergic blockade (metoprolol or esmolol) may be effective in terminating SVT as well. Esmolol has a short half-life of less than 10 minutes.

Electrophysiology

Table 9: Pharmacologic management for supraventricular tachycardia

Drugs	Mechanisms	Dosage	Side effects	Contraindications
Adenosine	Purinergic agonist Inhibition sinus node and AV node	6 mg by rapid IV. If ineffective,12 mg and 18 mg	Nausea, light-headedness, headache, flushing, chest pain, bradycardia, brief asystole	Persantine Cardiac transplant Bronchospasm
Verapamil	Slow or block AV nodal conduction and slow sinus rate	2.5–5 mg over 1–2 min	Negative inotropic effect, hypotension, cardiogenic shock, marked bradycardia	Hypotension Systolic dysfunction Atrial fibrillation with preexcitation
Diltiazem	Slow or block AV nodal conduction and slow sinus rate	0.25 mg/kg IV bolus then 5–15 mg/hour gtt	Negative inotropic effect, hypotension, bradycardia	Hypotension Systolic dysfunction Atrial fibrillation with preexcitation
Metoprolol	Block β-sympathetic nervous system at the receptor level Inhibitory effects on sinus node, AV node and myocardial contraction	2.5–5 mg 3x at 2-min interval	Negative inotropic effect, hypotension	Hypotension Cardiogenic shock Bradycardia Decompensated heart failure Bronchospasm
Esmolol	Inhibitory effects on sinus node, AV node and myocardial contraction	IV 500 mcg/min loading dose over 1 min before each titration	Negative inotropic effect, hypotension, peripheral ischemia, confusion, bradycardia, bronchospasm	Hypotension Cardiogenic shock Bradycardia Decompensated heart failure Bronchospasm
Digoxin	Na^+/K^+ ATPase inhibition Parasympathetic activation leading to sinus lowing and AV nodal inhibition	0.75–1.5 mg in divided doses over 12–24 hours	Nausea, vomiting, diarrhea, fatigue, confusion, colored vision, palpitation, arrhythmia, syncope	WPW syndrome Atrial fibrillation with preexcitation
Amiodarone	Class III AAD but with classes I, II and IV activity, block sodium, calcium and potassium channels	Oral: loading 1200–1600 mg daily, maintenance 200–400 mg daily IV: 150 mg over 10 min, then 360 mg over 6 hours, 540 mg over remaining 24 hours, then 0.5 mg/min	Thyroid abnormalities, pulmonary fibrosis, QT prolongation, liver function abnormalities	Severe sinus node dysfunction Hepatic dysfunction Pregnancy

FLOWCHART 7: Management of regular SVT in an acute setting

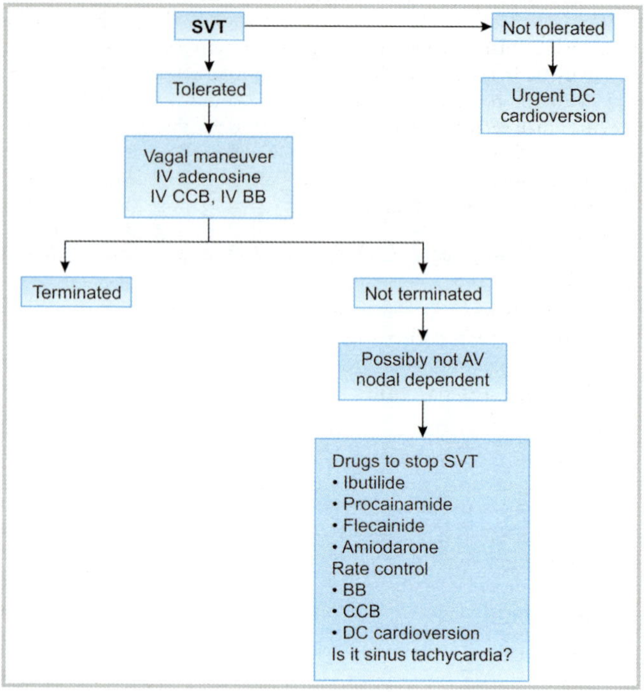

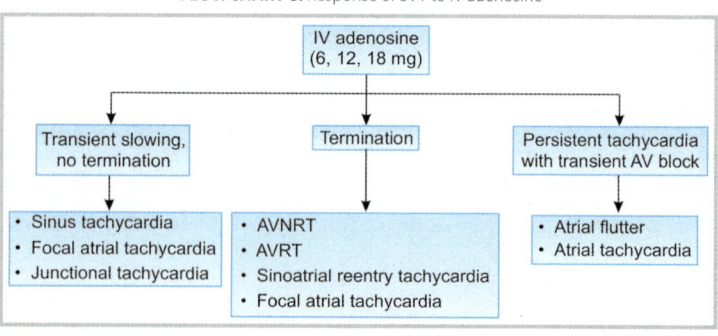

FLOWCHART 8: Response of SVT to IV adenosine

Metoprolol has a longer half-life but is less expensive. Both of these drugs have a negative inotropic effect and may cause hypotension. Beta blockade and intravenous digoxin are third line drugs for termination of AV nodal dependent SVT. The use of digoxin for the acute management of SVT is now rare.

AV Nodal Independent SVT

Intravenous beta-blockers, digoxin and/or calcium channel blockers can control the ventricular rate in patients who have atrial-based, AV nodal independent SVT (AT,

AFL and AFib). The one exception is SART that responds reliably to adenosine. The preference of the drug class is related to the underlying conditions, blood pressure and ventricular function. Betablockers (in combination with digoxin), for example, are useful in controlling the ventricular response rate in AFL and AFib, especially in the postoperative period. Intravenous diltiazem has less negative inotropic effect than verapamil and can be used to control the ventricular rate when there is borderline low blood pressure. Diltiazem also may be useful when there is concern about bronchospasm. Digoxin may require a large loading dose and a protracted period but is more useful for patients with ventricular dysfunction or hypotension.

The WPW syndrome, when it is manifest as rapid AFib, should be treated with a drug that blocks the accessory pathway: either procainamide or amiodarone. Digoxin, calcium channel blockers and beta-adrenergic blockers are strictly prohibited in these patients during acute management.

When to Use DC Cardioversion

Cardioversion is the best option for patients with an undiagnosed wide QRS complex tachycardia not tolerated hemodynamically and for any poorly tolerated (hemodynamic instability or evidence of heart failure or myocardial ischemia) SVT in which the rate cannot be controlled and the rhythm cannot be restored to sinus. In patients who have hemodynamic collapse due to any type of SVT other than sinus tachycardia, synchronized DC cardioversion is recommended.

Long-term Management

The long-term management of SVT depends on multiple factors, including the symptoms related to SVT, the recurrence rates, the underlying clinical conditions and the presence of structural heart disease. The choice of drug for long-term management of SVT depends on the mechanism of the SVT and the goal of treatment. For ATs, AFL and AFib a simple strategy is to control the ventricular rate instead of maintaining sinus rhythm. Beta-adrenergic blockers, calcium channel blockers and digoxin, in combination, can be effective. Antiarrhythmic drugs are often not effective for AFL and ablation may be necessary. Occasionally, the ventricular rate cannot be controlled and maintenance of sinus rhythm is not an option; in this case, AV nodal ablation with permanent pacemaker may be required.

Like AFib and AFL, ATs can increase the risk of thromboembolic events. Consideration must be given to the use of routine long-term anticoagulation for SVTs at risk for stroke. Similarly, there are no specific guidelines with respect to anticoagulation for AFL. Recent data indicate that AFL has a similar or slightly lower risk of thromboembolic risk when compared with AFib.

Catheter Ablation

Catheter ablation has emerged as a curative approach for the patients who have SVT. The mechanism by which catheter ablation may work is dependent upon the type of tachycardia. Catheter ablation involves the purposeful destruction or isolation of selective tissue responsible for the tachycardia. Delivery of heat to the tissue via RF energy remains the standard approach in the ablation of most arrhythmias. Cryoablation has been used with some success in selected patients who have arrhythmias. RF ablation can successfully cure AVNRT, AVRT, sinoatrial reentry, WPW, Mahaim tachycardias, focal AT, AFL, and even AFib. Additionally, ablation may be useful for JETs and occasionally for inappropriate sinus tachycardia.

Table 10: Complications of catheter ablation for SVT (depends on SVT type)	
Complications	Prevalence
AV block	0.67–1%
Cardiac tamponade	0.22–1.1%
Pericarditis	0.31%
Pneumothorax	0.15–0.22%
Tricuspid regurgitation	0.22%
Acute myocardial infarction	0.15%
Femoral artery pseudoaneurysm	0.15%
Death	0.1%

Complications in ablation include death (0.1%) (Table 10). There is approximately 0.4% risk of AV nodal block requiring a pacemaker with AVNRT "slow pathway" ablation. There are also risks of cardiac tamponade, pericarditis, hematoma and deep venous thrombosis. In general, the risks of the procedure are relatively low, and all risks are less than 1%.

❑ CONCLUSION

Supraventricular tachycardia remains a common and often symptomatic problem for many patients. A wide variety of types and clinical presentations of SVT exist. The diagnosis requires careful observation and interpretation of electrocardiographic recordings. Evaluation involves thoughtful assessment of the relationship between the tachycardia, hemodynamics, and symptoms. While rarely life-threatening, treatment is often required.

❑ SUGGESTED READINGS

Blomstrom-Lundqvist C, Scheinman MM, Aliot EM, et al. ACC/ AHA/ESC guidelines for the management of patients with supraventricular arrhythmias—executive summary: a report of the American College of Cardiology/American Heart Association Task Force on Practice Guidelines and the European Society of Cardiology Committee for Practice Guidelines (Writing Committee to Develop Guidelines for the Management of Patients With Supraventricular Arrhythmias). Circulation. 2003;108:1871-909.

Fuster V, Ryden LE, Cannom DS, et al. ACC/AHA/ESC 2006 guidelines for the management of patients with atrial fibrillation— executive summary: a report of the American College of Cardiology/ American Heart Association Task Force on Practice Guidelines and the European Society of Cardiology Committee for Practice Guidelines (Writing Committee to Revise the 2001 Guidelines for the Management of Patients with Atrial Fibrillation). J Am Coll Cardiol. 2006;48:854-906.

Gonzalez-Torrecilla E, Almendral J, Arenal A, et al. Combined evaluation of bedside clinical variables and the electrocardiogram for the differential diagnosis of paroxysmal atrioventricular reciprocating tachycardias in patients without pre-excitation. J Am Coll Cardiol. 2009;53:2353-8.

Olshansky B, Wilber DJ, Hariman RJ. Atrial flutter—update on the mechanism and treatment. Pacing Clin Electrophysiol. 1992;15:2308-35.

Rankin AC, Brooks R, Ruskin JN, et al. Adenosine and the treatment of supraventricular tachycardia. Am J Med. 1992;92:655-64.

Scheinman MM, Huang S. The 1998 NASPE prospective catheter ablation registry. Pacing Clin Electrophysiol. 2000;23:1020-8.

Scher DL, Arsura EL. Multifocal atrial tachycardia: mechanisms, clinical correlates, and treatment. Am Heart J. 1989;118:574-80.

Yusuf S, Camm AJ. The sinus tachycardias. Nat Clin Pract Cardiovasc Med. 2005;2:44-52.

3.6 Clinical Spectrum of Ventricular Tachycardia

❏ INTRODUCTION

As the field of invasive interventional electrophysiology has grown, interest in finding the cellular/molecular basis for arrhythmias has escalated. At this time, however, we clinically deal with myriad complex VTs, often with incomplete understanding and the desire to simplify information for clinical purposes.

Table 11 is an attempt to present a simple and clinically relevant classification. The usual first encounter for an arrhythmologist to a patient with documented VT is a rhythm strip, or, occasionally, a 12-lead ECG (Fig. 10) showing a monomorphic or polymorphic VT. This is a striking feature of VT and is seldom missed by a clinician, unless, in a given lead, the polymorphic nature of the VT is not appreciable. There can be serious consequences for not knowing polymorphic versus monomorphic VT (MMVT). Hence, it is prudent to emphasize at the outset that the distinction between the monomorphic and the polymorphic nature of the VT is important and can be deciphered by recording two leads perpendicular to each other.

Table 11: Clinical spectrum of ventricular tachycardia

	Monomorphic VT		Polymorphic VT	
SHD	No SHD	Long QT	Normal QT	Short QT
Myocardial fibrosis	RV outflow	Congenital (QT-1 to QT-12)	Brugada* (Type 1–3)	Short QT (1–5)
BBR (HPS disease)	Idiopathic LV-VT From sinus Valsalva,	Acquired: Drugs, electrolyte	Active ischemia	
ARVD (RV fatty infiltration) regional and familial forms of ARVD Naxos, Venetian	Mitral, pulmonic cusp Bidirectional Iatrogenic device leads		Myocardial hypertrophy LV Noncompaction Catecholaminergic PVT	
VT post surgical Scar			J-wave syndromes early repolarization syndrome hypothermia Idiopathic VF	

(Abbreviations: SHD: Structural heart disease; BBR: Bundle branch reentry; ARVD: Arrhythmic RV dysplasia; RV: Right ventricular; LV: Left ventricular; PVT: Polymorphic ventricular tachycardia; VF: Ventricular fibrillation).

*Regional expressions for Brugada-like syndromes:

— Thailand – Tai Lai (death during sleep)
— Phillipines – Bangungut (scream followed by sudden death-at night)
— Japan – Pokkuri – (unexpected sudden death at night)

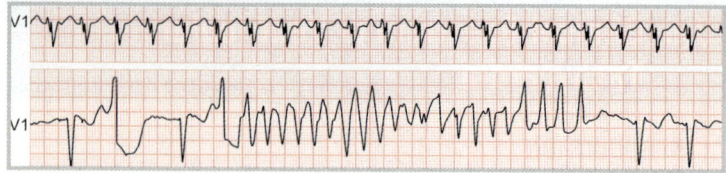

FIGURE 10: Rhythm strip (V1) shown. Note the monomorphic appearance of the VT in the top panel. P-wave is not clearly visible but its presence is suggested in some ST-T signals. The bottom tracing shows a prolongation of the QT interval, an episode of torsades de pointes, with rapid polymorphic VT of a constantly changing morphology that appears to be twisting around a central axis, which is the literal meaning of torsades de pointes (twisting of the points)

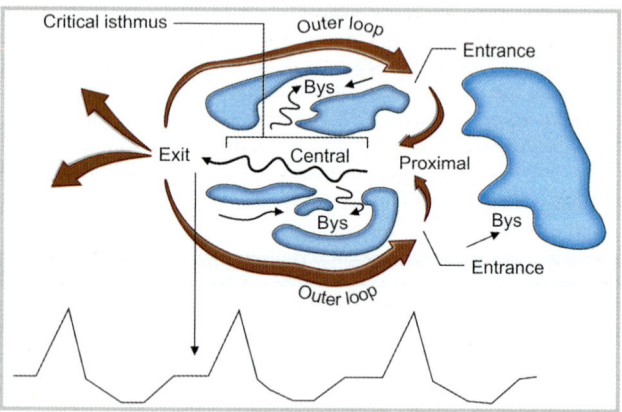

FIGURE 11: Classical model used to demonstrate reentry through the surviving muscle bands among the myocardial scar (shown as five islands). The QRS on the surface ECG starts where the impulse exits from the critical isthmus and turns around in a figure-of-eight fashion to reenter from the proximal end. Ablation at sites other than beside the central blue line is unlikely to be successful. This is why it is termed a critical area of slow conduction or as critical isthmus (*Source:* Modified from Stevenson W, Soejima K. Catheter ablation of ventricular tachycardia. In: Zipes DP, Jalife J (Eds). Cardiac Electrophysiology: From Cell to Bedside, 4th edition. Philadelphia: WB Saunders; 2004. pp. 1087-96)

❑ MONOMORPHIC VENTRICULAR TACHYCARDIA

Myocardial VT in Association with Structural Heart Disease

Myocardial VT in Association with Fibrosis/Scar (Table 11)

Coronary artery disease (CAD) remains the most common form of VT. Both monomorphic and polymorphic forms exist. However, the monomorphic forms are better understood and the underlying mechanism is easier to comprehend. Its distinction from other forms of wide QRS tachycardias has been extensively published. The classic model used to visualize this circuit of reentry is depicted in Figure 11. The fibrotic scar zone, shown as islands, the paths of impulse propagation in various directions, is indicated by arrows. On the surface ECG, QRS starts when the impulse exits from within the circuit. If one was to electrically stimulate this exit site, the surface ECG QRS would look identical to the spontaneous VT with a short stimulus artifact to QRS interval. Depending upon the geometry of the scar, the impulse could go in several directions, dictated by the shape of the scar and the state of the myocardium.

It should be pointed out that the diastolic interval between the QRS complexes is increased when the reentrant impulse is travelling through the isthmus (surviving muscle band, area of slow conduction), which is critical for the VT to continue. While this electrical activity is not visible on the surface ECG, it can be recorded by placing electrode catheters along the pathway. Penetration of this pathway occurs during sinus rhythm as well, and it can be recorded both by intracardiac recording techniques as well as from the surface by proper magnification and filters (the so-called signal-averaged ECG).

While the actual reentrant circuits may be more complex, the schema shown in Figure 11 gives one broad concept of how a VT can be mapped. When appropriate location of slow conduction is isolated, it leads to a successful ablation using radiofrequency or another form of energy. The baseline ECG is seldom normal in these patients, and likely to be suggestive of some cardiac pathology. Therapy for a scar-related VT can be manifold:

- In patients with an ejection fraction of less than 35%, implantable cardioverter defibrillator (ICD) is advised. The main reason is the prevention of sudden VT-related death from an existing or new arrhythmia . In many cases, particularly with slow VT (>280 ms), antitachycardia pacing will also terminate an organized MMVT, which is more comfortable for the patient
- With better left ventricular ejection fractions (LVEF), antiarrhythmic agents, particularly Class III drugs, such as sotalol, amiodarone and dronedarone, may be sufficient. In patients with CAD and VT, the addition of beta-blockers is beneficial because the role of ischemia in the initiation and maintenance of VT cannot be excluded with certainty at a given time. In high-risk patients post-myocardial infarction or cardiac surgery, an external defibrillator in the form of a life vest can be recommended
- When VT is incessant, endocardial and/or epicardial mapping and catheter ablation may be necessary
- Although surgical ablation is seldom necessary, it remains an option
- In rare situations, cardiac transplantation with or without ventricular assist devices may be the only option when there are no contraindications

Monomorphic VT Due to Bundle Branch Reentry

In this form of monomorphic VT, the underlying pathological substrate is the His–Purkinje system, which has markedly prolonged conduction time. More specifically, the right and left bundle branches are used for propagation to the ventricle via one bundle, returning to the His bundle through the contralateral bundle branch. Sometimes, the electrical circuit is localized to the two fascicles of the left bundle; in that case it is termed interfascicular reentry. The schema in Figure 12 depicts the reentry circuits and Figures 13A and B show bundle branch reentry (BBR)-VT, both a left bundle branch block (LBBB) pattern (A) and a right bundle branch block (RBBB) pattern (B). While the general incidence of BBR as the mechanism of MMVT is 6%, it is much higher in patients with idiopathic dilated cardiomyopathy and aortic valve disease. In patients with aortic valve disease, this is particularly common in the early post-surgical period. This form of VT is apparently a common finding in patients with myotonic dystrophy, when VT is observed in that population. The common theme among all of the above scenarios is the presence of His–Purkinje pathology manifested by

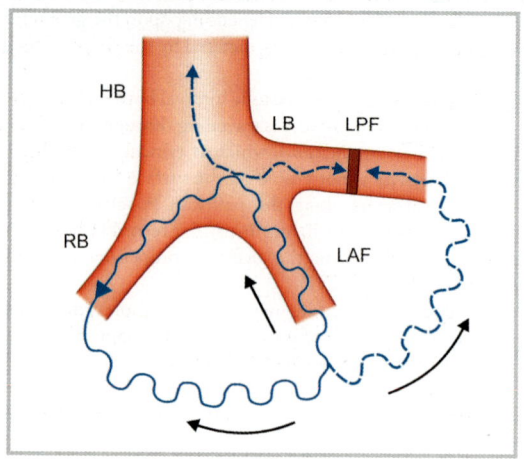

FIGURE 12: Schema demonstrates the circuit of bundle branch reentry VT. In this example, the impulse reaches the right ventricle via the right bundle (RB) and returns to the His bundle through the inferior fascicle of the left bundle (LB). While the same impulse approaches the His bundle via the superior fascicle, the two impulses will collide somewhere in that region. Activation of the His bundle will occur as a necessity since the left and right bundle are connected via the His bundle. The arrows depict the direction of impulse propagation. Tracings from top to bottom in each panel are surface ECG leads I, II and V1. The intracardiac tracings are HRA (high right atrial electrogram) and HB (His bundle electrogram). Time lines at the bottom are consecutive (Abbreviations: LAF: Left anterior fascicle; LPF: Left posterior fascicle)

nonspecific intraventricular conduction defect (IVCD), incomplete-to-complete bundle branch block on surface ECG with prolonged H-V interval on the His bundle electrogram recording.

Monomorphic VT in Association with Arrhythmogenic Right Ventricular Dysplasia

In arrhythmogenic right ventricular dysplasia (ARVD), the right ventricular (RV) muscle is replaced by fatty tissue, which in effect creates a model very similar to that shown in Figure 11. The disease may be patchy; affecting only RV apex, outflow or other parts, but may be quite extensive, replacing most RV myocardium with fatty infiltrates. At times the LV may also be affected.

For the most part, the main clinical problem these patients have is with nonsustained or sustained VT with a left bundle branch configuration with variable axis. While any axis may be noted, left bundle and left atrial (LA) morphology is very suggestive of ARVD; surface ECG also characteristically shows T-wave inversion in V1–V3 (Fig. 14) and may extend to V4 or V5. A late small deflection may be seen at the end of the QRS (epsilon wave) (Fig. 14 inset). Signal-averaged ECG is often positive. Diagnostic work should include magnetic resonance imaging (MRI), which is more sensitive than ultrasound, particularly in the early stages when the dysplasia is patchy.

Sotalol and amiodarone have been used to control VT. Catheter ablation is not encouraged due to the risk of perforation. The ICD therapy is recommended for the prevention of SCD.

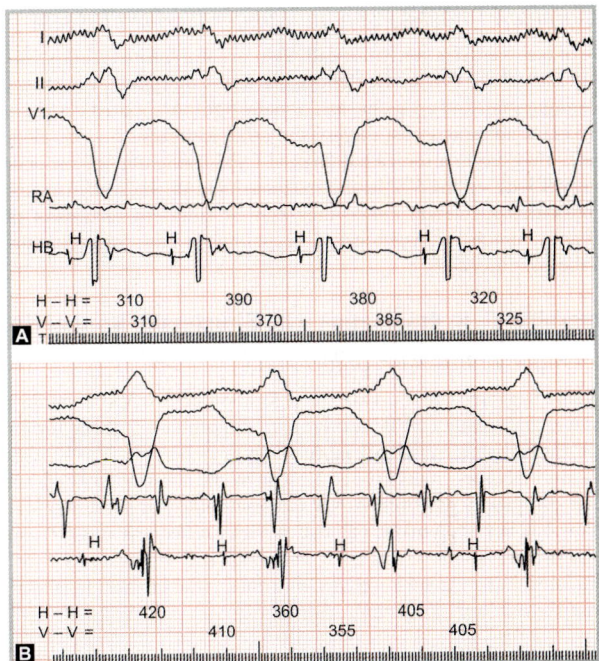

FIGURES 13A AND B: Bundle branch reentry with a left bundle branch block pattern (A) and right bundle branch block pattern (B) are shown. The axis is normal in A and leftward in B. The atrial rhythm is atrial fibrillation. Note that His deflection precedes the QRS and the change in the cycle length of H-H (labeled) precedes that of V-V (also labeled). In other words, the His bundle activation drives the ventricle, which is the opposite of what happens in myocardial VT, where the His bundle deflection follows the local V electrogram or is obscured by it. Nonetheless, the V-V cycle drives the H-H cycle in myocardial VT (*Source:* Blanck Z, Jazayeri M, Akhtar M. Facilitation of sustained bundle branch reentry by atrial fibrillation. J Cardiovasc Electrophysiol. 1996;7:348-52, with permission)

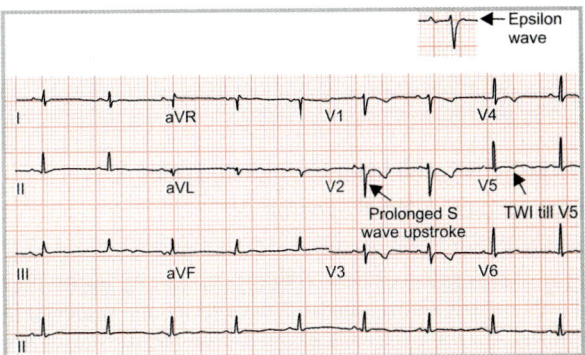

FIGURE 14: Twelve-lead ECG in arrhythmic right ventricular dysplasia (ARVD), the T-wave inversion V1–5 (usually up to V3) and late wave (epsilon wave in the insert) are characteristic findings in the baseline ECG of these patients (*Source:* Nasir K, Bomma C, Tandri H, et al. Electrocardiographic features of arrythmogenic right ventricular dysplasia/ cardiomyopathy according to disease severity: a need to broaden diagnostic criteria. Circulation. 2004;110:1527-34, with permission)

Monomorphic VT Post-surgery for Congenital Heart Disease

This type of tachycardia is mechanistically akin to a scar-related reentry. Since most of these incisional scars are in the right ventricle, the morphology is likely to be an LBBB configuration and a variable axis, usually right. Associated congenital heart disease (CHD), adhesions post surgery and other factors, such as development of thorax, etc., may create a somewhat atypical QRS configuration, but endocardial mapping will localize the VT in the neighborhood of the scar. Antiarrhythmic drugs and catheter ablation (while they may be sufficient to control the VT), concomitant pulmonary hypertension or pulmonic valve regurgitation would increase the risk for SCD.

Monomorphic VT in Association with Structurally Normal Heart

VT from Right Ventricular Outflow Tract

As the name suggests, the most common location of this VT is outflow which produces a characteristic LBBB and right atrial morphology. If the breakthrough occurs on the left side, an RBBB morphology may be seen. The baseline ECG is usually normal. The process could present in the form of isolated premature ventricular complexes, repetitive MMVT, nonsustained or sustained VT. When RV outflow VT is symptomatic, palpitation, lightheadedness and presyncope are common. Antiarrhythmic drugs, such as sotalol and amiodarone, may also be effective. Considering a good long-term outcome, catheter ablation is increasingly used as a preferred form of therapy.

Idiopathic Left Ventricle VT

The electrophysiologic basis of this VT is reentry within the peripheral Purkinje system. The QRS morphology is that of right bundle and LA, but other ranges of axis are occasionally observed. The baseline ECG and LVEF as a rule are normal. Intravenous verapamil will often terminate the VT but is less effective orally. Class III antiarrhythmic agents, such as amiodarone, are effective, but, at this time, catheter ablation is the first-line treatment considering this VT is easily inducible in the laboratory.

Aortic Sinus of Valsalva, Pulmonic, Mitral Cusp VT

Monomorphic VT with right axis occasionally arises from structures outside the traditional ventricular myocardium. While they mimic the outflow VT, awareness of these loci helps to improve mapping. Catheter ablation is the usual treatment.

PVT in Association with Long QT Interval (Table 11)

Congenital Long QT Interval Syndrome

At this writing, at least 12 entities (QT-1–12) have been described here briefly.

QT-1: QT-1 is the most common form [Fig. 15 (left panel)]. The PVT is typically triggered with physical activity, emotional stress, diving and swimming. Syncope, presyncope and SCD are the most serious clinical manifestations. The surface ECG shows a broad, prolonged T-wave and a long QT interval (Fig. 15). Early onset of symptoms, syncope, excessive QT prolongation is more than or equal to 550 msec in QT-1 and QT-2, and males with QT-3 are associated with a high risk of SCD (Fig. 15). Nonselective beta-blockers, such as propranolol and nadolol, are preferred, but others have been used.

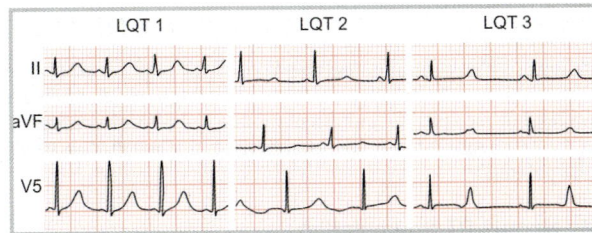

FIGURE 15: Congenital long QT (LQT). The three most common genetic varieties are shown. The corresponding chromosomes are labeled. See text for other details (*Source:* Moss AJ, Zareba W, Benhorin J, et al ECG T-wave patterns in genetically distinct forms of the hereditary long QT syndrome. Circulation. 1995;92:2929-34, with permission)

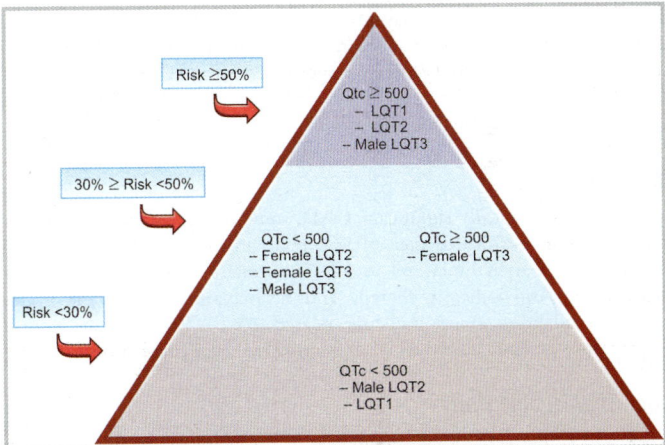

FIGURE 16: A pyramid showing risk stratification in congenital long QT (LQT) syndrome. (*Source:* Modified from Schwartz PJ, Priori SG. Long QT syndrome: genotype-phenotype correlations. In: Zipes DP, Jalife J (Eds). Cardiac Electrophysiology: From Cell to Bedside, 4th edition. Philadelphia: WB Saunders; 2004. pp. 651-9)

QT-2: QT-2 [Fig. 15 (middle panel)] is the second most common. The QT is prolonged as expected, but the T-wave is somewhat flat and less pronounced than QT-1. While adrenergic stress remains important, auditory stimuli in particular may trigger malignant arrhythmia.

QT-3: Compared to QT-1 and QT-2, QT-3 is less common but has a worse outcome. The QT-3 is prolonged [Fig. 15 (right panel)] due to increased inward Na^+ current. The ECG shows a prolonged ST segment, short T-wave and a long QT interval. Prognosis without therapy is poor, particularly in young males (Fig. 16). Risk stratification among patients with congenital long QT is shown in Figure 16.

Acquired Long QT Syndrome

Although the exact underlying etiology of acquired long QT is not understood, it is widely believed and sometimes reported that a genetic basis with low penetrance may account for some of these cases. An external trigger, such as an antiarrhythmic drug, electrolyte imbalance, etc., is required for the clinical manifestations of this form, i.e. prolongation of QT and torsades de pointes. Acute treatment is usually the administration of IV Mg^{++}, which often effectively halts torsades, but recognizing and discontinuing the offending agent is usually sufficient. Isoproterenol infusion and overdrive pacing are also used to stop the torsades de pointes.

PVT with Normal QT Prolongation

Brugada Syndrome

Brugada syndrome was initially described as the presence of an injury pattern in leads V1 and V2 with ST elevation followed by T-wave inversion and a history of syncope and SCD. Mostly seen in young males, death from PVT-VF occurs at night. The ECG abnormalities may not always be present. However, Class I agents, such as ajmaline and procainamide, can unmask the abnormality. Quinidine has been identified as a potentially effective agent to prevent SCD in this population. However, ICD remains the most reliable therapy to prevent PVT-VT related deaths in patients with Brugada syndrome.

Active Ischemia

In patients with clinically significant CAD, some degree of ischemia may exist at all times, but a critical degree of ischemia can induce a PVTVF. This is a highly malignant arrhythmia and usually fatal unless it stops spontaneously or is terminated. Anti-ischemic therapy and revascularization are the preferred treatment modalities. Acute ischemic-related PVT-VF should be addressed promptly since patients have died while waiting for revascularization.

Myocardial Hypertrophy

The VF and consequent SCD remain one of the main causes of cardiovascular death in patients with hypertrophic cardiomyopathy. Apical hypertrophy has a particularly malignant outcome. Syncope, near-syncope and nonsustained VT define a particularly high-risk population. The SCD is seen in both obstructive and nonobstructive forms. High-risk patients should be considered for ICD therapy, both for primary and for secondary prevention of SCD.

LV Noncompaction

Isolated LV noncompaction (LVNC) is a rare myopathy, primarily of autosomal inheritance. The main structural abnormality is intrauterine failure of LV muscle compaction. The main clinical manifestations are congestive heart failure and ventricular arrhythmias with around 20% incidence of SCD.

Catecholaminergic PVT

Catecholaminergic PVT (CPVT) can be a dominant or recessive inheritance, mostly manifested in childhood or young adults. The heart is structurally normal as is the baseline ECG. Adrenergic drive brings out characteristic bidirectional tachycardia or PVT. There is a high incidence of SCD (>30% mortality by age 30).

J-Wave Syndromes

This category includes several entities, where the individuals are prone to arrhythmic death. The primary defect seems to be imbalance of current during Phase 1 of the action potential producing Phase 2 reentry leading to VF. Some examples include Brugada syndrome, early repolarization, short QT syndrome and perhaps many cases of so-called idiopathic VF.

Idiopathic VF

This fascinating entity is described in greater detail by Belhassan and Viskin, and is associated with identifiable SHD. It is characterized by the occurrence of spontaneous VT with inducible PVT and VF, which respond to oral guideline both in the electrophysiology laboratory (i.e. not inducible after drug) and in the excellent clinical response seen over many years.

PVT in Association with Short QT Syndrome

This topic is somewhat new and with very limited experience and follow-up. At least five mutations have been described. The foregoing outline is a summary of VT as the subject is clinically viewed. For a comprehensive review and ACC/AHA/ESC guidelines on work-up and management of VT, the reader is referred to the most recent literature.

❏ SUGGESTED READINGS

Brugada P, Brugada J, Mont L, et al. A new approach to the differential diagnosis of a regular tachycardia with a wide QRS complex. Circulation. 1991;83:1649-59.

Brugada P, Brugada R, Brugada J. The Brugada syndrome. In: Saksena S, Camm AJ (Eds). Electrophysiological Disorders of the Heart. New York: Churchill Livingstone; 2005. pp. 697-703.

Epstein AE, DiMarco JP, Ellenbogen KA, et al. ACC/AHA/HRS 2008 Guidelines for Device-Based Therapy of Cardiac Rhythm Abnormalities: a report of the American College of Cardiology/ American Heart Association Task Force on Practice Guidelines (Writing Committee to Revise the ACC/AHA/NASPE 2002 Guideline Update for Implantation of Cardiac Pacemakers and Antiarrhythmia Devices) developed in Collaboration with the American Association for Thoracic Surgery and Society of Thoracic Surgeons. J Am Coll Cardiol. 2008;51:e1-e62.

Maron BJ, McKenna WJ, Danielson GK, et al. American College of Cardiology/European Society of Cardiology clinical expert consensus document on hypertrophic cardiomyopathy: a report of the American College of Cardiology Foundation Task Force on Clinical Expert Consensus Documents and the European Society of Cardiology Committee for Practice Guidelines. J Am Coll Cardiol. 2003;42: 1687-713.

Miller JM, Das MK, Arora R, et al. Differential diagnosis of wide QRS complex tachycardia. In: Zipes DP, Jalife J (Eds). Cardiac Electrophysiology: From Cell to Bedside, 4th edition. Philadelphia: W.B. Saunders; 2004. pp. 747-57.

Zipes DP, Camm AJ, Borggrefe M, et al. ACC/AHA/ESC 2006 Guidelines for management of patients with ventricular arrhythmias and the prevention of sudden cardiac death—executive summary: a report of the American College of Cardiology/American Heart Association Task Force and the European Society of Cardiology Committee of Practice Guidelines (Writing Committee to Develop Guidelines for Management of Patients with Ventricular Arrhythmias and the Prevention of Sudden Cardiac Death) Developed in collaboration with the European Heart Rhythm Association and the Heart Rhythm Society. Eur Heart J. 2006;27:2099-140.

3.7 Bradycardia and Heart Block

❏ INTRODUCTION

Bradycardia is generally defined as a heart rate less than 50 beats per minute. However, this simple definition is a gross oversimplification of what is a multifaceted and multifactorial issue. Bradycardia is a dichotomy of sorts, in some cases being a marker of excellent cardiovascular fitness, or conversely, a sign of cardiovascular disease, especially when it is symptomatic.

❏ BRADYCARDIA SYNDROMES/DISEASES

Iatrogenic and Noncardiac Causes

Before considering intrinsic conduction disease, in light of many patients living with multiple medical comorbidities as well as complex medical regimens being commonplace, it is of utmost importance to consider iatrogenic and noncardiac causes of bradycardia and heart block.

In terms of medications, the most common agents related to this issue are those already diagnosed for cardiovascular disease including tachycardias (Table 12). Noncardiac medications as culprits include lidocaine spray or topical, such as is used for endoscopic procedures, selective serotonin reuptake inhibitors (SSRIs), cholinesterase inhibitors (via enhancement of vagal tone) commonly used for treatment of Alzheimer's disease, and succinylcholine.

In terms of medical syndromes, potential causes include hypothyroidism, Lyme disease, endovascular cooling after cardiac arrest, and renal or hepatic disease. The latter two are more related to decreasing medication clearance and metabolism, thus increasing serum drug levels and potentiating a drug's effect. This is especially salient with digoxin and renally cleared BARBs, such as atenolol.

Familial

Development of the cardiac conduction system does not always occur in a normal fashion. When mutations occur, different syndromes may develop. One example of this (specifically related to sinus bradycardia) is familial sinus bradycardia.

Table 12: Common noncardiac and iatrogenic causes of bradycardia and heart block		
Cardiac medications	**Noncardiac medications**	**Medical disease**
BARBs (including eyedrops)	SSRIs	Lyme disease
Calcium channel blockers	Opiates	Renal/hepatic disease
Digoxin	Succinylcholine	Hypothyroidism
	Lithium	Carotid hypersensitivity
Amiodarone	Cholinesterase inhibitors (e.g. donepezil for Alzheimer's)	Renal/hepatic disease
Sotalol	Propofol	Endovascular cooling after cardiac arrest
Sodium channel blockers		
Clonidine		

Vagal Tone

Although the cardiac conduction system is primarily derived from myocardial cells and not neural crest cells (which differentiate into neural tissue), there is still a rich two-way interaction with the nervous system communication. Vasovagal reactions cause bradycardia in diverse situations and they may be triggered by psychiatric stressors like fear or sight of blood as well as volume depletion from multiple etiologies.

Interestingly, trained athletes, especially elite ones, frequently have asymptomatic bradycardia. Commonly, elite athletes may also have orthostatic hypotension. Rarely, vagally mediated bradycardia severe enough to cause presyncope or syncope may also (somewhat paradoxically) be seen in trained athletes, where high vagal tone assists in rapid post-exercise heart rate recovery, but in some cases may go too far in lowering heart rate, causing symptoms.

Cardiac Transplantation

In postcardiac transplant patients, bradycardia—specifically sinus bradycardia—occurs in approximately 18% of patients, and ultimately 4–7% require a permanent pacemaker. One of the primary risk factors for development of sinus bradycardia is ischemic time. Due to vagal and sympathetic denervation resulting from the surgical procedure, these patients have relative bradycardia and some degree of chronotropic incompetence but are somewhat shielded from bradycardia by the standard definition due to high intrinsic heart rate. The transplanted ventricle increases stroke volume to compensate for the lack of sympathetically increased heart rate with exercise; even though cardiac output may be normal at rest the transplant cannot increase HR enough to make up for the lesser heart rate with exercise. Reinnervation can occur, but the extent to which it happens varies from patient to patient.

❏ CLINICAL PRESENTATION

Depending on the patient's heart rate and robustness of so-called "back-up" pacemakers, patients may entirely be asymptomatic, symptomatic with exertion only or at rest. Common symptoms include light-headedness, dizziness, syncope, palpitations, shortness of breath at rest, dyspnea on exertion, angina, and progressive lower extremity edema.

❏ MEASUREMENT/DIAGNOSIS

The diagnosis of bradycardia, regardless of the mechanism, is primarily made by obtaining an ECG or rhythm strip from surface leads at the time of symptoms. Other times, bradycardia may be found serendipitously by an ECG or telemetry strip performed for other reasons. When a patient's symptoms suggest an arrhythmia of a low rate, occur paroxysmally, and the patient has a normal ECG or rhythm strip at presentation while asymptomatic, monitoring via a Holter may be appropriate. Another issue in diagnosing bradycardia is relative bradycardia, also known as chronotropic incompetence. This describes a scenario where at rest, the patient does not demonstrate significant symptoms, but with exertion, is unable to mount an appropriate heart rate to increase cardiac output appropriate for increased needs of exercise. Evaluation is primarily via exercise testing. In some cases, direct measurement of cardiac output is performed via right heart catheterization before, during and after temporary pacing at higher rates than baseline; if cardiac output significantly improves with a modest increase in heart rate, then chronotropic incompetence may be assumed.

❑ SINUS NODE DISEASE

Sick Sinus Syndrome

Sick sinus syndrome (SSS), in its most rudimentary sense, is defined as sinus node dysfunction, which results in an inadequate heart rate physiologically, and may include sinus bradycardia, sinus arrest, or sinus node exit block and may lead to takeover of cardiac pacemaking and atrial contraction by subsidiary intrinsic cardiac pacemaker sites. In patients with SA block and bradycardia–tachycardia syndrome, the SA node and AV node regions showed 70–80% decrease in nodal cells, infiltration of the SA node by connective tissue and left bundle branch (LBB) fibrosis.

The I(f) "funny" current has recently been found, albeit controversially, to have a significant role in spontaneous cardiac pacemaker activity. Recently, genetic factors related to this disease have been elucidated, specifically SCN5A mutation related functional loss of the sodium channel.

❑ AV NODE DISEASE

Pathology

The most common cause of permanent AV block is idiopathic bundle branch fibrosis. This may include the main AV bundle and LBB. Other etiologies include interruption of the AV node related to aortic or mitral valve calcification, myocardial infarction leading to ischemic damage to the AV node, or cardiomyopathy.

First-degree AV Block

Although a relatively common finding of a prolonged PR interval (>200 msec) on ECG, it has recently been postulated that this may precede more advanced AV block, and even itself serve as a marker of increased risk of other arrhythmic and mortality concerns.

Second-degree AV Block

Second-degree AV block is commonly divided into two varieties. Type I (Mobitz I, also "Wenckebach" second-degree AV block presents as a normal or near-normal PR interval (120–200 msec), which gradually prolongs with successive beats, until only a P wave is seen, and a "dropped" QRS occurs, which is the absence of AV conduction. After a brief reset, the next cycle begins, again with a normal PR interval, progressively lengthening again until a drop occurs. There may be the same number of beats prior to that which is dropped, or at times, variable numbers. Type I basically demonstrates AV nodal decremental conduction.

Type II (Mobitz II) second-degree AV block has dropped ventricular beats due to AV block. However, in this scenario, there is no PR lengthening, only dropped beats, which may occur after one, two or any number of normally conducted beats. An easy way to diagnose this mechanism is to evaluate the PR before and after the regular blocked P wave; if the PR after the block is not shorter by more than 20 msec then type II block must be considered. Patients with type II block also tend to have concomitant QRS prolongation.

A 2:1 AV block due to 2:1 conduction, may be type I or II, but which one is not able to be ascertained because there is no PR lengthening—or lack thereof— to be seen because block occurs after only one beat. It may be a progression from either. Anatomically, 80% of the time, 2:1 AV block occurs in the His-Purkinje system, and 20% in the AV node itself. The importance of differentiating type I versus type II AV block is that even if asymptomatic, the latter requires a permanent pacer, but in the former a permanent pacemaker is not needed unless symptoms are present.

Third-degree AV Block

Third-degree AV block is defined as a complete electrical dissociation of the atria and ventricles. The ventricular rhythm in this case, referred to as an escape rhythm, may either be a junctional, which is a normal, narrow-complex rhythm emanating more proximally to the AV node and generally faster (40–60 bpm), or ventricular where the rhythm is abnormal, wide complex and slower (<30 bpm). Rarely no escape rhythm is present whatsoever. Treatment entails eliminating or neutralizing reversible causes, such as AV nodal blockers (e.g. BARBs). If a patient has complete heart block, atropine should be given, especially if a junctional escape is present. If not effective, temporary pacing (first transcutaneous, then transvenous) is recommended. If the patient has what appears to be a permanent complete heart block, then permanent pacing is recommended.

Paroxysmal AV Block

Paroxysmal AV block has been as "a sudden," "paroxysmal pause-dependent phase 4 AV block occurring in diseased conduction system". It is essentially the change from 1:1 AV conduction, suddenly to complete heart block. There is no official definition for this type of AV block, and the prevalence may be underestimated because of this and difficulty in recording this arrhythmia. The most common risk factor is apparently right bundle branch (RBB) block. Treatment includes pacemaker implantation and removal of culprit AV nodal blocking agents if present.

❏ HEMIBLOCK

The hemiblocks are nevertheless important findings which may be intricately related to AV block. First of all, building on the concept of the right and left bundles in the His-Purkinje system, the LBB is generally found to divide into two discrete—yet somewhat interconnected— branches, the anterior and the posterior fascicles. Thus, the ventricular system, including the right bundle, is essentially trifasicular.

The left anterior fascicle, being anteriorly located, is the more vulnerable of the two LBBs. A left anterior hemiblock (LAH) (also known as a fascicular block) is defined as a leftward axis of less than −45 degrees, an "rS" pattern in II, III, aVF and with a narrow QRS complex. In the case of the latter two causes, the RBB is commonly affected concurrently, and by the nature of these progressive diseases, patients often eventually develop complete heart block. Generally, without significant coronary artery disease or infarction, the finding of isolated LAH does not appear to portend an increased risk of morbidity or mortality, although LAH is associated with risk of disease in the Framingham study.

The left posterior fascicle is supplied by both the anterior and the posterior descending coronary arteries. This dual blood supply makes it less prone to infarction and hemiblock. Left posterior hemiblock is defined as a rightward axis of greater than +100 degrees, narrow QRS and an rS in I and aVL. A pure left posterior fascicular block is rare, but tends to be found coexisting with a RBB block.

The concept of trifasicular block is uncommon and concomitant first-degree AVB, which is usually in the AVN. Patients with LAH and RBB block frequently have no symptoms or VT inducible. Differentiation from trifasicular block is usually easy (lack of symptoms) but exercise testing or EPS may be necessary, if a certain diagnosis is necessary.

❑ BUNDLE BRANCH BLOCK

The concept of the existence of the LBB and RBB coming off of the His was first published by Eppinger and Rothberger in 1909.

Left Bundle Branch Block

Left bundle branch (LBB) block is defined grossly as a QRS duration greater than or equal to 120 msec with left axis deviation. The most common cause is a left ventricular hypertrophy and/or enlargement (with associated increased weight of the heart), primarily due to hypertension or aortic valve disease. Other etiologies include myocardial infarction, electrolyte abnormalities, and fibrosis (Lev's and Lenegre's disease). A salient issue with LBB block is in myocardial infarction. It may be the presenting ECG finding for MI. If an old finding, it may hinder interpretation of the ECG in the setting of suspected acute coronary syndrome.

Right Bundle Branch Block

Right bundle branch (RBB) block is grossly defined as a QRS duration greater than or equal to 120 msec with right axis deviation, and commonly an RSR pattern in lead V1. Common causes or association with RBB block include pulmonary embolism (acute or chronic), pulmonary hypertension, left-sided heart failure causing RV volume or pressure overload, severe MR, pulmonic valve stenosis.

❑ TREATMENT

Treatment of bradycardia and heart block is primarily initiated if there are symptoms, such as syncope, lightheadedness, chest pain, shortness of breath and/or evidence of hemodynamic compromise or low cardiac output. Obviously, if offending agents should be discontinued, if possible. However, if this does not result in improvement, or drug therapy is needed for an indication, such as a tachyarrhythmia, then permanent pacing should be considered.

If cessation of an agent does not result in improvement, the next step would be pharmacologic therapy, such as atropine. There are special circumstances, such as BARB toxicity or digoxin toxicity where an antidote of sorts is available, such as glucagon or Digibind, respectively. For more acutely decompensated patients, beta-agonists, such as isoproterenol, may be required until pacing may be initiated. Beyond pharmacologic measures are the electromechanical therapies. External pacing is considered, but is only of benefit in a very short period of time due to the unpredictable transcutaneous capture and is poorly tolerated by the patient unless sedated, which itself may perpetuate bradycardia. Temporary pacing is indicated if the above noted therapies are unhelpful and the patient requires more time for conservative measures (holding medications, pharmacologic therapy) to work,

SUGGESTED READINGS

Baruscotti M, Robinson RB. Electrophysiology and pacemaker function of the developing sinoatrial node. Am J Physiol Heart Circ Physiol. 2007;293:H2613-23.

Cheng S, Keyes MJ, Larson MG, et al. Long-term outcomes in individuals with prolonged pr interval or first-degree atrioventricular block. JAMA. 2009;301:2571-7.

DiBiase A, Tse TM, Schnittger I, et al. Frequency and mechanism of bradycardia in cardiac transplant recipients and need for pacemakers. Am J Cardiol. 1991;67:1385-9.

Mark AL. The Bezold-Jarisch reflex revisited: clinical implications of inhibitory reflexes originating in the heart. J Am Coll Cardiol. 1983;1:90-102.

Miyamoto Y, Curtiss El, Kormos RL, et al. Bradyarrhythmias after heart transplantation. Incidence, time, course, and outcome. Circulation. 1990;82:IV313-7.

3.8 Arrhythmogenic Right Ventricular Dysplasia/Cardiomyopathy

INTRODUCTION

Arrhythmogenic right ventricular dysplasia/cardiomyopathy (ARVD/C) is a disease characterized histopathologically by progressive fibrofatty replacement of the myocardium, primarily of the right ventricle (RV). Affected individuals typically present between the second and the fourth decades of life with monomorphic ventricular tachycardia (VT) originating from the RV. ARVD/C can be the cause of sudden death in all stages of the disease but particularly in adolescence. From autopsy studies, it is known that fibrofatty tissue can replace major parts of normal myocardium in teenagers. Sudden death may occur in the early concealed phase of the disease.

MOLECULAR AND GENETIC BACKGROUND

Desmosome Structure and Function

The cellular adhesion junctions in the intercalated disk are vital for the structural and functional integrity of cardiac myocytes. Intercalated disks are located between cardiomyocytes at their longitudinal ends and contain three different kinds of intercellular connections: (i) desmosomes, (ii) adherens junctions, and (iii) gap junctions.

Desmosomes are important for cell-to-cell adhesion and are predominantly found in tissues that experience mechanical stress—the heart and the epidermis. They couple cytoskeletal elements to the plasma membrane. Figure 17 schematically represents the organization of the various proteins in the cardiac desmosome.

Cardiomyocytes are individually bordered by a lipid bilayer, which gives a high degree of electrical insulation. The electrical current that forms the impulse for mechanic contraction travels from one cell to the other via gap junctions. Gap junctions provide electrical coupling by enabling ion transfer between cells. The

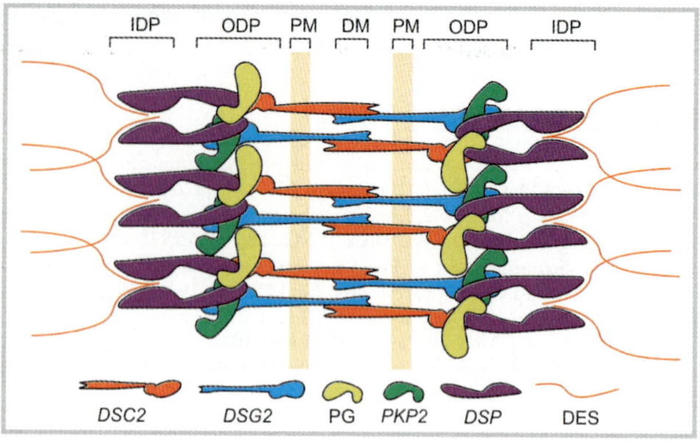

FIGURE 17: Schematic representation of the molecular organization of cardiac desmosomes. The plasma membrane (PM) spanning proteins desmocollin-2 (DSC2) and desmoglein-2 (DSG2) interact in the extracellular space at the dense midline (DM). At the cytoplasmic side, they interact with plakoglobin (PG) and plakophilin-2 (PKP2) at the outer dense plaque (ODP). The PKP2 and PG also interact with desmoplakin (DSP). At the inner dense plaque (IDP), the C-terminus of DSP anchors the intermediate filament desmin (DES) (*Source:* Modified from: Van Tintelen et al. Curr Opin Cardiol. 2007;22:185-92)

number, size and distribution of gap junctions all influence impulse propagation in cardiac muscle.

The intercalated disk is an intercellular structure, where desmosomes and adherens junctions not only provide mechanical strength but also protect the interspersed gap junctions, enabling electrical coupling between cells.

Desmosomal Dysfunction and ARVD/C Pathophysiology

It is not well known how mutations of desmosomal protein genes are related to the ARVD/C phenotype. Several mechanisms have been proposed. First, alterations in desmosomal proteins are thought to lead to mechanical uncoupling of myocytes at the intercalated disks, particularly under mechanical stress (e.g. exercise, sports activities, etc.). Mechanical uncoupling will be followed by (i) electrical uncoupling due to dysfunction of gap junctions and (ii) cell death with fibrofatty replacement.

Both electrical uncoupling and interconnecting bundles of surviving myocardium embedded in the fibrofatty tissue lead to lengthening of conduction pathways and load mismatch. This results in marked activation delay and conduction block that are pivotal mechanisms for reentry and thereby VT. Secondly, recent studies have shown that impairment of cell-to-cell adhesion due to changes in desmosomal components may affect the amount and distribution of other intercalated disk proteins, including connexin 43, the major protein forming gap junctions in the ventricular myocardium.

The third hypothesis involves the canonical Wnt/b-catenin signaling pathway. Plakoglobin can localize both to the plasma membrane and the nucleus. It was demonstrated that disruption of desmoplakin frees plakoglobin from the plasma membrane allowing it to translocate to the nucleus and suppress canonical Wnt/b-catenin signaling. Wnt signaling can inhibit adipogenesis by preventing mesodermal precursors from differentiating into adipocytes. Suppression of Wnt signaling by plakoglobin nuclear localization could, therefore, promote the differentiation to adipose tissue in the cardiac myocardium in patients with ARVD/C.

Autosomal Recessive Disease

In Naxos disease, affected individuals were found to be homozygous for a 2-base pair deletion in the *JUP* gene. All patients who are homozygous for this mutation have diffuse palmoplantar keratosis and woolly hair in infancy. Children usually have no cardiac symptoms but may have electrocardiographic abnormalities and nonsustained ventricular arrhythmias. A different autosomal recessive disease, Carvajal syndrome, is associated with a desmoplakin gene mutation. It manifests by woolly hair, epidermolytic palmoplantar keratoderma and cardiomyopathy..

Autosomal Dominant Disease

Mutations in the gene encoding the intracellular desmosomal component desmoplakin can cause "classic ARVD/C" with a clinical presentation of VT, sudden death as well as LV involvement as the disease progresses. Desmoplakin gene mutations have also been associated with predominantly left-sided ARVD/C and, as noted above, with autosomal recessive disease. Mutations in the *PKP2* gene as the most frequently observed genetic abnormality.

Other Nondesmosomal Genes

Mutations in the cardiac ryanodine receptor *RyR2*, which is responsible for calcium release from the sarcoplasmic reticulum, have been described in only one Italian ARVD/C family. Affected patients have exercise-induced polymorphic VT. Mutations in *RyR2* have primarily been associated with familial catecholaminergic polymorphic VT without ARVD/C. Although the general opinion is that *RyR2* mutations lead to catecholaminergic polymorphic VT without structural abnormalities, the mutations in ARVD/C have been advocated to act differently from those in familial polymorphic VT without ARVD/C.

❏ CLINICAL PRESENTATION

ARVD/C patients typically present between the second and the fourth decade of life with monomorphic VT originating from RV. However, in a minority of patients, sudden death, frequently at a young age, or RV failure are the first signs. Four different disease phases have been described for the classical form of ARVD/C, i.e. primarily affecting the RV (Table 13):
1. Early ARVD/C is often described as "concealed" owing to the frequent absence of clinical findings, although minor ventricular arrhythmias and subtle structural changes may be found.

Table 13: Different phases of disease severity	
Phase	**Characteristics**
1. Concealed	Asymptomatic patients with possibly only minor ventricular arrhythmia and subtle structural changes
2. Overt	Symptoms due to LBBB VT or multiple premature complexes, with more obvious structural RV abnormalities
3. RV failure	With relatively preserved LV function
4. Biventricular	Significant overt LV involvement

2. The overt phase follows, in which patients suffer from palpitations, syncope and ventricular arrhythmias of left bundle branch block (LBBB) morphology, ranging from isolated ventricular premature complexes to sustained VT and ventricular fibrillation (VF).
3. The third phase is characterized by RV failure due to progressive loss of myocardium with severe dilatation and systolic dysfunction in the presence of preserved LV function.
4. Biventricular failure occurs due to LV involvement at a later stage. This phase may mimic dilated cardiomyopathy (DCM) and may require cardiac transplantation.

❑ CLINICAL DIAGNOSIS

Diagnosis of ARVD/C can be very challenging. Although VF and sudden death may be the first manifestations of ARVD/C, symptomatic patients typically present with sustained VT with LBBB morphology, thus originating from the RV. The occurrence of VT episodes is usually induced by adrenergic stimuli mainly during exercise, especially competitive sports. The ARVD/C is a disease that shows progression over time. In clinical practice, diagnosis based on cardiac pathology is not practical. Endomyocardial biopsies have major limitations. Tissue sampling from the affected, often thin RV free wall is associated with a slight risk of perforation. Sampling from the interventricular septum is relatively safe. However, the septum is histopathogically rarely affected in ARVD/C. In addition, histology may be classified as normal due to the focal nature of the lesions.

Clinical diagnosis has been facilitated by a set of clinically applicable criteria for ARVD/C diagnosis defined by a Task Force based on consensus in 1994, and modified in 2010. The Task Force criteria included six different categories. They are derived into (i) global and regional dysfunction and structural alterations, (ii) tissue characterization, (iii) depolarization abnormalities, (iv) repolarization abnormalities, (v) arrhythmias, and (vi) family history, including pathogenic mutations.

Detailed history and family history, physical examination, 12-lead ECG, signal averaged ECG (SAECG), 24-hours Holter monitoring, exercise testing, and 2D echocardiography with quantitative wall motion analysis. When appropriate, detailed analysis of the RV can be done by cardiac magnetic resonance imaging (MRI). Invasive tests are also useful for diagnostic purposes.

Global and/or Regional Dysfunction and Structural Alterations

Evaluation of RV size and function can be done by various imaging modalities, including echocardiography, cardiac MRI, computed tomography and/or cineangiography. With RV cineangiography the finding of only regional akinesia, dyskinesia or aneurysm is considered sufficient for qualification as a major criterion. Cardiac MRI has the unique ability to characterize tissue composition, by differentiating fat from fibrous tissue.

Endomyocardial Biopsy

For reasons previously noted, undirected endomyocardial biopsies are infrequently diagnostic. However, it had been included as a major criterion by the Task Force. Diagnostic values according to the new Task Force criteria are considered major if histomorphometric analysis of endomyocardial biopsies shows that the number of residual myocytes is below 60% or below 50% by estimation, with fibrous replacement of the RV free wall in at least one sample, with or without fatty tissue replacement. If the number of residual myocytes is higher but still below 75% (morphometric) or below 65% (estimated), only a minor criterion is fulfilled.

ECG Criteria

Consistent with early electrical uncoupling, ECG changes and arrhythmias may develop before histologic evidence of myocyte loss or clinical evidence. ECG criteria on depolarization and repolarization have to be obtained during sinus rhythm and while off antiarrhythmic drugs.

Depolarization Abnormalities

The RV activation delay is a hallmark of ARVD/C. This delay is reflected by the presence of an epsilon wave, prolonged terminal activation duration (TAD) in the terminal part and after the QRS complex, and also by recording of late potentials on SAECG. Epsilon waves are defined as low amplitude potentials after and clearly separated from the QRS complex, in at least one of precordial leads, V1-V3. This highly specific major criterion is observed in only a small minority of patients.

Repolarization Abnormalities

In the new Task Force criteria, negative T waves in leads V1, V2 and V3 form a major ECG criterion in the absence of complete RBBB, and only if the patient is older than 14 years of age. Studies have reported variable prevalences of right precordial T wave inversion, ranging from 19 to 94%.
In the new Task Force criteria, two minor repolarization criteria were included:
1. Inverted T waves only in leads V1-V2 or in V4-V6 in individuals older than 14 years of age and in the absence of complete RBBB.
2. Inverted T waves in leads V1-V4 in individuals older than 14 years of age in the presence of RBBB. This was included since T wave inversion in RBBB seldom extends to V4 in otherwise healthy individuals.

Arrhythmias

In ARVD/C, ventricular arrhythmias range from premature ventricular complexes to sustained VT and VF, leading to cardiac arrest. Due to their typical origin in the RV, QRS complexes of ventricular arrhythmias show a LBBB morphology. Moreover, the QRS axis indicates the VT origin, i.e. superior axis from the RV inferior wall or apex (major criterion) and inferior axis (minor criterion) from the RV outflow tract (RVOT).

❏ NONCLASSICAL ARVD/C SUBTYPES

A variety of nonclassical ARVD/C subtypes have been identified and include:
1. Naxos disease.
2. Carvajal syndrome.
3. Left dominant arvd/c (ldac).

❏ MOLECULAR GENETIC ANALYSIS

It is important to realize that the clinical diagnosis of ARVD/C is based exclusively on fulfillment of the diagnostic Task Force criteria.

The strategy for genetic testing in ARVD/C is as follows:

Individuals with clinical diagnosis of ARVD/C are the first to be tested. The detection of a pathogenic mutation does not make a clinical diagnosis of ARVD/C. In contrast, if no mutation can be identified in a patient diagnosed with ARVD/C, the clinical diagnosis of ARVD/C is still applicable. If a pathogenic mutation is identified in the proband, parents, siblings and children of this patient can be tested for the mutation via the cascade method. When an (asymptomatic) relative is found to carry a pathogenic mutation, periodic cardiologic screening is required.

❏ PROGNOSIS AND THERAPY

The prognosis of classical ARVD/C is considerably better than that of patients with sustained VT from left ventricular structural heart disease. However, ARVD/C is a progressive disease and may lead to RV and also LV failure or sudden cardiac death. The death rate for patients with ARVD/C has been estimated at 2.5% per year. Electrophysiologic induction of VT with LBBB morphology and superior axis is a major diagnostic criterion. However, electrophysiologic studies have not proven to be useful in risk stratifying patients with ARVD/C.

Therapeutic options in patients with ARVD/C include antiarrhythmic drugs, catheter ablation and ICD. Patients with VT have a favorable outcome when they are treated medically and therefore pharmacologic treatment is the first choice. Since ventricular arrhythmias and cardiac arrest occur frequently during or after physical exercise or may be triggered by catecholamines, antiadrenergic β-blockers are recommended. Sotalol is the drug of first choice. Catheter ablation is an alternative in patients who are refractory to drug treatment and have frequent VT episodes with a predominantly single morphology. Although antiarrhythmic drugs and catheter ablation may reduce VT burden, there is no proof from prospective trials that these therapies will also prevent sudden death.

❏ SUMMARY

Arrhythmogenic right ventricular dysplasia cardiomyopathy is most often a genetically determined disease characterized by fibrofatty replacement of myocardial tissue. Primarily affecting the RV, but extension to the LV occurs, especially in more advanced stages of the disease. At the molecular level, both ventricles are affected, presumably in all stages of the disease. Its prevalence has been estimated to vary from 1:2000 to 1:5000. Patients typically present between the second and the fourth decade of life with exercises-induced tachycardia episodes originating from the RV. It is also a major cause of sudden death in the young and athletes.

❏ SUGGESTED READINGS

Basso C, Thiene G, Corrado D, et al. Arrhythmogenic right ventricular cardiomyopathy: dysplasia, dystrophy, or myocarditis? Circulation. 1996;94:983-91.

Corrado D, Basso C, Thiene G, et al. Spectrum of clinicopathologic manifestations of arrhythmogenic right ventricular cardiomyopathy/ dysplasia: a multicenter study. J Am Coll Cardiol. 1997;30:1512-20.

Marcus FI, McKenna WJ, Sherrill D, et al. Diagnosis of arrhythmogenic right ventricular cardiomyopathy/dysplasia: proposed modification of the task force criteria. Circulation. 2010;121:1533- 41, Eur Heart J. 2010;31:801-14.

McKenna WJ, Thiene G, Nava A, et al. Diagnosis of arrhythmogenic right ventricular dysplasia/cardiomyopathy. Task Force of the Working Group Myocardial and Pericardial Disease of the

European Society of Cardiology and of the Scientific Council on Cardiomyopathies of the International Society and Federation of Cardiology. Br Heart J. 1994;71:215-8.

Richardson P, McKenna W, Bristow M, et al. Report of the 1995 World Health Organization/International Society and Federation of Cardiology Task Force on the Definition and Classification of cardiomyopathies. Circulation. 1996;93:841-2.

Sen-Chowdhry S, Prasad SK, Syrris P, et al. Cardiovascular magnetic resonance in arrhythmogenic right ventricular cardiomyopathy revisited: comparison with task force criteria and genotype. J Am Coll Cardiol. 2006;48:2132-40.

Tandri H, Calkins H, Nasir K, et al. Magnetic resonance imaging findings in patients meeting task force criteria for arrhythmogenic right ventricular dysplasia. J Cardiovasc Electrophysiol. 2003;14:476-82.

3.9 Long QT, Short QT, and Brugada Syndromes

❑ INTRODUCTION

Over the past two decades, ample information has been accumulated on cellular mechanisms and genetics of arrhythmias in structurally normal heart. The basic pathogenic mechanism for these arrhythmias may involve hereditary disturbances in ionic currents at the cellular level while the heart remains grossly normal. The high rate of sudden death (especially in the young) due to congenital arrhythmias, coupled with the potential availability of preventive measures, mandate the need for higher awareness of the medical community of these potentially lethal arrhythmia syndromes.

❑ LQT SYNDROME

Jervell and Lange-Nielsen, in 1957, firstly described the congenital LQT syndrome. Jervell and Lange-Nielsen syndrome, is inherited in an autosomal recessive pattern. In 1995 and 1996, the first three genes associated with the most common forms of the LQT syndromes (types 1–3) were identified. Since then, the scientific and medical community has witnessed discovery of hundreds of variants in nearly a dozen genes associated with a wide variety of LQT or related arrhythmia syndromes.

Clinical Manifestations

The congenital LQT syndrome is a common identifiable cause of sudden death in the presence of structurally normal heart. The natural history of LQT syndrome is highly variable. The majority of patients may be entirely asymptomatic with the only abnormality being QT prolongation in the ECG. Some gene variant carriers of LQT syndromes may not even display the prolonged QT interval (silent carriers). Symptomatic patients typically present in the first two decades of life, including the neonatal period, with recurrent attacks of syncope precipitated by torsade de pointes type of ventricular arrhythmias.

Pathogenesis

As the QT interval represents a combination of action potential (AP) depolarization and repolarization, variations in QT interval may arise from the dysfunction of ion channel, responsible for the timely execution of the cardiac AP. A decrease in the outward repolarizing currents (mainly potassium currents) or an increase in the inward depolarizing currents (mainly sodium and calcium) may increase action potential duration (APD) and QT prolongation. The increases in APD result in lengthening of effective refractory period (ERP) that in turn predisposes to the occurrence of early afterdepolarizations (EADs), due to enhancement of the sodium–calcium exchanger (NCX) current and reactivation of the L-type calcium channels. These EADs are known to support ventricular arrhythmias.

Diagnosis

The typical case of LQTS, characterized by syncope or cardiac arrest associated with QT prolongation on ECG is fairly straightforward to diagnose. However, borderline cases may be more complex and pose a diagnostic challenge to the practicing clinician. Schwartz et al. devised a diagnostic criteria based on a scoring system first in 1985 and then, updated in 1993. Based on this scoring system, a score of one or less indicates low probability for LQTS; 2–3 denotes intermediate probability and higher than 3.5 indicates high probability for LQTS. If a patient receives a score of 2–3, serial ECG and 24-hour Holter monitoring may be obtained as the QT interval may vary from time to time. Short-term variability of QT interval has recently been demonstrated to correlate with high risk LQT syndrome.

Genetic Testing

The diagnostic criteria based on ECG and clinical history were primarily devised before the human genome project era and and QT interval (silent carriers). In select cases, genetic testing and molecular diagnostic methods may complement the ECG and clinical criteria; allowing for screening of proband family members to detect silent variant carriers that may predispose individuals to potential events. Identifying gene variants that promote arrhythmia susceptibility (either congenital or acquired) may provide important information to a physician in their clinical practice (i.e. avoiding QT prolonging drugs in patients harboring specific channel variants). It is important to note that current genetic testing for arrhythmias may harbor its own drawbacks. For example, false-negative results may occur when the patient has a variant in a gene not covered in the testing panel (the relevant gene or gene variant may not have even been discovered!). Moreover, the significance of a positive test result may often be difficult to ascertain.

Therapy

As the risk of cardiac events in LQTS is genotype, age and gender dependent, therapy should be carefully tailored to the individual patients according to their risk factors. According to a recently published study from the International LQTS Registry, beta-blocker therapy, significantly, reduces the risk of cardiac events in LQT1 and LQT2 patients. In contrast, beta-blockers may offer limited efficacy among LQT3 patients; as they display further QT prolongation at slower heart rates. Higher risk patients, such as LQT1 males and LQT2 females gain more benefit from beta-blocker therapy compared to lower risk subsets. Despite the significant risk reduction with beta-blocker therapy, high risk patients experienced considerable residual event rates.

ICD Therapy

Current guidelines recommend ICD therapy as a class IIa indication for primary prevention of cardiac events in LQTS patients who experience syncope or ventricular tachycardias during beta-blocker therapy. These guidelines provide a class IIb recommendation for ICD therapy in patients with risk factors for SCD, irrespective of medical therapy.

Left Cardiac Sympathetic Denervation

The left cardiac sympathetic denervation (LCSD) techniques use extrapleural approach and obviate the need for thoracotomy. LCSD may be considered in patients with recurrent syncope despite beta-blockade, and in patients, who experience arrhythmia storms with ICD therapy.

Genotype-specific Therapy

As cardiac events may be clustered around exercise or emotional stress in LQT1 patients, these individuals may be advised to avoid competitive sports and/or stressful situations. Beta blockers remain the mainstay of therapy in LQT1 syndrome.

In patients with LQT2, maintaining adequate serum potassium level is essential, as IKr activity may vary with serum potassium levels. Since arousal from sleep, especially with a sudden noise may be a triggering a risk factor in LQT2 patients, the use of alarm clock or telephone in the patient's bedroom should also be carefully considered.

Sodium-channel blockers have been proposed for gene-specific treatments in LQT3, which is associated with variants in the sodium channel gene (*SCN5A*). Early clinical studies demonstrated efficacy of mexiletine or flecainide in shortening of repolarization period and QT interval. Indeed, ACC/AHA 2006 guidelines for management of patients with ventricular arrhythmias and the prevention of sudden cardiac death recommended sodium-channel blockers for treatment of LQT3 patients as a class IIb indication.

SQT SYNDROME

SQT syndrome is a rare channelopathy associated with increased risk of atrial and ventricular arrhythmias. To date, the number of identified patients with SQT syndrome is low. However, with increasing awareness, the prevalence is expected to rise.

Clinical Manifestations

The clinical manifestations of SQT syndrome include propensity to AF, syncope and sudden death. In most reported cases, the QTc was less than 320 ms and often less than 340 ms. Therefore, it is prudent to suspect SQT syndrome in patients with a QT interval of less than 340 ms and personal and/or family history of lone AF, ventricular fibrillation, syncope, or sudden cardiac death.

Diagnosis

The precise cutoff point for QT interval in SQT syndrome is still somewhat debated. Currently, based on several reports, the upper limit of QT interval suggestive of SQT syndrome is considered 320–340 ms. However, the mere presence of SQT interval does not necessarily appear to be sufficient to make the diagnosis.

In addition patients may display a peculiar ECG morphology. Affected patients often demonstrate absent ST segment with the T-wave attached to the S-wave. A second finding, that is seen in at least about half of the patients, is a tall, peaked, narrow-based T-waves in the right precordial leads. Another distinctive ECG feature is the relatively prolonged T_{peak}-T_{end} interval which may indicate enhanced transmural dispersion of repolarization.

Therapy

Drugs that block outward potassium current and prolong repolarization seem attractive and have been tested in a limited number of cases. The class Ia antiarrhythmic agents, quinidine, and disopyramide have been demonstrated to prolong QT interval and ventricular ERP and reduce inducibility of ventricular arrhythmias. The high incidence of fatal cardiac events associated with SQT suggests the use of ICD therapy, early on, in the management of the symptomatic patients.

❑ BRUGADA SYNDROME

In 1992, Brugada and Brugada described a hereditary arrhythmia syndrome characterized by ST segment elevation in the right precordial leads, right bundle branch block and increased vulnerability to ventricular tachycardias and sudden death in the absence of any structural heart disease. Timely identification of symptomatic Brugada syndrome patients is important, as implantable cardioverter defibrillators (ICD) may be lifesaving in these individuals.

Clinical Manifestations

Brugada syndrome is characterized by the occurrence of polymorphic ventricular tachycardias in patients with the ECG patterns of a peculiar ST-segment elevation in right precordial leads and right bundle branch block (RBBB). An increased propensity to atrial fibrillation and supraventricular arrhythmias has also been reported. Patients with Brugada syndrome have structurally normal hearts; and are typically, otherwise healthy and active. Notwithstanding, recent research suggests that with the use of high resolution magnetic resonance imaging, subclinical structural abnormalities in right ventricle may be identified.

Diagnosis

Electrocardiographic signs of Brugada syndrome are classified into three types as follows:
- Type I: Coved ST-segment elevation greater than 2 mm followed by negative T-wave in greater than 1 mm right precordial lead (V1–V3)
- Type 2: Saddleback ST-segment elevation with a high takeoff ST-segment elevation of greater than 2 mm, a trough displaying greater than 1 mm ST-elevation followed by a positive or biphasic T-wave

- Type 3: Saddleback or coved appearance of ST-elevation less than 1 mm, present in greater than 1 mm right precordial lead (V1–V3).

Brugada syndrome is diagnosed on the basis of a spontaneous or drug-induced type 1 (coved-type), ST-segment elevation in the right precordial leads plus one of the following:
- Documented VF or polymorphic VT
- Unexplained syncope
- Nocturnal agonal respiration
- Inducibility of VT/VF with programmed electrical stimulation
- A family history of SCD at a young age (<45 years) or a coved-type ECG pattern.

Prognosis, Risk Stratification, and Therapy

The second consensus conference report on Brugada syndrome recommended electrophysiology studies (EPS) as a valuable tool in risk stratifying asymptomatic patients with spontaneous type 1 ECG pattern or with drug induced type 1 ECG pattern plus positive family history of SCD. Subsequent studies, however, have questioned the role of EPS in risk stratification of asymptomatic patients. Recently, the investigators of the FINGER Brugada syndrome registry demonstrated the following results:
- The risk of arrhythmic events is low in asymptomatic patients (0.5% event rate per year)
- The presence of symptoms and a spontaneous type 1 ECG are the only independent predictors of arrhythmic events
- Genders, family history of SCD, inducibility of ventricular tachyarrhythmias during EPS, and presence of a variant in the *SCN5A* gene, have no predictive value.

Recommendations to implant ICD at the present time may be limited to symptomatic patients with type 1 ECG pattern. To date, no pharmacologic intervention has been approved for the treatment of Brugada syndrome.

❏ SUGGESTED READINGS

Antzelevitch C, et al. Brugada syndrome: report of the second consensus conference: endorsed by the Heart Rhythm Society and the European Heart Rhythm Association. Circulation. 2005;111:659-70.

Epstein AE, et al. ACC/AHA/HRS 2008 Guidelines for Device- Based Therapy of Cardiac Rhythm Abnormalities: a report of the American College of Cardiology/American Heart Association Task Force on Practice Guidelines (Writing Committee to Revise the ACC/AHA/NASPE 2002 Guideline Update for Implantation of Cardiac Pacemakers and Antiarrhythmia Devices): developed in collaboration with the American Association for Thoracic Surgery and Society of Thoracic Surgeons. Circulation. 2008;117:e350-408.

Moss AJ, Schwartz PJ. Sudden death and the idiopathic long Q-T syndrome. Am J Med. 1979;66:6-7.

Patel U, Pavri BB. Short QT syndrome: a review. Cardiol Rev. 2009;17:300-3.

Schwartz PJ, et al. Diagnostic criteria for the long QT syndrome. An update. Circulation. 1993;88:782-4.

Schwartz PJ, Periti M, Malliani A. The long Q-T syndrome. Am Heart J. 1975;89:378-90.

Zipes DP, et al. Guidelines for management of patients with ventricular arrhythmias and the prevention of sudden cardiac death. Executive summary. Rev Esp Cardiol. 2006;59:1328.

3.10 Cardiac Resynchronization Therapy

❑ INTRODUCTION

Despite major advances in the treatment of systolic heart failure (HF), it continues to enact a large burden on healthcare systems around the world. Advances in pharmacological therapy, most notably the use of beta-blockers, ACE inhibitors, angiotensin receptor blockers, and aldosterone antagonists have reduced mortality in this population. The complexity of acute HF management has increased considerably over the past decades. In addition to an ever-expanding armamentarium of HF medications, device-based therapies have become more sophisticated with each generation. Thus, the need for clinicians who are well versed in all the aspects of HF management has never been greater.

❑ CRT: RATIONALE FOR USE

The contractile apparatus of the human heart is influenced by a myriad of factors, including the highly coordinated electrical activation of the atria and ventricles. Disruption to this activation pattern can impede ventricular performance. In advanced HF, it is common to see abnormal electrical conduction which promotes asynchronous activation of the ventricles, reduced cardiac output, and in the long-term, adverse ventricular remodeling. The term mechanical dyssynchrony has been used to describe the loss of synchronized contraction both between and within the right and left ventricles. This phenomenon, is usually but not always, the result of disorganized electrical activation.

❑ CRT IN PRACTICE

The CRT typically involves placing pacing leads in the right atrium, right ventricle and a branch of the coronary sinus (CS). The CRT implantation is performed using a transvenous approach whereby the CS is cannulated and a pacing lead is advanced into a lateral CS branch. The CS lead is also known as the LV lead, as it activates LV myocardium. Optimal lead placement is the subject of ongoing research and is dependent on many factors, including scar location and the regional mechanics of an individual's ventricle. To date, CRT has demonstrated a number of beneficial effects in patients with advanced systolic HF. Several studies have demonstrated its impact on physiologic endpoints such as improved hemodynamics, reduction in MR, increased ejection fraction, increased blood pressure and reverse remodeling. Table 14 illustrates the results of randomized clinical trials of CRT in patients with advanced HF. The following section will detail the results of three landmark trials involving CRT.

❑ SUMMARY OF CRT BENEFIT

Many trials have provided robust evidence that CRT has a favorable impact on many important physiologic and nonphysiologic end-points in HF. In addition, there is evidence that CRT alone (without back-up defibrillator) reduces mortality. There is some uncertainty about whether CRT coupled to ICD therapy confers additional mortality benefit. However, due to the wide range of benefits associated with CRT, it is reasonable to combine CRT and ICD therapy in patients who meet criteria for both. In accordance with this, the most recent ACC/AHA/HRS guidelines recommend CRT (with or without ICD) in patients who have left ventricular ejection fraction (LVEF) less than 35%, QRS duration more than 120 millisecond, and NHYA III or IV on optimal medical therapy.

Table 14: Randomized clinical trials of cardiac resynchronization therapy

Study	Design	No. of patients	Mean follow-up (months)	Results	P value
MUSTIC (NEJM 2001)	Crossover CRT vs no CRT in patients with CHF NYHA III, EF <35%, QRS >150 ms, LVEDD >60 mm, NSR	58	6	Improved 6 MWT QOL Hospitalization Peak VO_2	<0.001 <0.001 <0.05 <0.03
MIRACLE (NEJM 2002)	Parallel arms CRT vs no CRT in patients with CHF NYHA III, EF <35%, QRS >130 ms, LVEDD >55 mm, 6 MWT <450 m, NSR	453	6	Improved 6 MWT NYHA class QOL LVEF Peak VO_2	= 0.005 <0.001 = 0.001 <0.001 = 0.009
PATH-CHF (JACC 2002)	Crossover CRT (LV or BiV) vs no CRT in patients with CHF NYHA III-IV, EF <35%, QRS >120 ms, PR >150 ms, NSR	41	12	Improved 6 MWT Peak VO_2 QOL NYHA class LV and BiV had similar improvement	= 0.03 = 0.002 = 0.062 <0.001
MIRACLE ICD (JAMA 2003)	Parallel arms CRT + ICD vs CRT in patients with CHF NYHA III, EF <35%, QRS >130 ms, LVEDD >55 mm, cardiac arrest due to VT/VF, spontaneous VT or inducible VT/VF, NSR	369	6	Improved NYHA class QOL No change 6 MWT	= 0.007 = 0.02 = 0.36
CONTAK CD (JACC 2003)	Crossover, parallel controlled CRT vs no CRT in patients undergoing ICD implantation with CHF NYHA II-IV, EF <35%, QRS >120 ms, NSR, indications for ICD implantation	490	6	Improved 6 MWT Peak VO_2, LVEF LV volumes No significant change NYHA class QOL HF progression	= 0.043 = 0.030 <0.001 = 0.02 = 0.10 = 0.40 = 0.35
PATH-CHF II (JACC 2003)	Crossover CRT (LV only) vs no CRT in patients with CHF NYHA II-IV, EF <30%, QRS >120 ms, NSR, Peak VO_2 <18 ml/min/kg	86	6	Improved 6 MWT QOL Peak VO_2 No benefit in QRS 120–150 ms	= 0.021 = 0.015 <0.001

Contd...

Contd...

Table 14: Randomized clinical trials of cardiac resynchronization therapy

Study	Design	No. of patients	Mean follow-up (months)	Results	P value
COMPANION (NEJM 2004)	Parallel arms Optimal pharmacological therapy (OPT) vs CRT vs CRT + ICD (CRT-D) in patients with CHF NYHA III-IV, EF ≤ 35%, QRS > 120 ms	1520	16	Death or hospitalization for CHF reduced by 34% in CRT, 40% in CRT-D as compared to OPT All cause mortality reduced by 36% in CRT-D 24% in CRT	<0.002 <0.001 = 0.003 = 0.05
CARE-HF (NEJM 2005)	Open label, randomized Medical therapy vs Medical therapy + CRT in patients with CHF NYHA III-IV, EF ≤35%, QRS >120 ms with dyssynchrony (aortic pre-ejection > 140 ms, interventricular mechanical delay >40 ms, delayed activation of postlateral LV) QRS >150 ms (no dyssynchrony evidence needed)	814	Stopped early by DSMB 29.4	All cause mortality/hospitalization reduction by 37% in CRT All cause mortality reduced by 36% in CRT Improvement in QOL LVEF LVESV NYHA class	<0.001 <0.002 <0.01

(Abbreviations: 6 MWT: 6-Minute walking test; AF: Atrial fibrillation; CARE-HF: Cardiac resynchronization-heart failure study group; CHF: Congestive heart failure; CONTAK-CD: CONTAK-Cardiac defibrillator; COMPANION: Comparison of medical therapy, resynchronization, and defibrillation therapies in heart failure study group; CRT: Cardiac resynchronization therapy; DSMB: Data safety monitoring board; EF: Ejection fraction; ICD: Implantable cardioverter-defibrillator; JACC: Journal of American College of Cardiology; JAMA: Journal of American Medical Association; LVEDD: LV end diastolic diameter; LVESV: LV end systolic volume; MIRACLE: Multicenter insync randomized clinical evaluation trial; MUSTIC: Multisite stimulation in cardiomyopathies study group; NEJM: New England Journal of Medicine; NSR: Normal sinus rhythm; NYHA: New York Heart Association; QOL: Quality of life; PACE: Pacing and clinical electrophysiology; PATH-CHF: Pacing therapies in heart failure study group; VT: Ventricular tachycardia; VF: Ventricular fibrillation)

❑ PREDICTION OF RESPONSE TO CRT THERAPY

Response to CRT is dependant on the endpoint evaluated. When a clinical endpoint, such as NHYA classification, is used to determine response to CRT, there appears to be a consistent 20–30% nonresponder rate. However, when more objective measures, such as echocardiographic parameters, are employed, nonresponder rates may be closer to 40%. It remains unknown whether this discrepancy is related to the placebo effect from device implantation or for some other reason. An illustration of a step-by-step approach to CRT nonresponders is given in Flowchart 9.

FLOWCHART 9: Stepwise algorithm for management of heart failure patients who are nonresponders to CRT

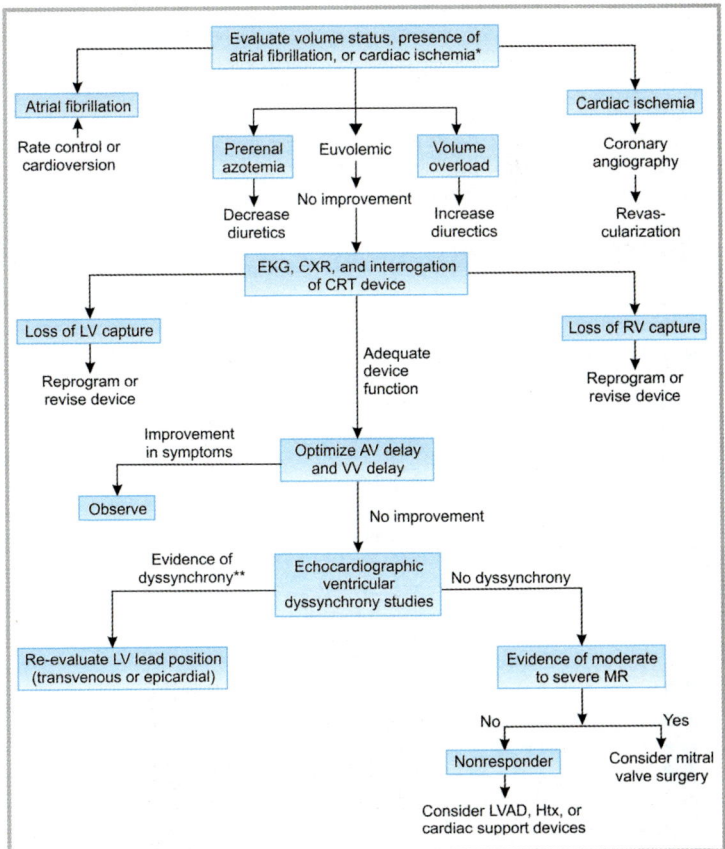

(Abbreviations: AV: Atrioventricular; CXR: Chest X-ray; EKG: Electrocardiogram; Htx: Heart transplant; LV: Left ventricular; LVAD: Left ventricular assist device; MR: Mitral regurgitation; RV: Right ventricular; VV: Interventricular). *Cardiac ischemia is evaluated in patients with ischemic cardiomyopathy. **Evidence of dyssynchrony includes septal to posterior wall motion delay ≥130 ms, intraventricular mechanical delay ≥40 ms and tissue Doppler imaging ≥65 ms. (*Source:* Modified from Aranda, et al, Management of heart failure after cardiac resynchronization therapy: integrating advanced heart failure treatment with optimal device function. J Am Coll Cardiol. 2005;46:2193-8)

❑ ROLE OF DYSSYNCHRONY IMAGING

Cardiac dyssynchrony can occur with respect to atrioventricular (A-V) VV delay (RV-LV) or LV. In general, patients with LV dyssynchrony are more likely to response to CRT. While QRS duration is a reasonable marker of VV (RV-LV) dyssynchrony; it does not predict LV dyssynchrony (as assessed by echocardiogram) with great accuracy. There have been a number of dyssynchrony criteria that have been shown to predict response to CRT. A complete review of dyssynchrony parameters is beyond the scope of this paper.

❑ DYSSYNCHRONY SUMMARY

Despite extensive research and the multitude of imaging modalities established to assess myocardial dyssynchrony, its role in CRT remains uncertain. No single dyssynchrony parameter has been shown to conclusively predict response to CRT. While many of the above techniques appear promising, conclusive large-scale trials will need to be performed before dyssynchrony assessment can be incorporated into routine clinical practice. Accordingly, neither the ACC/AHA/HRS guidelines for device-based therapy of cardiac rhythm abnormalities nor the ACC/AHA guidelines for the diagnosis and management of HF recommend the use of dyssynchrony imaging to establish candidacy for CRT

❑ CRT COMPLICATIONS

As with any implantable device there are a myriad of potential complications associated with CRT. In addition to standard device complications, such as infection and bleeding, there are several complications specific to CRT, including CS dissection and perforation, phrenic nerve stimulation and LV lead dislodgement. In major trials, LV lead dislodgement occurred in 4–6% of the patients. The CS sinus dissection or perforation ranged from 0.3 to 4% and 0.8 to 2%, respectively. Management for CS dissection or perforation is usually conservative and, in most instances, CS cannulation can safely be performed several weeks later.

❑ EMERGING CRT INDICATIONS

Though the benefits of CRT are well demonstrated in established conditions, a variety of new indications have emerged and are summarized in Table 15.

❑ SUMMARY

The advent of CRT has been an important development in the management of HF. The results of multiple large-scale clinical trials have consistently demonstrated its favorable impact on symptoms related to HF. In addition, there is mounting evidence that CRT is associated with mortality benefit. Current indications for CRT include patients with wide QRS and ejection fraction less than or equal to

Table 15: Emerging CRT indications

- Narrow QRS duration
- Atrial fibrillation
- Pacemaker dependant patients
- Minimally symptomatic heart failure
- CRT for acute decompensated heart failure

35% with advanced HF despite optimal medical management. Around 30–40% of the patients who are candidates for CRT do not respond. This can be improved by optimizing the device, using imaging to select patients based on dyssynchrony and optimal LV lead placement. In the future, indications for BIV implantation may expand to include select patients with systolic HF and narrow QRS and patients with normal ejection fraction who require chronic RV pacing.

MODIFIED SUMMARY OF GUIDELINES (ACC/AHA/HRS GUIDELINES FOR DEVICE-BASED THERAPY, JACC. 2008;51:E1-62)

Modified by Kanu Chatterjee

Class I: Conditions for which there is evidence and/or general agreement that a given procedure/therapy is useful and effective.

Class II: Conditions for which there is conflicting evidence and/or a divergence of opinion about the usefulness/efficacy of performing the procedure/therapy.

Class IIa: Weight of evidence/opinion is in favor of usefulness/efficacy.

Class IIb: Usefulness/efficacy is less well established by evidence/opinion.

Class III: Conditions for which there is evidence and/or general agreement that a procedure/therapy is not useful/effective and in some cases may be harmful.

Level A (highest): Derived from multiple randomized clinical trials.

Level B (intermediate): Data are on the basis of a limited number of randomized trials, nonrandomized studies or observational registries.

Level C (lowest): Primary basis for the recommendation was expert opinion.

Recommendations for Permanent Pacing in Sinus Node Dysfunction (SND)

Class I:
1. Permanent pacemaker implantation is indicated in symptomatic patients with symptomatic bradycardia including frequent symptomatic sinus pauses (Level of Evidence C).
2. Permanent pacemaker implantation is indicated for symptomatic chronotropic incompetence (Level of Evidence C).

Class IIa:
1. Permanent pacemaker implantation is reasonable for SND with heart rate less than 40/bpm, when a clear association between symptoms consistent with bradycardia and actual presence of bradycardia has not been documented (Level of Evidence C).
2. Permanent pacemaker implantation is reasonable in patients with unexplained syncope when SND is documented by electrophysiologic studies (Level of Evidence C).

Class IIb:
1. Permanent pacemaker therapy is reasonable in minimally symptomatic patients with chronic awake heart rate of less than 40/bpm (Level of Evidence C).

Recommendations for Acquired Atrioventricular Block in Adults

Class I:
1. Permanent pacemaker therapy is indicated in patients with third-degree and advanced second-degree AV block even in absence of symptoms (Level of Evidence C).
2. Permanent pacemaker therapy is indicated in patients with third-degree or advanced second-degree AV block in asymptomatic patients with documented period of asystole of 3 seconds or greater (Level of Evidence C).

3. Permanent pacemaker implantation is indicated in patients with third-degree or advanced second-degree AV block developing after AV nodal ablation (Level of Evidence C).
4. Permanent pacemaker therapy is indicated in postcardiac surgery AV block when AV block is unlikely to resolve (Level of Evidence C).
5. Permanent pacemaker treatment is indicated in patients with neuromuscular diseases (e.g. Duchane's and Baker's, limb girdle, peroneal muscular dystrophy) with third-degree or advanced second-degree AV block with or without symptoms (Level of Evidence B).
6. Permanent pacemaker therapy is indicated in symptomatic patients with any type of second degree AV block (Level of Evidence B).
7. Permanent pacemaker therapy is indicated in patients with systolic heart failure with third-degree or infranodal AV block in absence of symptoms related to heart block (Level of Evidence B).
8. Permanent pacemaker implantation is indicated in patients who develop second or third-degree AV block during exercise unrelated to myocardial ischemia (Level of Evidence C).

Class IIa:
1. Permanent pacemaker therapy is reasonable in asymptomatic patients with third-degree, or intra or infra Hisian AV block (Level of Evidence C).
2. Symptom limited exercise test at 3 to 6 weeks after discharge to assess prognosis, activity prescription or evaluation of medical therapy if early exercise test was submaximal.

Recommendations for Permanent Pacing in Chronic Bifascicular Block

Class I:
1. Permanent pacemaker therapy is indicated in patients with bifascicular block with advanced second-degree, intermittent third-degree or alternating bundle-branch block (Level of Evidence B).

Class IIa:
1. Permanent pacemaker implantation is reasonable in patients with bifascicular block with history of syncope when other causes have been excluded (Level of Evidence B).
2. Permanent pacemaker implantation is reasonable in patients with bifascicular block if HV interval is 100 ms or greater documented during electrophysiologic study (Level of Evidence B).

Recommendations for Permanent Pacing after the Acute Phase of Myocardial Infarction

Class I:
1. Permanent pacemaker therapy is indicated in post-ST elevation myocardial infarction with intermittent or persistent third-degree, advanced second-degree infranodal AV block or alternating bundle-branch block (Level of Evidence B).
2. Permanent pacemaker therapy is indicated in symptomatic second-degree or third-degree AV block (Level of Evidence C).

Recommendations for Permanent Pacing in Hypersensitive Carotid Sinus Syndrome and Neurocardiogenic Syncope

Class I:
1. Permanent pacemaker implantation is indicated in patients with recurrent syncope due to hypersensitive carotid sinus syndrome with ventricular asystole of 3 seconds or longer (Level of Evidence C).

Class IIa:
1. Permanent pacing is reasonable in patient with hypersensitive carotid sinus syndrome with cardioinhibitory response of 3 seconds or longer without provocative events (Level of Evidence C).

Class IIb:
1. In patients with neurocardiogenic syncope permanent pacemaker therapy may be considered associated cardioinhibitory response occurring spontaneously or during tilt-table test (Level of Evidence B).

Recommendations for Pacing After Cardiac Transplantation

1. Permanent pacemaker implantation is indicated for inappropriate heart rate response and for Class I indications as in nontransplant patients (Level of Evidence C).

Class IIb:
1. Permanent pacemaker therapy can be considered in postcardiac transplant patients with recurrent prolonged bradycardia or inappropriate heart rate response that limits rehabilitation (Level of Evidence C).

Recommendations for Pacing to Prevent Tachycardia

Class I:
1. Permanent pacemaker implantation is indicated for sustained pause-dependent ventricular tachycardia with or without QT prolongation (Level of Evidence C).

Class IIa:
1. Permanent pacemaker implantation is reasonable in high-risk patients with congenital Long QT syndrome (Level of Evidence B).

Class IIb:
1. Permanent pacing may be considered in patients with brady–tachy syndrome with recurrent atrial fibrillation (Level of Evidence B).
2. After discharge for activity counseling and/or exercise training as part of cardiac rehabilitation in patients who have undergone revascularization

Class IIb:
1. In patients with ECG abnormalities of LBBB, preexcitation syndrome, left ventricular hypertrophy, digoxin therapy, greater than 1 mm resting ST depression. Electronically paced ventricular rhythm.
2. Periodic monitoring in patients who continue to participate in exercise training or cardiac rehabilitation.

Class III:
1. Severe comorbidity likely to limit life expectancy and/or candidacy for revascularization.
2. To evaluate patients with acute myocardial infarction with uncompensated heart failure, cardiac arrythmia or noncardiac conditions that limit the ability to exercise (Level of Evidence C).
3. Predischarge exercise test in patients who had already cardiac catheterization (Level of Evidence C).

Asymptomatic Diabetic Patients

Class IIa:
1. Evaluation of asymptomatic patients with diabetes who plan to do vigorous exercise (Level of Evidence C).

Class IIb:
1. Evaluation of patients with multiple risk factors as guide to risk-reduction therapy.

2. Evaluation of asymptomatic men older than 45 years or women older than 55 years who plan to do vigorous exercise or who are involved in an occupation in which exercise impairment may impact public safety or who are at high-risk for CAD.

Class III:
1. Routine screening of asymptomatic men or women.

Patients With Valvular Heart Disease

Class I:
1. In patients with chronic aortic regurgitation for assessment of symptoms and functional capacity in whom it is difficult assess symptoms.

Class IIa:
1. In patients with chronic aortic regurgitation for evaluation of symptoms and functional capacity before participation in athletic activity.
2. In patients with chronic aortic regurgitation for assessment of prognosis before aortic valve replacement in asymptomatic or minimally symptomatic patients with left ventricular dysfunction.

Class IIb:
1. Evaluation of patients with valvular heart disease (see guide lines in valvular heart disease).

Class III:
1. For diagnosis of CAD in patients with moderate to severe valvular heart disease or with LBBB, electronically paced rhythm, preexcitation syndrome or greater than 1 mm ST depression in the rest ECG.

Patients With Rhythm Disorders

Class I:
1. For identification of appropriate settings in patients with rate-adaptive pacemakers.
2. For evaluation of congenital complete heart block in patients considering increased physical activity or participation in competitive sports (Level of Evidence C).

Class IIa:
1. Evaluation of patients with known or suspected exercise-induced arrhythmias.
2. Evaluation medical, surgical, or ablation therapy in patients with exercise-induced arrhythmias (including atrial fibrillation).

Class IIb:
1. Investigation of isolated ventricular ectopic beats in middle aged patients without other evidence of CAD.
2. For investigation of prolonged first-degree atrioventricular block or type I second degree Wenckebach, left bundle-branch block, right bundle-branch block or isolated ectopic beats in young persons considering participation in competitive sports (Level of Evidence C).

Class III:
1. Routine investigations of isolated ectopic beats in young patients.

❑ SUGGESTED READINGS

Auricchio A, Stellbrink C, Block M, et al. Effect of pacing chamber and atrioventricular delay on acute systolic function of paced patients with congestive heart failure. The pacing therapies for congestive heart failure study group. The guidant congestive heart failure research group. Circulation. 1999;99:2993-3001.

Epstein AE, Dimarco JP, Ellenbogen KA, et al. ACC/AHA/HRS 2008 guidelines for device-based therapy of cardiac rhythm abnormalities. J Am Coll Cardiol. 2008;51:e1-62.

Hjalmarson A, Goldstein S, Fagerberg B, et al. Effects of controlledrelease metoprolol on total mortality, hospitalizations and well-being in patients with heart failure: the Metoprolol CR/XL Randomized Intervention Trial in congestive heart failure (MERIT-HF). MERITHF Study Group. JAMA. 2000;283:1295-302.

Jessup M, Abraham WT, Casey DE, et al. Focused update: ACCF/ AHA guidelines for the diagnosis and management of heart failure in adults. J Am Coll Cardiol. 2009;119:1977-2016.

Lloyd-Jones D, Adams RJ, Brown TM, et al. Heart disease and stroke statistics 2010 update: a report from the American Heart Association. Circulation. 2010;121:e46-215.

3.11 Ambulatory Electrocardiographic Monitoring

❏ INTRODUCTION

Ambulatory electrocardiographic (AECG) monitoring, the recording of the electrocardiogram (ECG) over an extended period of time using a portable or implantable recording device, enables the clinician to study dynamic electrocardiographic changes during real-life activities. It is considered to be the cornerstone in the evaluation of patients with suspected cardiac arrhythmias. Currently available monitoring modalities include continuous or Holter monitors, external event (postevent and loop) recorders, implantable loop recorders (ILRs), and mobile cardiac outpatient telemetry (MCOT) (Fig. 18 and Table 16).

❏ HOLTER MONITORING

Ambulatory Holter monitoring is accomplished with portable battery-operated devices that continuously record multiple electrocardiographic channels, typically over a 24–48 hours period.. Holter monitors generally record two to three ECG leads. Although devices that allow for the recording of up to 12 ECG leads are

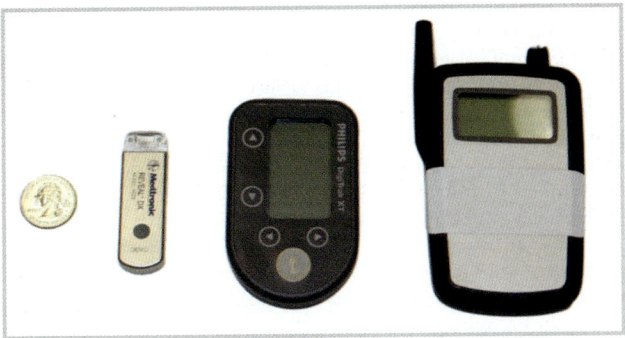

FIGURE 18: Examples of current monitoring devices are pictured next to a quarter, shown as a reference for size. From left to right: an implantable loop recorder; a Holter monitor and an event monitor. This model of the event monitor may also be used as mobile cardiac outpatient telemetry when programmed as such

Table 16: Characteristics of monitoring modalities

	Recording type	Monitoring period	Event activation	Transmission	Data analysis
Holter monitor	Continuous, full disclosure	Typically 24–48 hours	Manual	Typically none	Delayed
Loop recorder	Intermittent pre- and post-event	Typically up to 30 days	Manual and automatic	Dial-in trans-telephonic	Delayed
Event recorder	Intermittent post-event		Manual	Dial-in trans-telephonic	Delayed
ILR	Intermittent	Up to 3 years	Manual and automatic	Dial-in trans-telephonic or wireless	Delayed
MCOT	Continuous, full disclosure	Individualized, up to 30 days	Manual and automatic	Automatic and dial-in wireless	Immediate

(Abbreviations: ILR: Implantable loop recorder; MCOT: Mobile cardiac outpatient telemetry)

currently available, the clinical advantage of multichannel recordings is not well determined. Manually activated events are marked with time-stamps, which are linked to patient diaries in an attempt to correlate symptoms with an arrhythmia. Holter monitoring is generally utilized to detect a cause for symptoms and to diagnose rhythm disturbances that are expected to occur within a 24–48-hour monitoring period (Table 17). The major advantage of this modality is the continuous nature of the recording that provides "full disclosure" of the ECG during the monitoring period. This type of information is particularly useful for assessment of ventricular rate response in patients with atrial fibrillation or quantification of arrhythmia burden in patients with frequent ectopy.

Although an effective diagnostic modality in patients with daily symptoms, the diagnostic yield of a Holter monitor is likely to be low, as in the case of infrequent episodes of syncope or palpitations. Depending on patient selection and the length of monitoring, the likelihood of documenting cardiac rhythm during syncope is usually less than 20%; most of the captured events correlate with the absence of significant arrhythmia.

In addition to its diagnostic indications, Holter monitoring may be useful as a screening tool in identifying patients at increased risk for sudden death. The presence of asymptomatic non-sustained ventricular tachycardia may aid in risk stratification in patients with hypertrophic cardiomyopathy or ischemic heart disease and impaired left systolic ventricular function. Transient QT interval prolongation and macroscopic T wave alternans are recognized markers of risk for life-threatening ventricular arrhythmias in patients with long QT syndrome. While possible to ascertain from high quality Holter monitor recordings, the clinical utility of heart rate variability, SAECG, heart rate turbulence, microscopic T wave alternans and other complex methods of analyzing continuous ECG recordings remains controversial.

Detection of myocardial ischemia based upon variations in ST segments is another potential application of Holter monitoring. The ST segment changes on Holter recordings have been associated with adverse outcomes in patients with coronary artery disease in some series but not in others.

❏ EVENT RECORDERS

Similar to Holter monitors, event recorders are used to correlate symptoms to arrhythmias but over longer periods of time, usually up to one month. Unlike continuous monitors, these devices have limited memory capacity and are capable of storing only short intervals of ECG recordings related to manually or automatically activated events and, therefore, do not provide "full disclosure" data.

Event recorders are differentiated mainly by the presence or absence of the memory loop recording capability which allows for the storage of ECG recording immediately preceding a triggered event. A loop recorder continuously stores in internal loop memory several minutes of the most recent ECG by overwriting earlier data. Non-looping" or post-event monitors do not have internal loop memory and record ECG only prospectively following manual activation by the patient. These small handheld or wrist worn monitors that have "built-in" electrodes are applied directly to the skin for recording.

Event recorders are useful in the diagnosis of symptoms (such as palpitations, syncope or presyncope) suspected to be directly caused by an arrhythmia that occur at least monthly (Table 17). Extended surveillance with event recorders provides higher diagnostic yield than conventional short-term Holter monitoring and allows symptom-ECG correlation in up to twothirds of patients with frequent palpitations. Similarly, loop recorders have been shown to be superior to Holter monitors in the evaluation of patients with frequent syncope.

Table 17: Selection of monitoring modalities for common clinical indications

	Holter monitor	Event monitor		Implantable loop recorder	Mobile cardiac outpatient telemetry
		Looping	Non-looping		
Syncope					
≥1 episode/week	+				+
≥1 episode/month		+*			+
<1 episode/month				+	
Palpitations					
≥1 episode/week	+		+		+
≥1 episode/month		+	+		+
<1 episode/month			+	+	
Risk assessment (HCM, CAD, LQTS)	+		+*		
Atrial fibrillation					
Burden	+				+
Rate control	+	+*#			+
AAD monitoring	+*			+	

* With auto-trigger capability
# With an automatic atrial fibrillation algorithm
(Abbreviations: AAD: Antiarrhythmic drug; MCOT: Mobile cardiac outpatient telemetry; HCM: Hypertrophic cardiomyopathy; CAD: Coronary artery disease; LQTS: Long QT syndrome)

❏ MOBILE CARDIAC OUTPATIENT TELEMETRY

More recently, MCOT has been introduced into clinical practice. The devices used for MCOT are similar in size to conventional loop recorders and are capable of transmitting ECG data wirelessly, either directly or via a portable data manager (an external cellular telephone-sized device). Some providers use the same recorder which can be programmed either as a loop or MCOT monitor (Fig. 18). Potential advantages of MCOT over other modalities include continuous live ECG monitoring with automatic arrhythmia recognition and real-time ECG transmission to a central location that operates 24 hours a day and provides immediate notification of the ordering physician and patient about significant events based on prespecified notification criteria in addition to daily summary reports.

Initial experience suggests that MCOT may offer an improved diagnostic yield in patients with symptoms concerning for arrhythmia and may also potentially be useful for outpatient initiation of antiarrhythmic medications, thereby, obviating the need for hospitalization. Although there are potential advantages to this real-time approach to monitoring, more data are needed to define its role in the management of arrhythmia patients. The MCOT is a technologically and operationally demanding modality and, therefore, is substantially more expensive than conventional event recorders.

❏ IMPLANTABLE LOOP RECORDERS

Implantable loop recorders (ILRs) have extended diagnostic capabilities not afforded by external loop recorders and are generally indicated in patients with infrequent symptoms suspicious for cardiac arrhythmia. These small leadless devices are implanted subcutaneously, usually in the left pectoral area, and provide up to three years of continuous monitoring. They record a single bipolar ECG lead from a pair of electrodes embedded into the shell of the device. Despite relatively closely spaced electrodes, P waves and QRS complexes are generally visible. These devices have limited memory capacity (42–48 minutes of compressed ECG signals) and store only short intervals (seconds to minutes) of both patient and automatically activated ECG recordings based on prespecified parameters. Stored data can be retrieved either manually during interrogation with a standard pacemaker programmer or remotely over the phone.

The longer periods of monitoring afforded by ILRs compared to external loop recorders allow for better correlation of events with arrhythmias in patients with rare but serious symptoms. The reported diagnostic yield in symptom-ECG correlation is 30–88% depending on studied population of patients. Some data suggest that selected patients with unexplained syncopal events clinically suspicious for arrhythmia may benefit from relatively early utilization of these devices before embarking on the conventional diagnostic, particularly invasive, techniques provided that cardiac conditions associated with high risk of life-threatening arrhythmia are carefully excluded.

The ILRs play a relatively limited role in the evaluation of patients with palpitations as compared to syncope. Palpitations usually are a less severe symptom and are more likely to be diagnosed with external recorders or electrophysiologic testing. Some observational data suggest that ILRs may be useful in guiding pacemaker therapy in patients with severe and frequent episodes of neurocardiogenic syncope caused by significant bradycardia.

Disadvantages of ILRs exist. The major issue remains inappropriate detection of arrhythmia episodes secondary to either undersensing, most commonly due to loss of electrode contact within the device pocket or oversensing due to "noise". This may compromise automatic arrhythmia detection either by undersensing of tachyarrhythmia episodes or by saturation of the device memory with inappropriately sensed ECG recordings and thereby precluding storage of true arrhythmia episodes. An ILR is the most expensive of all available monitoring modalities and requires surgical implantation with inherent risk of pocket complications.

(AAA/AHA GUIDELINES FOR AMBULATORY ELECTROCARDIOGRAPHY: EXECUTIVE SUMMARY AND RECOMMENDATIONS, CIRCULATION. 1999;100:886-93) MODIFIED SUMMARY OF GUIDELINES

Modified by Kanu Chatterjee

Class I: Conditions for which there is evidence and/or general agreement that a given procedure/therapy is useful and effective

Class II: Conditions for which there is conflicting evidence and/or a divergence of opinion about the usefulness/efficacy of performing the procedure/therapy

Class IIa: Weight of evidence/opinion is in favor of usefulness/efficacy

Class IIb: Usefulness/efficacy is less well established by evidence/opinion

Class III: Conditions for which there is evidence and/ or general agreement that a procedure/therapy is not useful/effective and in some cases may be harmful

Level A (highest): Derived from multiple randomized clinical trials

Level B (intermediate): Data are on the basis of a limited number of randomized trials, nonrandomized studies or observational registries

Level C (lowest): Primary basis for the recommendation was expert opinion

Indications for Ambulatory Electrocardiography (AECG) to Assess Symptoms Possibly Related to Rhythmic Disturbances

Class I:
1. Patients with unexplained syncope, presyncope or episodic dizziness
2. Patients with unexplained recurrent palpitation

Class IIb:
1. Patients with unexplained episodic shortness of breath, chest pain, or fatigue
2. Patients with neurological events when transient atrial fibrillation or flutter is suspected
3. Patients with persistent symptoms after non-arrhythmogenic cause of syncope, presyncope dizziness or palpitation have been detected and treated

Class III:
1. Patients with symptoms of syncope, presyncope episodic dizziness or palpitation in whom other causes have been established
2. Patients with cerebrovascular accidents without other evidence of arrhythmia

Indications for AECG Arrhythmia Detection to Assess Risk for Future Cardiac Events in Patients without Symptoms from Arrhythmia

Class I: None

Class IIb:
1. Post-MI patients with LV systolic dysfunction (ejection fraction of 40% or less)

2. Patients with congestive heart failure
3. Patients with idiopathic hypertrophic cardiomyopathy

Class III:
1. Patients who have sustained myocardial contusion
2. Systemic hypertensive patients with LV hypertrophy
3. Post-MI patients with normal LV function
4. Preoperative arrhythmia evaluation of patients for noncardiac surgery
5. Patients with sleep apnea
6. Patients with valvular heart disease

Indications for measurement of Heart Rate Variability (HRV) to Assess Risk for Future Cardiac Events in Patients without Symptoms from Arrhythmia

Class I: None

Class IIb:
1. Post-MI patients with LV dysfunction
2. Patients with congestive heart failure
3. Patients with idiopathic hypertrophic cardiomyopathy

Class III:
1. Post-MI patients with normal LV function
2. Diabetic subjects to evaluate for diabetic neuropathy
3. Patients with rhythmic disturbances that preclude HRV analysis (i.e. atrial fibrillation)

Indications for AECG to Assess Antiarrhythmic Therapy

Class I: To assess antiarrhythmic drug response if required

Class IIa: To detect proarrhythmic response in patients at high risk

Class IIb:
1. To assess rate control during atrial fibrillation
2. To document recurrent or asymptomatic nonsustained arrhythmias in outpatients

Indications for AECG to Assess Pacemaker and ICD Function

Class 1:
1. In patients with frequent palpitation, syncope, or presyncope to assess device malfunction
2. To assess the response to adjunctive pharmacotherapy

Class IIb:
1. Evaluation of device function immediately after implantation
2. Evaluation of the rate of supraventricular arrhythmias

Class III:
1. Assessment of device malfunction when its diagnosis has been already established
2. For routine follow-up in asymptomatic patients

Indications for AECG for Ischemia Monitoring

Class IIa: Patients with suspected variant angina

Class IIb:
1. Evaluation of patients with chest pain who cannot exercise
2. Preoperative evaluation for vascular surgery who cannot exercise
3. Patients with known CAD and atypical chest pain syndrome

Class III:
1. Initial evaluation of patients with chest pain who are able to exercise
2. Routine screening of asymptomatic subjects

❏ SUGGESTED READINGS

Crawford MH, Bernstein SJ, Deedwania PC, et al. ACC/AHA Guidelines for Ambulatory Electrocardiography. A report of the American College of Cardiology/American Heart Association Task Force on Practice Guidelines (Committee to Revise the Guidelines for Ambulatory Electrocardiography). Developed in collaboration with the North American Society for Pacing and Electrophysiology. J Am Coll Cardiol. 1999;34:912-48.

Gibson TC, Heitzman MR. Diagnostic efficacy of 24-hour electrocardiographic monitoring for syncope. Am J Cardiol. 1984;53:1013-7.

Solano A, Menozzi C, Maggi R, et al. Incidence, diagnostic yield and safety of the implantable loop-recorder to detect the mechanism of syncope in patients with and without structural heart disease. Eur Heart J. 2004;25:1116-9.

3.12 Cardiac Arrest and Resuscitation

❏ INTRODUCTION

Cardiopulmonary resuscitation (CPR) guidelines are continuously changing as new evidence and techniques are developed and researched. Despite these advances, overall survival from sudden cardiac arrest remains low. The return of spontaneous circulation (ROSC) is directly related to adequate coronary perfusion, while good clinical outcomes are more closely related to adequate vital organ perfusion during and immediately after resuscitation.

Cardiopulmonary resuscitation is a relatively new concept. The idea of artificial blood flow with artificial respirations as a means to restore life, after what appears to be death, was not a concept that came easily. In the 1700s mouth-to- mouth resuscitation was recommended for drowning victims. Since then the AHA has established the standards of care for CPR. The AHA re-evaluates its recommendations and updates the guidelines as new information and research become available.

Cardiopulmonary Arrest

Sudden cardiac arrest is still a major public health problem and a leading cause of death in the United States. The epidemiologic definition of "sudden" is usually defined by less than 1 hour from onset of symptoms to terminal clinical event which could include death, loss of detectable pulse or cessation of breathing. This definition does not take into account unwitnessed events. The World Health Organization has included in its definition of "sudden" unwitnessed deaths that occur less than 24 hours prior to discovery of the victim. "Death" is defined as an absolute irreversible event; this is a biologic, legal and literal definition. "Cardiac arrest" can be reversible and is defined as the cessation of pump function. If the patient is unable to be resuscitated or resuscitation is not performed then the event becomes irreversible and is considered sudden cardiac death. Cardiovascular collapse is defined as loss of effective blood flow either due to cardiac dysfunction or loss of vascular function.

Based on research AHA change its recommendations for the 2010 guidelines to compression only CPR for witnessed out of hospital cardiac arrest victims. Two main conclusions can be currently drawn from these studies: (i) first and foremost

Table 18: Components needed for EMS system operation	
Regulation and policy	Legislation, regulations, and operational policies and procedures
Resource management	Lead agency identifies, categorizes, and coordinates resources
Human resources and training	Trained persons to perform required tasks
Transportation	Reliable and safe ambulances
Facilities	Proper and accessible with known hospital capabilities
Communication	Communication system for resource allocation
Trauma system	Predetermined for timely access
Public information and education	Public awareness/education for proper utilization of resources
Medical direction	Physician directed protocols and oversight
Evaluation	Provide improvement and implementation of new medical knowledge

CPR needs to be performed as quickly as possible and (ii) quality compressions with minimal interruption need to occur.

Emergency Medical Services

The credit for developing the first EMS system seems to go to Napoleon's Surgeon-in-Chief, Barron Jean Larrey. He noted that wounded soldiers were left unattended until the fighting ceased, after which rescue teams would enter the battlefield and care for the wounded. It has been a long way since then in ensuring that the citizens receive prompt emergency medical care. The basic components of an EMS system are described in Table 18.

❏ BASIC LIFE SUPPORT

Basic life support is the first step and the foundation for saving lives from sudden cardiac arrest. It involves immediate recognition, activation of emergency response system, performing high-quality CPR and rapid defibrillation when appropriate. The BLS also involves basic trauma and other medical techniques that have not been covered in this chapter.

Role of Bystanders

The role of bystanders in sudden cardiac arrest is extremely important in the "chain of survival". Bystanders can perform 3 of the 4 links in the chain of survival and greatly impact a victim's chance of survival with good neurologic outcome. Bystanders are important for recognition and EMS activation, perform immediate CPR and apply and use an AED for defibrillation. The new 2010 AHA guidelines for BLS emphasize immediate chest compressions without delay for rescue breathing and application of an AED as soon as it is available.

Emergency Medical Services Activation

Immediate activation of EMS is extremely important for the survival of sudden cardiac arrest victims. In many communities the time interval for EMS arrival is 7–8 minutes. This means that for the first several minutes the chances of survival for the victim is in the hands of bystanders. The sooner EMS can arrive at the scene the sooner victims can receive ACLS and postresuscitative care. The BLS algorithm has been simplified: immediate activation of the emergency response system and initiate chest compressions for any unresponsive adult victim who is not breathing normally. Lay rescuers should not attempt to check for a pulse as even trained healthcare providers often incorrectly assess the presence or absence of a pulse especially if blood pressure is extremely low.

Compression only Cardiopulmonary Resuscitation

Changing chest compression ratios, emphasizing more compressions and less ventilation was a controversial topic at the 2005 International Consensus Conference on Resuscitation and a major change to the AHA 2005 guidelines for CPR. During the time between 2005 and 2010 the AHA has been studying ways to simplify CPR and increase its use by laypersons due to the fact that survival rates of out of hospital cardiac arrest remain low. Compression only CPR for most adults for out of hospital cardiac arrest has been shown to achieve similar outcomes to those who receive standard CPR with rescue breathing. Thus, bystanders are encouraged and directed by dispatch to perform compression only CPR until the arrival of EMS. Starting the procedure with compressions only eliminates the step that most laypersons have difficulty with opening the airway and giving rescue breaths. However, children rarely arrest from a primary cardiac cause and thus for the pediatric cardiac arrest victim, rescue breathing may be much more important. Pediatric cardiac resuscitation has not been covered in this chapter.

Chest Compressions or Airway Management

The newest change to the AHA guidelines for CPR will be changing from "A-B-C" (airway, breathing, circulation) to "C-A-B" (chest compressions, airway, breathing). When a collapse is witnessed by a lone rescuer the AHA now advises to confirm unresponsiveness, activate the emergency response system and then begin chest compressions with a rate of 100 per minute for adults with a depth of at least 2 inches, allowing complete recoil of the chest after each compression. Proper hand position is two fingerbreadths above the xiphoid-sternal notch. For the lay person it is easier to understand "center of the chest between the nipples". The first compression cycle should be 30 compressions in length. Early application of an AED or defibrillator should be done as soon as another rescuer is available. Ventilations should be given with 2 breaths after 30 compressions with minimal interruption of compressions. Once a "shockable" rhythm is identified and a defibrillator or AED has been applied a shock should be delivered. After the shock is delivered CPR should be started immediately without checking for a pulse or rhythm. After 2 minutes of CPR there should be a pause for a rhythm and pulse check.

Mechanical Devices for Cardiopulmonary Resuscitation

Mechanical devices for adult CPR have been developed for several reasons. It is possible that mechanical devices may perform CPR better than standard CPR. Mechanical devices are also useful for long transports to prevent rescuer fatigue. The longer a rescuer performs CPR, the more the quality decreases as the rescuer becomes tired. Decreased quality of chest compressions with time is however well recognized. It is recommended that rescuers performing CPR change often during the resuscitation and if a long transport is to occur a mechanical device should be considered to be used to prevent rescuer fatigue as well as free up the rescuer to perform other duties.

Use of Automatic External Defibrillators

Automatic external defibrillators are small, portable, battery operated devices that allow providers to defibrillate cardiac arrest victims without interpretation of an electrocardiographic waveform. Laypersons can use the device with minimal or no training, as audible and visual prompts are incorporated into the machine. It is well known that the earlier a victim is defibrillated the better chance of survival. Most in-hospital defibrillators are now equipped with AED technology to help improve the time to first shock by allowing those untrained or uncertain to use the device.

When a victim is recognized and the emergency medical system is activated CPR should be started. Once the AED is available, the device should be placed by the patient's head for easy access and operation. The AED's power should be turned on which initiates a self check by the machine. The machine then instructs the user in its use. It will begin by advising to attach the electrode pads to the patient. There are pictures on the electrode pads for proper placement on the chest wall. The electrode pads should be placed on the right upper chest just below the clavicle and the left lower lateral chest below the nipple. The chest wall should be dry when the electrode pads are applied. The AED will then analyze the rhythm; some devices require a button to be pushed to analyze the rhythm. The CPR should continue uninterrupted as much as possible during set up and application of the electrode pads. During analysis of the rhythm, the patient should not be touched. The AED will then advise if a shock is indicated or if CPR should be continued. If shock is advised then the machine will indicate to "charge" then will wait for the user to push the "shock" button. Before the shock is initiated everyone must be clear of the patient. After the shock is initiated, CPR should be started immediately and not be delayed to analyze the rhythm and check for a pulse. This is a deviation from past AHA guidelines and if the AED is old it may not be programmed appropriately, but CPR should be initiated after the shock in any case. If return of circulation occurs then airway or breathing assistance should be maintained until more definitive care arrives. The cycle of shock, 2 minutes of CPR then rhythm or pulse check should continue until advanced interventions are available.

Pacemaker or Automatic Implantable Cardioverter Defibrillator Patient in Cardiac Arrest

If a patient has an implantable device, such as a defibrillator or pacemaker, care should be taken to avoid placing electrode paddles or pads on the device; placement should be at least 1 inch away to avoid any potential artifact interference during rhythm analysis and potential damage to the device from defibrillation. Pacemaker problems can occur from defibrillation or cardioverson, although this is rare, including damage to the circuitry resulting in complete dysfunction or inappropriate pacing or defibrillation. It is not necessary to turn off the devices during CPR; however, if it is indicated or to alleviate fears of the resuscitation team a circular magnet is needed. All patients who present with a cardiac dysrhythmia and have a pacemaker or AICD in place should receive an interrogation of the device by a cardiologist, trained nurse or technician following the resuscitation. This can be helpful in determining the cause of the arrest as well as ensuring proper pacemaker or AICD function and reprogramming.

Complications of Cardiopulmonary Resuscitation

Cardiopulmonary resuscitation is performed to save the life of the victim; however, it is not without complications. Resuscitation teams need to be aware of the potential complications in order to provide better care to a patient whose resuscitation is not going well or for those who deteriorate postresuscitation. The most common complication found was sternal and rib fractures with a rate of 25–30%. Other complications include anterior mediastinal hemorrhage, upper airway complications, abdominal organ injuries, and lung injuries.

If a patient during resuscitation becomes difficult to bag it is important to consider pneumothorax as the cause. If a pneumothorax occurs this can quickly lead to tension for patients who are receiving positive pressure ventilation. Abdominal organ injury from CPR is not a common complication, but can occur.

❏ ADVANCED CARDIAC LIFE SUPPORT

Advanced cardiac life support includes high quality BLS and interventions that can prevent cardiac arrest in the setting of ACSs, treat cardiac arrest and improve outcomes after the cardiac arrest patient is resuscitated. During any resuscitation the healthcare provider must recognize and treat reversible causes of cardiac arrest. The "5 Hs and 5 Ts" are known causes and possible complications of cardiac arrest. These are listed in Table 19.

Advanced Airway Management

The new 2010 AHA guidelines for ACLS have new recommendations for airway management that include: the use of quantitative waveform capnography for confirmation and continuous monitoring of endotracheal tube placement for adults, the use of supraglottic advanced airways as alternative to endotracheal intubation and they no longer recommend the routine use of cricoid pressure during airway management.

Endotracheal intubation is the recommended airway of choice for all patients needing invasive ventilation management or airway protection due to alteration in mentation, airway swelling or any other injuring that may compromise the upper airways. The possibility of spinal injury is a relative contraindication of direct laryngoscopy orotracheal intubation; however, if a patient requires endotracheal intubation for lifesaving reasons then one must perform the procedure with as much spinal immobilization as possible without interfering with the intubation procedure.

The difficult airway where intubation fails can be due to prominent upper incisors, inability to extend the neck, extremely large tongue, swelling, blood or

Table 19: Reversible causes of cardiac arrest	
Five Hs	**Five Ts**
Hypoxia	Toxins
Hypovolemia	Tamponade
Hydrogen ion (acidosis)	Tension pneumothorax
Hypokalemia/hyperkalemia	Thrombosis, pulmonary
Hypothermia	Thrombosis, coronary

(*Source:* Neumar RE, Otttto CS, Link MS, et al. Guidelines for cardiopulmonary resuscitation and emergency cardiovascular care. Part 8: Adult advanced cardiovascular life support. Circulation. 2010;122(Suppl. 3):S729-67)

Table 20: Medications which can be used during advanced cardiovascular life support

- Epinephrine
- Vasopressin
- Lidocaine
- Amiodarone
- Procainamide
- Atropine
- Magnesium sulfate
- Calcium chloride
- Morphine and oxygen

secretions in the airway, small lower jaw, inability to completely open the mouth, tumors or any other unusual anatomy. Good bag–valve–mask (BVM) ventilation is the first technique and probably the most important to know. BVM, however, can cause gastric distention and does not protect the airway from aspiration. An ideal airway should be rapidly and reliably inserted with minimal training, control ventilation, protect against aspiration and be able to be inserted with ongoing chest compressions.

Pharmaceutical Interventions

Pharmaceutical interventions for cardiac arrest victims are a controversial subject. There is no evidence that any medications given during cardiac arrest that have lead to any improvement in survival to hospital discharge. The most important factors in survival are high quality CPR and early defibrillation. The medications used during CPR should assist in potentiating the return of circulation, enhance cardiac function, support blood pressure and shunt blood toward vital organs. The AHA includes several medications in its advanced cardiovascular life support pulseless algorithm; these are mentioned in Table 20.

Defibrillation or Cardioversion

Defibrillation is a procedure where controlled electrical energy is applied to the myocardium either through the chest wall or through directly on the heart and is designed to terminate an unstable or pulseless rhythm. Defibrillators are divided into two main types: (i) Manual and (ii) Automatic.

Manual defibrillators require the provider to obtain and interpret an electrocardiogram and determine if (i) defibrillation is necessary, (ii) select an energy level, and (iii) decide if synchronization should be used. The goal of defibrillation is to uniformly depolarize a majority of the myocardium and terminate the abnormal dysrhythmia. Once electrical activity is reset and the myocardium regains its excitability, the SA node will presumptively reinitiate normal pacing and the myocardium can begin coordinated rhythmic contractions.

Defibrillators are classified by the type of waveforms they produce. Monophasic defibrillators send an electrical wave from one electrode to the other in only one direction. With biphasic defibrillators the electrode potential is reversed in midshock so the current reverses direction (Fig. 19).

While defibrillation is a lifesaving procedure it is not without risk. There are three basic risks: (i) risk to the patient, (ii) risk to the user, and (iii) risk to equipment or environment. Care must be taken to minimize these risks.

❑ RISKS

Defibrillators are equipped with "synchronization" mode which allows the user to avoid unintended delivery of a shock to the "T" wave of the ECG. The user must be sure, when using a manual defibrillator, to appropriately use the synchronization for

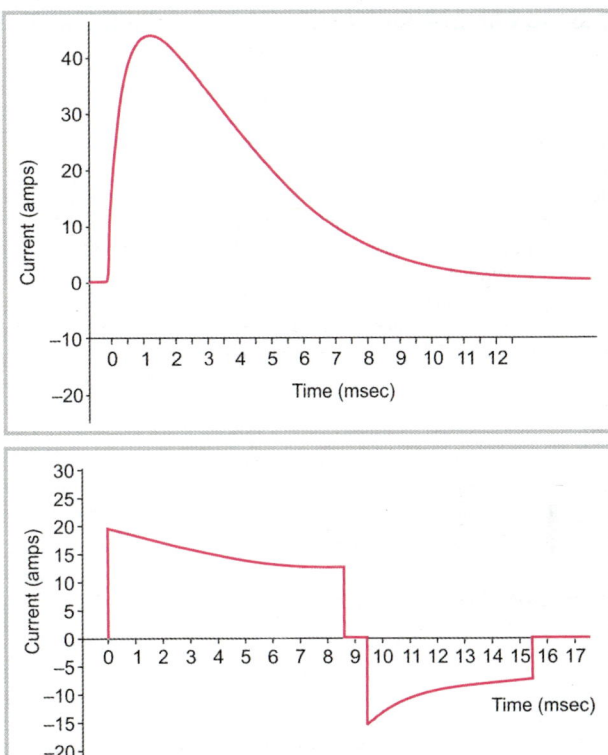

FIGURE 19: Monophasic vs biphasic waveforms. The monophasic waveform is damped and the biphasic waveform is truncated. (*Source:* Modified from Deakin CD, Nolan JP, Sunde KJ, et al. European resuscitation council guidelines for resuscitation 2010 Section 3. Electrical therapies: automated external defibrillation, cardioversion and pacing. Resuscitation. 2010;81:1293-304)

cardioversion of stable dysrhythmias but must avoid its use in unstable or pulseless rhythms, such as VF or polymorphic VT, where there will not be a discrete "R" wave to synchronize on and the device will not fire, thereby causing a delay until the synchronizer is disabled. The energy level applied to the myocardium from defibrillation can cause damage manifest as myocardial necrosis and functional damage evident as atrioventricular conduction disturbances. Incorrectly displayed asystole can occur when paddles or gel pads are used to display the ECG tracing due to electrical voltage "offset". This "false" asystole display can last long enough to mislead rescuers. If asystole is displayed, it must be confirmed immediately by attaching the standard ECG electrodes.

Risks to the rescuer during cardioversion or defibrillation are difficult to quantify. It is estimated that injury to paramedics was 1 per 1,700 without significant morbidity or mortality. It has been suggested that the traditional admonition to "clear" the patient before delivering a defibrillating shock is therefore unnecessary, providing gloves are worn and selfadhesive paddles are used. However the AHA recommends that all personnel stand clear during shock delivery.

❏ CESSATION OF RESUSCITATION

Termination of resuscitation is difficult for all providers of cardiac arrest patients but it can become especially difficult for emergency medical personnel in the prehospital setting. There are ethical, legal and cultural factors that need to be taken into consideration when deciding the need for termination of resuscitation. Initiation of resuscitation may conflict with a patient's desires or may not be in the best interest of the patient, and in some instances, resuscitation may not be the best use of limited resources. The public in general overestimates the probability of survival from cardiac arrest and even most physicians cannot accurately predict mortality rates of sudden cardiac arrest.

The AHA has developed the "BLS termination of resuscitation rule"; if all the following criteria are met then there is no indication for ambulance transport: (i) arrest was not witnessed by and EMS provider or first responder, (ii) no ROSC after three complete rounds of CPR and AED analysis, and (iii) no AED shocks delivered. The "ALS termination of resuscitation rule" states if all the following criteria are met then termination of resuscitation before transport is indicated: (i) arrest not witnessed by anyone, (ii) no bystander CPR provided, (iii) no ROSC after complete ALS care in the field, and (iv) no shocks delivered. Implementation of these rules usually includes contacting the EMS medical control. EMS providers should be trained in sensitive communication with family members about outcomes.

❏ POSTRESUSCITATION CARE

Postresuscitative care is a new section in the 2010 AHA guidelines for CPR. The goal is to emphasize an organized multidisciplinary program that focuses on optimizing neurologic, hemodynamic, and metabolic function that may provide an increase in survival to hospital discharge.

Once circulation is restored oxygen should be weaned down to lowest required to maintain oxygen greater than 94%, to avoid hyperoxia. With return of circulation a "post-arrest syndrome" often presents that requires proper inotropic support and monitoring. Standard vasopressor treatment is indicated to improve patient hemodynamics.

Cardiac interventions are aimed to prevent further myocardial necrosis and left ventricular dysfunction leading to heart failure. Percutaneous coronary intervention (PCI) will provide patients with ST elevation myocardial infarction the most favorable outcomes, even in out of hospital cardiac arrest where overall survival remains low. Early PCI following thrombolysis is associated with reduced recurrence of ischemia and reinfarction without increased risk of major hemorrhage.

❏ SUMMARY

Cardiopulmonary resuscitation from sudden cardiac arrest is challenging. Since 1960, our impact on patient survival from out of hospital cardiac arrest has changed very little. What we do know is that high quality, minimally interrupted CPR that is started immediately upon recognition is extremely important for improving patient survival. Rate and depth of compressions is the key to high quality CPR. Providers who do not perform CPR often should have frequent retraining. The AHA guidelines for 2010 have been simplified to help improve compliance and to emphasize compressions over other interventions in the field to help improve the number of patients who receives bystander CPR; this includes compression only CPR for those who may be unwilling or unable to perform conventional CPR.

❏ SUGGESTED READINGS

American Heart Association. History of CPR. Available from www.heart.org [Accessed October, 2010].

CPR and Sudden Cardiac Arrest Fact Sheet. American Heart Association. Available from www.heart.org [Accessed October, 2010].

Executive Summary: 2010 American Heart Association Guidelines for Cardiopulmonary resuscitation. Circulation. 2010. Available from www.circ.ahajournals.org [Accessed October, 2010]

Highlights of the 2010 American Heart Association Guidelines for CPR and ECC. Available from www.static.org/eccguidelines [Accessed December 2010].

Hinchey PR, Myers JB, Lewis R, et al. Improved out-of-hospital cardiac arrest survival after the sequential implementation of 2005 AHA guidelines for compressions, ventilations and induced hypothermia: the Wake County experience. Ann Emerg Med. 2010;56:358-61.

3.13 Risk Stratification for Sudden Cardiac Death

❏ INTRODUCTION

Sudden death is overwhelmingly a cardiac etiology [sudden cardiac death (SCD)] defined as unexpected death occurring within one hour of symptoms. The heart rhythm causing SCD is most frequently ventricular tachycardia (VT) or ventricular fibrillation (VF). Assessing risk is not trying to predict the future, but to plan for the possibility of this disaster with cost-effective strategies; the most comprehensive discussion of individual assessment was published almost a decade ago and yet is still largely valid.

Many noninvasive as well as invasive procedures are available to help the clinician to evaluate the risk of SCD. A partial list includes signal averaged electrocardiogram (ECG), heart rate variability and turbulence, and T-wave alternans. Unfortunately while these assessments have excellent basic background in theory, they do not pan out in studies of even the most common ischemic heart disease with congestive heart failure. However, we find studies revealing important simple clinical ways to help patients in specific categories. In general most SCDs involve patients with previous cardiac arrest or syncope or a family history of SCD.

❏ HEALTHY ATHLETES

Healthy athletes would a priori be the least likely to succumb to SCD. Surprisingly, there was a 2.5-fold increase in SCD in an Italian athletic population, compared to non-athletes. Symptoms of palpitations, syncope or seizure, especially during exercise, require further work up to identify the cause. Parenthetically, simple orthostatic dizziness due to vasodilatation is very common in elite athletes and needs to be separated from other symptoms. However, the European Society of Cardiology Consensus recommends routine ECGs, based on a reduction in SCD in athletes in Italy, but which is now reduced to the frequency observed in most other countries including the US. However, this reduction was an uncontrolled observation.

Athletes may by virtue of their training actually develop a unique set of cardiac findings, different from untrained persons of the same age, which need to be appreciated as normal for sport. These include asymptomatic slower heart rates and second degree AV block at rest, but normal rate and rhythm with exercise. Although we are only beginning to understand that ECG and echocardiographgic (ECHO) criteria may have to be altered in athletes such criteria change may depend on race. False-positive ECGs accounted for 98.8% of follow-up costs. Similar evaluation schemes have been used for soccer with similar outcomes. While 4.8% soccer players had potentially abnormal ECGs, only 1% had clearly abnormal evaluations preventing participation in the 2006 world cup.

❏ BRUGADA SYNDROME

Electrocardiogram (ECG) screening has the potential for identification of electrical disorders which could lead to SCD, although there is not much evidence that athletes would be affected by these entities. Brugada syndrome is one such disorder; it is an autosomal dominantly inherited disease producing a high-risk-associated ECG with a coved appearance of ST segment elevation (2 mm) in the right precordial leads; this pattern has (4.7-fold increase risk) predictive accuracy for SCD in meta analysis of 947 patients.

❏ LONG QT INTERVAL SYNDROME

Long QT interval syndrome has been well reviewed in general population as well as in athletes. New data collectively suggest that the magnitude of the QT prolongation is highly predictive. In adults, the diagnosis is made with a QTc > 480, but the risk in adults is incrementally greater with larger the QTc. In children, males are at higher risk, while after puberty females are at higher risk. Therapy with ICD is indicated if symptoms cannot be controlled with beta blocker therapy and or cervicothoracic sympathectomy. ICD may be appropriate if there is a strong family history of SCD or inability to take beta blockers.

❏ EARLY REPOLARIZATION

Early repolarization on the ECG has been implicated in the etiology of SCD although the mechanism is unclear. However, the occurrence of this finding in normal athletes with an apparently good prognosis make it a rather difficult risk assessment tool except perhaps when it is localized in the inferior leads in middle aged subjects.

❏ SHORT QT SYNDROME

Short QT syndrome known only since 2000 has little patient data from which to guide assessment. Certainly a patient with QTc less than 350 and resuscitated SCD should have a defibrillator, but even syncope is not predictive of SCD unless in the presence of a markedly positive family history.

❏ CATECHOLAMINE POLYMORPHIC VENTRICULAR TACHYCARDIA

Catecholamine polymorphic VT is a well studied and strikingly reproducible syndrome of exercise facilitated VT with multiple morphologies associated with mutations in ryanodine (autosomal dominant) or calsequestrin (autosomal recessive). Exercise-induced bidirectional ventricular ectopy and bidirectional VT makes the diagnosis and therapy with beta adrenergic blockers is indicated with ICD implantation if VT cannot be suppressed.

❑ WOLFF–PARKINSON–WHITE SYNDROME

Preexcitation of the ventricle by non-atrioventricular nodal structures when producing symptoms is called Wolff–Parkinson–White (WPW) syndrome. It is clear that patients with rapid tachycardia symptoms need therapeutic ablation. However, the recommendation for ablation in order for asymptomatic persons with preexcitation alone to participate in competitive athletics seems inappropriately invasive when the risk of preexcitation alone is unclear. Electrical syndromes, however, do not account for most of sudden deaths in young people.

❑ MARFAN'S SYNDROME

Marfan's syndrome is a connective tissue disorder caused by mutations in genes encoding supporting scaffold for elastin. Its prevalence is between 1 in 5,000 or 10,000. It causes SCD, produced by aortic dissection, rupture and pericardial tamponade. SCD without dissection are reported and ventricular arrhythmias are thought to be the cause; mitral valve prolapse is a common component of Marfan's syndrome but LV dilatation is the associated finding suggesting risk in Marfan's patients with ventricular ectopy and VT. Unfortunately, LV dilatation is not commonly found in sporadic cases of SCD with only MVP studied at autopsy. However, SD can occur without cardiac cause due to the elongated odontoid causing pressure on the cerebellum and medulla owing to alantoaxial hypermobility.

❑ CONGENITAL HEART DISEASE

Congenital heart disease (CHD) afflicts approximately 75 of 1,000 live births. Significant advances in the treatment of CHD over past 50 years have allowed the majority of afflicted children to reach adulthood. The number of adults with CHD now exceeds that of children. SCD is the most common cause of death in these patients. SCD is especially likely in patients with repaired cyanotic and left heart obstructive lesions. Predictors of mortality in patients with CHD include New York Heart Association (NYHA) functional class greater than one, cyanosis, age (postsurgical repair) and complexity of malformations. Patients with CHD presenting with cardiac arrest, sustained symptomatic VT or syncope and have significant systemic ventricular dysfunction are stratified as high-risk and ICD therapy is generally recommended. Three special groups are associated with the highest risk of SCD including patients treated with Mustard/Senning procedures, Fontan procedures and repaired tetralogy of Fallot (TOF). Although reduced left ventricular (EF < 35%) function is the strongest risk factor for SCD in ischemic heart disease (see below), there is debate as to whether such findings should be extended to patients with CHD. Systemic ventricular dysfunction (such as in corrected transposition) has been demonstrated in numerous observational studies and registries to identify CHD patients at risk for SCD.

❏ NONISCHEMIC CARDIOMYOPATHY

Nonischemic cardiomyopathy (NICM) is the primary etiology in 10–15% of SCDs and accounts for the second largest number of SCDs from cardiac causes behind coronary artery disease (CAD). NICM is characterized by biventricular dilatation and impaired ventricular contractility without CAD. Like ischemic heart disease, numerous diagnostic techniques exist to risk stratify without careful data to identify high-risk patients would benefit from existing interventions (ICDs); in fact, the majority of the major primary prevention trials enrolling patients with NICM failed to demonstrate definitive benefit to ICD therapy. The primary risk stratifying approach utilized was a combination of quantitative left ventricular function assessment and functional status based on NYHA functional class. Current guidelines recommend placement of ICDs in patients with NICM, EF less than 35% and NYHA Class II–III symptoms. A number of noninvasive diagnostic methods for risk stratifying patients with NICM have recently been reviewed with the exception of syncope, EF and NYHA functional class, no significant data exist for other methods of identifying patients that would benefit from available therapies.

❏ CORONARY ARTERY DISEASE

Coronary artery disease (CAD) accounts for (or is the underlying condition in) 65–80% of patients presenting with SCD. In recent years, the steady decrease in mortality due to CAD has correlated with the decrease in SCD, although the prevalence of CAD has increased. Medical therapy directed at treating CAD, in particular beta blockers and renin angiotensin system modifiers (ACE inhibitors ARBs, aldosterone antagonist) have been demonstrated to decrease the incidence of SCD.

Traditional risk factors of CAD (HTN, DM, smoking, hypercholesterolemia) identify patients at risk for ischemic heart disease and hence SCD (with obesity, DM and smoking showing an increased proportion of deaths that are sudden). NYHA functional class higher than 2, EF less than 35 and syncope identify patients who benefit from ICDs. Unlike NICM, there may be utility of invasive electrophysiologic

❏ SUMMARY

We have reviewed the available data on risk stratification in major entities encountered by clinicians. Generally good clinical judgment can be enhanced by the published knowledge; in addition to a history of SCD, symptoms of syncope or arrhythmogenic dizziness predict likely risk of SCD in most disorders. A family history of SCD may also inform, such an evaluation. An ECG abnormality coupled with the above may focus additional evaluation, such as exercise testing in appropriate patients. Documentation of structural heart disease by ECHO confirms risk in various population groups. Normal ECG and ECHO may exclude risk in many groups. Further research is needed to clarify the specific risk in more rare diseases. Unfortunately based on our experience with CAD, it is not likely we will find easy risk stratifiers in many disease states.

❏ SUGGESTED READINGS

Corrado D, Pelliccia A, Heidbuchel H, et al. Section of Sports Cardiology, European Association of Cardiovascular Prevention and Rehabilitation, Working Group of Myocardial and Pericardial Disease, European Society of Cardiology. Recommendations for interpretation of 12-lead electrocardiogram in the athlete. Eur Heart J. 2010;31:243-59.

Epstein AE, DiMarco JP, Ellenbogen KA, et al. ACC/AHA/HRS 2008 guidelines for device-based therapy of cardiac rhythm abnormalities: a report of the American College of Cardiology/American Heart Association Task Force on Practice Guidelines (writing committee to revise the ACC/AHA/NASPE 2002 guideline update for implantation of cardiac pacemakers and antiarrhythmia devices) developed in collaboration with the american association for thoracic surgery and society of thoracic surgeons. J Am Coll Cardiol. 2008;51:e1-e62.

European Heart Rhythm Association, Heart Rhythm Society, Zipes DP, et al. ACC/AHA/ESC 2006 guidelines for management of patients with ventricular arrhythmias and the prevention of sudden cardiac death: a report of the American College of Cardiology/ American Heart Association Task Force and the European Society of Cardiology Committee for Practice Guidelines (writing committee to develop guidelines for management of patients with ventricular arrhythmias and the prevention of sudden cardiac death). J Am Coll Cardiol. 2006;48:e247-e346.

Maron BJ, Doerer JJ, Haas TS, et al. Sudden deaths in young competitive athletes: analysis of 1866 deaths in the United States, 1980-2006. Circulation. 2009;119:1085-92.

Pelliccia A, Zipes DP, Maron BJ. Bethesda conference #36 and the european society of cardiology consensus recommendations revisited a comparison of U.S. and european criteria for eligibility and disqualification of competitive athletes with cardiovascular abnormalities. J Am Coll Cardiol. 2008;52:1990-6.

Priori SG, Aliot E, Blomstrom-Lundqvist C, et al. Task force on sudden cardiac death of the european society of cardiology. Eur Heart J. 2001;22:1374-450.

Chapter 4

Coronary Heart Diseases

4.1 Coronary Heart Disease: Risk Factors

❏ INTRODUCTION

Cardiovascular disease (CVD) remains the leading cause of death in the United States and many other parts of the world and results in substantial disability and loss of productivity. Coronary heart disease (CHD) and stroke are the leading contributors to this heavy CVD burden. The exact mechanisms underlying development of CVD still remain to be fully described. Multiple risk factors for the development of CVD have been identified. A risk factor is any personal, environmental, psychosocial, or genetic characteristic that gives an individual a higher likelihood of developing a particular disease. Cardiovascular disease risk factors are generally categorized into traditional/conventional and novel/emerging risk factors (Table 1). Risk factors can be inherited or acquired, some are modifiable and others are not. Risk factors may be defined dichotomously by their presence or absence or measured as a continuous variable.

Table 1: Risk factors for cardiovascular disease

Traditional risk factors

Modifiable	Nonmodifiable
• Hypertension • Diabetes • Hyperlipidemia • Obesity • Tobacco use • Physical inactivity	• Age (male ≥45 years, female ≥55 years) • Gender • Family history of premature coronary artery disease*

Selected emerging risk factors

- C-reactive protein
- Small LDL particles
- Lipoprotein(a)
- Homocysteine
- Lipoprotein-associated phospholipase A2
- Coagulation and hemostatic factors
- Apolipoproteins A and B
- White blood cell count

(*Definite myocardial infarction or sudden death before 55 years of age in father or other male first-degree relative or before 65 years of age in mother or other female first-degree relative)

❑ CHD SCREENING AND PREVENTION

The high lifetime risk of CHD warrants population wide screening for prevention and treatment. The long lag time between the onset of atherosclerosis and its related morbidity and mortality allows for detection and early intervention. Screening involves routine evaluation of asymptomatic people. Screening should be cost-effective with the goal of detecting, not excluding, disease. Using established risk factors, a significant percentage of 'at-risk' individuals can be screened as a target for preventive strategies.

❑ CLUSTERING AND MULTIPLICATIVE EFFECTS OF RISK FACTORS

Initially, risk factors for CHD, such as diabetes, hypertension, and hyperlipidemia, were targeted and treated individually. However, risk factors often occur in clusters and show a multiplicative effect rather than a simple additive effect. This has important implications for treatment. Most persons in a population have moderate elevation in multiple risk factors rather than an extremely high level of any single risk factor. Similarly, most cardiovascular events occur in individuals with mild to moderate abnormality in multiple risk factors. Targeting only high levels of individual risk factors will target only a small fraction of the population. Various expert groups stress the concept of 'comprehensive risk factor management'.

❑ CHD RISK ESTIMATION

Despite our knowledge and understanding of many CHD risk factors, a clinical challenge is to effectively predict risk of CHD in individuals to allow appropriate and cost-effective treatment. Risk estimates are also used to raise awareness about CHD, determine population attributable risk to target specific public health measures, and to communicate risk to patients. Coronary heart disease risk estimation measures the likelihood of a person developing a serious cardiovascular event over a specific follow-up time.

Framingham Risk Score (FRS)

FRS and National Cholesterol Education Program's Third Adult Treatment Panel update (NCEP ATP III) are the most widely used risk scores (Table 2). FRS predicts the 10-year risk of CHD using a multivariable mathematical model of risk. Absolute risk is divided into three risk categories: high, intermediate, and low risk (Table 3).

European Risk Scores

Since FRS is based on a North American sample, in Europe different risk scores were established including the Systematic Coronary Risk Evaluation (SCORE) project and the QRESEARCH cardiovascular RISK algorithm (QRISK). The SCORE has been adopted by the Joint European Societies' guidelines on CVD prevention. The SCORE risk prediction system uses only fatal CVD as the outcome measure. The risk chart provides more detail for middle-aged persons in whom the risk changes with age.

Table 2: Risk prediction scores for cardiovascular disease

Risk score (year)	Study summary	Variables	End point
Framingham Risk Score (1998)	5,209 men and women, ages 30–62 years Follow-up 10 years 10-year risk	Age, diabetes, smoking, hypertension, total cholesterol and LDL-C	All CHD
Framingham Risk Score for General Cardiovascular Disease (2008)	Men and women, ages 30–74 years without CVD at baseline Follow-up 12 years 10-year risk	Age, diabetes, smoking, treated and untreated systolic blood pressure, total cholesterol, HDL-C BMI replacing lipids in a simpler model	CVD (coronary death, myocardial infarction, coronary insufficiency, angina, ischemic stroke, hemorrhagic stroke, transient ischemic attack, peripheral artery disease, heart failure)
Reynolds Risk Score (2007)	24,558 women, age ≥45 years without CVD Median follow-up 10.2 years 10-year risk	Age, hemoglobin A_{1C}, smoking, systolic blood pressure, HDL-C, hs-CRP, total cholesterol, parental history of myocardial infarction at <60 years	Global CVD (composite end-point of cardiovascular death, myocardial infarction, ischemic stroke and coronary revascularization)
Reynolds Risk Score, men (2008)	10,724 men, ages 50–80 years 10-year risk	Age, hemoglobin A1C, smoking, systolic blood pressure, HDL-C, hs-CRP, total cholesterol, parental history of myocardial infarction at <60 years	Global CVD (composite end-point of cardiovascular death, myocardial infarction, ischemic stroke and coronary revascularization)
Third Report of NCEP Adult Treatment Panel (2002, Update 2004)	Uses Framingham Risk Score 10-year risk	Variables same as Framingham risk score. Diabetes is considered a CVD equivalent	Hard CHD (CHD death and nonfatal myocardial infarction)
SCORE (2003)	205, 178 persons, ages 45–64 years 10-year risk	Age, cholesterol, smoking, systolic blood pressure Individuals with >5% 10-year risk are defined as high risk	CVD death

Contd...

Contd...

Table 2: Risk prediction scores for cardiovascular disease

Risk score (year)	Study summary	Variables	End point
QRISK (2007)	Derivation cohort 1.28 million patients, age 35–74 years Median follow-up 6.5 years 10-year risk	Age, body mass index, ratio of total cholesterol to HDL-cholesterol, family history of premature cardiovascular disease, smoking, systolic blood pressure, deprivation score	CVD (myocardial infarction, ischemic stroke, transient ischemic attack and coronary heart disease)
Prospective cardiovascular Münster (PROCAM) (2002)	5,389 men, age 35–65 years 10-year follow-up	Age, LDL-C, smoking, HDL-C, systolic blood pressure, family history of premature myocardial infarction, diabetes mellitus, triglycerides Score 0 to > 60 with score > 53 defined as high risk (>20% 10-year risk of cardiac event)	Hard CHD (sudden cardiac death or a definite fatal or nonfatal myocardial infarction)
Rasmussen score (2003)	396 individuals	Blood pressure, N terminal proBNP, electrocardiogram, carotid intima-media thickness, microalbuminuria, treadmill exercise blood pressure, left ventricular ultrasound left ventricular mass index, small and large artery elasticity, optic fundoscopy for retinal vasculature	

(Abbreviations: CVD: Cardiovascular disease; CHD: Coronary heart disease; LDL-C: Low density cholesterol; HDL-C: High density cholesterol; hs-CRP: High-sensitivity C-reactive protein; NCEP: National cholesterol education program)

Table 3: Risk categories for 10-year risk of coronary heart disease

Risk category definition	
High risk	CHD or CHD risk equivalent* or ≥2 risk factors† and 10-year predicted risk of ≥20%
Moderately high risk	≥2 Risk factors and 10-year predicted risk of 10–20%
Moderate risk	≥2 Risk factors and 10-year predicted risk of ≥10%
Low risk	0–1 Risk factor

*Peripheral arterial disease, diabetes mellitus; †Risk factors include cigarette smoking, hypertension (blood pressure ≥140/90 mm Hg or on antihypertensive medication), low high-density lipoprotein cholesterol (<40 mg/dL), family history of premature CHD (CHD in male first-degree relative <55 years of age; CHD in female first-degree relative < 65 years of age) and age (men ≥ 45 years; women ≥55 years)

❏ TRADITIONAL CHD RISK FACTORS

Nonmodifiable Risk Factors for CHD

Certain risk factors for CHD are nonmodifiable including age, male gender and family history of CHD. Although these risk factors are nonmodifiable, they are an essential part of the risk prediction algorithms and identification of patients at higher risk for CHD events. Based on the Framingham Heart Study and NCEP ATP III recommendations, a positive family history of premature CHD is defined as a coronary event in parents before age 55 years in men and 65 years in women. Parental CHD, on an average, doubles the risk of CHD in an adult offspring. CVD in siblings also increases the risk of incident CVD even after adjustment for traditional risk factors and parental history of CVD.

Modifiable Risk Factors for CHD

Lifestyle Risk Factors

Lifestyle risk factors including physical inactivity, diet and psychosocial factors are established risk factors for CHD and carry considerable public health importance as targets for intervention. A healthy lifestyle, including eating fruits and vegetables, exercising regularly, and avoiding smoking led to 80% lower relative risk for myocardial infarction.

Smoking: Cigarette smoking is an important risk factor not only for CVD but also due to its impact on noncardiovascular morbidity and mortality. It is the single most important preventable cause of disease and early death. Smoking is a major public health threat in low-to-middle income countries where CVD is already on the rise.

In the clinical setting, it is important that every patient undergoes a full assessment of smoking status. Practitioners can use the clinical practice guidelines issued by the US Department of Health and Human Services to effectively intervene on tobacco users. The five steps recommended for intervention, referred to as the 5As, are summarized in Table 4.

Multiple options exist to help with smoking cessation including providing self-help materials to patients, behavioral counselling and group therapy. Support from spouse and family may also be important. Data regarding acupuncture and hypnotherapy for smoking cessation are inconsistent, and these are not currently recommended.

Table 4: The 5As for intervention for tobacco dependence*		
1.	Ask about tobacco use	Identify and document tobacco use status for every patient at every visit
2.	Advise to quit	In a clear, strong and personalized manner urge every tobacco user to quit
3.	Assess willingness to make a quit attempt	Is the tobacco user willing to make a quit attempt at this time?
4.	Assist in quit attempt	For the patient willing to make a quit attempt, use counseling and pharmacotherapy to help him or her quit
5.	Arrange follow-up	Schedule follow-up contact, preferably within the first week after the quit date

(*Fiore et al. Treating Tobacco Use and Dependence: Clinical Practice Guideline. Rockville, MD: US Dept of Health and Human Services; 2000)

Physical inactivity: Physical activity is any bodily movement that expends energy. It is generally measured by self-reporting or occasionally by activity monitors. Cardiorespiratory fitness is a physiological characteristic of a person measured by exercise testing.

Physical inactivity and excess caloric intake have greatly contributed to the global obesity epidemic. Physical activity exerts multiple cardiovascular benefits, including decreased risk of developing hypertension, insulin resistance, and dyslipidemia and beneficial effects on endothelial function and thrombogenesis. The minimum recommended level of physical activity includes moderate intensity exercise for 30 minutes on at least 5 days of the week. The daily 30 minutes can be accumulated in as little as 10-minute sessions and may include walking, cycling, gardening, elliptical, swimming, recreational sports, etc.

Nutrition: Diet is an important risk factor for CVD and also directly influences multiple CVD risk factors. Several dietary factors, including the intake of fruits, vegetables, fatty acids, fiber, alcohol, excess salt and the ratio of carbohydrates, fat and lipids have been studied in relation to CHD risk. Both epidemiological studies and intervention trials have demonstrated the importance of a balanced diet for CHD prevention.

Dietary lipids have an important role in the formation of atheromatous plaque. Diets, high in saturated and transfatty acids, are linked to higher rates of CHD. Saturated fatty acids increase low density lipoprotein cholesterol (LDL-C) concentration. anti-inflammatory, antiarrhythmic, and antithrombotic effects. Guidelines recommend less than 30% of total calories from dietary fat and less than 7% from saturated fats.

High sodium intake is linked to hypertension, CHD, and death. Current recommendations for the general population are to consume less than 5–6 gm of salt daily (equivalent of roughly 2,000–2,400 mg of sodium). A diet rich in fiber and natural products, fruits, and vegetables decreases risk of CHD.

Obesity: Obesity is an independent risk factor for CVD and increases mortality. Obesity is also associated with multiple other CVD risk factors, which in turn adversely affects the heart. Obesity has reached epidemic proportions in many industrialized countries and its prevalence continues to increase, posing a major global health problem. Prevalence of childhood and adolescent obesity is also on the rise. Sedentary lifestyle, ease of access to food, increase in portion size, and caloric intake are important reasons for the current obesity epidemic. Genetic factors and certain other environmental factors also predispose some individuals to excess weight. Obesity is defined as BMI of greater than or equal to 30 (Table 5). Other indexes of obesity include waist circumference and waist–hip ratio, increases in which are also linked to adverse cardiovascular outcomes. Different cutoffs for abnormal waist circumferences according to ethnicity are summarized in Table 6. Both BMI and waist circumference should be recorded for overall risk assessment and tracked over time as a vital sign.

Psychosocial factors: Several psychosocial factors are associated with increased risk of CVD, including depression, stress, anxiety, social isolation, lack of social support and stress at work. Depression especially after coronary events is not only common but also increases the incidence of recurrent coronary event by threefold. Lower socioeconomic class and adverse events in life are also associated with CVD. Poor socioeconomic status is linked to increased risk of CHD through multiple mechanisms, including unhealthy diet, lack of access to health care, excessive stress and tobacco use.

Type A behavior with associated hostility and anger raises the risk of CHD. Social isolation and lack of social support may increase the risk of CHD by 2–3-fold in men and 3–5-fold in women. Marital discord worsens prognosis in

Table 5: Classification of obesity by body mass index

Classification	Body mass index (kg/m^2)
Underweight	<18.5
Normal	18.5–24.9
Overweight	25.0–29.9
Obesity class	
— I	30.0–34.9
— II	35.0–39.9
— III	≥ 40

Table 6: Ethnic specific values for abnormal waist circumference

Ethnic group/region	Waist circumference	
North America	Male	≥102 cm
	Female	≥88 cm
Europe	Male	≥94 cm
	Female	≥80 cm
South Asians	Male	≥90 cm
	Female	≥80 cm
Chinese	Male	≥90 cm
	Female	≥80 cm
Japanese	Male	≥90 cm
	Female	≥90 cm
South and Central America	Use South Asian recommendations	
Middle East (Arab) and Eastern Mediterranean	Use European recommendations	

acute coronary syndrome. Psychosocial risk factors tend to cluster in the same individuals and groups; for instance, job stress is linked to depression, hostility, anger and social isolation. This compounds the risk of CVD.

Hypertension

Hypertension defined as a blood pressure of greater than or equal to 140/90 mm Hg is a major risk factor for CVD. In fact, there is a strong, graded relationship between blood pressure and fatal coronary events: risk doubles for every 20 mm Hg increase in systolic blood pressure or 10 mm Hg increase in diastolic blood pressure. Various mechanisms by which hypertension leads to coronary events include hemodynamic stress on blood vessels and heart, increased myocardial oxygen demand, diminished coronary blood flow and impaired endothelial function.

The seventh report of the Joint National Committee (JNC) on prevention, detection, evaluation, and treatment of high blood pressure recommends a treatment goal of less than 140/90 mm Hg for all individuals, however, in patients with CHD, renal insufficiency, congestive heart failure, peripheral vascular disease and diabetes a stricter goal of less than 130/80 mm Hg is recommended.

Hyperlipidemia

There is a strong positive association between total cholesterol and LDL-C and CVD risk. Elevated triglycerides and low HDL-C are also independent risk factors for CVD. Individuals with severely elevated levels of LDL-C due to genetic abnormalities show premature atherosclerosis. Different mechanisms by which LDL-C increases CHD include delivery of cholesterol to blood vessels, proinflammatory properties, role in plaque formation and plaque instability. High levels of HDL-C convey reduced risk of CHD. Low HDL-C and elevated triglycerides frequently occur with the presence of small dense LDL particles. This pattern of dyslipidemia is referred to as diabetic or atherogenic dyslipidemia.

Elevated LDL-C is the primary target for therapy and reduction in LDL-C substantially reduces CHD risk. In patients with elevated triglycerides (>200 mg/dL), non-HDL-C (total cholesterol minus HDL-C) is a secondary target for therapy due to a strong association with CHD risk. Non-HDL-C highly correlates with levels of apolipoprotein B, which is the major apolipoprotein of all major atherogenic lipoproteins. The non- HDL-C treatment goal is 30 mg/dL higher than LDL-C.

Diabetes Mellitus

Diabetes is a strong and independent risk factor for CVD. Whether diabetes confers a risk of events similar to that of established CHD is controversial, but current guidelines consider diabetes a CHD equivalent. Mechanisms by which diabetes causes CHD include increase in platelet aggregability, increase in inflammatory mediators, impaired endothelial function, dyslipidemia, increase in highly small, dense highly atherogenic LDL-C, among others.

Alcohol

Numerous prospective studies have suggested an inverse relation between moderate alcohol consumption (1–2 drinks per day) and CHD. Mechanisms by which alcohol may exert beneficial effects on CHD include antioxidant effects, increase in HDL-C and antithrombotic action. It is unclear if any particular type of alcoholic beverage is more protective.

❑ EMERGING RISK FACTORS

More than a hundred nontraditional or emerging risk factors have been reported. Whether they independently predict risk of CHD or add incremental information to existing risk factors continues to generate controversy and poses an obstacle to their incorporation into risk assessment and routine clinical practice. The emerging risk factors include both laboratory-based tests for biomarkers of atherosclerosis and noninvasive imaging modalities for detecting atherosclerosis. high-sensitivity C-reactive protein (hs-CRP), lipoprotein A, hyperhomocysteinemia, apolipoprotein B, and fibrinogen are some of the newly emerging markers. However, a recent US Preventive Services Task Force Recommendation Statement concludes that the current evidence is insufficient to assess the balance of benefits and harms of using non-traditional risk factors for screening asymptomatic men and women. Similarly, NCEP ATP III guidelines do not recommend routine use of emerging risk factors for risk assessment.

❑ SUBCLINICAL ATHEROSCLEROSIS

Detecting subclinical atherosclerosis with noninvasive imaging modalities has generated great interest. This is distinct from the general 'risk factor' concept. The presence of calcium in coronary arteries correlates with atherosclerosis and is measured using cardiac tomographic imaging. Coronary artery calcium (CAC) score, which quantifies the extent of coronary calcium, is reported as percentiles of calcification according to age and sex. A 'negative' test has a CAC score of 0 and is associated with a low risk of subsequent coronary events. To date, it is unclear whether CAC testing should lead to change in therapy if that results in a favorable impact on clinical outcomes.

Ankle brachial index is a noninvasive test to diagnose and assess the severity of peripheral vascular disease. It is the ratio of systolic blood pressure in the ankle, measured at the level of the posterior tibial or dorsalis pedis artery, to that of the brachial artery. A lower value of ankle brachial index is not only an indicator for the severity of peripheral vascular disease but also correlates independently with major coronary events and stroke. When used in conjunction with FRS, a low ankle brachial index (<0.90) approximately doubled the risk of cardiovascular events and death.

❑ TRANSLATING RISK FACTOR SCREENING INTO EVENT REDUCTION

It is our responsibility to fully implement strategies to ensure that any risk factors identified are fully treated. Barriers to such implementation exist at the physician, patient, system and societal level. Physicians can, through better communication and education, ensure better adherence to risk factor reduction strategies. Specific verbal and written instructions and prompt follow-up can help increase adherence. Monitoring progress goals and providing feedback can help patients stay on track, particularly with lifestyle modifications. There should be open communication between the specialists and primary care physicians. Enabling easy access to electronic medical records from index hospitalization as well as specialist visits should help primary care physicians to deliver risk factor reduction treatment on a long-term basis.

❏ SUGGESTED READINGS

Expert Panel on Detection, Evaluation and Treatment of High Blood Cholesterol in Adults. Executive Summary of the Third Report of the National Cholesterol Education Program (NCEP) Expert Panel on Detection, Evaluation, and Treatment of High Blood Cholesterol in Adults (Adult Treatment Panel III). JAMA. 2001;285:2486-97.

Grundy SM, Cleeman JI, Merz CN, et al. Implications of recent clinical trials for the National Cholesterol Education Program Adult Treatment Panel III Guidelines. J Am Coll Cardiol. 2004;44:720-32.

Kannel WB, Dawber TR, Kagan A, et al. Factors of risk in the development of coronary heart disease—Six-year follow-up experience. The Framingham Study. Ann Intern Med. 1961;55:33-50.

Pearson TA, Blair SN, Daniels SR, et al. AHA Guidelines for Primary Prevention of Cardiovascular Disease and Stroke: 2002 Update: consensus Panel Guide to Comprehensive Risk Reduction for Adult Patients Without Coronary or Other Atherosclerotic Vascular Diseases. American Heart Association Science Advisory and Coordinating Committee. Circulation. 2002;106:388-91.

US Preventive Services Task Force. Using nontraditional risk factors in coronary heart disease risk assessment: US Preventive Services Task Force Recommendation Statement. Ann Intern Med. 2009;151:1-38.

4.2 Acute Coronary Syndrome
(Unstable Angina and Non-ST-Segment Elevation Myocardial Infarction): Diagnosis and Early Treatment

❏ INTRODUCTION

Each year more than 1.3 million patients are admitted to hospitals throughout the United States with an acute coronary syndrome (ACS); unstable angina (UA) and non-ST-elevation myocardial infarction (NSTEMI) account for 60–70% of all those admissions. Recognizing that everyone with an ACS is not admitted to a hospital, one can appreciate the magnitude of this problem.

❏ UNSTABLE ANGINA AND NON-ST-SEGMENT

The UA/NSTEMI constitutes a subset of the clinical syndrome of ACS that is usually, but not always, caused by atherosclerotic coronary artery disease (CAD). In the spectrum of ACS, UA/NSTEMI is defined by an accelerated or unstable clinical syndrome consistent with angina, with electrocardiographic changes consistent with ischemia and/or positive biomarkers of necrosis (e.g. troponin), in the absence of ST-segment elevation.

❏ CLINICAL FEATURES

Anginal chest pain is the cardinal symptom of ischemic coronary disease. The pain is typically described as deep or poorly localized pain that is reproducibly associated with physical exertion or emotional stress, and is promptly relieved with rest or nitroglycerin. It may radiate to the jaw, neck, back or arm(s) and may be associated with shortness of breath, nausea, lightheadedness or diaphoresis. In patients with UA/NSTEMI, episodes of angina may be severe or prolonged, may be provoked by minimal exertion or may even occur at rest. Many patients do not describe angina as "chest pain" but may describe it as a discomfort; this distinction may be important while interviewing patients as they may deny having pain, but will admit to having discomfort. Atypical presentations may account for about one-third of all patients who present to the hospital with an ACS. Atypical symptoms are particularly common among the elderly, women, diabetics and patients with heart failure. It is important to recognize that the term "atypical" refers only to the reality that the symptoms are not classical/typical but does not exclude the diagnosis of ischemia as the etiology of these.

Physical Examination

A normal physical examination is common in patients with ACS and does not exclude this diagnosis. More importantly, findings on the physical examination can help to assess the hemodynamic impact of the ischemic insult. The signs and symptoms, such as cool, clammy skin, diaphoresis, sinus tachycardia, significant bradycardia, S3 or S4, mitral regurgitation murmur and bibasilar rales, may herald the onset of cardiogenic shock even before the development of frank hypotension. Occasionally, physical findings might suggest an alternative diagnosis, such as aortic dissection, pericarditis, cholecystitis, etc., and, therefore the importance of physical examination cannot be overemphasized.

Electrocardiogram

A 12-lead electrocardiogram (ECG) is an integral part of the initial evaluation of a patient with ACS. In addition to identifying candidates for reperfusion (e.g. STEMI patients), it also provides prognostic information. Typical ECG findings that are consistent with ischemia in patients with UA/NSTEMI include the presence of ST-segment depression (at least 0.5 mm in at least two contiguous leads), transient ST changes or presence of T wave inversions. However, up to 20% of patients with an NSTEMI, confirmed by cardiac enzymes, have no diagnostic ischemic ECG changes. While isolated T wave inversion is nonspecific, the finding of symmetric deep T wave inversion (>2 mm) in multiple precordial leads is usually associated with severe critical stenosis of the proximal left anterior descending artery (Wellen's syndrome) (Fig. 1). The finding of a normal initial ECG in a patient where the clinical suspicion is high should always prompt serial ECG evaluation (along with cardiac biomarker testing), especially if the ECG was obtained after the symptoms have resolved.

Biomarkers

Creatinine Kinase

Creatinine kinase (CK) has been the most commonly used biochemical markers among patients with ACS worldwide. The MB isoenzyme has greater specificity for myocardial tissue compared to total CK (which may be elevated in neurological or skeletal muscle disorders as well). The CK-MB levels peak at 10–18 hours after injury and usually remain elevated up to 72 (Fig. 2). Due to its shorter half-life, CK and CK-MB elevation is particularly useful in detecting episodes of reinfarction.

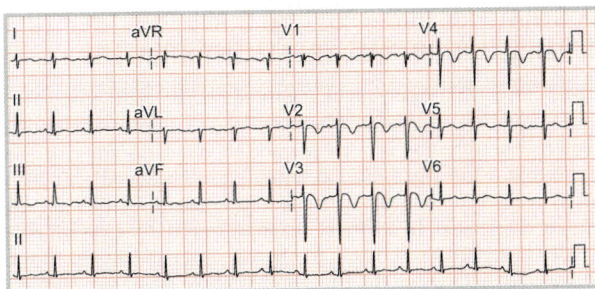

FIGURE 1: Symmetric deep T wave inversions involving multiple precordial leads (Wellen's syndrome). This patient had a 90% stenosis in his proximal left anterior descending artery stenosis. (*Source:* Modified from Rhinehardt J, Brady WJ, Perron AD, et al. Electrocardiographic manifestations of Wellen's syndrome. Am J Emerg Med. 2002;20: 638-43)

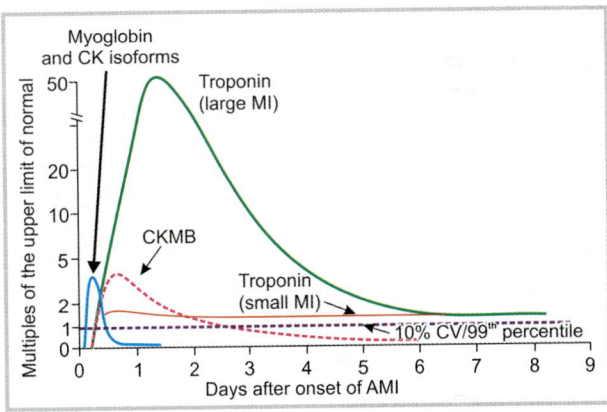

FIGURE 2: Timing of release of various biomarkers after acute ischemic myocardial infarction. (*Source:* Modified from Kumar, et al. Acute coronary syndromes: diagnosis and management, Part 1. Mayo Clin Proc. 2009;84(10):917-38)

Troponin

Cardiac troponins have gained widespread acceptance, and have largely replaced CK-MB as the biomarkers of choice for detecting myocardial injury. This is due to their high sensitivity and specificity to the heart muscle as well as the commercial availability of a rapid, inexpensive and reproducible test. Troponin is a multimer that is composed of three subunits: (i) Troponin (Tn) T, (ii) Tn I, and (iii) Tn C. Only Tn T and Tn I are commercially available as diagnostic tests. Since normal individuals should not have any detectable levels, levels higher than 99th percentile of a normal population of subjects are used as a cutoff for troponin elevation. Troponin levels do not increase until at least 6 hours after the onset of the infarct; therefore, a negative test during this period should be repeated after a period of 4–6 hours.

❑ RISK STRATIFICATION—PUTTING IT ALL TOGETHER TO DETERMINE THE OPTIMAL TREATMENT STRATEGY

Patients presenting with chest pain or angina equivalent, consistent with possible UA/NSTEMI are heterogeneous in terms of their risk of mortality. Therefore, appropriate risk stratification is of paramount importance. Early risk assessment must be twofold. Firstly, one must determine the likelihood that the clinical syndrome is related to coronary ischemia and evaluate whether the course of symptoms are accelerated. In addition, one must consider the overall risk factors that the individual patient will have CAD by assessing patient's risk factors. Next, one must consider findings on the ECG and available laboratory testing. Finally, one must consider the likelihood of alternative diagnoses.

Based upon this, a patient may be classified into one of the following groups:
- Definite ACS (clinical symptoms consistent with angina, and electrocardiogram (ECG) changes consistent with ischemia and/or positive troponin, or patients with known stable angina with acceleration in the pattern of the angina)
- Possible ACS (clinical symptoms consistent with angina, but lack of ECG changes or positive troponin)
- Stable angina (clinical symptoms consistent with angina, without a pattern of acceleration or instability)
- Noncardiac chest pain (clinical symptoms that are not consistent with angina and lack of ECG changes or positive troponins, especially with a documented noncardiac cause).

Several groups have developed comprehensive multivariable risk models that incorporate information from several predictor variables into a score for the purpose of determining intensity of initial treatment and prognosis. The most commonly used risk score in the United States is the thrombolysis in myocardial infarction (TIMI) risk score, which incorporates information from seven variables (Table 7). The TIMI risk score enables identification of high-risk patients that are at increased risk of death, and recurrent myocardial infarction (MI) and thus would benefit from aggressive therapies and early invasive treatment.

❑ EARLY MEDICAL THERAPY

The following section discusses early medical therapy in patients with ACS with special emphasis on UA/NSTEMI.

Based on the risk of future events, patients with a presumed diagnosis of UA/NSTEMI may be admitted to a coronary care unit (high risk), a telemetry unit (intermediate or low risk) or may be managed in a chest pain observation unit (low risk). Even though not rigorously studied, oxygen supplementation is

Table 7: TIMI risk score

- Age >65 years
- Chest pain in previous 24 hours
- Three major risk factors (diabetes, hypertension, hyperlipidemia, family history of ischemic heart disease and current smoking)
- Aspirin use in last 7 days
- Known coronary stenosis >50%
- ST segment deviation >0.5 mm or new left bundle branch block on initial ECG
- Elevated troponin level

(Score: One point is awarded for each parameter)

frequently used to provide adequate supply of oxygen, especially to the patients with oxygen saturations of 90% or below. The patients should be on bed rest during the early evaluation process.

Nitrates

These agents are donors of nitric oxide (NO), which causes activation of cyclic guanylylcyclase pathway resulting in an increase in intracellular cyclic guanosine monophosphate (cGMP). This leads to vasodilation, primarily in the venous bed with decrease in venous return and cardiac preload. Additional mechanisms include coronary vasodilation and improvement in blood flow to ischemic areas. Patients with ACS should receive a sublingual nitroglycerin (0.4 mg) or a buccal spray which may be repeated every 5 minutes for a total of 3 doses. If pain persists, then intravenous nitroglycerin should be initiated at a dose of 10 microgram/minute and rapidly titrated up (every 3–5 minutes) to achieve pain relief or until relative hypotension develops. Once the acute pain episode has resolved oral or, less commonly, topical nitrates may be used to prevent recurrences of symptomatic ischemic episodes.

Morphine

Morphine sulfate used in a dose of 1–4 mg intravenously is a useful adjunctive therapy for pain relief among patients with ACS. Some patients may develop hypotension which generally responds to supine positioning and/ or volume challenge. Rarely, respiratory depression may develop that responds to reversal with naloxone.

Beta Blockers

These drugs act by blocking the effect of catecholamines on β1-receptors of the heart which results in slowing of the heart rate, and reduction of contractility thereby reducing myocardial oxygen consumption. In the absence of contraindications, patients with ACS should be treated with β-blockers at initial presentation. Oral dosing is appropriate although it is reasonable to use intravenous dosing in patients who are persistently hypertensive.

Calcium Channel Blockers

These drugs inhibit the inward flux of calcium via L-type calcium channels and thus inhibit both myocardial and vascular smooth muscle contraction. Agents in this class have diverse effects—the dihydropyridines (nifedipine and amlodipine) predominantly cause vasodilation by relaxation of vascular smooth muscle; the nondihydropyridines (verapamil and diltiazem) have additional predominant negative inotropic and chronotropic actions. Calcium channel blockers that slow the heart rate may be used for the relief of angina in patients with angina refractory to nitrates and β-blockers, in patients with contraindications to β-blockers, in those with vasospastic angina, or in those with hypertension. The side effects include bradycardia, worsening of heart block, hypotension, and heart failure respectively.

Overall, the role of calcium channel blockers is primarily for symptomatic relief when β-blockers cannot be used or for the treatment of hypertension or persistent symptoms despite maximal therapy with β-blockers and nitrates.

Antiplatelet Agents

Potent antiplatelet therapy is the cornerstone of management of UA/NSTEMI given what has been previously described regarding the central role of platelets/thrombus in the pathophysiology of ACS.

Aspirin

For more than 50 years, aspirin has been the cornerstone of antiplatelet therapy and occupies a prominent role even today. It irreversibly acetylates the platelet enzyme COX-1 and thus prevents the generation of TXA2 from arachidonic acid thereby blocking the activation of platelets. The antiplatelet action lasts for the lifetime of the platelet (7–10 days), due to irreversible inhibition of COX-1 enzyme.

An initial dose of 162–325 mg daily followed by 75–162 mg daily for secondary prevention is recommended. Considerable controversy surrounds the optimal dose of aspirin for long-term use in patients for secondary prevention. However, all UA/NSTEMI patients should receive aspirin as soon as possible after hospital presentation and this should be continued indefinitely.

Adenosine Dinucleotide Phosphate Receptor Antagonists

The adenosine dinucleotide phosphate (ADP) is an important platelet agonist, which exerts its action by binding to the P2Y12 receptors on the surface of the platelets. The result of ADP signaling through the P2Y12 receptor pathway is the amplification of degranulation and ultimately platelet aggregation. This is achieved by enhanced surface expression and affinity of platelet glycoprotein IIb/IIIa protein which interacts with fibrinogen and vWF to result in platelet aggregation. Consequently, several drugs have been developed that target the inhibition of this pathway.

Clopidogrel

It is a thienopyridine that causes irreversible inhibition of the P2Y12 receptor and thus prevents ADP binding to its molecular target on the platelet surface. Clopidogrel has largely replaced ticlopidine (the first agent in this class, now rarely used) as the latter was associated with an increased risk of hematologic complications, such as neutropenia and thrombotic thrombocytopenic purpura.

Antiplatelet inhibition with clopidogrel is associated with an increased risk of major bleeding. This is of particular concern among patients who are identified as candidates for bypass surgery. It is recommended that clopidogrel be discontinued at least 5 days before planned/elective surgery, if possible. After bypass surgery, clopidogrel should be resumed whenever feasible and continued for a period of up to 1 year.

The antiplatelet response of clopidogrel shows considerable inter-individual variability. This may be overcome by higher loading doses. The variability in response is clinically relevant—patients who achieve lower platelet inhibition on clopidogrel (hyporesponders) have been shown to have an increased risk for adverse cardiac events including death. Clopidogrel is a prodrug that undergoes enzymatic conversion to its metabolically active form by the cytochrome P450 family of enzymes. As a result, polymorphism of the cytochrome P450 enzymes explains much of the observed variability in clopidogrel response in populations.

Newer Antiplatelet Agents

Prasugrel: Variability in the dose response of standard dose clopidogrel has led to an interest in the development of newer agents. Prasugrel is an oral thienopyridine drug and is less dependent on the cytochrome P450 enzymes for metabolic activation. After a loading dose of 60 mg, prasugrel reaches peak action within 30 minutes. Compared to clopidogrel (75 mg), prasugrel (10 mg) achieves more rapid and complete platelet inhibition with significantly less interindividual variability in its response; this is partly due to lesser dependence on the cytochrome P450 enzymes for metabolic activation; prasugrel is a reasonable alternative in patients with recurrent events on clopidogrel therapy.

Ticagrelor: Ticagrelor is a non-thienopyridine, directly acting oral ADP receptor antagonist that reversibly binds to the P2Y12 receptor, with a stronger and more rapid antiplatelet effect than clopidogrel. Unlike prasugrel and clopidogrel, it does not require metabolic activation, and its effect is reversed within 12–24 hours of drug discontinuation.

Glycoprotein IIb/IIIa inhibitors: These medications block the final common pathway of platelet activation and aggregation and thereby prevent platelet aggregation initiated from a variety of stimuli. Drugs which are currently available include the following: (1) Abciximab: A recombinant murine monoclonal antibody against the human GP IIb/IIIa receptor. Abciximab binds to this receptor tightly and inhibits platelet aggregation for days after the drug infusion is discontinued. (2) Eptifibatide: A cyclic peptide inhibitor with a rapid onset and short half-life (1–2.5 hours). Therefore it requires a continuous infusion for sustained response. (3) Tirofiban: A non-peptide Gp IIb/IIIa antagonist with a half-life of 4 hours.

The role of Gp IIb/IIIa inhibitors in the contemporary management of UA/NSTEMI continues to evolve. Currently, all three agents have been approved for use as adjunctive PCI therapy; however, only eptifibatide and tirofiban have been approved for use as upstream therapy. Concomitant use of aspirin and heparin is recommended with glycoprotein IIb/IIIa inhibitors. Since bleeding risk may be substantial, careful attention should be paid when using these drugs especially in patients who are at a heightened risk of bleeding (e.g. elderly, patients with renal disease, patients with small BMI, etc.).

Antithrombotic Agents

In addition to the medications that inhibit platelet activation and aggregation, medications that inhibit the coagulation cascade remain an important part of the treatment armamentarium.

Heparin

Unfractionated heparin (UFH) is the most commonly used medication in the setting of ACS. It is a glycosaminoglycan with polysaccharide side chains of varying lengths. It binds to antithrombin, which results in a conformational change in the latter, thereby inactivating factor IIa (thrombin) and Xa. In clinical practice, only one-third of a given dose of heparin binds to antithrombin. Heparin also binds to several other plasma proteins, which results in variability of dose response. Therefore, the anticoagulant effect of heparin should be closely monitored by measurement of activated partial thromboplastin time (APTT).

Low-molecular Weight Heparin

Low-molecular weight heparins (LMWH) are derived from heparin by chemical modification of the polysaccharide side chains. Enoxaparin is the most widely used LMWH in the United States. Compared to UFH, it is a more potent anti-Xa agent which inhibits generation of thrombin more effectively. Also, its greater bioavailability and lower plasma protein binding allows for a convenient subcutaneous dosing and predictable dose response and therefore does not require routine monitoring of anticoagulant effect. Anticoagulant activity of LMWH drugs cannot be reliably monitored using the APTT. Rather, it requires the measurement of anti-Xa activity and these assays are not as widely available. The standard dose of 1 mg/kg subcutaneous twice daily provides effective anticoagulant effect.

Fondaparinux

Fondaparinux is a synthetic pentasaccharide. It is an anti-Xa agent and does not have any direct effect on thrombin. This drug has predictable metabolism and can be conveniently dosed once a day by subcutaneous injection without any need for monitoring.

Direct Thrombin Inhibitors

Bivalirudin: Bivaliridin is a synthetic analog derived from hirudin. It has direct action on thrombin, and therefore differs from heparin in that it does not require a cofactor (antithrombin) for its action. It directly inactivates thrombin, including clotbound thrombin. It also does not bind any plasma proteins and therefore has predictable pharmacokinetics. It does not result in complications, such as thrombocytopenia.

Warfarin

Several studies have examined the role of warfarin in combination with aspirin in patients with ACS. More recent studies have suggested a benefit of carefully monitored oral warfarin at a goal INR of 2.0–2.5 along with aspirin in reducing the combined endpoint of death, MI or stroke. However, the contemporary role of warfarin is limited given the established role of clopidogrel in these patients particularly in those who receive PCI with a coronary stent. In the patient without a coronary stent, who may have another indication for warfarin, the combination of aspirin and warfarin may be preferable. The "triple" antithrombotic therapy (e.g. aspirin, clopidogrel and warfarin) has not been prospectively studied, and is likely to be associated with a greater risk of bleeding.

❑ EARLY INVASIVE OR INITIAL CONSERVATIVE STRATEGY

An early invasive strategy involves performing coronary angiography within the first 24–48 hours of admission with the intent of performing revascularization with PCI or CABG, as appropriate. An initial conservative strategy involves initial medical management as outlined below with coronary angiography reserved for patients who have recurrent ischemia or a high-risk stress test despite medical therapy.

The specific issues regarding PCI in patients with ACS, particularly those with NSTEMI are (i) the use of bare metal versus drug eluting stent at the time of PCI, and (ii) the timing of angiography and intervention. Existing data do not support a strategy for immediate intervention for patients with UA/NSTEMI (unlike that for STEMI). At the same time, there is no inherent benefit in delaying revascularization with PCI after a "cooling off" period.

❏ REVASCULARIZATION

Revascularization in patients with UA/NSTEMI may improve symptoms, quality of life, reduce ischemic complications or improve survival depending on the clinical circumstance. The need for revascularization depends on several factors which include patient age and more importantly functional status, serious comorbidities, expected survival, coronary anatomy, LV function and V, viability and severity of symptoms. Available alternatives for revascularization include PCI and CABG.

In general, the indications for revascularization (and for CABG vs PCI) for patients with UA/NSTEMI are similar to those in patients with stable angina, with the exception of patients who may be candidates for CABG, based on anatomy, but has urgent/emergent need for infarct-related artery (IRA) revascularization for poor TIMI flow or threatened closure of the vessel. In this instance, PCI of the IRA to stabilize the patient, with subsequent consideration of further need for revascularization, should be performed. The high-risk patients with left main (>50%) or three vessel disease, two-vessel disease with proximal LAD stenosis, diabetics with multivessel disease, and multivessel disease with LV dysfunction are better suited for CABG provided surgery can be performed with an acceptable risk (Flowchart 1).

FLOWCHART 1: Revascularization strategy in UA/NSTEMI

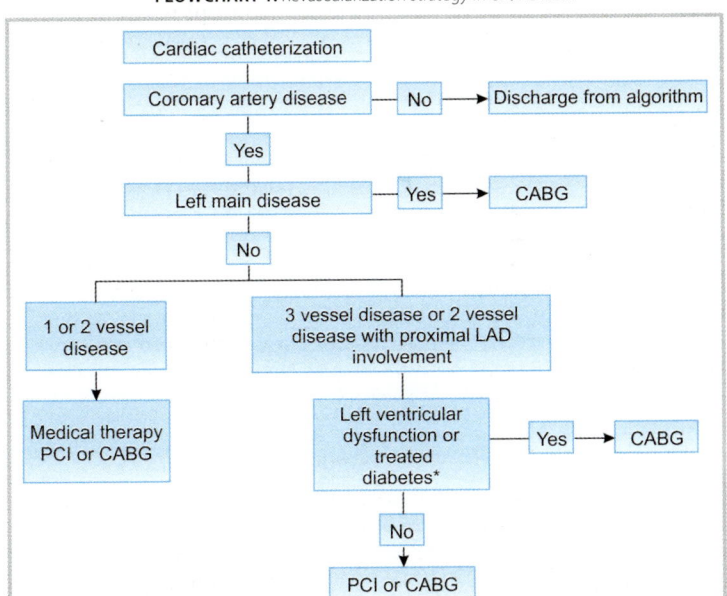

*There is conflicting information about these patients. Most consider CABG to be preferable to PCI
(*Source:* Modified from Anderson JL, Adams CD, Antman EM, et al. ACC/AHA 2007 guidelines for the management of patients with unstableangina/non ST-elevation myocardial infarction: a report of the American College of Cardiology/American Heart Association Task Force on Practice Guidelines. Circulation. 2007;116:e148-304)

❑ SUMMARY AND CONCLUSION

Over the past few years, there has been a tremendous growth in our understanding of the biology of atherosclerosis and the mechanisms that lead to ACS, one of the most dreaded consequences of coronary atherosclerosis. At the same time, important breakthroughs have emerged with development of new medications and treatment protocols that have improved patient outcomes. Diagnosis of ACS hinges on a careful assessment which includes a detailed history, physical examination, ECG and levels of cardiac biomarkers. The initial management of ACS includes initial medical stabilization with relief of pain, dual antiplatelet and antithrombotic therapy with consideration for early invasive treatment and revascularization. Revascularization should be considered in high-risk patients, and the choice of revascularization strategy and its timing depends on a patient's clinical condition, coronary anatomy and associated comorbidities.

❑ SUGGESTED READINGS

Anderson JL, Adams CD, Antman EM, et al. ACC/AHA 2007 guidelines for the management of patients with unstable angina/non ST-elevation myocardial infarction: a report of the American College of Cardiology/American Heart Association Task Force on Practice Guidelines (Writing Committee to Revise the 2002 Guidelines for the Management of Patients With Unstable Angina/Non ST-Elevation Myocardial Infarction): developed in collaboration with the American College of Emergency Physicians, the Society for Cardiovascular Angiography and Interventions, and the Society of Thoracic Surgeons: endorsed by the American Association of Cardiovascular and Pulmonary Rehabilitation and the Society for Academic Emergency Medicine. Circulation. 2007;116:e148-304.

Kushner FG, Hand M, Smith SC, et al. 2009 Focused Updates: ACC/ AHA Guidelines for the Management of Patients With ST-Elevation Myocardial Infarction (Updating the 2004 Guideline and 2007 Focused Update) and ACC/AHA/SCAI Guidelines on Percutaneous Coronary Intervention (Updating the 2005 Guideline and 2007 Focused Update): a report of the American College of Cardiology Foundation/American Heart Association Task Force on Practice Guidelines. J Am Coll Cardiol. 2009;54:2205-41.

Kushner FG, Hand M, Smith SC, et al. 2009 Focused Updates: ACC/ AHA Guidelines for the Management of Patients With ST-Elevation Myocardial Infarction (Updating the 2004 Guideline and 2007 Focused Update) and ACC/AHA/SCAI Guidelines on Percutaneous Coronary Intervention (Updating the 2005 Guideline and 2007 Focused Update): a report of the American College of Cardiology Foundation/American Heart Association Task Force on Practice Guidelines. J Am Coll Cardiol. 2009;54:2205-41.

Lloyd-Jones D, Adams RJ, Brown TM, et al. Heart disease and stroke statistics—2010 update: a report from the American Heart Association. Circulation. 2010;121:e46-215.

Naghavi M, Libby P, Falk E, et al. From vulnerable plaque to vulnerable patient: a call for new definitions and risk assessment strategies: Part II. Circulation. 2003;108:1772-8.

Patrono C, Baigent C, Hirsh J, et al. Antiplatelet drugs: American College of Chest Physicians Evidence-Based Clinical Practice Guidelines (8th Edition). Chest. 2008;133:199S-233S.

Smith SC, Feldman TE, Hirshfeld JW, et al. ACC/AHA/SCAI 2005 Guideline Update for Percutaneous Coronary Intervention: a report of the American College of Cardiology/American Heart Association Task Force on Practice Guidelines (ACC/AHA/SCAI Writing Committee to Update the 2001 Guidelines for Percutaneous Coronary Intervention). J Am Coll Cardiol. 2006;47:e1-121.

Smith SC, Feldman TE, Hirshfeld JW, et al. ACC/AHA/SCAI 2005 Guideline Update for Percutaneous Coronary Intervention: a report of the American College of Cardiology/American Heart Association Task Force on Practice Guidelines (ACC/AHA/SCAI Writing Committee to Update the 2001 Guidelines for Percutaneous Coronary Intervention). J Am Coll Cardiol. 2006;47:e1-121.

Wright RS, Anderson JL, Adams CD, et al. 2011 ACCF/AHA Focused Update of the Guidelines for the Management of Patients With Unstable Angina/Non-ST-Elevation Myocardial Infarction (Updating the 2007 Guideline): a report of the American College of Cardiology Foundation/American Heart Association Task Force on Practice Guidelines. Circulation. 2011

4.3 Acute Coronary Syndrome II (ST-Elevation, Myocardial Infarction, and Post-Myocardial Infarction): Complications and Care

❏ INTRODUCTION

ST-elevation myocardial infarction (STEMI) is a life-threatening event and a true medical emergency. The risk of morbidity and mortality associated with STEMI increases with greater amount of myocardium at risk, delay in reperfusion, lack of collaterals to the infarct related artery (IRA), previous cardiovascular disease comorbidities (e.g. diabetes, renal failure, etc.) and abnormal thrombolysis in myocardial infarction (TIMI) flow postreperfusion. The time from onset of symptoms to reperfusion is an extremely important factor on overall mortality. The success of restoration of normal flow in the IRA after primary percutaneous intervention was directly related to the ischemic time (i.e. symptom onset to initial balloon).

❏ CLINICAL PRESENTATION

Patients with diagnosis of STEMI will present with symptoms consistent with ACS. Those with STEMI, though, have a higher likelihood of early complications, including hemodynamic instability and shock, atrial and ventricular dysrhythmias and sudden cardiac death. Therefore, early evaluation, including prehospital evaluation and timely determination of optimal reperfusion is essential.

Prehospital Assessment

The advent of systems that allow for high quality digital transmission of a 12-lead electrocardiogram (ECG) from the field facilitates early recognition of STEMI and infield treatment, including thrombolysis. When a STEMI patient is to be transported to a facility with capability to perform primary angioplasty [percutaneous coronary intervention (PCI) center], activation of the cardiac catheterization laboratory team while the patient is in the field, decreases time to reperfusion, and improves likelihood of TIMI III flow in the IRA.

Emergency Room Evaluation

It is expected that when a patient presents to a facility with chest pain, or other symptoms consistent with MI, that an ECG be performed and read by a qualified physician as soon as possible, but always within 10 minutes of arriving at that facility. If the electrocardiogram (ECG) is not diagnostic but the clinical scenario is consistent, the ECG must be repeated in no more than 10 minutes to assess for changes or evolution. If EKG is consistent with a STEMI, then reperfusion must be the primary focus. A brief and rapid clinical evaluation must be performed.

Electrocardiogram

The ECG is the essential tool in the assessment and risk stratification of patients presenting with chest pain. The presence of ST-elevation on ECG denotes STEMI in greater than 80% of patients and can assist in the localization of the MI. It must be recognized that the clinical picture is very important in determining etiology of

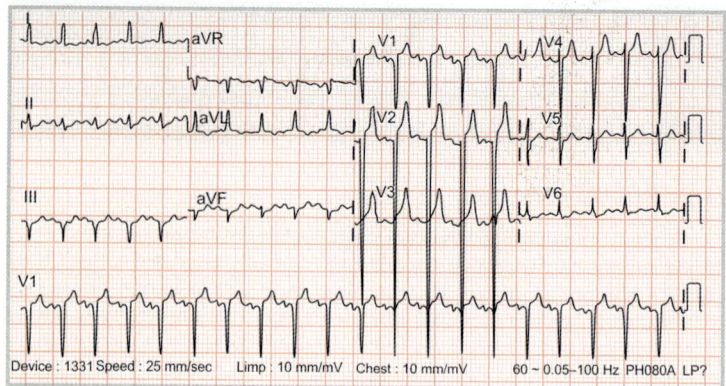

FIGURE 3: A 65-year-old patient who was in hospital undergoing evaluation for chest discomfort, developed recurrent chest pain and ECG was done within minutes. Patient has baseline j-point elevation in the anterior precordium likely due to LVH, but T waves are markedly different from previous and are tall and peaked consistent with hyperacute T waves. Note also the beginnings of subtle ST abnormalities in the inferior and lateral leads (V6 and aVF). Patient was taken to cardiac catheterization lab and had a thrombotic occlusion of the proximal left anterior descending (LAD) coronary artery

the ST-elevation, particularly when the ECG is not classic for STEMI (shape of ST segments, lack of reciprocal changes, etc.).

The first change in the ECG that occurs during vessel occlusion is upright, peaked and symmetric T waves (commonly referred to as hyperacute). The duration of this change, in the presence of persistent occlusion, is short (in minutes) and, therefore, is rarely seen clinically. If present, subtle reciprocal abnormalities may be seen increasing the suspicion for acute myocardial infarction (AMI) (Fig. 3). The subsequent evolution is to the development of ST-elevation. The shape of the ST-segment (coving or straightening of the segment compared to a normal concave upward segment), and the presence of reciprocal changes (ST-depressions) in the leads opposite the ST-elevation are strongly supportive of STEMI as the etiology of the ST-elevation.

Persistent ST elevation and the development of Q waves in the infarcted territory signals significant myocardial necrosis. ST-elevations that persist for days to weeks may signal the development of a ventricular aneurysm, defining nonviable myocardium. The lack of Q waves is in general a testament to early reperfusion and myocardial salvage.

Other Early Diagnostic Evaluation

Further evaluation with laboratory studies, portable chest X-ray, echocardiography, etc. should be done, if they do not delay reperfusion and if there is a clear clinical indication (evaluation for aortic dissection, etc.). Laboratory studies sent on arrival to the emergency room are helpful in assessing electrolytes (particularly potassium), renal function, hemoglobin, platelets and coagulation status. Urine toxicology screen should be considered on all patients, particularly those with few or no risk factors for CAD; this can be done after reperfusion. Biomarkers should be sent, but the reader must remember that elevation in the biomarker takes time and a normal initial troponin in a patient with is quite common. A bedside echocardiogram is helpful in patients in which the diagnosis is unclear or there is concern that anterior ST-depressions are a marker of posterior wall infarction.

❏ REPERFUSION

Reperfusion is the primary treatment of patients who present with STEMI. Medical therapy should be instituted as a reperfusion strategy is being put in place. The decision to perform primary PCI or administer a thrombolytic agent must be made and carried out rapidly in order to salvage as much myocardium as possible and, therefore, prevent morbidity and mortality. The standard of care is D2B (patient arrival to first balloon inflation in the catheterization laboratory) of less than 90 minutes and door to needle (patient arrival to administration of thrombolytic agent) of less than 30 minutes. Again, although these times are standards of care, the physician must aim for these times to be as low as is possible.

Thrombolysis

Available thrombolytics approved for use in STEMI have included: streptokinase, alteplase, reteplase and tenecteplase (TNK).
1. Streptokinase binds to plasminogen creating an active complex and thereby facilitates the transformation of plasminogen to plasmin resulting in fibrinolysis and proteolysis. It is therefore not specific to fibrin cleavage. It is antigenic and although significant allergic reactions are rare, repeat administration, even years after initial administration, increases the risk of serious allergic reaction.
2. Alteplase is fibrin specific (does not have proteolytic effects) and the bound alteplase or fibrin compound has a high affinity for plasminogen. It does not have the side effect of hypotension, and allergic reactions are rare. The half-life is short (3–4 minutes). The use of IV heparin with alteplase during STEMI results in increased patency and less reocclusion.
3. Reteplase is a recombinant plasminogen activator (rPA) that has less affinity for fibrin and a longer half-life than alteplase.
4. Tenecteplase (TNK-tPA) is a genetically engineered plasminogen activator. The half-life is longer allowing for single bolus dosing, which is advantageous in STEMI. In addition, it has less clinical intracranial bleeding than alteplase, though has been shown to have equal efficacy with respect to major adverse cardiac endpoints. Comparison and contrast of these four agents are provided in Table 8.

Facilitated Percutaneous Coronary Intervention

Facilitated percutaneous coronary intervention (PCI) (upstream administration of partial dose GpIIb/IIIa inhibitor or full or partial dose thrombolytic or a combination thereof with plan for emergent PCI), in ambulance or at a non-PCI center prior to transfer for planned immediate PCI, has not been shown to improve mortality and in many instances led to increased morbidity (increased need for revascularization, increased reinfarction rates, and increased major bleeding complications).

Full Dose Thrombolytic Agent

Full dose thrombolytic as primary reperfusion therapy has been shown to improve mortality in patients with STEMI, compared to standard medical therapy. Given the cost difference between streptokinase and t-PA and this apparent small benefit,

Table 8: Comparison of approved thrombolytic agents

	Streptokinase	Alteplase	Reteplase	Tenecteplase
Dose	1.5 MU over 30–60 minutes	Up to 100 mg in 90 minutes (weight based)	10 U × 2 each 30–50 mg over 2 minutes	Weight based
Bolus administration	No	No	Yes	Yes
Antigenic	Yes	No	No	No
Allergic reactions	Yes (hypotension)	No	No	No
Systemic fibrinogen depletion	Marked	Mild	Moderate	Minimal
~ 90 minutes patency rate	50%	75%	75%	75%
%TIMI 3 flow at 90 minutes	32	54	60	63
Approximate cost per dose (2004)	$613	$2974	$2750	$2833 for 50 mg (US$)

(*Source:* ACC/AHA guidelines for the management of patients with ST-elevation myocardial infarction. Circulation. 2004;110:588-636)

this study launched significant discussion regarding the cost or benefit of the use of accelerated t-PA over streptokinase, the financial impact this would have on hospitals, particularly smaller hospitals. Established contraindications are noted in Table 9.

Clinically, reperfusion after administration of thrombolytic is demonstrated when the patient has some or all of the following characteristics: resolution of ischemic symptoms, improvement in ST elevation by at least 50% and the presence of a notable reperfusion rhythm (accelerated idioventricular rhythm). Angiographically, reperfusion is noted with reestablishment of TIMI 3 (normal) flow in the IRA. Angiographically, failure of thrombolysis occurs in nearly 40% of patients treated with thrombolytics. Therefore, if reperfusion does not occur, it is essential that this be recognized and continued efforts to attain normal flow in the IRA be instituted. Rescue PCI is superior to both conservative medical therapy and repeat thrombolysis in patients who fail thrombolysis (with failure defined as reduction of <50% of the ST elevation at 90 minutes).

Elective Angiography and PCI after Successful Thrombolysis

In patients with apparent reperfusion after thrombolysis for STEMI, the consideration of invasive angiography and revascularization is based on the clinical features of the patient. Patients who develop recurrent ischemic symptoms or threatened reocclusion of the vessel have an increased mortality both at 30 days and at 2 years. During hospitalization PCI has been shown to decrease recurrent MI and 2-year mortality. Patients who develop shock, severe CHF, including pulmonary edema, or hemodynamically significant ventricular dysrhythmias during hospitalization should be considered for invasive angiography, and revascularization by PCI or coronary artery bypass grafting as appropriate. The issue of late (24 hours to 30 days) elective PCI of a persistently occluded IRA has been addressed. There is no data to suggest a benefit of this approach, in absence of symptoms.

Table 9: Contraindications and cautions for fibrinolysis in ST-elevation myocardial infarction

Absolute contraindications
- Any prior ICH
- Known structural cerebral vascular lesion (e.g. arteriovenous malformation)
- Known malignant intracranial neoplasm (primary or metastatic)
- Ischemic stroke within 3 months
- Suspected aortic dissection
- Active bleeding or bleeding diathesis (excluding menses)
- Significant closed-head or facial trauma within 3 months

Relative contraindications
- History of chronic, severe, poorly controlled hypertension
- Severe uncontrolled hypertension on presentation (SBP >180 mm Hg or DBP >110 mm Hg)†
- History of prior ischemic stroke greater than 3 months
- History of dementia, or known intracranial pathology not covered in contraindications
- Traumatic or prolonged (>10 minutes) CPR or major surgery (<3 weeks)
- Recent (within 2–4 weeks) internal bleeding
- Noncompressible vascular punctures
- For streptokinase: prior exposure (>5 days ago) or prior allergic reaction to these agents
- Pregnancy
- Active peptic ulcer
- Current use of anticoagulants: the higher the INR, the higher the risk of bleeding

(Abbriviations: ICH: Intracranial Hemorrhage; SBP: Systolic Blood Pressure; DBP: Diastolic Blood Pressure; CPR: Cardiopulmonary Resuscitation; INR: International Normalized Ratio; MI: Myocardial Infarction)

†Could be an absolute contraindication in low-risk patients with MI

(*Source:* Modified from ACC/AHA guidelines for the management of patients with ST-elevation myocardial infarction. Circulation. 2004;110: 588-636)

Primary Coronary Intervention

Reperfusion (vessel patency) can be accomplished at higher rates with primary coronary intervention than with thrombolysis in patients presenting with STEMI. Studies have shown that the majority of patients are candidates for this reperfusion strategy, and it is superior to full dose thrombolysis with statistically significant decrease in rates of death, nonfatal MI and stroke. Patients who have cardiogenic shock have the greatest benefit from primary coronary intervention versus thrombolysis.

❏ EARLY MEDICAL THERAPY

General Measures

As reperfusion therapy is being arranged, medical therapy must be initiated; this medical therapy mirrors that has been discussed for UA/NSTEMI in the section "Acute Coronary Syndrome I: Unstable Angina and Non-ST Segment Elevation Myocardial Infarction" in this chapter. Oxygen should be administered. Patients should be placed on continuous telemetry and all transport must be monitored with a defibrillator and emergency medications immediately available. As soon as STEMI is diagnosed, in a PCI center, preparation must be made for emergency transport into the cardiac catheterization laboratory.

Nitrates

In order to decrease the vasoconstriction, which is associated with STEMI, nitroglycerin (SL and IV as necessary) should be given. Care should be taken in the STEMI patient as abrupt changes in hemodynamics may occur.

Morphine

Morphine can serve as analgesia and thereby decreases the generalized anxiety and apprehension that is common in STEMI patients. One must be aware of the potential for hypotension associated with morphine dosing. Morphine will also have a positive effect on patients presenting with STEMI and pulmonary edema to decrease venous return and improve respiratory status.

Antiplatelet Agents

If not already given, the patient must receive aspirin therapy at a dose of 162–325 mg, chewed. The importance of aspirin cannot be underestimated, and therefore, if the physician is not certain that aspirin has been taken by the patient at home, or was given in the ambulance, it should be given without delay.

Thienopyridines are effective in decreasing MACE in patients presenting with STEMI as is seen in patients with UA/NSTEMI, and it is recommended to administer clopidogrel at arrival to all STEMI patients who are 75 years old or younger.

Unlike in the UA/NSTEMI patient, the benefit of upstream glycoprotein IIb/IIIA inhibitors has not definitively been demonstrated. These may be useful as adjunctive therapy during primary PCI for STEMI, although the most recent studies in which patients received dual oral antiplatelet therapy are small and fail to show a significant benefit.

Anticoagulation

Anticoagulation therapy should be administered in all STEMI patients who are without absolute contraindication. The choice of anticoagulant may be, in part, based on the reperfusion strategy, but in all cases full systemic anticoagulation with either unfractionated heparin or low molecular weight heparin or bivalirudin is beneficial. Anticoagulation should continue for 48 hours in patients treated with thrombolysis. In patients who undergo primary PCI, anticoagulation may be discontinued after the procedure, unless there is another indication (i.e. intra-aortic balloon pump, LV thrombus, mechanical valve, etc.).

Beta Blockers

Beta blockers should be given orally, with reservation of IV beta blockade for hypertensive or tachycardic patients with ongoing chest pain. Intravenous beta blockade should be avoided in patients at high risk for cardiogenic shock, those with systolic blood pressures below 105 mm Hg, and those who are more than 75 years old, due to a higher risk of hypotension and increased mortality.

❏ POSTMYOCARDIAL INFARCTION CARE

Assessment of Left Ventricular Ejection Fraction

All patients following an MI must have assessment of LV ejection fraction (LVEF). This not only guides medical therapy but also provides prognostic information. It has long been known that decreased LVEF post-MI and increased end systolic volume are markers for increased risk of development of CHF and death. Abnormal LVEF (<40%) portends an overall poor prognosis in the post-MI patient.

The choice of imaging modalities available today to assess EF include left ventriculography, transthoracic echocardiography, radionuclide imaging, CT and magnetic resonance imaging (MRI). Echocardiography offers the ability not only to assess the LVEF but also to assess for wall motion abnormalities in all territories, detects LV thrombus, ventricular septal defect, noninvasive estimate of pulmonary artery pressures, RV systolic function, pericardial effusion and importantly to assess for preexisting or post MI valvular abnormalities.

Stress Testing Prior to Discharge

Stress testing should be considered to assess areas of at-risk myocardium in the patient who has received successful thrombolysis, who presented late with presumed completed infarct and did not receive reperfusion therapy, who presented with ACS non-STEMI who has been chosen for a conservative medical therapy approach and in the patient who has an indeterminate lesion noted on coronary angiography during the index hospitalization. The choice of stress testing includes exercise treadmill testing with or without imaging (echocardiography or nuclear perfusion) or chemical stress testing with dobutamine or dipyridamole/adenosine/regadenosine (depending on the institutional practice) with echocardiography or nuclear perfusion.

Coronary Angiography and Revascularization

In patients who have not undergone early angiography, the need for angiography and possible intervention prior to discharge must be addressed. The potential contraindications should be evaluated and considered, including the patient's willingness to consent to both coronary angiography and potential revascularization. If no absolute or limiting relative contraindications exist, the following patients should be considered appropriate. In patients who present without STEMI, if any high-risk feature is identified on presentation, including accelerated or rest anginal symptoms, evidence of heart failure or hemodynamic instability, dynamic ECG changes or positive biomarkers for MI, one should strongly consider coronary angiography. In patients who have recurrent ischemic symptoms in hospital, particularly those who have angina at rest or are refractory to medical therapy, or those with post-infarction angina, coronary angiography is indicated. Patients with a decrease in EF or those with evidence of heart failure during hospitalization should undergo angiography.

Patients, who require revascularization, should undergo this without avoidable delay. The exception to this is in the patient who requires nonurgent CABG who has been given clopidogrel or prasugrel, who has acutely reversible renal failure, and who has had STEMI in which consideration of 3–7 days delay to CABG is recommended. There is an increase in hospital mortality early after MI in patients undergoing CABG with mortality rates of 11.8% if within 6 hours, 9.5% between 6 hours and 1 day and 2.8% after 1 day. The physician should recognize that although the bleeding risk in patients on clopidogrel and prasugrel is increased, there is no data to suggest that aspirin should be held at the time of CABG. As a matter of fact administration of aspirin in the patient's undergoing CABG is a Class I indication. Therefore, aspirin should be continued without interruption in all patients undergoing CABG.

❑ COMPLICATIONS

Right Ventricular Infarction

The involvement of the right ventricle in patients presenting with inferior wall STEMI portends a poor prognosis. Data suggest that in hospital mortality is increased from 5% (without RV infarct) to 31% (with RV infarct). In addition, the major complications of cardiogenic shock, high-grade AV block (both transient and requiring permanent pacemaker placement) and ventricular dysrhythmias, increased from 28% to 64% respectively.

Heart Failure or Cardiogenic Shock and Mechanical Complications after A Myocardial Infarction

The incidence of heart failure and frank shock is increased in patients presenting with STEMI, but is certainly a complication of NSTEMI as well. Patients with heart failure should have aggressive treatment of ischemia or infarct. As already described, patients with cardiogenic shock achieve greater benefit with primary PCI compared to thrombolysis. Assessment of LVEF early in treatment is necessary to determine if the clinical heart failure is secondary to systolic or diastolic dysfunction and to guide both medical and revascularization therapy.

Supplemental oxygen, morphine, nitrates and diuresis may improve symptomatic pulmonary edema. Beta blockers should be avoided early in acute heart failure complicating MI. The use of a pulmonary artery catheter may help guide medical therapy. An IABP may be necessary in patients with refractory heart failure or shock.

Dysrhythmias

In the early phase of STEMI (first 24–48 hours), ventricular dysrhythmias can occur related to the ischemic event. The patient should be supported during this time with the main goal being reperfusion, normalization of electrolytes and treatment of any heart failure. Cardioversion should be performed if the patient has ventricular fibrillation (VF), sustained and hemodynamically significant ventricular tachycardia (VT), or VT associated with angina or pulmonary edema. Recurrence may require antiarrhythmic therapy with IV amiodarone or IABP placement. The reader should recognize the benefit of IABP for the treatment of refractory ventricular dysrhythmias, particularly with patients with inferior MI (with or without RV infarction), bradycardia, and heart block may complicate the MI and require permanent pacemaker placement. Transient bradycardia or heart block should be treated supportively, and may require short-term temporary transvenous pacemaker placement if hemodynamically significant.

Recurrent Chest Discomfort

Recurrent ischemia or infarction must always be a consideration. The ECG evaluation during symptoms and monitoring of cardiac biomarkers of necrosis should be used for diagnosis of recurrent ischemia or reinfarction. Unfortunately, each of these presents a difficulty. Not uncommonly patients have a persistently abnormal ECG, or an ECG consistent with evolution of infarct, limiting the ability to confidently assess for acute or dynamic changes. In addition, the longer half-life of troponin prevents accurate determination of reinfarction in the first 10–14 days after MI; therefore, creatine kinase (CK and CK MB), which rises and falls more rapidly may be needed. Stress testing may be appropriate, if not of the American College of Cardiology Foundation/American Heart Association Task Force on Practice Guidelines. Circulation. 2009;120:2271-306.

Lloyd-Jones D, Adams RJ, Brown TM, et al. Heart disease and stroke statistics-2010 update: a report from the American Heart Association.Circulation. 2010;121:e46-215.

National Heart lung and Blood Institute. (2003).The Seventh Report of the Joint National Committee on Prevention, Detection, Evaluation, and Treatment of High Blood Pressure (JNC 7). [online] NHLBI website. Available from http://www.nhlbi.nih.gov/guidelines/hypertension/.

Wright RS, Anderson JL, Adams CD, et al. 2011 ACCF/AHA Focused Update of the Guidelines for the Management of Patients with Unstable Angina/Non-ST-Elevation Myocardial Infarction (Updating the 2007 Guideline). J Am Coll Cardiol. 2011;57:1920-59.

4.4 Management of Patients with Coronary Artery Disease and Stable Angina

❏ INTRODUCTION

Ischemic heart disease (IHD), usually due to underling coronary artery disease (CAD), remains the leading cause of mortality in the United States and in developed countries. In many patients with IHD, stable angina seems to be the initial clinical manifestation. Additionally, many patients who survive a nonfatal acute coronary syndrome (ACS), such as unstable angina or an acute myocardial infarction (MI), go onto experience anginal symptoms after such an acute event. Stable angina is important not only because of its high prevalence, but also because of its associated morbidity and mortality.

There two major goals of therapy in patients with chronic stable angina: relief of symptoms and reduction in cardiac morbidity and mortality. There are multiple medical and revascularization modalities available for treatment of anginal symptoms; however, recent data suggest that current therapies are not universally effective in controlling symptoms and most do not reduce cardiovascular events.

❏ CURRENT THERAPEUTIC APPROACHES FOR STABLE ANGINA

There are multiple therapeutic modalities currently available for treatment of anginal symptoms in patients with stable CAD. These include antianginal drugs and myocardial revascularization procedures. Until recently, the antianginal drug therapy primarily consisted of nitrates, beta-blockers and calcium channel blockers (CCB). Although antianginal drug therapy is effective in most patients, it is not infrequent that many patients are subjected to percutaneous or surgical revascularization.

❏ ANTIANGINAL DRUG THERAPY

Several antianginal agents primarily nitrates, beta-blockers and CCB (Table 10) have been used in the management of symptoms in patients with chronic CAD and stable angina pectoris. Although these drugs have been found to be effective antianginal agents, there is lack of data on the effect of such therapies on clinical for secondary prevention. Outpatient cardiac rehabilitation, also known as phase II, is a standard of care following MI, PCI, CABG surgery, valve surgery, heart transplant, and for those with stable angina.

Predischarge Education

Education must occur before discharge regarding importance of recurrence of symptoms, diet, exercise, smoking cessation, medication compliance and continuing cardiac rehabilitation as an outpatient. The patient must have a follow-up appointment scheduled prior to discharge. The timing of this appointment depends on the medical stability of the patient and can vary 1–6 weeks after discharge.

❑ SUMMARY

In summary, STEMI is a life-threatening event and a true medical emergency. It is important that physicians and patients alike recognize that time is muscle. At the time of arrival, the team must be prepared to rapidly evaluate the patient and make quick decisions regarding reperfusion. Protocols should be in place, and routinely reviewed, as this is an area of medicine where we as clinicians can make a great difference in the outcome of these patients. Recommendations should include lifestyle modification (diet, physical activity, smoking cessation), and medications to treat hypertension, hyperlipidemia, diabetes as well as the sequelae of the current insult (heart failure). Finally, we must prepare our patients to adapt to this changing event. Cardiac rehabilitation program is an important multidisciplinary intervention focused on exercise training, and lifestyle modification that can have a significant impact in returning patients back to a normal life and positively impact their outcomes.

❑ SUGGESTED READINGS

ACC ACC/AHA guidelines for the management of patients with STelevation myocardial infarction—executive summary: a report of the American College of Cardiology/American Heart Association Task Force on Practice Guidelines (Writing Committee to Revise the 1999 Guidelines for the Management of Patients with Acute Myocardial Infarction). Circulation. 2004;110:588-636.

Anderson JL, Adams CD, Antman EM, et al. ACC/AHA 2007 Guidelines of the Management of Patients with Unstable Angina/ Non-ST-Elevation Myocardial Infarction. A report of the American College of Cardiology/American Heart Association Task Force on Practice Guidelines (Writing Committee to Revise the 2002 Guidelines for the Management of Patients with Unstable Angina/ Non-ST-Elevation Myocardial Infarction). Circulation. 2007;116:e148-304.

Antman EM, Hand M, Armstrong PW, et al. 2007 Focused Update of the ACC/AHA 2004 Guidelines for the Management of Patients with ST-Elevation Myocardial Infarction. American College of Cardiology/American Heart Association Task Force on Practice Guidelines. Circulation. 2008;117:296-329.

Field JM, Hazinski MF, Sayre MR, et al. 2010 American Heart Association Guidelines for Cardiopulmonary Resuscitation and Emergency Cardiovascular Care Science. Circulation. 2010;122:S639-933.

Grundy SM, Cleeman JI, Merz CN, et al. Implications of recent clinical trials for the National Cholesterol Education Program Adult Treatment Panel III guidelines. Circulation. 2004;110:227-39.

Kushner FG, Hand M, Smith SC, et al. 2009 Focused Updates: ACC/ AHA Guidelines for the Management of Patients with ST-Elevation Myocardial Infarction (Updating the 2004 Guideline and 2007 Focused Update) and ACC/AHA/SCAI Guidelines on Percutaneous Coronary Intervention (Updating the 2005 Guideline and 2007 Focused Update): a report than 140/90 (with more stringent goal of <130/80 blood pressure in patients with diabetes mellitus or chronic kidney disease).

The use of an aldosterone antagonist has been well established in heart failure and has been shown to improve mortality and morbidity in patients who have had an AMI complicated by LV systolic dysfunction and heart failure.

Lipid Management

A majority of CAD patients are not able to either follow stringent diets or intense physical exercise regimens and are unable to attain their lipid goal with these lifestyle changes alone. Patients with recent ACS have the lowest target LDL, at less than 70 mg/dL, which is extremely difficult to achieve for most of the patients, without medications. Lipid lowering with 3-hydroxy-3-methyl-glutaryl-coenzyme A (HMG CoA) reductase inhibitors (statins) prevents cardiovascular events both primarily (prior to first event) and secondarily (after diagnosis of atherosclerotic cardiovascular disease).

It is recommended that a statin medication be initiated in patients who have no contraindication, early after the diagnosis of ACS (as early as day 1), and no later than at the time of discharge. Niacin has been shown to decrease the risk of recurrent nonfatal MI in patients with a previous history of MI, and is a consideration in the statin intolerant patient. Omega 3 fatty acids are beneficial in lowering triglycerides and thus raising HDL, both as an increase in dietary intake and as a supplement. The supplemental use of omega 3 fatty acids has been shown to prevent sudden cardiac death in patients with previous MI.

Smoking Cessation

Continued tobacco smoking in patients with CAD significantly increases the risk of reinfarcton and death. Compliance with smoking cessation increases when initiated at the time of an event (MI or CABG). Smoking cessation decreased the relative risk of mortality by 36% and significantly decreased the risk of nonfatal cardiac events, in a meta-analysis of studies performed in patients with previous cardiovascular events. The addition of pharmacotherapy to counseling is beneficial. Adding nicotine replacement therapy has been shown to increase the likelihood of cessation. Bupropion is at least as effective as nicotine replacement therapy in smoking cessation.

Cardiac Rehabilitation and Secondary Prevention of Coronary Heart Disease for Patients with Myocardial Infarction

Over the past two decades, there has been tremendous progress in pharmacological therapies, sophisticated technology-based diagnostic and therapeutic procedures for the treatment of cardiovascular diseases. Cardiac rehabilitation is a very important (and underutilized) multidisciplinary intervention that provides comprehensive services focused on exercise training and important lifestyle modifications for a patient with cardiovascular disease. It helps limit the functional and psychological impact of the illness and prevent future events.

Cardiac rehabilitation can begin as soon as an eligible inpatient stabilizes after AMI, PCI, CABG surgery, valve surgery, heart transplant or acute coronary syndrome. Inpatient rehabilitation, known as phase I, is intended to prevent deconditioning from hospitalization, ready the patient for referral to an outpatient cardiac rehabilitation program, assess for activity tolerance, prescribe activity for the period immediately following hospital discharge, and begin patient teaching previously performed and repetition of coronary angiography may be necessary to assess patency of stented vessels.

Post MI pericarditis may occur early after MI (within the first 4 days) or late, generally after discharge (Dressler's syndrome). It is diagnosed by characteristic pain, a pericardial rub on auscultation, ECG changes (which may be obscured in the early post MI period), presence of a small effusion on echocardiography and improvement with anti-inflammatory agents.

❑ SPECIAL CONSIDERATIONS

Diabetes

The diabetic population is unique with respect to ACS and have been shown to have worse short-term and long-term outcomes after an MI compared to non-diabetics. It is also known that they require more aggressive efforts at primary and secondary prevention. In addition, hyperglycemia during hospitalization has been associated with worse outcomes. Although the 2004 guidelines recommended aggressive glucose control with IV insulin to normalize blood glucose as a class I indication, that recommendation has been downgraded to a class II indication based on a recent study showing higher mortality in aggressively treated patients.

Women

In general, women present with ACS at an older age than men and have the potential to have a more atypical presentation. They should be treated in similar manner to their male counterparts in the setting of ACS. Many of the early trials for ACS did not include a significant percentage of women. Due to the smaller body size of women, there may be increased risk of bleeding with standard dosing of antiplatelet medications and anticoagulants. This should be considered when treating the female patient.

Elderly

Patients should not have care withheld or altered based on age alone. The recommendations made in this chapter and in the guidelines, in certain areas, are based on data from studies that suggested either a decreased benefit or an increased risk in patients who are elderly.

❑ CONTINUED MEDICAL THERAPY FOR PATIENTS WITH A MYOCARDIAL INFARCTION

Inhibition of the Renin–angiotensin–aldosterone Axis

Angiotensin-converting enzyme (ACE) inhibitors have been thoroughly studied in patients with heart failure. The data show that they are indicated and beneficial in patients post-MI who have a decreased LV systolic function (defined as LVEF >40%), or who have chronic kidney disease, diabetes or hypertension. The guidelines recommend against the routine use of IV ACE inhibitors, except in refractory hypertension.

Angiotensin receptor blockers should be considered in patients who are intolerant to ACE inhibitors (i.e. cough, angioedema, etc.) and have either a decrease in LVEF or who have hypertension requiring treatment, or as a primary option (versus ACE inhibitors) in these patients. The goal of blood pressure is less

Table 10: Pharmacologic actions of antianginal drugs					
Class	Heart rate	Arterial pressure	Venous return	Myocardial contractility	Coronary flow
β-blockers	↓	↓	↔	↓	↔
DHP CCB	↑*	↓	↔	↓	↑
Non-DHP CCB	↓	↓	↔	↓	↑
Long acting nitrates	↑/↔	↓	↓	↔	↑
Ranolazine†	↔	↔	↔	↔	↔

*Except amlodipine
†Late Na^+ channel blocker
(Abbreviations: ↓: Decrease, ↔: No effect; ↑: Increase

outcomes including MI and death in patients with chronic CAD and stable angina.

Nitrates

Nitrates exert their beneficial effects primarily by venodilatation resulting in venous pooling of blood, which reduces ventricular volume and cardiac work and chamber size. Nitrates are also systemic as well as coronary arterial vasodilators; however, to what extent these effects account for their antianginal efficacy is not well established (except in patients with coronary artery spasm). It is well established that sublingual nitroglycerine is the most effective therapy for relief of anginal symptoms and all patients with anginal symptoms should be given sublingual nitroglycerin. The long acting nitrates are often prescribed as prophylactic antianginal drugs. However, because of the problem of nitrate tolerance during long-term therapy, it is essential to use eccentric dosing scheme which provides a minimum of 10–12 hours nitrate free interval. Some of the important side effects/limitations of nitrates and other antianginal drugs in the treatment of stable angina are shown in Table 11.

Beta-blockers

Beta-blockers have been found to be effective antianginal therapy by increasing exercise tolerance and decreasing the frequency and severity of anginal episodes. Beta-blockers exert their effects through a reduction in myocardial oxygen demand which includes a decrease in ventricular inotropy, decreased heart rate and a decrease in the maximal velocity of myocardial fiber shortening. Therapy with beta-blockers has been associated with a reduced risk of death (sudden and nonsudden) and reduced risk of MI in patients who survived an acute MI. Table 11 illustrates some of the limitations/side effects of beta-blocker therapy in the treatment of stable angina.

Calcium Channel Blockers

Calcium channel blockers (CCB) are potent coronary and systemic arterial vasodilators, and these agents reduce blood pressure as well as cardiac contractility. CCBs have been shown to increase coronary blood flow and are highly effective antianginal agents in patients with coronary artery spasm. CCBs have become popular in treatment of patients with angina primarily because of the relatively lower incidence of side effects. The important side effects and limitation of CCB are shown in Table 11.

Table 11: Side effects, precautions, and contraindications of antianginal drugs

	Beta-blockers	Nitrates	Calcium channel blockers	Ranolazine
Side effects	• Hypotension • Syncope • Sexual dysfunction • Fatigue • Depression	• Hypotension • Syncope • Headache • Tolerance	• Hypotension • Flushing • Dizziness • Edema • Fatigue	• Dizziness • Headache • Constipation • Nausea
Precautions/contra-indications	• Bradycardia • AV conduction problems • Sick sinus syndrome • Peripheral vascular disease • COPD	• Left ventricular outflow tract obstruction • Erectile dysfunction (concomitant use of PDE5 inhibitors)	• Bradycardia • AV conduction problems • Sick sinus syndrome • Heart failure • LV dysfunction	• Use with QT prolonging • Drugs • Significant liver disease • Contraindicated with strong CYP3A4 inhibitors (ketoconazole, clarithromycin, or nelfinavir) and CYP3A inducers (rifampin, phenobarb)

❑ NEWER ANTIANGINAL DRUGS

Although there has been lack of development of newer antianginal drugs during the past 25 years, recently several new drugs with unique mechanism of action have been introduced for treatment of patients with stable angina.

Ranolazine

Ranolazine is the newest drug recently approved by the Food and Drug Administration (FDA) for use in the initial or supplementary treatment of patient with chronic angina. Although the precise mechanism of ranolazine is not established, it is thought to be related to selective late sodium channel blockade. Its antianginal effect is different than that of currently available conventional antianginal medications, as it is neither a coronary vasodilator, nor it is associated with reduction in hemodynamic parameters (e.g. heart rate, blood pressure, preload and inotropy) (Table 10).

Ranolazine is a safe and well-tolerated antianginal medication and is effective in patients who continue to experience angina despite optimized treatment with other conventional antianginal agents. Ranolazine can also be safely used in patients with compromised hemodynamic parameters (e.g. baseline bradycardia and/or risk of developing significant hypotension). Furthermore, ranolazine can be used safely in patients with diabetes, COPD, LV dysfunction/heart failure and in those patients requiring Phosphodiesterase-5 inhibitor, such as sildenafil. Compared to other antianginal drugs, ranolazine has fewer side effects (Table 11).

Ivabradine

Ivabradine is a newer drug that has been evaluated in patients with chronic CAD and stable angina. Ivabradine is a specific inhibitor of the I-f channels in the sinoatrial node. As a result, it is considered a pure heart rate lowering agent in patients with sinus rhythm. Ivabradine does not seem to have an effect on blood pressure, myocardial inotropy, intracardiac conduction, or ventricular repolarization. Ivabradine is an agent that seems effective in reducing myocardial ischemia, and in controlling symptoms in patients with chronic stable angina pectoris who are in sinus rhythm primarily by reducing heart rate. Ivabradine is effective in controlling anginal symptoms as well as increasing the exercise performance.

❏ COMBINATION THERAPY

Combination therapy is often necessary for adequate symptom control in many patients with stable angina. In general, combination therapy should utilize a beta-blocker with nitrate, or CCB based on patient's underlying comorbid conditions. Such combination may allow the clinician to use lower doses of each agent to achieve symptom control with minimal side effects. However, there has not been a systematic evaluation of combination therapy on hard clinical end points in patients with stable angina.

❏ OTHER DRUGS IN PATIENTS WITH STABLE ANGINA AND CHRONIC CAD

Angiotensin Converting Enzyme Inhibitors

Angiotensin converting enzyme inhibitors (ACEI) have well demonstrated vasculoprotective effects.

On the basis of available evidence, an ACEI should be considered in stable patients who are considered to be at high risk of cardiovascular events, and in patients with stable CAD and angina pectoris.

Lipid-lowering Therapy

Lipid-lowering therapy with statins not only reduces the risk of major acute coronary events (MACE), but it also reduces the need for revascularization as well as decreases the signs and symptoms of myocardial ischemia in patients with angina pectoris. It is recommended that all patients with chronic, stable angina should be treated with a statin to a goal of reducing LDL-C less than 70 mg/dL.

❏ ROLE OF MYOCARDIAL REVASCULARIZATION

Myocardial revascularization (revascularization) has been evaluated and compared to medical treatments in patients with chronic stable angina. Revascularization includes CABGS and PTCA with or without stent deployment [percutaneous revascularization (PCI)]. Although revascularization provides relief of anginal symptoms, it seems to abolish anginal episodes in a minority of patients. A significant proportion of patients will continue to experience anginal symptoms after revascularization. Furthermore, revascularization procedures are often performed in asymptomatic patients with the intent of reducing the incidence of coronary events and cardiac death in patients with stable CAD. However, little data exist to support such benefit.

❑ COMPARISON OF REVASCULARIZATION WITH PHARMACOLOGICAL ANTIANGINAL THERAPY

During the past four decades, several studies have compared the impact of pharmacological antianginal therapy versus revascularization in patients with chronic CAD and stable angina. In general, the results of these studies have shown that revascularization is usually more effective in symptom control compared to the conventional antianginal drug therapy. However, it is important to note that since the earlier time when many of the previous trials were conducted, the medical therapy of patients with stable angina has improved considerably with the routine use of beta-blockers, antiplatelet agents, ACEI and lipid lowering therapy particularly with statins, and as such the result of those earlier trials might not be applicable and pertinent today. A number of recent trials using these drugs have shown that medical therapy may be as effective as revascularization in controlling symptoms and, when aggressive risk factor modification is implemented, such strategy is also effective in reducing the risk of future coronary events in patients with chronic CAD and stable angina.

On the other hand, early as well as the recent revascularization trials in patients with stable CAD have provided data that confirm the impression that, compared to medical treatment, revascularization has resulted in similar rates of hard clinical outcomes in the main groups. The consistent benefit of revascularization, compared to medical treatment, appears to be a more striking, albeit temporary, improvement in anginal discomfort.

❑ CONCLUSION

There are many therapeutic options available for the treatment of anginal symptoms in patients with stable CAD. These options include nitrates, beta-blockers, CCB, and ranolazine. Although combination therapy is often necessary for symptomatic relief, there has been no evaluation of the effects of combination antianginal therapy on hard clinical end points in such patients. Recent trials have shown that medical therapy is as effective as revascularization in controlling symptoms and, along with aggressive risk factor modification, is highly effective in reducing the risk of future coronary events.

GUIDELINES: ACC/AHA/ACP-ASIM GUIDELINES FOR THE MANAGEMENT OF PATIENTS WITH CHRONIC STABLE ANGINA: EXECUTIVE SUMMARY AND RECOMMENDATIONS. CIRCULATION 1999;99:2829-48

Kanu Chatterjee

Class I: Conditions for which there is evidence and /or general agreement that a given procedure or treatment is useful and effective.

Class II: Conditions for which there is conflicting evidence and/or a divergence of opinion about the usefulness/efficacy of a procedure or treatment.

Class IIa: Weight of evidence/opinion is in favor of usefulness/efficacy.

Class IIb: Usefulness/efficacy is less well established by evidence/opinion.

Class III: Conditions for which there is evidence and/or general agreement that the procedure/treatment is not useful/effective and in some cases may be harmful.

Level of Evidence A: The presence of multiple randomized clinical trials.
Level of Evidence B: The presence of a single randomized trial or nonrandomized studies.
Level of Evidence C: Expert consensus.

Recommendations for Pharmacotherapy to Prevent MI and Reduce Symptoms

Class I
1. Aspirin in the absence of contraindications (Level of Evidence A).
2. Beta-blockers as initial therapy in absence of contraindications in patients with prior MI (Level of Evidence A).
3. Beta-blockers as initial therapy in absence of contraindications in patients without prior MI (Level of Evidence B).
4. Heart rate regulating calcium channel antagonists and/or long-acting nitrates as initial therapy when beta-blockers are contraindicated (Level of Evidence B).
5. Heart rate regulating calcium channel antagonists and/or long-acting nitrates in combination with beta-blockers when initial treatment with beta-blockers is not successful (Level of Evidence B).
6. Heart rate regulating calcium antagonists and/or long-acting nitrates as a substitute for beta-blockers if initial treatment with beta-blockers leads to unacceptable side effects (Level of Evidence C).
7. Sublingual nitroglycerin or nitroglycerin spray for the immediate relief of angina (Level of Evidence C).
8. Lipid-lowering therapy in patients with documented or suspected CAD and LDL cholesterol >130 mg/dl with a target LDL of <100 mg/dL (Level of Evidence A).

Class IIa
1. Clopidogrel when aspirin is absolutely contraindicated (Level of Evidence B).
2. Long-acting heart rate regulating calcium channel blocking agents instead of beta-blockers as initial therapy (Level of Evidence B).
3. Lipid-lowering therapy in patients with documented or suspected CAD and LDL cholesterol between 100 and 129 mg/dL, with a target of 100 mg/dL (Level of Evidence B).

Class IIb
1. Low-intensity anticoagulation with warfarin in addition to aspirin (Level of Evidence B).

Class III
1. Dipyridamole (Level of Evidence B).
2. Chelation therapy (Level of Evidence B).

❏ SUGGESTED READINGS

Abrams J, Thadani U. Therapy of stable angina pectoris: the uncomplicated patient. Circulation. 2005;112:e255-9.

Fox K, Ford I, Steg PG, et al. Ivabradine for patients with stable coronary artery disease and left-ventricular systolic dysfunction. (BEAUTIFUL): a randomised, double-blind, placebo-controlled trial. Lancet. 2008;372:807-16.

Fox K, Garcia MA, Ardissino D, et al. Guidelines on the management of stable angina pectoris: executive summary: the task force on the management of stable angina pectoris of the european society of cardiology. Eur Heart J. 2006;27:1341-81.

Gibbons R, Abrams J, Chatterjee K, et al.(2002). ACC/AHA 2002 guideline update for the management of patients with chronic stable angina: a report of the American College of Cardiology/American Heart Association Task Force on Practice Guidelines (Committee to update the 1999 guidelines for the management of patients with chronic stable angina). [online] Available from www.acc.org/clinical/ guidelines/stable/stable.pdf.

Stone PH. Ranolazine: new paradigm for management of myocardial ischemia, myocardial dysfunction, and arrhythmias. Cardiol Clin. 2008;26:603-14.

4.5 Cardiogenic Shock in Acute Coronary Syndromes

❏ INTRODUCTION

Cardiogenic shock, a syndrome of organ hypoperfusion secondary to cardiac failure, complicates ST-segment elevation myocardial infarction (STEMI) in 5–8% of cases. Hemodynamic features of this syndrome include hypotension, reduced cardiac output, and elevated right-or left-sided filling pressures (Table 12). Preshock or shock with end-organ hypoperfusion may be manifest as decreased urine output (oliguria), mental obtundation and/or cool extremities. Although shock is usually caused by left ventricular (LV) pump dysfunction secondary to a large area of LV ischemia or infarction, there is increasing data that neurohormonal or systemic inflammatory response syndrome (SIRS) may be a causative mechanism of shock in acute coronary syndromes (ACS). Other clinical entities must be considered when evaluating shock in the setting of ACS. Mechanical complications of myocardial infarction that can cause shock include right ventricular (RV) infarction, cardiac tamponade secondary to free wall rupture, papillary muscle ischemia or infarction and ventricular septal defect.

❏ PATHOPHYSIOLOGY

The primary cause of cardiogenic shock in ACS is LV dysfunction secondary to infarction and ischemia. Patients with predominantly diastolic dysfunction from ischemia may present with cardiogenic shock. When ischemia or infarction affects a large portion of the LV myocardium, stroke volume and consequently cardiac output decrease. With impairment in the pumping function of the left ventricle, tachycardia ensues to try to maintain cardiac output. However, due to inability to maintain cardiac output, hypotension ensues. In addition, LV filling pressures increase due to pump failure (Figs 4A to C). These compensatory mechanisms beget further ischemia as tachycardia decreases the diastolic filling of the coronary arteries, while hypotension and increased LV filling pressures decrease coronary perfusion pressure, which causes further ischemia leading to a downward spiral.

In addition to the hemodynamic effects of shock, decreased cardiac output stimulates increased sympathetic discharge. In addition, hypotension stimulates the release of renin and angiotensin. Catecholamine stimulation leads to

Table 12: Clinical and hemodynamic features of cardiogenic shock

Clinical
- Hypotension: Systolic blood pressure ≤90 mm Hg
- Impaired organ perfusion: Oliguria, cold clammy skin, mental obtundation

Hemodynamics
- Systolic blood pressure ≤90 mm Hg
- Cardiac index ≤2.2 L/min/m^2
- Primary LV failure: Pulmonary capillary wedge pressure ≥18 mm Hg with right atrial pressure lower than pulmonary capillary wedge pressure
- Primary RV failure: Right atrial pressure ≥15 mm Hg with pulmonary capillary wedge pressure less than right atrial pressure

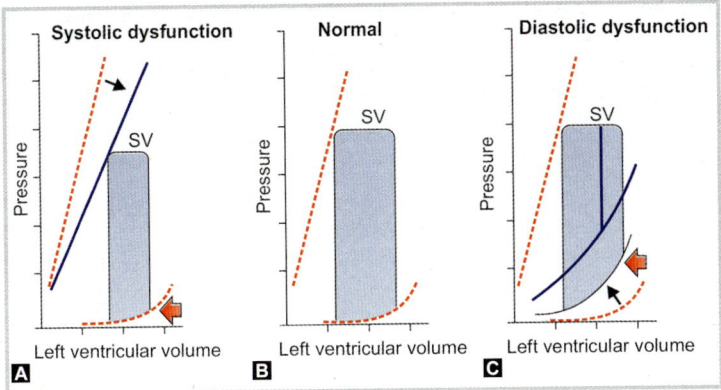

FIGURES 4A TO C: Schematic pressure-volume loops illustrate the mechanisms for increased LV diastolic pressure and lower cardiac output in systolic and diastolic dysfunction: (A) in cardiogenic shock patients with systolic dysfunction; (B) contractility is reduced compared to normals; and (C) cardiogenic shock patients with diastolic dysfunction, the major mechanism of increased diastolic filling pressure is increased ventricular stiffness resulting in an upward and leftward shift in the end-diastolic pressure-volume relationship (*Source:* Chatterjee K, McGlothlin D, Michaels A. Analytic reviews: Cardiogenic shock with preserved systolic function: A reminder. J Intensive Care Med. 2008;23:355-66)

tachycardia and increased systemic vascular resistance. Similarly, the renin-angiotension system causes deleterious affects by increasing systemic vascular resistance and by fluid retention, further compromising coronary blood flow and increasing filling pressures. These compensatory mechanisms exacerbate the physiology by increasing fluid retention and biventricular filling pressures, causing increased heart rate and systemic vascular resistance, further leading to worsening of the clinical picture.

❑ OTHER CARDIAC CAUSES OF CARDIOGENIC SHOCK

The evaluation of cardiogenic shock in ACS involves exclusion of other cardiac causes of shock in the setting of ACS, including RV infarction, ventricular septal rupture (VSR), ischemic mitral regurgitation, and cardiac rupture.

Right Ventricular Infarction

Right ventricular infarction may cause cardiogenic shock. Most commonly associated with inferior myocardial infarction, isolated RV infarction occurs in roughly 5% of cases of cardiogenic shock. There is typically RV volume overload with decreased LV preload. LV volume is not only decreased due to decreased RV function, but due to a shift of the interventricular septum to the LV from RV volume overload and increased end diastolic pressure.

Historically, treatment has been volume resuscitation; however, this may impair LV filling. Ideally, RV diastolic pressures should be maintained between 10 mm Hg and 14 mm Hg to maintain RV stroke index. The clinical presentation shows features of cardiogenic shock, evidence of right heart failure and the absence of pulmonary congestion. Elevated jugular venous pressure with a positive Kussmaul's sign, clear lungs, an RV S3 gallop and lack of increased intensity of P2, suggest RV infarct as the diagnosis. There is usually inferior ST elevation and elevation in V1 and V3R–V4R. Echocardiography usually reveals RV hypokinesis with dilatation, with relatively preserved LV ejection fraction. Treatment involves opening the infarct related artery and supportive medical measures

Ventricular Septal Rupture

Ventricular septal rupture is a rare complication of acute myocardial infarction. Risk factors for development of a post-MI VSD include older age, female sex, absence of previous angina or infarction, late time to revascularization and systemic hypertension. VSDs occur with either anterior or inferior myocardial infarctions. VSDs associated with anterior infarction are usually apical in location, whereas those associated with inferior infarction are in the basal septum. Rupture can occur within the first 24 hours in large infarctions associated with intramural hematomas, or 3–5 days later due to coagulation necrosis. Usually patients present with cardiogenic shock and biventricular failure with a loud holosystolic murmur that is heard best at the lower left sternal border often associated with a thrill. The defect can be diagnosed with echocardiography, ventriculography or catheterization to document a left-to-right shunt in the right ventricle.

Cardiac Rupture

Cardiac rupture occurs in less than 1% of patients who present with acute myocardial infarction. Cardiac rupture usually involves the anterior or lateral walls. Risk factors for cardiac rupture include female sex, advanced age, and systemic hypertension. Cardiac rupture usually occurs in patients without previous myocardial infarction who suffer a transmural infarct. Cardiac rupture usually occurs in the first 5 days after myocardial infarction but can occur up to 3 weeks after infarction. It is preceded by infarct expansion, with thinning of the necrotic area. Rupture can occur from a tear in the wall, or it can occur from a dissecting hematoma. Rupture usually leads to hemopericardium and death from cardiac tamponade. Patients can present with "pericardial" pain, nausea, hypotension and nonspecific symptoms. This is usually followed by pulseless electrical activity and death. Rupture can be diagnosed by transthoracic echocardiography.

Mitral Regurgitation

Acute severe mitral regurgitation from severe papillary dysfunction or papillary muscle rupture is a rare, life-threatening complication of acute myocardial infarction. This complication usually affects the posteromedial papillary muscle, which has its sole blood supply from the posterior descending artery. Sudden onset of severe mitral regurgitation is associated with decreased forward output and stroke volume, increased pulmonary venous congestion, pulmonary edema and signs of hypoperfusion. On examination, patients have a new holosystolic murmur, often with an associated palpable and audible S3 and S4. The murmur may not extend to the second heart sound due to reduction of regurgitation in late systole because of rapid equalization of LV and left atrial pressures. Echocardiography usually confirms the diagnosis. Pulmonary artery catheterization reveals a large V wave in the pulmonary capillary wedge tracing. Definitive surgical treatment with mitral repair or replacement should be performed.

❏ DIAGNOSTIC EVALUATION

Cardiogenic shock can often be suspected by the presence of signs of shock in the setting of acute myocardial infarction (Table 12). Further testing should be performed to confirm the diagnosis of cardiogenic shock given that there is considerable overlap with other causes of shock. Echocardiography is an invaluable tool for evaluating biventricular dysfunction and excluding mechanical complications of myocardial infarction as a cause of cardiogenic shock. Pulmonary artery catheterization is often useful, especially in patients who do not have prompt recovery from a shock state with reperfusion to guide further therapy. Invasive arterial monitoring is essential to guide further therapy

❏ MEDICAL MANAGEMENT

The mainstay of medical management for cardiogenic shock includes inotropic and vasopressor agents. Although dopamine and dobutamine improve the hemodynamics acutely in cardiogenic shock, there is no data to suggest that they improve survival. Norepinephrine is often a second-line agent given its potent alpha effects and is useful in patients who have a normal systemic vascular resistance in cardiogenic shock. Recent data suggest that the role of dopamine may need to be reconsidered as there is evidence that treatment with dopamine increases short-term mortality in comparison with those treated with norepinephrine. Vasodilators may be useful in preshock states; however, they are not recommended as lone agents once shock has ensued as they can lead to further hypotension, thus decreasing coronary blood flow. Vasodilators may be useful when used together with IABP or inotropes.

❏ MECHANICAL SUPPORT

Adjunctive mechanical circulatory support is often needed. Several devices are available for mechanical circulatory support in cardiogenic shock. They include IABP, TandemHeart (CardiacAssist, Inc., Pittsburgh, PA), Impella (Abiomed, Inc., Danvers, MA) and surgically implanted left ventricular assist devices (LVAD). While there are significant differences, the common objective is maintenance of adequate blood pressure, tissue perfusion and oxygenation.

❏ REVASCULARIZATION

Which particular method of mechanical coronary revascularization should be chosen for cardiogenic shock patients: PCI or CABG? PCI has the advantage of wider availability in the community and generally shorter reperfusion times. If successful, timely PCI confers a survival advantage, an important consideration since the SHOCK trial demonstrated a trend toward reduced clinical benefit if reperfusion was delayed. Nonetheless, a reduction in mortality was seen if revascularization was performed even after 48 hours from myocardial infarction and 18 hours after the onset of shock.

A history of previous myocardial infarction or failed thrombolysis is generally viewed as conferring a worse prognosis. Although some studies cite the presence of multivessel disease as being an adverse predictor, others do not.

CABG has historically been able to achieve complete revascularization in a larger proportion of patients. Outside of randomized studies, emergent CABG is much less likely to be used as an initial revascularization method (under 10%).

❑ SUGGESTED READINGS

Antman EM, Anbe DT, Armstrong PW, et al. ACC/AHA guidelines for the management of patients with ST-elevation myocardial infarction-executive summary: a report of the American College of Cardiology/American Heart Association Task Force on Practice Guidelines. Circulation. 2004;110:588-636.

Kushner FG, Hand M, Smith SC Jr, et al. 2009 focused updates: ACC/AHA guidelines for the management of patients with STelevation myocardial infarction (updating the 2004 guideline and 2007 focused update) and ACC/AHA/SCAI guidelines on percutaneous coronary intervention (updating the 2005 guideline and 2007 focused update): a report of the American College of Cardiology Foundation/American Heart Association Task Force on Practice Guidelines. Circulation. 2009;120:2271-306.

Lindholm MG, Kober L, Boesgaard S, et al. Cardiogenic shock complicating acute myocardial infarction; prognostic impact of early and late shock development. Eur Heart J. 2003;24:258-65.

Nieminen MS, Bohm M, Cowie MR, et al. Executive summary of the guidelines on the diagnosis and treatment of acute heart failure: the task force on acute heart failure of the European Society of Cardiology. Eur Heart J. 2005;26:384-416.

Reynolds HR, Hochman JS. Cardiogenic shock: current concepts and improving outcomes. Circulation. 2008;117:686-97.

Wong SC, Sanborn T, Sleeper LA. Angiographic findings and clinical correlates in patients with cardiogenic shock complicating acute myocardial infarction: a report from the SHOCK trial registry. Should we emergently revascularize occluded coronaries for cardiogenic shock? J Am Coll Cardiol. 2000;36:1077-83.

4.6 Acute Right Ventricular Infarction

❑ INTRODUCTION

Based on early experiments of right ventricular (RV) performance, it was felt for many years that RV contraction was unimportant in the circulation. However, recognition of the profound hemodynamic effects of RV systolic dysfunction became evident during the 1970s with the description of severe RV infarction (RVI), resulting in severe right heart failure, clear lungs and hypotension low output despite intact global left ventricular (LV) systolic function. Although the magnitude of hemodynamic derangements is related to the extent of RVFW contraction abnormalities, some patients tolerate severe RV systolic dysfunction without hemodynamic compromise whereas others develop life-threatening low output, emphasizing that additional factors modulate the clinical expression of RVI. Importantly, the term RV "infarction" is to an extent a misnomer. For in most cases acute RV ischemic dysfunction appears to represent viable myocardium, which recovers over time, especially following successful reperfusion and even after prolonged occlusion.

❑ PATTERNS OF CORONARY COMPROMISE RESULTING IN RVI

Significant RVI nearly always occurs in association with acute transmural inferior-posterior LV myocardial infarction (MI) and the RCA is always the culprit vessel, typically a proximal occlusion compromising flow to one or more of the major RV branches (Fig. 5). In contrast, distal RCA occlusions or circumflex culprits

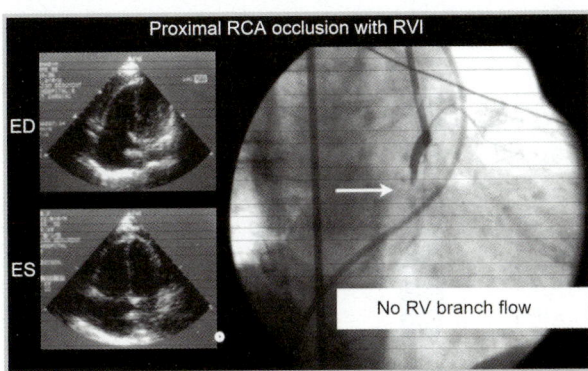

FIGURE 5: Patient with a proximal right coronary artery (right panel, arrow) compromising the right ventricular branches and resulting in severe RVI, indicated on echo as severe RV free wall dysfunction and depressed global RV performance at end systole (ES) and marked RV dilation at end diastole (ED)

that spare RV branch perfusion rarely compromise RV performance. Occasionally, isolated RVI may develop from occlusion of a nondominant RCA or selective compromise of RV branches during percutaneous interventions.

❏ EFFECTS OF ISCHEMIA ON RV SYSTOLIC AND DIASTOLIC FUNCTION

Proximal RCA occlusion compromises RVFW perfusion, resulting in RVFW dyskinesis and depressed global RV performance reflected in the RV waveform by a sluggish, depressed and systolic waveform. RV systolic dysfunction diminishes transpulmonary delivery of LV preload, leading to decreased cardiac output despite intact LV contractility. Biventricular diastolic dysfunction contributes to hemodynamic compromise. The ischemic RV is stiff and dilated early in diastole, which impedes inflow leading to rapid diastolic pressure elevation. Acute RV dilatation and elevated diastolic pressure shift the interventricular septum toward the volume-deprived LV, further impairing LV compliance and filling. Abrupt RV dilatation within the noncompliant pericardium elevates intrapericardial pressure, the resultant constraint further impairing RV and LV compliance and filling. These effects contribute to the pattern of equalized diastolic pressures and RV "dip-and-plateau" characteristic of RVI.

❏ EFFECTS OF REPERFUSION ON ISCHEMIC RV DYSFUNCTION

Although RV function may recover despite persistent RCA occlusion, acute RV ischemia contributes to early morbidity and mortality. Furthermore, spontaneous recovery of RV contractile function and hemodynamics may be slow. In patients, successful mechanical reperfusion of the RCA, including the major RV branches leads to immediate improvement in and later complete recovery of RVFW function and global RV performance. Reperfusion-mediated recovery of RV performance is associated with excellent clinical outcome (Fig. 6).

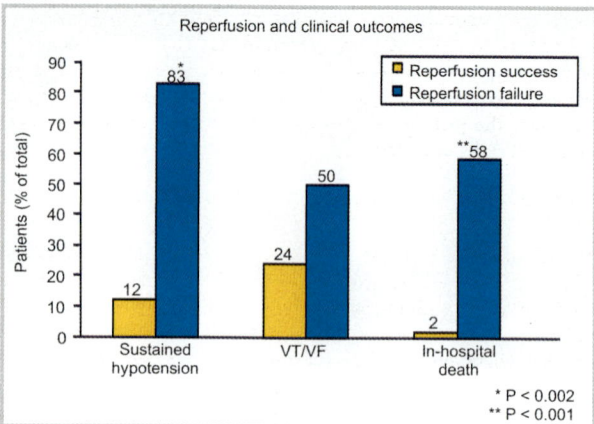

FIGURE 6: Bar graphs demonstrating benefits of successful reperfusion versus reperfusion failure with respect to reduced arrhythmias, sustained hypotension and inhospital survival. (*Source:* Bowers et al. N Eng J Med. 1998;338:933, with permission)

❏ RHYTHM DISORDERS AND REFLEXES ASSOCIATED WITH RVI

Bradyarrhythmias and Hypotension

Patients with acute RVI are at increased risk for both high-grade AV block and bradycardia-hypotension without AV block. During acute coronary occlusion, bradycardia-hypotension and AV block are far more common in patients with proximal RCA lesions inducing RV and LV inferior-posterior ischemia, compared to more distal occlusions compromising LV perfusion, but sparing the RV branches. These observations suggest that the ischemic right heart may elicit cardioinhibitory-vasodilator reflexes.

Ventricular Arrhythmias

Patients with RVI are prone to ventricular tachyarrhythmias, which should not be unexpected given that the ischemic RV is often massively dilated. In patients with RVI, VT/VF may develop in a trimodal pattern, either during acute occlusion, abruptly with reperfusion or later. However, successful mechanical reperfusion dramatically reduces the incidence of malignant ventricular arrhythmias, presumably through improvement in RV function, which lessens late VT/VF. Occasionally, RVI may be complicated by recurrent malignant arrhythmias and in some cases intractable "electrical storm", possibly due to sustained severe RV dilatation.

❏ CLINICAL PRESENTATIONS AND EVALUATION

Right ventricular infarction is often silent as only 25% of patients develop clinically evident hemodynamic manifestations. Patients with severe RVI but preserved global LV function may be hemodynamically compensated, manifest by elevated JVP but clear lungs, normal systemic arterial pressure and intact perfusion. When RVI leads to more severe hemodynamic compromise, systemic hypotension and hypoperfusion result. Patients with IMI may initially present without evidence of hemodynamic compromise, but subsequently develop hypotension precipitated by preload reduction attributable to nitroglycerin or associated with bradyarrhythmias. When RVI develops in the setting of global LV dysfunction, the picture may be dominated by low output and pulmonary congestion, with right heart failure.

❑ NONINVASIVE AND HEMODYNAMIC EVALUATION

Although ST segment elevation and loss of R wave in the rightsided ECG leads (V3R and V4R) are sensitive indicators of the presence of RVI, they are not predictive of the magnitude of RV dysfunction, nor its hemodynamic impact. Echocardiography is the most effective tool for delineation of the presence and severity of RV dilatation and depression of global RV performance. Echo also delineates the extent of reversed septal curvature that confirms the presence of significant adverse diastolic interactions, the degree of paradoxical septal motion indicative of compensatory systolic interactions, and the presence of severe RA enlargement which may indicate concomitant ischemic RA dysfunction and/or tricuspid regurgitation.

❑ DIFFERENTIAL DIAGNOSIS OF RVI

Important clinical entities to consider in patients who present with acute low output hypotension, clear lungs and disproportionate right heart failure include cardiac tamponade, acute pulmonary embolism, severe pulmonary hypertension, right heart mass obstruction and acute severe tricuspid regurgitation; entities including constrictive pericarditis or restrictive cardiomyopathy present a similar picture but are not acute processes (Table 13).

❑ THERAPY

Therapeutic options for the management of right heart ischemia include (Table 14). Treatment modalities include:
- Restoration of physiologic rhythm
- Optimization of ventricular preload
- Optimization of oxygen supply and demand
- Parenteral inotropic support for persistent hemodynamic compromise
- Reperfusion
- Mechanical support with intra-aortic balloon counterpulsation and RV assist devices.

Table 13: Differential diagnosis of hypotension with disproportionate right heart failure
- RVI
- Cardiac tamponade
- Acute pulmonary embolus
- Acute tricuspid regurgitation
- Pulmonary hypertension with RV failure
- Acute MI with LV failure
- Right heart mass obstruction
- Constriction/restriction

Table 14: RVI: Therapeutic algorithm

- Optimize oxygen supply and demand
- Establish physiological rhythm
- Optimize preload
- Inotropic stimulation for persistent low output
- Mechanical support devices:
  - IABP for refractory hypotension
  - RVAD
  - Reperfusion by primary PCI

❏ SUMMARY

Acute RCA occlusion proximal to the RV branches results in RVFW dysfunction. The ischemic, dyskinetic RVFW exerts mechanically disadvantageous effects on biventricular performance. Depressed RV systolic function leads to a diminished transpulmonary delivery of LV preload, resulting in reduced cardiac output. The ischemic RV is stiff, dilated and volume dependent, resulting in pandiastolic RV dysfunction and septally mediated alterations in LV compliance, exacerbated by elevated intrapericardial pressure. Under these conditions, RV pressure generation and output are dependent on LV septal contraction and paradoxical septal motion. Culprit lesions distal to the RA branches augment RA contractility and enhance RV filling and performance. Bradyarrhythmias limit the output generated by the rate-dependent ventricles. Ventricular arrhythmias are common, but do not impact short-term outcomes if mechanical reperfusion is prompt. Patients with RVI and hemodynamic instability often respond to volume resuscitation and restoration of physiologic rhythm. Vasodilators and diuretics should generally be avoided. In some patients, parenteral inotropes are required. The RV is relatively resistant to infarction and usually recovers even after prolonged occlusion. However, prompt reperfusion enhances recovery of RV performance and improves the clinical course and survival of patients with ischemic RV dysfunction.

❏ SUGGESTED READINGS

Gacioch GM, Topol EJ. Sudden paradoxic clinical deterioration during angioplasty of the occluded right coronary artery in acute myocardial infarction. J Am Coll Cardiol. 1989;14:1202-9.

Goldstein JA, Tweddell JS, Barzilai B, et al. Importance of left ventricular function and systolic interaction to right ventricular performance during acute right heart ischemia. J Am Coll Cardiol. 1992;19:704-11.

Jacobs AK, Leopold JA, Bates E, et al. Cardiogenic shock caused by right ventricular infarction: a report from the SHOCK registry. JAm Coll Cardiol. 2003;41:1273-9.

Lim ST, Marcovitz P, Pica M, et al. Right ventricular performance at rest and during stress with chronic proximal occlusion of the right coronary artery. Am J Cardiol. 2003;92:1203-6.

Ricci JM, Dukkipati SR, Pica MC, et al. Malignant ventricular arrhythmias in patients with acute right ventricular infarction undergoing mechanical reperfusion. Am J Cardiol. 2009;104:1678-83.

Chapter 5

Valvular Heart Diseases

5.1 Aortic Valve Disease

❏ AORTIC STENOSIS

Etiology

Calcific Aortic Stenosis

Otto et al. noted that the histology of the early lesion of aortic stenosis (AS) resembled that of the plaque of atherosclerosis, a disease that also leads to lesion calcification (Fig. 1). Hemodynamic shear stress likely plays a role in initiating AS, since calcium deposition is greatest on the aortic side of the valve where shear stress is the highest. Additionally, it is rare for all three aortic leaflets to be identical in size, and size difference likely causes inhomogeneity of stress across the valve, lending further credence to shear as one factor involved in the pathogenesis of AS. It is clear that inflammation also plays a major role in valvular calcium deposition. Once the inflammatory cascade is initiated myofibroblasts transdifferentiate in osteoblasts leading to calcium deposition and bone formation. Indeed lamellar bone, not just calcification is found in many stenotic aortic valves. Calcification is further facilitated by abnormalities of NOTCH1, a gene that represses calcification. Exactly how all of these abnormalities work in concert to cause valvular calcification and bone formation is unclear. One possible scheme is shown in Flowchart 1.

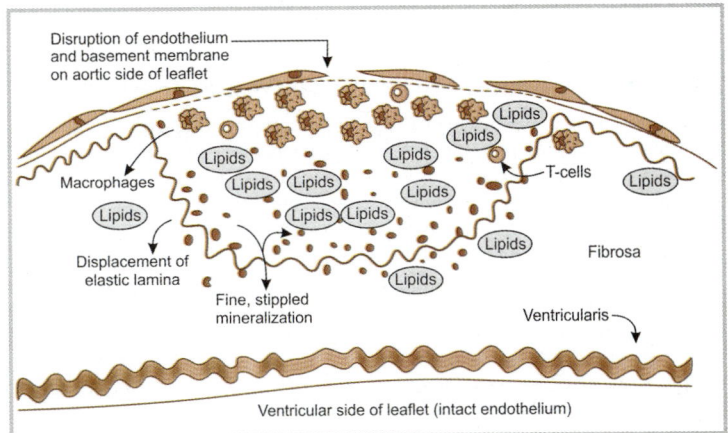

FIGURE 1: A diagram of the early lesion in AS is shown. Infiltration with lipids and inflammatory cells similar to the plaque of coronary disease is a prominent feature. (*Source:* Otto CM, Kuusisto J, Reichenbach DD, et al. Characterization of the early lesion of 'degenerative' valvular aortic stenosis: histological and immunohistochemical studies. Circulation. 1994;90:844-53, with permission)

FLOWCHART 1: A schema of a potential cascade of events leading to aortic valve calcification is shown

```
┌─────────────────────┐   ┌──────────────┐   ┌──────────────────────┐
│     INITIATORS      │   │ Effector cells│   │ Inflammatory agents  │
│                     │   │              │   │                      │
│ Oxidized LDL        │──▶│ Macrophages  │──▶│ NFkb                 │
│ Shear stress        │   │ Lymphocytes  │   │ IL 2,6               │
│ RAS                 │   │              │   │ TGF-β                │
│ Endothelial dysfunction│ │              │   │ TNF                  │
└─────────────────────┘   └──────────────┘   └──────────────────────┘
                                                        │
                                                        ▼
                    ┌──────────────────────────────────────┐
                    │ Myofibroblast transdifferentiation   │
                    │                                      │
                    │         Osteoblast                   │
                    │             │◀──── NOTCH 1 defect    │
                    │         Calcification                │
                    │             │                        │
                    │         Bone formation               │
                    └──────────────────────────────────────┘
```

Rheumatic Disease

Worldwide, rheumatic heart disease is a leading cause of aortic valvular inflammation leading to AS. Since rheumatic heart disease virtually always affects the mitral valve, the diagnosis of rheumatic AS should not be made in the presence of an anatomically normal mitral valve.

Other Causes

Congenital aortic cusp fusion resulting in AS is almost always diagnosed during childhood but occasionally the diagnosis is first made in the adult patient. Other rare causes of AS include chest irradiation and ochronosis.

Aortic Stenosis-induced Left Ventricular Pressure Overload

Aortic stenosis is the quintessential example of pressure overload. As the aortic orifice narrows, the left ventricle (LV) must generate increased force to drive blood past the narrowing, generating a pressure gradient between LV and aorta. This gradient is small until the aortic orifice becomes less than one half its normal 3 cm^2 orifice area. However, further narrowing causes a progressive and geometric increase in the transaortic valve gradient (Table 1). The gradient that develops between LV and aorta represents the pressure overload required for the LV to perform its task as a pump. Since ejection performance declines as afterload increases, concentric LVH has been considered a compensatory mechanism, allowing maintenance of normal afterload and ejection fraction.

The LVH may be beneficial by normalizing LV afterload, permitting normal LV ejection performance. However, in many cases LV is not adequate to normalize systolic wall stress, afterload increases and ejection fraction falls. Whether LVH does or does not normalize afterload, LVH often has deleterious consequences. These include myocardial ischemia, diastolic dysfunction, and decreased LV contractility, all potentiating the morbidity and mortality of AS.

Table 1: Relationship of gradient to AVA at a cardiac output of 6 L/min

AVA cm²	Mean gradient (mm Hg)
3.0	4
2.0	9
1.5	16
1.0	36
0.8	56
0.6	100

Natural History and the Role of Symptoms

Calcific AS is an invariably progressive disease, but on the other hand the rate of progression from patient to patient is extraordinarily variable. Progression in the decrease in valve area may be less than 0.1 cm² to as much as 0.3 cm² per year, while gradient may increase from less than 5 mm Hg to as much as 20 mm Hg per year. As shown in Figures 2A and B, the survival is nearly normal as long as the patient

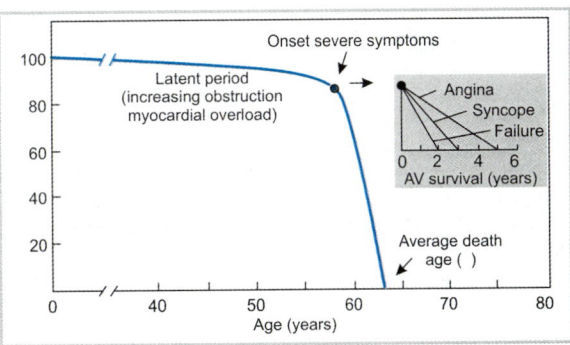

FIGURE 2A: The natural history of AS, as compiled primarily from autopsy studies performed in the sixties shows that survival is nearly normal until the classic symptoms of AS develop at which time mortality increases sharply (*Source:* Ross J Jr, Braunwald E. Aortic stenosis. Circulation. 1968;38(suppl. 1):61-7, with permission)

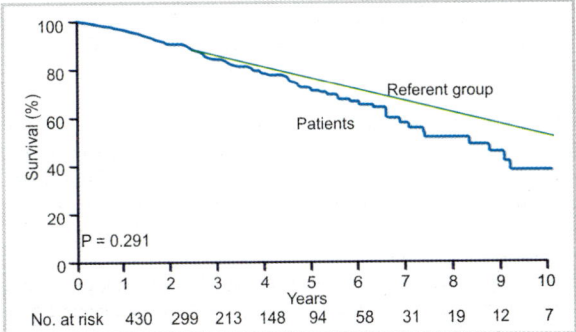

FIGURE 2B: The relative benignity of asymptomatic AS is confirmed 40 years later from follow-up of 622 patients with echo-proven severe AS. Survival is slightly but not significantly worse than an age-matched well population (*Source:* Ross J Jr, Braunwald E. Aortic stenosis. Circulation. 1968;38(suppl. 1):61-7, with permission)

is truly asymptomatic. However, once the classic symptoms of angina, syncope or the symptoms of heart failure develop the mortality rate soars to as much as 2% per month so that 3 years after the onset of symptoms, 75% of patients with AS will have died unless the aortic valve is replaced.

Physical Examination

Palpation of the carotid arteries finds their upstroke delayed in timing and reduced in volume (parvus et tardus Fig. 3). Palpation of the apical beat usually finds it in its normal position but increased in duration, width and forcefulness.

S1 that is usually normal in intensity; an S2 is often soft and single as the diseased aortic valve, neither opens nor closes, well leaving only the soft P2 component of S2. In cases of severe AS with LV dysfunction (or when left bundle branch block accompanies LVH), S2 may be paradoxically split. An S4 indicative of reduced LV compliance from LVH is usually present. The murmur of AS is often the physical finding that alerts the practitioners for the presence of the disease. It is a harsh systolic ejection murmur heard best in the aortic area, radiating to the neck. In mild to moderate disease, it typically peaks in mid-systole and is often accompanied by a thrill. As the disease becomes more severe, the murmur may lessen in intensity (as aortic flow diminishes) and the murmur reaches its peak intensity progressively later in systole.

Diagnosis

Electrocardiograph usually demonstrates the voltage criteria for the presence of LVH but the absence of this finding does not rule out the diagnosis of severe AS. *Chest X-ray* may show a boot shaped cardiac silhouette indicative of LVH. In extreme cases of aortic valve calcification, calcium may be seen deposited in the valve in the lateral view.

Echocardiogram is the modality of choice in diagnosing AS and in assessing its severity. The echocardiogram can evaluate the amount of LVH present, the effect of AS on LV systolic and diastolic function, estimate left atrial size and pulmonary artery pressure, and image the reduced movement of the aortic valve. Echocardiography can also estimate the amount of valvular calcification which can in turn be used as a prognostic factor in the progression of the disease. Importantly, echocardiography can also fairly precisely estimate the transvalvular gradient and the aortic valve area (Fig. 4), criteria for basing disease severity as categorized in Table 2.

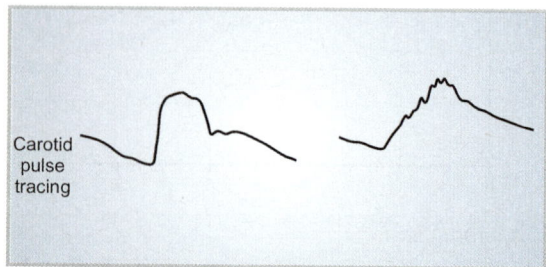

FIGURE 3: The normal carotid upstroke (left) is compared to the classic delayed and reduced (parvus et tardus) carotid upstroke of severe AS (right)

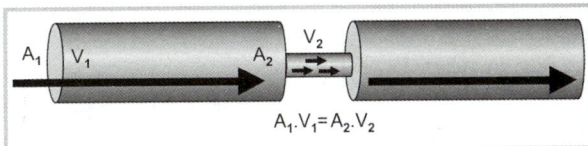

FIGURE 4: A schematic explaining the continuity equation is shown. As the area at the aortic valve decreases from stenosis, velocity must increase to maintain equal (continuous) flow on both sides of the valve. *Source:* Modified from Carabello

Table 2: Classification of the severity of aortic stenosis in adults			
	Aortic stenosis		
Indicator	Mild	Moderate	Severe
Jet velocity (m per second)	Less than 3.0	3.0–4.0	Greater than 4.0
Mean gradient (mm Hg)	Less than 25	25–40	Greater than 40
Valve area (cm^2)	Greater than 1.5	1.0–1.5	Less than 1.0
Valve area index (cm^2 per m^2)			Less than 0.6

Calcium Scoring can be done by cardiac computed tomography (CT) and electron-beam imaging and is helpful in predicting the rapidity of disease progression. However, aortic valve calcium scoring is not universally accepted as a surrogate for other imaging studies in assessing AS severity.

Natriuretic peptides are likely to become useful in monitoring the patient with AS, but only after prospective studies arrive at specific levels indicating when the patient is approaching the need for valve replacement.

Treatment

Medical Therapy

There is no effective chronic medical therapy for AS. Aortic valve replacement (AVR) is life saving and is the only long-term therapy that affects outcome. Diuretics can be used cautiously to treat heart failure acutely. Nitrates can be used to treat angina episodically.

AVR for Symptomatic AS

Figure 5 demonstrates the dramatic difference in survival for symptomatic patients undergoing AVR versus those who refused surgery. The advent of percutaneously and/or transapically placed stented aortic valves [transcutaneous aortic valve implantation (TAVI)] represents a sea change in the therapy for patients deemed too high risk for standard AVR. In this procedure a stented valve is delivered into the aortic annulus percutaneously or transapically after the calcified native valve is pushed aside by prior balloon dilatation. As shown in Figures 6A to D, the survival benefit is striking.

AVR in Asymptomatic AS

This small but definite risk raises the issue of performing AVR in asymptomatic patients where the risk of surgical mortality is also low, approximately 1% or less in expert hands. Thus, there is a small but definite risk of waiting for symptoms and a

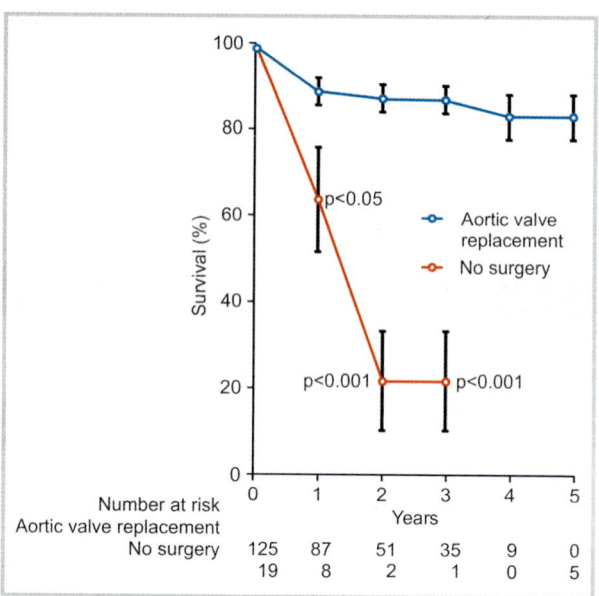

FIGURE 5: The large survival benefit is shown for patients with severe symptomatic AS who underwent AVR versus those who refused surgery. (*Source:* Schwarz F, Baumann P, Manthey J, et al. The effect of aortic valve replacement on survival. Circulation. 1982;66(5):1105-10, with permission)

small but definite risk of proceeding to AVR, a situation with no clear cut proper course of action. A reasonable solution to this conundrum is to identify a high risk group of asymptomatic AS patients for whom AVR is preferable to waiting for symptoms to develop. Several data lend themselves to implementing this strategy. First, when transvalvular jet velocity exceeds 4.0 m/sec, there is a 70% likelihood that symptoms will develop in 2 years; if jet velocity exceeds 5.5 m/sec, there is a 70% chance that symptoms will develop in 1 year (Fig. 7).

High jet velocity, along with declining LV function, heavy valve calcification, a rapid increase in gradient, severe LVH and a rising BNP level are associated with a high risk of symptom development and might be indication for early AVR. All of the foregoing must be tempered by patient preference and the existence of comorbidities that alter the risk and benefit of AVR.

❑ AORTIC REGURGITATION

Etiology

Bicuspid aortic valve noted above to cause AS, may also be the cause of aortic regurgitation (AR). While sometimes involving leaflet pathology, bicuspid valve is also frequently associated with a dilated aortic root. Extreme dilatation of the aorta may lead to aortic dissection, and thus this pathology must be viewed as a duel problem that includes the consequences of valvular AR as well as the potential of aortic dissection. Other diseases of the aortic root leading to AR include Ehlers-Danlos syndrome, Marfan's syndrome, ankylosing spondylitis, hypertension, and syphilis.

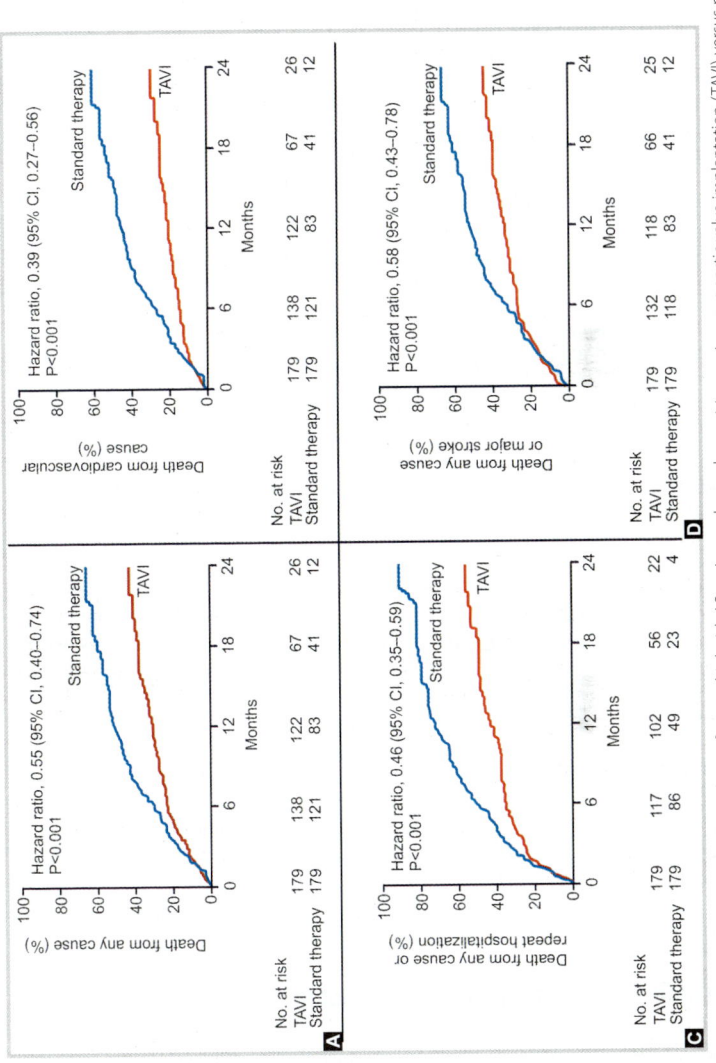

FIGURES 6A TO D: Four different analyzes of survival are shown for very high risk AS patients who underwent transcutaneous aortic valve implantation (TAVI) versus medical therapy in a randomized trial. The benefit from TAVI is striking

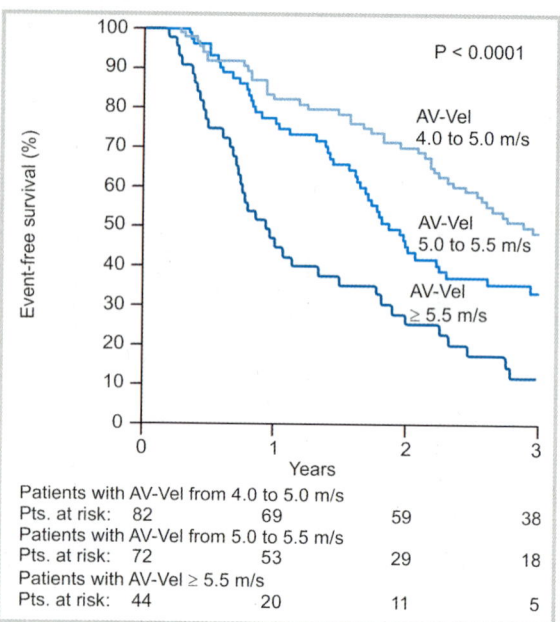

FIGURE 7: Event free survival for asymptomatic AS patients is segregated by transaortic jet velocity (*Source:* Rosenhek R, Zilberszac R, Schemper M, et al. Natural history of very aortic stenosis. Circulation. 2010;121:(1):151-6, with permission)

The most common leaflet abnormality leading to severe AR in developed nations is leaflet destruction from infective endocarditis. In other parts of the world rheumatic heart disease causing leaflet scarring and retraction is still a leading cause of AR.

Pathophysiology

Aortic regurgitation produces a combined volume and pressure overload on the LV. The blood volume regurgitated into the LV during diastole is lost to forward flow. This loss is compensated by eccentric LVH whereby new sarcomeres are laid down in series, increasing myocyte length and LV chamber volume. Normal ejection of an increased end-diastolic volume enables total stroke volume to increase (Figs 8A to E).

Natural History and the Role of Symptoms

From the time of diagnosis of severe AR, progression to the need for surgery (see below) occurs at a rate of about 4% per year, roughly half the rate of MR progression. The symptoms for AR are similar to those of AS but the frequency distribution is different in that syncope and angina are relatively rare in AR and heart failure is much more common. Heart failure develops from both diastolic and systolic LV dysfunction.

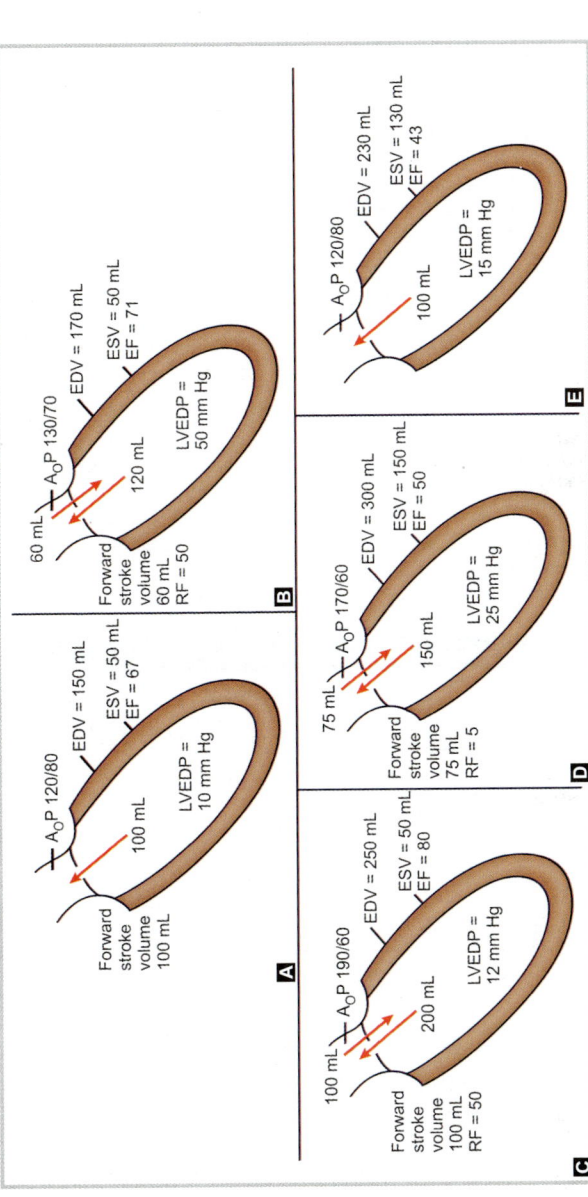

FIGURES 8A TO E: The pathophysiologic stages or AR are depicted here. (A) Shows a normal LV. (B) Depicts acute AR. Increased sarcomere stretch (preload) increases end diastolic volume slightly so that total stroke volume increases slightly. However regurgitation of 50% of the total stroke volume decreases forward stroke volume from 100 cc to 60 cc. The LV volume overload greatly increases LV end-diastolic pressure. (C) Shows chronic compensated AR. LV dilatation has permitted an increase in both total and forward stroke volume while allowing LV filling pressure to return toward normal. (D) LV contractile dysfunction has ensued. End-systolic volume has increased greatly as the weakened myocardium in concert with increased afterload curtail LV emptying. In turn stroke volume has fallen and LV filling pressure has increased. (E) Depicts the beneficial effects of AVR (Abbreviations: EDV: End diastolic volume; ESV: End systolic volume; LVEDP: Left ventricular end diastolic pressure)

Physical Examination

The apical beat is forceful and displaced downward and to the left of the midclavicular line. The typical murmur is diastolic, has a blowing quality, and is heard best at the left lower sternal border with the patient sitting up and leaning forward. This AR murmur may be associated with a diastolic mitral rumble (Austin Flint) caused by impingement of the AR jet upon the mitral valve, partially closing the mitral valve while causing it to vibrate. This murmur is a sign that the AR is severe. The AR causes a large total stroke volume to be ejected into the aorta, in turn causing a widened pulse pressure. These act in concert to cause a myriad of physical signs. The carotid pulse is brisk in upstroke and collapses rapidly (Corrigan's pulse). The pulse may cause the head to bob with each cardiac cycle (De Musset's sign). The stethoscope placed over the femoral artery may detect a sound similar to a pistol shot, or when the bell is pressed into the femoral artery, a to and fro murmur (Duroziez's sign) may be heard. Traction on the nailbed may cause systolic plethora and diastolic blanching of the bed (Quincke's pulse). Systolic blood pressure in the leg may be augmented by greater than 40 mm Hg compared to brachial pressure (Hill's sign).

Diagnosis

Echocardiography forms the mainstay of diagnosis. Left ventricular size and function can be quantified. Valve and root anatomy are assessed to yield the etiology of the patient's AR. The AR jet is visualized and used to determine disease severity (Table 3). Echocardiography is also useful in assessing the degree of aortic root dilatation when aortopathy is the cause of AR.

Table 3: Classification of the severity of aortic regurgitation in adults

	Aortic regurgitation		
	Mild	**Moderate**	**Severe**
Qualitative			
Angiographic grade	1+	2+	3–4+
Color Doppler jet width	Central jet, width less than 25% of LVOT	Greater than mild but no signs of severe AR	Central jet, width greater than 65% LVOT
Doppler vena contracta width (cm)	Less than 0.3	0.3–0.6	Greater than 0.6
Quantitative (cath or echo)			
Regurgitant volume (mL per beat)	Less than 30	30–59	Greater than or equal to 60
Regurgitation fraction (%)	Less than 30	30–49	Greater than or equal to 50
Regurgitant orifice area (cm^2)	Less tha 0.10	0.10–0.29	Greater than or equal to 0.30
Additional essential criteria			
Left ventricular size			Increased

Cardiac magnetic resonance imaging provides accurate assessment of AR severity, of LV volumes and mass and of aortic root dimensions.

Exercise testing in asymptomatic patients is advisable to gain insight into the patient's exercise tolerance and as an objective method for assessing symptomatic status because the presence or absence of symptoms represents a key determinant of the natural history of the disease.

Cardiac catheterization may yield important diagnostic information if the degree of AR severity is still unclear following noninvasive testing.

Treatment
Medical Therapy
Asymptomatic Patient with Normal LV Function
Therapy to reduce aortic impedance is logical both to reduce afterload and to increase forward flow while decreasing regurgitant flow. Several observational studies have suggested benefit to this approach in patients with severe asymptomatic disease while relatively small randomized trials have generated disparate results, making it impossible to make any firm recommendation regarding medical therapy for patients with AR.

Symptomatic AR Patients or Those with LV Dysfunction
AR patients with heart failure should presumably be treated with standard therapies for heart failure including ACE inhibitors and beta-blockers, with questions on the safety of both classes of drugs. Moreover, the only accepted therapy for symptomatic patients with severe AR is AVR or valve repair.

Surgery and the Timing of AVR
Occasionally, the aortic valve can be repaired but usually therapy requires AVR. Currently there is no indication for correcting less than severe disease, as defined in Table 3 above, because there is no evidence that mild to moderate AR is harmful unless it worsens. Prognosis for patients with severe AR is excellent until either symptoms or asymptomatic LV dysfunction develops, and prognosis remains excellent as long as AVR is performed promptly when these triggers for surgery arise. Six to twelve months clinical and echocardiographic follow-up is indicated to survey for the onset of symptoms and to assess changes in LV size and function. If EF is falling toward 50–55% or end systolic dimension is increasing toward 50–55 mm, AVR is indicated.

Acute Severe AR: A Dangerous Masquerade
In many respects, acute severe AR as might occur from leaflet perforation due to infective endocarditis is almost a different disease from severe chronic AR. In acute AR, there has been no time for LV enlargement to occur and thus total stroke volume and pulse pressure are not increased. Therefore, most of the signs leading to the dramatic physical examination of the patient with chronic AR are absent, and physical examination is often misleadingly bland. In severe acute AR any sign of heart failure or mitral valve preclosure is an indication for urgent AVR. While there is often concern of reinfection of the prosthetic valve used to correct acute AR, this in fact only occurs rarely. Further, there is no proven effective medical therapy for acute severe AR other than appropriate antibiotic coverage.

❏ SUGGESTED READINGS

Angiography and Interventions and the Society of Thoracic Surgeons. Circulation. 2006;114:e84-231.

Bonow RO, Carabello BA, Kanu C, et al. ACC/AHA 2006 guidelines for the management of patients with valvular heart disease: a report of the American College of Cardiology/American Heart Association Task Force on Practice Guidelines (writing committee to revise the 1998 Guidelines for the Management of Patients With Valvular Heart Disease): developed in collaboration with the Society of Cardiovascular Anesthesiologists: endorsed by the Society for Cardiovascular

Carabello BA, Crawford MH. Aortic stenosis. In: Crawford MH (Ed). Current Diagnosis and Treatment in Cardiology, 2nd edition. New York: McGraw-Hill Professional; 2003. pp. 108-20.

Carabello BA. Aortic valve disease. In: Taylor GJ (Ed). Primary Care Management of Heart Disease. St. Louis: Mosby; 2000. p.236. Carabello BA. Progress in mitral and aortic regurgitation. Prog Cardiovasc Dis. 2001;43:457-75.

Grande KJ, Cochran RP, Reinhall PG, et al. Stress variations in the human aortic root and valve: the role of anatomic asymmetry. Ann Biomed Eng. 1998;26:534-45.

Otto CM, Kuusisto J, Reichenbach DD, et al. Characterization of the early lesion of 'degenerative' valvular aortic stenosis: histological and immunohistochemical studies. Circulation. 1994;90:844-53.

Owens DS, Katz R, Takasu J, et al. Incidence and progression of aortic valve calcium in the multi-ethnic study of atherosclerosis (MESA). Am J Cardiol. 2010;105:701-8.

Pellikka PA, Sarano ME, Nishimura RA, et al. Outcome of 622 adults with asymptomatic, hemodynamically significant aortic stenosis during prolonged follow-up. Circulation. 2005;111:3290-5.

Rajamannan NM, Subramaniam M, Springett M, et al. Atorvastatin inhibits hypercholesterolemia-induced cellular proliferation and bone matrix production in the rabbit aortic valve. Circulation. 2002;105:2260-5.

Rosenhek R, Zilberszac R, Schemper M, et al. Natural history of very severe aortic stenosis. Circulation. 2010;121:151-6.

Ross J Jr, Braunwald E. Aortic stenosis. Circulation. 1968;38:61-7.

Schwarz F, Baumann P, Manthey J, et al. The effect of aortic valve replacement on survival. Circulation. 1982;66:1105-10.

5.2 Mitral Valve Disease

❏ INTRODUCTION

Normal mitral valve (MV) function depends on the structural integrity and coordinated action of the anatomic components of the mitral apparatus (Fig. 9). The MV is a complex structure formed by four elements. The annulus is asymmetrical, with a fixed portion (corresponding to the anterior leaflet) shared with the aortic annulus and a dynamic portion (corresponding to the posterior leaflet) that represents most of the circumference of the annulus.

❏ RHEUMATIC HEART DISEASE

In the developed countries of the world, the incidence of RF has fallen markedly during the last century. This decrease in incidence preceded the introduction of antibiotics and is a reflection of improved socioeconomic standards, less overcrowded housing and improved access to medical care.

Valvular Heart Diseases

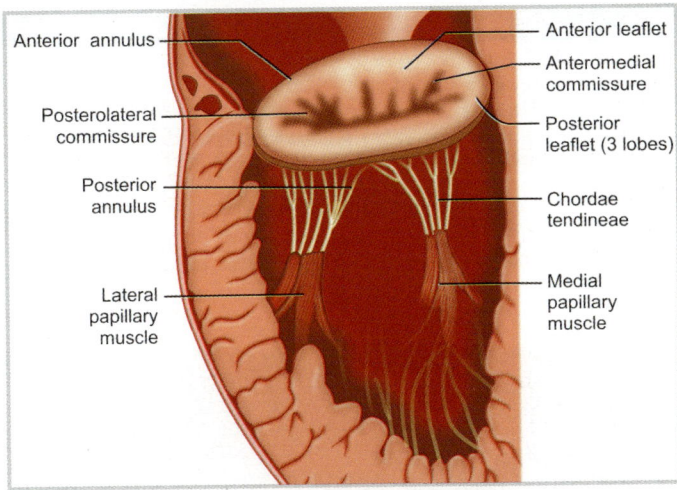

FIGURE 9: Mitral valve apparatus

FLOWCHART 2: Preventive and therapeutic strategies in rheumatic fever and rheumatic heart disease

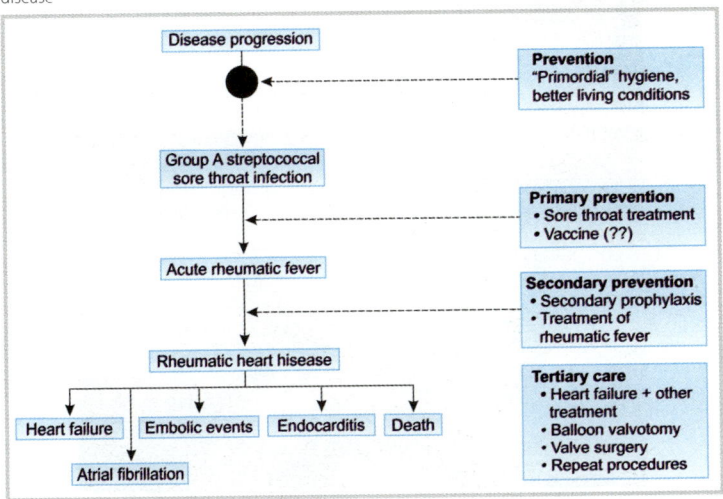

As shown in Flowchart 2, the sequelae of RF and chronic RHD are devastating and contribute to a large financial burden on the individual, family and the society.

❑ MITRAL STENOSIS

Etiology and Pathology

In clinical practice, the predominant cause of mitral stenosis (MS) is RF. Congenital MS is rare and is typically diagnosed in infancy or early childhood. Various causes of MS are listed in Table 4.

Table 4: Causes of mitral stenosis

- Rheumatic fever
- Degenerative mitral annular calcification
- Congenital (parachute valve, DOMV, as a part of HLHS)
- Rare causes: malignant carcinoid disease, systemic lupus erythematosus, rheumatoid arthritis, mucopolysaccharidoses of Hunter–Hurler phenotype, Fabry disease, Whipple disease
- Conditions mimicking MS: left atrial tumors, cor triatriatum, ball valve thrombus, infective endocarditis with large vegetation

(Abbreviations: DOMV: Double orifice mitral valve; HLHS: Hypoplastic left heart syndrome; MS: Mitral stenosis)

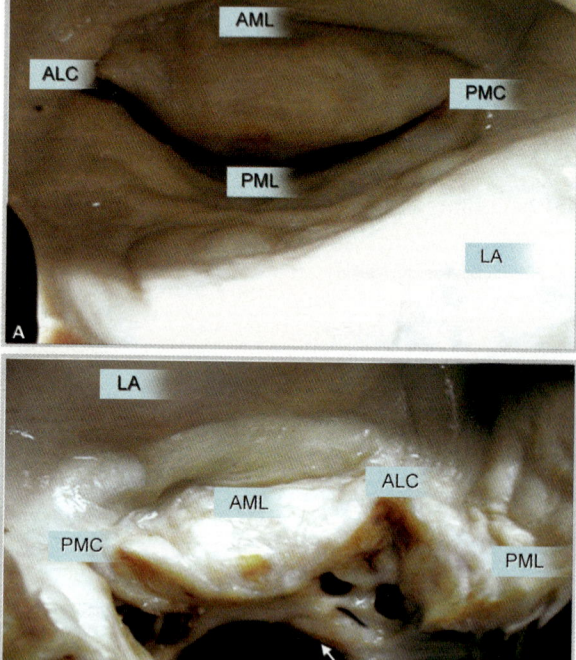

FIGURES 10A AND B: Pathology of mitral stenosis: (A) Mitral valve viewed from left atrial (LA) aspect shows crescentic appearance of the valve orifice; (B) The opened out valve highlights the commissural and chordal fusion (arrow) and leaflet thickening. (Abbreviations: AML: Anterior mitral leaflet; PML: Posterior mitral leaflet; ALC: Anterolateral commissure; PMC: Posteromedial commissure; LV: Left ventricle)

Rheumatic MS results from the affection of commissures, cusps, chordae and the PMs (Figs 10A and B). Fibrotic process tends to involve all the structures resulting in a funnel shaped mitral orifice. In severe forms of MS, fibrosis is so intense that the leaflets, chordae and the PMs become a single mass, hence making it difficult to differentiate at what level one component of the MV ends and the other component begins. Secondary pathological changes include left atrial (LA) hypertrophy and dilatation, LA thrombi and changes of venous, and arterial hypertension in the pulmonary vasculature with secondary right ventricular (RV) hypertrophy.

Clinical Diagnosis

The interval between the initial episode of RF and MV obstruction is variable. Female gender is predominantly affected. Patients frequently adapt to their level of functional capacity and deny symptoms despite objective effort limitation. Anemia, fever, infection, pregnancy, undue exertion or onset of AF often precipitates pulmonary edema. The hemodynamic basis and mechanism of symptoms are summarized in Table 5.

Clinical findings are influenced by severity of MS, presence and severity of PH, rhythm, morphology of the valve and associated valve lesions. The physical findings seen in MS are shown in Table 6.

Table 5: Symptoms in mitral stenosis

Hemodynamic/other mechanism	Symptoms
Elevated PWP	Dyspnea, orthopnea, PND, pulmonary edema
↑ PAP, RVF, low cardiac output	Fatigue, chest pain, dyspnea, pain abdomen, pleural effusion, edema feet, ascites
Atrial fibrillation	Palpitations, precipitation of heart failure, systemic emboli, tachycardiomyopathy (rare)
Dislodgement of LA thrombi	Systemic emboli (stroke, limb ischemia, saddle emboli, etc.)
Multifactorial	Hemoptysis
Compression of recurrent laryngeal nerve by LA or PA	Hoarseness of voice (Ortner's syndrome)

(Abbreviations: PWP: Pulmonary wedge pressure; PND: Paroxysmal nocturnal hyspnea; PAP: Pulmonary artery pressure; RVF: Right ventricular failure; LA: Left atrial (atrium); PA: Pulmonary artery)

Table 6: Physical examination in mitral stenosis

Pulse	Normal, low volume, AF
JVP	Normal, "a" wave (if PH), signs of TR
Palpation	Tapping apex, parasternal heave, palpable P2
Auscultation	Loud S1, OS, diastolic murmur with presystolic crescendo component, loud P2, RV S3, TR, PR (rare)
Assessment of severity	A2-OS interval, length of murmur, signs of PH
Assessment of valve morphology	Intensity of S1, and OS
Associated valve lesions	Murmurs of AR, MR, AS, organic tricuspid valve disease

(Abbreviations: JVP: Jugular venous pulse; PH: Pulmonary hypertension; TR: Tricuspid regurgitation; P2: Pulmonic component of second heart Sound; S1: First heart sound; RV-S3: Right ventricular gallop; PR: Pulmonary regurgitation; AR: Aortic regurgitation; MR: Mitral regurgitation; AS: Aortic stenosis; OS: Opening snap)

Investigations

Electrocardiogram can be completely normal especially in those with mild MS. Patients in sinus rhythm usually show evidence of LA enlargement. Right axis deviation, RV hypertrophy and right atrial enlargement are seen in patients with PH.

Chest X-ray can be normal but usually reflects the hemodynamic changes of pulmonary venous hypertension. Calcification of MV is uncommon in young patients.

Two-dimensional (2D) transthoracic echocardiography (TTE) with Doppler assessment helps in confirming the diagnosis, evaluating the valve area, transvalvar gradient, valve morphology, estimates of PH and LV function. Presence of LA thrombus or rare occurrence of vegetation on the MV can also be diagnosed by TTE. However, sensitivity of transesophageal echocardiogram (TEE) is much more as compared to TTE in diagnosing LA thrombi or MV vegetations. Simple echocardiogram scoring system designed by Wilkins et al. based on the amount of thickening, degree of pliability, severity of subvalvar affection and presence and extent of calcification helps in deciding whether or not the valve is suitable for BMV (Figs 11A and B).

Treadmill stress testing or bicycle ergometry may provide a useful objective assessment of functional capacity in patients whose symptoms are equivocal or discordant with the severity of MS. Exercise echocardiography can also be used to assess the evolution of mitral gradient and PASP in patients with doubtful symptoms.

Coronary angiography is required for exclusion of atherosclerotic coronary artery disease (CAD) either prior to surgery or during balloon mitral valvotomy (BMV).

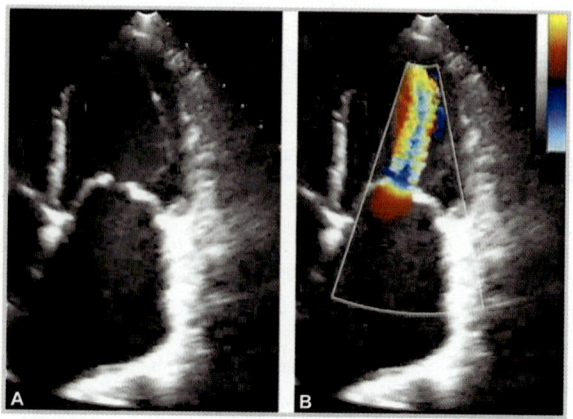

FIGURES 11A AND B: 2D echocardiography and color Doppler in mitral stenosis. 2D echocardiography with color flow mapping during diastole in a patient with mitral stenosis showing thickened, but pliable leaflets and severe flow acceleration across the stenosed valve. The valve morphology is ideally suited for a balloon mitral valvotomy

Management

Medical Treatment

There is a limited role for medical therapies especially for those who are in sinus rhythm. Treatment of precipitating factors, like anemia, infection, AF and electrolyte imbalance, can help in relieving the symptoms. In general, all patients should receive the recommended rheumatic prophylaxis, such as injection of benzathine penicillin or other suitable agent. All patients should receive appropriate antibiotic prophylaxis for those procedures known to cause bacteremia. Diuretics are often recommended for relieving the congestive symptoms. The role of digoxin in patients with sinus rhythm remains controversial. With its modest inotropic effect, digoxin seems to be of some value in patients with PH and RV failure.

Atrial ectopic per se do not need any treatment although they usually precede AF. The contributors to AF in RHD are LA size, pressure, fibrosis and persistent rheumatic activity. Acute AF is often associated with a rapid ventricular response. Cordarone is effective in rhythm control but in the presence of unrelieved MS, maintaining sinus rhythm is difficult. If patient is hemodynamically unstable, immediate direct current cardioversion is indicated. Generally, low molecular weight heparin or unfractionated heparin is administered initially to be followed by oral anticoagulation. Chronic rate control for these patients is achieved with the use of digoxin, a beta-blocker, a calcium channel blocker or a combination of these agents.

Mechanical Relief of Obstruction

Mitral stenosis results in a mechanical obstruction to forward flow and available therapies are aimed at relieving this obstruction. Four procedures are effective in providing the desired palliation. These are percutaneous BMV, closed surgical commissurotomy, open surgical commissurotomy, and MV replacement.

The timing of intervention is guided by the observational data. Figure 12 shows that the survival benefits with mechanical relief of obstruction (surgical

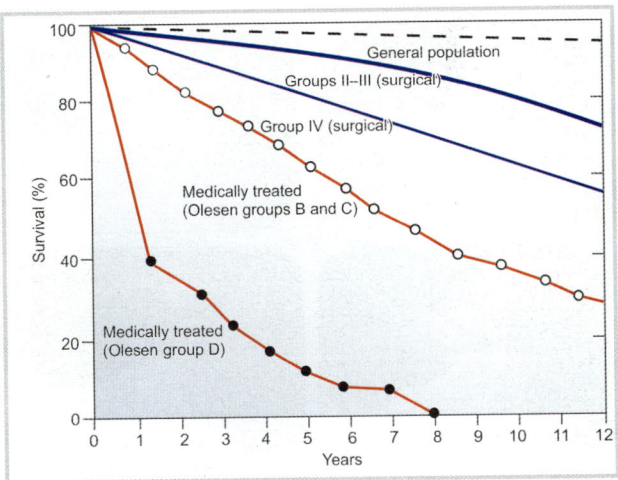

FIGURE 12: Survival according to therapy and symptomatic status for patients with MS. Groups II, III and IV equivalent to NYHA classifications II, III and IV are approximately similar to the groups B, C, and D respectively. Class IV patients had improved survival when treated surgically

commissurotomy in this series) compared with medical therapy are greater in patients with advanced symptoms. It seems reasonable to provide mechanical relief once more than mild symptoms are present. PH increases the risk of surgery, and it is advisable to relieve the mechanical obstruction prior to development of significant PH.

Percutaneous BMV is currently the technique of choice. Percutaneous BMV has been found to be equal or superior in safety and efficacy to closed or open surgical commissurotomy, acutely as well as in long-term. Figure 13 shows MV area at base line and during the study period with the three techniques in prospective randomized trials conducted in India. The technique and device developed by Inoue (Figs 14A to E) remains the preferred approach all over the

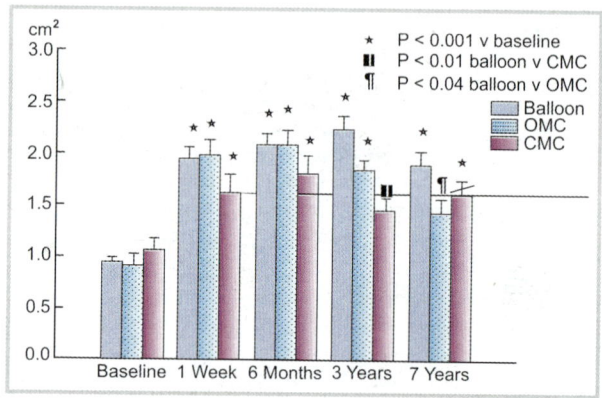

FIGURE 13: Mitral valve area following balloon, open mitral commissurotomy (OMC) and closed mitral commissurotomy (CMC). Mitral valve area at base line, 1 week, 6 months, 3, and 7 years after balloon dilation, CMC or OMC, in prospective randomized trials conducted in Hyderabad, India

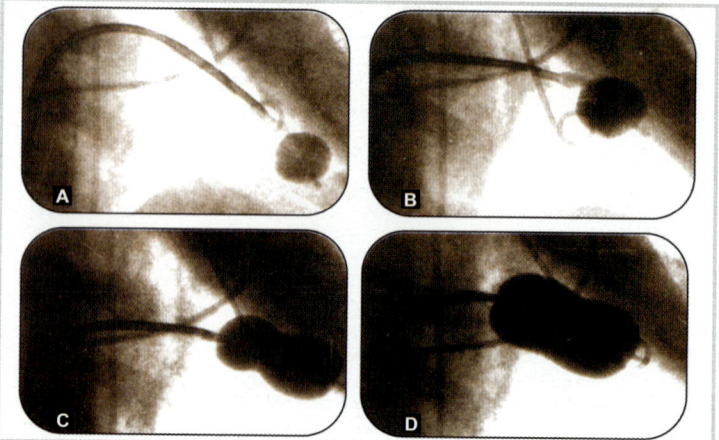

FIGURES 14A TO D: The BMV using Inoue balloon technique. Steps in BMV using Inoue balloon: (A) Balloon inserted in left ventricle (LV) through left atrium (LA) after trans-septal puncture; (B) Balloon positioned at mitral valve; (C) Waist in partially inflated balloon across the narrowed valve, and (D) Fully inflated balloon with disappearance of waist indicating relief of obstruction

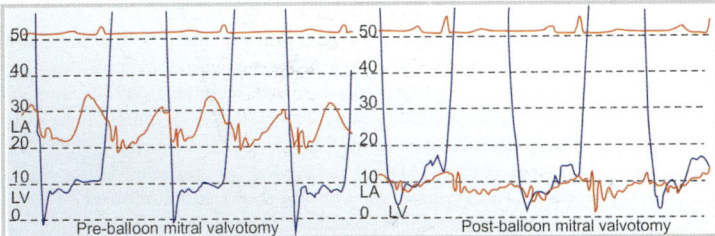

FIGURE 14E: Hemodynamic traces during BMV using Inoue balloon technique. Simultaneously recorded LV, LA pressures show remarkable reduction in gradient after BMV

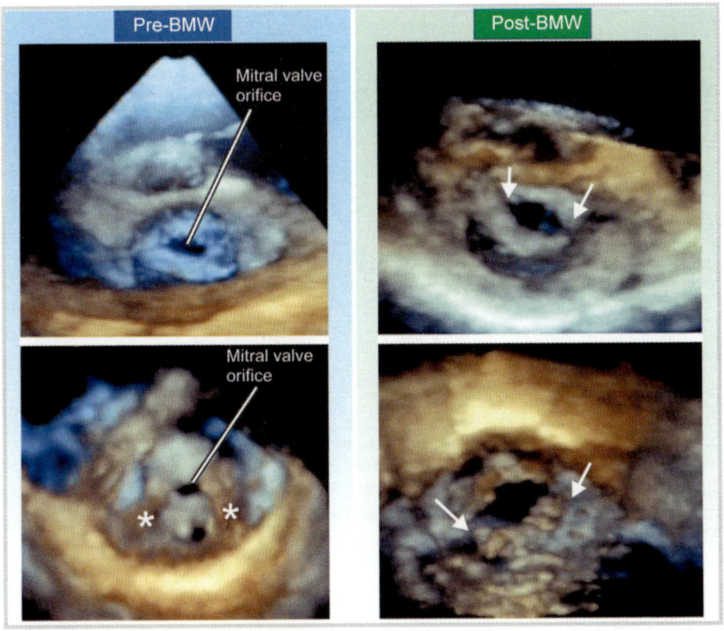

FIGURE 15: Three-dimensional echocardiography preballoon mitral valvotomy and postballoon mitral valvotomy. Three dimensional (3D) echocardiographic images recorded in diastole from atrial (upper panel) and ventricular aspect (lower panel) before (left panel) and after (right panel) Inoue balloon mitral valvotomy (BMV) in mitral stenosis. These images demonstrate commissural splitting (short white arrows) as the mechanism of benefit after BMV. The restricted leaflet motion due to fibrosis in chordopapillary apparatus (stars) remains unchanged

world. The predominant mechanism of benefit following BMV as demonstrated by 2D or three dimensional (3D) echocardiography is commissural splitting (Fig. 15). The other possible mechanisms for relief of obstruction are stretching of the valve orifice and cracking of valvular calcifications. The procedure typically results in a doubling of the MV area (on average from 1.0 cm^2 to 2.0 cm^2) with a 50% reduction in gradients. The success rate is 80–95% and is defined as the MV area increasing to greater than 1.5 cm^2 and LA pressure decreasing to less than 18 mm Hg without major complications.

Open mitral valvotomy is reserved for patients judged to be unsuitable for percutaneous procedures because of calcification, thrombus or associated regurgitation. The operation consists of dealing with cusps, commissures and subvalvar apparatus by use of fairly standardized techniques. Open surgical commissurotomy is currently indicated in patients with LA thrombus, poor valve morphology and for technical failures with BMV.

Mitral valve replacement (MVR) is needed in patients where valve morphology precludes valve conservation and in those with combined MS and MR. Emergency valve replacement is needed, if severe acute MR occurs during BMV.

❑ MITRAL REGURGITATION

Etiology

The MR is classified in several ways, i.e. depending on the presentation, mechanism (primary or secondary), etiology and the component of MV apparatus it involves. A distinction is made between primary (organic) and secondary (functional) MR. In primary MR, there is derangement of one or more components of the valve apparatus, permitting back flow, causing LV volume overload. If this overload is severe and prolonged, it results in LV remodeling, dysfunction, PH, heart failure and eventually death. Correction of primary MR in a timely fashion reverses these consequences; thus, there is an unchallenged cause and effect relationship between the primary MR and its effect on the LV.

In secondary MR, the valve itself is usually normal. However, LV previously damaged by infarction develops papillary muscles (PMs) displacement and annular dilatation, causing the MV to leak (Figs 16A and B).

The MR can result from involvement of any of its components, e.g. valve leaflets, chordae tendineae, PMs and annulus (Table 7), and the presentation can be acute or chronic.

The etiology of MR is changing the world over. The RHD still remains a leading cause of MR in the developing countries, whereas degenerative MR is the most common etiology in the Europe and the USA. An etiological classification of MR is shown in Table 8.

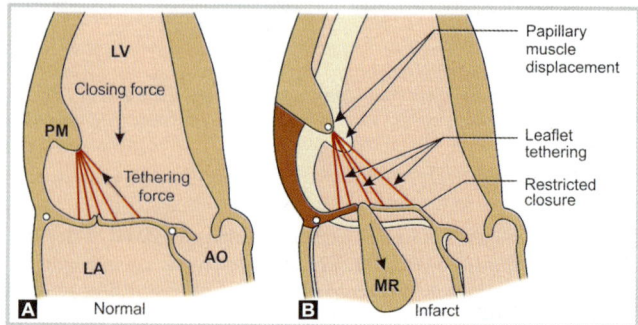

FIGURES 16A AND B: Mechanism of secondary mitral regurgitation. Balance of forces acting on mitral leaflets in systole (A) and effect of papillary muscle (PM) displacement (B). Dark shading indicates myocardial infarction; light shading indicates normal baseline (Abbreviations: AO: Aorta; LA: Left atrium; LV: Left ventricle; MR: Mitral regurgitation)

Table 7: Causes of mitral regurgitation according to involvement of valve structures

Structure	Etiology
Valve leaflets	Rheumatic, degenerative, IE, trauma (surgery, BMV, others), congenital (cleft, arcade, DOMV), SLE, tumors
Chordae tendineae (rupture/abnormal insertion)	Degenerative, IE, trauma, RHD, congenital anomalies, Marfan's, Ehlers–Danlos syndrome
Annulus disorders	Degenerative, calcification, IE (abscess), trauma (surgery)
Annular dilatation	Degenerative, dilated cardiomyopathy, submitral aneurysm, other causes of LV dilatation
Papillary muscle	CAD, cardiomyopathy, trauma, infiltrative disease, Kawasaki's disease, congenital

(Abbreviations: IE: Infective endocarditis; BMV: Balloon mitral valvotomy; DOMV: Double orifice mitral valve; SLE: Systemic lupus erythematosus; RHD: Rheumatic heart disease; LV: Left ventricular; CAD: Coronary artery disease)

Table 8: Etiology of mitral regurgitation

Inflammatory	RHD, SLE, nonspecific aortoarteritis, Kawasaki's disease, scleroderma
Degenerative	Degenerative (MVP, flail, Barlow's disease) Marfan's, Ehlers–Danlos syndrome, pseudoxanthoma elasticum, calcification of MV annulus
Infective	IE affecting normal or abnormal valve
Congenital	MV cleft, parachute MV, MR in association with atrioventricular septal defect, CTGA, anomalous origin of coronary artery from left pulmonary artery
Traumatic	Surgery, balloon valvotomy, chest trauma

(Abbreviations: RHD: Rheumatic heart disease; SLE: Systemic lupus erythematosus; MVP: Mitral valve prolapse; MV: Mitral valve; IE: Infective endocarditis; MR: Mitral regurgitation; CTGA: Corrected transposition of great arteries)

Table 9: Causes of acute mitral regurgitation

- Infective endocarditis (leaflet perforation, chordal rupture, abscess formation)
- Chordal rupture (degenerative disease, spontaneous, Marfan's, RHD, IE)
- Papillary muscle dysfunction/rupture
- Leaflet tear during balloon mitral valvotomy, surgery
- Trauma (Blunt chest trauma, penetrating injuries, surgical technical problems)

(Abbreviations: IE: Infective endocarditis; RHD: Rheumatic heart disease)

Acute MR usually results from chordal rupture, PM dysfunction or rupture, leaflet tear or perforation and often presents as an emergency. The causes of acute MR are diverse and represent acute manifestations of disease processes that may under other circumstances, cause chronic MR (Table 9).

Clinical Diagnosis

Patients with chronic MR remain asymptomatic for several years due to the ease with which the LA and LV accommodate the volume overload. The regurgitation volume is initially less than the forward stroke volume. However, as the regurgitant volume exceeds the forward stroke volume, the effective forward cardiac output

Table 10: Symptoms in chronic and acute mitral regurgitation

Hemodynamics/other mechanism	Symptoms
Chronic MR	
LVVO, AF, VPB	Palpitations
LV dysfunction	Dyspnea, PND, orthopnea
PH, RVF	Fatigue, dyspnea, edema, pain abdomen
Compression of recurrent laryngeal nerve by LA	Hoarseness of voice
Acute MR	
Elevation of LA, PA pressure	Acute onset dyspnea, PND, orthopnea, pulmonary edema

(Abbreviations: LVVO: Left ventricular volume overload; AF: Atrial fibrillation; VPB: Ventricular premature beat; LV: Left ventricle; PND: Paroxysmal nocturnal dyspnea; PH: Pulmonary hypertension; RVF: Right ventricular failure; LA: Left atrium; PA: Pulmonary artery)

Table 11: Physical signs in mitral regurgitation

Category	Findings
Chronic severe MR	Cardiomegaly, LV apex, LA pulsations, apical grade 3–4/6, holosystolic murmur, MDM, S3, signs of PH, AF
Acute MR	Normal heart size, apical low pitched soft systolic murmur, S4, PH-TR
Specific signs for rheumatic MR	Findings of associated MS, aortic valve involvement
Specific signs for degenerative MR	Mid systolic click, late systolic murmur, findings of flail leaflet
Specific signs for secondary MR	Cardiomegaly, S3, early systolic murmur

(Abbreviations: LV: Left ventricle; LA: Left atrium; MDM: Mid diastolic murmur; PH: Pulmonary hypertension; AF: Atrial fibrillation; TR: Tricuspid regurgitation)

falls and symptoms appear. The hemodynamic basis of symptoms in chronic and acute MR is shown in Table 10.

The etiological differentiation of rheumatic MR from other causes like degenerative disease or functional MR is made on the basis of the typical clinical features of each entity (Table 11).

Investigations

Electrocardiogram is frequently normal in patients with mild or moderate chronic MR. The LA and LV enlargement occurs with increasing severity and duration of MR. The AF is frequent and the incidence varies with the etiology, age and severity of MR. In secondary MR, electrocardiography shows Q waves, most frequently in the inferior and/or lateral leads and a left bundle branch block.

Chest X-ray is usually normal in patients with mild MR. Cardiomegaly is often seen in patients with chronic severe MR and is contributed by enlargement of LV and LA (Fig. 17). In severe acute MR, despite marked elevation of PASP, the cardiac size is usually normal and only mild enlargement of LA is seen. Signs of pulmonary venous congestion are often prominent.

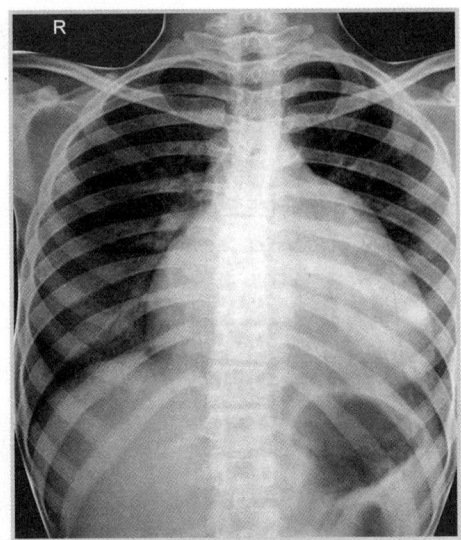

FIGURE 17: Roentgenogram of chest posteroanterior view. X-ray in a patient with chronic severe mitral regurgitation shows prominent left atrial appendage and cardiomegaly

Echocardiography also provides information regarding etiology and severity thereby helping and deciding the time and type of intervention (e.g. valve repair or replacement). The TEE is superior to TTE for defining the anatomy of the MV, for detection of vegetation especially if the valve is calcific and to interrogate the LA appendage. It is extremely useful in those with suboptimal TTE window. The 3D echocardiography provides superior imaging of the MV components and is currently utilized intraoperatively. Stress echocardiography is emerging as a useful modality.

It can help distinguish among rheumatic MR (thickened leaflets with restricted motion, calcification, and chordal shortening) (Fig. 18), degenerative disease 16–18 (characterized by thickened and redundant leaflets with excessive motion and prolapse) (Figs 19A and B) and congenital heart disease (cleft valve) and rule out secondary MR due to ischemic or nonischemic LV dysfunction.

Echocardiography guides the timing of surgical intervention especially in those patients with chronic MR who are asymptomatic by estimating the severity of regurgitation, LV function and size, LA size, PA pressure, LA volume, LV end systolic and end diastolic volumes, stroke volume, EF, and regurgitant fraction.

In acute MR, echocardiography shows little increase in internal diameter of either the LA or LV. Characteristic features of Doppler echocardiography are the wide jet of MR and elevation of the PASP. It demonstrates structural abnormality like chordal rupture, flail leaflet or PM rupture depending on the etiology and dictates the need of early surgery.

Coronary angiography is required in patients who have known or suspected CAD, risk factors for CAD or in ischemic MR.

64-slice multislice computed tomography (MSCT) has been utilized to provide anatomic and geometric information about the MV apparatus. The technique may be of value to guide surgical treatment of MR.

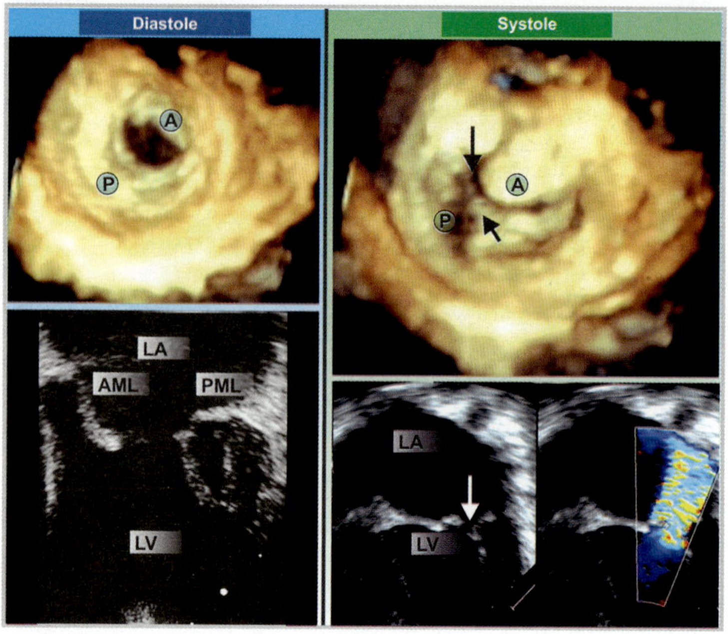

FIGURE 18: Three-dimensional (3D) echocardiography, two-dimensional (2D) echocardiography, and color Doppler in mitral regurgitation (MR). The 3D echocardiography and 2D echocardiography images of the mitral valve (MV) in diastole and systole reveal in a 10-year-old boy with rheumatic MR. The 3D diastolic frame reveals adequate mitral valve orifice from the left atrial (LA) aspect. The 2D image in diastole reveals restricted posterior mitral leaflet (PML) motion, thickened subvalvar structures which are hallmarks of rheumatic affection. The 2D systolic frame shows incomplete coaptation of the MV leaflets with posteriorly directed mitral regurgitation jet. The true crescentic regurgitant orifice is obvious only on 3D systolic frame

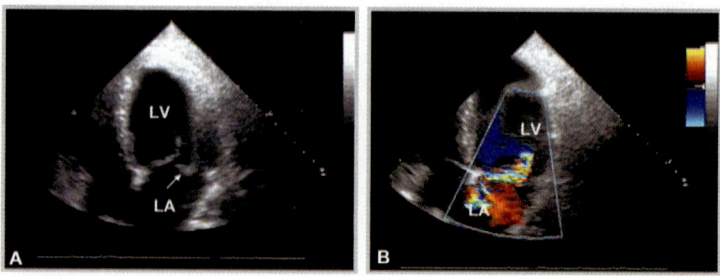

FIGURES 19A AND B: Echocardiography in degenerative mitral valve disease. (A) Two dimensional echocardiography images in apical four chamber view showing prolapse of the posterior mitral leaflet (arrow); (B) Color flow showing images severe mitral regurgitation (Abbreviations: LV: Left ventricle; LA: Left atrium)

Cardiovascular magnetic resonance imaging has recently been used to identify MVP and show regurgitant jets. It can match the diagnostic sensitivity and specificity of TTE. This technique, in addition, can measure LV volumes, identify myocardial scar and detect fibrosis involving the PMs.

Management

Medical Treatment

There is no proven medical therapy for the treatment of chronic MR. In MR, secondary to RHD, rheumatic prophylaxis using benzathine penicillin or other suitable agent is recommended. The infective endocarditis (IE) prophylaxis is often warranted. The vasodilators are useful in stabilizing patient with acute MR by reducing regurgitant fraction. Role of vasodilator in chronic, asymptomatic MR with preserved LV function is debatable. However, angiotensin converting enzyme inhibitors (ACEI) or angiotensin receptor blockers (ARB) are certainly recommended for the treatment of heart failure. Diuretics are useful in patients with congestive symptoms.

Surgical Treatment

The definitive treatment of hemodynamically significant MR is the surgical correction of MR. Three different MV operations are currently used for correction of MR: (i) Repair, (ii) MVR with preservation of part or all of the mitral apparatus, and (iii) MVR with removal of the valve apparatus.

According to American College of Cardiology/American Heart Association guidelines (2006), surgery is recommended for the management of chronic severe MR in symptomatic patients and asymptomatic patients with evidence of LV dysfunction, defined as an LVEF of 30–60% and LV end-systolic dimension of 40 mm or greater. The guidelines mention that patients with a severely reduced LVEF (<30%) may not benefit from surgery. Other reasonable indications for surgery in asymptomatic patients include elevation of PA pressure and new onset AF. The management of asymptomatic patients with normal LVEF remains controversial.

The MVR in which MV apparatus is resected is often performed in RHD where the valve apparatus is severely distorted by the disease process. The advantages of MVR with preservation of the chordal apparatus are that this operation preserves LV function, enhances postoperative survival compared with MVR, in which the apparatus is disrupted.

The MV repair has a clear advantage over replacement, as it preserves LV systolic function, obviates the need for oral anticoagulation and improves survival. Figure 20 shows lower operative mortality and better survival rates at 10 years

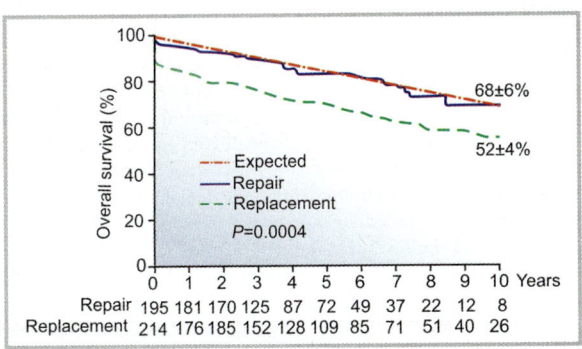

FIGURE 20: Postoperative survival. Following mitral valve repair, postoperative survival is ompared to that mitral valve replacement. (*Source:* Modified from Carabello BA)

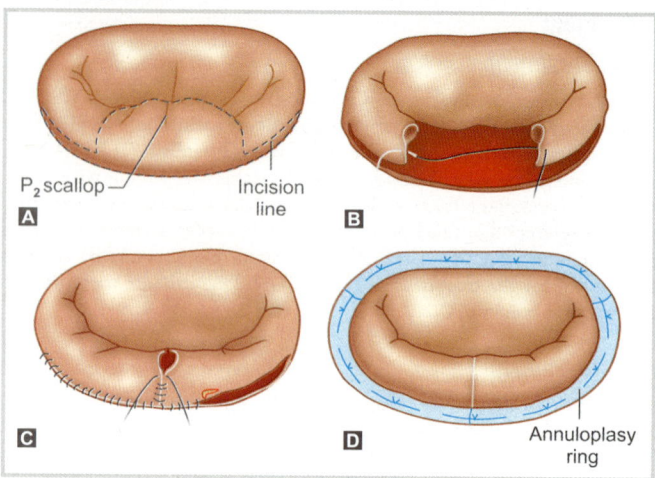

FIGURES 21A TO D: Steps for surgery for mitral valve prolapse. (A) Shows the surgeon's view, from the atrium of a valve with a flail P2 scallop. Dashed line shows the planned incision of ruptured and elongated chordae. (B) View after resection of the diseased portion. (C) Re-apposition of the leaflet edges. (D) Reconstructed valve with a annuloplasty ring

by valve repair compared with MVR. It is currently the operation of choice for MR secondary to degenerative valve disease. Valve repair with artificial chordal reconstruction is occasionally feasible in rheumatic MR. Prosthetic ring or band annuloplasty restores the normal circumference and shape of the MV annulus and is a mainstay of all repair procedures regardless of the technique employed (Figs 21A to D).

Minimally invasive valve surgery refers to a constellation of surgical techniques/technologies that minimize surgical trauma through smaller incisions compared with a conventional sternotomy. The most common minimally invasive approach for MV repair, MVR includes a right thoracotomy, a robotically assisted right thoracic approach, and a partial sternotomy. In highly experienced centers, minimally invasive surgery is safe, efficient treatment option providing greater patient satisfaction and fewer complications.

Percutaneous MV repair is a new technique which has been investigated for treatment of MR due to degenerative valve disease and secondary MR using a clip (Evalve MitraClip) (Fig. 22) made of a cobalt-chromium alloy and Dacron. The edge-to-edge technique (Fig. 23) mimics the surgical procedure introduced by O Alfieri, which creates a double mitral orifice by means of a few stitches securing the two leaflets together at their mid part. The current experience in more than 500 patients suggests that the technique although demanding, is feasible and safe in experienced hands. The immediate outcomes are favorable with 30 day mortality in 0–2% and functional improvement in 66–90% of patients at 30 days.

Surgery in IE is indicated for those with acute MR secondary to chordal rupture or leaflet perforation, uncontrolled heart failure, large and mobile vegetation and when intensive specific antibiotic therapy, fails to control infection. The MVR has been the standard surgical therapy but recent reports suggest that repair is feasible depending on the degree of tissue destruction.

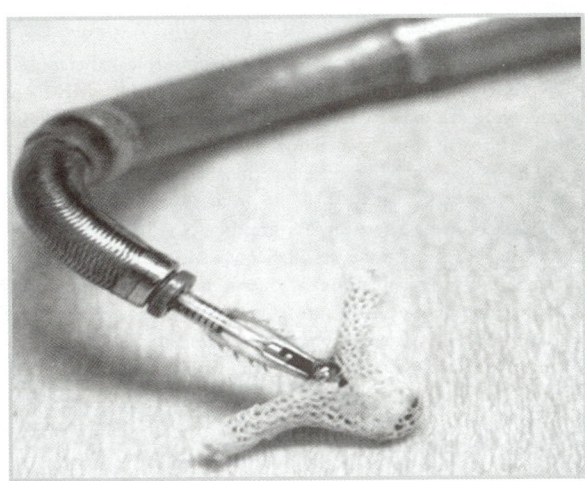

FIGURE 22: MitraClip device. This device is covered with polyester fabric to facilitate tissue ingrowth. The distal gripping element helps with leaflet fixation. The clip delivery system exits through a guide catheter. (*Source:* Feldman T, Kar S, Rinaldi M, et al. Percutaneous mitral repair with the MitraClip system: safety and midterm durability in the initial EVEREST (Endovascular Valve Edge-to-Edge REpair Study) cohort. J Am Coll Cardiol. 2009;54(8):686-94, with permission)

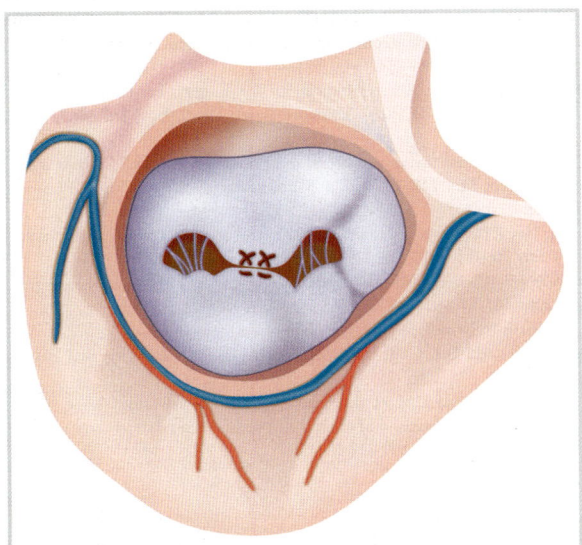

FIGURE 23: Double orifice mitral valve (MV) surgical repair. The MV is viewed from the left atrial side. The middle scallops of the anterior and posterior leaflets have been sutured together, which creates a double orifice, edge-to-edge, or bow-tie repair. (*Source:* Modified from Feldman T)

Treatment of Secondary Mitral Regurgitation

The therapeutic options in functional MR include medical therapy, devices and surgery. The ACE inhibitors and beta blockers which reduce MR by progressive reverse remodeling are indicated. Digoxin, diuretics, nitrates and spironolactone are also useful. Cardiac resynchronization therapy (CRT) is beneficial in selected patients and has been shown to reduce functional MR.

The failing ventricle usually benefits from relief of severe MR. Several procedures like coronary artery bypass grafting (CABG), MVR with chordal sparing, MV repair (surgical or percutaneous) and ventricular remodeling are available. There are several unanswered questions regarding appropriate patient selection, acceptable perioperative mortality, long-term survival benefit and the choice of the operation. Percutaneous MV repair using MitraClip has recently been shown to be feasible and safe in patients with functional MR secondary to severe LV dysfunction. The precise indications and long-term follow-up remain uncertain. The role of percutaneous ring annuloplasty to reduce annular dilatation is also being investigated.

❏ SUGGESTED READINGS

Bach DS, Awais M, Gurm HS, et al. Failure of guideline adherence for intervention in patients with severe mitral regurgitation. J Am Coll Cardiol; 2009. pp. 860-5.

Bonow R, Carabello BA, Kanu C, et al. ACC/AHA 2006 guidelines for the management of patients with valvular heart disease: a report of the American College of Cardiology/American Heart Association task force on practice guidelines (writing committee to revise the 1998 guidelines for the management of patients with valvular heart disease): developed in collaboration with Society of Cardiovascular Anesthesiologists: endorsed by Society for Cardiovascular Angiography and Interventions and Society of Thoracic Surgeons. Circulation. 2006;114:e84-231.

Carabello BA. Mitral valve disease: indications for surgery. In: Yusuf S, Cairns JA, Camm AJ, Fallen EL, Gresh BJ (Eds). Evidence-Based Cardiology, 3rd edn. Hoboken: Wiley-Blackwell; 2010.

Carabello BA. The current therapy for mitral regurgitation. J Am Coll Cardiol. 2008;52:319-26.

Di Salvo TG, Acker MA, Dec GW, et al. Mitral valve surgery in advanced heart failure. J Am Coll Cardiol. 2010;55(4):271-82.

Marsan NA, Bax JJ. Changes in functional mitral regurgitation after cardiac resynchronization therapy. Eur Heart J. 2010;31:2323-5.

Otto CM. Clinical practice. Evaluation and management of chronic mitral regurgitation. N Engl J Med. 2001;345:740-6.

Roy SB, Gopinath N. Mitral stenosis. Circulation. 1968;38:68-76.

Schmitto JD, Mokashi SA, Cohn LH. Minimally-invasive valve surgery. J Am Coll Cardiol. 2010;56:455-62.

Sharma S, Loya YS, Desai DM, et al. Percutaneous mitral valvotomy using Inoue and double balloon technique: comparison of clinical and hemodynamic short term results in 350 cases. Cathet Cardiovasc Diagn. 1993;29:18-23.

5.3 Tricuspid Valve Disease: Evaluation and Management

❏ INTRODUCTION

Tricuspid valve (TV) is often described as the forgotten valve deserving of more respect. The TV disease is generally classified as primary or intrinsic valve pathology or secondary or functional valve dysfunction. The primary valve disease results from structural abnormality of the valve apparatus. The secondary or functional TV disease results from the factors that generally lead to tricuspid annular dilatation commonly from left heart disease and resulting RV hypertension, dilatation and dysfunction (Flowchart 3).

❏ ETIOLOGY OF TRICUSPID VALVE DISEASE

Primary Tricuspid Valve Disease

These are characterized by intrinsic pathology of the valve apparatus:
- Congenital
  - Ebstein's anomaly
  - Congenital cleft valve
  - Congenital tricuspid stenosis
  - Tricuspid atresia
- Acquired
  - Rheumatic
  - Infective endocarditis
  - Degenerative: tricuspid valve prolapse

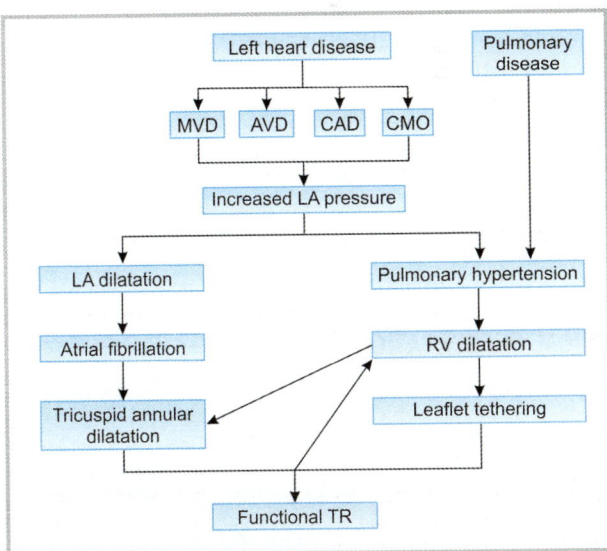

FLOWCHART 3: Functional TR—pathogenesis

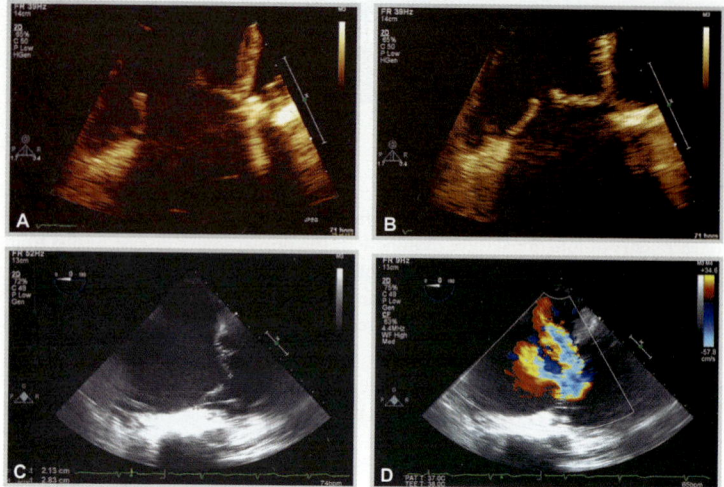

FIGURES 24A TO D: Functional tricuspid regurgitation. (A) Tricuspid valve in diastole in fully open position; (B) Tricuspid valve in systole exhibits incomplete closure with central orifice of regurgitation; (C) Transesophageal echocardiography cross-section exhibits dilated annulus (4.9 cm), and systolic tethering distance of 1.6 cm with incomplete valve closure; (D) Transesophageal echocardiography cross-section with prominent central jet of tricuspid regurgitation

- Carcinoid heart disease
- Toxic [e.g. phen-fen or methysergide valvulopathy (?)]
- Tumors (e.g. fibroelastoma, myxoma)
- Trauma (e.g. pacemaker lead trauma, or use of biopsy instrument)
- Radiation injury.

Secondary or Functional Tricuspid Valve Disease

These are characterized by normal valve apparatus aside from abnormal annular dilatation and tethering of leaflets in systole (Figs 24A to D):
- RV dilatation (e.g. atrial septal defect, pulmonary regurgitation)
- RV hypertension (e.g. pulmonary hypertension, pulmonary stenosis)
- RV dysfunction (e.g. cardiomyopathy, myocarditis)
- Segmental RV dysfunction (e.g. ischemia or infarction, endomyocardial fibrosis, arrhythmogenic RV dysplasia). Asymmetric tethering with segmental pathology may lead to an eccentric jet
- Chronic atrial fibrillation (with right atrial and annular dilatation).

❏ CLINICAL PRESENTATION

The abnormal valve function may be in the form of: (i) pure or predominant tricuspid stenosis, (ii) pure or predominant TR, or (iii) mixed.

The symptoms specific to advanced TV disease are related to: (i) decreased cardiac output, for example, fatigue, and (ii) right atrial hypertension, for example, liver congestion resulting in right upper quadrant discomfort, or gut congestion with symptoms of dyspepsia, indigestion, or fluid retention with leg edema and ascites. It may be emphasized that significant TV disease may not be associated

Table 12: Clinical signs of severe tricuspid regurgitation

- Venous pulse: Prominent systolic (C-V) wave
- Holosystolic murmur increasing in intensity with inspiration (Carvallo's sign)
- Hepatomegaly with systolic pulsation
- Parasternal lift especially with right ventricular hypertension

Note:
- The classic systolic V wave is present in less than 75% of patients
- The murmur is heard in less than 20% of patients
- Hepatomegaly is noted in 90%, but systolic pulsation is inconsistent
- Parasternal lift also occurs with severe mitral regurgitation, being late systolic

with any symptoms until a late stage of the disease involving progressive RV dysfunction. Physical signs of TR are listed in Table 12.

❏ LABORATORY DIAGNOSIS

Electrocardiogram

There are no specific markers of TV disease, although the following clues may be present: (i) RV hypertrophy and "strain" with right QRS axis and (ii) right atrial enlargement with prominent P waves. Specific electrocardiograph signs of primary etiology may be noted, such as left axis deviation and complete right bundle branch block in AV canal defect associated with cleft valve, and Ebstein's anomaly may exhibit wide QRS.

Chest Radiograph

Cardiomegaly associated with prominent right heart borders may be noted. There are no specific findings to suggest a diagnosis of TV disease.

Echocardiography

Two-dimensional echocardiogram combined with spectral and color flow Doppler evaluation provides the most accurate laboratory test in detection and quantitation of TV disease. In addition, the TV morphology provides clues of underlying etiology and pathophysiology of valve dysfunction (Figures 25 and 26). Echocardigraphy findings of severe TR are listed in Table 13.

Transesophageal Echocardiography

The TTE is often of diagnostic quality because the TV and the right ventricle are closer to the anterior chest wall and several parasternal, apical and subcostal views are used to image these structures. However, TTE is indicated for better anatomic definitions of the valve lesions or precise measurement of the tricuspid annulus. The assessment of severity of tricuspid stenosis or TR is generally more accurate with TTE. In the intraoperative setting, TEE is especially used for measuring the tricuspid annulus diameter.

Cardiac Catheterization and Selective Angiography

Diagnostic cardiac catheterization should rarely, if ever, be undertaken for the diagnosis or quantitation of TV disease.

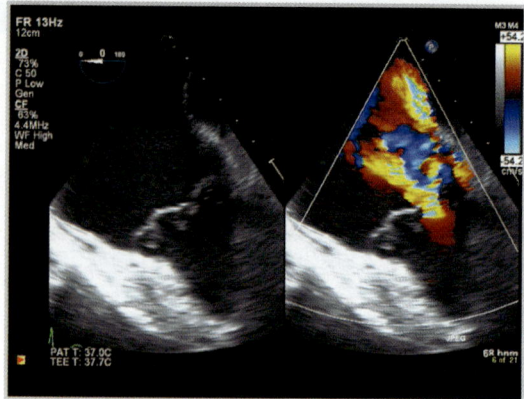

FIGURE 25: Transesophageal echocardiography image of tricuspid valve in systole exhibits billowing valve prolapse and multiple jets of regurgitation

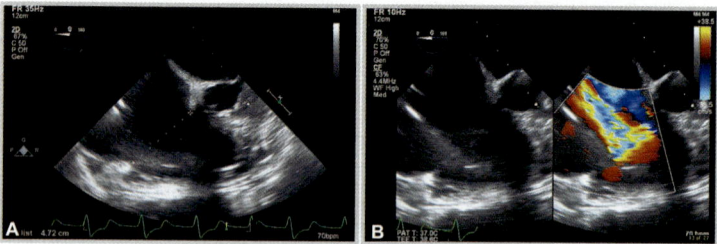

FIGURES 26A AND B: Transesophageal echocardiography cross sections of tricuspid valve restricted by pacemaker lead resulting in severe regurgitation and secondary annular dilatation. (A) Tricuspid annulus measures at 4.7 cm; (B) Pacemaker lead restricting the leaflet with severe regurgitation

Table 13: Echocardiography: diagnosis of severe tricuspid regurgitation

- Regurgitant jet area greater than 10 cm^2 (least utilized)
- PISA: radius greater than 9 mm with aliased scale adjusted to peak TR velocity
- Continuous wave Doppler velocity profile with early peak and rapid deceleration indicative of high right atrial LV wave
- Hepatic vein flow: systolic flow reversal in both respiratory phases

(Abbreviations: PISA: Proximal isovelocity surface area; TR: Tricuspid regurgitation; LV: Left ventricular)

❑ TREATMENT

The treatment of TV disease must entertain two important considerations, namely the appropriate timing and the appropriate management strategy.

Appropriate Timing

As an isolated lesion, mild or moderate TV disease does not need to be treated. Mild or even moderate TR may be observed using current echo-Doppler techniques in normal subjects. In the absence of structural changes, such as annular dilatation or leaflet disruption, such lesions are not known to progress. Chronic severe regurgitation often begets more regurgitation. For isolated severe TV disease, intervention should be considered as earliest signs of RV and/or hepatic dysfunction develop.

The rules governing management are different when moderate TV dysfunction is associated with other valvular or myocardial disorders. The timing of intervention is generally dictated by considerations relating to accompanying left heart disease. Approximately 40% of patients exhibit regression of TR following mitral valve surgery with reduction in pulmonary hypertension. There is no reliable criterion to predict as to which patients are likely to regress. Since it fails to regress in nearly 60% of patients and reoperations tend to carry higher morbidity and mortality, it is a recommended practice to treat tricuspid lesion more aggressively during the mitral valve surgery.

Management Strategies

Medical Treatment

The TR secondary to pulmonary hypertension may be treated by medical management of underlying etiology, when feasible. Thus, appropriate treatment of myocarditis or depressed left ventricular function may result in amelioration of functional TR. Similarly, improvement in lung function in chronic obstructive lung disease or appropriate control of sleep apnea may improve the associated TR. It is worth emphasizing that functional TR may be dynamic, being load dependent. Intensive medical treatment of heart failure may substantially improve the severity of TR.

Surgical Treatment

Tricuspid stenosis: Rheumatic tricuspid stenosis is nearly always associated with rheumatic mitral valve disease. Successful mitral and tricuspid repair may be carried out; however, long-term results are poor. Mitral valve replacement with TV replacement may be considered in patients unwilling to entertain a risk of reoperation. These patients will require mechanical prosthesis being in younger age group.

Tricuspid regurgitation: Since the most commonly observed TR undergoing surgery is functional or secondary to mitral, aortic or ischemic heart disease; the surgical approaches will be considered in some detail. Significant TR is often a marker of adverse outcome. A variety of techniques for valve repair have been used over the years. These fall broadly into two categories: (i) suture techniques and (ii) annuloplasty techniques (Table 14).

Tricuspid Valve Replacement

Although most studies have reported a better early and long-term outcome with valve repair, there are some cases with marked distortion of the annulus and severe tethering of the leaflets where valve replacement may be necessary. Generally bioprosthetic valves are preferred, since valve thrombosis and infection following mechanical valve replacement are distinct risks.

Residual regurgitation following TV replacement is lower than after valve repair; however, the perioperative midterm survival and event free survival is better with valve repair (Table 15).

The 2006 American College of Cardiology/American Heart Association (ACC/AHA) Guidelines for management of patients with valvular heart disease pertaining to TV are summarized in Table 16.

Table 14: Surgical approaches for secondary or functional

- Suture techniques
  - DeVega purse string suture repair
  - Suture plication of posterior leaflet
  - Edge-to-edge suture technique
- Annuloplasty techniques
  - Carpentier ring annuloplasty
  - Duran flexible ring annuloplasty
  - MC3 partial ring devised to replicate tricuspid geometry
  - Peri-Guard annuloplasty
  - Other rings and bands
- Valve replacement
  - Bioprosthesis
  - Mechanical valve

Table 15: Tricuspid valve repair versus replacement: mid-term outcomes

Study design		Retrospective analysis; a single center experience
Patient groups		178 with TV repair; 72 with TV replacement (54 bioprosthesis, 18 mechanical)
Type of follow-up		Clinical and echocardiographic
Duration of follow-up		5.2 ± 4.1 years
In hospital deaths		Repair, 4%; Replacement, 22%
Survival	5 years	Repair, 90 ± 3%; Replacement, 63 ± 6%
	10 years	Repair, 76 ± 5%; Replacement, 55 ± 6%

Table 16: The 2006 American College of Cardiology/American Heart Association (ACC/AHA) guidelines for management of patients with valvular heart disease

Class	Management
Class I	TV repair is beneficial for severe TR in patients with MV disease requiring MV surgery (level of evidence: B)
Class IIa	TV replacement or annuloplasty is reasonable for severe primary TR when symptomatic (level of evidence: C)
	TV replacement is reasonable for severe TR secondary to diseased/abnormal TV leaflets not amenable to annuloplasty or repair (level of evidence: C)
Class IIb	Tricuspid annuloplasty may be considered for less-than-severe TR in patients undergoing MV surgery when there is pulmonary hypertension or tricuspid annular dilatation (level of evidence: C)
Class III	TV replacement or annuloplasty is not indicated in asymptomatic patients with TR whose pulmonary artery systolic pressure is less than 60 mm Hg in the presence of a normal MV (level of evidence: C)
	TV replacement or annuloplasty is not indicated in patients with mild primary TR (level of evidence: C)

(Abbreviations: MV: Mitral valve; TR: Tricuspid regurgitation; TV: Tricuspid valve)

The current approaches to surgical treatment of TV disease at time of mitral and/or aortic valve surgery are summarized in Table 17.

Table 17: Indication for TV surgery during mitral and/or aortic valve surgery			
	Intraoperative transesophageal echocardiography		
Severe TR			TV Repair
Mild-to-moderate TR	Prior known severe TR		TV Repair
	No prior severe TR	Annulus diameter ≥40 mm	TV Repair
		Annulus diameter 35–39 mm PASP >50 mm Hg	TV Repair
		Annulus diameter <35 mm	No need for repair

(Abbreviations: PASP: Pulmonary artery systolic pressure; TR: Tricuspid regurgitation; TV: Tricuspid valve)

❏ SUGGESTED READINGS

Bonow RO, Carabello BA, Chatterjee K, et al. ACC/AHA 2006 guidelines for the management of patients with valvular heart disease: a report of the American College of Cardiology/American Heart Association task force on practice guidelines (writing Committee to Revise the 1998 guidelines for the management of patients with valvular heart disease) developed in collaboration with the Society of Cardiovascular Anesthesiologists endorsed by the Society for Cardiovascular Angiography and Interventions and the Society of Thoracic Surgeons. Circulation. 2006;114:e84-231.

Dreyfus GD, Corbi PJ, Chan KM, et al. Secondary tricuspid regurgitation or dilatation: which should be criteria for surgical repair? Ann Thorac Surg. 2005;79:127-32.

Shiran A, Sagie A. Tricuspid regurgitation in mitral valve disease incidence, prognostic implications, mechanism, and management. J Am Coll Cardiol. 2009;53:401-8.

Singh SK, Tang GH, Maganti MD, et al. Midterm outcomes of tricuspid valve repair versus replacement for organic tricuspid disease. Ann Thorac Surg. 2006;82:1735-41.

Skudicky D, Essop MR, Dareli P. Efficacy of mitral balloon valvotomy in reducing the severity of associated tricuspid valve regurgitation. Am J Cardiol. 1994;73:209-11.

Tei C, Shah PM, Cherian G, et al. Echocardiographic evaluation of normal and prolapses tricuspid valve leaflets. Am J Cardiol. 1983;52:796-800.

Waller BF, Howard J, Fess S. Pathology of tricuspid valve stenosis and pure tricuspid regurgitation—Part III. Clin Cardiol. 1995;18: 225-30.

5.4 Congenital Pulmonic Stenosis

❏ INTRODUCTION

Congenital pulmonic stenosis is a congenital obstruction above, at, or below the pulmonary valve and does not include extrinsic obstruction to the right ventricular outflow tract from mediastinal masses or internal obstruction from tumors. In 90% of patients the pulmonary valve is stenotic. The anomaly is common, with an incidence per million live births of 532 (median) to 836 (75th percentile). It constitutes about 7% of all congenital heart diseases.

❏ VALVAR PULMONIC STENOSIS

The stenosis is usually isolated but can occur with almost any other form of congenital heart disease; a secundum atrial septal defect or a patent foramen ovale is a common association. The stenosis may occur in siblings or successive generations. It is seen occasionally in patients with Noonan or Williams–Beuren syndromes, or neurofibromatosis. Chromosome 22q11 deletion (CATCH 22 syndrome, DiGeorge syndrome) is an occasional association.

Most patients are asymptomatic at rest and on exercise except for neonates with critical stenosis or the older adult with severe obstruction and myocardial damage. Even those with severe stenosis can be asymptomatic, but some, however, have fatigue, cyanosis, congestive heart failure, or even classical angina pectoris on exertion.

Physical Examination

Body habitus and growth are usually normal. Some patients have a pentagonal or moon-shaped face. Patients with severe stenosis may show cyanosis and clubbing. If right ventricular end-diastolic pressure is raised, the jugular vein has a prominent "a" wave, but mean venous pressure is usually normal. There may be a prominent right ventricular heave at the lower left sternal border, and a systolic thrill can often be felt at the upper left sternal border.

The mainstay of clinical diagnosis is auscultation. To understand how auscultation helps assess severity, consider the pressure tracings shown in Figure 27.

In pulmonic stenosis (right panel), however, the pressure gradient between right ventricle and main pulmonary artery is prolonged, with a triangular right ventricular pressure wave, and the associated systolic murmur, also diamond shaped, is longer and ends close to the second heart sound.

With more severe stenosis, right ventricular pressure increases, and ejection lengthens. The murmur is therefore prolonged and its peak intensity occurs beyond mid-systole, and the murmur may even end after the aortic component of the second heart sound (Fig. 28). The murmur is usually quite loud, grade 3/6 or more.

The degree of splitting of the second heart sound increases as stenosis severity increases (Fig. 28), with the measured splitting (taken during held expiration) given to the right of each phonocardiogram in milliseconds. Auscultation can assess severity by the length of the systolic murmur and the position of its maximal intensity, the width of splitting of the second sound, and the frequency of the murmur. Another prominent auscultatory feature, shown well in the middle panel of Figure 28, is the early systolic ejection click. This click is louder during expiration and is more marked in mild or moderate than severe stenosis.

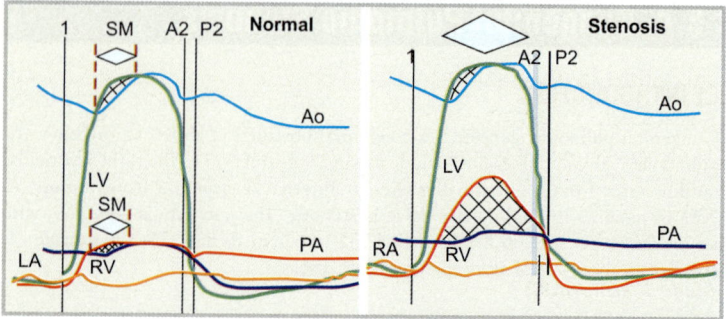

FIGURE 27: Pressure tracings in normal subjects and subjects with aortic or pulmonic stenosis. (Abbreviations: SM: Systolic murmur; LV: Left ventricle; RV: Right ventricle; LA: Left atrium; RA: Right atrium; PA: Main pulmonary artery; Ao: Aorta; A1: Aortic first heart sound; A2: Aortic second heart sound; P2: Pulmonic second heart sound)

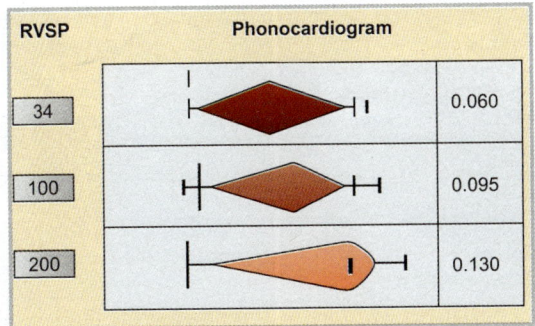

FIGURE 28: Selected phonocardiograms based on a series published by Gamboa et al. The three phonocardiograms represent mild, moderately severe, and very severe stenosis (Abbreviation: RVSP: Right ventricular systolic pressure)

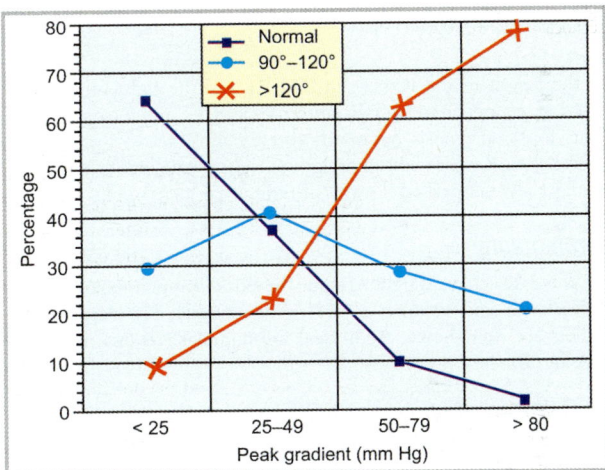

FIGURE 29: Relationship between peak gradient and severity of stenosis. The percentage in each severity group is shown for normal (QRS axis < 90°, mild right axis deviation of 90–120°, and marked right axis deviation > 120°)

Laboratory Investigations

Chest Roentgenogram

This is typical beyond the neonatal period. Even mild stenosis produces poststenotic dilatation of the main pulmonary artery. If the right ventricle is hypertrophied, then the heart has a more rounded right heart border, but is not enlarged except in some patients with severe stenosis or congestive heart failure.

Electrocardiogram

Right ventricular hypertrophy produces increased anterior and rightward forces. Figure 29 shows the relationship between peak pressure gradient and mean frontal axis deviation as shown by Ellison et al. Right ventricular hypertrophy enlarges R wave in lead V1 and the S wave in leads V5 and V6. There is a very rough correlation

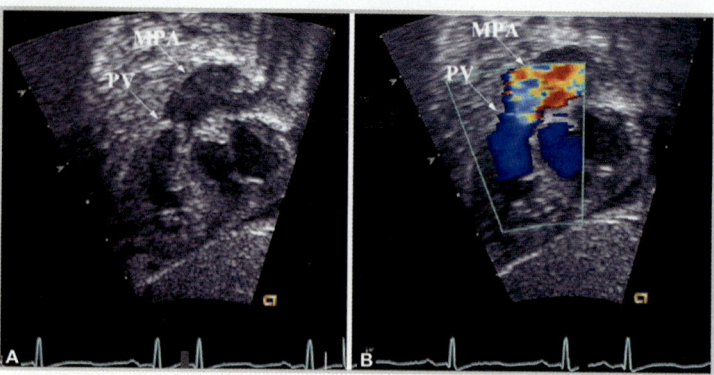

FIGURES 30A AND B: (A) 2D echocardiogram to show doming pulmonary valve with tiny central orifice, and marked poststenotic dilatation. (B) Doppler study shows turbulence beyond the valve, and hints at the narrow orifice. (Abbreviations: PV: Pulmonary valve; MPA: Main pulmonary artery). (*Source:* Echocardiograms by Dr Paul Stanger)

between the height of the R wave in lead V1 and the right ventricular systolic pressure. Most patients have an rsR' pattern in lead V1 and reference to standards is necessary for the diagnosis, but in very severe stenosis lead V1 may show either a pure R wave or a qR wave—absolute signs of right ventricular hypertrophy. Severe stenosis may show tall peaked P waves of right atrial hypertrophy.

Echocardiography

M-mode and 2-D echocardiograms show the thickened pulmonary valve, changes in wall thickness and volume of the right ventricle. Dysplastic myxomatous valve leaflets are well shown. Additional infundibular stenosis may be detected (Figs 30A and B).

Cardiac Catheterization

This has been replaced almost entirely by echocardiography. Pressures are measured in the right ventricle and right atrium, and with a slow careful pullback from the pulmonary artery the site of obstruction is identified. If right ventricular systolic pressure is very high, no attempt should be made to enter the pulmonary artery lest the orifice be completely obstructed. Angiography demonstrates the site(s) of obstruction, and the doming valve with a jet passing through the narrowed orifice (Figs 31A to C).

Differential Diagnosis

In addition to congenital pulmonic stenosis, an ejection murmur at the base is often due to
- An innocent pulmonary flow murmur which is seldom more than grade 2/6 in intensity, and ends by mid-systole.
- Atrial septal defect; the can be distinguished from pulmonic stenosis because an atrial septal defect has palpable hyperactivity of the right ventricle and wide fixed splitting of the second heart sound, and often a mid-diastolic rumble over the tricuspid area.
- Aortic stenosis murmur is often lower, and the narrow splitting of the second heart sound is incompatible with a loud ejection murmur of pulmonic stenosis.

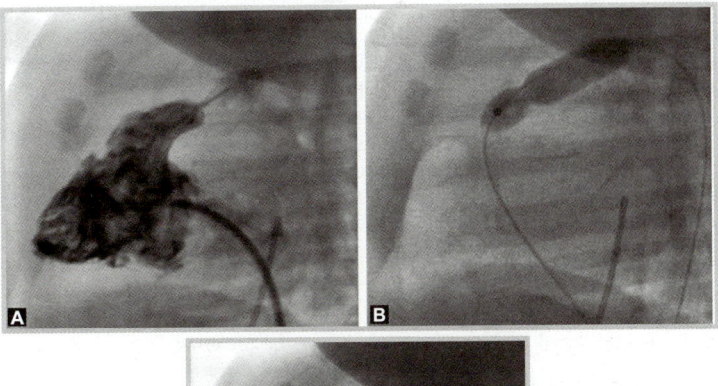

FIGURES 31A TO C: Angiograms (lateral view) in an infant with severe valvar pulmonic stenosis. (A) Angiogram shows doming valve and narrow jet through tiny orifice; (B) Angiogram shows dilating balloon in valve, with almost no waist, indicating enlargement of orifice; (C) Angiogram shows wider outflow orifice after balloon valvotomy, as well as well-marked poststenotic dilatation of the main pulmonary artery. (Source: Dr David Teitel. Same patient as shown in Figure 30)

- Massive dilatation of the main pulmonary artery associated with no or minimal stenosis at the pulmonic valve may be deceptive.

Treatment

Any patient with symptoms or severe stenosis (right ventricular systolic pressure >100 mm Hg), with or without symptoms, requires valvotomy. Patients with right ventricular systolic pressure less than 50 mm Hg do not need treatment, although if untreated they should evaluated periodically for changes in pressure or ventricular function. For those with intermediate pressures, the decision to treat is made easier by the introduction of balloon valvotomy.

Surgery

Sir Russell Brock first opened the stenotic valve by passing a dilator through the right ventricular wall and then blindly dilating the stenotic pulmonic valve. This was followed by opening the valve under direct vision during brief hypothermic circulatory arrest, and later with cardiopulmonary bypass. However, blind valvotomy has still been used successfully in neonates to avoid complications of cardiopulmonary bypass.

Surgical valvotomy has an in-hospital mortality of 10–40% in neonates, but only 0–6% beyond that period. The pressure gradient across the valve and right ventricular systolic pressure decrease, even in neonates, although there are usually residual gradients of 10–30 mm Hg. Long-term postoperative survival up to 40 years after operation is excellent (~95%), except for neonates and older adults, and is close to that for the normal population.

Some patients need reoperation, occasionally to repair an associated lesion, such as an atrial or ventricular septal defect, or a tricuspid valve lesion, but most often for marked pulmonic regurgitation or for residual or recurrent pulmonic stenosis.

Balloon Valvotomy

This was introduced by Kan et al. and is now the preferred form of treatment unless there are other intracardiac lesions that need correction at the same time. The procedure is performed at cardiac catheterization under anesthesia or deep sedation. If the annulus is very wide, a double balloon technique can be used. In experienced hands the procedure is safe and effective.

Failure to dilate the valve occurred in less than 10% of patients, many of whom had dysplastic valves. Balloon dilatation has been successful in adults (including one octogenarian), even with calcified valves. Deaths from the procedure are rare, with rates of 0.15% and 0.2% in two large collaborative studies. Since these reports included some of the early procedures, the rate is probably lower today.

The results in general are good. About 7% of the patients (64 out of 860) needed intervention for restenosis. Pulmonic regurgitation was seen in most patients after balloon valvotomy.

Critical stenosis of neonates and infants has also been treated successfully by balloon valvotomy. The early mortality is higher in younger children than in older children due to the severity of the illness and the associated lesions, but survivors do fairly well.

❑ ISOLATED INFUNDIBULAR STENOSIS

Infundibular stenosis not secondary to pulmonic valve stenosis is usually associated with a ventricular septal defect or tetralogy of Fallot. In fact, some of the patients who present with isolated infundibular stenosis are known to have had a ventricular septal defect that closed spontaneously. Nevertheless, some do not have this association. Isolated infundibular stenosis is rare. The natural history is unknown. Patients present at ages between 2 and 63 years, and about half are children.

History and physical examination are the same as for valvar pulmonic stenosis except that there is no early systolic ejection click, and the pulmonic component of the second heart sound is not softened.

Chest Roentgenogram differs from that in valvar stenosis in that there is no poststenotic dilatation of the main pulmonary artery. Electrocardiogram is same as described for valvar pulmonic stenosis.

Echocardiogram is diagnostic in showing an obstruction of the infundibulum and a normal pulmonary valve. Cardiac Catheterization is performed carefully with a very slow pull back from the main pulmonary artery to the right ventricle, shows the level and degree of obstruction.

As the pulmonary valve is normal, the surgeon can excise the fibromuscular obstruction widely to reduce the risk of recurrence while not running the risk of pulmonary regurgitation. Short-term results have been excellent, and should parallel those for valvar stenosis of equivalent degree and age.

❑ SUPRAVALVAR STENOSIS

Stenosis above the valve may occur in the main pulmonary artery, at the bifurcation with extension into the right and left pulmonary arteries, in multiple peripheral pulmonary arteries, or combinations of these sites. Most supravalvar stenosis is associated with tetralogy of Fallot and pulmonary atresia, or after various operations on the main pulmonary artery, including aortopulmonary shunts and arterial switch procedures. Peripheral pulmonary artery stenosis due to rubella embryopathy is rare today.

Supravalvar stenoses occur as part of the Williams–Beuren syndrome due to a contiguous gene deletion at 7q11.23 that affects elastin formation, or the Alagille syndrome (arteriohepatic dysplasia) due to a heterozygous mutation of the JAG1 gene on chromosome 22.

Other family members may be affected in both syndromes. Symptoms depend upon the severity of the stenosis and whether other organ systems are involved.

The stenotic murmur may be heard better in the axillae if the stenosis is in a peripheral pulmonary artery but otherwise cannot be differentiated from murmurs at other sites of obstruction. There is no early systolic ejection click. As diastolic pressure in the pulmonary artery is low, the pulmonic second heart X-ray may show right ventricular hypertrophy, but there is never poststenotic dilatation of the main pulmonary artery. If stenosis predominantly affects one lung, there may be reduced vascular markings on that side. Electrocardiogram shows typical features of right ventricular hypertrophy. Echocardiogram may show stenosis in the main pulmonary artery or near the bifurcation but is unhelpful with intraparenchymal stenoses. It is useful, however, in excluding stenosis at or below the pulmonary valve and in evaluating right ventricular function. Other imaging methods, such as magnetic resonance imaging or angiography, are used to examine intrapulmonary arterial stenosis. Cardiac catheterization allows assessment of pressures and sites of obstruction and with associated angiography can evaluate the peripheral arteries.

Treatment

Williams–Beuren Syndrome

Surgery is preferred if the stenosis is severe and in the main pulmonary artery or at the bifurcation, and also if other cardiac lesions are to be repaired at the same time. The stenotic segments are excised with an end-to-end anastomosis if short, but more often are incised longitudinally and a patch is inserted. Residual or recurrent stenosis is common in those severely affected. If the stenosis is in the intrapulmonary arteries, the only option is to dilate the narrowed region with a balloon, or sometimes with a cutting balloon, and maintain the dilatation with a stent.

Stamm et al. observed about 80% survival at 20 years. The reoperation rate over 20 years was about 15% for those with right ventricular systolic pressure below aortic pressure, almost all within the first 2 years, but about 85% for those whose initial right ventricular systolic pressures were suprasystemic.

Alagille Syndrome

The mainstay of treatment is liver transplantation, and if necessary correction of associated cardiac or pulmonary arterial lesions. In one study, 20-year survival after liver transplantation was 80% without and 40% with associated cardiovascular disease are usually complex.

❏ SUGGESTED READINGS

Brock RC. Pulmonary valvulotomy for the relief of congenital pulmonary stenosis. Br Med J. 1948;1:1121-6.

Earing MG, Connolly HM, Dearani JA, et al. Long-term follow-up of patients after surgical treatment for isolated pulmonary valve stenosis. Mayo Clin Proc. 2005;80:871-6.

Ellison RC, Freedom RM, Keane JF, et al. Indirect assessment of severity in pulmonary stenosis. Circulation. 1977;56(Suppl. 1):I14-20.

Emerick KM, Rand EB, Goldmuntz E, et al. Features of Alagille syndrome in 92 patients: frequency and relation to prognosis. Hepatology. 1999;29:822-9.

Franch RH, Gay BB Jr. Congenital stenosis of the pulmonary artery branches. A classification, with postmortem findings in two cases. Am J Med. 1963;35:512-29.

Gay BB Jr, French RH, Shuford WH, et al. The roentgenologic features of single and multiple coarctations of the pulmonary artery and branches. Am J Roentgenol Radium Ther Nucl Med. 1963;90:599-613.

Goudevenos J, Wren C, Adams PC. Balloon valvotomy of calcified pulmonary valve stenosis. Cardiology. 1990;77:55-7.

Hoffman JI, Kaplan S. The incidence of congenital heart disease. J Am Coll Cardiol. 2002;39:1890-900.

Hoffman JIE. The Natural and Unnatural History of Congenital Heart Disease. Oxford: Wiley-Blackwell; 2009.

Ikkos D, Jonsson B, Linderholm H. Effect of exercise in pulmonary stenosis with intact ventricular septum. Br Heart J. 1966;28:316-30.

Johnson GL. Pulmonary valve stenosis. In: Moller JH (Ed). Surgery of Congenital Heart Disease: Pediatric Cardiac Care Consortium 1984-1995. Armonk NY; Futura Publishing Company Inc; 1998. pp. 165-78.

Kan JS, White RI Jr, Mitchell SE, et al. Percutaneous balloon valvuloplasty: a new method for treating congenital pulmonary-valve stenosis. N Engl J Med. 1982;307:540-2.

Milo S, Yellin A, Smolinsky A, et al. Closed pulmonary valvotomy in infants under 6 months of age: report of 14 consecutive cases without mortality. Thorax. 1980;35:814-8.

Stamm C, Friehs I, Moran AM, et al. Surgery for bilateral outflow tract obstruction in elastin arteriopathy. J Thorac Cardiovasc Surg. 2000;120:755-63.

Swan H, Zeavin I, Blount SG Jr, et al. Surgery by direct vision in the open heart during hypothermia. J Am Med Assoc. 1953;153:1081-5.

5.5 Catheter-based Treatment of Valvular Heart Disease

❏ INTRODUCTION

Valvular heart disease is an important cause of mortality and morbidity and has been successfully treated with cardiac surgery. However, a large proportion of patients with valvular disease do not undergo surgical treatment due to advanced age, multiple comorbidities and excessive operative risk. Most recently, major advances in percutaneous repair and replacement of cardiac valves have the potential to revolutionize the field of interventional cardiology.

❏ CATHETER-BASED TREATMENT OF MITRAL VALVE DISEASE

Percutaneous Balloon Mitral Valvuloplasty

Percutaneous balloon mitral valvuloplasty (PMV) is an alternative to surgical mitral valve commissurotomy in patients with symptomatic mitral stenosis. The goal of the procedure is to produce a controlled tear of the fused valve commissures toward the mitral annulus, resulting in commissural widening, thereby relieving the signs and symptoms of mitral stenosis. The procedure provides excellent early hemodynamic effects and a low rate of residual stenosis and restenosis in appropriate candidates. Long-standing hemodynamic and clinical outcomes have been reported to be comparable to surgical commissurotomy. This is a widely used, safe procedure with a low complication rate and is currently the preferred therapy for selected patients with mitral stenosis.

Transthoracic and transesophageal echocardiography is the most widely used method to assess the mitral valve apparatus. Several echocardiographic scores have been generated to predict the success of a balloon valvuloplasty. The Wilkins score is an anatomic classification of the mitral valve based leaflet mobility, valvular and subvalvular thickening and valvular calcification. A number of observational studies have shown that a Wilkins valve score of less than or equal to 8 (maximum of 16) is predictive of low success with percutaneous valvuloplasty.

There are several contraindications for percutaneous mitral valvuloplasty including the presence of left atrial thrombus, massive or bicommissural calcification, greater than 2+ mitral regurgitation, severe aortic valve or tricuspid valve disease and severe concomitant coronary artery disease requiring bypass surgery.

Procedure

Invasive hemodynamic assessment is routinely performed, including left and right heart pressure measurements, as well as cardiac output prior and immediately after the procedure. The Gorlin formula is used to calculate the mitral valve area and, typically, the severity of mitral regurgitation is assessed with a left ventriculography before and after the procedure. Most of the described techniques of percutaneous mitral balloon valvuloplasty use the antegrade transseptal approach. A retrograde approach has also been described. The antegrade transseptal method can be accomplished by using a single-balloon (Inoue technique) or double-balloon technique via the femoral vein and a transseptal puncture. The Inoue balloon is advanced across the stenotic valve; this balloon is a self-positioning, hourglass shaped device that centers itself in the stenotic orifice of the mitral valve (Figs 32A and B). The balloon is then inflated in a stepwise manner with hemodynamic

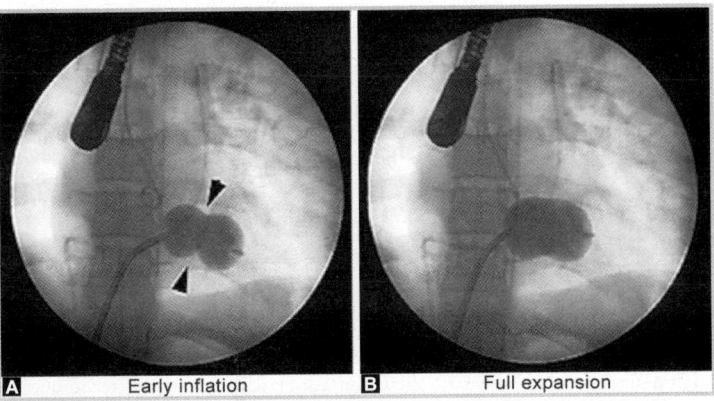

FIGURES 32A AND B: Percutaneous balloon valvotomy (PMV) for mitral stenosis with the Inoue technique. Fluoroscopic images showing the balloon across the mitral valve during (A) early inflation and (B) full expansion.

measurements repeated after each inflation to minimize the risk of damaging the mitral leaflets leading to mitral regurgitation. In the retrograde approach, the balloon catheter is advanced over a guidewire that has been inserted through the femoral arteries and snared in the descending aorta with catheters that have been advanced from the femoral vein to the right atrium and transseptally to the left atrium and left ventricle. When using the two-balloon system the cylindrical balloons are inflated simultaneously. There is no significant difference of long-term follow-up results between the two techniques. The increase in the mitral valve area is directly related to balloon size. In addition to these techniques, a nontransseptal retrograde technique has also been described. Cribier et al., more recently, introduced a metallic valvulotome device that produces results similar to the balloon devices. The valvulotome can be resterilized and reused, thereby decreasing procedural cost, which is particularly important in developing countries where rheumatic heart disease is most prevalent.

Failure rates of PMV are variable and highly dependent on the operator's experience and center volume. Success rates range from greater than 95% in ideal patients to less than 50–60% in patients with suboptimal anatomy. Overall mortality is low and is reported to be from 0% to 3% and the incidence of major complications has been reported up to 12%. Three well-described major complications have been associated with mitral valvuloplasty: (i) hemopericardium resulting in pericardial tamponade, (ii) embolic events and (iii) severe mitral regurgitation. Minor complications may include vasovagal reactions, prolonged hypotensive episodes, arrhythmias requiring treatment, significant atrial septal defect and, rarely, conduction abnormalities including complete heart block. Criteria that have been suggested for terminating the procedure include mitral valve area greater than 1.0 cm^2 per square meter of body surface area, complete opening of at least one commissure or the appearance of increase in mitral regurgitation.

Mitral Valvuloplasty in Pregnancy

Pregnant women with severe symptomatic mitral stenosis represent a highly select patient subgroup. The narrowed mitral valve orifice causes a limitation in cardiac output and an increase in left atrial pressure, which can result in pulmonary edema. Hemodynamic changes associated with pregnancy such as increase in circulating blood volume and cardiac output may lead pregnant women to develop decompensated symptoms. The PMV is a safe and effective therapy, and appears to be preferable for the fetus, compared with open mitral valve surgery during pregnancy in patients that do not respond to conservative management. The success rate of this procedure is very high, although there are concerns about the effects of the radiation exposure to the fetus during the procedure.

Percutaneous Therapies for Mitral Regurgitation

The preferred surgical approach for mitral regurgitation is mitral repair combined with mitral valve annuloplasty or MVR with a prosthetic valve. According to the European Heart Survey, up to one half of patients with severe symptomatic mitral regurgitation did not undergo surgery largely due to advanced age, presence of comorbidities or impaired left ventricular function. These data highlight the need for less invasive alternatives to open heart surgery. Transcatheter techniques of mitral leaflet repair and annuloplasty have evolved over the last few years although all remain under investigation.

Percutaneous Mitral Annuloplasty

A simplified interventional approach to simulate surgical annuloplasty has been to utilize devices to, geometrically, deform the antero-posterior or septal-lateral dimension of the mitral annulus. Devices are in development to perform percutaneous annuloplasty either from within the coronary sinus (indirect annuloplasty) or direct approaches to the mitral annulus (direct annuloplasty) via the cavity surface. These techniques are in the early stages of clinical trials.

Percutaneous Mitral Leaflet Repair

The MitraClip valve repair system (Abbott Vascular, Santa Clara, CA) utilizes a technique that is designed to treat degenerative and functional mitral regurgitation, is analogous to the Alfieri surgical procedure. A small clip is delivered with a transaxial steerable delivery system during transseptal catheterization. The anterior and posterior leaflets are then, securely attached together (edge to edge), which creates a double orifice inlet valve that improves leaflet coaptation and thus, decreases mitral regurgitation. This device has now been shown to be feasible and safe in the Endovascular Valve Edge-to-Edge Repair Study (EVEREST) and is approved for use in Europe.

❏ CATHETER-BASED TREATMENT OF PULMONARY VALVE DISEASE

Percutaneous Pulmonic Balloon Valvuloplasty

In the past, surgical valvotomy was the treatment of choice for pulmonary stenosis; however, balloon valvuloplasty has now gained acceptance as first line treatment strategy. Percutaneous balloon pulmonic valvuloplasty is highly effective and the pulmonic valve gradient, typically, is reduced by greater than 50%. Major complications of PPV are rare and more frequent in the younger pediatric population. The complications are similar to those of a right heart catheterization in addition to mild pulmonary valve insufficiency without significant hemodynamic consequences. Right ventricular outflow tract (RVOT) perforation and vessel trauma have been reported in the neonatal population. Restenosis following PPV is uncommon and less likely to occur, if the final gradient after PPV is less than 30 mm Hg.

Percutaneous Pulmonary Valve Implantation

Recently, transcatheter options have become available for replacement of the pulmonic valve. These treatments may become attractive options for patients at increased risk of operative repair. The bovine jugular Melody valve (Medtronic, Inc. Minneapolis, MN) is the first transcatheter heart valve approved in the United States. It is approved for placement in dysfunctional RVOT conduits. The PPVI has shown promising early results in managing dysfunctional right ventricle-to-pulmonary artery conduits in patients with congenital heart disease. This device has been approved as an alternative to surgery in pediatric and adult patients with RVOT conduits from previous congenital heart disease surgery and either moderate to severe PR or an RVOT stenosis with a mean gradient of greater than or equal to 35 mm Hg.

❑ CATHETER-BASED THERAPIES FOR AORTIC STENOSIS

Surgical aortic valve replacement for critical aortic stenosis has excellent outcomes and is the treatment of choice for the vast majority of symptomatic, severe aortic stenosis patients. However, perioperative complication rates and associated mortality increase with patient related factors such as advanced age and age-related increase in comorbidities.

Percutaneous Aortic Balloon Valvuloplasty

The modern procedure is most commonly performed with a retrograde approach to the valve via transfemoral arterial access (Figs 33A to D), transvenous antegrade, transseptal approach. A pulmonary artery catheter is placed for hemodynamic measurements, including measurement of cardiac output before and after completion of the procedure. When the retrograde technique is used, the left ventricular cavity is entered by advancing a catheter through the stenotic aortic valve over a guide wire. With the antegrade technique, the left atrium is entered using transseptal catheterization and a sheath. A guidewire is then manipulated across the stenosed valve to provide support for the balloon catheter. An appropriately sized dilating balloon catheter is then advanced over the guidewire and rapidly inflated to open fused commissures followed by rapid deflation to limit adverse hemodynamic

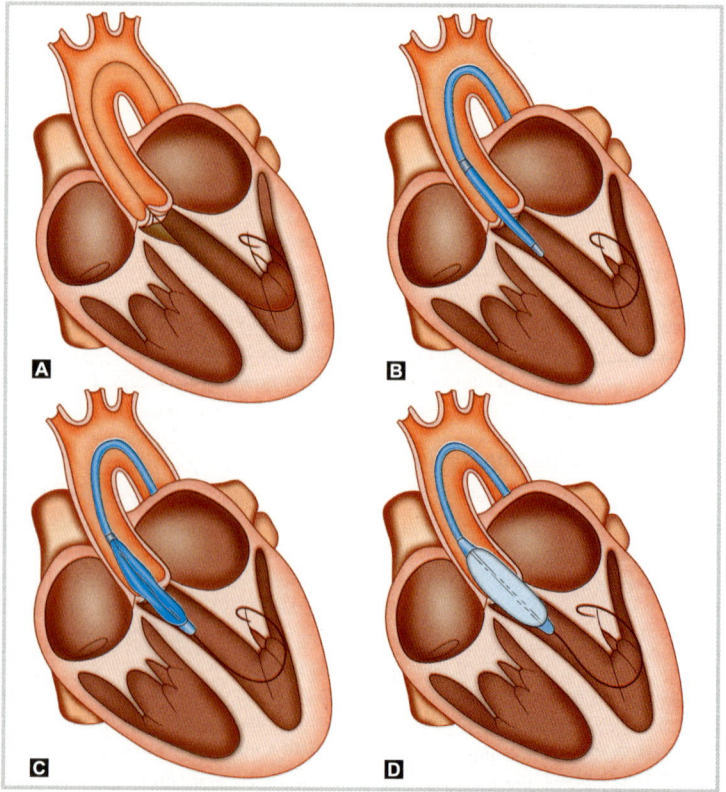

FIGURES 33A TO D: Retrograde technique of balloon aortic valvuloplasty

effects of valve obstruction. Balloon inflations are performed with or without rapid ventricular pacing. Rapid pacing via a transvenous pacing catheter can effectively, limit stroke volume and help stabilize balloon position during inflation. As the balloon obstructs flow through the valve, a significant fall in blood pressure occurs and the procedure requires rapid inflation and deflation to prevent hemodynamic collapse. After the valvuloplasty, the resultant valve area is calculated using the Gorlin equation. Left ventricular ejection fraction and degree of any resultant aortic insufficiency is assessed by contrast ventriculography or echocardiography. Further inflations with larger diameter balloons can be performed, if the result is unsatisfactory and aortic insufficiency has not, significantly, worsened. Although balloon aortic valvuloplasty results in immediate reduction in the transvalvular gradient, a high incidence of restenosis that leads to recurrent clinical symptoms has caused the procedure to fall out of favor.

Aortic Valvuloplasty in Special Circumstances

The prognosis for a patient in cardiogenic shock secondary to critical aortic stenosis is poor and surgical aortic valve replacement can be life-saving. However, evidence of multiorgan failure and hemodynamic instability may preclude these patients from an immediate operation. Moreno et al. showed that emergency percutaneous aortic balloon valvuloplasty could be performed successfully, as a bridge to ultimate surgical therapy or as a palliative treatment in critically ill patients, although morbidity and mortality remains high, despite a successful procedure.

Severe symptomatic aortic stenosis in the pregnant woman is poorly tolerated, if left unrelieved. Altered hemodynamics during pregnancy combined with a relatively fixed cardiac output caused by the stenotic valve leads to a significant risk of maternal death. Experience with balloon aortic valvuloplasty in pregnancy is limited and restricted to case reports, all of which had good results and outcomes for the mother.

Percutaneous Aortic Valve Implantation

A large portion of patients with symptomatic, severe aortic stenosis present a prohibitive risk for surgical aortic valve replacement and balloon valvuloplasty offers limited long-term results. The TAVI has emerged as a promising technology for providing treatment to this group of patients. A number of percutaneous valves and delivery devices are under development and in early clinical trials. In contrast to surgical replacements, these devices are all placed without removing the native diseased valves. Currently, there are two major technologies that have passed the preclinical development stage: (1) the self-expanding CoreValve ReValving system (Medtronic, Inc., Minneapolis, MN) and (2) the balloon expandable Edwards SAPIEN valve (Edwards Lifesciences Corp, Irvine, CA). The CoreValve prosthesis is a porcine trileaflet valve mounted on a self-expanding stent that is implanted via the transfemoral approach, whereas the Edwards SAPIEN valve is a bovine pericardial tissue valve mounted in a balloon expandable stainless steel stent placed either via transfemoral or transapical approaches. There is increasing evidence that TAVI may be an attractive option for AS patients with high operative risk and may become the standard of care for inoperable patients. Early results from cohort A from the PARTNER trial show promising results comparing TAVI to AVR in high surgical risk patients with severe aortic stenosis. However, long-term data is lacking including the durability of the valve and significance of paravalvular leak. This technique and the device are still considered first generation and rapid evolvement may be expected.

GUIDELINES
SELECTED AMERICAN HEART ASSOCIATION/AMERICAN COLLEGE OF CARDIOLOGY GUIDELINES

Aortic Balloon Valvotomy

Class IIb:
- Aortic balloon valvotomy might be reasonable as a bridge to surgery in hemodynamically unstable adult patients with aortic stenosis who are at high risk for aortic valve replacement.
- Aortic balloon valvotomy might be reasonable for palliation in adult patients with aortic stenosis in whom aortic valve replacement cannot be performed because of serious comorbid conditions.

Class III:
- Aortic balloon valvotomy is not recommended as an alternative to aortic valve replacement in adult patients with aortic stenosis; certain younger adults without valve calcification may be an exception.

Indications for Percutaneous Mitral Balloon Valvotomy

Class I:
- Percutaneous mitral balloon valvotomy is effective for symptomatic patients (New York Heart Association functional class II, III, or IV), with moderate or severe mitral stenosis and valve morphology favorable for percutaneous mitral balloon valvotomy in the absence of left atrial thrombus or moderate-to-severe mitral regurgitation
- Percutaneous mitral balloon valvotomy is effective for asymptomatic patients with moderate or severe mitral stenosis, and valve morphology that is favorable for percutaneous mitral balloon valvotomy who have pulmonary hypertension (pulmonary artery systolic pressure greater than 50 mm Hg at rest or greater than 60 mm Hg with exercise) in the absence of left atrial thrombus or moderate-to-severe mitral regurgitation.

Class IIa:
- Percutaneous mitral balloon valvotomy is reasonable for patients with moderate or severe mitral stenosis who have a nonpliable calcified valve, are in New York Heart Association functional class III–IV, and are either not candidates for surgery or are at high risk for surgery.

Indications for Balloon Valvotomy in Pulmonic Stenosis

Class I:
- Balloon valvotomy is recommended in adolescent and young adult patients with pulmonic stenosis who have exertional dyspnea, angina, syncope, or presyncope and an RV-to-pulmonary artery peak-to-peak gradient greater than 30 mm Hg at catheterization.
- Balloon valvotomy is recommended in asymptomatic adolescent and young adult patients with pulmonic stenosis and RV-to-pulmonary artery peak-to-peak gradient greater than 40 mm Hg at catheterization.

❏ SUGGESTED READINGS

Bonow RO, Carabello BA, Chatterjee K, et al. 2008 focused update incorporated into the ACC/AHA 2006 guidelines for the management of patients with valvular heart disease: a report of the American College of Cardiology/American Heart Association task force on practice guidelines (writing committee to revise the 1998 guidelines for the management of patients with valvular heart disease). Endorsed by the Society of Cardiovascular Anesthesiologists, Society for Cardiovascular Angiography and Interventions, and Society of Thoracic Surgeons. J Am Coll Cardiol. 2008;52:e1-142.

Feldman T, Kar S, Rinaldi M, et al. Percutaneous mitral repair with the MitraClip system: safety and midterm durability in the initial EVEREST (Endovascular Valve Edge-to-Edge REpair Study) cohort. J Am Coll Cardiol. 2009;54:686-94.

Grube E, Laborde JC, Gerckens U, et al. Percutaneous implantation of the CoreValve self-expanding valve prosthesis in high-risk patients with aortic valve disease: the Siegburg first-in-man study. Circulation. 2006;114:1616-24.

Herrmann HC, Wilkins GT, Abascal VM, et al. Percutaneous balloon mitral valvotomy for patients with mitral stenosis. Analysis of factors influencing early results. J Thorac Cardiovasc Surg. 1988;96:33-8.

Inoue K, Owaki T, Nakamura T, et al. Clinical application of transvenous mitral commissurotomy by a new balloon catheter. J Thorac Cardiovasc Surg. 1984;87:394-402.

Pepine CJ, Gessner IH, Feldman RL. Percutaneous balloon valvuloplasty for pulmonic valve stenosis in the adult. Am J Cardiol. 1982;50:1442-5.

Vahanian A, Baumgartner H, Bax J, et al. Guidelines on the management of valvular heart disease—the task force on the management of valvular heart disease of the European society of cardiology. Eur Heart J. 2007;28:230-68.

5.6 Infective Endocarditis

❏ INTRODUCTION

In contrast to improved outcomes with other types of heart disease, the prognosis of infective endocarditis (IE) has appreciably not changed in the last few decades, with inhospital mortality ranging from 15% to 30%. The increasing prevalence of healthcare-associated endocarditis, coupled with the rise of antibiotic-resistant microbial pathogens, means that endocarditis will continue to be associated with high morbidity and mortality in the foreseeable future.

Among adults, endocarditis can be broadly divided into four major groups at risk of disease: (i) native valve endocarditis, (ii) prosthetic valve endocarditis, (iii) endocarditis in illicit drug users, and (iv) healthcare-associated endocarditis. These four categories have significantly different predisposing factors, microbiologic patterns and outcomes (Table 18). Endocarditis has also been categorized clinically as "acute" or "subacute", a distinction that more often reflects the infecting organism (e.g. *Staphylococcus aureus* causing acute endocarditis) and the course of disease rather than the epidemiologic subgroup.

Endocarditis in children occurs primarily in infancy and adolescence, reflecting newborns with predisposing factors and late sequelae of congenital heart disease. Approximately 40% of children with endocarditis have pre-existing heart disease; indwelling venous catheters and premature birth are the other major epidemiologic factors associated with childhood endocarditis. Staphylococcal infections are the most frequent etiologic organism, with viridans group streptococci being second most common.

Table 18: Risk factors, microbiologic patterns and outcomes of endocarditis

	Types of endocarditis			
	Native valve	**Prosthetic valve**	**Illicit drug use**	**Healthcare associated**
Risk factors	Mitral valve prolapse Rheumatic heart disease Congenital heart disease Chronic kidney disease Diabetes	Prior endocarditis Risk is higher during first 12 months for mechanical valve, greater for bioprosthesis after 12 months	Injection drug use (especially heroin)	Recent hospitalization or interaction with healthcare system
Most common microbiologic patterns	*Viridans* group *Streptococci* *Staphylococcus aureus* *S. gallolyticus* (formerly *bovis*) *Enterococci*	Early: *S. aureus* Coagulase-negative *Staph* *Enterococcus* *Streptococci* Late: Coagulase-negative *Staph* *S. aureus* *Enterococcus*	*S. aureus* *Streptococci*	*S. aureus* *Enterococci* Coagulase-negative *Staph* *Streptococci*
Inhospital mortality	15–20%	20–30%	5–10%	20–30%

Endocarditis in adults has four major patterns of presentation: (i) native valve endocarditis, (ii) prosthethic valve endocarditis, (iii) endocarditis associated with illicit drug use, and (iv) healthcare-associated endocarditis. These subgroups are associated with different risk factors, microbiologic patterns and mortality

❏ PATHOGENESIS

Patient and microbial factors both contribute to the propensity for development of endocarditis. Patient factors include preexisting cardiac conditions that cause abnormal pressure-flow dynamics, leading to endothelial injury and development of nonbacterial thrombotic endocarditis (NBTE) or sterile vegetation, which is composed of a platelet-fibrin network at sites of endothelial injury. Sites of NBTE provide a nidus for bacterial adhesion and invasion, and microbial factors determine the likelihood of bacterial persistence and sustained infection. A working model for this process is shown in Flowchart 4. Patient factors and microbial factors interact to lead to develop endocarditis. Injury to the valvular endothelium from trauma, turbulence or metabolic changes leads to platelet-fibrin deposition and formation of NBTE. Trauma to mucous membranes or other compromised tissue allows bacterial entrance to the circulation and bacteremia. Bacterial adhesion factors promote adherence to NBTE, promoting further platelet aggregation, coverage of the bacteria by a platelet fibrin meshwork, and formation of mature vegetation.

Once a vegetation is established, multiple mechanisms lead to pathologic sequelae of disease, including valve destruction and periannular extension, embolization of the vegetation or parts of the vegetation with end-organ damage or abscess formation, metastatic foci of infection from bacteremic seeding and deposition of immunologic complexes that result in further end-organ damage.

FLOWCHART 4: Proposed pathogenesis of infective endocarditis

```
Valvular            Mucous membranes
endothelium         or other
                    colonized tissue
     │                   │
     │    Trauma         │   Local ecological factors
     │    Turbulence     │   Bacteriocins
     │    Metabolic changes   IgA protease
     │                   │   Bacterial adherence
     ↓                   ↓
Platelet-fibrin       Trauma
deposition              │
     ↓                  ↓
Nonbacterial         Bacteremia
thrombotic
endocarditis (NBTE)         Complement
                            antibody
         ↓
      Adherence
         ↓
     Colonization
                     Bacterial division
                     Fibrin deposition
                     Platelet aggregation
                     Extracellular proteases
                     Protection from neutrophils
         ↓
       Mature
     vegetation
```

Microbiology

The microbiology of endocarditis varies widely depending on the presence of a native (Table 19) or prosthetic valve and whether the patient is an injection illicit drug user. These epidemiologic factors have important implications for empiric therapy of endocarditis. Culture-negative endocarditis accounts for 5–10% of cases and usually is due to administration of antibiotics prior to obtaining blood cultures. Culture-negative endocarditis may also be caused by fastidious organisms that grow poorly in blood culture, as well as by diseases that may mimic IE.

Streptococci and staphylococci account for 80–90% of cases of native valve endocarditis. Streptococci were until recently the most common cause of endocarditis in the absence of drug use, but staphylococci have become increasingly common due to healthcare-associated infections. The majority of endocarditis cases in injection drug users are caused by S. aureus, but important albeit less frequent organisms also contribute to the microbiology of intravenous drug use-associated endocarditis.

Prosthetic valve endocarditis has a distinct microbiology depending on the timing of presentation (Table 20). Endocarditis occurring within 60 days of valve implantation is categorized as "early" prosthetic valve endocarditis and is considered nosocomial in etiology. Endocarditis occurring more than 1 year post-implantation is categorized as "late" and more generally reflects community acquisition. Cases

Table 19: Epidemiology and microbiology of native valve endocarditis

Etiologic organism	Epidemiologic notes
Streptococci (25–35%)	
Viridans group *streptococci*	Most common cause of endocarditis
S. gallolyticus (formerly *bovis*)	Associated with colonic malignancy
S. pneumoniae	Highly virulent
Strep. groups B, C and D	Group B associated with emboli
Staphylococci (30–40%)	
S. aureus	Highly invasive
Coagulase-negative *Staph.*	Associated with indwelling catheters
Enterococcus (10–15%)	
E. faecalis	
E. faecium	
Gram-negative (2–3%)	
E. coli	
Salmonella	Also associated with parenteral drug use
Haemophilus	
Neisseria	
HACEK group	Previously considered culture-negative
Gram-positive rods (1–2%)	
Corynebacterium	More commonly seen in prosthetic valve endocarditis
Listeria	
Fungi/yeast (1–2%)	
Candida	Fungemia often persistent
Aspergillus	Difficult to isolate
Histoplasma	
Culture-negative (3–5%)	
T. whippelei	Causative microbe of Whippelei's disease
C. burnetii	Causative microbe of Q fever
Bartonella	*B. henselae* associated with cats
	B. quintana associated with homelessness

occurring between 60 days and 1 year have microbiologic patterns that overlap with early and late prosthetic valve endocarditis.

Culture-negative endocarditis occurs in 5–10% of cases of suspected endocarditis. The most common reason for negative blood cultures is that the patient has received antibiotics prior to obtaining blood cultures. The organisms in most of these "culture-negative" cases are probably viridans group streptococci or HACEK species, as these are relatively fastidious organisms that are easily inhibited by antimicrobial agents. Staphylococci and enterococci, in contrast, are hardy organisms that better tolerate exposure to antibiotics. The other reason

Table 20: Epidemiology and microbiology of prosthetic valve endocarditis. Early prosthetic valve endocarditis is defined as endocarditis occurring within sixty days of prosthetic valve implantation

Early prosthetic valve endocarditis	
Etiologic microorganism	**Prevalence (%)**
Staph aureus	36
Coagulase-negative Staph.	17
Culture negative	17
Fungal	9
Enterococcus	8
S. gallolyticus	2
Viridans group streptococci	2
E. coli	2
Pseudomonas	2
Serratia marcescens	2
Late prosthetic valve endocarditis	
Coagulase-negative Staph	20
Staph aureus	18
Enterococcus	13
Culture negative	12
Viridans group streptococci	10
S. gallolyticus	7
Fungal	2
Polymicrobial	2
Other streptococci	2
Listeria	1
Mycobacteria	1

for negative blood cultures is that the endocarditis is caused by an organism that grows poorly or not all in artificial media and requires serologic diagnosis or special culture techniques. Noninfectious causes of apparent endocarditis must also be considered when cultures are negative. A history of occupational or environmental exposures may provide clues to the diagnosis. For example, a history of exposure to cats is suggestive of *Bartonella hensalae*; homelessness, alcoholism, and exposure to body lice is associated with *Bartonella quintana*. Contact with psittacine birds is associated with *Chlamydophila psittaci*, whereas occupational exposure to animals (e.g. veterinarians, farmers, residence on or visitor to a farm) or unpasteurized milk or milk products is a risk factor for *Brucella* spp. or *Coxiella burnetii*, the agent of Q fever. Diagnosis of endocarditis caused by these agents requires serological testing, polymerase chain reaction (PCR) or use of special culture media.

Legionella is a cause of culture-negative, nosocomial prosthetic valve endocarditis. Aspergillus, the second most common cause of fungal endocarditis after *Candida*, causes an endocarditis characterized by bulky vegetations on echocardiogram in which systemic embolization is a prominent feature; diagnosis usually requires culture or histopathological diagnosis of valvular vegetation or a thromboembolus.

Whipple's disease is caused by *Tropheryma whippelei*. Endocarditis may occur as part of a systemic disease, or endocarditis may be the only presentation or infection. In cases of systemic disease, biopsy of another affected tissue (e.g. small bowel) followed by periodic-acid Schiff staining and PCR analysis may aid in diagnosis.

❏ PRESENTATION AND DIAGNOSIS

The symptoms and signs of endocarditis may be related to the valve infection itself, embolic phenomena and immunologic effects of prolonged infection. In straightforward cases, the presence of fever, a murmur, positive blood cultures and echocardiographic visualization of vegetation confirms the diagnosis.

The modified Duke criteria are a widely accepted set of criteria for establishing a diagnosis of endocarditis. These criteria categorize endocarditis as definite, possible or rejected based on certain clinical findings principal among which is a new regurgitant murmur, blood cultures or serologies, and echocardiography (Table 21).

Blood Culture

Blood cultures at the first suspicion of endocarditis and before administration of antibiotics are paramount in making the diagnosis. Three sets of blood cultures, both aerobic and anaerobic, should be drawn within the first 24 hours. If initial cultures are negative, the microbiology laboratory should also be informed of the suspicion for endocarditis, in order to facilitate further subculture.

Since the bacteremia of endocarditis is continuous in most cases, the majority and typically all blood cultures will be positive. In the absence of prior antibiotics, one of the first two cultures is positive in 95–98% of cases.

The modified Duke criteria define a positive blood culture as two separate cultures obtained at different times and from different sites that are positive for a typical causative agent of endocarditis [e.g. infection with viridans group streptococci, *S. gallolyticus* (formerly *bovis*), *S. aureus*, *Enterococcus* or HACEK organisms]. In the case of blood cultures positive for other organisms, the requirement is for two blood cultures more than 12 hours apart, all three of the initial cultures positive or the majority of more than four cultures positive in the first 24 hours. If none of these criteria are met and infectious endocarditis still suspected, a positive blood culture may still be considered a minor criteria toward diagnosis (Table 21).

Echocardiography

Echocardiography is integral to the diagnosis and prognostic assessment of endocarditis. The modified Duke major criteria for the diagnosis of IE include echocardiographic evidence of vegetation, annular abscess, dehiscence of a prosthetic valve, or new valvular regurgitation.

The views obtained with transthoracic echocardiography (TTE) are often inadequate for clear visualization of valvular structures, including the periannular tissues. TEE is performed with higher imaging frequencies and therefore has better spatial resolution and consequently improved detection of small vegetations. In addition, there are fewer impediments between the probe and the cardiac

Table 21: Modified Duke criteria for diagnosis of endocarditis

Definite endocarditis
Pathological criteria
- Microorganisms demonstrated by culture or histological culture of a vegetation, embolism or abscess OR
- Pathological lesions; vegetation or intracardiac abscess confirmed by histology showing active endocarditis

Clinical criteria
- 2 major criteria OR
- 1 major criterion and 3 minor OR
- 5 minor criteria

Possible endocarditis
- 1 major and 1 minor criterion OR
- 3 minor criteria

Rejected endocarditis
- Firm alternate diagnosis OR
- Resolution of endocarditis syndrome after 4 days or less of antibiotics OR
- No pathologic evidence for endocarditis at surgery or autopsy, if 4 days or less of antibiotics OR
- Does not meet criteria for possible endocarditis

Major criteria
Blood cultures positive
- Typical microorganisms consistent with endocarditis from 2 separate blood cultures:
  - *Viridans* group streptococci
  - *S. gallolyticus*
  - HACEK organisms
  - *Staphylococcus aureus*
  - Community-acquired *Enterococcus* (in absence of primary focus)
- Microorganisms consistent with endocarditis from persistently positive blood cultures, defined as:
  - at least 2 blood cultures drawn >12 hours apart or all of 3 or majority of ≥4 separate cultures of blood (with first and last sample drawn at least an hour apart)
- Single blood culture positive for *C. burnetii* or anti-phase I IgG antibody titer >1:800

Evidence of endocardial involvement
- Positive echocardiogram:
  - Oscillating intracardiac mass on valve or supporting structures, in the path of regurgitant jets, or on implanted prosthetic material in absence of an alternative anatomic explanation
- Abscess
- New partial dehiscence of a prosthetic valve
- New valvular regurgitation (worsening, changing or preexisting murmur not sufficient)

Minor criteria
- Predisposition, predisposing heart condition or parenteral drug use
- Fever, temperature >39°C
- Vascular phenomena, major arterial emboli, septic pulmonary infarcts, mycotic aneurysm, intracranial hemorrhage, conjunctival hemorrhages and Janeway's lesions or Osler's nodes
- Immunologic phenomena: glomerulonephritis, Roth's spots and rheumatoid factor
- Microbiologic evidence: positive blood culture but does not meet a major criterion as above or serological evidence of active infection with an organism consistent with endocarditis

structures to obscure findings. The TEE is usually the only modality that can clearly demonstrate perivalvular extension of infection, fistulae and abscess formation (Figs 34A to C).

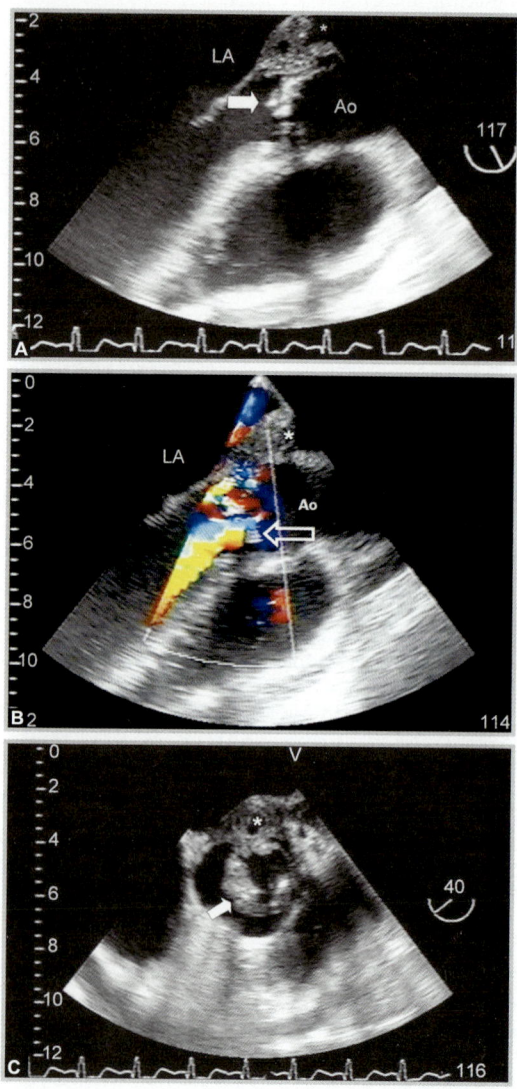

FIGURES 34A TO C: Aortic valve endocarditis with paravalvular abscess. (A and C). Transesophageal two-dimensional and (B) color Doppler flow imaging views of aortic valve endocarditis. Vegetation (open arrow) and paravalvular abscess (asterisk) are seen in the long axis and short axis views (A and C); the abscess comprises irregular tissue and fluid filled cavities in the periannular region between the aorta and the left atrium. Color Doppler flow imaging demonstrates a wide jet of severe aortic valve regurgitation in diastole (open arrow) (Abbreviations: LA: Left atrium; Ao: Ascending aorta)

The choice between initial TTE and TEE echocardiography must be based on the initial clinical suspicion of IE. If the suspicion is relatively low (perhaps due to an alternative site of infection or the absence of predisposing factors for endocarditis), TTE may be an adequate first diagnostic test. For low-likelihood patients with excellent image quality, a negative TTE may be sufficient. A high quality study that demonstrates neither vegetation nor valvular dysfunction does not definitively "rule out" endocarditis, but does effectively risk stratify the patient if they do have IE by other clinical criteria. Initial imaging with TEE should be performed in patients with high-risk clinical features, such as new atrioventricular block or *S. aureus* bacteremia, in patients with prosthetic valves (where the infection is likely to involve perivalvular extension) and in patients where chest wall imaging will likely result in low quality images. If a TEE cannot be obtained within the first 24 hours, an initial TTE should be performed in the interim to avoid missing an opportunity to recognize a large vegetation or significant valvular insufficiency that might predict embolism or need for early surgery.

Other Diagnostic Studies

In cases of initially culture-negative endocarditis, testing for *C. burnetii* serologies may establish Q fever as an etiology, and this is now considered a major criterion for the diagnosis of endocarditis.

In cases of suspected fungal endocarditis, testing for *Candida* antigenemia or *Aspergillus*-associated galactomannan levels may aid in diagnosis. Culture, histopathologic examination or PCR-based assays of explanted heart valve tissue may be useful for identification of the causative microorganism in cases where blood cultures were negative.

Other imaging modalities may complement echocardiography in diagnosis of endocarditis. A study of multislice CT in a population of patients at moderate or high risk of IE suggested that CT has similar sensitivity and specificity to that of TEE in identifying large vegetations and perivalvular extension of infection. Cardiac CT may be useful in evaluating presence of coronary artery disease in patients requiring surgery for endocarditis, especially if there is concern about causing iatrogenic vegetation embolism during cardiac catheterization. Combining anatomic data from CT with gallium-67 SPECT imaging of inflammation may also assist in localizing infection.

❏ MANAGEMENT

Medical therapy with antibiotics targeted to the infectious organism is the mainstay of treatment for endocarditis. When medical therapy fails or in certain clinical circumstances, surgical excision and replacement of the infected valve is the treatment of choice. Other important clinical considerations include management of persistent fever and, especially in subjects with prosthetic valves, whether to continue anticoagulation.

Medical Therapy

Empiric therapy may be withheld in a patient who is not acutely ill in order to obtain blood cultures and even while awaiting results of those cultures. It also may be appropriate to discontinue empiric antimicrobial therapy in a stable patient in order to obtain blood cultures and observe the patient if pre-treatment blood cultures were not obtained or are negative. Empiric antimicrobial therapy should be initiated as soon as possible after three blood cultures have been obtained for acutely ill patients, including those who are hemodynamically unstable, those who have evidence of heart failure or end-organ dysfunction, or those who appear septic.

Empiric therapy for native-valve endocarditis should provide coverage for staphylococci, streptococci, enterococci, and HACEK organisms, as these are the most likely infectious etiologies. Two commonly recommended regimens are nafcillin plus penicillin plus gentamicin and vancomycin plus gentamicin, but given the prevalence of methicillin-resistance among *S. aureus* strains, vancomycin plus gentamicin is preferable. An alternative regimen that avoids the issue of aminoglycoside toxicity is vancomycin plus ceftriaxone. Vancomycin plus gentamicin is the preferred regimen for the patient with serious allergy to beta-lactam antibiotics. The recommended empiric regimen for the patient with suspected prosthetic valve endocarditis is vancomycin plus rifampin plus gentamicin.

Once a causative organism for endocarditis has been identified and its antimicrobial susceptibility determined, a standardized regimen should be used to treat the patient (Table 22). A betalactam antibiotic, the preferred agent for treatment of endocarditis, should be used whenever possible.

Table 22: Antimicrobial therapy of bacterial endocarditis*

Clinical setting	Regimens	Comments
Empirical therapy, once blood cultures have been obtained	Vancomycin 15 mg/kg IV q12h + gentamicin 3 mg/kg IV q24h OR Vancomycin 15 mg/kg IV q12h + ceftriaxone 2g IV q24h OR Nafcillin 2g IV q4h + penicillin 3 million units IV q4h + gentamicin 3 mg/kg IV 24h	Not recommended if MRSA is a consideration
Viridans group streptococci or *S. gallolyticus* (formely *bovis*), penicillin MIC ≤0.12 µg/mL, native valve	Ceftriaxone 2 gm IV q24h for 4 weeks OR Penicillin 3 million units IV q4h for 4 weeks OR Vancomycin 15 mg/kg IV q12h for 4 weeks OR Penicillin 3 million units IV q4h for 2 weeks + gentamicin 3 mg/kg IV q24h for 2 weeks OR Ceftriaxone 2 gm IV q24h for 2 weeks + gentamicin 3 mg/kg IV q24h for 2 weeks	Vancomycin should be used only if a beta-lactam cannot be used Two-week gentamicin combination regimen not recommended for elderly patients; patients with underlying renal disease, impaired hearing or other eight cranial nerve deficit; patients with complicated endocarditis; target peak gentamicin serum concentration of 3–4 µg/mL and trough of <1 µg/mL
Viridans group streptococci or *S. gallolyticus*, penicillin MIC >0.12 and ≤0.5 µg/mL, native valve	Ceftriaxone 2 gm IV q24h for 4 weeks + gentamicin 3 mg/kg IV q24h for 2 weeks OR Penicillin 3 million units IV q4h for 4 weeks + gentamicin 3 mg/kg IV q24h for 2 weeks OR Vancomycin 15 mg/kg IV q12h for 4 weeks	See above for target gentamicin concentrations Vancomycin should be used only if a beta-lactam cannot be used

Contd...

Contd...

Table 22: Antimicrobial therapy of bacterial endocarditis*

Clinical setting	Regimens	Comments
Viridans group streptococci or *S. gallolyticus*, penicillin MIC >0.5 µg/mL, native valve	Ampicillin 2 gm IV q4h for 4–6 weeks + gentamicin 1 mg/kg IV q8h for 4–6 weeks OR Penicillin 4 million units IV q4h for 4–6 weeks + gentamicin 1 mg/kg IV q8h for 4–6 weeks OR Vancomycin 15 mg/kg IV q12h for 6 weeks + gentamicin 1 mg/kg IV q8h for 6 weeks	Vancomycin should be used only if a beta-lactam cannot be used
Viridans group streptococci or *S. gallolyticus* (formely *bovis*), penicillin MIC ≤0.12 mg/mL, prosthetic valve	Penicillin 4 million units IV q4h for 6 weeks OR Ceftriaxone 2 gm IV q24h for 6 weeks OR Vancomycin 15 mg/kg q12h IV for 6 weeks	Although some authorities recommend addition of gentamicin 3 mg/kg IV/IM q24h to penicillin or ceftriaxone, evidence of improved outcome is lacking Vancomycin should be used only if a beta-lactam cannot be used
Viridans group streptococci or *S. gallolyticus* (formely *bovis*), penicillin MIC >0.12 µg/mL, prosthetic valve	Ceftriaxone 2 gm IV q24h for 6 weeks + gentamicin 1 mg/kg IV q8h for 6 weeks OR Penicillin 4 million units IV q4h for 6 weeks + gentamicin 1 mg/kg IV q8h for 6 weeks OR Vancomycin 15 mg/kg q12h IV for 6 weeks	Vancomycin should be used only if a beta-lactam cannot be used
S. pneumoniae, beta-hemolytic *streptococci*, native valve	Ceftriaxone 2g IV q24h for 4 weeks OR Penicillin 4 million units IV q4h for 4 weeks OR Vancomycin 15 mg/kg q12h IV for 4 weeks	Vancomycin should be used only if a beta-lactam cannot be used
Staphylococcus aureus, or coagulase-negative staphylococci, methicillin susceptible, native valve	Nafcillin or oxacillin 2 gm q4h IV for 4–6 weeks OR Cefazolin 2 gm q8h IV for 6 weeks OR Vancomycin 15–20 mg/kg q8–12h IV for 6 weeks	Two weeks of nafcillin or oxacillin therapy may be sufficient in patients with isolated tricuspid valve endocarditis and no metastatic foci of infection Vancomycin should only be used if a beta-lactam is contraindicated; target trough concentrations of 15–20 µg/mL
Staphylococcus aureus or coagulase-negative staphylococci, methicillin susceptible, prosthetic valve	Nafcillin (or oxacillin) 2 gm q4h IV for 6 weeks + rifampin 600–900 mg in two divided doses for 6 weeks + gentamicin 1 mg/kg q8h for 2 weeks OR	Use vancomycin only if use of nafcillin or oxacillin is contraindicated; target vancomycin trough concentrations of 15–20 µg/mL

Contd...

Contd...

Table 22: Antimicrobial therapy of bacterial endocarditis*

Clinical setting	Regimens	Comments
	Vancomycin 15–20 mg/kg q8h–12h IV for 6 weeks + rifampin 600–900 mg in two divided doses for 6 weeks + gentamicin 1 mg/kg q8h IV for 2 weeks	
Staphylococcus aureus, or coagulase-negative staphylococci, methicillin resistant native valve	Vancomycin 15–20 mg/kg q8–12h IV for 6 weeks OR Daptomycin 6 mg/kg IV q24h for 6 weeks	Target vancomycin trough concentrations of 15–20 µg/mL Equivalent to vancomycin for right-sided endocarditis; not FDA approved for left-sided endocarditis
Staphylococcus aureus or coagulase-negative staphylococci, methicillin resistant prosthetic valve	Vancomycin 15–20 mg/kg q8h–12h IV for 6 weeks + rifampin 600–900 mg in two divided doses PO/IV for 6 weeks + gentamicin 1 mg/kg q8h IV for 2 weeks	
Enterococcus faecalis or *E. faecium*, susceptible to penicillin, gentamicin, and vancomycin; native or prosthetic valve	Ampicillin 2g q4h IV for 4–6 weeks + gentamicin 1 mg/kg q8h IV for 4–6 weeks OR Penicillin 4 million units q4h IV for 4–6 weeks + gentamicin 1 mg/kg q8h IV for 4–6 weeks OR Vancomycin 15 mg/kg q12h IV for 6 weeks + gentamicin 1 mg/kg q8h IV for 6 weeks	6 weeks of therapy recommended for prosthetic valve infection Use of vancomycin not recommended unless penicillin or ampicillin cannot be used
Enterococcus faecalis or *E. faecium*, susceptible to penicillin and vancomycin, resistant to gentamicin; native or prosthetic valve	Ampicillin 2 gm q4h IV or penicillin 4 million units q4h IV for 4–6 weeks+ streptomycin 7.5 mg/kg q12h IV for 4–6 weeks OR Vancomycin 15 mg/kg q12h IV for 6 weeks + streptomycin 7.5 mg/kg q12h IV for 6 weeks	6 weeks of therapy recommended for prosthetic valve infection Confirm susceptibility to streptomycin; if resistant then use ceftriaxone 2g q12h IV instead of streptomycin and treat for a total duration of 8 weeks
Enterococcus faecalis or *E. faecium*, susceptible to vancomycin and gentamicin, resistant to penicillin; native or prosthetic valve	Vancomycin 15 mg/kg q12h IV for 6 weeks + gentamicin 1 mg/kg q8h IV for 6 weeks	
E. faecium resistant to penicillin, vancomycin, gentamicin, native or prosthetic valve	Linezolid 600 mg q12h IV/PO at for least 8 weeks OR Quinupristin-dalfopristin 7.5 mg/kg q8h IV for at least 8 weeks	Cure rates <50% with medical therapy alone; valve replacement therapy may be necessary for cure

Contd...

Contd...

Table 22: Antimicrobial therapy of bacterial endocarditis*		
Clinical setting	**Regimens**	**Comments**
E. faecalis resistant to penicillin, vancomycin, gentamicin, native or prosthetic valve	Ampicillin 2 g q4h IV for at least 8 weeks + ceftriaxone 2 g q12h IV for at least 8 weeks	
HACEK	Ceftriaxone 2g q24h IV for 4 weeks OR Ciprofloxacin 500 mg q12h PO or 400 mg q12h IV for 4 weeks	
Culture-negative endocarditis, native valve	Ampicillin-sulbactam 3 g q6h IV for 4–6 weeks + gentamicin 1 mg/kg q8h IV for 4–6 weeks OR Vancomycin 15 mg/kg q12h IV for 4–6 weeks + gentamicin 1 mg/kg q8h IV for 4–6 weeks + ciprofloxacin 500 mg q12h PO or 400 mg q12h IV for 4–6 weeks	
Culture-negative endocarditis, prosthetic valve, implanted ≤1 year	Vancomycin 15 mg/kg q12h IV for 6 weeks + gentamicin 1 mg/kg q8h IV for 2 weeks + cefepime 2 gm IV 8h for 6 weeks + rifampin 600–900 mg in two divided doses PO/IV for 6 weeks	
Culture-negative endocarditis, prosthetic valve, implanted >1 year	Ampicillin-sulbactam 3 g q6h IV for 4–6 weeks + gentamicin 1 mg/kg q8h IV for 4–6 weeks OR Vancomycin 15 mg/kg q12h IV for 4–6 weeks + gentamicin 1 mg/kg q8h IV for 4–6 weeks + ciprofloxacin 500 mg PO q12h or 400 mg IV 12h for 4–6 weeks	

*Recommended doses for patients with normal renal function.

Surgical Therapy and Timing of Surgery

In the recent international collaboration on endocarditis study, 40% of patients underwent surgical therapy during the index hospitalization. Despite the increasing utilization of surgery, there remains significant uncertainty regarding optimal timing of surgery and identification of subgroups that preferentially benefit from early surgical intervention. The decision to proceed with surgery is complex. The major indications for surgery are development of heart failure, a structural deterioration of the valve, annulus, or prosthesis, and failure of antibiotic therapy. Relative indications include embolization and large vegetation size (Table 23, Fig. 35).

The continued high mortality of endocarditis despite improved diagnostic tools and aggressive antibiotic therapy has led investigators to examine whether early surgery might confer a mortality benefit in patients with endocarditis. Analysis of

> **Table 23: Indications for surgical therapy of endocarditis**
>
> - Indications
>   - Worsening heart failure
>   - Failure of antibiotic therapy: especially fungal infection, left-sided infection with gram-negative bacteria or persistently positive blood cultures after >1 week of antibiotics
>   - Disrupted valve or prosthesis: valve perforation, annular extension, fistula or unstable prosthesis
> - Relative indications
>   - Risk of embolization: large vegetation >10 mm, persistent vegetation after embolization, or enlarging vegetation despite antimicrobial therapy

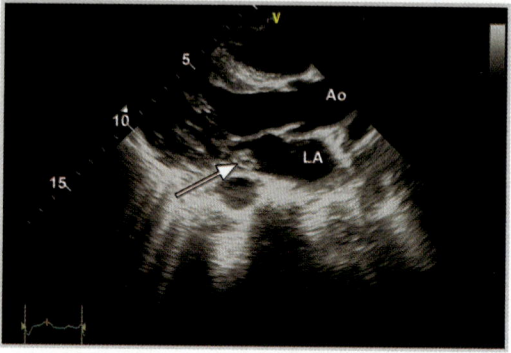

FIGURE 35: Mitral valve endocarditis. Transthoracic echocardiography demonstrates a large, 1.6 mm diameter vegetation (arrow) on the mitral valve in a 23-year-old patient with methicillin-resistant *Staphylococcus aureus* endocarditis

this question is difficult due to lack of randomized data and the inherent survivor bias of surgery (i.e. patients who live longer are more likely to undergo surgery). Propensity analyses addressing early use of surgery have yielded conflicting results, with some studies suggesting no benefit to surgery and others suggesting significant benefit of early surgery. The largest of these studies found that surgery performed during the initial hospitalization was associated with decreased mortality among patients with paravalvular complications, stroke, systemic embolization, and *S. aureus* endocarditis.

Persistent Fever

Continued fever despite antibiotic administration often raises the issue of possible failure of medical therapy. Fifty percent of patients will become afebrile within three days of antimicrobial therapy; fever of more than two weeks' duration should raise suspicion for periannular extension, secondary seeding, or an alternative diagnosis.

Anticoagulation

Anticoagulation in the presence of a prosthetic valve is controversial and requires balancing the risk of valve thrombosis with intracranial bleeding from subclinical emboli. With a rate of 50% for stroke or intracranial hemorrhage and a 70%

mortality rate in patients with *S. aureus* prosthetic valve endocarditis, strong consideration should be given to discontinuation of anticoagulation during the early, septic phase of the infection.

In the presence of known intracranial embolization, anticoagulation should be discontinued for a minimum of two weeks. Anticoagulation in the presence of native valve endocarditis has never been shown to reduce the risk of embolization. Although aspirin had apparent benefit in preventing embolization in animal models of endocarditis, randomized trials showed no benefit and suggested an increased risk of intracranial bleeding. For this reason, antiplatelet agents should be stopped in a patient with infectious endocarditis unless there is a clinical indication (e.g. recent intracoronary stenting).

Prevention of Endocarditis

Current AHA and ACC/AHA prophylaxis guidelines are based on these human studies, combined with the lack of prospective evidence supporting periprocedural antibiotic prophylaxis of endocarditis. Antibiotic prophylaxis is recommended based on patient-specific risk of poor IE outcome, rather than based on the lifetime incidence of IE (Table 24). Antibiotics are recommended only for dental surgery, and no longer for gastrointestinal or genitourinary procedures (Table 25). The

Table 24: ACC/AHA guidelines for antibiotic prophylaxis for the prevention of endocarditis

- Class I: No class I guidelines for antibiotic prophylaxis
- Class IIa: It is reasonable to administer antibiotics to the following group of patients prior to a dental procedure that involves manipulation of the gingival tissues, periapical region of the teeth, or perforation of the oral mucosa:
    - Patients with prosthetic cardiac valves or prosthetic material used for cardiac valve repair
    - Patients with previous infective endocarditis
- Patients with congenital heart disease, unrepaired congenital heart disease, including palliative shunts and conduits, completely repaired congenital heart defect repaired with prosthetic material or device, whether placed by surgery or by catheter, during the first 6 months post-procedure. Repaired congenital heart disease with residual defects at the site of or adjacent to the site of a prosthetic patch or prosthetic device
- Cardiac transplant recipients with valve regurgitation due to a structurally abnormal valve

Table 25: Antibiotic regimens for prevention of endocarditis during dental procedures

Clinical situation	Antibiotic	Adult	Children
Able to take oral antibiotics	Amoxicillin	2 grams	50 mg/kg
Unable to take oral medication	Ampicillin OR	2 grams IM or IV	50 mg/kg IM or IV
	Cefazolin OR	1 gram IM or IV	50 mg/kg IM or IV
	Ceftriaxone	1 gram IM or IV	50 mg/kg IM or IV
Allergic to penicillins or ampicillin—oral	Cephalexin OR	2 grams	50 mg/kg
	Clindamycin OR	600 mg	20 mg/kg
	Azithromycin OR	500 mg	15 mg/kg
	Clarithromycin	500 mg	15 mg/kg
Allergic to penicillins or ampicillin—unable to take oral medications	Cefazolin OR	1 gram IM or IV	50 mg/kg IM or IV
	Ceftriaxone OR	1 gram IM or IV	50 mg/kg IM or IV
	Clindamycin	600 mg IM or IV	20 mg/kg IM or IV

clinical strategy for avoiding endocarditis in patients at more than baseline risk for endocarditis hinges on maintenance of excellent oral health, and advice to contact the health care provider for sustained fever before beginning antibiotic therapy, so that reliable blood cultures can be obtained if endocarditis is suspected.

❑ SUGGESTED READINGS

Blumberg EA, Robbins N, Adimora A, et al. Persistent fever in association with infective endocarditis. Clin Infect Dis. 1992;15: 983-90.

Cabell CH, Abrutyn E, Fowler VG Jr, et al. Use of surgery in patients with native valve infective endocarditis: results from the International Collaboration on Endocarditis Merged Database. Am Heart J. 2005;150:1092-8.

Day MD, Gauvreau K, Shulman S, et al. Characteristics of children hospitalized with infective endocarditis. Circulation. 2009;119: 865-70.

Lalani T, Cabell CH, Benjamin DK, et al. Analysis of the impact of early surgery on in-hospital mortality of native valve endocarditis: use of propensity score and instrumental variable methods to adjust for treatment-selection bias. Circulation. 2010;121:1005-13.

Li JS, Sexton DJ, Mick N, et al. Proposed modifications to the Duke criteria for the diagnosis of infective endocarditis. Clin Infect Dis. 2000;30:633-8.

Murdoch DR, Corey GR, Hoen B, et al. Clinical presentation, etiology, and outcome of infective endocarditis in the 21st century: the International Collaboration on Endocarditis-Prospective Cohort Study. Arch Intern Med. 2009;169:463-73.

Nishimura RA, Carabello BA, Faxon DP, et al. ACC/AHA 2008 Guideline update on valvular heart disease: focused update on infective endocarditis: a report of the American College of Cardiology/ American Heart Association Task Force on Practice Guidelines endorsed by the Society of Cardiovascular Anesthesiologists, Society for Cardiovascular Angiography and Interventions, and Society of Thoracic Surgeons. J Am Coll Cardiol. 2008;52:676-85.

Reynolds HR, Jagen MA, Tunick PA, et al. Sensitivity of transthoracic versus transesophageal echocardiography for the detection of native valve vegetations in the modern era. J Am Soc Echocardiogr. 2003;16:67-70.

Tleyjeh IM, Steckelberg JM, Murad HS, et al. Temporal trends in infective endocarditis: a population-based study in Olmsted County, Minnesota. JAMA. 2005;293:3022-8.

Wang A, Athan E, Pappas PA, et al. Contemporary clinical profile and outcome of prosthetic valve endocarditis. JAMA. 2007;297: 1354-61.

Werner AS, Cobbs CG, Kaye D, et al. Studies on the bacteremia of bacterial endocarditis. JAMA. 1967;202:199-203.

Wilson W, Taubert KA, Gewitz M, et al. Prevention of infective endocarditis: guidelines from the American Heart Association: a guideline from the American Heart Association Rheumatic Fever, Endocarditis, and Kawasaki Disease Committee, Council on Cardiovascular Disease in the Young, and the Council on Clinical Cardiology, Council on Cardiovascular Surgery and Anesthesia, and the Quality of Care and Outcomes Research Interdisciplinary Working Group. Circulation. 2007;116:1736-54.

Yavari A, Ayoub T, Livieratos L, et al. Diagnosis of prosthetic aortic valve endocarditis with gallium-67 citrate single-photon emission computed tomography/computed tomography hybrid imaging using software registration. Circ Cardiovasc Imaging. 2009;2:e41-3.

5.7 Prosthetic Heart Valves

❏ RISK OF VALVE REPLACEMENT

A number of risk models for predicting operative mortality for valve replacement include the EuroSCORE, the New York Model and the Society of Thoracic Surgeons (STS) Database. The EuroSCORE model has been shown to over predict risk, presumably since other models are more recent and reflect improvements in valve surgery. The New York Model may need regional correction to maintain its accuracy.

The STS Database has identified clinical variables that independently influence operative mortality (Table 26). According to STS data from 2002 to 2006 (including 67,292 isolated aortic valve replacements and 21,229 isolated mitral valve replacements), unadjusted operative mortality for isolated valve procedures was 3.4%. The unadjusted hospital morbidity rates ranged from 0.3% for deep sternal wound infection to 11.8% for prolonged ventilation. A model for predicting risk for patients undergoing combined valve surgery and coronary artery bypass grafting has also been reported using data (i.e. 101,661 procedures) from the same time period. An online risk calculator is available through a link from the STS website.

Table 26: Clinical variables that influence valvular heart surgery risk estimated by the Society of Thoracic Surgery database

- Status of procedure (i.e. elective, urgent, emergent)
- Age
- Gender
- Race/ethnicity
- Diabetes mellitus and whether therapy is diet, oral agent or insulin
- Creatinine level
- Dialysis
- Hypertension
- Infectious endocarditis
- Chronic obstructive pulmonary disease and severity
- Peripheral vascular disease
- Immunosuppressive therapy
- Cerebrovascular disease
- Prior cardiac surgery
- Preoperative myocardial infarction
- Presentation with acute coronary syndrome (e.g. unstable angina, non-ST elevation myocardial infarction, ST elevation myocardial infarction)
- Congestive heart failure and New York Heart Association functional class
- Preoperative inotropes
- Intra-aortic balloon pump
- Atrial fibrillation/flutter or other arrhythmias
- Number of diseased coronary arteries at cardiac catheterization
- Left ventricular ejection fraction
- Severity of regurgitant valve lesions (mitral, aortic or tricuspid valves)
- Severity of stenotic valve lesions (aortic or mitral valves)

Adapted from: www.sts.org/sections/stsnationaldatabase/riskcalculator/

Operative mortality in high-risk patients undergoing combined coronary revascularization and valve surgery can be reduced by "hybrid" operations of percutaneous coronary intervention followed by the valve surgery.

❏ TYPES OF PROSTHETIC VALVES

The ideal valve prosthesis should have excellent hemodynamics, long durability, high thromboresistance and excellent implantability. The currently available prostheses are not ideal.

Examples of mechanical and biologic valves are given in Figures 36A to H.

Mechanical Valves

Mechanical valves have three key components: occluder (i.e. the closure mechanism), housing and sewing ring. All have some degree of regurgitant flow (i.e. the washing jet) that prevents thrombus formation on the surface of the valve. Mechanical valves are durable but require chronic anticoagulation because of thrombogenicity.

Bioprosthetic Valves

Bioprosthetic valves are considered heterograft (i.e. from porcine or bovine tissue) or homograft (i.e. human cadaver). Porcine valves may be stented with the valve tissue mounted on supportive prosthetic material or stentless in the aortic position with the valve tissue supported by the donated annulus and aortic root. Bovine pericardial valves are manufactured from sheets of bovine pericardium mounted inside or outside of a supporting stent.

Biological valves do not require anticoagulation (unless there are other compelling reasons, such as atrial fibrillation) but durability is limited.

❏ SELECTING THE OPTIMAL PROSTHESIS

Optimal valve prosthesis is characterized by excellent hemodynamics, long durability, high thromboresistance and ease of implantability. Unfortunately, none of the currently available prostheses have all these features and the selection of a prosthetic valve for the individual is determined by the relative importance of these characteristics.

Improved mortality with mechanical valves compared to porcine valves has been demonstrated in early randomized trials. In a more recent randomized trial comparing contemporary mechanical and bioprosthetic aortic valves, the differences in mortality were not significant at 13 years. There was no difference in cardiac related mortality between newer generation bioprostheses (i.e. C-E SAV and pericardial) and mechanical bileaflet valves implanted between 1995 and 2003 with a mean follow-up of 106 months.

Nonrandomized trials demonstrate that the survival rates and risk of complications are dependent on patient-related factors, such as age, left ventricular dysfunction, heart failure, coronary artery disease, coronary artery bypass grafting, arrhythmias, pulmonary hypertension, and coexistent conditions, such as renal failure, lung disease, hypertension and diabetes. Thus, comparison of outcomes between mechanical and biological valves requires caution unless baseline characteristics of patients are similar. However, the choice between mechanical and bioprosthetic valves is largely related to a trade-off between the durability advantages of mechanical valves compared to lower bleeding risk of bioprostheses (Table 27).

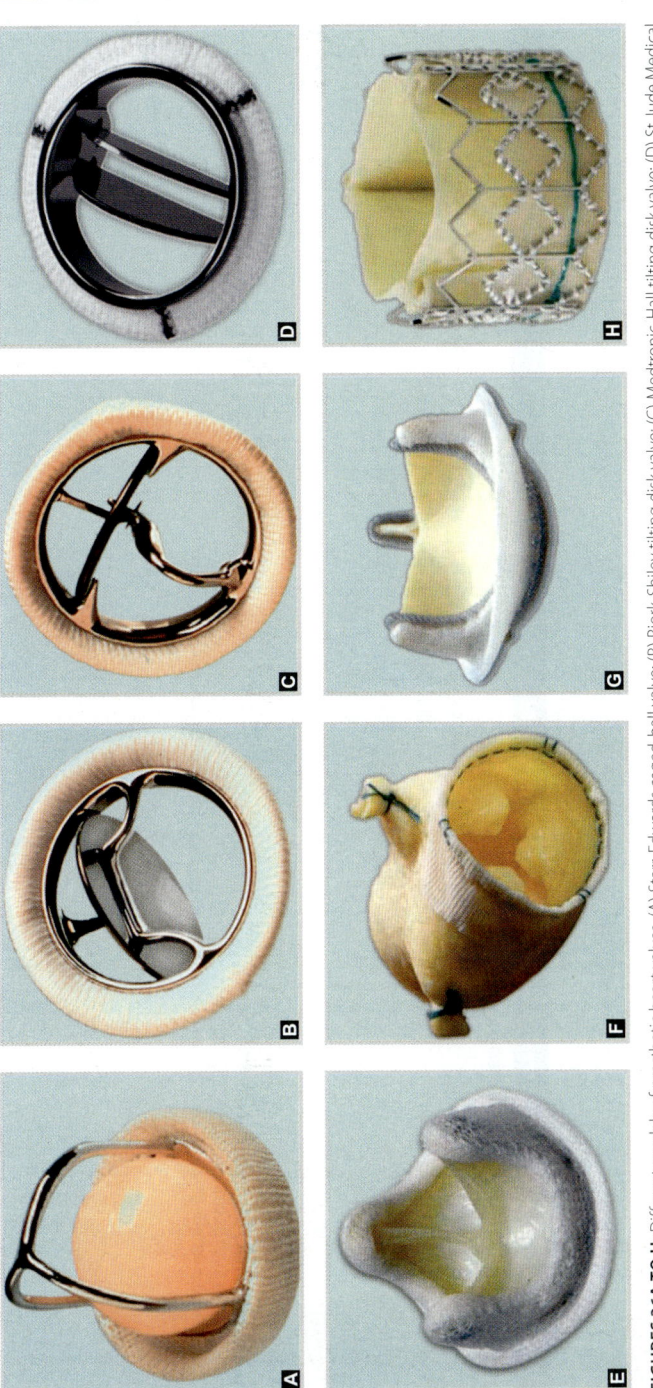

FIGURES 36A TO H: Different models of prosthetic heart valves. (A) Starr-Edwards caged-ball valve; (B) Bjork-Shiley tilting disk valve; (C) Medtronic-Hall tilting disk valve; (D) St Jude Medical bileaflet valve; (E) Medtronic Hancock II porcine valve; (F) Medtronic Freestyle porcine valve; (G) Carpentier-Edwards Perimount bovine pericardial valve; (H) Edwards SAPIEN transcatheter pericardial aortic valve (*Source:* Sun JCJ, Davidson MJ, Lamy A, et al. Antithrombotic management of patients with prosthetic heart valves: current evidence and future trends. Lancet. 2009;374:565-76)

Table 27: Comparison of complications in patients with mechanical and biological prostheses in randomized trials

	Systemic emboli				Bleeding				Reoperation			
	Aortic		Mitral		Aortic		Mitral		Aortic		Mitral	
Study	Mech	Bio	Mech	Bio	Mech	Bio	Mech	Bio	Mech	Bio	Mech	Bio
VA (%)	18 ± 4	18 ± 4	18 ± 5	22 ± 5	51 ± 4**	30 ± 4	53 ± 7*	31 ± 6	10 ± 3	29 ± 5*	25 ± 6	50 ± 8
Edinburgh (%)	24 ± 6	39 ± 9	53 ± 7	32 ± 6	61 ± 8**	42 ± 12	53 ± 8	37 ± 11	7 ± 3	56 ± 8***	13 ± 4	78 ± 7***
Tassano (Linearized rate, %/pt-yr)	0.54	0.24			1.47†	0.72			0.62	2.32**		

(Abbreviations: Mech: Mechanical valve, Bio: Biological valve)
*0.001 < p ≤ 0.01, **0.0001 ≤ p < 0.001, ***p < 0.0001
†21% in the bioprosthesis group were taking warfarin. Bleeding occurred in 3.4% of bioprosthesis patients not taking warfarin, compared to 12.7% of patients with mechanical valves (p = 0.001)

FLOWCHART 5: Algorithm for the selection of the optimal prosthesis in the individual patient

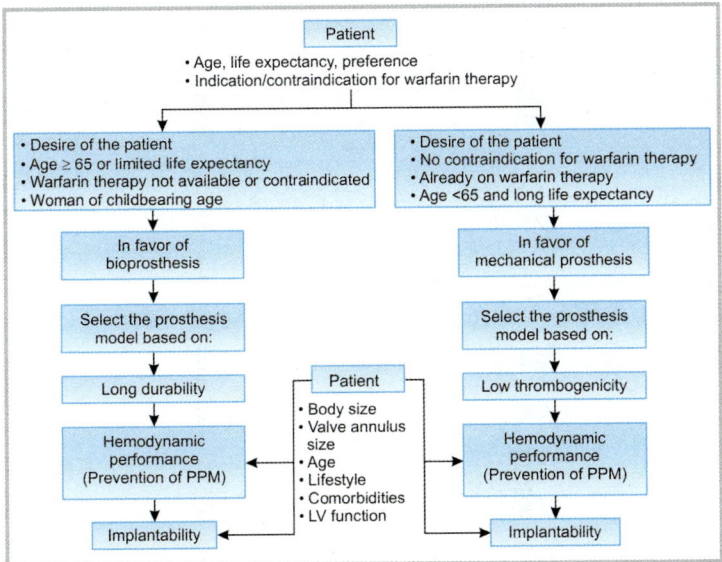

(*Source:* Pibarot P, Dumesnil JG. Prosthetic heart valves: selection of the optimal prosthesis and long-term management. Circulation. 2009;110:1034-48)

The selection of prosthetic heart valves for women of childbearing age is difficult. Mechanical bileaflet valves may be favored because of durability. They may be a reasonable choice for women who are compliant and committed to careful anticoagulation. However, a biological valve prosthesis may be preferred in young women who are not interested in anticoagulation or for whom close follow-up is not possible. Unfortunately, pregnancy in a woman with a bioprosthetic valve is associated with SVD and the incidence may average 24% during or shortly after the pregnancy.

The selection of the optimal prosthesis depends on a number of clinical variables including age, ability to tolerate full dose oral anticoagulation, comorbidities, LV function, body size and valve annulus size (Flowchart 5).

❏ PROSTHESIS-PATIENT MISMATCH

Prosthesis-patient mismatch (PPM) occurs when the effective orifice area (EOA) of a normal functioning valve is too small in relation to the patient's body size and cardiac output requirements, resulting in abnormally high transvalvular gradients. Criteria for PPM have been established and are based on the EOA indexed for body surface area. The projected indexed EOA is typically determined from reference values published by echocardiography laboratories (Tables 28 and 29).

Severe PPM is estimated to occur in 2–10% of patients and is defined as an EOA/m^2 less than or equal to 0.65 for aortic valve prostheses and less than or equal to 0.9 for mitral. Moderate PPM may be frequent in both the aortic (20–70%) and mitral (30–70%) positions and is defined as EOA/m^2 of less than or equal to 0.85 for aortic valve prostheses and less than or equal to 1.2 for mitral.

Table 28: Normal reference values of EOAs for aortic prostheses

	19	21	23	25	27	29
Stented porcine						
Mosaic (Medtronic)	...	1.4 ± 0.4	1.5 ± 0.4	1.8 ± 0.5	1.9 ± 0.1	2.1 ± 0.2
Hancock II (Medtronic)	...	1.3 ± 0.4	1.3 ± 0.4	1.6 ± 0.4	...	1.6 ± 0.2
Intact (Medtronic)	...	1.6 ± 0.4	1.6 ± 0.4	1.7 ± 0.3	...	...
Biocor (St Jude Medical)	...	...	1.3 ± 0.3	1.7 ± 0.4	2.2 ± 0.4	...
C-E Standard (Edwards Lifescience)	0.9 ± 0.2	1.5 ± 0.3	1.7 ± 0.5	1.9 ± 0.5	2.3 ± 0.6	2.8 ± 0.5
C-E Supra-annular	1.1 ± 0.1	1.4 ± 0.9	1.6 ± 0.6	1.8 ± 0.4	1.9 ± 0.7	...
Stented bovine						
C-E Perimount	1.1 ± 0.3	1.3 ± 0.4	1.5 ± 0.4	1.8 ± 0.4	2.1 ± 0.4	2.2 ± 0.4
C-E Perimount Magna	1.3 ± 0.3	1.7 ± 0.3	2.1 ± 0.4	2.3 ± 0.5	...	...
Mitroflow (Sorin)*	1.1 ± 0.1	1.3 ± 0.1	1.5 ± 0.2	1.8 ± 0.2	...	...
Labcor-Santiago	1.2 ± 0.1	1.3 ± 0.1	1.8 ± 0.2	2.1 ± 0.3	...	...
Stentless bioprosthesis						
Freestyle (Medtronic)	...	1.4 ± 0.3	1.7 ± 0.5	2.1 ± 0.5	2.5 ± 0.1	...
Toronto SPV (St Jude Medical)	...	1.3 ± 0.6	1.6 ± 0.6	1.8 ± 0.5	2.0 ± 0.3	2.4 ± 0.6
O'Brien (Cryolife)	1.5 ± 0.3	1.7 ± 0.4	2.3 ± 0.2	2.6 ± 0.2	2.8 ± 0.3	...
Prima (Edwards)	...	1.4 ± 0.7	1.5 ± 0.3	1.8 ± 0.5	...	...
Pericarbon (Sorin)	1.2 ± 0.5	1.3 ± 0.6	1.5 ± 0.5	...	...	...
Caged-ball mechanical						
Starr-Edwards	...	...	1.1 ± 0.2	1.1 ± 0.3	...	...
Single leaflet tilting disk mechanical						
Bjork-Shiley	...	1.1 ± 0.3	1.3 ± 0.3	1.5 ± 0.4	1.6 ± 0.3	...
Medtronic-Hall	...	1.1 ± 0.2	1.4 ± 0.4	1.5 ± 0.5	1.9 ± 0.2	...
Bileaflet tilting disk mechanical						
Standard (St Jude Medical)	1.5 ± 0.1	1.4 ± 0.4	1.6 ± 0.4	1.9 ± 0.5	2.5 ± 0.4	2.8 ± 0.5
Regent (St Jude Medical)	1.6 ± 0.4	2.0 ± 0.7	2.3 ± 0.9	2.5 ± 0.8	3.6 ± 0.5	...
CarboMedics standard (Sorin Group)	1.0 ± 0.3	1.5 ± 0.4	1.4 ± 0.3	1.8 ± 0.4	2.2 ± 0.2	3.2 ± 1.6
Top Hat CarboMedics (Sorin Group)	...	1.2 ± 0.3	1.4 ± 0.4	1.6 ± 0.3	...	...
ATS Standard (ATS)	1.1 ± 0.3	1.4 ± 0.5	1.7 ± 0.5	2.1 ± 0.7	2.5 ± 0.1	3.1 ± 0.8
On-X (MCRI)	1.5 ± 0.2	1.7 ± 0.4	1.9 ± 0.6	2.4 ± 0.6	...	...

*Data limited

Table 29: Normal reference values of EOAs for mitral prostheses

	23	25	27	29	31	33
Stented porcine						
Hancock I or not specified (Medtronic)	...	...	1.3 ± 0.8	1.5 ± 0.2	1.6 ± 0.2	1.9 ± 0.2
Hancock II (Medtronic)	...	...	2.2 ± 0.1	2.8 ± 0.1	2.8 ± 0.1	3.1 ± 0.2
Mosaic (Medtronic)	...	1.5 ± 0.4	1.7 ± 0.5	1.9 ± 0.5	1.9 ± 0.5	...
Stented bovine						
Carpentier-Edwards Perimount*	...	1.6 ± 0.4	1.8 ± 0.4	2.1 ± 0.5	...	...
Single leaflet tilting disk mechanical						
Bjork-Shiley	...	1.7 ± 0.6	1.8 ± 0.5	2.1 ± 0.4	2.2 ± 0.3	...
Bileaflet tilting disk mechanical						
Standard (St Jude Medical)	1.0	1.3 ± 0.2	1.7 ± 0.2	1.8 ± 0.2	2.0 ± 0.3	...
CarboMedics Standard (Sorin Group)	...	2.9 ± 0.8	2.9 ± 0.7	2.3 ± 0.4	2.8 ± 1.1	...
On-X (MCRI)	...	1.9 ± 1.1	2.2 ± 0.5	2.2 ± 0.5	2.5 ± 1.1	2.5 ± 1.1

*Data limited

PPM in the aortic position is associated with less improvement in symptoms and functional class, less regression of LV hypertrophy and more adverse cardiac events including mortality. Preoperative left ventricular function is predictive of a combined endpoint of increased incidence of heart failure symptoms or death related to heart failure at three years in patients with moderate PPM after aortic valve replacement.

PPM in the mitral position can be equated to residual mitral stenosis with similar consequences (i.e. persistence of abnormally high mitral gradients and increased left atrial and pulmonary arterial pressure). Pulmonary pressures are higher in patients with severe PPM. Unfortunately, when PPM after mitral valve replacement is predicted on the basis of projected EOA, options are limited. No alternative techniques exist to implant a larger prosthesis and durability of homografts and stentless valves are not optimal.

Management of PPM is directed at avoiding severe mismatch in patients undergoing aortic and mitral valve replacement and avoiding moderate mismatch in patients with preexisting LV dysfunction and/or severe LV hypertrophy and in patients engaging in regular and/or intense physical activity (especially younger patients).

If the projected indexed EOA predicts significant PPM in the aortic position, an alternate prosthesis or aortic root enlargement provide options. Several approaches (Figs 37A and B) for posterior aortic root enlargement have been described and both involve suturing a pericardial patch to the posterior root to allow enlargement of the annulus without compromising the coronary ostia. In addition to aortic root enlargement, alternate procedures include a supra-annular stented bioprosthesis, stentless bioprosthesis, newer generation mechanical valve, homograft or the Ross operation.

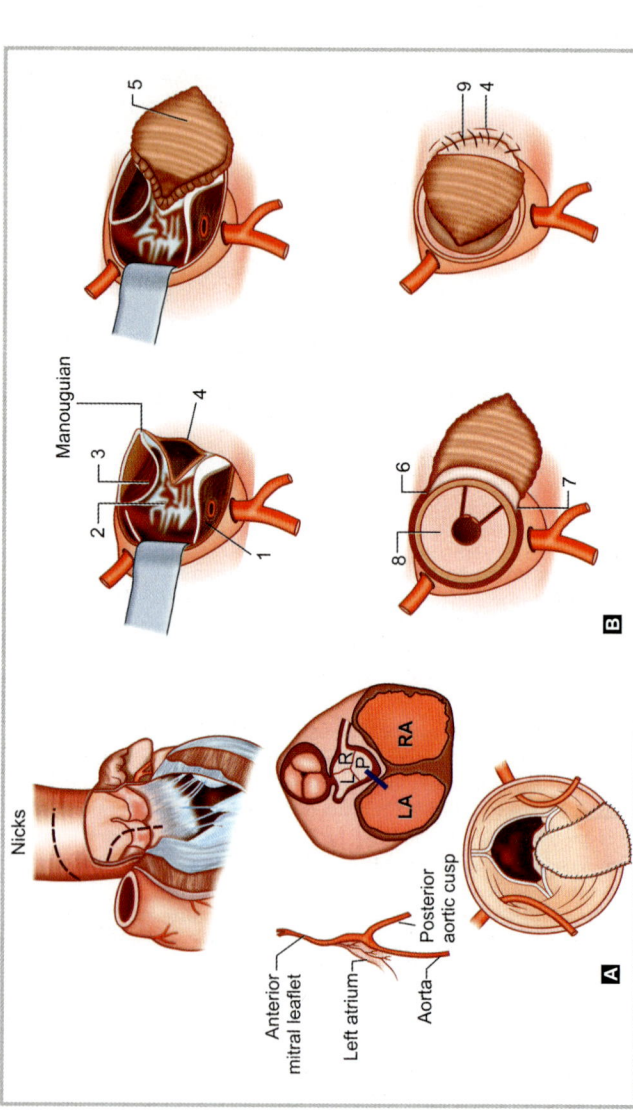

FIGURES 37A AND B: In posterior root enlargement techniques, the aorta is excised posteriorly across the aortic annulus to the anterior leaflet of the mitral valve. The defect is closed with autologous or bovine pericardium is placed as a patch. The Nicks enlargement (A) involves extension of an oblique aortotomy and the Manouguian enlargement (B) involves extension of a transverse aortotomy. The valve prosthesis is sutured in a supra-annular position (*Source:* Dhareshwar J, Sundt TM, Dearani JA, et al. Aortic root enlargement: what are the operative risks? J Thorac Cardiovasc Surg. 2007;134:916-24)

❏ LONG-TERM MANAGEMENT

Antithrombotic Therapy

General Management

Mechanical valves are prone to thrombus formation and all such patients require warfarin therapy. Mitral prostheses have increased risk of thromboembolic events compared to aortic valves. In addition, the risk of a thromboembolic event is higher in the initial three months of implantation (before the valve is endothelialized) compared to later. Risk factors associated with an increased risk of thromboembolism include atrial fibrillation, LV dysfunction, left atrial dilation, previous history of thromboembolism and hypercoagulable condition.

Current ACC/AHA guidelines recommend a relatively low goal INR of 2.0–3.0 for bileaflet or Medtronic-Hall single leaflet aortic valve prostheses, when no risk factors, for thromboembolism are present. During the initial 3 months however, a goal INR of 2.5–3.5 can be considered (due to the increased risk of thromboembolism early after valve replacement). A goal INR of 2.5–3.5 is recommended if patients with these valves have risk factors associated with increased thromboembolism (Flowchart 6).

In those patients with a high-risk of thromboembolism and in whom aspirin cannot be used, there is a suggestion of benefit for INR goals of 3.5–4.5 or to add clopidogrel to warfarin therapy. However, the higher INR goal is associated with an increased risk of bleeding. Aspirin is recommended in a dose of 75–100 mg a day as an addition to warfarin in patients with mechanical heart valves.

Pregnancy

The embryopathy can be prevented if warfarin is not taken during the first trimester and fetal complications are less common with warfarin doses under 5 mg per day. Three anticoagulation regimens have been proposed in the ACC/AHA Valvular Heart Disease Guidelines for use in pregnant patients with mechanical valves as an alternative to warfarin:

- Continuous, intravenous dose-adjusted unfractionated heparin (UFH). While the fetal risk is lower compared to the other regimens, the maternal risks of prosthetic valve thrombosis, systemic embolization, infection, osteoporosis, and heparin-induced thrombocytopenia are relatively higher
- Subcutaneous dose-adjusted unfractionated heparin with the PTT at least twice control. Heparin is initiated at 17,500 to 20,000 U every 12 hours with PTT check at 6 hours.
- Subcutaneous dose-adjusted low molecular weight heparin (LMWH) administered twice daily to maintain the anti-Xa level between 0.7 and 1.2 U per mL 4 hours after administration.

The suggested dosing regimens are:
- Either LMWH or UFH between 6 and 12 weeks and close to term only, with warfarin at other times
- Aggressive, dose-adjusted UFH throughout pregnancy
- Aggressive, dose-adjusted LMWH throughout pregnancy. Besides, the addition of low-dose aspirin (i.e. 75–100 mg per day) in the second and third trimesters of pregnancy is reasonable

For women with high-risk mechanical valves (e.g. older generation valve in the mitral position or history of thromboembolism), the American College of Chest Physicians Practice Guidelines suggest the use of oral anticoagulants over heparin, in an effort to avoid maternal complications, recognizing the potential

FLOWCHART 6: Algorithm for antithrombotic therapy for prosthetic heart valves. Risk factors: atrial fibrillation, previous thromboembolism, left ventricular ejection fraction <35% and hypercoagulable state

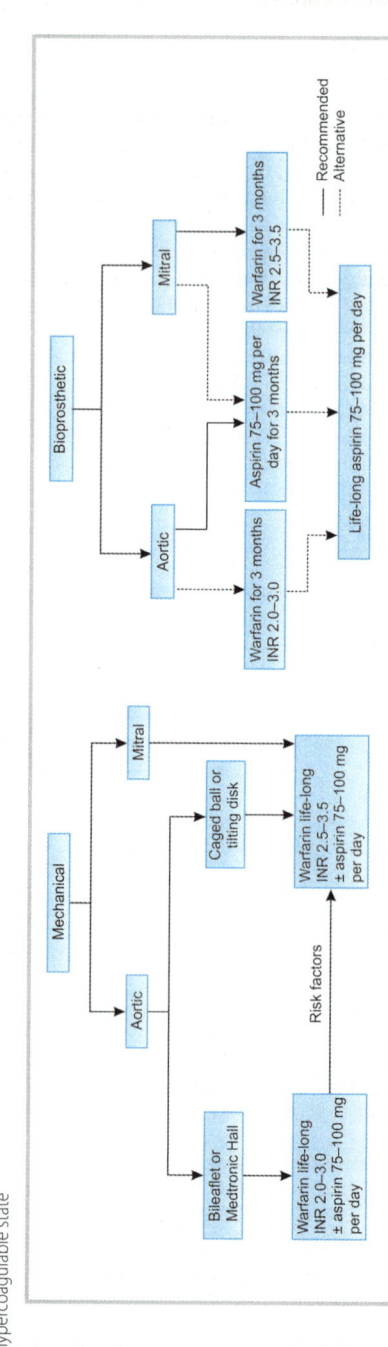

risk of fetal complications. During warfarin use in pregnancy, the INR goal is 3.0 (range 2.5–3.5).

Noncardiac Surgery

Bridging therapy with intravenous anticoagulation may be needed in patients with mechanical valves who require interruption of warfarin therapy for noncardiac surgery, invasive procedures, or dental care. However, antithrombotic therapy should not be stopped for procedures in which bleeding would be unlikely or inconsequential.

In patients at low-risk of thrombosis, defined as those with a bileaflet mechanical AVR with no risk factors for increased risk of thromboembolism, it is recommended that warfarin be stopped 48–72 hours before the procedure (so the INR falls to less than 1.5) and restarted within 24 hours after the procedure since intravenous heparin is usually unnecessary. In patients at high-risk of thrombosis, therapeutic doses of intravenous UFH should be started when the INR falls below 2.0 (typically 48 hours before surgery), stopped 4–6 hours before the procedure, restarted as early after surgery as bleeding stability allows, and continued (with a goal PTT of 55–70 seconds) until the INR is again therapeutic with warfarin therapy.

In the event of emergency surgery, it is reasonable to give fresh frozen plasma to patients with mechanical valves who require interruption of warfarin. Fresh frozen plasma is preferable to high dose vitamin K, which may create a hypercoagulable state.

Echocardiography Follow-up

After valve surgery, current guidelines recommend an echo Doppler at the first postoperative visit (i.e. 2–4 weeks after discharge) if a baseline study was not obtained during hospitalization. The echocardiogram in addition to an interval or complete history and physical examination indicates laboratory evaluation (e.g. complete blood count, BUN, creatinine, electrolytes, LDH or INR). Routine visits annually are recommended, but with a repeat echocardiogram only if there is a change in clinical status (e.g. new murmur, concern for prosthetic valve or LV dysfunction). However, an annual echocardiogram may be considered in patients with a bioprosthetic valve after the first 5 years.

Echo parameters of interest include leaflet morphology and mobility, as well as measurement of transprosthetic gradients and EOA, estimation of the degree of regurgitation, evaluation of LV size and function and calculation of pulmonary arterial systolic pressure. Quantitative Doppler parameters are useful in determining the intrinsic gradient of the valve, providing a comparison for subsequent studies (Table 30).

When an elevated gradient is obtained, the differential diagnosis is Flowchart 7:
- Pathological valve obstruction
- LV outflow tract obstruction
- PPM
- High flow state
- Localized high gradient in presence of bileaflet mechanical valve.

In general, the criteria for grading severity of regurgitant lesions in prosthetic valves (Tables 31 and 32) are similar to native valves largely related to the paucity of studies in patients with prosthetic valves.

Table 30: Parameters for evaluation of the severity of prosthetic aortic valve regurgitation

Parameter	Mild	Moderate	Severe
Valve structure and motion	Usually normal	Abnormal*	Abnormal*
LV size	Normal	Normal or mildly dilated	Dilated
Color Doppler jet width of central jets (% LVOT diameter)	Narrow (<25%)	Intermediate (26–64%)	Large (>65%)
Jet density of CW Doppler spectrum	Incomplete or faint	Dense	Dense
Jet deceleration rate (PHT, ms) by CW Doppler	Slow (>500)	Variable (200–500)	Steep (<200)
LVOT flow vs pulmonary flow by PW Doppler	Slightly increased	Intermediate	Greatly increased
Diastolic flow reversal in the descending aorta by PW Doppler	Absent or brief early diastolic	Intermediate	Prominent, holodiastolic
Diastolic flow reversal in the descending aorta by PW Doppler	Absent or brief early diastolic	Intermediate	Prominent, holodiastolic
Regurgitant volume (mL/beat) by Doppler	<30	30–59	> 60
Regurgitant fraction (%) by Doppler	<30	30–50	> 50

*Abnormal: Dehiscence or rocking, immobile mechanical occluder, thickened or prolapse of bioprosthetic leaflets
Abbreviations: PHT: Pressure half-time; LVOT: Left ventricular outflow tract

❑ LONG-TERM COMPLICATIONS

Thromboembolic and Bleeding Complications

When a patient has a systemic embolic event, the adequacy of anticoagulation control should be assessed. If inadequate, therapy is adjusted to maintain therapeutic goals. If anticoagulation is adequate, the dosage of antithrombotic therapy should be increased, when clinically safe.

Obstruction of a prosthetic valve may be caused by thrombus, pannus ingrowth or a combination of both. Recommendations for management have been provided by the ACC/AHA Guidelines on Valvular Heart Disease. Emergency operation is reasonable for patients with a thrombosed left-sided prosthetic valve and NYHA functional class III–IV symptoms or a large clot burden. However, operative mortality approaches 15–20% with functional class IV patients. Thrombolytic therapy is an alternative to surgery in left sided valve thrombosis, but there is a 12–15% risk of systemic embolism and a 5% risk of major bleeding. The repeat thrombosis rate is as high as 15–20%. An algorithm for management was recently proposed by Pibarot and Dumesnil (Flowchart 8).

Valvular Heart Diseases

FLOWCHART 7: Algorithm for the interpretation of high transprosthetic gradients.

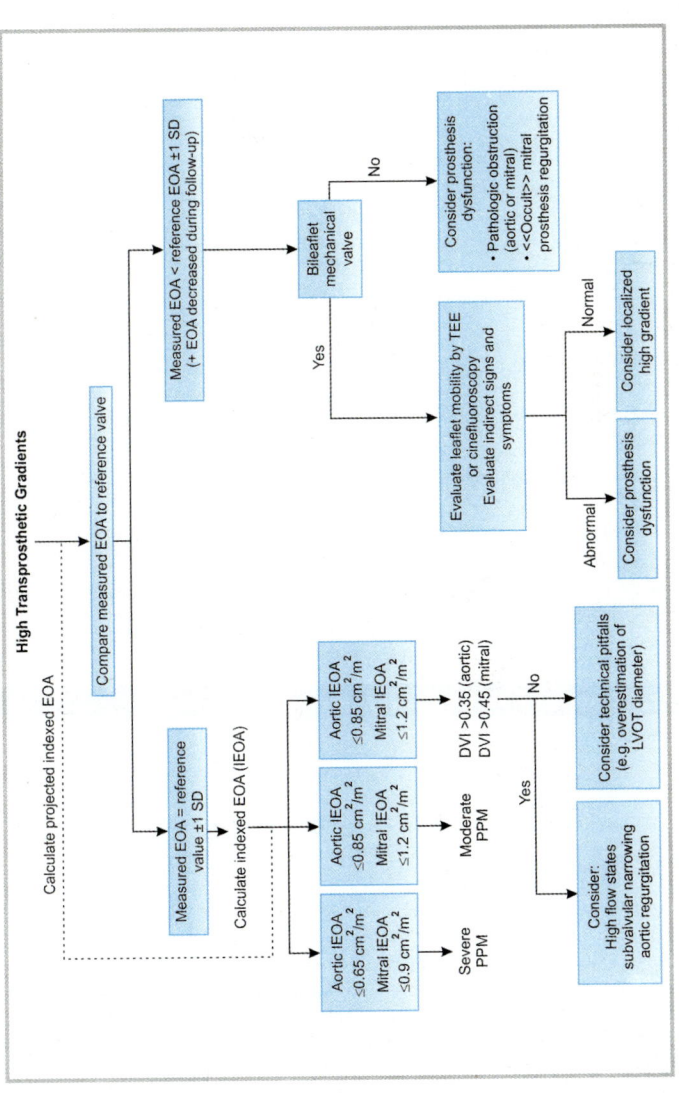

IEOA: indexed effective orifice area
(*Source:* Pibarot P, Dumesnil JG. Prosthetic heart valves: selection of the optimal prosthesis and long-term management. Circulation. 2009;119:1034-48)

Table 31: Parameters for evaluation of the severity of prosthetic mitral valve regurgitation

Parameter	Mild	Moderate	Severe
Valve structure and motion	Usually normal	Abnormal*	Abnormal*
LV size	Normal	Normal or dilated	Usually dilated
Jet area by color Doppler (cm^2)	<4 sq cm or <20% of LA area	Variable	>8 sq cm or >40% of LA area (if central jet)
Flow convergence (at Nyquist limit of 40 cm/s)	None or minimal i.e. (radius <4 mm)	Intermediate	Large (i.e. radius >9 mm)
MR Jet density on CW Doppler	Incomplete or faint	Dense	Dense
Jet contour on CW Doppler	Parabolic	Usually parabolic	Early peaking, triangular
Pulmonary venous flow	Systolic dominance	Systolic blunting	Systolic flow reversal
Vena Contracta width by color Doppler (cm)	<0.3	0.3–0.59	≥0.6
Regurgitant volume (mL/beat) by Doppler	<30	30–59	≥60
Regurgitant fraction (%) by Doppler	<30	30–49	≥50
Effective regurgitant orifice area (cm^2)	<0.20	0.20–0.49	≥0.50

*Abnormal: Dehiscence or rocking, immobile mechanical occluder, thickened or prolapse of bioprosthetic leaflets

Table 32: Doppler parameters of prosthetic aortic and mitral valve stenosis

Parameter	Normal	Possible stenosis	Suggests significant stenosis
Aortic valve			
Peak velocity (m/sec)	<3	3–4	>4
Mean gradient (mm Hg)	<20	20–35	>35
DVI	≥0.30	0.25–0.29	<0.25
EOA (cm^2)	>1.2	0.8–1.2	<0.8
Jet contour	Triangular, early peaking	Triangular to intermediate	Rounded, symmetrical contour
AT (ms)	<80	80–100	>100
Mitral valve			
Peak velocity (m/sec)	<1.9	1.9–2.5	≥2.5
Mean gradient (mm Hg)	≤5	6–10	>10
EOA (cm^2)	>2.0	1.0–2.0	<1.0
PHT (ms)	<130	130–200	>200

Valvular Heart Diseases

Table 33: Recommendations for managing elevated INRs or bleeding in patients receiving warfarin: Clinical practice guidelines from the American College of Chest Physicians

INR more than therapeutic range but <5.0; no significant bleeding	Lower dose or omit dose; monitor more frequently and resume at lower dose when INR therapeutic; if only minimally above therapeutic range, no dose reduction may be required
INR ≥5.0, but <9.0; no significant bleeding	Omit next one or two doses, monitor more frequently, and resume at an appropriately adjusted dose when INR in therapeutic range. Alternatively, omit dose and give vitamin K (1–2.5 mg po), particularly if at increased risk of bleeding. If more rapid reversal is required because the patient requires urgent surgery, vitamin K (≤ 5 mg po) can be given with the expectation that a reduction of the INR will occur in 24 hours. If the INR is still high, additional vitamin K (1–2 mg po) can be given
INR ≥ 9.0; no significant bleeding	Hold warfarin therapy and give higher dose of vitamin K (2.5–5 mg po) with the expectation that the INR will be reduced substantially in 24–48 hours. Monitor more frequently and use additional vitamin K if necessary. Resume therapy at an appropriately adjusted dose when INR is therapeutic.
Serious bleeding at any elevation of INR	Hold warfarin therapy and give vitamin K (10 mg by slow IV infusion), supplemented with FFP, PCC, or rVIIa, depending on the urgency of the situation; vitamin K can be repeated every 12 hours
Life-threatening bleeding	Hold warfarin therapy and give FFP, PCC, or rVIIa supplemented with vitamin K (10 mg by slow IV infusion). Repeat, if necessary, depending on INR
Administration of vitamin K	In patients with mild to moderately elevated INRs without major bleeding, give vitamin K orally rather than subcutaneously

FLOWCHART 8: Algorithm for the management of patients with left-sided prosthetic valve thrombosis

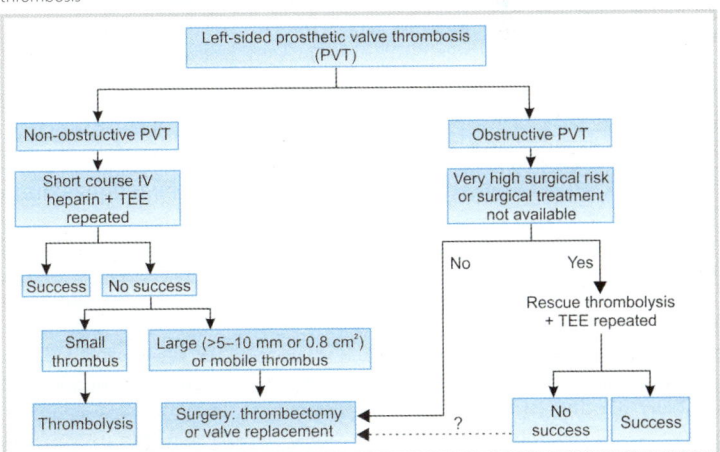

(*Source:* Pibarot P, Dumesnil JG. Prosthetic heart valves: selection of the optimal prosthesis and long-term management. Circulation. 2009;119:1034-48)

Table 34: Differentiating thrombus from pannus formation (data from 24 obstructed valves in 23 patients)			
	Thrombus	Pannus	P
Duration from implant to reoperation (days)	62	178	0.0006
Duration of symptoms to reoperation (days)	9	305	0.0006
Rate of adequate anticoagulation (%)	21	89	0.003
Aortic position (%)	21	70	0.035
Abnormal valve motion on TEE (%)	100	60	0.021
Length (cm)	2.8 ± 2.5	1.2 ± 0.04	0.038
Soft ultrasound density (%)	92	29	0.007
Videointensity (mass/prosthesis)	0.46 ± 0.14	0.71 ± 0.17	0.006

Bleeding is often due to excessive anticoagulation and can be managed by withholding warfarin and monitoring the level of anticoagulation with serial INR determinations. Guidelines for managing bleeding complications are provided by the American College of Chest Physicians (Tables 33 and 34).

Structural Valve Deterioration

Mechanical prostheses have excellent durability, and SVD is rare with contemporary valves. The SVD after bioprosthetic valve replacement begins at about 5 years for mitral position and at about 8 years for aortic position. Risk factors associated with bioprosthetic SVD include:
- Younger patients, related to the heightened and more effective immune response in response to residual animal antigens. However, very early SVD of bioprostheses can occur in elderly patients
- Mitral position which is related to higher closure pressure and increased stress on the valve
- Renal insufficiency
- Hyperparathyroidism
- Hypertension: In the aortic position, SVD of bioprostheses may be related to stress from elevated diastolic BP.

A diagnosis of infective endocarditis (IE) is based on the presence of either major or minor clinical criteria. Overall, *S. aureus* is the most common causative organism of prosthetic valve endocarditis (PVE) followed by coagulase-negative staphylococci, streptococci and enterococci. However, the microbiology varies according to time of developing endocarditis after valve surgery. In patients with PVE within 1 year of surgery and no drug abuse, methicillin-resistant coagulase negative staphylococcus was the most common organism in a recent series, followed by *S. aureus*.

Medical therapy alone is more likely to succeed in late PVE and non-staphylococcal infections. Antibiotic treatment regimens are summarized in Table 35. The ACC/AHA 2008 update on IE recommended antibiotic prophylaxis of endocarditis for dental procedures in prosthetic valve patients that involve manipulation of either gingival tissue or the periapical region of teeth or perforation of oral mucosa. In addition, prophylaxis is no longer recommended for procedures that involve the respiratory tract, unless the procedure involves incision

Table 35: Antibiotic regimens for treating prosthetic valve endocarditis

1. Viridans group *Streptococcus* and *Streptococcus bovis*
    A. Penicillin-susceptible strains (minimum inhibitory concentration ≤0.12 μg/mL)
       Aqueous crystalline penicillin G sodium
       or ceftriaxone x 6 weeks,
       with or without gentamicin x 2 weeks
       Vancomycin x 6 weeks (if unable to tolerate penicillin or ceftriaxone)
    B. Penicillin relatively or fully resistant strains (minimum inhibitory concentration > 0.12 μg/mL)
       Aqueous crystalline penicillin G sodium
       or ceftriaxone x 6 weeks,
       plus gentamicin x 6 weeks
       Vancomycin x 6 weeks (if unable to tolerate penicillin or ceftriaxone)

2. *Staphylococcus*
    A. Oxacillin-susceptible strains
       Nafcillin or oxacillin x ≥6 weeks (penicillin G may be substituted if penicillin susceptible [i.e. minimum inhibitory concentration ≤0.1 μg/mL]),
       plus rifampin x ≥ 6 weeks,
       plus gentamicin x 2 weeks
       For penicillin allergic: Substitute cefazolin (if nonanaphylactoid reaction) or vancomycin (if anaphylactoid reaction)
    B. Oxacillin-resistant strains
       Vancomycin x ≥6 weeks,
       plus rifampin x ≥6 weeks,
       plus gentamicin x 2 weeks

3. Enterococcal
    A. Susceptible to penicillin, gentamicin and vancomycin
       Ampicillin or aqueous crystlalline penicillin G x ≥6 weeks,
       plus gentamicin x ≥6 weeks
       Vancomycin x 6 weeks (if unable to tolerate penicillin or ampicillin),
       plus gentamicin x 6 weeks
    B. Susceptible to penicillin, streptomycin and vancomycin, but resistant to gentamicin
       Ampicillin or aqueous crystalline penicillin G x ≥6 weeks,
       plus streptomycin x ≥6 weeks
       Vancomycin x 6 weeks (if unable to tolerate penicillin or ampicillin),
       plus streptomycin x 6 weeks
    C. Susceptible to aminoglycoside and vancomycin, but resistant to penicillin
        1. β-lactamase producing strain
           Ampicillin-sulbactam plus gentamicin x 6 weeks (if gentamicin resistant, then >6 weeks of ampicilin-sulbactam will be needed)
           Vancomycin plus gentamicin x 6 weeks (if unable to tolerate ampicillin-sulbactam)
        2. Intrinsic penicillin resistance
           Vancomycin x 6 weeks,
           plus gentamicin x 6 weeks
    D. Resistant to penicillin, aminoglycoside and vancomycin
        1. *E. faecium:* Linezolid x ≥8 weeks or quinupristin-dalfopristin x ≥8 weeks
        2. *E. faecalis:* Imipenem/cilastatin plus ampicillin sodium x ≥8 weeks
           or ceftriaxone sodium plus ampicillin sodium x ≥8 weeks

4. HACEK microorganisms
   Ceftriaxone or ampicillin-sulbactam or ciprofloxacin (if unable to tolerate ceftriaxone or ampicillin-sulbactam) x 6 weeks

Contd...

Contd...

Table 35: Antibiotic regimens for treating prosthetic valve endocarditis

5. Culture negative
   A. Early (≤1 year)
      Vancomycin x 6 weeks,
      plus gentamicin x 2 weeks,
      plus cefepime x 6 weeks,
      plus rifampin x 6 weeks
   B. Late (>1 year)
      Ampicilin-sulbactam x 6 weeks,
      plus gentamicin x 6 weeks,
      plus rifampin x 6 weeks
      Vancomycin x 6 weeks (if unable to tolerate penicillin),
      plus gentamicin x 6 weeks,
      plus ciprofloxacin x 6 weeks,
      plus rifampin x 6 weeks
   C. *Bartonella*
      1. Suspected
         Ceftriaxone x 6 weeks,
         plus gentamicin x 2 weeks,
         with or without doxycycline
      2. Documented, culture positive
         Doxycycline x 6 weeks,
         plus gentamicin x 2 weeks

of the respiratory tract, such as tonsillectomy and adenoidectomy. Prophylaxis is no longer recommended for GI or GU procedures, including diagnostic esophagogastroduodenoscopy or colonoscopy.

Regimens for prophylaxis are administered 30–60 minutes before the procedure and they include amoxicillin 2 gm PO. For penicillin allergic patients, the recommendation is to substitute cephalexin 2 gm (although cephalosporins are not recommended if allergy is manifest as anaphylaxis), clindamycin 600 mg, azithromycin 500 mg or clarithromycin 500 mg. If the patient is NPO, cefazolin or ceftriaxone 1 gm IM/IV or clindamycin 600 mg IM/IV can be given.

Paravalvular Regurgitation

Small paravalvular jets are common on intraoperative TEE, occurring in 10–25% of cases. These leaks typically resolve with healing and less than 1% require reoperation at 1–2 years. Moderate or severe regurgitation on postoperative TEE is rare (i.e. 1–2%) and requires correction, which can be performed by repair alone in about 50% of cases.

Hemolysis

Hemolysis is usually associated with either structural deterioration or paravalvular leak and due to turbulence through the valve or between the sewing ring and the native ring. A paravalvular leak may be visualized with TEE. The hallmark of mechanical hemolytic anemia is the presence of fragmented erythrocytes in the peripheral blood smear. Medical management is limited but there are reports of benefit with beta-adrenergic blockers, presumed related to reduced shearing forces on the erythrocytes. Pentoxifylline may reduce hemolysis by improving erythrocyte deformability. Iron, folate and erythropoietin supplementation may be necessary.

❏ SUGGESTED READINGS

Baddour LM, Wilson WR, Bayer AS, et al. Infective endocarditis. Diagnosis, antimicrobial therapy and management of complications. Circulation. 2005;111:e394-e433.
Barbetseas J, Nagueh SF, Pitsavos C, et al. Differentiating thrombus from pannus formation in obstructed mechanical prosthetic valves: an evaluation of clinical, transthoracic and transesophageal echocardiographic parameters. J Am Coll Cardiol. 1998;32:1410-17.
Bonow RO, Carabello BA, Chatterjee K, et al. ACC/AHA 2006 guidelines for the management of patients with valvular heart disease: executive summary. Circulation. 2006;114:450-527.
Hannan El, Wu C, Bennett EV, et al. Risk index for predicting in hospital mortality for cardiac valve surgery. Ann Thorac Surg. 2007;83:921-30.
Lopez J, Revilla A, Villacosta I, et al. Definition, clinical profile, microbiological spectrum and prognostic factors of early-onset prosthetic valve endocarditis Eur Heart J. 2007;28:760-5.
Nishimura RA, Carabello BA, Faxon DP, et al. ACC/AHA 2008 Guideline update in valvular heart disease: focused update on infective endocarditis. J Am Coll Cardiol. 2008;52:676-85.
O'Brien SM, Shahian DM, Filardo G, et al. The Society of Thoracic Surgeons 2008 Cardiac Surgery Risk Models: part 2—Isolated valve surgery. Ann Thorac Surg. 2009;88:S23-S42.
Pibarot P, Dumesnil JG. Prosthetic heart valves: selection of the optimal prosthesis and long-term management. Circulation. 2009;119:1034-48.
Ruel M, Al-Faleh H, Kulik A, et al. Prosthesis-patient mismatch after aortic valve replacement primarily affects patients with pre-existing left ventricular dysfunction: impact on survival, freedom from heart failure and left ventricular mass regression. J Thorac Cardiovasc Surg. 2006;131:1036-44.
Salem DN, O'Gara PT, Madias C, et al. Valvular and structural heart disease. American College of Chest Physicians evidence-based clinical practice guidelines. Chest. 2008;133:593S-629S.
van Gameren M, Kappetein AP, Steyerberg EW, et al. Do we need separate risk stratification models for hospital mortality after heart valve surgery. Ann Thorac Surg. 2008;85:921-31.
www.sts.org/sections/stsnationaldatabase/riskcalculator/

5.8 Antithrombotic Therapy in Valvular Heart Disease

❏ INTRODUCTION

A major component of the management of patients with valvular heart disease is the prevention of distal emboli of thrombotic or platelet rich material by the use of antithrombic therapy. The risk of thromboembolic events is related to patient specific factors and valve characteristics. Patient factors include atrial fibrillation, heart failure and left atrial size, which are frequently associated with valvular heart disease (Table 36). Some of these factors or combinations of them may be indications for antithrombic therapy regardless of the presence of valve disease. In native valve disease with normal sinus rhythm, antithrombic therapy would not be considered unless other high-risk features are present.

Prosthetic valves fall into two broad categories: (i) biological valves and (ii) mechanical valves; although the former often have nonbiological components. In general, biological valves are less thrombogenic and less durable. Mechanical valves are more durable, but more thrombogenic (Table 37). Annuloplasty rings and

Table 36: Patient factors that increase the risk of thromboembolism in valvular heart disease

- Advanced age
- Atrial fibrillation
- Heart failure
- Reduced left ventricular systolic performance
- Enlarged atria
- Previous thromboembolic events
- Coagulation abnormalities

Table 37: Relative thrombogenicity of prosthetic valves

Prosthesis category	Valve type	Thrombosis risk
Mechanical	Caged-ball	High
	Mono-disk	Intermediate
	Bileaflet	Intermediate
	Annuloplasty ring	Low
Biological	Heterograft	Low
	Homograft	Low
	Percutaneous valve	Low

Table 38: Factors that increase the risk of bleeding on anticoagulants

- Bleeding diatheses
- History of GI bleeding
- Genetic variations in warfarin metabolism
- Advanced age
- History of hemorrhagic stroke
- Chronic kidney disease
- Excess alcohol use
- High risk for trauma
- Diabetes
- Unreliable in taking medications

the sewing rings of most prosthetic valves require up to 3 months to endothelialize and then the risk of thrombosis decreases. Valvuloplasty and valve repair damage valve surfaces which creates a short-term concern for thrombus formation.

❏ PROPHYLACTIC ANTITHROMBIC THERAPY

The major risk of anticoagulant therapy is bleeding, and this risk needs to be balanced against the potential benefits. Some of the risk factors that increase the likelihood of bleeding on anticoagulant therapy are shown in Table 38. They mitigate against antithrombic therapy in borderline cases, but in certain types of valvular heart disease, antithrombic therapy is mandatory.

Several new oral anticoagulants are being tested, and there is hope that a better agent will be available soon. Several studies have shown that warfarin is significantly superior to antiplatelet agents, such as aspirin, dipyridamole and pentoxifylline, either used singularly or in combinations. Thus, these agents would only be used in situations where there was a very high risk of bleeding on warfarin,

Table 39: Chronic anticoagulation recommendations and INR range for the following native valve diseases

Valve disease	INR
Mitral stenosis and high-risk factors	2–3
Mitral regurgitation and high-risk factors	2–3
Mitral valve prolapse and TIA or stroke	2–3
Valve disease and atrial fibrillation	2–3
Valve disease and prior embolic event	2–3
Mitral valvuloplasty, 1 month before and after	2–3

or when antiplatelet therapy alone was felt to be adequate. Often warfarin needs to be combined with antiplatelet therapy due to other comorbidities such as coronary artery disease.

Table 39 shows the recommended anticoagulation intensity by INR for the various valve diseases which are discussed below.

❏ RHEUMATIC VALVULAR HEART DISEASE

The most common condition associated with thrombotic emboli in rheumatic valvular disease is patients with mitral valve disease. The risk is greatest in patients with mitral stenosis and atrial fibrillation. Rheumatic mitral regurgitation is known to have a lower risk of thrombotic complications unless there is concomitant mitral stenosis. Due to this low risk in pure rheumatic mitral regurgitation, there is no recommended prophylactic antithrombotic treatment regimen for this condition. However any rheumatic mitral valve disease in the presence of atrial fibrillation or a prior embolic event would require anticoagulation with warfarin, with a target INR of 2–3. If, on this therapy, there is any recurrence of thrombi, it would be appropriate to add an antiplatelet agent such as aspirin, dipyridamole or clopidogrel. In rheumatic mitral stenosis patients who are perivalvuloplasty, anticoagulation is usually done for 3 weeks prior to the procedure and for 4 weeks afterward.

❏ MITRAL VALVE PROLAPSE

Embolic phenomena are uncommon in this, often hereditary, degenerative valvular disease. There have been reports of amaurosis fugax, transient ischemic attacks (TIA) or frank strokes in patients with mitral valve prolapse in the absence of atrial fibrillation. For asymptomatic mitral valve prolapse patients, no specific prophylactic therapy is recommended. Those who have had TIA or stroke should receive aspirin or another antiplatelet agent. If recurrent cerebral events occur then anticoagulation is recommended to an INR of 2–3. Prophylactic therapy should be indefinite and probably should be continued after valve repair in those with a prior history of TIA or stroke.

❏ CALCIFIED OR DEGENERATIVE VALVULAR DISEASE

The incidence of calcific valve disease is most common in the aortic and secondly in the mitral valve. Both can lead to systemic emboli, either from calcium or thrombotic material. The past occurrence of calcific emboli can sometimes be detected by examination of the eyegrounds. If thrombotic emboli are suspected or proven then anticoagulation with an INR of 2–3 is recommended. Patients with atherosclerosis and associated valvular calcifications are often on aspirin or other antiplatelet therapy and this should be continued.

❏ PROSTHETIC VALVES

Mechanical Valves

In general, the risk of thrombus formation is highest in mechanical prosthetic valves as compared to bioprosthetic valves. As a general rule, all mechanical prosthetic heart valves in any valvular position in the heart are anticoagulated, unless there is a contraindication. The guidelines for anticoagulation of mechanical prosthetic valves varies somewhat between Continental Europe, the United Kingdom and the United States, possibly due to variations in the predominant valves available in the different locals and differences in the coumarins that are used. The recommendations below and in Table 40 are based upon the American College of Cardiology and American Heart Association Guidelines. If patients are at particularly high risk for thrombus, have had recurrent thrombosis or have coronary artery disease, then aspirin or another antiplatelet agent should be added. If aspirin cannot be taken, then clopidogrel is a reasonable alternative, or some have suggested increasing the INR to the 3–4 range.

❏ BIOPROSTHETIC VALVES

Bioprosthetic valves generally have a lower risk of thrombosis than mechanical valves. The highest risk of thrombosis is early after surgery due to the sewing ring. Since complete endothelialization of the sewing ring may take up to 3 months, it is recommended that bioprosthetic valves receive anticoagulation for the first 3 months at an INR of 2–3. It is also recommended that heparin bridging be started as soon as feasible after surgery and continued until the INR is above 2. This approach is always taken in the mitral position, but some surgeons do not anticoagulate aortic bioprosthetic valves given the lower incidence of thrombus with them. Long-term anticoagulation is not indicated for these valves unless there

Table 40: Recommended chronic anticoagulation INR range for the following valve prostheses	
Valve type	INR
Mechanical valves:	
Aortic caged-ball	3–4
Aortic mono-disk	2–3
Aortic bileaflet	2–3
Mitral caged-ball	3–4
Mitral mono-disk	2.5–3.5
Mitral bileaflet	2.5–3.5
Annuloplasty ring	
First 3 months	2–3
Biological valves	
First 3 months	2–3

is a high-risk situation such as atrial fibrillation. However aspirin is recommended for all patients with bioprosthetic valves, unless they cannot take aspirin. There are no recommendations for percutaneously delivered bioprosthetic aortic valves, but most operators put them on lifelong aspirin. Some use aspirin plus clopidogrel for the first month.

❑ VALVULOPLASTY AND VALVE REPAIR

Percutaneous mitral balloon valvuloplasty for mitral stenosis is a high-risk situation for dislodging any atrial thrombi. Consequently, patients should be anticoagulated prior to the procedure for 3–4 weeks. Prior to atrial puncture a transesophageal echocardiography (TEE) should be done to confirm that no thrombi are present. Heparin should be given during the procedure and long-term anticoagulation should be given if indicators are present. Mitral valve repair almost always includes placement of an annuloplasty ring, which is similar to the sewing ring of a prosthetic valve. Most recommend anticoagulation for 6 weeks to 3 months after mitral valve repair. Long-term anticoagulation would depend on other risk factors.

❑ MANAGEMENT ISSUES

Diagnosis of Thrombotic Valve Complications

Echocardiography is the key to the diagnosis of thrombotic complications of valvular heart disease. Patients at high risk for intracardiac thrombosis, who have known or suspected valvular disease, should have echocardiographic imaging, even if treatment is indicated without such imaging, because it is useful to have baseline images to compare subsequent images taken when thrombotic events are suspected. Computed tomography (CT) scans and magnetic resonance imaging (MRI) can also be used to detect intracardiac thrombi. Both require contrast administration and CT involves exposure to radiation. Both are expensive relative to echocardiography. Thus, they are usually used in special circumstances, where this type of imaging would be expected to be superior to echocardiography, or when echocardiographic images are not adequate to resolve the clinical issue. Cardiac fluoroscopy is also useful for detecting thrombus induced mechanical valve dysfunction. The mechanical leaflet apparatus is radiopaque, and derivations from normal positions during the cardiac cycle can readily be detected.

Valve Thrombosis

The development of thrombus can obstruct a mechanical prosthetic valve or prevent its closure resulting in regurgitation. The differential diagnosis includes pannus formation, which is a form of exuberant scar tissue around the sewing ring which encroaches on the valve orifice and sometimes impinges on leaflet function. Also, infective endocarditis should be excluded because treatment would be different.

Thrombus can often be treated medically, whereas pannus ingrowth would require repeat surgery. Thrombus may respond to an infusion of heparin, and this would be indicated for patients without symptoms or hemodynamic compromise who have demonstrated valve thrombus. The risk of thrombolysis in addition to bleeding is breaking up of the thrombus, resulting in emboli. The protocol used for thrombolysis of a thrombosed valve is the same as the protocol for pulmonary embolus. Do not use the protocol for myocardial infarction. The overall efficacy of thrombolysis for thrombosed prosthetic valves is about 80%, but complications occur in 15–20% and mortality in 3–12%. However surgical mortality has been reported to be 12–46%.

Pregnancy

The ideal management of pregnancy in patients, who need to be on chronic oral anticoagulation, is to switch them to heparin preconception, and either continue it throughout pregnancy or switch to warfarin after the first trimester. In high risk patients for whom it is necessary, aspirin is acceptable during pregnancy. Anticoagulation with warfarin should be discontinued prior to delivery, which is easy to do if the delivery is planned. If it is not going to be an induced delivery, the patient should switch to heparin for the last 6 weeks then resume warfarin after delivery. Heparin can be stopped just prior to delivery or reversed with protamine if necessary.

Elective Surgery

Since surgery induces a hypercoagulable state, the risk of thrombosis is elevated during surgery. All mechanical prosthetic valve patients, including those with aortic bileaflet valves, are at intermediate to high risk of having thrombosis and heparin bridging is required. This is accomplished by discontinuing warfarin for 4 days prior to surgery, starting heparin 2 days later and stopping it 4 hours prior to surgery, then restarting it as soon as it is safe postoperatively. In patients at especially high risk one can monitor the INR and start the heparin as soon as it hits 2.0, rather than just starting the heparin arbitrarily on day 2. In case of emergency surgery, warfarin should be discontinued and fresh frozen plasma or prothrombin concentrate administrated. Do not use vitamin K as this might induce a prothrombotic state, unless heparin is coadministrated.

Endocarditis

Anticoagulation in infective endocarditis patients is controversial. This is a situation where the risk versus potential benefits need to be carefully weighed. In general, patients at high risk of emboli to the systemic circuit should be continued on anticoagulation even if they develop infective endocarditis. Such patients include those with mitral stenosis and atrial fibrillation, mechanical prosthetic valves, and previous embolic strokes. However careful attention should be given to keeping the INR in the recommended range, if patients are on warfarin or keeping the activated clotting time in the therapeutic range, if they are on heparin, is important. As soon as antibiotic therapy is started in infective endocarditis the risk of stroke decreases quickly and is low after 2 weeks of effective treatment. In patients who have cerebral embolism it would be prudent to stop anticoagulation for 7–14 days to reduce the likelihood of massive intracerebral bleeding.

In marantic endocarditis, emboli are frequent. The basic treatment is trying to control the underlying disease, but if emboli occur, then heparin therapy is indicated unless there is a contraindication, such as a recent intracerebral bleed. Whether long-term anticoagulation therapy with warfarin is indicated for such patients after they leave the hospital is unclear. This decision would require the careful balancing of potential benefits versus risks with the physician who is taking care of the patients underlying disease.

❑ SUGGESTED READINGS

Bates SM, Greer IA, Hirsh J, et al. Use of antithrombotic agents during pregnancy: the seventh ACCP conference on antithrombotic and thrombolytic therapy. Chest. 2004;126:627S-44S.

Bonow RO, Carabello B, de Leon, et al. ACC/AHA guidelines for the management of patients with valvular heart disease. Executive summary. A report of the American College of Cardiology/American Heart Association task force on practice guidelines (Committee on management of patients with valvular heart disease). J Heart Valve Dis. 1998;7:672-707.

Douketis JD, Berger PB, Dunn AS, et al. The perioperative management of antithrombotic therapy: American College of Chest Physicians evidence-based clinical practice guidelines (8th edition). Chest. 2008;133:299S-339S.

Goldsmith I, Turpie AG, Lip GY. Valvuar heart disease and prosthetic heart valves. BMJ. 2002;325:1228-31.

Little SH, Massel DR. Antiplatelet and anticoagulation for patients with prosthetic heart valves. Cochrane Database Syst Rev. 2003;(4):CD003464.

Sun JC, Davidson MJ, Lamy A, et al. Antithrombotic management of patients with prosthetic heart valves: current evidence and future trends. Lancet. 2009;374:565-76.

Vahanian A, Baumgartner H, Bax J, et al. Guidelines on the management of valvular heart disease: the task force on the management of valvular heart disease of the European Society of Cardiology. Eur Heart J. 2007;28:230-68.

Chapter 6

Vascular Diseases

6.1 Evaluation and Management of the Patient with Essential Hypertension

❑ EVALUATION OF THE PATIENT WITH HYPERTENSION

In most patients with systemic hypertension, there are no clinical manifestations other than the elevated blood pressure. Therefore, unless blood pressure is measured routinely in all patients, hypertension will remain unrecognized.

Physical Findings

The classification of blood pressure measurement and severity of pressure elevation are presented in Table 1. The small vessels of the optic fundus provide an excellent means to assess the degree of systemic vasoconstriction; this examination should be performed routinely. The earliest state (Group 1) of hypertensive vascular disease is recognized by increased arterial tortuosity and mild constriction. Coexisting arteriosclerotic changes are manifested by the discontinuity of the arterioles at arteriovenous (AV) crossings (i.e. AV nicking; Group II). Appearance of exudates and hemorrhages (Group III) represents accelerated hypertension and/or renal disease. The appearance of papilledema (Group IV) permits the diagnosis of malignant hypertension.

One should always compare the simultaneous palpations of femoral and brachial arterial pulsations in all patients with hypertension in a search for a delay in the propagation of the aortic pulse wave as a manifestation of coarctation of the aorta (particularly in young patients) or, for evidence of atherosclerotic occlusive processes in older patients. Auscultation of the carotid arteries (for bruits) may provide signs of preventable strokes and transient ischemic attacks. Funduscopic examination may reveal cholesterol emboli in the retinal arterioles. Renal arterial bruits on examination of the abdomen, flanks and back provide an important sign of occlusive renal arterial disease and renovascular hypertension.

The earliest clinical index of cardiac involvement in hypertension is left atrial enlargement, which may be suspected by an atrial diastolic gallop rhythm (fourth heart sound). This auscultatory finding is highly concordant with at least two of four conventional electrocardiographic criteria of left atrial abnormality (Table 2).

As LVH becomes more evident by chest roentgenogram and electrocardiogram, a louder aortic component of the second heart sound is heard, the fourth heart sound is almost always present, and there is a palpable and sustained left ventricular lift. Clearly, the presence of a third heart sound, this ventricular diastolic gallop rhythm, connotes the presence of left ventricular failure.

Table 1: Classification of blood pressure for adults

Class	Systolic pressure (mm Hg)	Diastolic pressure (mm Hg)
Normal	<120	and <80
Prehypertension	120–139	or 80–89
Stage 1	140–159	or 90–99
Stage 2	>160	or >100

Table 2: Clinical classification of hypertensive heart disease

Stage 1
Normal-sized heart without evidence of cardiac enlargement (by chest film, electrocardiogram, or echocardiogram)

Stage II
Early left ventricular hypertrophy as detected by a fourth heart sound and two of the following ECG criteria:
- P wave in lead II ≥0.3 mV and ≥0.12 sec Bipeak interval in notched P wave ≥ 0.04 sec
- Ratio of P wave duration to PR segment ≥1.6 (lead II)
- Terminal (negative) atrial forces (in V) ≥0.04 sec
- Echocardiography of LVH

Stage III
Clinically evident left ventricular hypertrophy as evidenced by:
- ECG criteria of LVH
- Sum of tallest R and deepest S waves ≥ 4.5 mV (precordial)
- LV "strain"—that is QRS and T wave vectors 180° apart
- QRS frontal axis <0°
- All three ECG criteria (above)
- Echocardiographic evidence of LVH

Stage IV
- Left ventricular failure
- Systolic or diastolic dysfunction with preserved systolic function

Laboratory Studies

It is important for the physician to discuss the appropriate preparation for laboratory tests with the patient (Tables 3 to 5). If possible, these should be done with the patient of all medications.

The following discussion is offered to provide a rationale for interpretation of those laboratory studies that may be ordered in the evaluation of the patient with hypertension. Clearly, not all of these studies are necessary in the routine evaluation of a patient with hypertension; however, this discussion is offered to permit a means for understanding and evaluating a patient with hypertension. It is also for the pertinence and significance for the patient who may have one or more of those diseases that frequently coexist with hypertension. For the uncomplicated patient, the minimal evaluation, usually, includes complete blood count (without differential); determination of serum creatinine, potassium blood sugar, uric acid and cholesterol (with high and low density cholesterol) concentrations; and an electrocardiogram. It is clear that the fewer the number of laboratory studies, the more cost effective, but there are certain studies that will enhance the evaluation.

Table 3: Laboratory studies that may be of value in the evaluation of the patient with hypertension

I. Complete blood count:
   - White blood cell count (and differential)
   - Hemoglobin concentration
   - Hematocrit
   - Adequacy of platelets
II. Blood chemistries:
   - Glucose (fasting, 2-hour postprandial, or glucose tolerance test)
   - Hemoglobin A1c
   - Uric acid
   - Cholesterol concentration (total, high-density lipoprotein, and low-density lipoprotein fractions)
   - Renal function (serum creatinine and/or blood urea concentrations)
   - Serum electrolytes (Na, K, Cl, CO_2) concentrations
   - Calcium and phosphorus concentrations
   - Total protein and albumin concentration
   - Hepatic function (alkaline phosphatase, bilirubin, serum glutamic oxaloacetic transaminase)
   - Serum glutamic pyruvic transaminase, lactic acid dehydrogenase)
III. Urine studies:
   - Urinalysis
   - Urine culture
   - A 24-hour collection (protein, Na, K, creatinine)

Table 4: Factors responsible for hypokalemia

I. Dietary sodium excess associated with diuretic therapy
II. Chronic gastrointestinal potassium losses
   - Vomiting
   - Diarrhea
   - Laxative abuse
   - Pyloric obstruction
   - Nasogastric suction
   - Villous adenoma (colon)
   - Malabsorption syndrome
   - Ureterosigmoidoscopy
III. Adrenocortical excess
   - Primary aldosteronism (adenoma or hyperplasia)
   - Cushing's syndrome and disease
   - Other adrenal steroidal hormone excess
IV. Drug therapy and food
   - Diuretics
   - Licorice
   - Adrenal steroids
   - Salicylate intoxication
   - Outdated tetracycline
V. Renal disease (chronic)
   - Potassium-wasting nephropathy
   - Nephrotic syndrome
   - Renal tubular acidosis
VI. Secondary hyperaldosteronism
   - Renal arterial disease
   - Congestive heart failure
   - Cirrhosis
VII. Diabetes mellitus (acidosis)
VIII. Primary periodic paralysis (hypokalemic type)

Table 5: Specialized studies of value in evaluating patients with hypertension	
Study	**Indications**
Intravenous urography	• Consideration of renal parenchymal disease • History of urinary tract infections, renal stones or obstructive uropathy • Persistence of hypertension after toxemia of pregnancy
Renal arterography	• Abdominal, flank or back bruit (see text) • Sudden onset of hypertension • Sudden severity of known hypertension (loss of blood pressure control on prior adequate therapy) • Disparity in renal lengths (by urography or scintigraphy) of ≥1 cm • Renal venous renin activities functional assessment of the arterial lesions(s) at the time of selective renal arteriography • Noninvasive arteriograms demonstrating renal arterial disease • Evaluation of progression of known renal arterial disease
Isotope renography and renal scans	• Follow-up of patient with renal arterial disease (e.g. to assess reduction in renal size or to compare postoperative to preoperative studies) • Postoperative assessment of the patency of renal blood supply • Use in conjunction with digital subtraction arteriography
Plasma renin activity (peripheral venous blood)	• Assessment of low-renin forms of hypertension (e.g. primary aldosteronism, volume-dependent hypertension) • Assessment of high-renin forms of hypertension in association with pharmacologic provocative studies to aid in selecting therapeutic programs
Hormonal studies	• Catecholamines for pheochromocytoma or with clonidine suppression test • Aldosterone levels for hyperaldostronism aldosteronism • Corticosteroid levels for Cushing's disease or syndrome • Thyroid function studies for hyperthyroidism or hypothyroidism • Parathormone for hyperparathyroidism • Growth hormone for acromegaly • Insulin levels for associated diabetes mellitus
Blood (i.e. plasma) volume	• Determination of volume expansion and confirmation of "Pseudotolerance" to antihypertensive therapy • Preoperative assessment of patient with pheochromocytoma

Chest Roentgenogram

It permits recognition of cardiac enlargement, the stigmata of aortic coarctation (rib notching), and complications of hypertension (e.g. pulmonary congestion, aortic widening). It also provides evidence for associated diseases. The extent of cardiac enlargement is easily quantified by chest film and electrocardiogram, thus, providing a means to assess changes with therapy.

Electrocardiography

As indicated, left atrial abnormality is the first electrocardiographic sign of cardiac enlargement. Although the electrocardiographic literature is replete with criteria for diagnosis of LVH, each criterion has its own false-negative and false-positive results. The McPhie criterion (the sum of the tallest R-wave and deepest S-wave in any of the precordial leads achieving a total voltage of 4.5 mV) has the lowest false-positive result (1.5%). The criteria that we have used are detailed in Table 2, and when used with measurements determined from chest roentgenograms are of value in classifying the severity of hypertensive heart disease.

There is a large variety of specialized diagnostic tests available to evaluate the patient with hypertension. As a rule, none needs to be performed routinely. However, the major specialized tests are presented in Table 5, each with its major indications.

❏ ANTIHYPERTENSIVE THERAPY

Lifestyle Management

At present, the non-drug treatments of lifestyle modifications have been increasingly emphasized in specific clinical recommendations and/or disease guidelines, and they have been emphasized as well, in public education and publications in the lay-media. They include recommendations for the management of overweight/obesity, dietary salt (i.e. sodium) excess, tobacco smoking, alcohol abuse, a regular exercise program, the role of potassium and other electrolyte substances, and the adverse effects of nonantihypertensive drugs on blood pressure. Moreover, they add to the antihypertensive effectiveness of prescribed antihypertensive agents in the overall management of hypertensive patients.

Pharmacological Therapy

In Table 6, JNC-7 provides a detailed listing of all the available antihypertensive drugs, their respective classes, the different agents and their respective trade names with their usual doses prescribed.

Table 6: Classes of antihypertensive agents

Diuretics
- Thiazide congeners
- Loop-acting agents
- Potassium-sparing agents
- Aldosterone antagonists
- Sodium pump inhibitors

β-Adrenergic receptor antagonists
- Cardioselective (β_1) inhibitors
- Nonspecific ((β_1, β_2) inhibitors
- Complex molecules
- α-β-blockers
- β-blockers-vasodilators

Adrenergic inhibitor
- Centrally acting agents
- Peripherally acting agents
- α-Adrenergic receptor antagonists
- Complex molecules (central and peripheral actions)

Direct-acting vasodilators
- Direct vascular smooth muscle relaxing agents act primarily on arteriolar or smooth muscle

Renin–angiotensin system inhibitors
- Agents that inhibit renin release from the kidney
- Inhibitors of the angiotensin converting enzyme
- Angiotensin II receptor antagonists
- Renin inhibitors

Calcium antagonists
- Agents that inhibit calcium entry into cardiac and vascular myocytes
- Agents that inhibit calcium entry into vascular myocytes

❏ HEMODYNAMIC CONCEPTS

The hemodynamic hallmark of hypertensive disease is an increased total peripheral resistance throughout the organ circulations. Increased venular smooth muscle tone serves to redistribute the circulating intravascular volume from the peripheral to the central (i.e. cardiopulmonary) circulation. Thus, early in the development of hypertension, this intravascular volume shift is manifested by an increased cardiac output. Later, in more established hypertension, the cardiac output returns toward the normal and the regional or organ blood flows are normal and may even become reduced. As hypertensive disease progresses in severity, vascular resistance increases, thereby, raising the arterial pressure further. Two primary cardiovascular adaptations result from these changes. First, the heart and vessels adapt structurally to their increasing workloads, thereby increasing cardiac (i.e. left ventricular) mass and vascular wall thickness. The second adaptive change is a further contraction of intravascular (i.e. plasma) volume in most nonvolume dependent forms of hypertension. When the heart and vessels, no longer can adapt structurally and functionally, secondary humoral and/or hormonal mechanisms (e.g. renin angiotensin- aldosterone, vasopressin, catecholamines) come into play. Eventually, cardiac and circulatory failure ensues with an associated further expansion of effective circulating blood volume and its attendant impaired renal excretory function.

❏ CLINICAL PHARMACOLOGIC CONCEPTS

An "ideal" antihypertensive agent should be one that (i) reduces vascular smooth muscle tone in order to reduce total peripheral and organ vascular resistances, (ii) maintains cardiac output and organ blood flows (especially to the heart, brain and kidneys) at normal levels, (iii) does not inordinately, reflexively, stimulate the heart (in response to the induced hypotension) to increase its rate, contractility or ejection, and metabolism, and (iv) does not expand intravascular volume in response to the reduced hydrostatic and renal perfusion pressures.

Diuretics

Currently, the diuretic is not necessarily prerequisite for beta-blocker, calcium antagonist, ACE inhibitor, ARB or renin inhibitor to be included in the antihypertensive therapeutic program.

Thiazides and Congeners

The thiazides and their congeners produce natriuresis through inhibition of carbonic anhydrase as well as by active sodium reabsorption in the proximal and distal renal tubules. With resulting natriuresis, diuresis and volume contraction, the enzyme renin is released from the juxtaglomerular apparatus resulting in the generation of angiotensin II and the adrenal cortical release of aldosterone, thereby providing a negative feedback mechanism for the natriuretic stimulus. Further, potassium, magnesium and chloride ions are also lost concurrently in the urine, thus, inducing a hypokalemic alkalosis (and secondary hyperaldosteronism) that may be confused with other causes of the other forms of hyperaldosteronism (e.g. primary aldosteronism, renal arterial disease, and cardiac failure).

A major side effect associated with the thiazides is that of hypokalemia (Table 4). In this regard, is the consequence of excessive dietary sodium intake associated with acceptable doses of the thiazides that produce hypokalemia.

Reduction of the dietary sodium intake will facilitate the overall effectiveness of the diuretic and minimizes concern for the induced hypokalemia. Another concept related to the diuretics is their potential to produce cardiac dysrhythmias (and, perhaps, sudden death) resulting from the induced hypokalemia and possibly, also hypomagnesemia.

The thiazides increase the tubular reabsorption of urate and, hence, affect plasma uric acid concentration. If the hyperuricemia is severe enough, it should be monitored intermittently during treatment, anticipating potential gout. If the uric acid concentration exceeds levels that may produce symptomatic gout, specific therapy may be prescribed. The thiazdes may also induce carbohydrate intolerance or hyperglycemia of varying degrees. When using lower dosages, risk of development of diabetes requiring hypoglycemic therapy may not be any greater than with other antihypertensive drug classes. Other metabolic side effects related to the thiazide diuretics and congeners include hypercalcemia, hypomagnesemia, hyperlipidemia and, of course, dehydration and thirst.

Loop Diuretics

Furosemide is the most common loop acting diuretic in clinical use, and, unlike the thiazides, they promote natriuresis by inhibiting sodium transport at the ascending limb of the loop of Henle. Since, more of the filtered sodium is delivered to the distal tubule for exchange; a greater amount of potassium wastage will result naturally. The onset of action is more immediate (frequently within 20 minutes) and, consequently, the initial diuresis is more rapid than the thiazides, rebound sodium and water retention is more pronounced, and there may be greater potassium wastage. Thus, these agents should be reserved for intravenous necessities, patients with renal functional impairment or cardiac failure, or when the thiazides cannot be administered.

Potassium-sparing Agents (Spironolactone and Eplerinone)

They act by inhibiting the distal tubular action of aldosterone of sodium-for-potassium inhibition. Since, much of the obligate sodium ion transport occurs at the level of the proximal tubule; their potency is not as great as the thiazides. Thus, they are particularly useful, alone or when combined with a thiazide, for patients with primary or secondary hyperaldosteronism; and they are particularly effective in patients with cardiac failure.

Particular care should be emphasized clearly that when using these (and other) potassium sparing agents in patients predisposed to develop hyperkalemia. This caution should be heeded particularly in those patients with impaired renal function or with cardiac failure, especially, if these patients are receiving an ACE inhibitor or an ARB or if they are receiving supplemental potassium.

Amiloride and Triamterene

These two agents are structurally related and act on the same non aldosterone-dependent sodium-for-potassium renal tubular transport mechanism. Both of these agents reduce pressure with a thiazide and are frequently jointly compounded to preserve potassium.

Beta-adrenergic Receptor Blockers (Beta-blockers)

Although they were found first to be effective for the treatment of patients with angina pectoris, not all patients with hypertension responded to beta-blocker monotherapy with a meaningful pressure reduction. In particular, they were found to be most effective in younger patients, especially those with a hyperkinetic circulation, and for patients with such comorbid diseases as coronary arterial disease (with or without myocardial infarction) or when used with a diuretic.

The hemodynamic actions of the various beta-blockers presently available are listed in Tables 7 and 8. The arterial pressure reduction produced by most beta-blockers is often associated with a decreased cardiac output, although the calculated total peripheral resistance may increase. With this class of agents, heart rate, myocardial tension and contractility and metabolism are usually reduced.

The authors believe that the beta-blockers are indicated in the hypertensive patients with a hyperdynamic beta-adrenergic circulation or other hyperkinetic circulatory states. These are also indicated certainly in patients with hypertension and a prior myocardial infarction, those with cardiac dysrhythmias responsive to beta-blockers (e.g. catecholamines), idiopathic mitral prolapse syndrome and the patients who are already receiving a beta-blocker in lower doses than for treating hypertension (e.g. migraine, muscle tremor, glaucoma). Sweeping conclusions as to the merits (or lack thereof) of any drug class are not at all justified.

Table 7: Beta-adrenergic receptor blockers

Generic name	Trade name	Pharmacologic and clinical features
Acebutolol	Sectral	Cardioselective; possesses intrinsic sympathomimetic activity
Atenolol	Tenormin	Cardioselective; given once daily
Metoprolol	Lopressor	Cardioselective; may be given once daily
Nadolol	Corgard	Nonselective; given once daily
Pindolol	Visken	Nonselective; possesses intrinsic sympathomimetic activity
Propranolol	Inderal	Nonselective; available longest; may be given once daily; approved for angina pectoris, migraine
Timolol	Blocadren	Nonselective; approved for glaucoma and prevention of myocardial reinfarction
Labetalol	Normodyne; trandate	Nonselective; α-β-blockade
Carvedilol	Coreg	Once daily; generic twice daily (also probable endothelial action)
Bistolic	Nebibolol	Once daily

Table 8: Postulated antihypertensive mechanism of β-blocking drugs

- Reduced cardiac output
- Readjustments of blood flow
- Preferential responses of component regional circulations
- Total body autoregulation ("reverse Guyton")
- Reduced vessel distention ("reverse Bayliss")
- Readjusted baroreceptors
- Altered high-pressure cardiovascular reflexes
- Reduced plasma rennin activity
- Altered catecholamine biosynthesis
- Inhibited presynaptic β-receptors
- Central action of an active metabolite of the agent

Calcium Antagonists

Calcium antagonists act by inhibition of availability of the calcium ions cardiac and vascular smooth muscle cells that serve to inhibit myocytic contractility and reducing heart rate (particularly, the dihydropyridines).

All calcium antagonists reduce arterial pressure without expanding intravascular volume, explaining why they may be used as a monotherapeutic agent without a diuretic. The natriuretic effect of the calcium antagonists is explained, in part, due to their ability to inhibit renal sodium reabsorption through the sodium-for-calcium exchange mechanism. The foregoing statement should not be construed to relate to the development of pedal edema with higher doses of the calcium antagonists to renal sodium and fluid retention. Another common side effect of the calcium antagonists is gingival hyperplasia.

Calcium antagonists are of particular value for initial treatment when there is need for immediate pressure reduction, for promotion of coronary vasodilation in patients with angina pectoris unresponsive to beta-adrenergic receptor blockade; when an ACE inhibitor or ARB is contraindicated due to occlusive bilateral renal arterial disease or unilateral arterial disease of a solitary kidney. The authors have found that rather than increasing the dose of one calcium antagonist to control pressure better, the addition of a second calcium antagonist may obviate development of peripheral edema. Finally, the calcium antagonists have been formulated with ACE inhibitors and ARBs and more recently with a third agent, the diuretic.

Angiotensin Converting Enzyme (ACE) Inhibitors

The ACE inhibitors are also effective for monotherapy with all degrees of severity, including refractory hypertension, severe cardiac involvement (including LVH, angina pectoris, cardiac failure, and for secondary prevention and death after myocardial infarction), and for prevention of end-stage renal disease (particularly in patients with diabetes mellitus). These agents work by inhibiting the ACE, thereby, reducing the generation of angiotensin II as well as the inactivation of the very potent vasodilator bradykinin (which may explain another antihypertensive action).

Hemodynamically, the ACE inhibitors reduce arterial pressure though arteriolar dilation and consequent reduction of total peripheral resistance without associated increased cardiac output, reflexively. Renal blood flow increases through reduction of pre- and postglomerular arteriolar resistances and, thereby decreases glomerular hydrostatic pressure. Additionally, it inhibits the mitogenic effects of angiotensin II and reduces cardiac remodeling and apoptosis, thereby explaining its usefulness in preventing and/or reducing severity of cardiac failure.

A number of ACE inhibitors are available and their antihypertensive effects are enhanced by diuretics which are frequently provided when coformulated. It is worthwhile to emphasize the potential of this combination to augment pressure reduction and postural hypotension. Their side effects, notably, are few.

Angiotensin II Receptor Blockers (ARB) or Antagonists

These agents act by inhibiting the type 1 angiotensin II receptors' action in vascular smooth muscle, heart, kidney, adrenal cortex, brain and other organs. The ARBs, like the ACE inhibitors, have similar clinical indications and have been useful, particularly in those patients who cannot use the ACE inhibitor due to side effects (most notably, angioneurotic edema and the cough produced by ACE inhibition). Controversy currently, exists as to whether there are quantitative or synergistic clinical benefits of the ARB when used concurrently with the ACE inhibitor. A number of ARBs are available clinically and are active orally. As with the ACE inhibitors, the action of the ARBs are markedly enhanced when given with a diuretic and several compounds are available when coformulated. The antihypertensive and hemodynamic effects of these compounds are very similar to the ACE inhibitors.

Renin Inhibitors

At present, there is only one renin inhibitor available for clinical use (aliskiren). The agent directly inhibits the rate-limiting biochemical step in angiotensin II generation by impairing the action of renin that leads to the subsequent conversion of angiotensin I. This agent has been shown to be useful in patients with essential hypertension, with renal protection in patients with proteinuria, diabetes and cardiac failure.

Others

Although some of the subgroups of adrenergic inhibitors still have some clinical pertinence today, they are primarily of historical importance. Ganglion blockers were the mainstay of treatment of severe hypertension many years ago; they are now used rarely, usually with intravenous formulations for immediate and controlled hypotension in certain severe hypertensive emergencies or for control of arterial pressure during certain operative (e.g. neurosurgical) procedures.

Rauwolfia alkaloids are a group of drugs with varying potency to deplete brain, adrenal glands and postganglionic sympathetic nerve ending of their natural biogenic amines (catecholamines and serotonin). These agents were used with great frequency in the early years of antihypertensive drug therapy and are still, commonly used in many areas around the world. When given by injection (e.g. reserpine 1.0–5.0 mg) they have been useful in treating hypertensive emergencies and the cardiovascular related symptoms of thyrotoxicosis.

Guanethidine and guanadrel are postganglionic neuronal depletors. The former agent has been available for 50 years for treatment of patients with severe hypertension. It has a prolonged delay (48–72 hours) in action; and, once achieved, its hypotensive action may persist for days or weeks (and as much as one month) after discontinuance. When these agents are discontinued, the arterial pressure may fall precipitously.

Centrally Acting Postsympathetic Alpha-adrenergic Agonists

Methyldopa has been available for clinical use for almost 50 years and is still used widely, throughout the world. Present concept of its hypotensive action is by false neurotransmission that stimulates postsynaptic alpha-adrenergic receptor sites in brain, thereby, reducing adrenergic outflow from brain medullary centers to the cardiovascular system and kidney. As a result, arteriolar resistance falls, and a reduced venous resistance results in reduced venous return to the heart although cardiac output and renal blood flow are not reduced as much as the foregoing described sympatholytics.

Clonidine, although chemically different from methyldopa, shares certain pharmacological actions. They reduce arterial pressure through a decreased vascular resistance as a result of central stimulation of alpha-adrenergic receptor sites in medullary centers and reducing brain adrenergic outflow. The more recent availability of the clonidine patch has apparently reduced the occurrence of the rebound phenomena.

Postsynaptic (Peripheral) Alpha-receptor Antagonists

When presynaptic alpha-2 receptors are stimulated further release of norepinephrine from the nerve ending into the synaptic cleft is inhibited, making alpha-1 receptor blockers (doxazosin, prazosin, terazosin) not to prevent alpha-2 receptor stimulation. These agents reduce arterial pressure as a result of a decreased vascular resistance (without associated increased heart rate, cardiac output or myocardial contractility). As a result, they may produce postural hypotension (often after the first dose administered), strongly suggesting that this first dose should be the lowest dose available and cautionary advice to the patient (most frequently the man with prostatic hyperplasia) who takes this medication at bedtime.

Smooth Muscle Vasodilators

These agents (hydralazine and minoxidil) have been used with a resurgence associated with the introduction of the beta-blockers and with varying success rates in patients with cardiac failure. They reduce blood pressure associated with a fall in vascular resistance and reflexive stimulation of the heart by increasing heart rate, myocardial contractility and increased myocardial oxygen demand.

❏ TREATMENT ALGORITHMS ADVOCATED OVER THE YEARS

Stepped Care Approach

The historical background to this approach dates back to the multicenter and placebo-controlled Veterans Administration Cooperative Study, which was the first study to demonstrate the efficacy and safety of an antihypertensive drug therapy. This concept of introducing therapy with the simplest agent and later, with other agents that acted additively or synergistically, was employed by other specialties in medicine for its simple rationale and effectiveness.

Individualized Stepped-care Approach (Table 9)

Later, as other agents became available which, by practicality, they were used by adding to the diuretic (if not initially), and with the addition of other agents. This therapeutic concept was presented in the later JNC recommendations and a very practical approach to the management of the hypertensive patient was practicable. Thus, a nonpharmacological or lifestyle management approach to treatment was advocated for all patients (even if normotensive, but with a strong family history of hypertension, "high normal" blood pressures, and more recently with those patients with prehypertension). If this nondrug treatment

Table 9: Individualized stepped-care approach to antihypertensive therapy	
Nonpharmacologic approaches (baseline) initial selection	
Adequate response	Inadequate response
Increase dosage	Add second agent
Substitute another agent	Add third (or more) agents

was found to be adequate, the patient would be followed carefully with periodic monitoring of blood pressure. If, however, this approach was found to be of an inadequate response, introduction of a pharmacological agent was instituted. Usually, this would be a diuretic, although with the introduction of one of the newer antihypertensive agents (calcium antagonist, ACE inhibitor, ARB, and more recently, the renin inhibitor). If a second or third agent were indicated, this might be done first with the addition of the drug or, later, with a combination drug. Experience has taught us that following this approach upward of 85% of patients would respond to this approach.

❑ SUGGESTED READINGS

Chobanian AV, Bakris GL, Black HR, et al. Seventh report of Joint National Committee on prevention, detection, evaluation, and treatment of high blood pressure (JNC-7). JAMA. 2003;289:2560-72.

Frohlich ED, Gifford R, Horan M, et al. Nonpharmacologic approaches to the control of high blood pressure: report of the subcommittee on non-pharmacologic therapy of the Joint national committee on detection, evaluation, and treatment of high blood pressure. Hypertension. 1986;8:444-67.

Frohlich ED, Sasaki O, Chien Y, et al. Changes in cardiovascular mass, left ventricular pumping ability, and aortic distensibility after calcium antagonist in Wistar-Kyoto and spontaneously hypertensive rats. J Hypertens. 1992;10:1369-78.

Frohlich ED. Promise of prevention and reversal of target organ involvement in hypertension. Journal of Renin Angiotensin Aldosterone System. 2001;2:S4-9.

Frohlich ED. Role of beta-adrenergic receptor blocking agents in hypertensive diseases: personal thoughts as the controversy persists. Ther Adv Cardiovasc Dis. 2009;3:455-64.

Multicenter Diuretic Cooperative Study Group. Multiclinic comparison of amiloride, hydrochlorothiazide and hydrochlorothiazide plus amiloride in essential hypertension. Arch Intern Med. 1981;141:482-6.

Susic D, Varagic J, Ahn J, et al. Crosslink breakers: a new approach to cardiovascular therapy. Current opinion in cardiology. 2004;19:336-40.

Veterans Administration Cooperative Study Group on Antihypertensive Agents. Effects of treatment on morbidity in hypertension. II. Results in patients with diastolic blood pressure averaging 90 through 114 mm Hg. JAMA. 1970;213:1143-52.

6.2 Peripheral Vascular and Cerebrovascular Disease

❑ INTRODUCTION

Peripheral vascular disease (PVD) includes myriad pathophysiological syndromes that affect arterial, venous and lymphatic circulation, essentially all vascular disease that alters end-organ perfusion. In contrast, peripheral arterial disease (PAD) involves disorders that jeopardize blood supply to the upper or lower extremities. The most common cause of PAD is atherosclerosis, although it less commonly results from embolism, vasculitis, fibromuscular dysplasia (FMD), entrapment, or thrombosis.

❑ PERIPHERAL ARTERIAL DISEASE

The prevalence of PAD based on ankle-brachial index (ABI) varies from 3 to 11% in adults who are more than 40 years old and increases to 14.5–20% in the elderly (Fig. 1) and 12.6–30.9% in patients with risk factors for CAD. Prevalence is even higher (up to 40%) in patients with established vascular disease other than PAD.

Patients often underreport symptoms that may give a clue to the diagnosis of PAD. American College of Cardiology/American Heart Association (ACC/AHA) guidelines strongly recommend a comprehensive review of systems with a focus on the vascular system in individuals at risk or with symptoms suggestive of underlying vascular disease. Table 10 represents the key points in review and physical examination of the vascular system.

The major risk factors for PAD are the same as for coronary artery disease (CAD) and include age more than or equal to 50 years (striking evidence, see

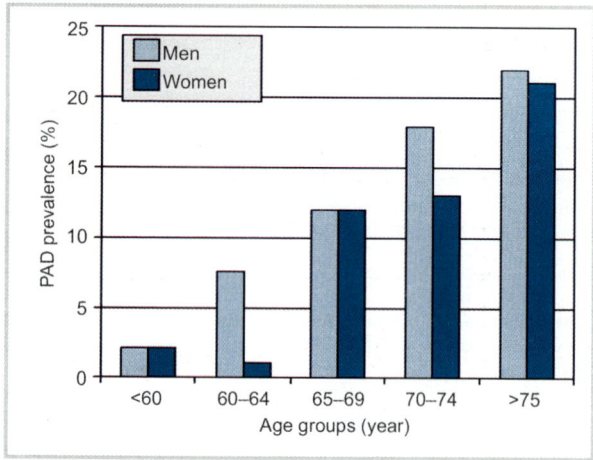

FIGURE 1: Prevalence of large-vessel peripheral arterial disease (PAD) by age. (*Source:* Modified from Criqui MH, Fronek A, Barrett-Connor E, et al. The prevalence of peripheral arterial disease in a defined population. Circulation. 1985;71:510-5)

Table 10: Focused review of system and vascular examination	
Review of system	
Exertional lower extremity pain or impairment	• Can be described as: fatigue, aching, numbness or pain • Primary site: buttock, thigh, calf or foot
Nonhealing ulcer	(See critical limb ischemia section)
Postprandial abdominal pain	• Provoked by eating and is associated with weight loss (mesenteric ischemia)
Physical examination	
Blood pressure	• In both arms and notation of asymmetry. Difference >20 mm Hg indicates innominate, subclavian or axillary disease

Contd...

Contd...

Table 10: Focused review of system and vascular examination

Palpation of carotid pulse and notation of the carotid upstroke and presence of bruit	• Carotid bruit should be described as systolic, diastolic or both • Sensitivity of bruits is low in detecting high-grade lesion in asymptomatic patients (56%) and slightly better in symptomatic patients (63%) • Carotid bruit is a poor predictor of underlying carotid stenosis and risk of stroke in asymptomatic patients • Carotid bruit is a prognostic indicator of cardiovascular death and myocardial infarction
Auscultation of flank and abdomen	• Prevalence of bruit in general population: 6.5–27% • Sensitivity for detection of renal artery stenosis: 39–77.7%
Allen test	• False-positive result with overextension of the wrist
Abdominal palpation	• Sensitivity for detection of AAA is 33%. Even lower in obese patients
Physical examination of lower-extremity PAD	
Inspection	• Gangrene, ulcers with necrotic base involving distal foot • Distal hair loss, atrophic skin changes and foot discoloration (All low yield for clinical diagnosis of PAD)
Palpation of pulses	• Brachial, radial, ulnar, femoral, popliteal, dorsalis pedis and posterior tibial site • Pulse intensity should be recorded numerically: 0 = absent; 1 = diminished; 2 = normal; 3 = bounding • Abnormal pedal pulses have high specificity for presence of PAD • In a small number of normal individuals, dorsalis pedis pulse is absent (debranching from anterior tibial at the ankle) • Patients with isolated occlusion of internal iliac may present with impotency, buttock claudication • (Leriche's syndrome) and sometimes normal femoral and pedal pulses • Absent of pedal pulses: physicians tend to overdiagnose PAD
Buerger test	• Elevate the supine patient's foot perpendicular to the horizontal plane, which will cause foot pallor in those with vascular disease. Then, by slowly lowering the limb, record the angle at which a reddish hue returns (resolution of pallor below the horizontal plane is considered abnormal) • Low sensitivity
Capillary refill test	• Digital pressure to the plantar skin of the distal great toe for 5 minutes, local pallor >5 seconds is regarded as delayed refill • Low yield for diagnosis of PAD
Auscultation of both femoral arteries	• For detection of bruits

(Abbreviations: AAA: Abdominal aortic aneurysm; PAD: Peripheral arterial disease)

epidemiology section), male gender, race, smoking, diabetes mellitus, dyslipidemia and hypertension (HTN). Odds ratios for the major risk factors of PAD are depicted in Figure 2.

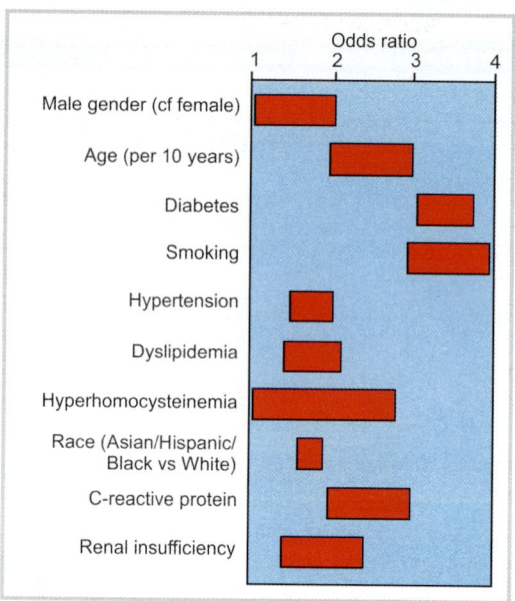

FIGURE 2: Approximate odds ratio for risk factors for symptomatic peripheral arterial disease. (*Source:* Modified from Norgren L, Hiatt WR, Dormandy JA, et al. Inter-Society Consensus for the Management of Peripheral Arterial Disease (TASC II). J Vasc Surg. 2007;45:S5-67)

Clinical Presentation and Natural History

Clinical presentation, natural history and outcome of patients with PAD are summarized in Flowchart 1.

The term "claudication" is derived from the Latin word *caudicatio*, translated as "to limp," in vascular medicine it is defined as fatigue, discomfort or pain that occurs in specific limb muscle groups during exertion due to exercise-induced ischemia. Most patients with PAD are asymptomatic (defined as absence of claudication), and among those with leg symptoms, the majority have atypical symptoms; and only less than 20% of patients present with classic intermittent claudication (IC).

Critical limb ischemia (CLI) is defined as chronic ischemic rest pain (more than two weeks), ulcers or gangrene attributed to objectively proven PAD (abnormal ABI <0.5; toe pressure <50 mm Hg; transcutaneous O_2 <30 mm Hg). The clinical severity of ischemia can be classified according to either Fontaine or Rutherford classifications (Table 11). Ischemic foot ulcers are painful (not so in diabetic neuropathy), cold, pale and have irregular margins (Figs 3A and B). Acute limb ischemia (ALI) is defined as any sudden decrease in limb perfusion causing a potential threat to limb viability. Causes for ALI include native thrombosis, embolism primarily from cardiac source and graft thrombosis. Physical findings of ALI may include the 5 Ps: Pain, Pulselessness, Pallor, Paresthesia and Paralysis (poor prognostic sign).

FLOWCHART 1: Fate of claudication over 5 years

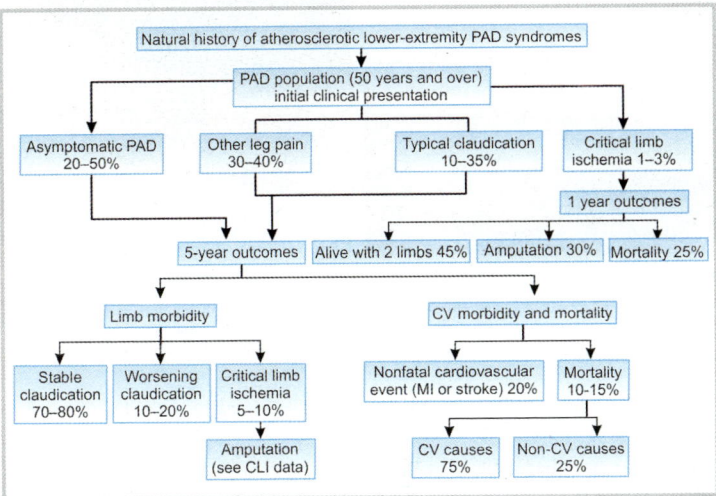

(Abbreviations: CLI: Chronic limb ischemia; CV: Cardiovascular; MI: Myocardial infarction; PAD: Peripheral arterial disease). (*Source:* Reproduced with permission from Hirsch AT, Haskal ZJ, Hertzer NR, et al. ACC/AHA 2005 guidelines for the management of patients with peripheral arterial disease (lower extremity, renal, mesenteric, and abdominal aortic): executive summary a collaborative report from the American Association for Vascular Surgery/Society for Vascular Surgery, Society for Cardiovascular Angiography and Interventions, Society for Vascular Medicine and Biology, Society of Interventional Radiology, and the ACC/AHA Task Force on Practice Guidelines (Writing Committee to Develop Guidelines for the Management of Patients with Peripheral Arterial Disease) endorsed by the American Association of Cardiovascular and Pulmonary Rehabilitation; National Heart, Lung, and Blood Institute; Society for Vascular Nursing; TransAtlantic Inter-Society Consensus; and Vascular Disease Foundation. J Am Coll Cardiol. 2006;47:1239-312, and Weitz JI, Byrne J, Clagett GP, et al. Diagnosis and treatment of chronic arterial insufficiency of the lower extremities: a critical review. Circulation. 1996;94:3026-49)

Table 11: Classification of peripheral arterial disease (PAD): Fontaine's stages and Rutherford's categories

Fontaine		Rutherford		
Stage	Clinical	Grade	Category	Clinical
I	Asymptomatic	0	0	Asymptomatic
IIa	Mild claudication	0	1	Mild claudication
IIb	Moderate-to-severe claudication	I	2	Moderate claudication
		I	3	Severe claudication
III	Ischemic rest pain	II	4	Ischemic rest pain
IV	Ulceration or gangrene	III	5	Minor tissue loss
		III	6	Major tissue loss

(*Source:* Reproduced with permission from Norgren L, Hiatt WR, Dormandy JA, et al. Inter-Society Consensus for the Management of Peripheral Arterial Disease (TASC II). J Vasc Surg. 2007;45:S5-67)

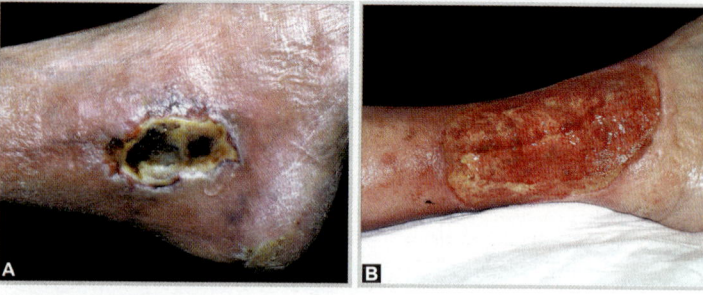

FIGURES 3A AND B: (A) Ischemic ulcers are usually painful, cold and pale with irregular margins; (B) Ulcers secondary to venous insufficiency are usually painless, with regular margins located in medial malleolar (Photographs Courtesy of Dr Jeffrey Niezgoda)

Screening for PAD

Despite the fact that patients with asymptomatic PAD have a threefold to six fold increased risk of death from CAD and CVD, there is no general agreement among major professional organizations. However, based on the Inter-Society Consensus for PAD (TASC II), ACC/AHA guidelines and American Diabetes Association (ADA) guidelines, screening ABI is strongly recommended for the following populations:

- Leg symptoms suggestive of IC or rest ischemia
- All patients with abnormal pedal pulses
- All patients between 50 years and 69 years of age who have a cardiovascular risk factor (particularly diabetes and smoking)
- All patients age more than or equal to 70 years regardless of risk factor status
- All patients with Framingham score 10–20%
- All patients with diabetes and age less than 50 years, if they have at least one additional cardiovascular risk factor
- Known CAD, carotid artery stenosis (CAS) or renal artery stenosis (RAS).

Diagnosis

Ankle–brachial Index

The ankle–brachial index (ABI) is a simple, noninvasive test that is used for both screening and establishing diagnosis of PAD with a high degree of accuracy. It is simply calculated by dividing the highest ankle pressure (mm Hg) by highest arm pressure (mm Hg) in both limbs. In normal individuals without PAD, ankle systolic pressure is usually 10–15 mm Hg higher than arm brachial pressure due to the effect of pulse wave reflection. A truly normal ABI is greater than 1.10 and abnormal ABI is defined as less than or equal to 0.90.

In patients with diabetes or renal insufficiency, measured ABI level could be falsely high (>1.40), mainly due to calcified vessels. In this situation toe–brachial index (TBI) can be measured. The abnormal value for TBI is less than 0.70 because toe pressure is approximately 30 mm Hg less than ankle pressure. Exercise testing is recommended in patients with high pretest probability of PAD and a normal resting ABI. A decrease in ABI of 15–20% from baseline would be diagnostic for PAD.

Other Noninvasive Vascular Modalities

- Duplex ultrasound (DUS): Doppler velocity consists of three waveforms: a systolic peak, early diastole reversal flow and forward flow in late diastole. In severe PAD, there is a decrease in peak systolic flow, absence of reversal flow and increase of flow in late diastole
- Computed tomography angiogram (CTA): The primary limitation is in the evaluation of severely calcified lesions. Other limitations include the use of a relatively large amount of IV contrast
- Magnetic resonance angiogram (MRA): It cannot be used in patients with contraindication to magnetic resonance (e.g. those with defibrillator, pacemaker, or metallic stents, coils and clips). Finally, the US Food and Drug Administration (FDA) has issued a warning on the use of gadolinium for patients with renal impairment because it has been linked to the development of nephrogenic systemic fibrosis, also known as nephrogenic fibrosing dermopathy
- Digital subtraction angiography (DSA): It is considered the "gold standard" imaging test. A direct assessment of pressure gradient (more than 5–10 mm Hg) across the stenotic lesion will provide more information regarding the need for intervention. In patients with ALI, angiography remains the procedure of choice for intra-arterial lytic therapy. On the other hand, angiography is an invasive procedure and carries certain risk (e.g. mortality, dissection, bleeding, renal failure), and it should only be performed in appropriate clinical scenarios.

Management

A summary of recommended interventions with supporting data is depicted in Table 12. The PAD is considered a CAD "risk equivalent," therefore aggressive risk-factor modification is strongly recommended.

Both ACC/AHA and TASC II strongly recommend supervised exercise as initial treatment for all patients with PAD (Class I, Level of evidence: A). A review of 22 randomized controlled trials with 1,200 participants with PAD showed that an exercise program significantly improves maximal pain-free walking time and distance irrespective of symptoms (Table 13).

Table 12: Summary of medical management for PAD	
Management of athero-sclerotic risk factors	**Recommendation/Comment**
Smoking cessation	- Physician advice - Nicotine replacement therapy - Bupropion - Improvement of leg symptoms and preventing systemic complication - Associated with significant reduction in all-cause mortality, rate of amputation, progression of PAD and graft failure
Lipid-lowering therapy (statins)	- Dietary modification - LDL goal <70 mg/dL - Benefit beyond LDL level
Blood pressure lowering drugs	- BP goal <140/90 mm Hg, or <130/80 mm Hg in patients with DM and CKD - Benefit of ACE-I beyond antihypertensive effect - Consider using beta-blockers in patients with PAD and CAD (No data supporting worsening of symptoms with its use)

Contd...

Contd...

Table 12: Summary of medical management for PAD

Management of atherosclerotic risk factors	Recommendation/Comment
Antithrombotic therapy	• Aspirin (81–325 mg) as first choice, consider clopidogrel (75 mg) as suitable alternative • No benefit with combination of aspirin and clopidogrel unless for patients undergoing stenting • Reduce risk of ischemic stroke, myocardial infarction or vascular death • Warfarin: No proven benefit except for IC
Management of symptoms	
Exercise therapy	• Strong data based on randomized controlled trials • Consider supervised exercise therapy three times per week for 30–60 minutes as initial treatment for all patients with PAD • Maintain high physical activity during daily life
Cilostazol	• Use in all patients with life-limiting intermittent claudication • Improves symptoms and increases pain-free walking distance • Avoid in patients with congestive heart failure* • Increased plasma concentration with concomitant use of CYP450 3A4 inhibitors • Proven benefit over pentoxifylline
Pentoxifylline	• The benefit is marginal • Tachyphylaxis with long-term use • Not commonly used in US

*As noted by a US Federal Drug Administration black box warning. Abbreviations: ACE-I: Angiotensin-converting enzyme inhibitor; CAD: Coronary artery disease; CKD: Chronic kidney disease; DM: Diabetes mellitus; IC: Intermittent claudication; LDL: Low-density lipoprotein; MI: Myocardial infarction; PAD: Peripheral arterial disease

Table 13: Exercise regime compared to usual care

Outcome or subgroup title	No. of studies	No. of participants	Mean difference (95% CI)
Maximum walking distance (m)	6	391	113.20 (94.96–131.43)
Pain-free walking distance (m)	6	322	82.19 (71.73–92.65)
Maximal walking time (min)	7	255	5.12 (4.51–5.72)
Pain-free walking time (min)	3	150	2.91 (2.51–3.31)

(Abbreviations: CI: Confidence interval; m: Meter; min: Minute). (*Source:* Watson L, Ellis B, Leng GC. Exercise for intermittent claudication. Cochrane Database Syst Rev. 2008;CD000990)

Cilostazol (Pletal) is a phosphodiesterase type-3 inhibitor with vasodilator and mild antiplatelet properties. The superiority of cilostazol in increasing maximal and pain-free walking distance is established in randomized trials. Current guidelines recommend the use of cilostazol 100 mg twice daily in all patients with PAD and lifestyle-limiting claudication in the absence of heart failure to improve symptoms and walking distance. Pentoxifylline (Trental) is a methylxanthine derivative with hemorheological properties. Available data indicate that the benefit of pentoxifylline is marginal and is not well established. The ACC/AHA guidelines assign a class IIb indication for the use of pentoxifylline (400 mg twice daily) as a second-line alternative to cilostazol.

Revascularization

There are three clear indications for revascularization in patients with PAD:
1. Life-limiting claudication despite aggressive risk-factor modification, supervised exercise program and trial of cilostazol.
2. Critical limb ischemia and limb salvage, and
3. Acute limb ischemia.

Endovascular interventions for revascularization include angioplasty, stent, stent grafts, plaque-debulking procedure, thrombolysis and percutaneous thrombectomy. Surgical options include autogenous or synthetic bypass, endarterectomy or an intraoperative hybrid procedure.

Endovascular therapy offers several distinct advantages over open-surgical intervention for selected lesions. Lower morbidity and mortality rates, shorter hospital stay and patient preference, along with remarkable technological advances (especially stents), have all resulted in the selection of endovascular therapy as a first-line invasive strategy in suitable lesions. In addition, use of endovascular therapy generally does not preclude or alter subsequent surgery, if needed. Surgical intervention is reserved for lesions that are not amenable to percutaneous intervention. As a general rule, a bilateral surgical bypass from the infrarenal abdominal aorta to both femoral arteries is usually recommended for diffuse disease throughout the aortoiliac system. While aortobifemoral bypass sustains the highest patency rate, patency rate is significantly lower in infrainguinal and post-extra-anatomic bypasses.

Once the diagnosis of acute arterial occlusion has been made, immediate administration of IV unfractionated heparin (UH) followed by continuous UH infusion is recommended per TASC II. Time is crucial; the decision to administer UH is based on the clinical evaluation and should not be delayed awaiting results of further diagnostic procedures. Following the initiation of heparin, treatment varies depending on the viability of the limb. Patients with ALI should undergo intervention to restore flow. Options include surgery and catheter-directed thrombolysis (CDT) therapy. TASC II recommends CDT as the method of choice in patients in whom the degree of severity allows this more time-consuming approach (Category I: viable; Category IIa: marginally threatened), whereas a surgical approach is recommended in patients with profound limb ischemia (Category IIb: immediately threatened).

❑ CAROTID ARTERY DISEASE

Stroke is the third-leading cause of death just after heart disease and cancer. The majority of strokes are caused by embolic events due to atheroemboli from the carotid artery, the ascending aorta and arch vessels, or cardiac thromboembolism from the left atrium or ventricle. It is estimated that carotid artery stenosis (CAS) is responsible for 15–20% of all strokes, depending upon population studied.

Atherosclerosis is the most common disease of the carotid circulation. Other conditions associated with cerebral ischemia and infarction include diseases of the aorta (dissection, aneurysm and aortitis), arteritis, FMD, dissection, primary vascular tumors, trauma and complication of head and neck cancer. Risk factors for CAS are the same as risk factors in other vascular beds and carries the same risk for future cardiac events as the presence of coronary heart disease (CHD); thus, it is classified as CHD equivalent.

Screening

Currently, there is no consensus to support routine screening of asymptomatic patients with noninvasive modalities, except for patients undergoing coronary artery bypass graft (CABG). A carotid DUS is recommended prior to CABG in asymptomatic patients age more than 65 years or with left main coronary stenosis, PAD, history of smoking, TIA or stroke, or carotid bruits. Patients with ischemic stroke and those with both CAS and a high CHD risk factor based on the Framingham algorithm (>20%) should undergo noninvasive evaluation to rule out significant underlying obstructive epicardial disease.

Diagnosis

Noninvasive Testing

DUS, computed tomography angiography and magnetic resonance angiography are recommended by ACC/AHA guidelines as Class I (Level of evidence: A) for the initial evaluation of carotid artery disease in patients presenting with acute stroke. DUS is considered as the first choice in most centers. In asymptomatic patients, MRA or CTA could be considered, if results from DUS are inconclusive.

Conventional Angiogram

Cerebral angiogram is considered the gold standard for imaging carotid arteries. Development of digital subtraction angiography reduces the dose of contrast and shortens the length of the procedure. On the other hand, it carries a higher cost and estimated risk of neurological complication, and death is reported as 4% and 1%, respectively. With the advance of noninvasive modalities, cerebral angiogram is rarely used as the first diagnostic approach nowadays.

Management

Treatment of CAS includes risk-factor modification and medical treatment alone, medical treatment plus carotid endarterectomy (CEA) or medical treatment plus carotid stenting.

Antiplatelets, Dipyridamole, and Warfarin

Initial therapy for all patients with noncardiac ischemic stroke should involve aspirin (ASA 50–325 mg) or the combination of ASA and extended-release dipyridamole, or clopidogrel monotherapy (Class I, Level of evidence: A). Asymptomatic patients with one or more atherosclerosis risk factors should be started on antiplatelets as well. In symptomatic patients, ASA results in relative risk reduction of 16% for fatal stroke and 28% for nonfatal stroke, while extended-release dipyridamole plus ASA is shown to be superior to ASA alone for secondary prevention in patients with minor stroke or TIA. Clopidogrel has largely replaced ticlopidine due to its superior safety profile and once-daily dosing. The combination of ASA and clopidogrel carries no additional benefit for secondary prevention of stroke. Regarding warfarin, there is no data suggesting benefit over ASA in patients with noncardioembolic stroke.

Carotid Endarterectomy

In patients with symptomatic moderate-to-severe CAS, carotid endarterectomy (CEA) is recommended for prevention of future ipsilateral ischemic stroke. The

AHA recommends CEA in symptomatic and asymptomatic patients with stenosis of 50–99% and 60–99%, if the risk of perioperative stroke or death is less than 6% and 3% (life expectancy at least 5 years), respectively.

Carotid Stenting

New advances in self-expanding stents and the recent adoption of embolic protection devices (EPDs), in addition to patient preference, resulted in carotid artery stenting becoming an emerging and less-invasive revascularization method to prevent stroke, especially in patients at high risk for surgery. Based on the 1-year result of SAPPHIRE trial, the US FDA granted approval for the stent and protection devices used in SAPPHIRE, but only for symptomatic patients with high risk features for CEA.

❏ RENAL ARTERY STENOSIS

Renal artery stenosis (RAS) is the most common cause of secondary hypertension and is described as a narrowing of one or both renal arteries or their branches. Atherosclerosis involving the ostium and proximal third of the main renal artery and perirenal aorta accounts for 90% of cases of RAS and is called atherosclerotic renal artery stenosis (ARAS). Less frequently, RAS is caused by FMD. ARAS and FMD have distinct presentation and clinical consequences (Table 14).

Patients with ARAS have a markedly lower rate of survival, partly due to their extensive vascular comorbidities. Progression of stenosis is reported in one-third to one-half of ARAS cases, primarily in patients with bilateral RAS, with occlusion occurring in 10–15% of cases. In contrast, the likelihood of progression is lower in patients with FMD, and occlusion is rare. The RAS is also associated with loss of renal size and function.

Screening and Diagnostic Tests

Clinical situations suggesting high likelihood of RAS include:
- Onset of hypertension before age 30 or after 55 years
- Accelerated, resistant or malignant HTN
- Development of new azotemia or worsening renal function after administration of an angiotensin-converting enzyme (ACE) inhibitor or angiotensin receptor blocking (ARB) agent
- Unexplained atrophic kidney or asymmetry in renal sizes is more than 1.5 cm
- Recurrent episodes of acute (flash) pulmonary edema, in the presence of normal left ventricular ejection fraction
- Refractory angina or unexplained congestive heart failure.

Table 14: Characteristics of atherosclerotic renal artery stenosis and fibromuscular dysplasia		
Variable	**Atherosclerosis**	**Fibromuscular dysplasia**
Age at presentation	Older (>50 years)	Usually young (<40 years)
Sex	Either	Usually female
Lesion location	Ostial, proximal, middle*	Middle or distal
Blood pressure response to revascularization	Unclear	Normotension in most patients

*Locations are listed in descending order of likelihood (*Source*: Dworkin LD, Cooper CJ, et al. Clinical practice. Renal-artery stenosis. N Engl J Med. 2009;361:1972-8)

Current ACC/AHA guidelines recommend screening for renovascular disease only if finding of significant stenosis would change the management (i.e. a corrective procedure will be undertaken). Once RAS is suspected, it is confirmed by imaging. Captopril renal scintigraphy, selective renal vein renin measurements, and plasma renin activity are not useful screening tools for RAS. Digital subtraction angiography remains the gold standard imaging modality for diagnosis of RAS. Noninvasive imaging modalities have been introduced for detection of RAS. DUS provides a functional assessment of the severity of stenosis, and higher velocity correlates with a greater stenosis.

Medical Management

Pharmacologic therapy for HTN in patients with ARAS and FMD should follow the Joint National Committee (JNC7) guidelines. Use of renin–angiotensin–aldosterone inhibitors can be associated with acute renal failure, especially in patients with bilateral RAS, advanced kidney disease or high-grade stenosis in one kidney. The probability of the latter complication is low and, in most cases, reversible with discontinuation of treatment. ACE inhibitors also have shown mortality benefit in a large cohort study; therefore, the presence of RAS is not a contraindication for the use of renin-angiotensin inhibitors if patients are carefully monitored.

Revascularization

Angioplasty and/or stenting have become the procedure of choice over surgical approach for ARAS revascularization. In patients with FMD, when the lesion meets clinical criteria for intervention, angioplasty is the procedure of choice as it is associated with low mortality and morbidity. The use of stents in patients with FMD has been reserved as a "bailout" procedure for suboptimal results when dissection occurs after PTA. In contrast, balloon angioplasty alone has resulted in suboptimal results in patients with ARAS and ostial renal lesion compared to stenting, with a higher rate of restenosis in long-term followup. Therefore, renal stent placement is indicated for ostial ARAS lesions that meet the clinical criteria for intervention.

Based on ACC/AHA guidelines on RAS, percutaneous intervention should be considered for the following scenarios only when medical management fails:
- Class I: Unexplained congestive heart failure of recurrent pulmonary edema
- Class IIa: Accelerated, malignant or resistant HTN HTN with medication intolerance or unilateral small kidney
  Chronic renal failure with bilateral RAS or unilateral solitary kidney
  Recurrent unstable angina
- Class IIb: Asymptomatic bilateral or solitary viable kidney with severe RAS
  Asymptomatic unilateral significant RAS in a viable kidney
  RAS and chronic renal failure when unilateral stenosis is present.

❏ SUBCLAVIAN ARTERY STENOSIS

Atherosclerosis is the most common cause of subclavian artery stenosis (SAS). Other causes should be included in differential diagnosis such as vasculitis, congenital malformations (e.g. following surgical repair of aortic coarctation), thoracic outlet syndrome, or sequel from radiation. Hemodynamically significant SAS proximal to ipsilateral vertebral artery results in lower pressure in distal subclavian artery. As a consequence, with repetitive arm movement, reversal of flow occurs from the contralateral vertebral artery and brain stem, resulting in neurological symptoms (e.g. drop attacks, dizziness). This is referred to as "subclavian steal syndrome."

Physical examination in patients with SAS typically reveals a significant difference in brachial systolic blood pressure (>15 mm Hg differential) between the affected and normal arms and lower amplitude with delayed pulse in the affected arm. While DUS, MRA and CTA are postulated as diagnostic tools for detection of hemodynamically significant SAS, contrast angiography is considered the gold standard and "confirmatory" procedure of choice in this population. The surgical approach for treatment of symptomatic SAS has shown reasonable long term patency but, among other complications, carries a mortality rate of about 2% and a stroke rate of about 3%. Percutaneous intervention with stenting has shown high procedural success rate with good long-term patency rate and lower rate of major complications; therefore, it should be considered as the primary treatment in patients who need revascularization for SAS.

❏ MESENTERIC ISCHEMIA

Mesenteric ischemia is caused by reduction in intestinal blood flow due to occlusion, vasospasm or hypoperfusion of mesenteric vasculature. Acute mesenteric ischemia (AMI) most commonly occurs due to emboli or thrombosis of mesenteric arteries and could result in a mortality rate exceeding 60%. Risk factors for developing AMI include advanced age, atherosclerosis, cardiac arrhythmias, low cardiac output state, valvular heart disease, recent myocardial infarction, and intraabdominal malignancy.

Diagnosis of AMI depends on strong clinical suspicion, especially in patients with risk factors. Classically, patients present with rapid onset of severe preumbilical pain, which is often out of proportion to findings on physical examination. In contrast, the pain may occur more insidiously (hours to days) in patients with thrombotic causes, vasculitis or nonocclusive ischemia. Mesenteric angiography remains the gold standard diagnostic study for AMI, and has resulted in the decline in mortality of patients with AMI over the past 30 years. On the other hand, CTA appears to be an acceptable alternative in settings where obtaining angiography is impractical or there is only moderate suspicion of AMI. The ultimate goal of treatment in patients with AMI is to restore intestinal flow as rapidly as possible. Initial management should include aggressive hemodynamic monitoring and support, gastric decompression, broad-spectrum antibiotics, correction of acidosis and systemic anticoagulation. Vasoconstricting agents and digitalis should be avoided. Patients suspected of having intestinal infarction or perforation should undergo surgery on an emergency basis regardless of the cause for AMI, whereas the endovascular approach (including transcatheter thrombolytic therapy, balloon angioplasty and stenting) is reserved for patients with AMI in the absence of peritoneal signs or subjects with peritoneal signs who are poor candidates for surgery.

Chronic mesenteric ischemia (CMI) (also called intestinal angina) refers to episodic or constant intestinal hypoperfusion. Typical patients have history of smoking and underlying atherosclerotic vascular disease and classically complain of dull, crampy, postprandial epigastric pain that increases after large meals with high fat content. Other symptoms include nausea, vomiting, early satiety, weight loss and cachexia. The diagnosis of CMI is supported by the demonstration of high-grade stenosis in multiple mesenteric vessels in patients with unexplained chronic abdominal pain, weight loss and food aversion. Angiography is currently considered to be the gold standard diagnostic test. Therapeutic options for patients with CMI include surgical reconstruction or PTA with or without placement of stents. Current ACC/AHA practice guidelines recommend percutaneous endovascular approach as a Class I indication for treatment of CMI.

❑ SUGGESTED READINGS

Adams RJ, Albers G, Alberts MJ, et al. Update to the AHA/ASA recommendations for the prevention of stroke in patients with stroke and transient ischemic attack. Stroke. 2008;39:1647-52.

American Diabetes Association. Peripheral arterial disease in people with diabetes. Diabetes Care. 2003;26:3333-41.

Beebe HG, Stark R, Johnson ML, et al. Choices of operation for subclavian-vertebral arterial disease. Am J Surg. 1980;139:616-23.

Criqui MH, Fronek A, Barrett-Connor E, et al. The prevalence of peripheral arterial disease in a defined population. Circulation. 1985;71:510-5.

Hirsch AT, Haskal ZJ, Hertzer NR, et al. ACC/AHA 2005 guidelines for the management of patients with peripheral arterial disease (lower extremity, renal, mesenteric, and abdominal aortic): executive summary a collaborative report from the American Association for Vascular Surgery/Society for Vascular Surgery, Society for Cardiovascular Angiography and Interventions, Society for Vascular Medicine and Biology, Society of Interventional Radiology, and the ACC/AHA Task Force on Practice Guidelines (Writing Committee to Develop Guidelines for the Management of Patients with Peripheral Arterial Disease) endorsed by the American Association of Cardiovascular and Pulmonary Rehabilitation; National Heart, Lung, and Blood Institute; Society for Vascular Nursing; TransAtlantic Inter-Society Consensus; and Vascular Disease Foundation. J Am Coll Cardiol. 2006;47:1239-312.

Latchaw RE, Alberts MJ, Lev MH, et al. Recommendations for imaging of acute ischemic stroke: a scientific statement from the American Heart Association. Stroke. 2009;40:3646-78.

McDermott MM, Liu K, Greenland P, et al. Functional decline in peripheral arterial disease: associations with the ankle brachial index and leg symptoms. JAMA. 2004;292:453-61.

McKinsey JF, Gewertz BL. Acute mesenteric ischemia. Surg Clin North Am. 1997;77:307-18.

National Cholesterol Education Program (NCEP) Expert Panel on Detection, Evaluation, and Treatment of High Blood Cholesterol in Adults (Adult Treatment Panel III). Third Report of the National Cholesterol Education Program (NCEP) Expert Panel on Detection, Evaluation, and Treatment of High Blood Cholesterol in Adults (Adult Treatment Panel III). Circulation. 2002;106:3143-421.

Norgren L, Hiatt WR, Dormandy JA, et al. Inter-Society Consensus for the Management of Peripheral Arterial Disease (TASC II). J Vasc Surg. 2007;45:S5-67.

Sacco RL, Adams R, Albers G, et al. Guidelines for prevention of stroke in patients with ischemic stroke or transient ischemic attack: a statement for healthcare professionals from the American Heart Association/American Stroke Association Council on Stroke: cosponsored by the Council on Cardiovascular Radiology and Intervention: the American Academy of Neurology affirms the value of this guideline. Stroke. 2006;37:577-617.

Selvin E, Erlinger TP. Prevalence of and risk factors for peripheral arterial disease in the United States: results from the National Health and Nutrition Examination Survey, 1999-2000. Circulation. 2004;110:738-43.

U.S. Preventive Services Task Force. (2007). Screening for Carotid Artery Stenosis. [online] U.S. Preventive Services Task Force website. Available from http://www.uspreventiveservicestaskforce.org/uspstf/uspsacas.htm.

Watson L, Ellis B, Leng GC. Exercise for intermittent claudication. Cochrane Database Syst Rev. 2008;CD000990.

6.3 Aortic Dissection and Aneurysm

AORTIC DISSECTION

❏ INTRODUCTION

Acute aortic dissection (AAD) is a catastrophic illness that occurs with an incidence of 5–30 cases per million people per year leading to at least 7,000 cases per year in the United States. The major predisposing factors are atherosclerosis and inherited diseases. The majority of the cases are sporadic, but more than 20% are inherited as a single gene disorder. The most common familial thoracic aortic aneurysms and dissections (TAAD) is Marfan's syndrome which is caused by mutations in fibrillin-1 gene (FBN-1), the less common Loeys–Dietz syndrome (caused by mutations in TGFBR1 and 2) as well as the non-syndromic thoracic aortic aneurysm. The mode of inheritance in most cases is autosomal dominant with variable penetrance.

Aortic dissection occurs secondary to different mechanisms. Either it is related to a tear in the intima, which directly opposed a diseased medial layer (commonly called cystic medial degeneration) or from intramural hemorrhage and hematoma formation in the media subsequently followed by perforation of the intima or, it could be secondary to a perforating penetrating ulcer. Cystic medial degeneration is an intrinsic feature of several hereditary defects of connective tissue disease, notably Marfan and Ehlers–Danlos syndromes, and is also common in patients with bicuspid aortic valve (Fig. 4). Chest traumas as well as pregnancy in the third trimester and early postpartum period are also risk factors for aortic dissection.

❏ CLASSIFICATION

The Stanford, DeBakey and anatomical classifications have been shown in Table 15 and Figure 5.

New studies have demonstrated that intramural hematoma and aortic ulcers may be signs of evolving dissections or dissections subtypes. A new differentiation of acute aortic syndromes has thus been proposed by the following classes:
- Class I: Aortic dissection with a flap
- Class II: Intramural hematoma
- Class III: Subtle-discrete aortic dissection
- Class IV: Plaque Ulceration

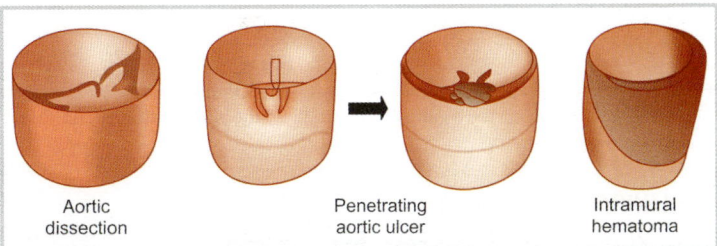

FIGURE 4: Aortic dissection, penetrating aortic ulcer, intramural hematoma. (*Source:* Ramanath VS, et al. Acute aortic syndromes and thoracic aortic aneurysm. Mayo Clin Proc. 2009;84:465-81)

Table 15: Commonly used classification systems to describe aortic dissection

Type	Site of origin and extent of aortic involvement
DeBakey	
Type I	Originates in the ascending aorta, propagates at least to the aortic arch and often beyond it distally
Type II	Originates and is confined to the ascending aorta
Type III	Originates in the descending aorta and extends distally down the aorta or, rarely, retrograde into the aortic arch
Stanford	
Type A	All dissections involving the ascending aortal, regardless of the site of origin
Type B	All dissections not involving the ascending aorta
Descriptive	
Proximal	Includes DeBakey types I and II or Stanford type A
Distal	Includes DeBakey type III or Stanford type B

(*Source:* Libby P. Braunwald's Heart Disease: A Textbook of Cardiovascular Medicine, 8th edn.)

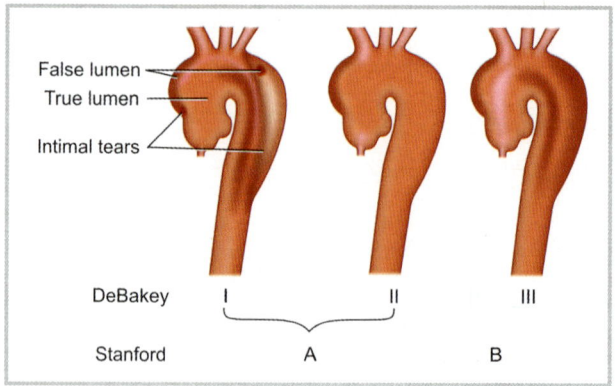

FIGURE 5: Anatomy and classification of aortic dissection (*Source:* Libby P. Braunwald's Heart Disease. A Textbook of Cardiovascular Medicine, 8th edn)

- Class V: Blunt chest trauma usually causes dissection of the ascending aorta and/or the region of the ligamentum botalli at the aortic isthmus and due to iatrogenic dissection.

❏ CLINICAL EXAMINATION

Aortic dissection is characterized by sudden onset of chest pain present in nearly 90% of the cases. The chest pain is described as sharp more often than tearing, ripping or stabbing. In proximal dissections, the chest pain is usually located proximally, whereas distal dissections are characterized by interscapular as well as back pain. The chest pain of aortic dissection may migrate from the point of origin to other sites, following the path of the extension of the dissection. Migratory pain is found in 17% of the cases. The presence of any neck, jaw and throat pain is highly suggestive of proximal dissection whereas pain involving the back, abdomen and lower extremities is suggestive of dissection involving the descending aorta. In some cases, the patient will present with pleuritic chest pain secondary to hemorrhage or inflammation in the pericardial space from the dissected aorta. Chest pain may be absent, and this is usually indicative of chronic aortic dissection or occurs in a patient with prior cardiac surgery.

Other symptoms present at presentation but less frequent are: syncope (13%), cerebrovascular accident (6%), congestive heart failure (7%), ischemic peripheral neuropathy or paraplegia, cardiac arrest and death.

Hypotension occurs more commonly in patients with proximal aortic dissection whereas hypertension occurs in patients with distal aortic dissection. Other clinical findings are pulse deficits related to the extension of aortic dissection found in 20% of the cases, a murmur of aortic valve regurgitation is seen in 40–50% of the cases of type A dissection. Congestive heart failure may occur secondary to acute valve aortic regurgitation.

Other associated clinical findings include pleural effusions seen on the left side, hemothorax secondary to the rupture of the aortal into the pleural space, hemoptysis and hematemesis secondary to rupture in the tracheobronchial tree or in the esophagus, superior vena cava syndrome, Horner's syndrome and unexplained fever due to the release of pyogenic substances from the aortic wall.

❏ DIAGNOSIS

Chest X-ray

The most common abnormality seen on chest X-ray is mediastinal enlargement seen in 60–90% of the cases. If calcification of the aortic knob is present, separation of the intimal calcification from the outer aortic soft tissue border by more than 1 cm is called the "calcium sign" and is suggestive of aortic dissection.

Electrocardiography

The electrocardiography (ECG) is frequently abnormal, showing signs of left ventricular hypertrophy, myocardial ischemia, nonspecific ST-T wave deviations, or myocardial infarction, more frequently involving the inferior wall. The association of chest pain without any ischemic changes should prompt one to consider aortic dissection in the differential diagnosis.

D-dimer

D-dimer was markedly elevated in patients with AAD. The cutoff level of 500 ng/mL used to "rule out" pulmonary embolism was also reliable to rule out AAD. At this cutoff level, sensitivity was 96.6% (95% CI, 90.3, 99.3) and specificity 46.6% (95% CI, 25.1, 54.6). While D-dimer was found to be very sensitive it is not specific for the diagnosis of AAD. A new biomarker calponin, a troponin counterpart of smooth vessel, has potential for the early diagnostic study of AAD within 24 hours of presentation. Acidic calponin has a sensitivity of 58% and specificity of 72% at 24 hours and basic calponin has a sensitivity of 50% and specificity of 66% at 24 hours.

Imaging

Transthoracic Echocardiogram

Transthoracic echocardiogram (TTE) has a sensitivity of 60–85% and specificity of 93–96% for the involvement of the ascending aorta. The value of TTE is limited in patients with abnormal chest configuration, obesity, emphysema and in patients on mechanical ventilation.

Transesophageal Echocardiogram

Transesophageal echocardiogram (TEE) has a sensitivity of 90% in patients with type A aortic dissection and sensitivity of only 80% in type B. Although TEE can be performed quickly in the emergent setting, it should only be interpreted by an experienced echocardiographer. Dissection extending to the ostium of coronary arteries can be visualized in TEE (Fig. 6).

CT Angiogram

In CT angiogram (CTA), AAD is diagnosed by the presence of two different lumina separated by an intimal flap. Helical CT has improved CT diagnostics because it minimizes motion artifacts and eliminates respiratory misregistration. The diagnosis is based on the demonstration of an intimal flap which separates the true from the false lumen.

Magnetic Resonance Imaging

Although magnetic resonance imaging (MRI) is both highly sensitive and specific in the diagnosis of AAD, the technique is not always available on an emergency basis and is difficult to execute on a hemodynamically unstable patient. The MRI sensitivity exceeds 90%. Despite its accuracy, artifacts might occur in as many as 64% of the cases. The MRI demonstrates the extent of the disease, pericardial involvement and aortic valve regurgitation.

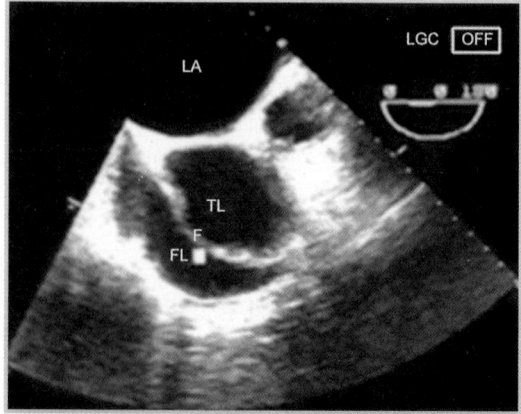

FIGURE 6: TEE of dissection of descending aorta in the horizontal plane (*Source:* Khan IA, Nair CK. Clinical diagnosis and management perspective of aortic dissection. Chest. 2002;122:311-28)

Aortography

The angiographics signs of aortic dissection include visualization of two lumina or an intimal flap, or indirect findings, such as deformity of the aortic lumen, thickening of the aortic walls, branch vessels abnormalities and aortic regurgitation. The true lumen is typically compressed and tends to adopt a spiral configuration down the aorta. Injections in false lumen are characterized by the absence of branch vessels. Contrast aortography accurately identifies branch vessel involvement. Aortography had long been considered the diagnostic standard for the evaluation of aortic dissection. However, prospective studies have shown that the sensitivity of aortography is 88% and falls to 77% when the definition of aortic dissection includes intramural hematoma and noncommunicating disease. The specificity of aortography is 94%.

Coronary Angiography

Although new imaging techniques are gaining an emerging role in the assessment of coronary ostial involvement by the dissecting flap, coronary angiography remains the gold standard of evaluation of coronary arteries.

❏ TREATMENT

Initial Treatment

Admission to ICU, blood pressure regulation and hemodynamic stabilization are critical in the initial treatment of aortic dissection. The initial goal should be to reduce the blood pressure to 100–120 mm Hg (mean 60–75 mm Hg) or the lowest level commensurate with adequate vital organ function (cardiac, cerebral, and renal) perfusion. Beta-blockers and vasodilators are the two medications used to control the blood pressure and to reduce the force of left ventricular ejection (dp/dt). Vasodilators should not be used as monotherapy because they can abruptly raise dp/dt, potentially worsening the dissection. The use of long acting ? blockers should be avoided in patients who are surgical candidates secondary to untoward influences intraoperative blood pressure which could be complicated. A short-acting beta-blocker, such as esmolol, would be more appropriate in this case. Nitroprusside sodium and labetalol are very helpful agents. If beta blockers are contraindicated, then a calcium channel blocker, such as verapamil ordiltiazem, is frequently used.

Hypotension should raise the suspicion of cardiac tamponade or aortic rupture. Pseudohypotension resulting from altered arm circulation due to the dissection should always be excluded. In the case of hypotension, volume expansion should be initiated. If hypotension persists, pressors of choice are norepinephrine or phenylephrine. Dopamine should be reserved for improving renal perfusion and only at low doses given the fact that it may raise the dp/dt and theoretically extend the dissection.

Cardiac Tamponade

Urgent pericardiocentesis may be harmful rather than beneficial because it can precipitate hemodynamic collapse and death. If the patient is relatively stable, emergent surgery with intraoperative pericardium decompression is the treatment of choice. However, if the patient has marked hypotension, aspiration of the minimum volume of fluid to raise the blood pressure to the lowest level acceptable should be the treatment of choice.

Type A Acute Aortic Dissection

At 24 hours of presentation, medical management alone results in mortality rate of 20%, 30% at 48 hours of presentation and 50% at 1 month. Patients with intramural hematoma of the ascending aortal should be treated surgically. Current surgical techniques include resection of the intima tear, replacement or resuspension of the aortic valve if it has been disrupted by the dissection, coronary artery bypass if necessary and replacement of the ascending aorta. If the dissection involves the aortic arch, partial or total replacement of the aortic arch may be necessary. After the diseased segment containing the intimal tear is resected, aortic continuity is reestablished by interposing a prosthetic sleeve graft between the two ends of the aorta.

Type B Acute Aortic Dissection

Patients with uncomplicated type B acute aortic dissection and intramural hematoma of the descending aorta are typically managed medically. These patients have a high surgical mortality rate due to comorbidities and underlying atherosclerosis which is often present. Aggressive medical management consists of maintaining the systolic blood pressure at or below 120 mm Hg with beta-blockers and other agents. Surgical treatment is indicated in patients presenting with complications as refractory pain, malperfusion of vital organs, dissection progression, aneurysm expansion and refractory hypertension.

Endovascular Repair

Endovascular repair may retard the progression of disease in patients who are not open surgical candidates or who refuse open surgical repair. Endovascular repair has no role in the management of aortic dissection involving the arch and ascending thoracic aorta (type A) which often originates close to the sinotubular junction and often propagates proximally into the aortic root, causing coronary occlusion, aortic regurgitation and pericardial tamponade. The treatment is prompt surgical repair under hypothermic circulatory arrest. Endovascular treatment also has a limited role in the management of uncomplicated acute aortic dissection involving the descending thoracic and abdominal aortic segments of the aorta (type B). The primary treatment is medical using combinations of beta-blockers and vasodilators. Endovascular intervention is however indicated for the treatment of acute type B dissection (less than 2 weeks) complicated by visceral malperfusion, rupture, rapid false lumen expansion, or unremitting pain. Endovascular repair is also used to treat cases of chronic type B dissection in which the false lumen has dilated to the point of aneurysm formation.

Regardless of whether treatment occurs in the acute or chronic phase, the goal of endovascular repair is true lumen expansion and false lumen thrombosis. In this regard the endovascular repair of acute dissection is more likely to succeed that endovascular repair of chronic dissection; hence, the argument for treating acute dissection even in the absence of complications in the hope of preventing aneurysm formation.

Acute Type B Dissection

Endovascular intervention for acute type B dissection usually entails endovascular stent graft implantation, fenestration or some combination of the two. The goal of endovascular stent graft implantation is to close the inter-luminal connections (tears or fenestrations) and channel flow away from the false lumen into the true lumen. The goal of fenestration is to open interluminal connections, provide a route of egress for false luminal flow, and equalize pressure between the true and false lumens. Although some authors endeavor to eliminate false lumen flow completely using stent grafts in the aorta and stents within the visceral branches, a more typical approach is to use endovascular aortic repair and interluminal fenestration in different segments of the aorta. Endovascular repair is often confined to the proximal descending thoracic aorta where the dissection originates and where aneurysms occur most often, whereas fenestrations are confined to the proximal abdominal aorta where the visceral arteries preclude the implantation of an unbranched aortic stent graft. It is still unclear whether endovascular intervention has a role in the management of uncomplicated acute type B dissection. However, intervention can be life-saving when acute type B dissection is complicated by rupture or, more commonly, visceral malperfusion.

Chronic Type B Dissection

The excess mortality seen in the years after aortic dissection is attributable to false lumen dilatation and rupture. These false lumen aneurysms are slightly more likely to rupture and far more difficult to treat that atherosclerotic aneurysms of similar size. The aortic dissection usually extends into the abdominal aorta with multiple fenestrations at the level of the visceral arteries. Implantation of the stent graft into the true lumen of the supraceliac aorta leaves the false lumen as a potential route of retrograde flow into the aneurysm. More complete aneurysm exclusion requires thoracoabdominal repair, which can be difficult to accomplish by endovascular means when the true lumen is small and the false lumen gives rise to some of the branches.

Nevertheless, unbranched repair of the proximal aortic true lumen may have a role when only the proximal portion of the lumen often perfuse well through a newly pressurized true lumen. Nevertheless, persistent obstruction of a visceral artery may require the insertion of a stent. If the goal is to completely isolate the false lumen from the circulation, covered stents can bridge the gap between the true lumen of the aorta and the true lumen of the branch. These may be inserted at a second operation, based on the findings of the first postoperative computed tomographic angiography (CTA).

AORTIC ANEURYSM

❏ INTRODUCTION

Although aortic aneurysm sometimes causes aortic dissection and visa versa, these are two very different diseases. What they have in common is structural failure of the aortic wall. Of the two, aneurysm is less likely to present as an acute aortic emergency and more likely to be treated by endovascular means. Aneurysms are caused by proteolytic degradation of adventitial elastin, among other things. The weakened aortic wall dilates, increasing wall tension, accelerating dilatation and increasing the risk of rupture. In most cases, the process is painless up to the point of rupture, hemorrhage and death.

❏ TREATMENT

The goal of aneurysm repair is to connect the non-dilated segments proximal and distal to the aneurysm using an impervious conduit, which isolates the aneurysm from flow and pressure, thereby preventing dilatation and rupture. In the elective setting, this is a prophylactic operation with no short-term benefits, only risks. The long-term benefit, freedom from risk of rupture, depends on the size of the aneurysm and the life expectancy of the patient, together with the efficacy and durability of the repair.

❏ ANATOMIC SUBSTRATE FOR ENDOVASCULAR ANEURYSM REPAIR

The basic requirements for successful endovascular aneurysm repair include: a route of aortic access through the iliac arteries and nondilated implantation sites of sufficient length between the aneurysm and the orifices of indispensable arteries. Whatever the device, straight wide iliac arteries are less likely to impede device insertion and long cylindrical implantation sites are less likely to disrupt the seal. Various authors have tried to categorize arterial anatomy as a way to predict the likelihood of complications. However, the threshold values that divide favorable anatomy from unfavorable anatomy are always arbitrary and nonpredictive for several reasons. The anatomic selection criteria described in the instructions for use should not be regarded as absolute requirements for safe effective aneurysm repair, but they cannot be ignored because they defined the patient populations of industry-sponsored IDE studies, and those studies provided much of the published literature on device performance.

❏ ADJUNCTIVE DEVICES AND TECHNIQUES

Aneurysms fall into four groups depending on the state of the neck proximally and the iliac arteries distally:
1. Treatable using standard stent grafts.
2. Treatable using standard stent grafts with the help of additional devices and techniques.
3. Treatable using complex fenestrated or branched stent grafts.
4. Untreatable by purely endovascular means.

In the days of aorto-aortic AAA repair, 80–90% of cases were in group 4, but the number has been dwindling steadily with every advance in the field. These days, few patients lack the anatomic substrate for some form of endovascular repair. However, the laudable desire to spare the patient the discomfort, morbidity and disability of conventional open repair can be carried to excess. In most high volume centers, the open surgical repair of juxtarenal and pararenal aortic aneurysms is associated with low mortality rates and predictable long-term efficacy. In contrast, less than a dozen centers have the means to perform complex endovascular repairs and the long-term results of these investigational procedures are unknown.

❏ ENDOLEAK

Since the primary goal of endovascular aneurysm repair is to isolate the aneurysm from the circulation, persistence of perigraft perfusion (endoleak) has to be regarded as a sign of failure. However, an endoleak's effect on sac pressure, dilatation and risk of rupture depends very much on the source.

In the absence of an endoleak, the sac pressure is low, the aneurysm shrinks and there is no risk of rupture. Untreated leakage directly into the aneurysm either around the end of the stent graft (type I) or through a defect in the wall of the stent graft (type III) is associated with high sac pressure, rapid dilatation, and a high rate of rupture. Leakage into the aneurysm sac by an indirect route through lumbar or inferior mesenteric branches (type II) occupies an intermediate position between direct leakage and no leakage. Most type II endoleaks resolve spontaneously within 6 months, and in the absence of aneurysm dilatation, rupture is rare. Moreover, type II endoleaks are notoriously difficult to treat by transarterial means, especially when the lumbar arteries are involved. Type IV endoleak is a form of type III endoleak through tiny defects in the graft which sealed upon heparin reversal. However, continued transmission of pressure to the aneurysm sac often leads to aneurysm dilatation (type V endoleak, or endotension). The substitution of a more tightly woven graft fabric seems to have eliminated this complication of repair with the AneuRx stent graft. Graft porosity on a microscopic level appears to have been responsible for a similar phenomenon following repair with the original excluder stent graft, requiring changes in the graft fabric.

❏ LATE-OCCURRING COMPLICATIONS OF ENDOVASCULAR ANEURYSM REPAIR

Although modern stent grafts appear to be more durable than their predecessors, the complications of stent graft instability will continue to be present for years as patients outlast their devices.

Migration

Since the cross-sectional area of the trunk of a bifurcate stent graft is larger than the cross-sectional area of the limbs, pressure-related forces push the bifurcation in a caudal direction. Bends in the trunk or limbs of a stent graft tend to generate transaxial forces, pulling the center of the stent graft toward the anterior wall of the aneurysm and the ends of the neck and common iliac arteries. Experience has shown that friction, arterial ingrowth, and column strength provide little protection against migration. The most stable stent grafts have barbs, suprarenal stents and a long-body/short-leg configuration. If detected in its early stages, the problem is easy to correct using a stent graft extension with active, barb-mediated attachment proximally and a long overlap with the original graft distally.

Endotension

Aneurysm dilatation in the absence of endoleak (endotension) was a common problem after endovascular repair using first generation AneuRx and Exluder stent grafts, but they are not the only stent grafts to fail in this way. Endotension occurs with increasing frequency once any stent graft has been in place 5 years, or more. It is managed by treating both potential causes of aneurysm pressurization, because perigraft perfusion raises the possibility of true hemorrhagic rupture.

Neck Dilatation

For self-expanding stent grafts, the amount of neck expansion depends on the degree of oversizing. When the diameter of the neck equals the unconstrained diameter of the stent graft (full expansion) dilatation ceases and the diameter plateaus. One occasionally sees stent migration in patients with neck dilatation, but most such cases occur following repair with a device that lacks active barb-mediated fixation.

Balloon-expanded stent grafts behave differently. Balloon driven expansion initially stretches the neck, but then neck diameter stablizes because the balloon-expanded stent will expand no further. In addition, uncovered portions of a balloon-expanded stent often become incorporated into the surrounding aortic tissue, stabilizing the dimensions of the proximal part of the implantation site.

❑ FOLLOW-UP IMAGING

The purpose of follow-up imaging is to detect impending failure while the underlying problem remains amenable to endovascular correction. The choice of imaging modality and follow-up interval depends on the late failure mode of the particular stent graft. Contrast-enhanced CT scan is not the only suitable means of surveillance. Significant migration is always associated with anterior displacement of the graft within the aneurysm, which can be seen by comparing serial non-contrast CT scans or lateral X-rays of the abdomen.

❑ SUGGESTED READINGS

Chuter TA, Gordon RL, Reilly LM, et al. An endovascular system for thoracoabdominal aortic aneurysm repair. J Endovasc Ther. 2001;8:25-33.

Conners MS, Sternbergh WC, Carter G, et al. Endograft migration 1 to 4 years after endovascular abdominal aortic aneurysm repair with the AneuRx device: a cautionary note. J Vasc Surg. 2002;36:476-84.

Keramati AR, Sadeghpour A, Farahani MM, et al. The non-syndromic familial thoracic aneurysms and dissections maps to 15q21 locus. BMC Med Genet. 2010;11:143.

Lebreton G, Litzler PY, Bessou JP. Acute aortic syndome: a 'last glance' before incision. Interact Cardio Vasc Thorac Surg. 2010;11: 357-9.

Libby P, Bonow RO, Mann DL, et al. Braunwald's Heart Disease. A Textbook of Cardiovascular Medicine, 8th edn.

May J, White GH, Yu W, et al. Importance of graft configuration in outcome of endoluminal aortic aneurysm repair: a 5-year analysis by the life table method. Eur J Vasc Endovasc Surg. 1998;15:406-11.

Mikich M. Dissection of the aorta: a new approach. Heart. 2003;89: 6-8.

Nienaber CA, Eagle K. Aortic dissection: new frontiers in diagnosis and management. Therapeutic management and follow-up. Circulation. 2003;108:772-8.

Suzuki T, Distante A, Zizza A, et al. Preliminary experience with the smooth muscle troponin-like protein calponin as a novel biomarker for diagnosing acute aortic dissection. Eur Heart J. 2008;29:1439-45.

White GH, Yu W, May J, et al. Endoleak as a complication of endoluminal grafting of abdominal aortic aneurysms: classification, incidence, diagnosis, and management. J Endovasc Surg. 1997;4:152-68.

6.4 Autonomic Dysfunction and the Cardiovascular System

❏ INTRODUCTION

The functions of our autonomic nervous system (ANS) are often taken for granted. And yet, every time we rise from a recumbent to a standing position, our cardiovascular system must undergo instantaneous adaptations, otherwise we will faint and fall. Besides maintaining hemodynamic competency during postural changes, the ANS continuously responds to a variety of internal and external cues to regulate other equally vital physiological functions—most of which occurs without us being conscious of it. These include such important homeostatic functions as regulation of blood pressure, circulatory volume, respiration, temperature, gastrointestinal activity and metabolism.

❏ AUTONOMIC REGULATION OF THE CARDIOVASCULAR SYSTEM

Classically, the ANS can be divided into three components: (1) the sympathetic, (2) parasympathetic and (3) enteric systems. More recently, it has been appreciated that sensory input from various organs and tissues via afferent neuronal pathways is a critical component of autonomic function. Afferent neurons possess special receptive terminals that sense mechanical forces (such as pressure, stretch, shear, etc.), or the chemical milieu (such as pH, PO_2, PCO_2, noxious irritants, etc.). In humans, the major centers of cardiovascular autonomic nervous integration and control are in the medulla and include the nucleus tractus solitarii (NTS) as well as motor output centers in the brainstem. In addition, feedback regulatory loops also occur at more peripheral sites including the spinal cord and autonomic ganglia. The two principle efferent pathways that control the cardiovascular system—the sympathetic and parasympathetic pathways—often, but not always, have opposite influences on target tissues; and the resultant effect on cardiovascular responses represents the relative balance between the two pathways.

Regulation of Blood Pressure

One of the most critical functions of the ANS is to maintain adequate blood flow to the various organs and tissues of the body, and to do so, the mean systemic arterial pressure must be regulated within an optimal range. Long-term regulation of arterial pressure—on the time scale of hours to days—involves humoral regulation of the effective circulatory volume; although neural actions on the kidney also play a role. On the other hand, short-term regulation of arterial pressure—on the time scale of seconds to minutes—is almost exclusively under autonomic control. Collectively, the principle autonomic reflexes that regulate blood pressure are referred to as the baroreflex.

Arterial baroreceptors are specialized stretch-activated sensory nerves located on the carotid sinuses and the aortic arch that sense distension of the vessel wall induced by pressure changes (Fig. 7). The carotid sinuses are highly compliant portions of the internal carotid arteries located at the branching of the internal and external carotid arteries, and the aortic arch distends with each ejection of blood from the left ventricle. Distension of these arterial walls causes depolarization

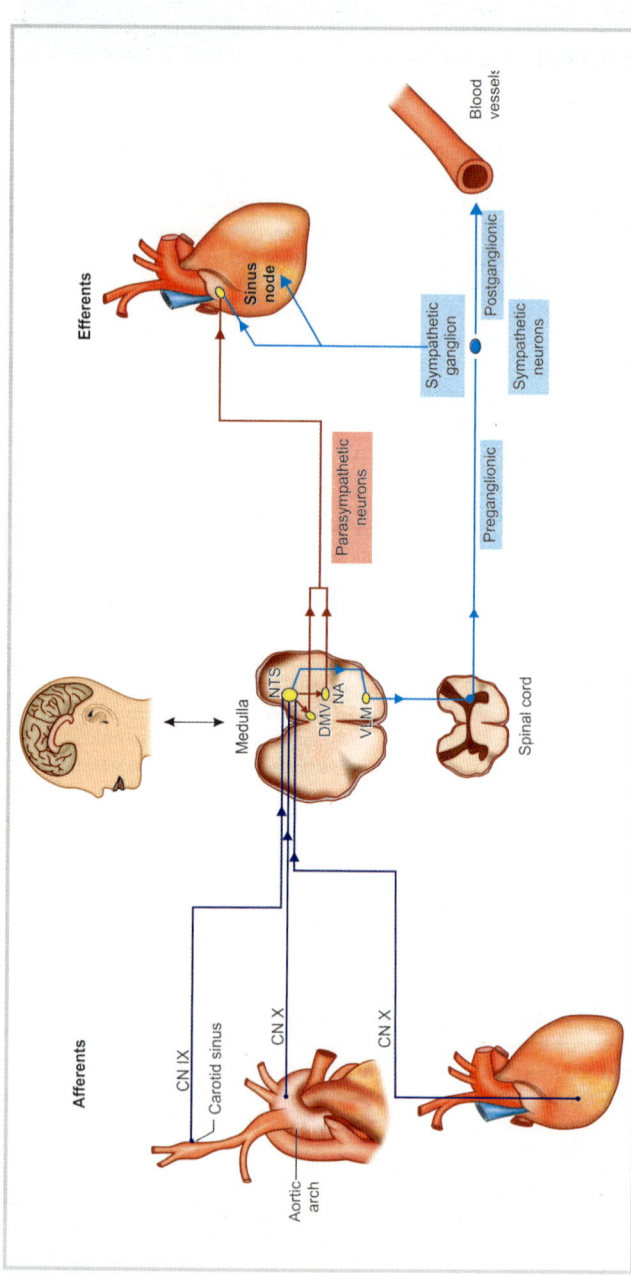

FIGURE 7: Schematic representation of the baroreflex. Afferent pathways (blue) from arterial and cardiopulmonary baroreceptors follow the glossopharyngeal (CN IX) and vagus (CN X) nerves to the NTS in the medulla. Excitatory interneurons project from the NTS to the cardioinhibitory regions, including the DMV and NA which mediate parasympathetic output (brown pathways) to the heart. The NTS also sends projections to the vasomotor and cardioacceleratory regions in the VLM which control sympathetic output (sky blue pathways) to the vasculature and heart respectively (Abbreviations: CN: Cranial nerve; NTS: Nucleus tractus solitaries; NA: Nucleus ambiguous; DMV: Dorsal motor nucleus of the vagus; VLM: Ventrolateral medulla)

of stretch-activated baroreceptor nerve terminals, which then generate action potentials of varying firing frequency.

Heart Rate Control

A denervated heart, such as occurs with a transplanted heart, has an intrinsic sinus nodal heart rate of approximately 100 beats/minute. Deviations from this intrinsic rate are primarily under the influence of the ANS. When a healthy person is at rest, parasympathetic efferent input to the sinus node lowers the average heart rate to 60–70 beats/min, and the sympathetic input to the sinus node is essentially silent. Rapid changes in heart rate, such as occur with the respiratory cycle (sinus arrhythmia) and those induced by the baroreflex, are mediated by fluctuating parasympathetic input. During stress or exercise, sympathetic input to the heart becomes dominant and heart rate rises accordingly.

Chemoreflex Influence on Heart Rate and Blood Pressure

The chemoreceptors, which consist of both peripheral and central components, are the major sensors that regulate respiration. However, chemoreflexes also influence both blood pressure and heart rate, and have a particularly important modulatory effect in some disease conditions such as sleep apnea. The peripheral chemoreceptors which primarily sense hypoxemia reside in the carotid bodies located near the carotid sinuses at the branching of the internal and external carotid arteries. The central chemoreceptors are located in the medulla, and they primarily sense hypercapnea or acidosis.

❑ AUTONOMIC TESTING

The functional effects of the ANS on the cardiovascular system can be tested by a variety of means. Some of these tests can be performed at the bedside or in the outpatient office setting; others require more sophisticated equipment and are primarily performed at specialized clinics and research centers of autonomic dysfunction.

Orthostatics

Measurement of orthostatic blood pressure and heart rate response at the bedside is a simple and useful test that often recapitulates a patient's symptoms, and provides insight into the underlying pathophysiology. Orthostatic hypotension is a fall of systolic blood pressure of at least 20 mm Hg or a fall of diastolic blood pressure of at least 10 mm Hg within 3 minutes of standing or head-up tilt on a tilt table. After careful measurement of supine blood pressure and heart rate, the patient is asked to stand, or sit with feet dangling over the bedside if standing is not possible. Blood pressure and heart rate is measured when the patient becomes symptomatic or at 3 minutes.

Valsalva Maneuver

The valsalva maneuver is typically performed in a supine position and patient is asked to blow into a closed tube at 40 mm Hg, or exhale forcefully against a closed glottis and maintain the strain for 10–15 seconds while blood pressure waveform and heart rate are analyzed. The normal blood pressure and heart rate responses are divided into four phases. Phase 1 is associated with a brief increase in blood pressure. Blood pressure falls during the early part of phase 2, and the later part of phase 2 is associated with a return of blood pressure and an increase in heart rate. Blood pressure then briefly falls in phase 3, and then is followed by a "blood pressure overshoot" in phase 4 that represents a normalization of venous return to the heart in the setting of persistently elevated sympathetic tone. The normal heart rate responses during Valsalva maneuver reflect baroreflex responses; the falls in blood pressure during phases 2 and 3 trigger an increase in heart rate, whereas the increase in blood pressure during phases 1 and 4 are accompanied by decrease in heart rate. The most commonly seen abnormalities in patients with autonomic dysfunction are failure to correct hypotension in phase 2 and/ or failure to overshoot blood pressure in phase 4.

Resting Heart Rate

One of the simplest measures of autonomic function is resting heart rate, and it has gained increasing appreciation as an important prognostic indicator. Low resting heart rates are commonly seen in competitive athletes and are indicative of high parasympathetic tone. Conversely, higher resting heart rate is associated with multiple cardiovascular disease conditions, and it is characterized by loss of parasympathetic, and increasing sympathetic activity.

Baroreflex Sensitivity

As previously described, the baroreceptor reflex is the principal neural mechanism involved in short-term (seconds to minutes) blood pressure regulation. A sudden increase in blood pressure evokes a reflex increase in cardiovagal activity and a corresponding decrease in heart rate (or increase in R–R interval recorded with electrocardiography). Computer analysis of spontaneous fluctuations in blood pressure and heart rate enables calculations of spontaneous baroreceptor sensitivity. The most common analysis method (sequence method) involves identifying sequences of three or more consecutive beats where systolic blood pressure and R–R interval are positively correlated. "Up" sequences are defined by an increase in blood pressure and R–R interval, while "down" sequences represent a decrease in blood pressure and R–R interval. The average of the slopes for changes in blood pressure and R–R interval relationships define the baroreceptor sensitivity.

Heart Rate Variability

Today, it is recognized that these normal R–R interval changes (decrease during inspiration and increase with expiration—the so-called respiratory "sinus arrhythmia") are predominantly mediated by oscillations in parasympathetic activity to the sinus node. In addition, heart rate variability is also under the control of other autonomic and homeostatic mechanisms. Heart rate variability measurement requires continuous electrocardiographic recording to measure R–R intervals over a period of time, and generally utilizes computer software for analysis by either time-domain or frequency-domain methods. Like baroreceptor sensitivity, heart rate variability diminishes with increasing age and it has been used to predict adverse outcomes in cardiovascular disease.

Heart Rate Recovery

During exercise, the heart rate rises from both parasympathetic withdrawal and sympathetic activation. The rapid fall in heart rate that occurs within 30 seconds after stopping exercise is predominantly a function of the reactivation of the parasympathetic nervous system, and is termed heart rate recovery.

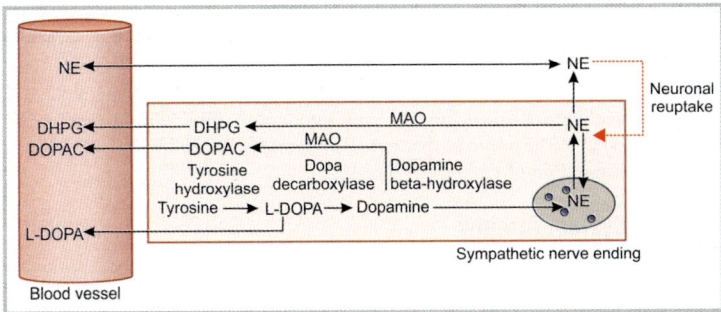

FIGURE 8: Major sources of plasma catecholamines, their precursors and metabolites. Within sympathetic nerves, tyrosine undergoes hydroxylation to dihydroxyphenylalanine (L-DOPA; levodopa), which is decarboxylated to dopamine and further hydroxylated to norepinephrine (NE). NE that enters the plasma is mainly from synaptic vesicle release; although the vast majority of NE is taken back up into the nerve terminals via an uptake-1 mechanism. Dopamine is metabolized to dihydroxyphenylacetic acid (DOPAC), and NE to dihydroxyphenylglycol (DHPG) through monoamine oxidase (MAO) activity

Catecholamine Blood Measurement

Measuring plasma catecholamine levels is an important adjunct in diagnosing autonomic dysfunction. The most relevant endogenous catecholamines, their precursors and metabolites that can be detected in human plasma are 3,4-dihydroxy-L-phenylalanine (dopa), norepinephrine, dihydroxyphenylacetic acid (DOPAC) and dihydroxyphenylglycol (DHPG), as depicted on Figure 8.

Cardiac Sympathetic Imaging

Imaging of the postganglionic sympathetic catecholamine cardiac innervation has been used with increasing frequency both in research and clinical practice. The most commonly used radiotracer is 123I-metaiodobenzylguanidine (123I-MIBG), a sympathomimetic agent that is taken up into sympathetic nerves by the uptake-1 process and sequestered in storage vesicles. However, since it is not degraded like norepinephrine, it can be measured using single proton emission tomography (SPECT). The 123I-MIBG was first used in diagnosing and localizing pheochromocytoma, neuroblastoma and carcinoid tumors. More recently, it has been used to determine cardiac sympathetic innervation and function, and has prognostic significance in a variety of cardiac diseases.

❑ PRIMARY CHRONIC AUTONOMIC FAILURE

Chronic autonomic dysfunction or failure most commonly occurs as a secondary manifestation of other diseases that lead to peripheral neuropathy, such as diabetes, amyloidosis or immune-mediated neuropathies. The term primary chronic autonomic failure is reserved for those rare cases where autonomic dysfunction dominates the clinical presentation, in the absence of an underlying cause.

Pure Autonomic Failure

Pure autonomic failure is a rare, sporadic disorder characterized by orthostatic hypotension as well as bladder and sexual dysfunction—in the absence of other neurological deficits. It generally presents in individuals in their sixties, is slowly progressive, and the prognosis is generally good. The dysfunction in pure autonomic failure occurs at the level of peripheral autonomic neurons, and low norepinephrine levels due to inadequate sympathetic neuronal release are a defining characteristic. Neuropathological abnormalities have been described in both preganglionic and postganglionic sympathetic neurons in pure autonomic failure, and the presence of Lewy bodies led to the proposal that pure autonomic failure might be a peripheral, or early manifestation of Parkinson's disease.

Multiple System Atrophy

The term multiple system atrophy was introduced to combine the entities of striatonigral degeneration, olivopontocerebellar ataxia, and Shy-Drager syndrome. As with pure autonomic failure, the autonomic dysfunction associated with multiple system atrophy is characterized by profound orthostatic hypotension and urogenital dysfunction. However, unlike pure autonomic failure, patients with multiple system atrophy also develop severe movement disorders, which manifest as either Parkinsonism or cerebellar ataxia. The pathological features of multiple system atrophy include neuronal degeneration in the central nervous system, including preganglionic central autonomic neurons, while sparing peripheral postganglionic autonomic neurons. In addition to neuronal degeneration, the diagnostic hallmark of multiple system atrophy is glial cytoplasmic inclusion bodies. The clinical diagnosis requires a reduction in systolic blood pressure of 30 mm Hg systolic or diastolic pressure of 15 mm Hg (note that this is a more pronounced decrease of blood pressure than recommended previously in the American Autonomic Society consensus statement on the definition of orthostatic hypotension).

❏ SECONDARY AND CONGENITAL AUTONOMIC FAILURE

Autonomic failure most commonly occurs in the setting of underlying systemic disease, with diabetes mellitus being the most common cause. Autonomic failure is predominantly a manifestation of a more generalized peripheral neuropathy, and similarly it generally begins distally and progresses proximally. The vagus nerve is the longest autonomic nerve, and the earliest manifestations of diabetic autonomic neuropathy are usually associated with parasympathetic denervation. A relative increase in sympathetic/parasympathetic balance ensues leading to an increase in resting heart rate, a decrease in heart rate variability, and blood pressure dysregulation due to baroreflex abnormalities. Sympathetic denervation usually presents in a later stage of the disease and manifests as a further decline in exercise tolerance, and ultimately to the development of orthostatic hypotension.

❏ CHRONIC ORTHOSTATIC INTOLERANCE

Postural Orthostatic Tachycardia Syndrome

One of the most frequent complaints of patients that present to autonomic clinical centers is intolerance of postural changes. Yet, unlike the disorders of autonomic failure described previously, most patients do not, in fact, have orthostatic hypotension. Nevertheless, these patients do have autonomic abnormalities and the hallmark of this disorder is an exaggerated increase in heart rate upon standing or head-up tilt. The disorder has been termed postural orthostatic tachycardia syndrome or POTS. The symptoms associated with POTS are varied but most commonly include lightheadedness or dizziness, weakness, fatigue, blurred vision and possible presyncope, as well as palpitations, tremulousness and anxiety.

Gastrointestinal symptoms are frequent, which include nausea, bloating, diarrhea and constipation. The most commonly used diagnostic criteria for POTS include a sustained increase in heart rate of more than 30 beats/minute, or tachycardia more than or equal to 120 beats/minute within 10 minutes of standing or upright tilting, in the absence of orthostatic hypotension.

Treatment of Orthostatic Hypotension/Intolerance

Treatment of chronic orthostatic hypotension due to autonomic dysfunction is challenging. Because in most patients normotension cannot be usually restored, the goal of treatment is to improve quality of life by ameliorating symptoms using a combination of both non-pharmacological and pharmacological interventions.

Nonpharmacologic Therapy

The first step in dealing with patients with orthostatic hypotension is to carefully review all medications and eliminate those that can potentially exacerbate symptoms; these include antihypertensive drugs, diuretics, nitrates and antidepressants. In particular, patients should be educated to arise slowly from supine to seated or standing position. Leg-crossing is another maneuver that has been shown to prolong the standing time in patients with autonomic disturbances. Patients should learn to avoid certain triggers, including prolonged coughing, straining or walking in hot and humid weather. Regular exercise training involving aerobic exercise and lower limb resistance can increase sympathetic tone, promote blood volume expansion and reverse deconditioning.

Pharmacologic Therapy

Pharmacologic therapies for chronic orthostatic hypotension and POTS syndrome are similar, and they will be discussed together. Although there are many drugs and supplemental agents available, mineralocorticoids, followed by sympathomimetics are the first line of therapy. Midodrine is a peripheral selective alpha-1-adrenergic agonist that was approved in 1996 for the treatment of symptomatic orthostatic hypotension. Other sympathomimetics, such as ephedrine, pseudoephedrine, and phenylpropanolamine have also been used, but they are generally less effective. Some patients with POTS, particularly those troubled by prominent adrenergic symptoms, may benefit from low dose beta-blocking agents; however, they should be avoided in patients with chronic orthostatic hypotension.

❏ SUGGESTED READINGS

Consensus statement on the definition of orthostatic hypotension, pure autonomic failure, and multiple system atrophy. The ConsensusCommittee of the American Autonomic Society and the American Academy of Neurology. Neurology. 1996;46:1470.

DiBona GF. Physiology in perspective: the wisdom of the body. Neural control of the kidney. Am J Physiol Regul Integr Comp Physiol. 2005;289:R633-41.

Goldstein DS, Holmes C, Sharabi Y, et al. Plasma levels of catechols and metanephrines in neurogenic orthostatic hypotension. Neurology. 2003;60:1327-32.

Management of Autonomic Disorders. In: Robertson D, Low PA, Polinsky RJ (Eds). Primer on the Autonomic Nervous System. San Diego: Academic Press; 1996. p. 319.

Pinna GD, La Rovere MT, Maestri R, et al. Comparison between invasive and non-invasive measurements of baroreflex sensitivity; implications for studies on risk stratification after a myocardial infarction. Eur Heart J. 2000;21:1522-9.

Pop-Busui R. Cardiac autonomic neuropathy in diabetes: a clinical perspective. Diabetes Care. 2010;33:434-41.

Smit AA, Halliwill JR, Low PA, et al. Pathophysiological basis of orthostatic hypotension in autonomic failure. J Physiol. 1999;519:1-10.

Chapter 7

Heart Failure

7.1 Diagnosis

The diagnosis of heart failure, irrespective of its etiology, should begin with taking history followed by clinical examination, and noninvasive and if required invasive tests.

❑ ANALYSIS OF SYMPTOMS

Dyspnea is the most common presenting symptom of heart failure. The typical history of paroxysmal nocturnal dyspnea is the characteristic of cardiac dyspnea. Orthopnea and exertional dyspnea have less diagnostic value. The Framingham criteria for diagnosis of heart failure are summarized in Table 1.

Chest pain is an uncommon symptom of heart failure. However typical angina and atypical chest pain are present in some patients with heart failure with or without coronary artery disease. Patients with chronic heart failure do not usually present with history of frank syncope. However, in patients with previously undiagnosed left ventricular systolic dysfunction, syncope resulting from ventricular tachyarrhythmias may occur as the initial manifestation of heart failure.

Exertional fatigue is a common presenting symptom of patients with heart failure. However, like exertional dyspnea, it has a relatively low positive predictive value. The other occasional symptoms of chronic heart failure are nocturnal cough, nocturia, right upper quadrant pain if hepatomegaly is present, and disordered sleep.

Table 1: Criteria of congestive heart failure—Framingham study

Major criteria
- Paroxysmal nocturnal dyspnea or orthopnea increased venous pressure >6 cm
- Neck-vein distention
- Rales
- Cardiomegaly (circulation time >25 sec)
- Hepatojugular reflux
- Acute pulmonary edema
- S3 gallop

Minor criteria
- Ankle edema
- Night cough
- Dyspnea on exertion
- Pleural effusion
- Decreased vital capacity
- Sinus tachycardia (120 bpm or higher)

Major or minor criteria
- Weight loss >4.5 kg in five days in response to treatment
- Two major or one major and two minor

❏ PHYSICAL EXAMINATION

The presence of abnormal physical findings not only establishes the diagnosis but also provides clues regarding the etiology of heart failure. Elevated jugular venous pressure has a specificity of 97%, sensitivity of 10%, and a positive predictive value of 2% (Fig. 1).

Lower extremity edema has a specificity of 99%, sensitivity of 13%, and the positive predictive value of 6%. The S3 gallop sound in patients older than 45 years has a specificity of 95%, sensitivity of 31% and a positive predictive value of 61%. Thus, the presence of the S3 gallop sound has a significant diagnostic relevance. The S3 gallop sound is associated with increased left ventricular end-diastolic pressure, and increased levels of B-type natriuretic peptide (BNP).

A gallop rhythm almost always indicates heart failure with reduced ejection fraction (HFREF) due to dilated cardiomyopathy with increased end-systolic and end-diastolic volumes and end-diastolic pressure. Presence of pulsus alternans is diagnostic of systolic heart failure (HFREF) (Fig. 2). Similarly, a positive

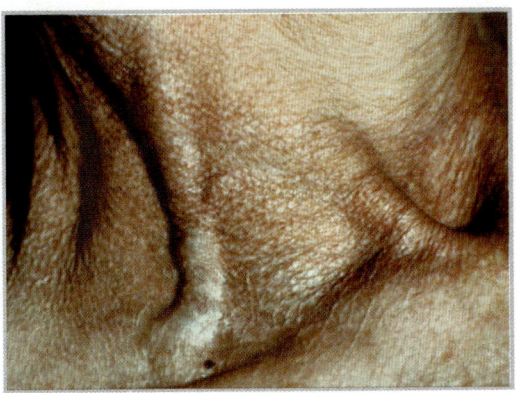

FIGURE 1: Distended right external and internal jugular veins in a patient with heart failure

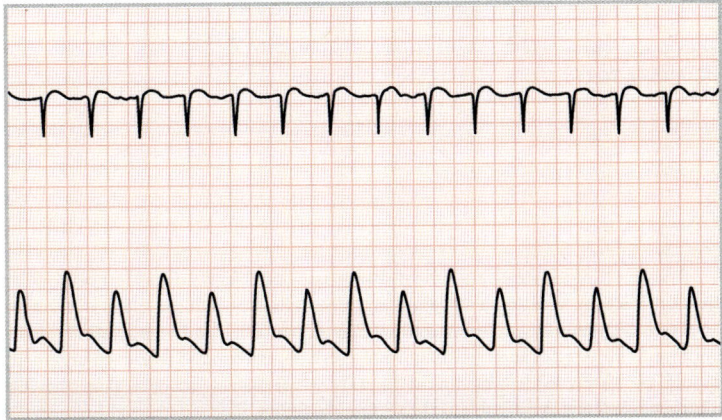

FIGURE 2: Direct arterial pressure recording showing pulsus alternans in a patient with systolic heart failure (HFREF)

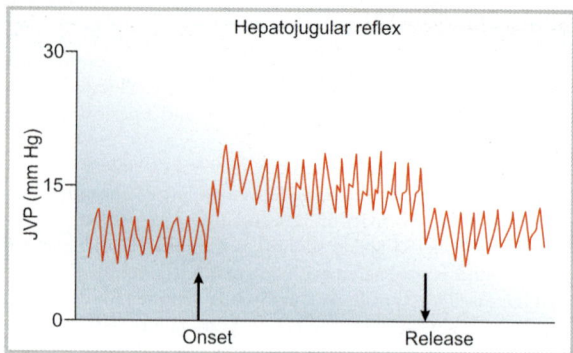

FIGURE 3: Schematic illustration of positive hepatojugular reflux which usually indicates systolic heart failure (HFREF) (*Source:* Published with permission from Ewy GA. Ann Intern Med. 1998;109:456)

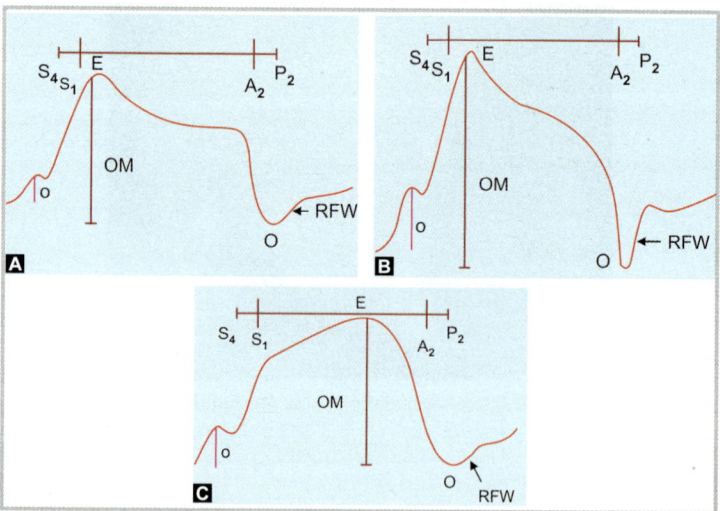

FIGURES 4A TO C: Schematic illustrations of a normal (A), hyperdynamic (B), and sustained (C) left ventricular apical impulse. (Abbreviations: OM: Outward movement; A2: Aortic component of the second heart sound; P2: Pulmonic component of the second heart sound; O: Opening of the mitral valve; RFW: Rapid filling wave; A: A wave; S1: First heart sound; S4: Fourth heart sound; E: E point). The illustrations represent apex cardiogram

hepatojugular reflux is also very suggestive of systolic heart failure (HFREF) (Fig. 3).

A normal apical impulse is almost always associated with normal left ventricular ejection fraction, whereas a sustained impulse indicates reduced ejection fraction or severe left ventricular hypertrophy (Figs 4A to C). The hyperdynamic apical impulse is also associated with normal ejection fraction. Cardiac enlargement should be suspected if the apical impulse is displaced laterally past the left midclavicular line. A palpable right ventricular heave (left parasternal lift) usually indicates right ventricular failure and may be present in patients with advanced heart failure.

Table 2: New York Heart Association functional classification

1. No limitations on physical activity, no symptoms with ordinary activities
2. Slight limitation, symptoms with ordinary activities
3. Marked limitation, symptoms with less than ordinary activities
4. Severe limitation, symptoms of heart failure at rest

Symptoms: Fatigue, dyspnea, palpitations, or angina

Table 3: Heart failure: new classification not based on the severity of symptoms

Stage A: At high risk for HF but without structural heart disease or symptoms of HF
Stage B: Structural heart disease but without symptoms of HF
Stage C: Structural heart disease with prior or current symptoms of HF
Stage D: Refractory HF requiring specialized interventions

Table 4: A few causes of "giant T wave" inversions are summarized

- Intermittent left bundle branch block
- Post-pacing T wave changes (cardiac memory, Chatterjee syndrome)
- Post ablation of accessory pathway
- Subarachnoid hemorrhage
- Apical hypertrophic cardiomyopathy
- Hypertrophic obstructive cardiomyopathy
- Markedly prolonged QT
- Post Stokes–Adams–Morganni syndrome
- Post-right coronary artery contrast injection

The signs of pulmonary arterial hypertension, such as an increased intensity of the pulmonic component of the second heart sound (P2), may be detected during auscultation. It can be present both in patients with systolic or diastolic heart failure. Auscultatory signs of mitral regurgitation, when detected, usually indicate systolic heart failure. Tricuspid regurgitation is usually secondary to pulmonary hypertension and may be present both in systolic and diastolic heart failure.

During clinical evaluation, it is highly desirable to assess the severity of symptoms and the stages of heart failure. To assess the functional class, the New York Heart Association (NYHA) classification is used (Table 2). Determination of functional class is important to assess prognosis. For the diagnosis of the potential etiology and the stages of heart failure the recommendations in the ACC/AHA guidelines are employed (Table 3).

❏ ELECTROCARDIOGRAM

The characteristic electrocardiographic features in this condition are large QRS voltage in the lateral precordial leads with deep T wave inversions (giant T wave inversions). It should be appreciated that heart failure is much less common in apical hypertrophic cardiomyopathy than in hypertrophic obstructive cardiomyopathy. Giant T wave inversions may also be observed in hypertrophic obstructive cardiomyopathy. The causes of giant T wave inversions are summarized in Table 4.

An electrocardiogram should be obtained in all patients. It may reveal arrhythmias, evidence of previous myocardial infarction (Fig. 5), and left ventricular hypertrophy (Figs 6 and 7).

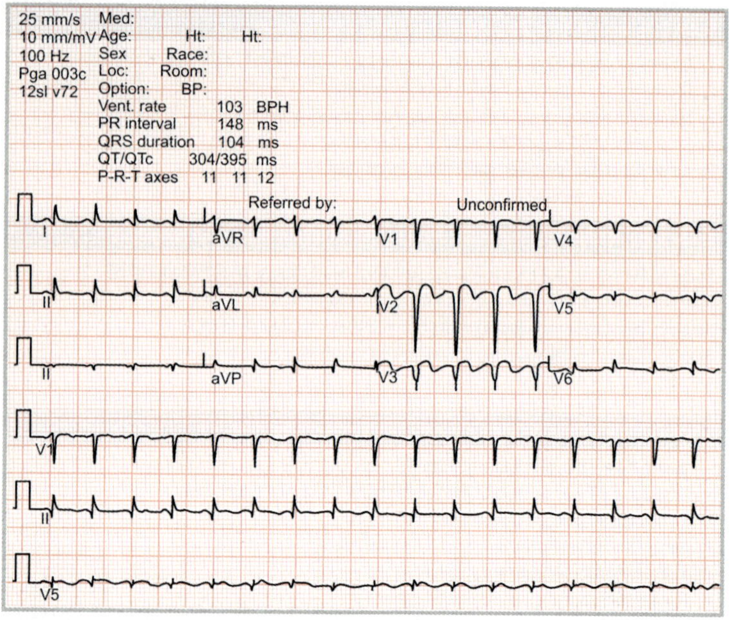

504 Manual of Cardiology

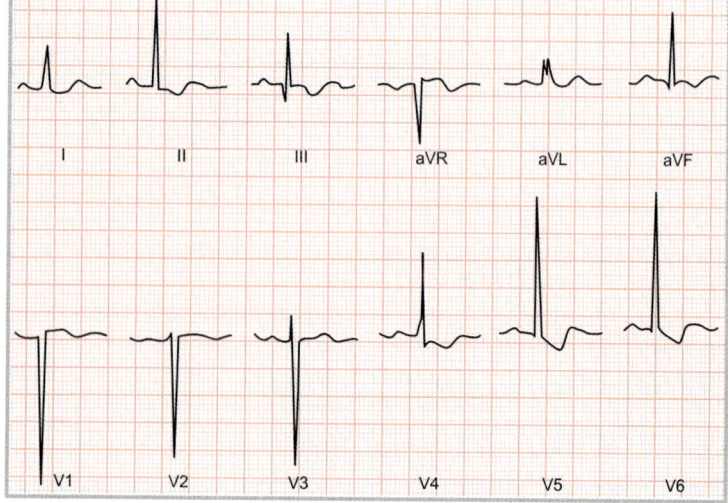

FIGURE 5: The electrocardiographic features of chronic left ventricular aneurysm are illustrated. Anterolateral myocardial infarction with Q waves in leads V2–V6 with persistent ST segments elevations are present. Localized slurring of QRS in V5 lead suggests periinfarction block of "GRANT"

FIGURE 6: The electrocardiographic features of concentric left ventricular hypertrophy are illustrated. Left ventricular hypertrophy with repolarization abnormalities and normal frontal plane QRS axis are evident

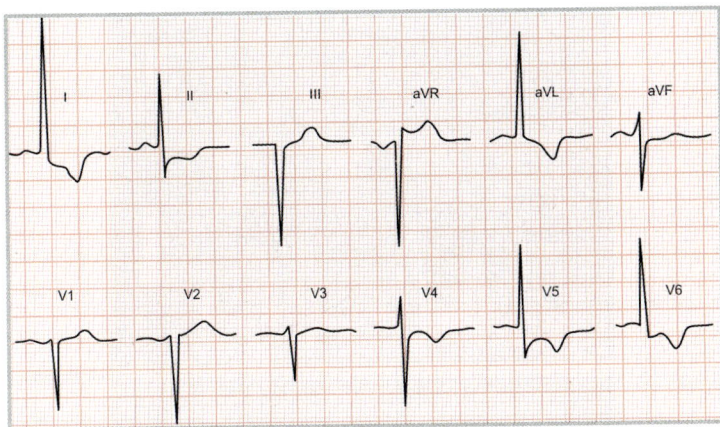

FIGURE 7: The electrocardiographic features of eccentric left ventricular hypertrophy are illustrated. Left ventricular hypertrophy with repolarization changes and left axis deviation of QRS complex are evident

❑ CHEST RADIOGRAPH

The diagnosis of heart failure can be established if the radiologic findings of hemodynamic pulmonary edema are present. However, even in patients with decompensated chronic heart failure, the chest radiograph may be normal. The radiologic findings of hemodynamic pulmonary edema, such as prominent upper lobe vessels, perihilar haziness and Kerley's B lines, may be absent.

❑ ECHOCARDIOGRAPHY

The guidelines recommend that echocardiography is appropriate for evaluation of cardiac dyspnea and other symptoms of heart failure. Echocardiography is useful to distinguish between systolic and diastolic heart failure. In systolic heart failure left ventricle is dilated, end-diastolic and end systolic volumes are increased and the ejection fraction is reduced (Fig. 8). An ejection fraction of less than 45% by echocardiography is used for the diagnosis of systolic heart failure. Left ventricular ejection fraction of 45% or greater is used for the diagnosis of diastolic heart failure. In diastolic heart failure left ventricular size is normal and its wall thickness is increased (Fig. 9). Atrial enlargements can be present in both systolic and diastolic heart failure.

Doppler echocardiography is essential to assess left ventricular diastolic function. An early left ventricular diastolic dysfunction is characterized by a decrease in peak transmitral E-velocity, an increase in atrial-induced A-velocity and a decrease in E/A ratio. The early abnormal filling pattern is related to impaired left ventricular relaxation. In patients with advanced heart failure, the "restrictive filling pattern" is observed. A marked increase in E/A ratio with a short E deceleration time is the major Doppler echocardiographic features of "restrictive filling pattern" (Fig. 10). The abbreviated duration of E wave velocity is related to elevated left ventricular end-systolic pressure and a rapid decrease in the transmitral pressure gradient during left ventricular filling. The moderate left ventricular diastolic dysfunction is characterized by normal E/A ratio—"the pseudo-normalized filling pattern."

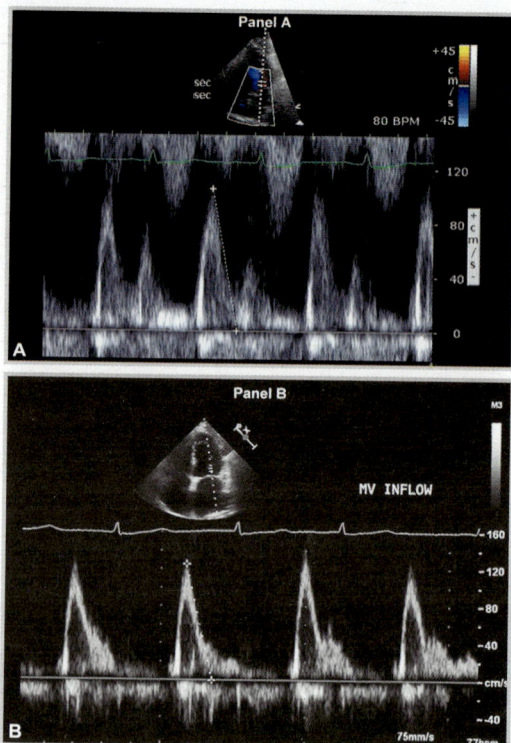

FIGURE 8: Transthoracic echocardiogram of a patient with systolic heart failure due to dilated cardiomyopathy (Panel A and B). The left ventricle is dilated and its wall appears thinner than normal

This pattern can be distinguished from normal filling pattern by demonstrating the reduced E-velocity by Tissue Doppler Imaging. It should be appreciated that the abnormal left ventricular transmitral filling patterns can be present in both systolic and diastolic heart failure.

❏ CARDIAC MAGNETIC RESONANCE AND CARDIAC TOMOGRAPHY

Cardiac magnetic resonance (CMR) imaging can also be used to assess left ventricular volumes and ejection fraction (Fig. 11). In patients with systolic and diastolic heart failure the left ventricular volumes, size and ejection fraction can be determined by CMR. With the use of contrast agents, such as gadolinium the other morphologic changes such as left ventricular mass and magnitude of fibrosis can be more accurately assessed by this technique.

The electron beam computed tomography (EBCT) is useful for the diagnosis of presence of coronary artery calcium. A high coronary calcium score is associated with a greater likelihood of atherosclerotic coronary artery disease. The contrast enhanced multislice computed tomographic coronary angiography is being increasingly used not only for detection of presence of coronary artery disease

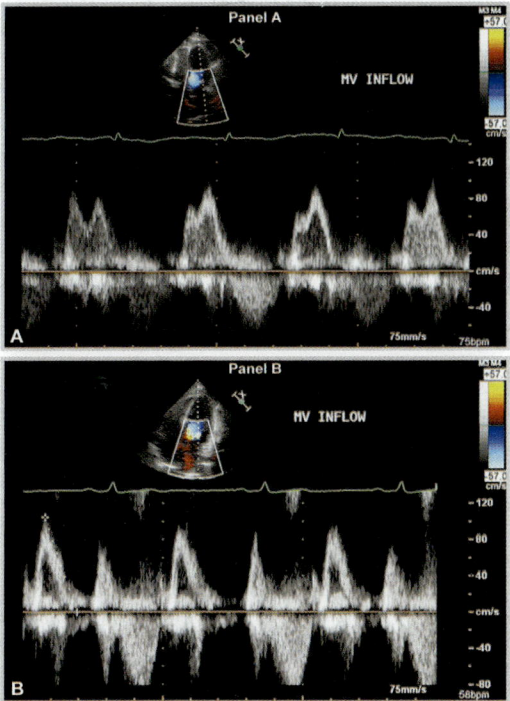

FIGURE 9: Transthoracic echocardiogram of a patient with diastolic heart failure is illustrated. The left ventricular cavity size is normal and its wall thickness is increased. Doppler echocardiographs show dominant "A" wave. Panel B shows normal transmitral flow pattern

but also for diagnosis of ischemic and nonischemic dilated cardiomyopathy. The contrast CT can be used for distinguishing between restrictive cardiomyopathy and constrictive pericarditis (Fig. 12).

❏ BIOMARKERS

A number of biomarkers can be elevated in heart failure (Table 5). Natriuretic peptide serum levels, particularly of BNP or its counterpart aminoterminal pro-B-type natriuretic peptide (NT-proBNP), should be determined in all patients with suspected or established heart failure. The measurement of serum BNP and NT-proBNP is most useful in distinguishing between cardiac and non-cardiac dyspnea. The levels of serum concentration of BNP are directly related to the severity of congestive heart failure. Both in males and females, the BNP levels progressively increase with the increasing severity of NYHA functional class (Fig. 13).

Troponins I and T are cardiac specific regulatory proteins. After myocardial damage they are released into circulation and their levels can be detected within 3–12 hours of myocardial injury. Troponins are released in patients with chronic heart failure even in absence of coronary artery disease. Troponins are also elevated

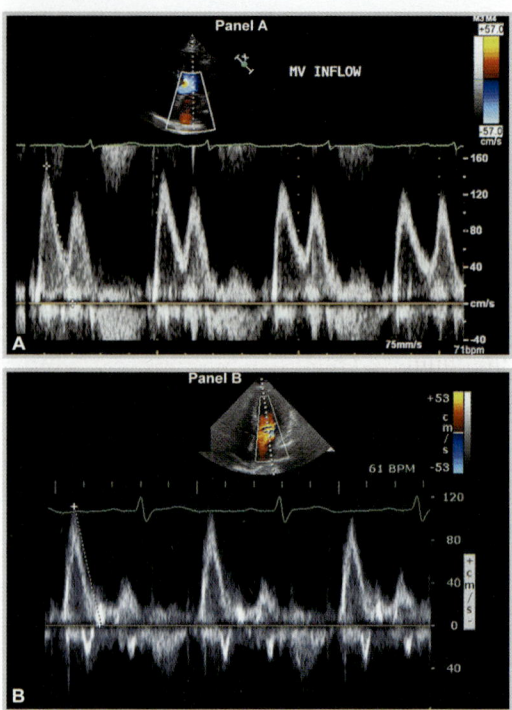

FIGURE 10: Doppler echocardiography of a patient with systolic heart failure. It shows pseudonormalization of transmitral flow pattern

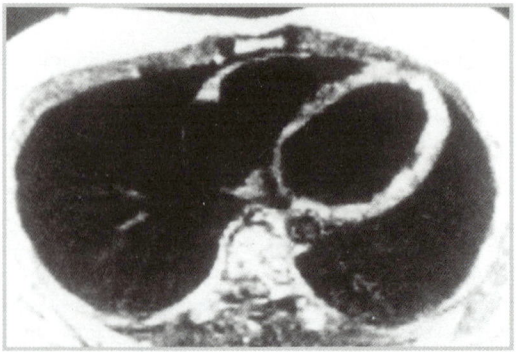

FIGURE 11: Cardiac magnetic resonance image of a patient with systolic heart failure. The left ventricle is dilated and its wall is thin

in patients with acute decompensated heart failure. Myocyte damage is the principal mechanism for the elevated troponins in heart failure.

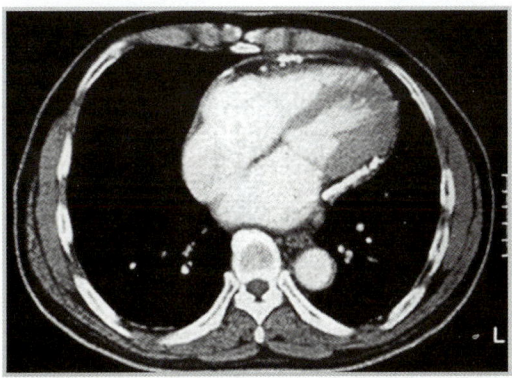

FIGURE 12: Computed tomographic image of a patient with constrictive pericarditis. The calcium in the pericardium is evident

Table 5: Biomarkers in heart failure

Neurohormones
- Natriuretic peptides (ANP, BNP, CNP)
- Plasma renins and angiotensins
- Catecholamines
- Endothelins
- Arginine vasopressins
- Adrenomedullin

Cardiac injury biomarkers
- Troponins
- Heart-type fatty acid binding protein
- Apoptotic protein
- Growth differentiating factor-15

Inflammatory markers
- Tumor necrosis factor-alpha
- C-reactive protein

Matrix remodeling markers
- Matrix metalloproteinases
- Tissue inhibitors of metalloproteinases
- Telopeptides and propeptides of collagen types I and III
- Galectin

Oxidative stress markers
- Oxidized low-density lipoproteins
- Myeloperoxidase
- Plasma malondialdehyde
- Serum uric acid

Although a large number of biomarkers are elevated in heart failure, for its diagnosis, only measurement of BNP or NT-proBNP is necessary. The ACC/AHA guidelines for indications of measurement of natriuretic peptides are summarized in Table 6.

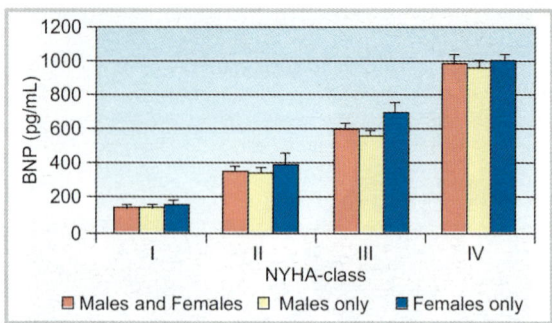

FIGURE 13: The relations between BNP levels and the severity of heart failure. Both in men and women, BNP levels increase with increasing NYHA class (*Source:* Modified from Maisel AS et al. N Engl J Med. 2002;347:161-7)

Table 6: ACC/AHA and HFSA guidelines on the use of natriuretic peptide measurement in patients with heart failure	
ACC/AHA 2009 Heart Failure Guideline Update	**HFSA 2006 Practice Guideline: Acute Heart Failure Diagnosis**
Measurement of natriuretic peptides [B-type natriuretic peptide (BNP) and NT-proBNP] can be useful in the evaluation of patients presenting the urgent care setting in whom the clinical diagnosis of heart failure is uncertain. Measurement of natriuretic peptides (BNP and NT-proBNP) can be helpful in risk stratification (Level of evidence: A)	The diagnosis of decompensated heart failure should be based primarily on signs and symptoms (Level of evidence: C)
The value of serial measurements of BNP to guide therapy for patients with heart failure is not well established.	When the diagnosis is uncertain, determination of plasma BNP or NT-proBNIP concentration should be considered in patients being evaluated for dyspnea who have signs and symptoms compatible with HF (Level of evidence: A)

❑ EXERCISE TESTS AND SIX-MINUTE WALK TEST

Reduced exercise tolerance is one of the major symptoms of heart failure. Although exercise tests are not necessary for the diagnosis of heart failure, they are useful to assess the functional class and prognosis. The NYHA classification is most frequently used to determine the functional class (Table 6). The prognosis is worse in class IV patients than in patients in classes II and III.

The six-minute walk test measures the total distance that a patient can walk on the level surface with their maximal capacity in six minutes. This test is most applicable to distinguish between patients with NYHA classes III and IV heart failure. It correlates well with the NYHA functional class for the assessment of prognosis but correlates less well, with VO_2 particularly in patients in the NYHA functional Classes I and II. It should be appreciated that exercise test is not essential for the diagnosis of heart failure, but it is useful to assess the exercise capacity and prognosis.

❏ MYOCARDIAL ISCHEMIA

In patients with heart failure, with known or suspected coronary artery disease presence of myocardial ischemia should be assessed. Many noninvasive imaging techniques are available for the detection of myocardial ischemia, which includes pharmacologic or exercise stress thallium or Tc-99m sestamibi tomographic perfusion imaging (Fig. 14), and positron emission tomography (Fig. 15). Cardiac

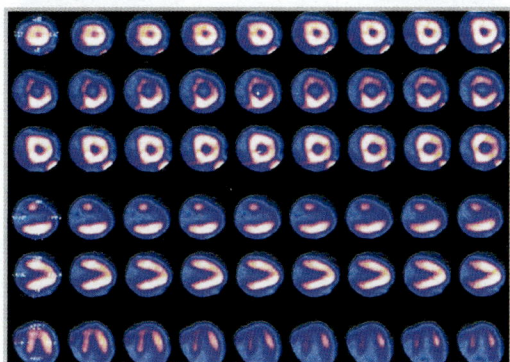

FIGURE 14: Gated perfusion single photon emission computed tomography dual isotope imaging using thallium-201 (rest, even rows) technetium-99m sestamibi (stress-related, odd rows) to detect the presence and extent of ischemic myocardium. The first four rows from the top show short axis slices from apex (left) to base (right). Rows 5 and 6 show vertical long axis slices from septum (left) to lateral wall (right) and rows 7 and 8 show horizontal long axis slices from inferior wall (left) to anterior wall (right). A large reversible perfusion defect in the anterolateral wall of the left ventricle (left anterior descending coronary artery territory) is evident, indicating the presence of ischemic myocardium (*Source:* Dr Eli Botvinick, University of California/San Francisco)

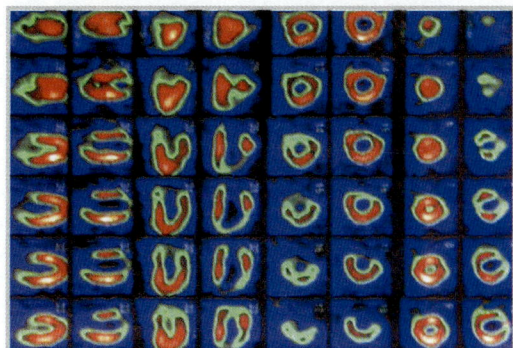

FIGURE 15: Radionuclide (scintigraphic) evaluation of the presence of ischemic but viable myocardium by positron emission tomography (PET) is illustrated. Short axis slices (rows 1–4), vertical long axis slices (rows 5 and 6), and horizontal long axis slices (rows 7 and 8) are shown. The resting perfusion images with rubidium-82 (rows 1, 3, 5 and 7) demonstrate a large lateral perfusion defect, but other areas take up rudium-82 indicating that these myocardial segments are perfused and viable. The fluorodeoxyglucose images (rows 2, 4, 6 and 8) show complementary uptake which indicates active myocardial metabolism and thus viability. (*Source:* Dr Eli Botvinick, University of California/San Francisco)

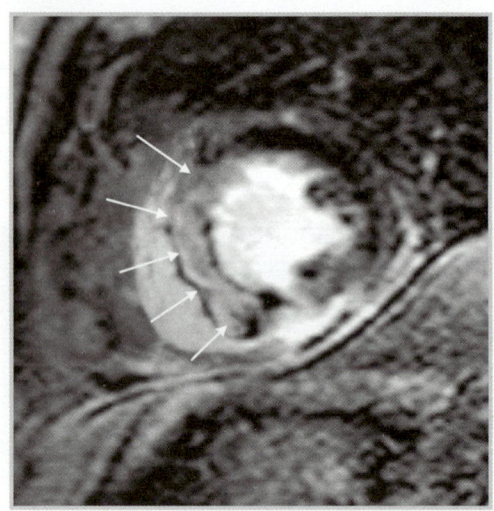

FIGURE 16: Cardiac magnetic resonance imaging with the use of the contrast gadolinium in a patient with heart failure is illustrated. The delayed enhancement image shows area of myocardial fibrosis (arrows)

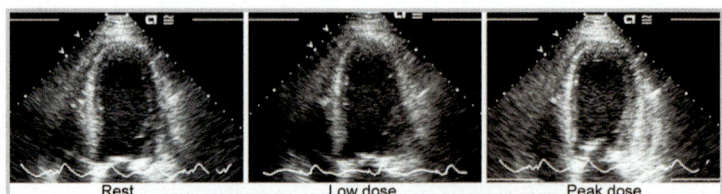

FIGURE 17: Dobutamine stress echocardiogram in a patient with systolic heart failure is illustrated. With the low dose of dobutamine there was thickening of the anteroapical segment of left ventricle. With larger doses, there was thinning of the same segments

magnetic resonance imaging (CMRI) with the use of contrast agent, such as gadolinium, can demonstrate myocardial fibrosis (Fig. 16). Dobutamine stress echocardiography can be used for the diagnosis of myocardial ischemia (Fig. 17).

❑ GENETIC STUDIES

The guidelines recommend genetic evaluation in patients with suspected nonischemic dilated cardiomyopathy. It should include obtaining careful family history of the patient, screening family members, genetic counseling, and genetic testing.

Approximately mutations of 30 genes have been identified in patients with familial dilated cardiomyopathy. However, it remains unclear whether genetic studies provide any benefit in the management of these patients. In clinical practice routine genetic studies are not necessary.

❏ SUGGESTED READINGS

Bellenger NG, Davies LC, Francis JM, et al. Reduction in sample size for studies of remodeling in heart failure by the use of cardiovascular magnetic resonance. J Cardiovasc Magn Reson. 2000;2:271-8.

Douglas PS, Khandheria B, Stainback RF, et al. ACCF/ASE/ASNC/ SCAI/SCCT/SCMR 2007 appropriateness criteria for transthoracic and transesophageal echocardiography: a report of the American college of cardiology foundation quality strategic directions committee criteria working group, American society of echocardiography, American college of emergency physicians, American society of nuclear cardiology, society of cardiovascular computed tomography and the society for cardiovascular magnetic resonance endorsed by the American college of chest physicians and the society of critical care medicine. J Am Coll Cardiol. 2007;50:187-204.

Harlan WR, Oberman A, Grimm R, et al. Chronic congestive heart failure in coronary artery disease: clinical criteria. Ann Intern Med. 1977;86:133-8.

Hershberger RE, Lindenfeld J, Mestroni L, et al. Genetic evaluation of cardiomyopathy: a Heart Failure Society of America practice guideline. J Card Fail. 2009;15:83-97.

Maisel AS, Krishnaswamy P, Nowak RM, et al. Rapid measurement of B-type natriuretic peptide in the emergency diagnosis of heart failure. N Eng J Med. 2002;347:161-7.

Marcus GM, Michaels AD, De Marco T, et al. Usefulness of the third heart sound in predicting an elevated level of B-type natriuretic peptide. Am J Cardiol. 2004;3:1312-3.

Masson S, Latini R, Anand IS. An update on cardiac troponins as circulating biomarkers in heart failure. Curr Heart Fail Rep. 2010;7:15-21.

McKee PA, Castelli WP, McNamara PM, et al. The natural history of congestive heart failure: the Framingham study. N Engl J Med. 1971;285:1441-6.

Nagarajan V, Tang WH. Biomarkers in advanced heart failure: diagnosis and therapeutic insights. Congestive Heart Failure. 2011;17:169-74.

7.2 Systolic Heart Failure (Heart Failure with Reduced Ejection Fraction)

❏ INTRODUCTION

The clinical definition of systolic heart failure is a "syndrome which results from reduced left ventricular ejection fraction". It should be appreciated that ejection fraction is not independent of loading conditions. A markedly reduced preload and increased afterload is associated with reduced ejection fraction without any changes in contractile function. A number of risk factors for developing systolic heart failure have been identified (Table 7).

Table 7 Risk factors for developing systolic heart failure
Hypertension
Coronary artery disease
Diabetes
Insulin resistance
Smoking
Cardiotoxins
Family history of cardiomyopathy

❏ VENTRICULAR REMODELING

In systolic heart failure, the left ventricle is dilated and becomes more spherical. This altered shape and geometry is the principal mechanism for secondary mitral regurgitation without any structural changes of the mitral valve leaflets. The left ventricular wall thickness either remains unchanged or decrease compared to normal controls (Fig. 18). The left ventricular cavity size is substantially increased. As a result, left ventricular wall stress is increased, which contributes to reduced ejection fraction. There is an inverse relation between wall stress and ejection fraction.

Both end-diastolic and end-systolic volumes are increased, but there is a greater increase in end-systolic than in end-diastolic volumes which is contributory to reduced ejection fraction. In systolic heart failure left ventricular hypertrophy is eccentric. The echocardiographic left ventricular volumes, ejection fraction and mass in patients with systolic heart failure compared to normal controls are summarized in Table 8. Some of the features of left ventricular remodeling in systolic heart failure are summarized in Table 9. The cellular and molecular changes in systolic heart failure are summarized in Table 10.

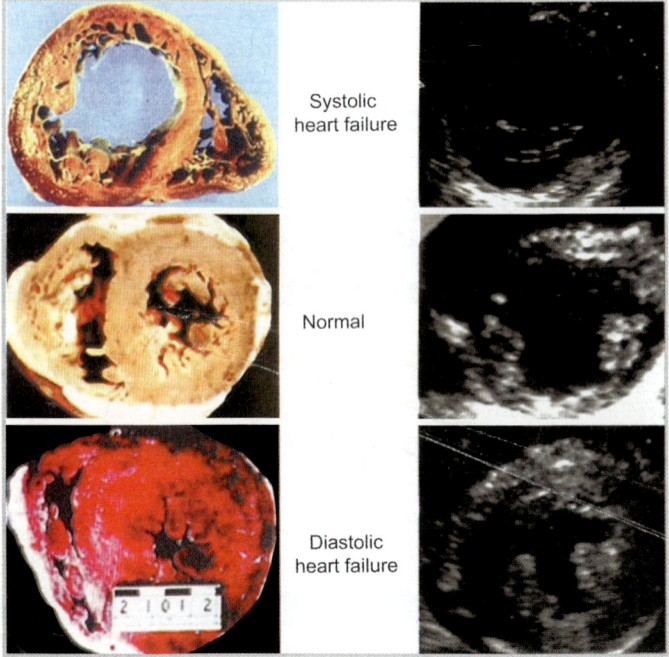

FIGURE 18: The left hand panel illustrates the transverse sections of the heart in a heart and in severe systolic heart failure, with diastolic heart failure. In the right hand panel two-dimensional echocardiographic cross-sectional views of the heart are shown. Compared to normal, in systolic heart failure, the left ventricle is dilated and spherical. The wall thickness is not increased. In diastolic heart failure, the left ventricular cavity is smaller than normal, and the left ventricular wall thickness is markedly increased (*Source:* MA Konstam. JCF. 2003;9:1-3)

Table 8: Systolic heart failure

	Controls	SHF
LVEDV	102	192
LVESV	46	137
LVEF	54	31
LVM	125	230
LVM/V	1.49	1.22

(Abbreviations: LVEDV: Left ventricular diastolic volume; LVESV: Left ventricular end systolic volume; LVEF: Left ventricular ejection fraction; LVM: Left ventricular mass; LVM/V: Left ventricular mass/volume ratio)

Table 9: Systolic heart failure remodeling

- Usually eccentric hypertrophy
- Disproportionate increase in ventricular cavity size
- Increased ventricular mass
- Cavity/mass ratio increased
- Wall thickness—decreased or unchanged
- Increased wall stress
- Reduced ejection fraction
- Altered ventricular shape and geometry
- Frequent mechanical dyssynchrony with or without electrical dyssynchrony

Table 10: Systolic heart failure

Myocyte	
Hypertrophy	+
Apoptosis	+
Necrosis	+
Fibrosis	+
Ca Regulation	−
MMPs/TIMPs	+
Collagen	
Cross-links	−
Titin isoforms	
N2BA/N2B	+

+: Increased; −: Decreased
(Abbreviations: Ca: Calcium; MMPs: Matrix metalloproteinases; TIMPs: Tissue inhibitors of metalloproteinases)

Neurohormonal activation has been shown to be a major contributing mechanism for progression of heart failure. In systolic heart failure plasma levels of many neurohormones are elevated. Moreover, if there is more activation of neurohormones with the potential to produce adverse remodeling, progression of heart failure occurs (Table 11).

The adverse vascular and cardiac effects of angiotensin are mediated by activation of angiotensin subtype 1 (AT1) receptors. Activation of angiotensin subtype 2

Table 11: Adverse effects of neurohormonal activation

- Adverse hemodynamic effects
- Vascular remodeling
- Ventricular remodeling
  - Myocyte hypertrophy
  - Extracellular matrix changes
- Promotes atherothrombosis
- Increased oxidative stress
- Endothelial dysfunction
- Myocardial necrosis
- Apoptosis

Table 12: Arginine vasopressin (AVP) in heart failure

AVP* is a nonapeptide secreted from the posterior pituitary gland
- Stimuli for secretion
  - A decrease in blood pressure
  - A reduction in circulating blood volume
  - Arterial underfilling
  - A rise in plasma osmolality
- Activation of V_{1a} receptors
  - Vascular bed
    - Systemic arterial vasoconstriction
    - Increased SVR, increased LV afterload
    - Systemic venoconstriction—increased preload
    - Coronary vasoconstriction—myocardial ischemia
  - Myocardium
    - Myocyte hypertrophy
- Activation of V_{1b} receptors (anterior pituitary)
  - Increased release of ACTH
  - Increased release of aldosterone
    - Adverse vascular remodeling
    - Myocardial hypertrophy and fibrosis
    - Impaired renal water and sodium excretion
- Activation of V_2 receptors in renal collecting ducts and distal tubule
  - Activation of water channel aquaporin-2
  - Decreased water permeability in collecting duct
  - Increased water retention
  - Volume overload
  - Hyponatremia

*Also known as antidiuretic hormone (ADH)

(AT2) receptors produce counter regulatory effects such as vasodilatation, decreased vascular smooth muscle cell proliferation and decreased myocardial hypertrophy. Both angiotensin I and angiotensin II can generate angiotensin (I-VII), which also cause vasodilatation and decrease growth. Endothelins are potent vasoconstrictors and are produced by vascular smooth muscle cells. Although its blood levels are increased in chronic systolic heart failure, the significance of increased endothelin remains uncertain.

The plasma arginine vasopressin levels are increased in patients with heart failure and the levels are higher in patients with symptomatic than in patients with asymptomatic left ventricular systolic dysfunction. The pathophysiologic effects of arginine vasopressin in heart failure are summarized in Table 12.

Table 13: Circulating catecholamines and hemodynamics in patients with and without heart failure (HF)

	Patients with HF (n = 63)	Patients without HF (n = 26)
Norepinephrine (pg/mL)	665 ± 510*	184 ± 135
Dopamine (pg/mL)	407 ± 405†	197 ± 259
Epinephrine (pg/mL)	73 ± 98^{NS}	55 ± 73
SWI (gm/m^2)	21 ± 9*	53 ± 13
PCWP (mm Hg)	27 ± 8*	11 ± 3

*p < .01
†p < .05

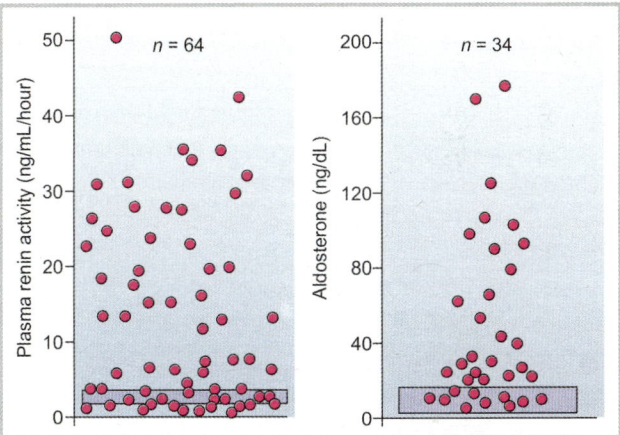

FIGURE 19: Changes in plasma rennin activity and aldosterone levels in patients with systolic heart failure are illustrated

In systolic heart failure, sympathoadrenergic activity is increased. The plasma levels of norepinephrine are substantially elevated (Table 13). The level of norepinephrine is higher in patients with more severe heart failure.

Aldosterone level is elevated in systolic heart failure (Fig. 19). Increased levels of aldosterone are associated with water and salt retention and worsening heart failure. There is increased loss of potassium and magnesium which is associated with increased risks of arrhythmia. The potential adverse effects of aldosterone are summarized in Table 11 (Fig. 20).

Activation of cytokines, such as tumor necrosis factor-alpha and interleukin-1, may be contributory to the progression of heart failure. These cytokines have the proinflammatory and prothrombotic properties, and they are also produced in the myocardium. They may cause direct toxic effects on the myocytes and cause myocyte necrosis and apoptosis. They also exert adverse effects on extracellular matrix and promote adverse ventricular remodeling. Increased levels of these cytokines may cause impairment of left ventricular function. However, that any beneficial effect of pharmacologic interventions to counteract the adverse effects of these inflammatory cytokines has not been documented.

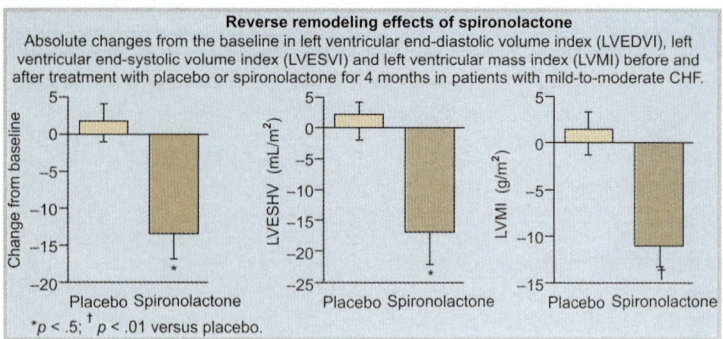

FIGURE 20: The effects of aldosterone on ventricular remodeling (*Source:* Modified from Tsutamoto, et al. J Am Coll Cardiol. 2001;37:1228-33)

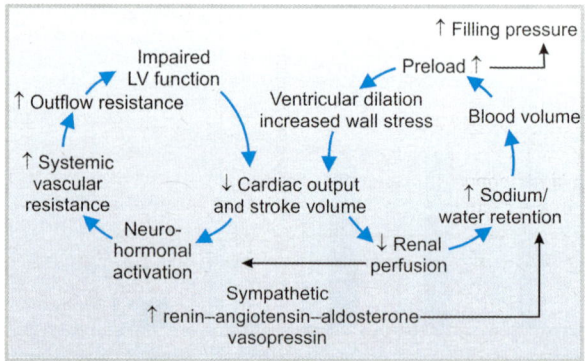

FIGURE 21: The vicious cycle of adverse left ventricular remodeling in systolic heart failure initiated by impaired systolic function is illustrated

The counterregulatory neurohormones are activated as a compensatory mechanism to reduce the risks of adverse left ventricular remodeling. The brain natriuretic peptides (B-type) and atrial natriuretic peptides are activated to counteract the deleterious effects of renin-angiotensin and adrenergic systems on ventricular and atrial remodeling. The natriuretic peptides decrease myocyte hypertrophy, fibrosis and collagen synthesis. Atrial natriuretic peptides decrease atrial remodeling and B-type natriuretic peptides reduce adverse ventricular remodeling. The vasodilator prostacyclins, nitric oxide, and endogenous antioxidants are increased in heart failure, and they have the potential for decreasing adverse ventricular remodeling. The other neurohormones, such as adrenomedullin, which also has the potential to reduce progression of heart failure, have not been adequately investigated.

The impaired left ventricular systolic function can establish a vicious cycle of adverse remodeling (Fig. 21).

The ischemic heart disease is the most common cause of systolic heart failure. In acute coronary syndromes, ventricular remodeling is initiated soon after the

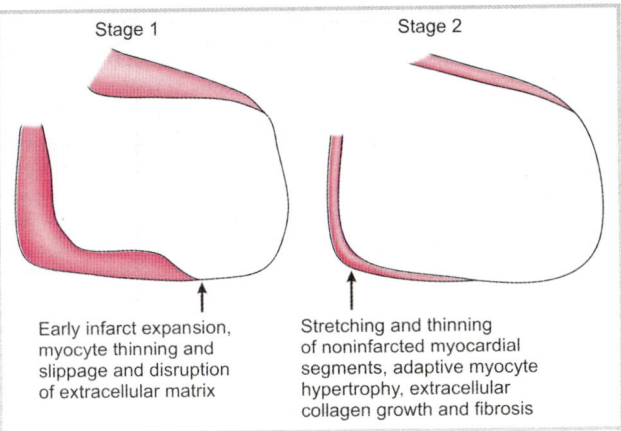

FIGURE 22: Schematic illustrations of left ventricular remodeling soon after acute myocardial infarction (stage 1) and late after myocardial infarction (stage 2) are shown

onset of myocardial infarction. The features of the postinfarction left ventricular remodeling are illustrated in Figure 22.

It should be appreciated that the adverse left ventricular remodeling can occur despite adequate recanalization of the infarct related artery but a threshold magnitude of myocardium needs to be damaged. It is uncommon for the adverse remodeling to occur, if the left ventricular ejection fraction is greater than 40%, and the infarct size is relatively small.

❏ FUNCTIONAL DERANGEMENTS AND HEMODYNAMIC CONSEQUENCES

The principal myocardial dysfunction in systolic heart failure is impaired left ventricular contractility. The analysis of left ventricular pressure volume loop demonstrates a rightward and downward shift of the left ventricular end-systolic pressure volume line indicating reduced contractile function. The stroke volume declines, and there is an increase in end-systolic and end-diastolic volumes. With a further deterioration of ventricular function; however, stroke volume declines and there is an increase in residual volumes. The increase in left ventricular volume is associated with increased wall stress (afterload), which causes further impairment of left ventricular systolic function.

The hemodynamic consequences of impaired pump function in systolic heart failure are characterized by decreased stroke volume and cardiac output and increased left ventricular diastolic pressure. There is a passive increase in left atrial and pulmonary venous pressures which is associated with increased pulmonary artery pressure. The pulmonary arterial hypertension is predominantly post capillary. However, in chronic severe systolic heart failure, there is also an increase in pulmonary vascular resistance. This mixed type of pulmonary arterial hypertension increases right ventricular afterload and induce right ventricular failure. Thus there is an increase in systemic venous pressure with its hemodynamic consequences such as lower extremity edema.

❏ INITIAL TREATMENT OF SYSTOLIC HEART FAILURE

Except age and gender, the other risk factors are modifiable and every effort should be made to treat these risk factors (Table 14). The patients in stage B have structural heart disease and have asymptomatic left ventricular systolic dysfunction. In time, these asymptomatic patients develop overt heart failure. The rate of development of symptomatic heart failure in untreated patients is approximately 10% per year.

Large clinical trials have demonstrated that treatment with angiotensin-converting enzyme inhibitors in these patients is associated with decreased cardiovascular mortality and morbidity. The beta-blocker therapy also decreases morbidity and mortality in patients with acute coronary syndromes irrespective of the symptomatic and functional status (CAPTICORN trial).

The treatment with aldosterone antagonist in post-infarction patients is also associated with decreased risks of developing heart failure, cardiovascular mortality, sudden cardiac death and ventricular remodeling (EPHESUS trial). The treatment of the risk factors for developing heart failure such as management of hypertension, diabetes and obesity are similar to those in patients in stage A heart failure (Table 15).

The controlled studies have reported that adequate treatment of hypertension is associated with approximately 50% reduction of the risks of developing new heart failure. For the treatment of hypertension, the use of angiotensin-converting enzyme inhibitors or angiotensin receptor blocking agents are preferable to alpha adrenergic blocking agents for reduction of the risk of development of heart failure. In patients with diabetes with or without hypertension, treatments with angiotensin-converting enzyme inhibitors or angiotensin receptor blocking agents should be considered not only to reduce the risk of end organ damage but also to reduce the risk of development of heart failure. The metabolic syndrome is associated with increased risk of developing heart failure. Hyperlipidemia is one of the major risk factors of atherosclerotic vascular disease. In patients with history of myocardial infarction, adequate control of lipids particularly with the

Table 14: Systolic heart failure management

- Stage A—treat hypertension
    - Encourage smoking cessation
    - Treat lipid disorders
    - Encourage regular exercise
    - Discourage alcohol abuse
    - Discourage illicit drug use
    - Angiotensin inhibition in appropriate patients
- Stage B—treatment for stage A
- Angiotensin inhibition in appropriate patients
- Beta-blockers in appropriate patients

Table 15: Systolic heart failure stage C

- Angiotensin inhibition therapy
- Adrenergic blocking agents
- Aldosterone antagonists in severe heart failure
- Hydralazine-isosorbide dinitrate, in self-reported blacks
- Diuretics to relieve congestive symptoms
- Digitalis in selected patients
- Treatments for stage A

use of "statins" has the potential to decrease the risk of death and development of heart failure. There is controversy regarding the use of aspirin concurrently with angiotensin-converting enzyme inhibitors.

❏ SYMPTOMATIC SYSTOLIC HEART FAILURE

Pharmacologic Treatments

In patients in stage C heart failure, angiotensin-converting enzyme inhibitors or angiotensin receptor blocking agents and beta-blocking agents are indicated. These therapies have been documented not only to ameliorate symptoms but also to improve morbidity and mortality (Figs 23 and 24) (Table 11). The use of angiotensin-converting enzyme inhibitors is associated with reverse ventricular remodeling, improved ventricular function and decrease in morbidity and mortality. The commonly used angiotensin inhibitors and their doses are summarized in Table 16.

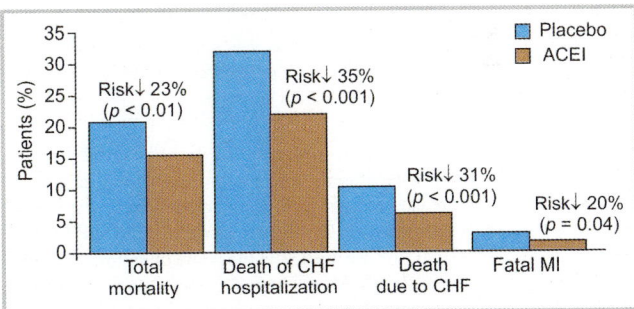

FIGURE 23: The effects of angiotensin-converting enzyme inhibitors on the mortality and morbidity of patients with systolic heart failure are illustrated. Compared to placebo there is a reduction in total mortality, death or hospitalizations for heart failure, death due to heart failure and fatal myocardial infarction (Abbreviations: ACEI: Angiotensin-converting enzyme inhibitor; MI: Myocardial infarction). (*Source:* Modified from Garg, et al. JAMA. 1995;273:1450-6)

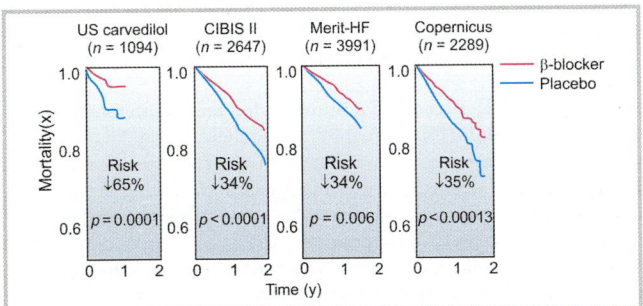

FIGURE 24: The mortality benefit of beta-blocker treatment in the United States. Carvedilol, MERIT-HF, CIBIS-II and COPERNICUS trials are illustrated (Abbreviations: CIBIS: Cardiac insufficiency bisoprolol study; MERIT-HF: Metoprolol CR/XL randomized intervention trial in congestive heart failure; COPERNICUS: Carvedilol prospective randomized cumulative survival trial)

Table 16: Angiotensin inhibitors used in the treatment of heart failure

Agent	Total daily dose (mg)	Frequency
ACEI		
Captopril	75–150	Thrice daily
Enalapril	10–40	Twice daily
Fosinopril	10–40	Once daily
Lisinopril	10–40	Once daily
Quinapril	10–40	Once or twice daily
Ramipril	2.5–20	Once or twice daily
Trandolapril	1–4	Once daily
ARB		
Losartan	25–50	Twice daily
Valsartan	150–300	Once daily
Candesartan	4–16	Once daily

(Abbreviations: ACEI: Angiotensin-converting enzyme inhibitor; ARB: Angiotensin receptor blocking agent)

In patients intolerant to angiotensin-converting enzyme inhibitors or with contraindications for their use, angiotensin receptor blocking agents should be considered. The angiotensin receptor blocking agents exert their beneficial effects by blockade of the angiotensin II receptor subtype I and the angiotensin-converting enzyme pathway is not involved. The blockade of angiotensin receptors is associated with increased levels of angiotensin-converting enzyme due to activation of the negative feedback loop.

The rational of beta-blocker therapy in systolic heart failure is to decrease the adverse effects of increased adrenergic activity. It should be appreciated that initially with introduction of beta-blocker therapy there may be deterioration of hemodynamics, and left ventricular function due to decrease in the contractile function. However, usually in 6–8 weeks, there is improvement in symptoms and left ventricular function. Several prospective randomized trials have documented symptomatic improvement and prognosis with beta-blocker therapy (Fig. 24)

The aldosterone receptor antagonists spironolactone and eplerenone are effective in producing left ventricular reverse remodeling and improving prognosis of patients with systolic heart failure.

The angiotensin II is the major stimulus for the aldosterone release. Thus theoretically inhibition of the formation of angiotensin may be associated with decreased level of aldosterone. However, the effects of aldosterone antagonists are not diminished with the concurrent use of angiotensin converting enzyme inhibitors or angiotensin receptor blocking agents. Aldosterone antagonists decrease myocyte and vascular smooth muscle cell hypertrophy and decrease myocardial fibrosis, the principal mechanisms of their beneficial effects on ventricular remodeling.

It is suggested that the starting dose of aldosterone antagonists should be low and the electrolytes and renal function should be evaluated at 1 week and then at 2 weeks before increasing the dose. After increasing the dose, the electrolytes and renal function should be repeated again after 1 and 2 weeks. It is advisable to monitor renal function and electrolytes more frequently in patients with relative hypotension and more severe heart failure. It is also important not to use aldosterone antagonists in patients with serum creatinine greater than 2.5 mg/dL or serum potassium greater than 5.0 mEq/l.

Omega-3 fatty acids have the potential to improve left ventricular ejection fraction and promote reverse remodeling in patients with non-ischemic systolic heart failure. Hydralazine and nitrates are effective in improving symptoms and prognosis of patients with severe heart failure. A number of randomized clinical trials have been performed to assess effects of combination of hydralazine and isosorbide dinitrate on survival of patients with systolic heart failure. It has been postulated that the increased nitric oxide availability may be contributory to the beneficial effects of hydralazine and nitrates-combination therapy. The guidelines recommend the use of hydralazine and nitrate combination therapy for all patients, irrespective of race or gender, with severe systolic heart failure who remain symptomatic despite standard therapy.

There is no indication for use of amlodipine, a dihydropyridine calcium-channel blocker in patients with systolic heart failure except for the treatment of associated hypertension or angina. Diuretics are essential to relieve congestive symptoms. In patients with signs and symptoms of pulmonary and systemic venous congestion, initially loop diuretics are used. The loop diuretics that are used in clinical practice are furosemide, ethacrynic acid, bumetanide and torsemide. Although furosemide is the most frequently used diuretic, it should be appreciated that when it is administered orally its bioavailability is only 50%. The absorptions of torsemide and bumetanide are greater and more predictable.

The more severe the heart failure is, the more likely that it will be necessary to use combination of diuretics with different sites of action on the nephrons. The loop diuretics are combined with thiazide diuretics and then with potassium sparing diuretics. The most frequently used oral thiazide diuretic is metolazone, at a dose between 2.5 mg and 20 mg daily. Acetazolamide is a proximal tubular diuretic, but it is less potent than the loop diuretics. It is seldom used except for severe diuretic induced metabolic alkalosis.

The inadequate response to diuretics in heart failure is often called diuretic resistance or cardiorenal syndrome. A number of factors appear to be contributory to the development of cardiorenal syndrome.

- Decreased renal perfusion due to low cardiac output, renal vasoconstriction, and redistribution of cardiac output
- Inappropriate systemic and renal neuroendocrine activation
- Vasodilatation of the afferent renal arterioles, partly mediated by prostaglandins and nonsteroidal anti-inflammatory agents (NSAIDS), which block the prostaglandins reduce the efficacy of the diuretics
- The efferent arteriolar vasoregulation, mediated by the renin-angiotensin system and the use of angiotensin inhibitors, which are indicated for the treatment of heart failure may contribute to deteriorating renal function in heart
- Decreased sodium load to the tubules due to low cardiac output and a marked reabsorption of sodium.

In patients with obvious volume overload and resistance to diuretic therapy, mechanical means for fluid removal may be employed. In patients with refractory heart failure, intravenous vasodilators are often used to improve hemodynamics and cardiac function. The intravenous vasodilators that are used in clinical practice are sodium nitroprusside, nitroglycerine, and nesiritide. In patients with advanced heart failure, the positive inotropic agents are used when there is poor response to standard pharmacologic treatments. Oral digoxin has been employed to improve hemodynamics and left ventricular function in patients with systolic heart failure.

Intravenous catecholamines and vasopressors are used as supportive treatments in patients with severe refractory heart failure (stage D).

Dobutamine is predominantly a beta-1 adrenoreceptor agonist. It also stimulates beta-2 adrenergic receptors. The hemodynamic effects of dobutamine are characterized by an increase in stroke volume and cardiac output and a modest decrease in mean arterial pressure. Dopamine stimulates dopaminergic receptors (DA1 and DA2), and adrenergic receptors (beta-1, beta-2, and alpha). Neuronal release of norepinephrine and its reduced neuronal reuptake occur with dopamine. Thus, circulating norepinephrine levels are substantially increased. The hemodynamic effects of dopamine are related to its dose. The hemodynamic effects with higher doses are characterized by increased, systemic vascular resistance, arterial pressure and no further increase in cardiac output. Pulmonary capillary wedge and pulmonary artery pressures may also increase. To increase arterial pressure with dopamine, it is necessary to use the alpha receptors stimulating doses.

Norepinephrine and phenylephrine are also used in hypotensive patients to maintain arterial pressures. They increase systemic vascular resistance and arterial pressure without inducing tachycardia. Stroke volume and cardiac output may decrease due to increased left ventricular afterload.

The relatively cardiospecific phosphodiesterase inhibitors (phosphodiesterases III and IV), milrinone and amrinone exert positive inotropic effect and increase stroke volume and cardiac output. Systemic vascular resistance and mean arterial pressure may decrease. There is also a substantial reduction of systemic and pulmonary venous pressures. However, these agents increase ventricular arrhythmias and may increase mortality. The phosphodiesterase type V inhibitors are systemic and pulmonary vasodilators and are widely used for the treatment of precapillary pulmonary arterial hypertension and for erectile dysfunction. Preliminary studies indicate that these agents may be beneficial in patients with pulmonary hypertension due to left ventricular dysfunction.

Levosimendan is an intravenous calcium sensitizing agent and has been shown to produce beneficial hemodynamic effects, which consist of increase in cardiac output and decrease in pulmonary capillary wedge pressure. However, in a randomized clinical trial comparing levosimendan and dobutamine, there was no survival benefit with levosimendan.

❏ NONPHARMACOLOGIC TREATMENTS

A number of nonpharmacologic treatments have been attempted for the treatment of refractory systolic heart failure (Table 17).

Table 17: Nonpharmacologic interventions

- LV volume reduction surgery
  - Batista, Dore, Saver procedures
- Mitral valve repairs
- DDD-pacing with short P–R interval
- Ventricular assist devices
- Passive ventricular constraint devices
  - Myosplints
  - Mesh jacket
- Cardiac transplantation
- Revascularization in ischemic cardiomyopathy
- Resynchronization with or without ICD

❏ FOLLOW-UP EVALUATION

It has been suggested that patient education, evidence-based, guideline-recommended treatments should be initiated in the hospitals prior to discharge of the patients. Heart failure disease management programs should be established and the team should include pharmacists. Multidisciplinary chronic heart failure management programs should be established which allow implementation of appropriate therapy. The team should consist of nurses trained in management of heart failure, heart failure specialists and pharmacists. Some programs also include exercise and rehabilitation specialists. Exercise training is recommended in NYHA class II and III patients with chronic heart failure. Regular exercise can improve symptoms, exercise capacity, and quality of life. It can be associated with reduced hospitalization rates. The potential mechanisms of the benefits of exercise training in heart failure are summarized in Tables 18 and 19.

Table 18: Potential mechanisms of benefits of exercise training in heart failure

- Reduction in sympathetic activity, increase in parasympathetic activity
- Decrease in circulating deleterious neurohormones
- Decrease generation of reactive oxygen species (ROS)
- Restore endothelial function
- Generation of more nitric oxide (NO)
- Exerts anti-inflammatory effect by reducing inflammatory cytokines, platelet-related inflammatory mediators and peripheral markers of endothelial dysfunction

Table 19: Potential mechanisms of benefits of exercise training in heart failure

- Improves oxygen consumption, and lactate threshold, delays onset of anaerobic metabolism in skeletal muscle
- Decreases systemic vascular resistance
- Decreases end-diastolic and end-systolic volumes and increases left ventricular ejection fraction

❏ SUGGESTED READINGS

1. Bolognese L, Neskovic AN, Parodi G, et al. Left ventricular remodeling after primary coronary angioplasty: patterns of left ventricular dilatation and long term prognostic implications. Circulation. 2002;106:2351-7.
2. Francis GS, Benedict C, Johnstone DE, et al. Comparison of neuroendocrine activation in patients with left ventricular dysfunction with and without congestive heart failure. A substudy of the Studies of Left Ventricular Dysfunction (SOLVD). Circulation. 1990;82: 1724-9.
3. Hunt SA, Abraham WT, Chin MH, et al. 2009 focused update incorporated into the ACC/AHA 2005 Guidelines for the Diagnosis and Management of Heart Failure in Adults. A Report of the American College of Cardiology Foundation/American Heart Association Task Force on Practice Guidelines Developed in Collaboration with the International Society for Heart and Lung Transplantation. Circulation. 2009;53:e1-90.
4. Kitzman DW, Little WC, Brubaker PH, et al. Pathophysiological characterization of isolated diastolic heart failure in comparison to systolic heart failure. JAMA. 2002;288:2144-50.
5. Konstam MA. Systolic and diastolic dysfunction in heart failure? Time for a new paradigm. J Cardiac Fail. 2003;9:1-3.
6. Mann DL. Inflammatory mediators and the failing heart: past, present and the foreseeable future. Circ Res. 2002;91:988-98. Med. 2001;344:1651-8.
7. Packer M, Bristow MR, Cohn J, et al. The effects of carvedilol on morbidity and mortality in patients with chronic heart failure. U.S. Carvedilol Heart Failure Study Group. N Engl J Med. 1996;334:1349-55.

8. Packer M, Coats AJ, Fowler MB, et al. Effect of carvedilol on survival in severe chronic heart failure: results of the Carvedilol Prospective Randomized Cumulative Survival (COPERNICUS) study. N Engl J
9. Pitt B, Remme W, Zanand F, et al. Eplerenone, a selective aldosterone blocker, in patients with left ventricular dysfunction after myocardial infarction. N Engl J Med. 2003;348:1309-21.
10. Pitt B, Zannad F, Remme WJ, et al. For the Randomized Evaluation Study Investigators. The effect of spironolactone on morbidity and mortality in patients with severe heart failure. N Engl J Med. 1999;341:709-17.
11. Taylor AL, Ziesche S, Yancy C, et al. Combination of isosorbide dinitrate and hydralazine in blacks with heart failure. N Engl J Med. 2004;351:2049-57.
12. Vantrimpont P, Rouleau JL, Wun CC, et al. Additive beneficial effects of beta blockers to angiotensin-converting enzyme inhibitors in the Survival and Ventricular Enlargement (SAVE) study. J Am Coll Cardiol. 1997;29:229-36.

7.3 Diastolic Heart Failure (Heart Failure with Preserved Ejection Fraction)

❑ DEFINITION

One of the pathophysiologic definitions, as proposed by Brutsaert et al. is that it is "a condition resulting from an increased resistance to filling of one or both ventricles leading to symptoms of congestion due to an inappropriate upward shift of the diastolic-pressure-volume relation (i.e. during the terminal phase of the cardiac cycle). Another proposed pathophysiologic definition is that it is a condition in which the "ventricular chamber is unable to accept an adequate volume of blood during diastole at normal diastolic pressures and at volumes sufficient to maintain an appropriate stroke volume". Although these definitions describe the pathophysiologic characteristics of diastolic heart failure, they cannot be used in clinical practice.

In clinical practice most commonly used definition of diastolic heart failure (HFNEF) is when "the symptoms and signs of heart failure are present, and the ejection fraction is greater than 45%".

It should be appreciated that EF is load dependent. A lower preload and a higher after load are associated with a lower EF.

❑ EPIDEMIOLOGY AND RISK FACTORS

The incidence and prevalence of diastolic heart failure have been studied in a number of epidemiologic studies and have estimated the prevalence of diastolic heart failure between 50% and 55%. The prevalence increases with age, and it is more common in women than in men. The risk factors for diastolic heart failure are similar to those of systolic heart failure (Table 20).

❑ PATHOPHYSIOLOGY

Ventricular Remodeling

The morphologic changes in diastolic heart failure are summarized in Tables 21 and 22. Tissue Doppler imaging (TDI) studies have reported the prevalence of

Table 20: Systolic vs diastolic heart failure

ADHERE—All enrolled discharges		
Profile	SHF	DHF
EF	(59,523)	(50,497)
EF	<40%	>40%
Age	69.9	74.2*
Female	39%	62.2%*
CAD	63%	54%*
Diabetes	42%	46%*
AF	29%	33%*
BNP	1486	925*

*< 0.0001
(Abbreviations: EF: Ejection fraction; CAD: Coronary artery disease; AF: Atrial fibrillation; SHF: Systolic heart failure; DHF: Diastolic heart failure)

Table 21: Diastolic heart failure—remodeling

- Ventricular hypertrophy, usually concentric
- Increased ventricular mass
- Increased ventricular wall thickness
- Little or no increase in the cavity size
- Increased mass/cavity ratio
- Decreased wall stress
- Maintained ejection fraction
- Little or no change in ventricular shape
- Mechanical dyssynchrony with or without electrical dyssynchrony— present in approximately 1/3rd of patients

Table 22: Diastolic heart failure

	Controls	DHF
LVEDV	102	87
LVESV	46	37
LVEF	54	60
LVM	125	160
LVM/V	1.49	2.12

(Abbreviations: LVEDV: Left ventricular end diastolic volume; LVESV: Left ventricular end-systolic volume; LVEF: Left ventricular ejection fraction; LVM: Left ventricular mass; LVM/V: Left ventricular mass/volume ratio; DHF: Diastolic heart failure). (*Source:* Adapted from Kitzman DW, et al. JAMA. 2002;288:2144)

dyssynchrony in over 30% of patients with diastolic heart failure. In patients with diastolic heart failure left ventricular mechanical dyssynchrony may occur with or without electrical dyssynchrony.

The distinctive features of left ventricular remodeling in isolated diastolic and systolic heart failures are illustrated in Figure 18. In this example, compared to a normal heart, the left ventricular wall thickness in diastolic heart failure is markedly increased and the cavity is small. In contrast, in systolic heart failure the thickness of left ventricular wall is decreased and the cavity is dilated compared to normal wall.

Compared to normal myocyte, the myocyte in diastolic heart failure is thicker and there is increase in diameter without an increase in its length. The length/width ratio is decreased. There is increased myocyte protein synthesis. In systolic heart failure the myocyte length is increased without changing its diameter. The length/width ratio is increased. Left ventricular endomyocardial biopsy in patients with symptomatic diastolic and systolic heart failure demonstrates distinctive features in myocardial structure.

In both diastolic and systolic heart failure the collagen volume is increased. In diastolic heart failure, the thickness of the collagen bundles and the continuity of the fibrillar components of the extracellular matrix surrounding the myocytes are increased. In systolic heart failure, there is degradation and disruption in collagen. The collagen cross links are increased in diastolic heart failure. The matrix metalloproteinases (MMPs) are reduced and the endogenous tissue inhibitors of metalloproteinases (TIMPs) are increased. Abnormal calcium regulation has been observed in diastolic heart failure. Myocardial ischemia impairs myocardial relaxation due to abnormality of calcium regulation. There is reduced reuptake of the cytosolic calcium by the sarcoplasmic reticulum. Ischemia may induce myocyte necrosis and apoptosis. The changes in myocytes and extracellular matrix are summarized in Table 23.

Neurohormonal Changes

The plasma norepinephrine levels, circulating levels of interleukin-6 and interleukin-8, and of tumor necrosis factor-alpha (TNF-α) are increased. These may contribute to myocyte hypertrophy and myocardial inflammatory changes, which may be associated with myocyte necrosis and apoptosis. The counter regulatory hormone B-type natriuretic peptide (BNP) is also increased. Despite increased levels of BNP, ventricular remodeling continues.

Table 23: Diastolic heart failure

	DHF
Myocyte	
hypertrophy	+
apoptosis	+
necrosis	+
Fibrosis	+
Ca regulation	−
MMPs/TIMPs	−
Collagen	
cross-links	+
Titin isoforms	
N2BA/N2B	−

(Abbreviation: DHF: Diastolic heart failure)
+: Increased; −: Decreased

Heart Failure

Functional Derangements

The principal functional abnormality in diastolic heart failure is increased stiffness and decreased compliance of the left ventricle. The diastolic pressure-volume relation shifts upward and to the left. As a result, there is a disproportionate increase in left ventricular diastolic pressure for any increase in left ventricular diastolic volume (Figs 25A and B and 26A to C). Myocardial hypertrophy, fibrosis and ischemia contribute to increased left ventricular fibrosis.

Due to the upward and leftward shift of the diastolic pressure-volume relation, left ventricular diastolic pressure is increased and there is a passive increase in

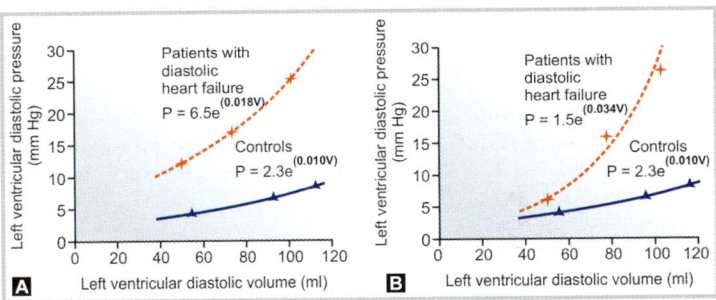

FIGURES 25A AND B: The changes in left ventricular diastolic pressure (mm Hg) (y-axis) and changes in left ventricular diastolic volume (mL) (x-axis) in groups of patients with diastolic heart failure and matched controls are illustrated. In patients with diastolic heart failure, the left ventricular pressure volume relation is shifted upward and to the left (*Source:* Zile et al. N Engl J Med. 2004;350:1953-9, with permission)

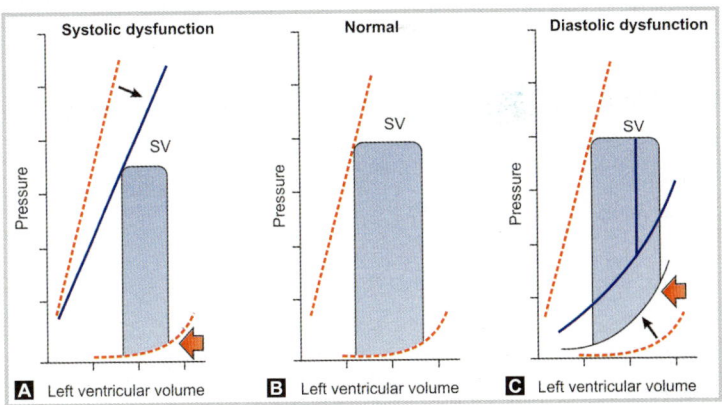

FIGURES 26A TO C: Schematic diagram of pressure-volume relations in Normal (B), Systolic dysfunction (A) and Diastolic dysfunction (C) are illustrated. In systolic heart failure, the end-systolic pressure-volume relation line (solid line) is shifted downward and to the right indicating reduced contractile function compared to normal (dashed line). In diastolic heart failure, there is no shift in the end systolic pressure-volume line indicating no change in contractile function. With a marked upward and leftward shift of the diastolic pressure-volume relation there is not only increased in left ventricular diastolic pressure but also a decrease in stroke volume (SV) (*Source:* Modified from GP Aurigemma. N Engl J Med. 2004;35:1097, with permission)

pulmonary venous pressure with signs and symptoms of pulmonary venous congestion. With a further upward shift of the diastolic pressure volume relation left ventricular filling is compromised which is associated with decreased stroke volume and cardiac output (Fig. 26A to C).

Hemodynamic Consequences

The hemodynamic consequences of advanced diastolic heart failure are characterized by an increase in left ventricular diastolic pressure and a passive increase in left atrial and pulmonary venous pressures. There is an obligatory increase in pulmonary arterial pressure, which is associated with increased right ventricular afterload. Thus, right ventricular failure ensues with clinical manifestations, such as dependent peripheral edema.

Clinical Presentation

Asymptomatic left ventricular diastolic dysfunction is far more common than symptomatic diastolic heart failure. However, in symptomatic patients, the signs and symptoms of overt diastolic heart failure are similar to those of systolic heart failure (Table 24).

Diagnosis

The diagnosis of heart failure is made by the clinical evaluations, and the Framingham criteria are used for diagnosis.
- EF assessment is done by transthoracic echocardiography; however, radionuclide imaging and contrast angiography may be employed

Table 24: Prevalence of specific symptoms and signs in systolic vs diastolic heart failure		
	Diastolic HF (EF >50%)	**Systolic HF (EF <50%)**
Symptoms		
Dyspnea on exertion	85%	96%
Paroxysmal nocturnal dyspnea	55%	50%
Orthopnea	60%	73%
Physical examination		
Jugular venous distension	35%	46%
Rale	72%	70%
Displaced apical impulse	50%	60%
S3	45%	65%
S4	45%	66%
Hepatomegaly	15%	16%
Edema	30%	40%
Chest radiograph		
Cardiomegaly	90%	90%
Pulmonary venous hypertension	75%	80%

(Abbreviation: HF: Heart failure).
(*Source:* Zile MR, Brutsaert DL. Circulation. 2002;105:1387-93)

- Cardiac magnetic resonance imaging (CMRI) has also been used to assess diastolic function
- Assessment of myocardial ischemia due to obstructive coronary artery disease is desirable; stress radionuclide imaging or stress echocardiographic studies can be employed to assess myocardial ischemia. Presently, coronary angiography is the gold standard. The contrast computerized tomographic studies (contrast CTA) is being increasingly used to exclude clinically significant obstructive coronary artery disease
- Measurement of BNP or N terminal pro-BNP is useful in excluding the diagnosis of heart failure
- The routine hemodynamic measurements are not indicated for the diagnosis of heart failure.

If a patient has signs and symptoms of heart failure and the left ventricular EF is normal or near normal and there is evidence of diastolic dysfunction diagnosis of diastolic heart failure is established. Cardiopulmonary exercise or six-minute walk tests are not necessary for the diagnosis of heart failure but they are performed to assess the results of therapy.

Treatment Strategies

The principal objectives of the treatment of diastolic heart failure are to relieve symptoms, improve quality of life and decrease mortality and morbidity. The majority of patients with diastolic heart failure present with symptoms of systemic and pulmonary venous congestion, for which diuretics are necessary. In the Hong Kong Diastolic Heart Failure Study, the patients were randomized to receive diuretics alone, diuretics and ramipril or diuretics and irbesartan. In all three groups, hospital admission rates decreased and exercise tolerance improved. Addition of ramipril or irbesartan resulted in a decrease in NT-proBNP. This study suggests that diuretics alone are effective to ameliorate congestive symptoms. The nitrates decrease right atrial and pulmonary capillary wedge pressures and can relieve symptoms of systemic and pulmonary venous congestion.

Angiotensin blockade by either angiotensin-converting enzyme inhibitors (ACEIs) or angiotensin receptor blocking agents (ARBs) that is of proven benefit in systolic heart failure are also being used for management of diastolic heart failure. The rationale for considering the use of angiotensin inhibitors is that these agents have the potential to improve diastolic function and also modify the risk factors for development of diastolic heart failure. Angiotensin-converting enzyme inhibitors can cause regression of left ventricular hypertrophy and improve diastolic function in patients with hypertensive heart disease. ACEIs can also decrease myocardial stiffness. Intracoronary infusion of enalaprilat, in a dose that does not reduce blood pressure, was associated with improved left ventricular diastolic compliance and relaxation in patients with left ventricular hypertrophy due to aortic stenosis. The mechanism of the beneficial effect was assumed to be decreased production of myocardial angiotensin II.

The rationale for the use of ARBs is similar to that of ACEIs. Angiotensin II subtype 1 receptor blocking agents decrease left ventricular hypertrophy and improve diastolic function. Losartan has been reported to decrease myocardial fibrosis and improve left ventricular compliance. The randomized clinical trials, however, have failed to demonstrate a substantial benefit of ARBs in patients with diastolic heart failure.

The beneficial effects of beta blockers have not been documented in patients with diastolic heart failure as compared to that seen in systolic heart failure. The rational for the use of beta blockers is to decrease heart rate which improves ventricular filling which is impaired in diastolic heart failure. Furthermore, beta-blockers have the potential to decrease myocardial ischemia which is associated with diastolic dysfunction.

Aldosterone antagonists are beneficial in patients with systolic heart failure as they decrease adverse ventricular remodeling and improve prognosis. However, in patients with diastolic heart failure, such benefits have not been documented. In a small clinical trial, patients with diastolic heart failure were randomized to receive selective aldosterone antagonist, eplerenone or placebo. The majority of patients in both groups were receiving beta-blockers and angiotensin inhibitors. During 12 months of follow-up in the placebo group, there was a progressive increase in the markers of collagen turnover and inflammation and deterioration of diastolic function. With eplerenone treatment, there was no increase in type III collagen aminoterminal peptide. There was also no decrease in brain-natriuretic peptide levels. With eplerenone treatment there was only a modest improvement in diastolic function without any change in other clinical variables. This study suggests that diastolic heart failure is a progressive disease.

A small randomized trial was performed to assess the clinical and hemodynamic effects of a phosphodiesterase-5 inhibitor sildenafil (50 mg three times daily) in patients with diastolic heart failure. All patients had pulmonary hypertension. The etiology of diastolic heart failure was hypertensive heart disease. Evaluations were repeated at 6 and 12 months. With sildenafil treatment, there was a significant reduction in pulmonary artery pressure, pulmonary vascular resistance and right atrial pressure. The reduction in pulmonary vascular resistance suggests pulmonary vasodilatation by sildenafil. There was also a reduction in pulmonary capillary wedge pressure and an increase in cardiac output. There was an improvement in pulmonary function along with a decrease in lung-water. Reduction in right atrial and pulmonary capillary wedge pressures along with an increase in cardiac output suggest an improvement in right and left ventricular function with sildenafil therapy. In the placebo treated patients, there was either no change or deterioration in hemodynamics and in right and left ventricular function. With sildenafil therapy, there was also improvement in quality of life. The mechanism of the beneficial effect of sildenafil appears to be due to increased cGMP by inhibition of phosphodiesterase-5.

Amiodarone and dronedarone are the pharmacologic agents of choice in case of atrial fibrillation in heart failure (30%). If atrial fibrillation is permanent, adequate control of ventricular rate should be attempted with beta-blockers and heart rate regulating calcium channel blockers. Digoxin should be avoided if possible. If the ventricular rate cannot be adequately controlled pharmacologically, atrioventricular nodal ablation and pacemaker therapy should be considered. It is preferable to assess heart rate response during activity and not on resting heart rate to adjust pharmacologic therapy for rate control.

Non-pharmacologic treatments, such as chronic resynchronization therapy (CRT), have not been shown to be of any benefit in the management of patients with diastolic heart failure, although dyssynchrony is present in approximately 30% of patients. The treatment strategies of diastolic heart failure are summarized in Table 25.

❏ FUTURE DIRECTIONS

There have been considerable advances in the understanding of the structural and functional abnormalities in diastolic heart failure. However, there has been very

Table 25: Diastolic heart failure—management strategies

- Diuretics and/or nitrates to relieve congestive symptoms
- Digitalis may be effective in selected patients
- Reduction in heart rate is beneficial in diastolic heart failure
- Adequate treatment of hypertension, diabetes, obesity
- Treatments to reduce determinants of myocardial ischemia and to increase coronary blood flow
- Restoration and maintenance of sinus rhythm in patients with atrial fibrillation
- Implantable cardioverter—defibrillator in the survivors of sudden cardiac death
- Cardiac transplantation in selected patients
- Exercise training
- Counseling of the patient and the family of the disease, treatment options, and prognosis
- Regular follow-up evaluation preferably by the heart failure team

Table 26: Diastolic heart failure

- New potential therapies
    - Modulation of collagen cross-links
    - Modulation titin isoforms
    - Modulation of MMP/TIMP
- Reduction of matrix fibrosis
    - Chymase antagonists
    - TGF-beta
- Improved relaxation
    - Phospholamban inhibition
    - D-ribose
    - Levosimendan (calcium sensitizer)
    - PDE-5 inhibitors
    - To decrease myocardial deposition of AGEs
    - To enhance myocardial NO

(Abbreviations: MMP/TIMP: Matrix metalloproteinase/tissue inhibitor of metalloproteinase ratio; TGF: Transforming growth factor; D-Ribose: Dextro-ribose; AGE: Acylate glycation end product; PDE: Phosphodiesterase; NO: Nitric oxide)

little or no advances in therapy. It appears that the initiating pathophysiologic mechanisms for the structural and functional abnormalities continue and progressively worsening heart failure develops. Thus, research should continue for novel therapies for management of diastolic heart failure. The new potential therapies are summarized in Table 26.

❏ SUGGESTED READINGS

Brutsaert DL, Sys SU, Gillebert TC. Diastolic failure: pathophysiology and therapeutic implications. J Am Coll Cardiol. 1993;22:318-25.

Gary R, Davis L. Diastolic heart failure. Heart Lung. 2008;37:405-16.

Guazzi M, Vicenzi M, Arena R, et al. Pulmonary hypertension in heart failure with preserved ejection fraction. A target of phosphodiesterase -5 inhibition in 1-year study. Circulation. 2011;124:164-74.

Mak GJ, Ledwidge MT, Watson CJ, et al. Natural history of markers of collagen turnover in patients with early diastolic dysfunction and impact of eplerenone. J Am Coll Cardiol. 2009;54:1674-82.

Owan TE, Hodge DO, Herges RM, et al. Trends in prevalence and outcomes of heart failure with preserved ejection fraction. N Engl J Med. 2006;355:251-9.

Solomon SD, Janardhanan R, Verma A, et al. Effect of angiotensin receptor blockade and antihypertensive drugs on diastolic function in patients with hypertension and diastolic dysfunction: a randomized trial. Lancet. 2007;369:2079-87.

Sweitzer NK, Lopatin M, Yancy CW, et al. Comparison of clinical features and outcomes of patients hospitalized with heart failure and normal ejection fraction (> or = 55%) versus those with mildly reduced (40% to 55%) and moderately to severely reduced (< 40%) fractions. Am J Cardiol. 2008;101:1151-6.

van Heerebeek L, Borbély A, Niessen HW, et al. Myocardial structure and function differ in systolic and diastolic heart failure. Circulation. 2006;113:1966-73.

Yip GW, Wang M, Wang T, et al. The Hong Kong diastolic heart failure study: a randomised controlled trial of diuretics, irbesartan and ramipril on quality of life, exercise capacity, left ventricular global and regional function in heart failure with a normal ejection fraction. Heart. 2008;94:573-80.

Zile MR, Brutsaert DL. New concepts in diastolic dysfunction and diastolic heart failure: part I: diagnosis, prognosis and measurements of diastolic function. Circulation. 2002;105:1387-93.

7.4 Cardiorenal Syndrome: The Interplay between Cardiac and Renal Function in Patients with Congestive Heart Failure

❑ DEFINITION OF THE CARDIORENAL SYNDROME

The definition of the cardiorenal syndrome (CRS) is described as concomitant dysfunction of the heart and kidneys in which an acute or chronic dysfunction in one organ may result in an acute or chronic dysfunction in the other organ, worsening renal function (WRF) during acute heart failure (HF) treatment or diuretic resistance. Ronco et al. have suggested that the CRS should be characterized according to whether the impairment of each organ is primary, secondary or whether abnormal heart and kidney functions occur simultaneously as a result of a systemic disease. The direct and indirect effects of each dysfunctional organ can initiate and perpetuate the combined disorder of the two organs through complex neurohormonal feedback mechanisms. Consequently, the subdivision of CRS into five different subtypes may facilitate care of individual patients (Table 27).

The kidney receives 20% of CO; thus, the function of the heart and kidney are closely intertwined. Changes in volume and pressure in the cardiac atria initiate atrial–renal reflexes, which alter renal function (Flowchart 1).

Role of Decreased Cardiac Output

The role of decreased CO in the pathogenesis of the cardiorenal syndrome is more complex than it would first appear. A seminal study by Ljungman clearly demonstrates the powerful autoregulatory ability of the kidney to maintain renal perfusion even with significant reductions in CO. However, the same study found that when the cardiac index fell below 1.5 L/min/m^2 renal perfusion was reduced with a significant fall in GFR (Fig. 27). Finally, marked cardiorenal dysfunction can be reversed in some patients when CO is restored using a left ventricular assist device. In general, the data suggest that very low CO may impair renal function in selected patients but other factors clearly play a role.

Table 27: Cardiorenal syndrome

Type	Name	Description
Type 1	Acute cardiorenal syndrome	Abrupt worsening of cardiac function (e.g. acute cardiogenic shock, or acutely decompensated heart failure) leading to acute kidney injury
Type 2	Chronic cardiorenal syndrome	Chronic abnormalities in cardiac function (e.g. chronic heart failure) causing progressive and potentially permanent chronic kidney disease
Type 3	Acute renocardiac syndrome	Abrupt worsening of renal function (e.g. acute kidney ischemia or glomerulonephritis) causing acute cardiac disorders (e.g. heart failure, arrhythmia, ischemia)
Type 4	Chronic renocardiac syndrome	Chronic kidney disease (e.g. chronic glomerular or interstitial disease) contributing to decreased cardiac function, cardiac hypertrophy and/or increased risk of adverse cardiovascular events
Type 5	Secondary cardiorenal syndrome	Systemic conditions (e.g. diabetes mellitus, sepsis) causing both cardiac and renal dysfunction

FLOWCHART 1: Development of the cardiorenal syndrome is complex and still poorly understood. Intrinsic renal disease and impaired renal perfusion are important physiologic components of the syndrome. Renal blood flow is not only dependent on CO but is affected by high venous pressures as well. Patients may have worsening renal function due to multiple intrinsic and extrinsic renal factors

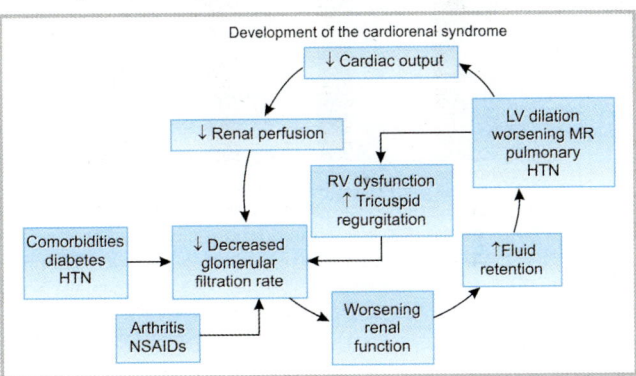

Role of Elevated Central Venous Pressure

Recent studies however have lent support to this concept. Mullens in a study of severely ill HF patients found that CVP was the best predictor of the percentage who would go on to develop renal insufficiency. The same group has advanced the concept of a related parameter, namely increased intraabdominal pressure as risk factor for renal insufficiency (Figs 28 and 29). In the Figure 8, the technique for measuring intraabdominal pressure at the bedside with the use of a modified urinary catheter is illustrated. They also have reported that in patients admitted with decompensated HF serum creatinine levels are significantly higher when intra-abdominal pressure was greater than 8 mm Hg (Fig. 29). They also have shown that reduction of intra-abdominal pressure either by paracentesis when ascites is present or by ultrafiltration may at times result in improved renal function.

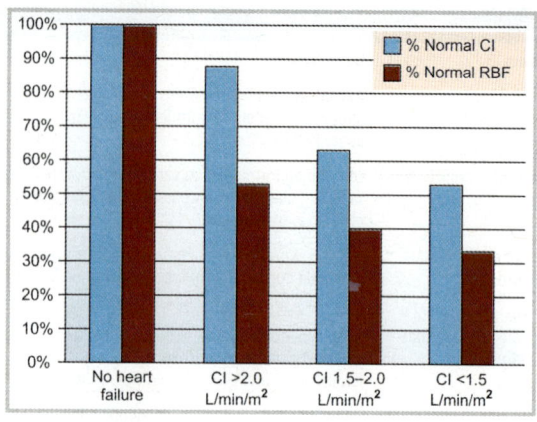
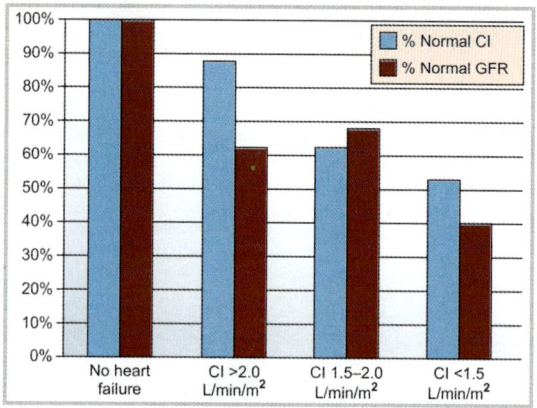

FIGURE 27: Data from Ljungman et al. evaluating the effect of CO on renal function. There was a stepwise decrease in renal blood flow as cardiac index declined with worsening heart failure. Of note, however, GFR is relatively maintained until cardiac index falls below a critical level of 1.5 L/min/m². (*Source:* Modified from Ljungman S, et al. Drugs. 1990;39:10-21)

❑ ROLE OF EVIDENCE-BASED THERAPIES IN PATIENTS WITH HEART FAILURE AND THE CARDIORENAL SYNDROME

Diuretics

Diuretics form the cornerstone of therapy for patients with HF who are hospitalized for symptoms of volume overload and are also important for maintenance of euvolemia in the outpatient setting.

Furosemide, torsemide, bumetanide, and ethacrynics are amongst the most potent agents for stimulating diuresis and natriuresis through inhibition of the $Na^+/K^+/2Cl^-$ cotransporter on the luminal side of the thick ascending limb of the loop of Henle. Since 25% of the filtered load of sodium chloride is normally reabsorbed here, loop diuretics can cause profound diuresis and natriuresis. Nevertheless, loop diuretics often lower GFR via adenosine release and stimulation of the renin–angiotensin–aldosterone system (RAAS). Loop diuretics decrease pulmonary

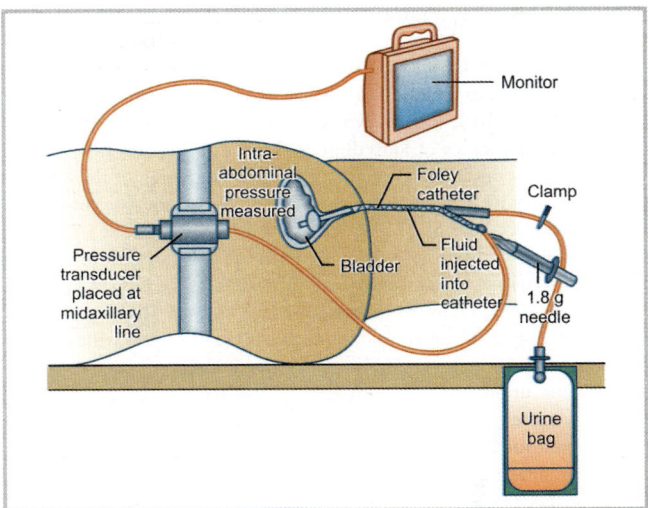

FIGURE 28: Technique for measuring intra-abdominal pressure at the bedside using a modified urinary catheter. When filled with fluid the bladder pressure is at equilibrium with the intra-abominal pressure and can be measured using a standard transducer leveled at the midaxillary (midabdominal) line. (*Source:* Modified from Mullens W, et al. J Am Coll Cardiol. 2008;51:300-6)

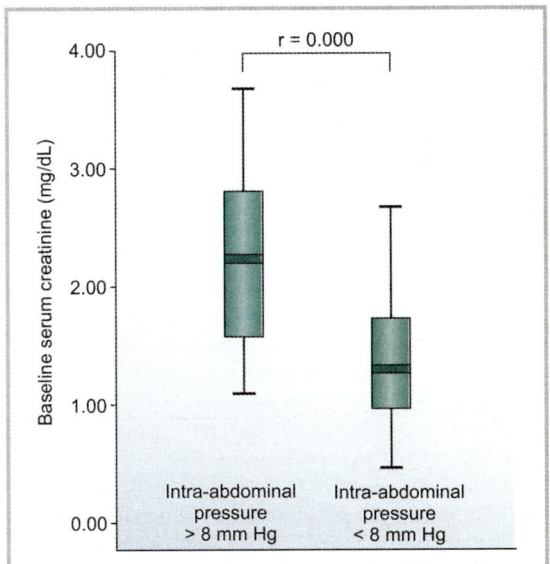

FIGURE 29: Levels of intra-abdominal pressure greater than 8 mm Hg were associated with significantly higher serum creatinine levels in patients admitted with severe decompensated heart failure (*Source:* Modified from Mullens W, et al. J Am Coll Cardiol. 2008;51:300-6)

congestion and lower left ventricular filling pressures prior to the onset of their diuretic effects.

Thiazide and thiazide-like agents have greatest utility in CHF when used concomitantly with loop diuretics. In advanced HF the combination of decreased renal blood flow (RBF), progressive renal dysfunction and RAAS activation may render maximal doses of loop diuretic therapy ineffective. In the setting of acute and chronic loop diuretic therapy, functional adaptation of the distal tubule with compensatory increases in sodium reabsorption (or diuretic resistance) and the effects of extracellular fluid volume depletion have also been well described. Simultaneous use of high-dose loop diuretics and a thiazide or metolazone inhibits sodium transport in the ascending thick limb of the loop of Henle as well as the compensatory sodium reabsorption in the early distal convoluted tubule. Most thiazide drugs also directly inhibit carbonic anhydrase, which minimizes compensatory sodium reabsorption in the proximal tubule.

The diuretic utility of potassium sparing diuretics, such as spironolactone, eplerenone, triamterene and amiloridein HF is to counteract potassium wasting and hypokalemic metabolic alkalosis associated with loop and thiazide diuretic use. High doses of potassium-sparing diuretics should be avoided or used with caution in patients with CHF and renal dysfunction as development of dose- dependent hyperkalemia is common in this setting. However, in some instances of marked diuretic resistance; high dose spironolactone when used with careful monitoring has been found to augment diuresis.

Effect of Diuretic Use on Morbidity and Mortality

The use of loop diuretics is associated with further deterioration of renal function, and this is observed more frequently among patients receiving combination loop diuretic and metolazone therapy. Furthermore, higher doses of loop diuretics are associated with higher serum creatinine and reduced survival and an increased risk of hospitalization and death related to CHF compared to those not taking these medications. While the use of diuretics is essential for most patients with CHF, there are adverse outcomes associated with worsening renal and left ventricular function.

Spironolactone and eplerenone are currently the only diuretics, which have been shown to reduce mortality in HF, and this is probably not related to the agents' diuretic effect.

The largest diuretic trial to date, the diuretic optimization strategies evaluation (DOSE) in acute heart failure trial brings a new perspective to the debate on dose and route of administration of diuretics in HF. In this trial, patients were randomized into four groups who received substantially different diuretic regimens. The high doses of furosemide were associated with slightly higher serum creatinine levels at 48 hours, but these were not statistically significant. This change was greatest at day 4 and resolved by day 60. There was a greater total urine output at 48 hours in the high dose groups. There was no statistically significant difference in the combined endpoint of death, rehospitalization or emergency department visit at 60 days between the groups. The DOSE study is perhaps our best look at different diuretic regimens and their outcomes, but it has important limitations in that it was underpowered to evaluate mortality differences and perhaps the low dose regimen was too low to be effective. Nonetheless, it demonstrated that mild WRF that was seen early in hospitalization usually resolved after discharge without long-term consequences.

ACE-I and ARB

The beneficial effects of ACE-I and ARB treatment in patients with CKD (with or without HF) are related to their hemodynamic actions and a wide range of neurohumoral, cellular, and vascular actions. The frequency with which renal function changes in HF patients treated chronically with ACE-I was reported in the studies of left ventricular dysfunction (SOLVD). Decreased renal function was defined as a rise in serum creatinine of greater than 0.5 mg/dL above baseline. More patients randomly assigned to enalapril had a decrease in renal function compared with controls (16% vs 12%). Older age, diuretic therapy and diabetes were associated with a greater likelihood of a negative renal function change, whereas beta-blocker treatment and a higher ejection fraction were renoprotective in all patients irrespective of therapy. Renal function can also deteriorate suddenly when ACE-I or ARB therapy is first begun, or it can acutely change in patients receiving chronic therapy. In most patients who experience ARF with ACE-I or ARB therapy, one or more mechanisms are typically implicated (Table 28).

Nonetheless, RAAS blockade should be continued when at all possible as mortality is very high when ACE-I/ARBs are stopped for renal reasons and the inability to maintain the use of these agents is a marker for very poor prognosis. In HF increased angiotensin II levels cause constriction of the efferent arteriole which elevates glomerular filtration pressure and helps to preserve GFR. Reversal of these elevated pressures in the CKD patient with either ACE-I or ARB therapy will generally lead to an initial fall in GFR around 10–20% (Fig. 30). Such small increases in serum creatinine should not prompt discontinuation of the RAAS blocking drug. The risk of ACE-I or ARB WRF is greater in patients with CKD of any cause than in those with normal renal function.

Table 28: Principles of ACE-I or ARB therapy: renal considerations

- ACE inhibitors and ARBs improve RBF and stabilize glomerular filtration rate in most patients with HF unless they adversely affect cardiac hemodynamics
- ACE inhibitor and ARB therapy is indicated in patients with diabetic nephropathy and in patients with nondiabetic nephropathies when protein excretion exceeds 1 g/d. Concurrent primary renal diseases are not uncommon in the HF patient
- A rise in serum creatinine may occur after initiation of RAAS inhibitor therapy in patients with HF. This rise usually occurs shortly after initiation of therapy, is in the 10–20% range, is not progressive and is of renal hemodynamic origin. Renal function often stabilizes and may decline thereafter
- Although there is no serum creatinine level per se that contraindicates ACE inhibitor therapy, greater increases in serum creatinine occur more frequently when ACE inhibitors are used in patients with underlying chronic kidney disease
- The occurrence of AKI should prompt a search for systemic hypotension (MAP < 65 mm Hg), ECF volume depletion or nephrotoxin administration and attempts to correct/remove these factors. Consideration should also be given to searching for high-grade bilateral renal artery stenosis or stenosis in a solitary kidney
- ACE inhibitors should be temporarily discontinued when AKI occurs and precipitating factors for AKI corrected; an ARB or a DRI is not an appropriate substitute under these conditions. Once AKI has resolved with correction of the precipitating factors, ACE inhibitor therapy can be cautiously reintroduced

(*Source*: Sica DA. The use of ACE inhibitors and angiotensin receptor blockers in patients with coexistent renal disease and heart failure. In: Heywood JT, Burnett J (Eds). The Cardiorenal Syndrome: A Clinician's Guide to Pathophysiology and Management. Cardiotext Publishing; 2011)

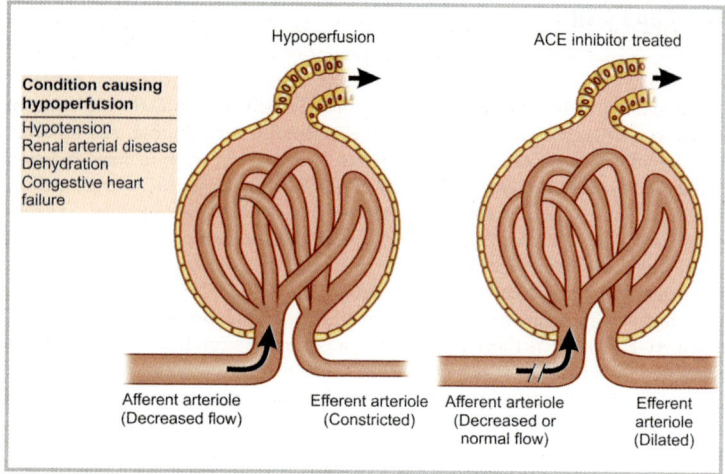

FIGURE 30: Glomerular filtration is regulated in part by changes in vascular tone in the afferent and efferent arterioles. Angiotensin II (ANG II) is a potent vascular smooth muscle constrictor and preferentially constricts the efferent arteriole leaving the glomerulus more than the afferent arteriole entering the glomerulus. Therefore higher levels of ANG II tend to preserve GFR. When ACE-I or ARB are used for heart failure ANG II is reduced or its effects are blocked at the receptor site with resulting efferent arteriolar dilation and reduced pressure in the glomerulus. This causes a physiologic and expected small decline in GFR and rise in serum creatinine (*Source:* Modified from Schoolwerth AC, et al. Circulation. 2001;104:1985-91)

Inotropes

These drugs are recommended in patients with fluid overload if they respond poorly to intravenous diuretics or have diminished or WRF, but the effects of these drugs on the kidney in patients with HF have not been clearly defined. Despite its potential to aid renal perfusion, clinical studies suggest that dobutamine has little effect on renal vascular resistance and indices of renal function, such as GFR. Clinically dobutamine may improve renal function when CO in significantly reduced. Dopamine exhibits a graded pharmacological response with a dose-dependent predominant activation of dopaminergic receptors, beta-receptors, and alpha-receptors.

Milrinone confers its positive inotropic effect through antagonism of the phosphodiesterase III (PDE) enzyme, resulting in cyclic adenosine monophosphate (cAMP) mediated increases in cardiomyocyte intracellular calcium concentrations.

Levosimendan, an inodilator, is approved for acutely decompensated HF in Europe. Unlike catecholamine and phosphodiesterase III inhibitors, its inotropic effects are achieved without an increase in intracellular calcium. The levosimendan infusion versus dobutamine (LIDO) compared the effects of levosimendan and dobutamine on hemodynamic performance and clinical outcome in patients with low-output HF and demonstrated that in patients with severe, low-output HF, levosimendan improved hemodynamic performance more effectively than dobutamine. This benefit was accompanied by lower mortality in the levosimendan group than in the dobutamine group for up to 180 days.

❏ ROLE OF ULTRAFILTRATION ON DIURETIC RESISTANCE AND THE CARDIORENAL SYNDROME

Intravenous treatment with diuretics may initially facilitate fluid loss and improve symptoms, but their use is associated with increased neurohormonal activation, intravascular volume depletion, hemodynamic impairment, and renal function decline. Alternative therapeutic strategies like ultrafiltration are needed to counteract development of diuretic refractoriness, particularly in those cases in which progressively increasing diuretic doses are required.

Reduction of extravascular lung water with ultrafiltration allows the rapid improvement of respiratory symptoms (dyspnea and orthopnea), pulmonary gas exchanges, lung mechanics and radiological signs of pulmonary vascular congestion, and alveolar and interstitial edema. Removal of systemic extravascular water allows resolution of peripheral edema and, when present, ascites and pleural effusions. The subtraction of extravascular pulmonary water, by reducing the intrathoracic pressure and, thus, the diastolic burden on the heart, exerts a positive influence on cardiac dynamics. The hemodynamic improvement following ultrafiltration is the result of both the reduction of the extracardiac constraint and the optimization of circulating volume. In addition to edema removal, ultrafiltration allows for other effects that are particularly useful in patients with advanced HF and associated CKD:

- Correction of hyponatremia
- Restoration of urine output and diuretic responsiveness
- Reduction of circulating levels of neurohormones, and
- Removal of other cardiac depressant mediators.

Recovery of diuretic responsiveness is a major clinical effect because it allows for maintenance and even improvement in the following days and months, of the clinical benefits achieved at the end of a single session of ultrafiltration. Moreover, it permits the use of lower dosages of diuretics, with potentially fewer side effects. Studies are needed to confirm the positive clinical impact of ultrafiltration, to better define protocols and more appropriate renal replacement modalities, to identify patients and clinical settings in which the greatest benefit can be obtained and, finally, to definitively establish the effect of ultrafiltration on hard clinical endpoints.

❏ TREATMENT OF THE CARDIORENAL SYNDROME: AN APPROACH TO THE INDIVIDUAL PATIENT

A systematic approach to the HF patient presenting with WRF has been devised and in order to focus the evaluation, five key questions must be answered about the patient at hand.

1. What is the volume status of the patient, i.e. hypovolemic, hypervolemic, or euvolemic?
2. Is there systemic hypotension (systolic BP <80 mm Hg)?
3. Is the central venous pressure markedly elevated?
4. What is the cardiac output?
5. Is there evidence for intrinsic renal disease?

Evaluation of volume status and the early recognition of hypovolemia are important because intercurrent gastrointestinal illness and iatrogenic volume depletion are common yet rapidly correctable. The recognition of hypovolemia is critical because rapid volume replacement of 500–1000 cc of normal saline can improve CO by restoring normal preload, and hence blood pressure and renal perfusion. Hemodynamic monitoring to determine volume status may be necessary in some circumstances when uncertainty remains (Table 29).

Table 29: Management of the cardiorenal syndrome

Cause of the cardiorenal syndrome	Volume status	Cardiac output	SVR	Treatment
Hypovolemia	↓↓	↓	↓ or normal	• Stop diuretic • Volume replacement
Excess vasoconstriction	↑ or normal	↓↓	↑↑	• ↑ RAS blockade • Nitroprusside • Nesiritide • Nitroglycerin
Cardiogenic shock	↑ or normal	↓↓	↑ or normal	• Dobutamine • Dopamine • Norepinephrine • LVAD
Excessive vasodilation	↑ or normal	↓ or normal	↓↓	• Dopamine • Norepinephrine • Vasopressin • LVAD
Diuretic resistance	↑↑	↓ or normal	normal	• Diuretic infusion • Diuretic combination • Ultrafiltration • Nesiritide
Intrinsic renal disease	↑↑	Normal	normal	• Diuretic Infusion • Ultrafiltration • Hemodialysis • Renal transplantation

Once hypovolemia has been ruled out or corrected, then systolic hypotension should be addressed. In patients with less severe hypotension, blood pressure may be restored with dobutamine if there is a history of severe LV dysfunction. Profound hypotension may require pressor support with norepinephrine and/or epinephrine. The appearance of the cardiorenal syndrome coupled with hypotension is a true medical emergency that requires rapid action but also hemodynamic data to address the underlying CV abnormality. Knowing the CO can be important for decision making for several reasons. When the cardiac index is below 1.5 L/min/m^2 then renal function is difficult to maintain. The use of dobutamine or milrinone in this instance can rapidly improve renal function and stabilize the patient. The resolution of renal dysfunction by improving CO with inotropes demonstrates adequate renal reserve and confirms a cardiac basis for the cardiorenal syndrome. Due to the problematic long-term outcomes with inotropes and poor prognosis associated with renal dysfunction, strong consideration should be given to more definitive therapy such as cardiac transplantation or left ventricular assist device (LVAD) placement. Use of an LVAD can restore renal function and is associated with improved prognosis.

A small minority may have hypotension without profound reduction of CO; hence calculated SVR is very low due to peripheral vasodilation, mimicking septic shock. Kanu Chatterjee has coined the phrase "pseudosepsis syndrome" to describe this syndrome in HF patients, often with renal dysfunction. The etiology of the syndrome is unclear but appears to result in renal hypoperfusion from low blood pressure and shunting of blood to the periphery. This syndrome may be

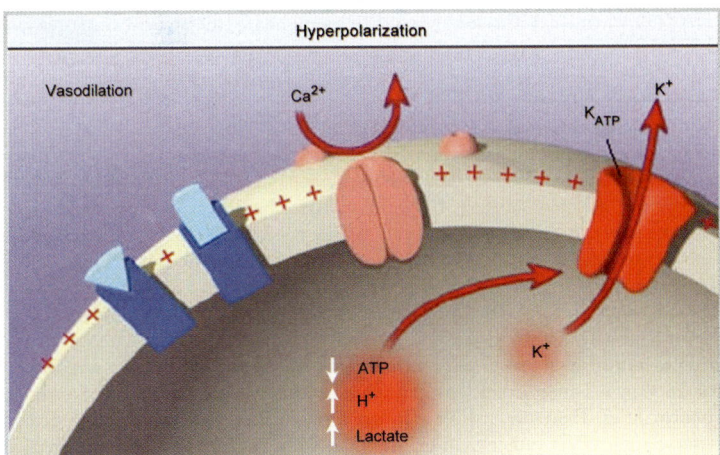

FIGURE 31: Vasodilation lactic acidosis produces vasodilatation via KATP channels. Potassium leaves smooth muscle cells via the K_{ATP} channels, resulting in plasma membrane hyperpolarization. This leads to inactivation of the voltage-gated calcium channels and prevents a rise in the cytoplasmic calcium concentration and so prevents arteriolar smooth muscle constriction (*Source:* Modified from Landry DW, et al. N Engl J Med. 2001;345:588-95)

seen after bypass surgery in patients with marked LV dysfunction and is often resistant to norepinephrine infusion. There is a beneficial response to vasopressin infusions in such patients with improved blood pressure and reduced requirements for norepinephrine. Due to hypotension and vasodilation, ACEI, ARB or other vasodilators should be discontinued in these patients until blood pressure stabilizes without pressor support (Fig. 31).

On the other hand, patients may present with the cardiorenal syndrome with low normal blood pressure coupled with a very elevated SVR. Although much less common in the era of ACE-I, it can be seen when ACE-I are not used out of concern for renal dysfunction or when an intercurrent gastrointestinal illness results in an abrupt withdrawal of ACE inhibition. Patients present with poor urine output, WRF, and cold extremities. Vasodilators are critical here because of the profound vasoconstriction, producing increased afterload and reduced CO. Intravenous vasodilators such as nitroprusside or nesiritide may be employed until the patient can be placed on ACE inhibitors. Some may require short-term inotropic support as vasodilators are added. The role of nesiritide in the management of decompensated HF is controversial. The drug may be beneficial in some patients with the cardiorenal syndrome, especially perhaps those with vasoconstriction.

An important practical consideration is the method used to measure CO. The gold standard remains invasive monitoring with a pulmonary artery catheter. Recent concerns about complications and the publication of the ESCAPE trial have led to a dramatic reduction in its use. This does not mean it should never be used, and the hemodynamic information it provides can be invaluable in managing critically ill HF patients. In the patient with cardiorenal syndrome a single measurement of CO may be sufficient to determine hemodynamics and guide initial therapy. In this instance a bedside echocardiographic determination of CO can be quicker, less expensive and noninvasive. The most accurate technique involves pulsed Doppler interrogation of the LV Outflow Tract and Measuring the Time-Velocity Integral

(LVOT-TVI cm/sec). This number is then multiplied by the outflow tract area just below the aortic valve (cm^2) to determine the stroke volume, LVOT-TVI × LVOT area = stroke volume (cm^3/sec). The stroke volume is then multiplied by the heart rate to determine CO.

Once the kidney has been identified as the cause of the renal dysfunction there are important implications for therapy. Diuretics can be used as long as the patient remains volume overloaded, although meticulous care should be taken to avoid overdiuresis and hypotension. In some instances bumetanide or torsemide may be more effective than furosemide and may be tried if urine output is inadequate. Another technique to deal with renal resistance is the addition of a distal tubular diuretic to block sodium reuptake in this area of the nephron. With prolonged use of loop diuretics distal tubular hyperplasia and increased reabsorption of sodium may occur with resulting diuretic resistance (Figs 32A to C). Metolazone or hydrochlorothiazide can be used to mitigate this effect. However, the response to this therapy is unpredictable and can result in tremendous diuresis and electrolyte abnormalities. Therefore, it is best to use a single dose of these agents and then observe their effect rather than giving them daily. An intravenous form thiazide (chlorothiazide) is available for those who cannot take oral agents.

When renal dysfunction is profound then the option of dialysis is available as either a temporary or permanent therapy for the cardiorenal syndrome. Short of dialysis for patients who do not respond adequately to diuretics, ultrafiltration is an important option. In selected patients renal transplantation should be considered as the ultimate therapy for the kidney centered cardiorenal syndrome.

The CV system evolves to maintain a balanced milieu, and HF develops when the system fails, usually because of CV disease, to regulate this balance. Present therapies can restore this balance in many patients, but not in all, especially when the kidney, a much more complex organ than the heart, is responsible. If the progress made in HF is to be continued, the kidney should be a major focus of research, and if renal function could be restored and GFR increased reliably, then care of patients with the cardiorenal syndrome would be greatly improved.

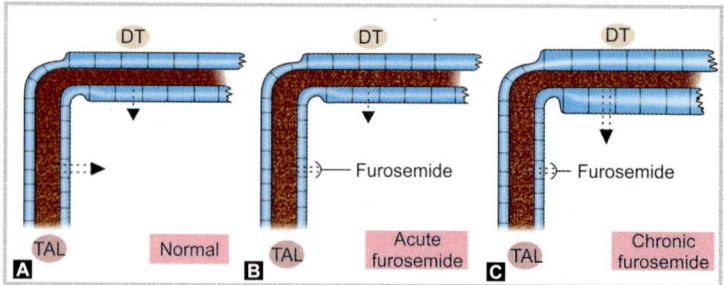

FIGURES 32A TO C: (A) In normal circumstances Cl$^-$ is reabsorbed actively with passive Na$^+$ reabsorption in the thick ascending limb of Henle (TAL). Sodium and chloride are also reabsorbed in the distal tubule (DT) but to lesser extent than in the TAL; (B) When furosemide is given initially, it blocks Cl$^-$ transport from the lumen of the TAL and is reabsorbed with Na$^+$ into the vascular bed in the medulla. As a consequence, more NaCl is delivered to the DT with more than normal reabsorption. However, net NaCl excretion is increased; (C) With chronic administration of furosemide the increased concentration of NaCl in the DT results in hypertrophy of the DT cells with enhanced Na+ reabsorption. Therefore, net excretion of NaCl is reduced. The addition of a second diuretic acting at the DT can restore furosemide-induced NaCl excretion (*Source:* Modified from Ellison DH. The physiologic basis of diuretic drug action and synergism. Principles of medical biology. Molecular and Cellular Pharmacology. JAI Press Inc. 1997. pp. 577-99)

❑ SUGGESTED READINGS

Ellison DH. The physiological basis of diuretic drug action and synergism. In: Bittar EE, Bittar N (Eds). Principles of Medical Biology. JAI Press; 1997. pp. 577-99.

Follath F, Cleland JG, Just H, et al. Efficacy and safety of intravenous levosimendan compared with dobutamine in severe low-output heart failure (the LIDO study): a randomised double-blind trial. Lancet. 2002;360:196-202.

Hampton JR, van Veldhuisen DJ, Kleber FX, et al. Randomised study of effect of ibopamine on survival in patients with advanced severe heart failure. Second Prospective Randomised Study of Ibopamine on Mortality and Efficacy (PRIME II) Investigators. Lancet. 1997;349:971-7.

Hernandez AF. Acute Study of Clinical Effectiveness of Nesiritide in Decompensated Heart Failure (ASCEND HF) Paper presented at: American Heart Association; November 14, 2010; Chicago, Illinois.

Knight EL, Glynn RJ, McIntyre KM, et al. Predictors of decreased renal function in patients with heart failure during angiotensin converting enzyme inhibitor therapy: results from the studies of left ventricular dysfunction (SOLVD). Am Heart J. 1999;138:849-55.

Ljungman S, Laragh JH, Cody RJ. Role of the kidney in congestive heart failure. Relationship of cardiac index to kidney function. Drugs. 1990;39:10-21; discussion 22-4.

Mullens W, Abrahams Z, Francis GS, et al. Importance of venous congestion for worsening of renal function in advanced decompensated heart failure. J Am Coll Cardiol. 2009;53:589-96.

Mullens W, Abrahams Z, Francis GS, et al. Prompt reduction in intraabdominal pressure following large-volume mechanical fluid removal improves renal insufficiency in refractory decompensated heart failure. J Card Fail. 2008;14:508-14.

Pitt B, Remme W, Zannad F, et al. Eplerenone, a selective aldosterone blocker, in patients with left ventricular dysfunction after myocardial infarction. N Engl J Med. 2003;348:1309-21.

Pitt B, Zannad F, Remme WJ, et al. The effect of spironolactone on morbidity and mortality in patients with severe heart failure. Randomized Aldactone Evaluation Study Investigators. N Engl J Med. 1999;341:709-17.

Rimondini A, Cipolla CM, Della Bella P, et al. Hemofiltration as short-term treatment for refractory congestive heart failure. Am J Med. 1987;83:43-8.

Ronco C, House AA, Haapio M. Cardiorenal syndrome: refining the definition of a complex symbiosis gone wrong. Intensive Care Med. 2008;34:957-62.

Winton FR. The influence of venous pressure on the isolated mammalian kidney. J Physiol. 1931;72:49-61.

7.5 Acute Heart Failure Syndromes

❑ INTRODUCTION

Acute heart failure syndromes (AHFS) have been defined as new onset or gradual or rapidly worsening heart failure (HF) signs and symptoms requiring urgent therapy. Regardless of the underlying etiology for HF or the precipitant for acute decompensation, patients are characterized by pulmonary and systemic congestion due to elevated ventricular filling pressures with or without low cardiac output.

Approximately 80% of AHFS patients have worsening chronic HF requiring hospitalization, of which only a small subset (~5%) present with advanced or end-stage HF. The remaining 20% of admissions have *de novo* or HF for the first time. Of these patients, approximately 50% have a relatively preserved ejection fraction, what has been termed diastolic dysfunction, HF with normal ejection fraction, HF with preserved systolic function or heart failure with preserved ejection fraction (HFPEF). The mean age is 75 with a nearly equal split between males and females. For HFPEF, patients are slightly older with a greater predominance of women. Dyspnea, or breathlessness, is the most common symptom at the time

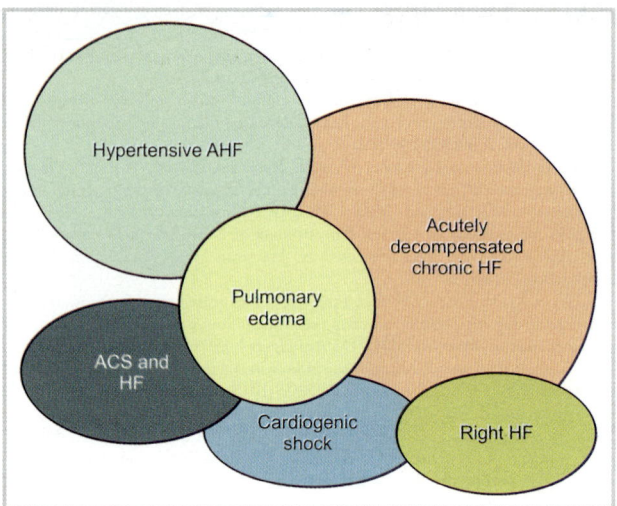

FIGURE 33: The European Society of Cardiology classification based on presenting profiles (*Source:* Reproduced with permission from Filippatos G, Zannad F. An introduction to acute heart failure syndromes: definition and classification. Heart Fail Rev. 2007;12:87-90)

of presentation, with classic HF signs, such as jugular venous distention, peripheral edema and rales, commonly seen. Nearly 50% of patients will have systolic blood pressure of 140 mm Hg or greater at the time of presentation, with less than 10% of patients hypotensive. The AHFS patient has substantial cardiac and noncardiac comorbidities. Several unique differences are noted between patients with reduced systolic function and those with HFPEF, namely a history of hypertension and atrial arrhythmias.

The European Society of Cardiology classification based on presenting profiles is shown in Figure 33. Patients may also be divided based on the presence or absence of chronic HF. Another scheme classifies patients based on the potential to restore cardiac function. Patients may be broadly divided into two groups: (i) those with end-stage or advanced HF and (ii) those in whom a restoration of cardiac function is possible.

❑ PATHOPHYSIOLOGY

There are multiple overlapping pathophysiologic mechanisms, with some playing a greater role in certain patients than others. Pulmonary and systemic congestion resulting from high left ventricular (LV) diastolic filling pressures are a pathophysiologic feature common to nearly all AHFS patients (Table 30). Hemodynamic congestion, resulting from an increase in left ventricular filling pressure (LVFP) commonly results in signs and symptoms of clinical congestion, namely JVD, peripheral edema and/or an increase in body weight (Table 31). These high filling pressures lead to further activation of neurohormones, may cause subendocardial ischemia, as well as changes in LV geometry resulting in mitral insufficiency, all of which may contribute to worsening HF.

Troponin release, in the absence of clinical ACS, is a well documented phenomenon in HF and a negative prognostic marker. While the exact

Table 30: Assessment of congestion

Body weight	Increase in BW predicts hospitalization. However, a reduction in BW in response to different therapies may not necessarily result in decreased hospitalization or mortality
Arrhythmias	Both bradyarrhythmias and tachyarrhythmias can contribute to congestion
Blood pressure	Either no change in BP or an increase in BP from supine to the upright position or valsalva manuever usually reflects a relatively high LV filling pressure
Jugular venous pressure	Equals RA pressure. In a chronic state, the RA pressure correlates with PCWP/LVDP
Rales	Associated with increase in PCWP when present with other signs of elevated filling pressure (e.g. JVD, S3), but is non-specific by itself
Edema	Peripheral edema, only when associated with JVD, indicates right-sided failure that is usually associated with left sided HF. During hospitalization, may move from dependent periphery to the sacral area
Orthopnea test	Patients often do not tolerate lying flat when there is a rapid increase in filling pressure. However, in a chronic state, this position may be tolerated in spite of a relatively high filling pressure
BNP/NT-proBNP	Marker of increased filling pressures
Chest X-ray	Pulmonary congestion (cephalization, interstitial edema, alveolar edema, pleural effusions) may be absent in spite of a very high PCWP, even in patients with severe, but chronic HF. However, when present, indicates a high PCWP

(Exercise testing to assess functional classification might aid in assessment of residual congestion)
(Abbreviations: BW: Body weight; BP: Blood pressure; HF: Heart failure; PCWP: Pulmonary capillary wedge pressure; LVDP: Left ventricular diastolic pressure; BNP: B-type natriuretic peptide. (*Source:* Georghiade M, Pang PS. Acute heart failure syndromes. J Am Coll Cardiol. 2009;53:557-73, with permission)

Table 31: Hemodynamic versus clinical congestion

- *Hemodynamic congestion* refers to the state of volume overload resulting in increased left ventricular filling pressure
- *Clinical congestion* refers to the constellation of signs and symptoms that result from increased left ventricular filling pressure
- Clinical congesting can be thought to consist of cardiopulmonary congestion (respiratory distress, third heart sound, rales, interstitial/alveolar edema, chest X-ray findings) and systemic congestion (jugular venous distention, peripheral edema)
- Hemodynamic congestion precedes cardiopulmonary congestion by several days
  - In its preclinical state, hemodynamic congestion can exist without clinical manifestation
  - Intervention in preclinical hemodynamic congestion may prevent development of clinical congestion that generally requires hospitalization contributing to heart failure progression
- Resolution of clinical congestion can occur with persistent hemodynamic congestion.

(*Source:* Gheorghiade M, Filippatos G, De Luca L, et al. Congestion in acute heart failure syndromes: an essential target of evaluation and treatment. Am J Med. 2006;119:S3-10, with permission)

pathophysiologic mechanisms are not fully known, troponin release likely occurs due to a supply/demand mismatch (increased myocardial oxygen demand and decreased coronary perfusion). Myocardial injury in AHFS remains an area of investigation; likely new insights will emerge, given the continued development of high sensitivity troponin assays.

Approximately 90% of AHFS patients have renal impairment at hospital admission, defined by eGFR <90 mL/min/m^2. Hemodynamic abnormalities, such as low cardiac output, high venous pressure, neurohormonal disturbances, untoward drug effects (e.g. high dose loop diuretics or ACEI), may all contribute to renal impairment. In addition, patients have significant comorbid conditions, such as diabetes and hypertension, which play a role in renal impairment.

Fluid overload is the clinical hallmark of AHFS. However, it has been suggested that total volume increase may not be the predominant pathophysiologic result for all patients; rather fluid redistribution may be a significant driver of pulmonary congestion.

The improper availability, metabolism and/or utilization of substrates to fuel the energy needs of the heart have been proposed as another pathophysiologic contributor to HF. Whether supplemental nutrition to augment or replenish the fuel needs of the heart, in addition to the other benefits of nutritional supplementation, improves outcomes in AHFS is an area of ongoing research.

Although traditional therapies improve signs and symptoms, they have also been associated with undesirable effects:
- Nonpotassium sparing IV loop diuretics have been associated with electrolyte abnormalities, further activation of neurohormones and worsening renal function
- High-dose diuretic therapy has been associated with worse outcomes [diuretics optimization strategies evaluation (DOSE) trial]
- Commonly used inotropes, such as dobutamine and milrinone (and levosimendan in Europe) increase myocardial oxygen consumption in the face of inadequate reserves. In addition, they have also been commonly called inodilators; these vasodilatory effects may impair coronary and renal perfusion, initiating or amplifying injury or dysfunction.

Viable but dysfunctional myocardium is most commonly associated with chronic ischemia (i.e. hibernation); yet, patients without CAD have also been shown to exhibit viable but dysfunctional myocardium. Excessive sympathetic stimulation (as seen in Takotsubo cardiomyopathy) or micronutrient deficiencies are two other potential mechanisms contributing to viable but dysfunctional tissue in HF patients. The hemodynamic and neurohormonal stress of AHFS may further jeopardize this viable tissue.

❑ ACUTE HEART FAILURE SYNDROMES MANAGEMENT

For the vast majority of patients, hospital management begins in the emergency department (ED). As patients progress through their hospital stay, on an average around 6 days (median = 4 days), management goals also change. The AHFS care can broadly be divided into three main phases (Table 32):
1. Stabilization
2. Evidence-based management
3. Reconstruction

Stabilization Phase

Definitive airway management, assessment and support of breathing, and circulatory support as needed (the A, B, C's) remain essential principles of initial assessment and resuscitation. Other life-threatening conditions, such as STEMI, papillary muscle rupture, malignant arrhythmias and hypertensive emergencies, should be promptly identified and treated. In patients who present in extremis,

Table 32: Phases of AHFS management

Phases	Goals	Available tools
Initial or emergency department phase of management	Treat life-threatening conditions	e.g. STEMI -> reperfusion therapy
	Establish the diagnosis	History, physical exam, EKG, X-ray, natriuretic peptide level
	Determine the clinical profile	BP, HR, signs (e.g. pulmonary edema), ECG, X-ray, laboratory analysis, echocardiography
	Identify and treat precipitant	History, physical exam, X-ray, ECG, laboratory analysis
	Disposition	No universally accepted risk-stratification method
In-hospital phase	Monitoring and reassessment	Signs/symptoms, HR, SBP, ECG, orthostatic changes, body weight, laboratory analysis (BUN/Cr, electrolytes), potentially BNP
	Assess right and left ventricular pressures	SBP (orthostatic changes, valsalva maneuver), echocardiography, BNP/NT-proBNP, PA catheter
	Assess and treat (in the right patient) other cardiac and non-cardiac conditions	Echo-Doppler, cardiac catheterization, electrophysiology testing
	Assess for myocardial viability	MRI, stress testing, EKG, radionuclear studies
Discharge phase	Assess functional capacity	6-minute walk test
	Re-evaluate exacerbating factors (e.g. non-adherence, infection, anemia, arrhythmias, hypertension) and treat accordingly	Examples: physical therapy, education for diet control and medication, evaluation for sleep apnea
	Optimize pharmacologic therapy	ACCF/AHA and ESC guidelines
	Establish post-discharge planning	Discharge instructions including body weight monitoring, smoking cessation, medication adherence, follow-up

(*Source:* Khan SS, Gheorghiade M, Dunn JD, et al. Managed care interventions for improving outcomes in acute heart failure syndromes. Am J Manag Care. 2008;14:S273-86; quiz S287-91, with permission)

diagnosis and treatment occur in parallel. A proposed algorithm for treatment is presented in Flowcharts 2 to 5.

Patients' initial management should be guided by their predominant clinical profile (Fig. 33). For example, vasodilators should promptly be considered for those who present with a hypertensive profile. The goals are to improve hemodynamic and volume status, leading to symptom improvement. However prudent attention to vital signs is warranted. Identification and treatment of the precipitant for decompensation is essential (Table 33).

Patients at higher risk for morbid events or with high-risk clinical or laboratory features have been relatively well defined (Table 34). While the unstable patient warrants intensive care admission, clear guidelines for ICU versus step-down or intermediate care versus general ward have not been well established. Importantly, absence of high-risk features does not equal low-risk.

FLOWCHART 2: Suggested initial triage in patients with suspected heart failure syndromes

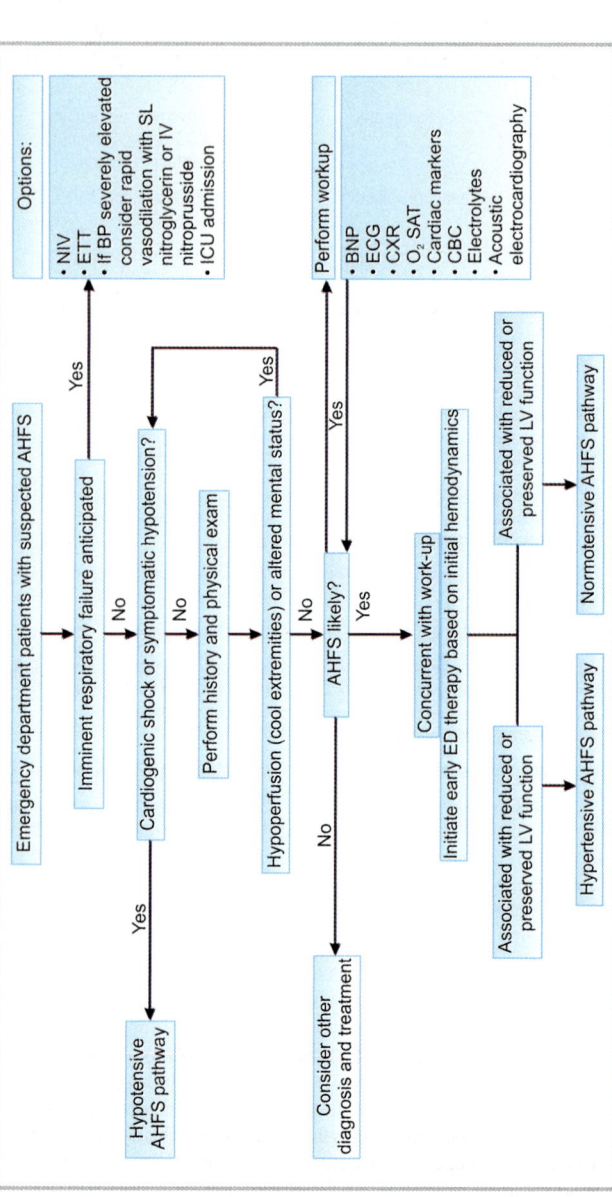

(Abbreviations: AHFS: Acute heart failure syndrome; NIV: Noninvasive ventilation; ETT: Endotracheal intubation; BP: Blood pressure; SL: Sublingual; BNP: B-type natriuretic peptide; CXR: Chest X-ray; O_2 SAT: Oxygen saturation; LV: Left ventricular) (*Source:* Reproduced with permission from Collins S, Storrow AB, Kirk JD, et al. Beyond pulmonary edema: diagnostic, risk stratification, and treatment challenges of acute heart failure management in the emergency department. Ann Emerg Med. 2008;51:45-57)

FLOWCHART 3: Suggested treatment algorithm for patients with hypotensive acute heart failure syndromes

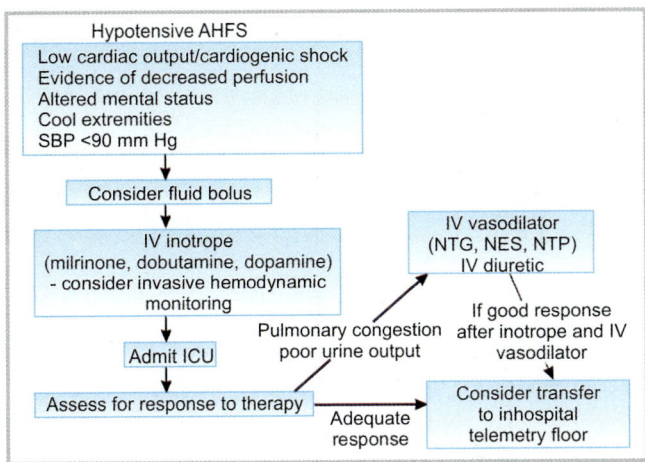

(Abbreviations: NTG: Nitroglycerin; NES: Nesiritide; NTP: Nitroprusside) (*Source:* Reproduced with permission from Collins S, Storrow AB, Kirk JD, et al. Beyond pulmonary edema: diagnostic, risk stratification, and treatment challenges of acute heart failure management in the emergency department. Ann Emerg Med. 2008;51:45-57)

Goals of Stabilization Phase

After addressing any immediate life-threats, improving symptoms, hemodynamic and volume status, along with identification and treatment of precipitants of decompensation are the initial stabilization phase goals.

Transition to Evidence-based Phase

Once stabilized, they transition back to chronic HF management, where evidence-based management is robust. However, translational gaps between evidence and daily practice have been noted, with variations seen by age, race, geographic region and comorbid conditions. When compared to guidelines for reduced EF patients, the evidence is limited for those patients with HFPEF. For HFPEF, management of comorbid conditions is strongly recommended.

Goals of Transitional Phase

During hospitalization, attempts to resolve or either return to baseline status prior to hospitalization is an important goal. Optimization of hemodynamic status and return to euvolemia should ideally be achieved prior to discharge. A strategy of earlier discharge with mild signs and symptoms and close follow-up may also be considered; however, further research is needed. Unless clearly contraindicated and/or the cause for decompensation, outpatient chronic HF medications (such as beta-blockers) should be continued. Initiation or assessment for implementation of guideline-based therapies should occur during the hospital setting. Use of biomarker guided strategies to facilitate management decisions appear promising, however further studies in the hospital setting are needed prior to universal recommendations. Finally, a clear post-discharge plan with reconciliation of all

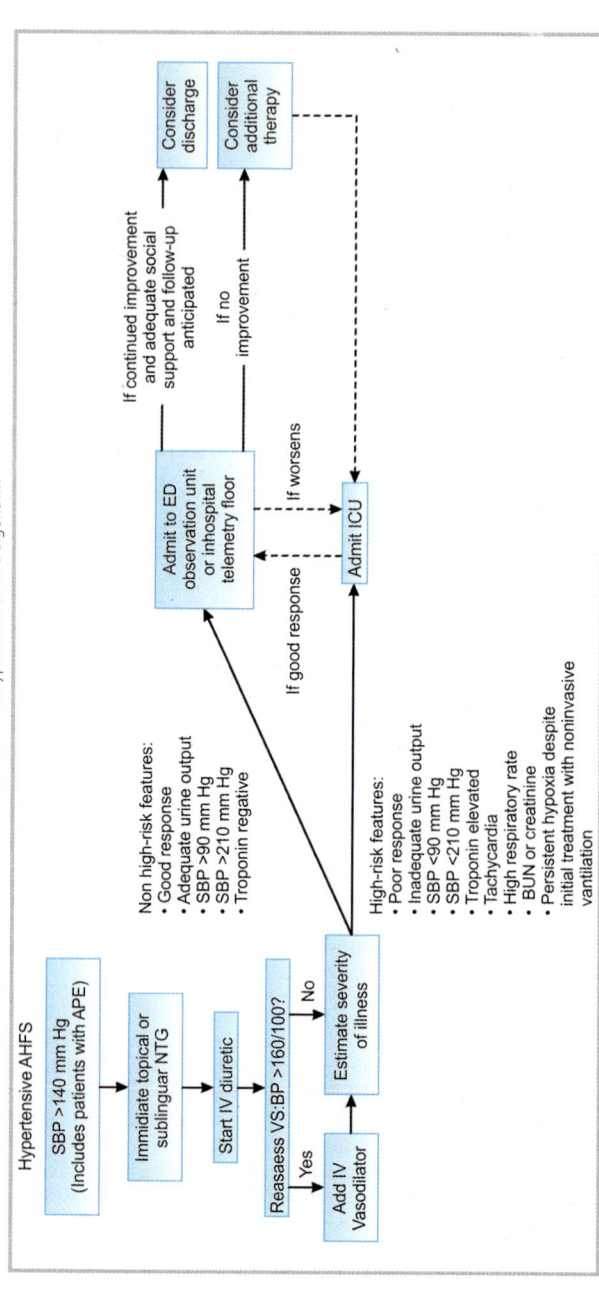

FLOWCHART 4: Hypertensive AHFS algorithm

(Abbreviations: SBP: Systolic blood pressure; NTG: Nitroglycerin; IV: Intravenous; VS: Vital signs; BP: Blood pressure; ED: Emergency department; ICU: Intensive care unit). (*Source:* Reproduced with permission from Collins S, Storrow AB, Kirk JD, et al. Beyond pulmonary edema: diagnostic, risk stratification, and treatment challenges of acute heart failure management in the emergency department. Ann Emerg Med. 2008;51:45-57)

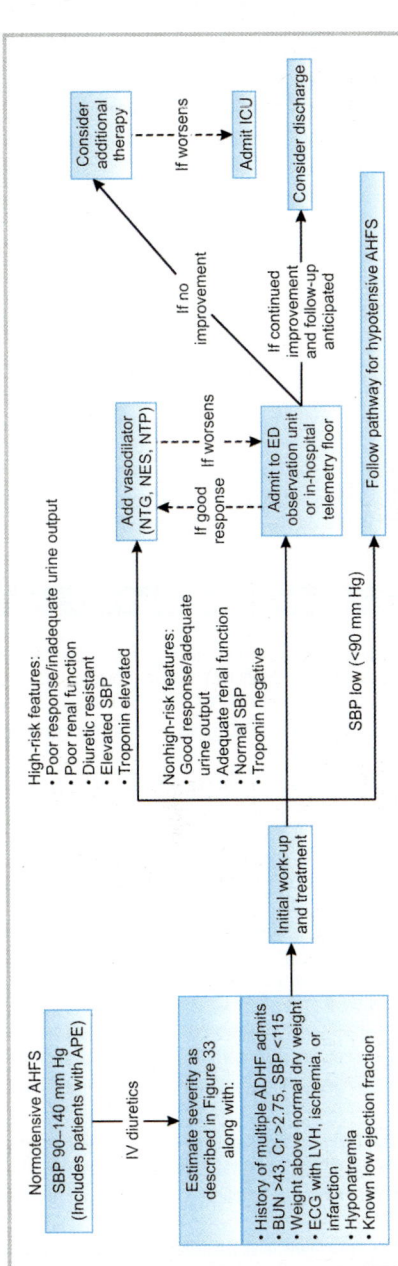

FLOWCHART 5: Normotensive AHFS Algorithm

(Abbreviations: SBP: Systolic blood pressure; APE: Acute pulmonary edema; ADHF: Acute decompensated heart failure; LVH: Left ventricular hypertrophy; NTG: Nitroglycerin; NES: Nesiritide; NTP: Nitroprusside; ED: Emergency department; AHFS: Acute heart failure syndromes; ICU: Intensive care unit). (*Source:* Reproduced with permission from Collins S, Storrow AB, Kirk JD, et al. Beyond pulmonary edema: diagnostic, risk stratification, and treatment challenges of acute heart failure management in the emergency department. Ann Emerg Med. 2008;51:45-57)

Table 33: Precipitating factors for HF hospitalization and their association with in-hospital mortality

Factor	No. of patient	Adjusted length of stay ratio	p value	In hospital mortality	
				Adjusted odds ratio (95% confidence interval)	p value
Ischemia/acute coronary syndrome	7155	0.99	.22	1.20 (1.03-1.40)	.02
Arrhythmia	6552	1.04	<.001	0.85 (0.71-1.01)	.07
Nonadherence to diet	2504	0.96	.01	0.69 (0.48-1.00)	.05
Uncontrolled hypertension	5220	.096	<.001	0.74 (0.55-0.99)	.04
Nonadherence to medications	4309	0.96	<.001	0.88 (0.67-1.17)	.39
Pneumonia/respiratory process	7426	1.08	<.001	1.60 (1.38-1.85)	<.001
Worsening renal function	3304	1.09	<.001	1.48 (1.23-1.79)	<.001
Other	6171	0.99	.23	1.15 (0.97-1.36)	.10

(*Source:* Fonarow GC, Abraham WT, Albert NM, et al. Factors identified as precipitating hospital admissions for heart failure and clinical outcomes: findings from OPTIMIZE-HF. Arch Intern Med. 2008;168:847-54, with permission)

Table 34: Prognostic indicators as potential targets of therapy in AHFS*

Systolic blood pressure	Admission and early post-discharge SBP inversely correlates with post-discharge mortality. The higher the BP, the lower both in-hospital and post-discharge mortality. However, the readmission rate of ~30% is independent of the SBP at time of admission
Coronary artery disease	Extent and severity of CAD appears to be a predictor of poor prognosis
Troponin release	Results in threefold increase in in-hospital mortality, twofold increase in post-discharge mortality and athreefold increase in the rehospitalization rate
Ventricular dyssynchrony	Increase in QRS duration occurs in ~40% of patients with reduced systolic function and is a strong predictor of early and late post-discharge mortality and rehospitalization
Renal impairment	Associated with a 2–3-fold increase in post-discharge mortality. Worsening renal function during hospitalization or soon after discharge is also associated with an increase in inhospital and post-discharge mortality (REF LBCT)
Hyponatremia	Defined as serum sodium <135 mmol/L, occurs in ~25% of patients, and is associated with a 2–3-fold increase in post-discharge mortality
Clinical congestion at the time of discharge	An important predictor of postdischarge mortality and morbidity
Ejection fraction	Considered adverse prognostic marker. Similar postdischarge event rates and mortality between reduced and preserved EF19
BNP/NT-proBNP	Elevated natriuretic peptides associated with increased resource utilization and mortality
Functional capacity at the time of discharge	Predischarge functional capacity, defined by the 6-minute walk test, is emerging as an important predictor of post-discharge outcomes

(*Source:* Gheorghiade et al. Circulation. 2005, with permission)
*This is not an all-inclusive list

medications, comprehensive understanding from the patient's perspective and a resilient transition of care plan is needed prior to discharge.

Reconstruction Phase

As HF is both progressive and irreversible, the concept of cardiac reconstruction is controversial. Yet, the vast majority of patients do not have end-stage HF, improvement or restoration of cardiac function has been observed in a sizable number of patients and, most importantly, many patients have potential targets that, if treated per guidelines, may improve cardiac performance.

Vulnerable Phase

The early postdischarge period may also be called a vulnerable phase, as patients demonstrate continued changes in signs and symptoms, worsening neurohormonal profile, and changes in renal function, despite evidence-based therapy. As optimization of guideline therapies and/or implementation of other therapies that require optimal medical management (e.g. cardiac resynchronization therapy) may be difficult to achieve during a short hospital stay, comprehensive assessment and implementation of known lifesaving therapies during the early postdischarge period may improve outcomes (Fig. 34).

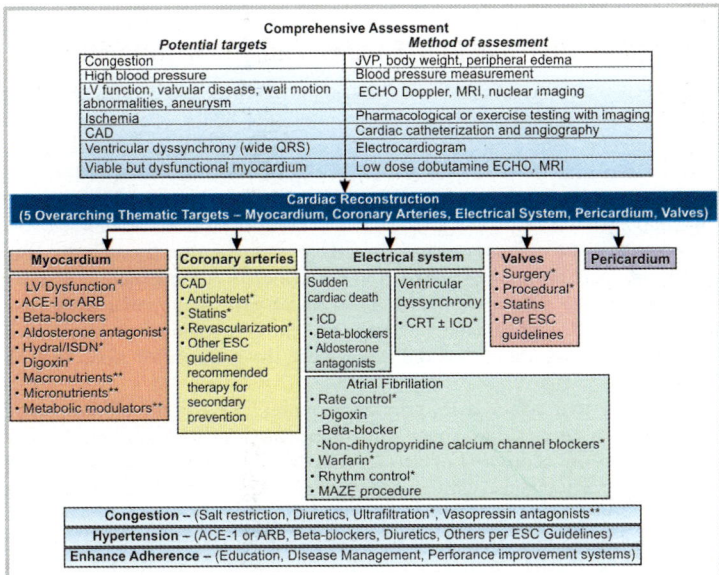

FIGURE 34: Comprehensive assessment and cardiac reconstruction (Abbreviations: AHFS: Acute heart failure syndromes; JVP: Jugular venous pulse; LV: Left ventricle; CAD: Coronary artery disease; ACE-I: Angiotensin converting enzyme inhibitor; ARB: Angiotensin receptor blocker; ICD: Implantable cardiac defibrillator; CRT: Chronic resynchronization therapy; Hydral: Hydralazine; ISDN: Isosorbide dinitrate; CABG: Coronary artery bypass grafting; AF: Atrial fibrillation)
*Select patients
**Investigational agents
#Viable but dysfunctional myocardium
(*Source:* Modified and reproduced with permission from Gheorghiade M, Pang PS. Acute heart failure syndromes. J Am Coll Cardiol. 2009;53:557-73)

Table 35: The translational phase 1 of development

T1 Concept

- A more thorough understanding of all a molecule's effects on the heart (effects on viable but noncontractile myocardium, coronary profusion, diastolic function, etc.) is important
- Reproduce the results obtained in large animal HF models in homogeneous group of patients taking into account systolic and diastolic dysfunction, extent and severity of CAD, viable but dysfunctional myocardium, etc.
- These in depth evaluations should take advantage of recent progress made in noninvasive methods of assessment of cardiac function and structure (echocardiography, MRI spectroscopy, etc.)
- These studies would also expand our understanding of the pharmacokinetic and pharmacodynamic properties of novel molecules as, unlike animal models to date, patients with HF are commonly on background therapy for HF and have substantial comorbid conditions that might influence safety, efficacy and outcomes
- These studies should be conducted in dedicated centers that have the patient population, technology and the expertise to conduct such technically challenging studies

(*Source:* Gheorghiade M, Pang PS, O'Connor CM, et al. Clinical development of pharmacologic agents for acute heart failure syndromes: a proposal for a mechanistic translational phase. Am Heart J. 2011;161:224-32, with permission)

❑ CLINICAL TRIALS IN ACUTE HEART FAILURE SYNDROMES

Only one new therapy for AHFS has been approved in the last decade, nesiritide, whose primary benefit was improved dyspnea at 3 hours when compared to regular therapy excluding nitroglycerin. Retrospective analyses regarding the safety of nesiritide led to the acute study of clinical effectiveness of nesiritide in decompensated heart failure (ASCEND-HF) trial, the largest AHFS clinical trial conducted to date. Although the safety of nesiritide was well established, the efficacy coprimary endpoint—death or HF rehospitalisation through 30 days; or dyspnea score at 6 and 24 hours—was not achieved. A more modest dyspnea improvement was seen as compared to vasodilation in acute congestive heart failure (VMAC), approximately 2% improvement over standard therapy, which was statistically significant but did not achieve the prespecified alpha level of 0.025.

Only one trial achieved its primary endpoint; the efficacy of vasopressin antagonism in heart failure study with tolvaptan (EVEREST) clinical status trials, which were comprised of two identical short-term trials. The composite primary endpoint of global clinical status and body weight was reached; however, this was driven entirely by the body weight component. A key secondary endpoint, dyspnea reduction at day one was also seen in both trials, however, the absolute clinical benefit was modest; approximately 6–7% compared to standard therapy. Although no long-term benefit was seen, there was also no evidence of long-term harm.

T1 Translational Phase

This terminology has been adopted specifically to HF clinical development, as a more focused and rigorous approach during earlier stages of development may better identify promising novel therapies. In addition, this approach would allow for discontinuation of programs that have little chance of success (Table 35).

❑ SUGGESTED READINGS

Adams KF, Fonarow GC, Emerman CL, et al. Characteristics and outcomes of patients hospitalized for heart failure in the United States: rationale, design, and preliminary observations from the first 100,000 cases in the Acute Decompensated Heart Failure National Registry (ADHERE). Am Heart J. 2005;149:209-16.

Collins SP, Storrow AB. Acute heart failure risk stratification: can we define low risk? Heart Failure Clinics. 2009;5:75-83.

Dickstein K, Cohen-Solal A, Filippatos G, et al. ESC Guidelines for the diagnosis and treatment of acute and chronic heart failure 2008: the Task Force for the Diagnosis and Treatment of Acute and Chronic Heart Failure 2008 of the European Society of Cardiology. Developed in collaboration with the Heart Failure Association of the ESC (HFA) and endorsed by the European Society of Intensive Care Medicine (ESICM). Eur Heart J. 2008;29:2388-442.

Felker GM, Lee KL, Bull DA, et al. Diuretic strategies in patients with acute decompensated heart failure. N Engl J Med. 2011;364:797-805.

Fonarow GC, Heywood JT, Heidenreich PA, et al. Temporal trends in clinical characteristics, treatments, and outcomes for heart failure hospitalizations, 2002 to 2004: findings from Acute Decompensated Heart Failure National Registry (ADHERE). Am Heart J. 2007;153:1021-8.

Gheorghiade M, Braunwald E. Reconsidering the role for digoxin in the management of acute heart failure syndromes. JAMA. 2009;302:2146-7.

Gheorghiade M, Gattis Stough W, Adams KF, et al. The Pilot Randomized Study of Nesiritide Versus Dobutamine in Heart Failure (PRESERVD-HF). Am J Cardiol. 2005;96:18G-25G.

Gheorghiade M, Konstam MA, Burnett JC, et al. Short-term clinical effects of tolvaptan, an oral vasopressin antagonist, in patients hospitalized for heart failure: the EVEREST Clinical Status Trials. JAMA. 2007;297:1332-43.

Hernandez AF, O'Connor CM, Starling RC, et al. Rationale and design of the Acute Study of Clinical Effectiveness of Nesiritide in Decompensated Heart Failure Trial (ASCEND-HF). Am Heart J. 2009;157:271-7.

Heywood JT, Fonarow GC, Costanzo MR, et al. High prevalence of renal dysfunction and its impact on outcome in 118,465 patients hospitalized with acute decompensated heart failure: a report from the ADHERE database. J Card Fail. 2007;13:422-30.

Ingwall JS, Weiss RG. Is the failing heart energy starved? On using chemical energy to support cardiac function. Circ Res. 2004;95:135-45.

Jondeau G, Neuder Y, Eicher JC, et al. B-CONVINCED: Beta-blocker CONtinuation Vs. INterruption in patients with Congestive heart failure hospitalizED for a decompensation episode. Eur Heart J. 2009;30:2186-92.

Pang PS, Komajda M, Gheorghiade M. The current and future management of acute heart failure syndromes. Eur Heart J. 2010;31:777-83.

7.6 Cardiopulmonary Exercise Testing and Training in Heart Failure

❏ INTRODUCTION

Exercise capacity (functional capacity) in patients with heart failure (HF) has prognostic value, and objective testing becomes an important tool to assess patients for mortality risk. Oxygen uptake is the product of the central cardiovascular system and the peripheral expressed as cardiac output × the arteriovenous difference (Flowcharts 6A and B). This equation is derived from the Fick principle. Maximal oxygen uptake (VO_{2max}) is defined as the maximal amount of oxygen that the organism can "uptake" and even if workload is increased, no further increases in oxygen uptake are noted. Thus the ability to increase one's VO_2 is related to the ability of the heart to increase its cardiac output in response to the demand of muscles and the ability of muscles to extract more oxygen from the oxygenated blood. In the normal adult cardiac output can increase by 400–500% of baseline by a 2–4-fold rise in heart rate and a more modest but significant increase in stroke

FLOWCHARTS 6A AND B: Maximal oxygen uptake (VO_{2max}) = C.O. (HR × SV) × Δ(A-V)O_2. Mechanisms to augment cardiac output (C.O.) in (A) healthy persons without HF and (B) patients with HF. VO_{2max} = CO (HR × SV) × ▲A-V O_2. CO indicates cardiac output

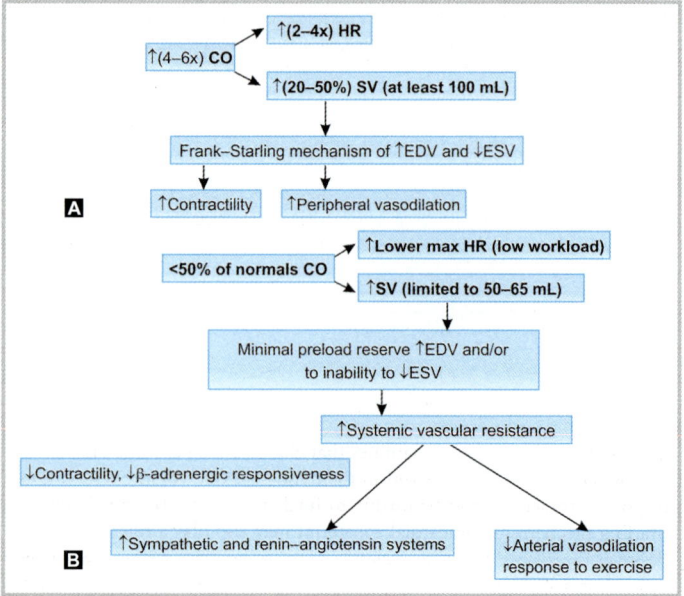

(Abbreviations: HR: Heart rate; SV: Stroke volume; ▲A-VO_2: Arteriovenous oxygen difference; EDV: End-diastolic volume; ESV: End-systolic volume) (*Source:* See text from: Piña. Circulation. 2003;107:1210-1225)

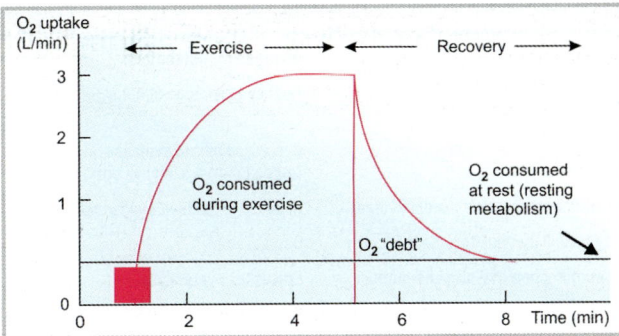

FIGURE 35: Oxygen uptake during exercise and recovery

volume of 20–50%. The Frank–Starling mechanism is responsible for the increase in end-diastolic volume and coupled with increased inotropism and a lower end-systolic volume, the stroke volume increases (Flowchart 6).

The term "peak VO_2" is often used rather than "maximal VO_2" to define the last VO_2 recorded at the highest workload of exercise, leaving the definition of "maximal" to obtaining a plateau effect at high levels of work. The cardiovascular response to exercise is dependent on age, gender, level of fitness and genetic factors. The type of exercise and posture that is performed and the number of skeletal muscles involved also affect the VO_2. Figure 35 illustrates the VO_2 curve as it increases with increased workload, plateaus at maximal exercise and drops in recovery. The area under the exercise curve is the oxygen consumed and that of the area under the recovery portion is the oxygen debt. Baseline VO_2 is the value at rest and often referred to as 1 MET or "metabolic equivalent". Generally, this value is approximately 3.5 mL/kg/min.

❑ EXERCISE RESPONSE IN HEART FAILURE

The cardiac output may appear to be relatively normal at rest, but cannot increase adequately with even mild exertion in HF patients and therefore exercise capacity is reduced even in mild HF. In general, the source of exercise intolerance is multifactorial (the central and peripheral factors have been described in Subchapter 2.4: ECG Exercise Testing.

Central Factors

- The heart rate and inotropic responses to circulating catecholamines are impaired, partly due to downregulation of beta receptors due to the chronically increased circulating catecholamines that characterized chronic HF
- HF patients may already be within their end-diastolic volume reserve coupled to poor contractility, and be unable to further increase stroke volume via the Starling mechanism. Pericardial constraint may also play a role
- Exercise is associated with an elevation in the pulmonary wedge pressure which can exacerbate pulmonary congestion, thereby causing dyspnea and limiting exercise capacity. The high left-sided pressure is accompanied by equalization with right atrial pressure, probably due to pericardial constraint in addition to increased blood return to the right side of the heart

Table 36: Skeletal muscle changes in heart failure	
Changes in structure	**Changes in metabolism**
Loss of type I (slow twitch) fibers (endurance fibers)	Reduced glycogen content
Increase in type II (fast twitch) fibers (easily fatigued)	Decreased citrate synthase (mitochondrial oxidative enzyme)
Decreased fiber size (cross-sectional area)	Increase in reactive oxygen species
Decreased capillary density	Decreased pH
Decreased mitochondrial size and number	Ergoreflex overactivity
Apoptosis	

- As ventricular dilatation worsens, mitral regurgitation may occur due to stretching of the mitral annulus and contribute to the poor forward cardiac output. Vasodilators may improve peak forward cardiac output by decreasing the regurgitant jet.

Peripheral Factors

- Blood flow is impaired in HF due to vasoconstriction due to the neurohormonal responses (angiotensin II, endothelin) coupled with impaired cardiac output and abnormal vasodilatation due to abnormal release of vasoactive substances. Nitric oxide secretion is also impaired as is the vasodilatory response to it.
- Patients with HF have a lower percentage of type I oxidative skeletal muscle fibres and an increase in the more glycolytic type IIb when compared to normal subjects. This fiber "switch" can account for peripheral muscle fatigue. Intramuscular acidosis is due to early and increased anaerobic metabolism with exercise leading to increased lactic acid levels. Table 36 lists the skeletal muscle changes in HF.
- In general, capillary density is also lower in patients with HF when compared to normal healthy subjects. Oxidative enzymes, such as citrate synthase, succinate dehydrogenase and others, are also decreased in patients with HF.

❑ CARDIOPULMONARY EXERCISE TESTING

Understanding the link between the pulmonary system and the cardiovascular system is necessary to fully comprehend the mechanism of cardiopulmonary testing (Fig. 36).

Exercise capacity is an important prognostic indicator in patients with HF and is frequently used to gauge the severity of the patient's symptoms. Measuring the maximal oxygen uptake in HF patients has become a common clinical practice. It provides an objective measure of the HF patient's functional status and helps in monitoring the response to treatment as well as making decisions in terms of various interventions, including referral for heart transplantation.

Exercise testing can be administered using various modalities, e.g. treadmill or bicycle, adjusted to patient level of ability and modified with the use of imaging to improve accuracy. When oxygen uptake measurements are added, exercise testing can add much information to the ordinary exercise test. Cardiopulmonary exercise (CPX) testing with metabolic parameters has been used in fitness testing of athletes to determine true maximum function and to study exercise physiology.

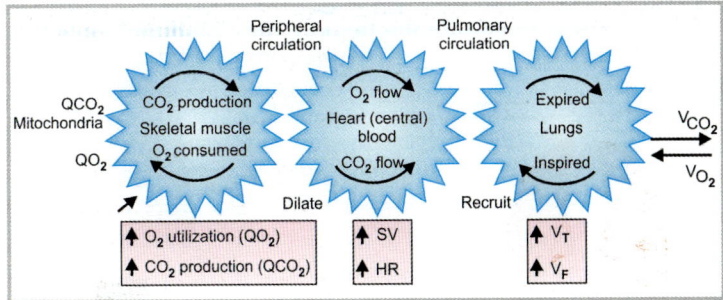

FIGURE 36: Cardiopulmonary unit

CPX testing is the most accurate exercise test to determine true functional capacity and in the case of HF patients, to predict prognosis. With the advent of modern testing systems that integrate breath by breath technology, computerized systems and patient-friendly mouthpiece and tubing, CPX testing has become accessible for broader use.

CPX can measure the VO_2 and the CO_2 production by quantifying gases at the mouth with the use of a pneumotachometer to measure air flow. Therefore, CPX is an indirect measure of what is occurring at the tissue level by gas detection at the mouth.

Technical Aspects

The pneumotach measures airflow across a membrane and converts it to a digital signal for minute ventilation (VE) (Fig. 37). Rapid gas analyzers include a heated zirconium for O_2 where the gradient between room air (adjusted to temperature, humidity and barometric pressure) is measured and converted to a digital signal for O_2 consumed (VO_2). The CO_2 analyzer is infrared since CO_2 absorbs infrared light and the amount is converted to a digital signal for the VCO_2 in the sample air. Some of the parameters that can be measured or derived by CPX have been listed in Table 37.

Oxygen Uptake

Exercise capacity can be quantitated clinically by measurement of oxygen uptake (VO_2), carbon dioxide production (VCO_2) and minute ventilation. VO2 is usually expressed as "peak" or "maximal" in L/min or normalized by body weight to mL/kg/min. Weber and Janicky have divided the levels of VO_2 in HF patients by class of A-D based on testing with hemodynamic parameters. Class A has the least impairment as shown in Table 38.

Ventilatory Threshold or Anaerobic Threshold

The ventilatory threshold (VT), formerly referred to as the anaerobic threshold (AT), is defined as the point at which minute ventilation increases disproportionately relative to VO_2, a response that is generally seen at 60–70% of VO_{2max}. The VT is a reflection of the disproportionate increase in lactic acid production by working muscles. It can be used to distinguish between non-cardiac (pulmonary or musculoskeletal) and cardiac causes of exercise limitation, since

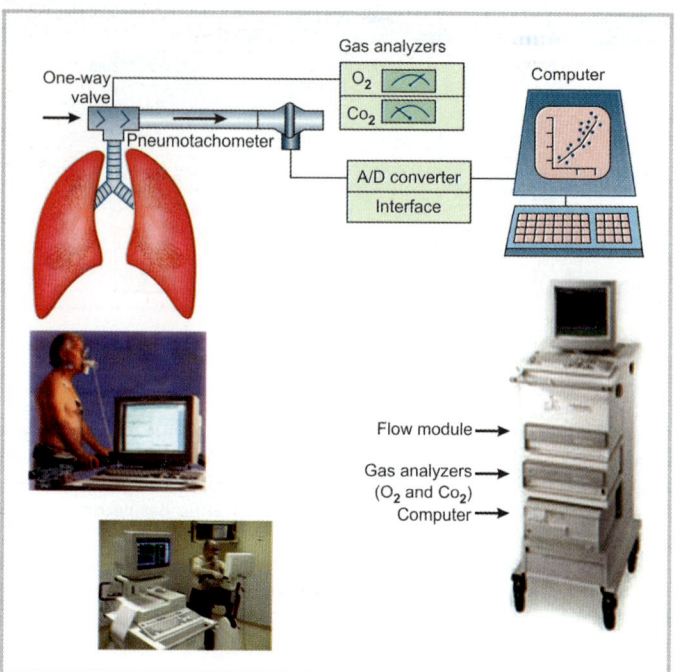

FIGURE 37: Technical components

Table 37: Parameters measure or derived from CPX	
Parameter	Expressed as units of measure
Oxygen uptake	VO_2 L/min or mL/kg/min
Carbon dioxide production	CO_2 L/min or mL/kg/min
Ventilatory (anaerobic) threshold	VT or AT mL/kg/min or % peak VO_2
Respiratory exchange ratio (RER)	VCO_2/VO_2
Oxygen pulse	VO_2/heart rate
Ventilatory equivalent for O_2	VEO_2
Ventilatory equivalent for CO_2	$VECO_2$
Minute ventilation	VE
Ventilatory efficiency	VE/VCO_2

patients who fatigue prior to reaching VT are likely to have a noncardiac problem. It has been suggested that the VT might be more predictive than the peak VO_2 because it is less prone to error or to patient effort. Figure 38 illustrates the VT choice using the VCO_2-VO_2 slope method. Most current CPX systems have this algorithm built into the software.

Table 38: Functional impairment during incremental treadmill testing the Weber classification

Class	Severity	Peak VO$_2$ (mL/kg/min)	AT	CI max (L/min/m$_2$)
A	Mild to none	>20	>14	>8
B	Mild to moderate	16–20	11–14	6–8
C	Moderate to severe	10–16	8–11	4–6
D	Severe	6–10	5–8	2–4
E	Very severe	<6	<4	<2

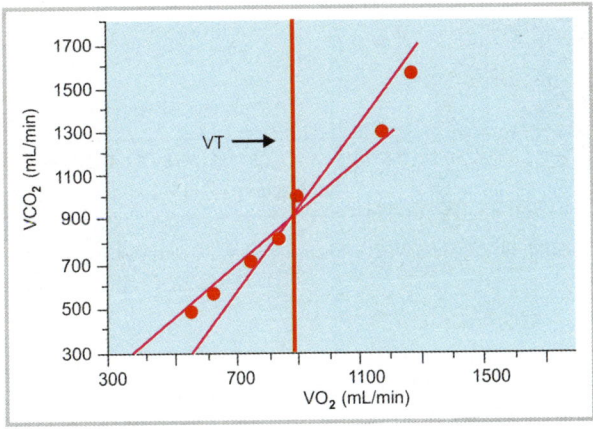

FIGURE 38: VT choice using the VCO$_2$–VO$_2$ slope method

Oxygen Pulse

The Peak VO$_2$ divided by the heart rate (PeakVO$_2$/HR) is called the oxygen pulse and is an indirect measure of stroke volume. The relationship between cardiac output and VO$_2$ also forms the basis for the Fick equation used to measure cardiac output.

Respiratory Exchange Ratio (RER)

This value is equal to the VCO$_2$/VO$_2$ and is an indirect measure of effort. As exercise progresses, and VCO$_2$ exceeds the rate of VO$_2$ increase, the RER will increase beyond 1.0. As VT approaches, the RER is usually greater than 1.1. The RER can help the professional who administers the test to gauge the level of patient effort and compare to the level of perceived exertion.

Ventilatory Efficiency

A possible alternative in HF patients who cannot achieve a true VO$_2$max is the measurement of the ventilatory efficiency, i.e. ventilation-to-CO$_2$ production ratio in early exercise. During CPX a close linear relationship exists between the production of CO$_2$ (VCO$_2$) and minute ventilation (VE). The slope of the regression line relating CO$_2$ production and minute ventilation (VE/VCO$_2$) can

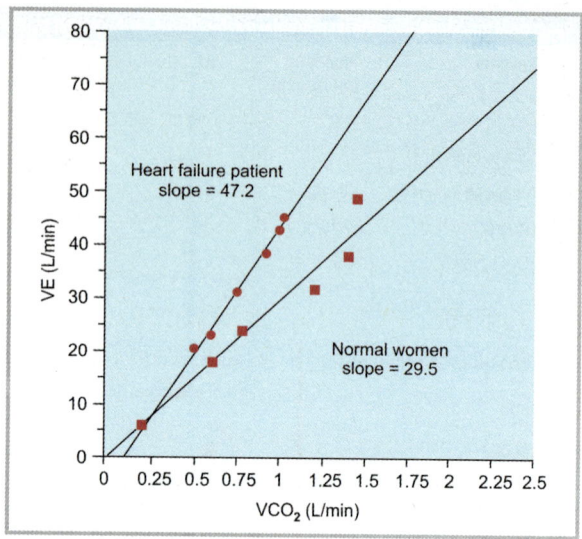

FIGURE 39: Slope of VE/VCO$_2$ in a normal woman and a man with heart failure

be used to describe the ventilatory response to exercise. In patients with HF, the VE/VCO$_2$ slope is easier to obtain than parameters of maximal exercise capacity and may be an additional predictor of outcome. In HF, the VE/VCO$_2$ slope is higher than in normal (Fig. 39). A VE/VCO$_2$ regression line slope of greater than 34 is associated with reduced cardiac output during exercise, increased pulmonary artery wedge pressures and reduced survival.

Ventilation

A patient with primarily lung disease may exhibit a low VO$_2$ due to ventilatory limitations which impair the exercise response prior to achieving a cardiovascular limit. It is recommended that if testing a patient with known lung disease, a full pulmonary function test be performed and these results should be evaluated in conjunction with the CPX findings.

Conducting the Exercise Test

The protocol most commonly used for testing of patients with HF is the modified Naughton protocol. However, with CPX, most protocols can work well. It is important, as a good testing format, to choose a protocol that fits with the patient's ability to walk or bike. Choosing an acceptable protocol tailored to a patient can make a great difference in cooperation and feeling of comfort and trust. Since actual measurements of effort (RER) and function (VO$_2$) are being collected, the choice of protocol is not as salient. A warm-up period is recommended especially for patients who are fairly sedentary. This warm-up period will also allow to quality check the CPX gases for accuracy, drift and potential troubleshooting.

Table 39: Indications for CPX testing in heart failure
• Prognostic implications
• The presence and nature of ventilatory limitations
• The presence and nature of cardiovascular limitation with heart failure
• The extent of conditioning or deconditioning
• The maximum tolerable workload and safe levels of daily exercise to give recommendations
• The extent of disability for rehabilitation purposes
• Oxygen desaturation and appropriate levels of supplemental oxygen therapy if lung disease is present

❏ INDICATIONS FOR CPX TESTING IN HEART FAILURE

Common indications for CPX testing in patients with HF have been listed in Table 39.

Peak VO_2 and Prognosis

The values of peak VO_2 were illustrated in a report of 114 consecutive ambulatory patients with advanced disease referred for possible cardiac transplantation to a large academic medical center and were prospectively divided into three groups:

- Group 1: Patients who were accepted as transplant candidates (peak VO_2 ≤14 mL/kg/min)
- Group 2: Patients who were considered too well for transplantation (peak VO_2 >14 mL/kg/min)
- Group 3: Patients who were rejected for transplantation due to various reasons such as malignancy or age (peak VO_2 ≤14 mL/kg/min).

Keeping in mind that a normal person can achieve higher than 20 mL/kg/min, these values were considered low and demonstrated impaired functional capacity. The 1-year survival of the healthier patients in group 2 was 94%, an outcome that was similar to that in transplanted patients in group 1. The prognosis was the poorest in group 3, although survival varied with the peak VO_2 in this group. Patients with a value less than or equal to 10 mL/kg/min had the lowest survival, while those between 10–14 mL/kg/min had an outcome that was only slightly worse than patients in group 1. Based on this study, many transplant centres have used 14 mL/kg/min as a cutoff point for listing patients for transplantation. However it does not take into consideration the lower peak VO_2 that occurs with age alone without disease or gender.

The HF-ACTION trial tested over 2,000 patients with NYHA Classes II and III HF, 50% ischemics and reported a mean peak VO_2 of 14.9 mL/kg/min. Therefore, the "magic number" of 14 mL/kg/min should be reconsidered in light of this new and extensive database.

Evaluation of Dyspnea: Presence of Ventilatory Limitations

Flowchart 2 is an algorithm to help interpret the ventilation and the VO_2 parameters when dyspnea is a symptom. A peak VO_2 of below 85% predicted for age and gender is low and requires looking carefully at the VT. The VT should be approximately 60–70% of the peak VO_2. An early VT may indicate circulatory issues. Ventilatory impairment is usually indicated by a breathing reserve of less than 30%. If this is suspected, the CPX test could be accompanied by a pulse oximeter looking for desaturation. If the RER is less than 1.0, the patient may have exerted a poor effort or was experiencing anxiety.

Extent of Deconditioning and Deriving: An Exercise Prescription

Patients often cut down activities that would cause symptoms and answer negatively to symptoms of dyspnea or fatigue. A CPX can help to determine the true level of deconditioning versus limitation due to disease. The CPX test can help to better delineate patients for safe level of exercise training using either a heart rate or a perceived level of effort. Determination of VT can assure that training is prescribed at a level below it by encouraging RER to greater than 1.0 during the exercise test. In the era of beta blockers, a rate of perceived exertion (RPE) below the VT may serve as an adequate intensity where heart rate may be blunted during the CPX test.

❏ EXERCISE TRAINING IN HEART FAILURE

Bed rest is deleterious to normal subjects, and it is certainly deleterious to patients with HF. Functional capacity can decrease by as much as 8.4% in men and 6.8% in women and total exercise tolerance decreases by 8.1% in men and 7.3% in women by 10 days. Peak heart rate increases in both men and women with bed rest alone. Inactivity also increases submaximal heart rate with a decrease in vagal tone, increased sympathetic catecholamine secretion, and enhanced beta-receptor sensitivity to circulating catecholamines. Added to this deconditioning, clinicians may recommend bed rest in an effort to not "push" the heart.

Exercise training does not improve cardiac function at rest, as estimated from left ventricular ejection fraction, baseline cardiac output or wedge pressure. Training, however, has been reported to affect the following:

- Increased peak VO_2, peak cardiac output, and leg blood flow during exercise
- Improved muscle energetics so that oxygen utilization becomes more efficient
- Partial reversal of the abnormalities in mitochondrial density and ultrastructure and on fiber type distribution in skeletal muscle seen with HF
- Improvement of peripheral endothelial dysfunction with restoration of endothelium-mediated flow-dependent dilation, possibly due to enhanced endothelial release of nitric oxide
- These benefits can result in a greater amount of work performed externally with less work internally
- Potential for reduction in sympathetic tone and an increase in vagal tone at rest, thereby restoring autonomic cardiovascular control toward normal.

The HF-ACTION demonstrated the safety of training in this population. To date, HF-ACTION is the largest study to prospectively ask the question about benefits on exercise training in HF on mortality and morbidity. The trial showed a modest reduction in the primary endpoint of all cause mortality or all cause hospitalization [hazard ratio (HR) 0.93, 95% (CI 0.84–1.02), p _0.13

Guideline Recommendation

The European Society of Cardiology has added exercise training to the latest chronic HF guidelines stating that "regular, moderate daily activity is recommended for all patients with HF" and has given it a class I, level of evidence B. The guidelines also state that "exercise training is recommended, if available, to all stable chronic HF patients. There is no evidence that exercise training should be limited to any particular HF patient subgroups (etiology, NYHA class, LVEF or medication). Exercise training programs appear to have similar effects whether provided in a hospital or at home (Class of recommendation I, level of evidence A").

In 2009, the AHA/ACC updated the chronic HF guidelines and stated that: "Exercise training should be considered for all stable outpatients with chronic HF who are able to participate in the protocols needed to produce physical conditioning. Exercise training should be used in conjunction with drug therapy. Exercise training is beneficial as an adjunctive approach to improve clinical status in ambulatory patients with current or prior symptoms of HF and reduced LVEF" (Class I, level of evidence: B).

❏ SUGGESTED READINGS

Coats AJ, Adamopoulos S, Radaelli A, et al. Controlled trial of physical training in chronic heart failure: exercise performance, hemodynamics, ventilation, and autonomic function. Circulation. 1992;85:2119-31.

Convertino VA. Cardiovascular consequences of bed rest: effect on maximal oxygen uptake. Med Sci Sports Exerc. 1997;29:191-6.

Dickstein K, Cohen-Solal A, Filippatos G, et al. ESC Guidelines for the diagnosis and treatment of acute and chronic heart failure 2008: the Task Force for the Diagnosis and Treatment of Acute and Chronic Heart Failure 2008 of the European Society of Cardiology. Developed in collaboration with the Heart Failure Association of the ESC (HFA) and endorsed by the European Society of Intensive Care Medicine (ESICM). Eur Heart J. 2008;29: 2388-442.

Hambrecht R, Gielen S, Linke A, et al. Effects of exercise training on left ventricular function and peripheral resistance in patients with chronic heart failure: a randomized trial. JAMA. 2000;283:3095-101.

Hunt SA, Abraham WT, Chin MH, et al. Focused update incorporated into the ACC/AHA 2005 guidelines for the diagnosis and management of heart failure in adults: a report of the American College of Cardiology Foundation/American Heart Association Task Force on Practice Guidelines. Circulation. 2009;119:e391-479.

O'connor CM, Whellan DJ, Lee KL, et al. Efficacy and safety of exercise training in patients with chronic heart failure: the HFACTION randomized controlled trial. JAMA. 2009;301: 1439-50.

Pina IL, Apstein CS, Balady GJ, et al. Exercise and heart failure: a statement from the American Heart Association Committee on exercise, rehabilitation, and prevention. Circulation. 2003;107:1210-25.

Pina IL, Kokkinos P, Kao A, et al. Baseline differences in the HFACTION trial by sex. Am Heart J. 2009;158(Suppl. 4):S16-S23.

Riegel B, Moser DK, Anker SD, et al. State of the science: promoting self-care in persons with heart failure: a scientific statement from the American Heart Association. Circulation. 2009;120:1141-63.

Wasserman K, Hansen JE, Sue DY, et al. Principles of Exercise Testing and Interpretation, 2nd edition. Philadelphia: Lea and Febiger; 1994. p. 127.

7.7 Advanced Cardiac Therapies for End-stage Heart Failure: Cardiac Transplantation and Mechanical Circulatory Support

❏ INTRODUCTION

Treatment of end-stage heart failure (HF) now exploits both organ transplant and circulatory pump strategies with good results, even if the goal of full rehabilitation remains elusive for most. Heart transplantation and left ventricular assist device (LVAD) implantation have well-established benefit over medical therapy for palliation of advanced heart failure in well-selected individuals. Survival with heart transplantation is about 88% in the first year and 50% at the end of 10 years (Fig. 40). Likewise, with improved durable LVADs, the survival is remarkable at 66% at the end of 2 years (Fig. 41). These therapies offer almost an absolute survival

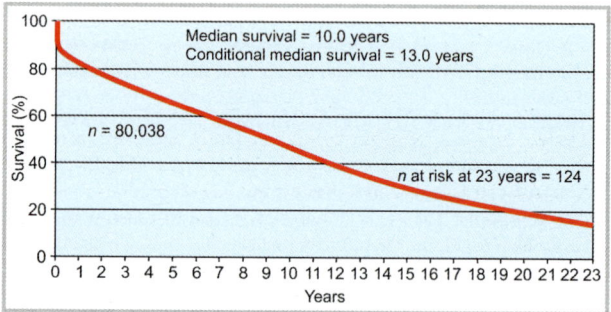

FIGURE 40: Long-term survival of patients undergoing heart transplantation. (*Source:* Modified from ISHLT registry)

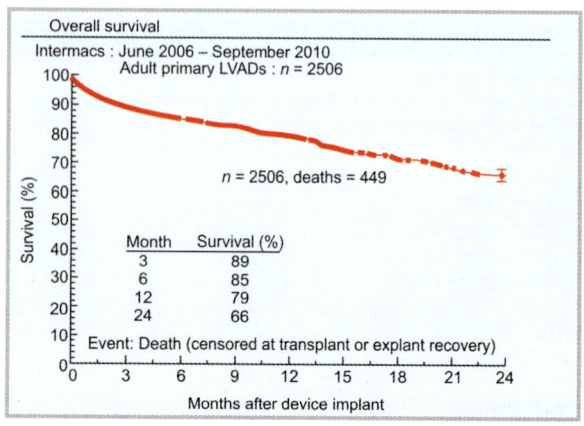

FIGURE 41: Medium-term survival after LVAD implantation. (*Source:* Modified from INTERMACS registry)

improvement of 150% at the end of 1 year in appropriately selected heart failure patients when compared to conventional medical management.

❑ IDENTIFYING CANDIDATES FOR ADVANCED CARDIAC THERAPIES

Recognition of Advanced Heart Failure with Poor Prognosis

For patients with end stage HF, prognosis remains guarded without advanced cardiac therapies and recognition of these patients is important to triage into appropriate care strategies. Determination of prognosis in heart failure has evolved from recognizing different patient characteristics, which are associated with poor prognosis to prospectively validated risk scores that are able to predict short-term and long-term survival, and morbidity better.

Prognostic Determinants and Risk Scores in Heart Failure

Many individual patient characteristics, which are determinants of the prognosis in heart failure, have been identified (Table 40). Of all these individual characteristics New York Heart Association (NYHA) classification, serum sodium and creatinine have been long recognized as important indicators of severity of heart failure.

Prognostic Scores

Heart failure survival score (HFSS) was one of first scores developed to predict survival of patients on the transplant list. Subsequently, Seattle heart failure model (SHFM) and MUerte Subita en Insuficiencia Cardiaca (MUSIC) score have been developed as prognostic tools. These three major prognostic systems have been validated in populations receiving optimal medical therapy and have been compared in Table 41.

A prognostic risk model has been developed to predict the probability of sudden cardiac death. The model consists of increased cardiothoracic ratio, QRS dispersion, QTc dispersion and nonsustained ventricular tachycardia as independent predictors of sudden death, and these have been combined in a score. Such a risk score is especially important in resource poor societies to decide on

Table 40: Poor prognostic indicators in patients with heart failure

Demographic/patient indicators
- Advancing age
- Female gender
- Diabetes mellitus
- Presence of coronary artery disease
- Worsening NYHA class
- Increasing heart rate

Laboratory/electrocardiogram/echocardiogram indicators
- Rising serum creatinine
- Anemia
- Prolonged QT interval
- NT Pro-BNP
- LV mass
- LV ejection fraction

(Abbreviations: LV: Left ventricular; NYHA: New York Heart Association; NT Pro-BNP: N-terminal prohormone brain natriuretic peptide)

Table 41: Comparison of heart failure prognostic risk scores

Risk scoring system	Variables included	Advantages	Disadvantages
Heart failure survival score	- Ischemic cardiomyopathy - Resting heart rate - LVEF - Mean BP - Interventricular conduction - delay (IVCD) - Peak VO_2 - Serum sodium	- Extensively validated in the current era - Useful in low-risk and high-risk group	- For moderate-risk group patients other factors need to be considered before deciding on transplant listing - Validated in patients waiting for transplant - Lack of validation in patients in racial groups in whom isosorbide dinitrate and hydralazine combination has been shown to be beneficial
Seattle heart failure model	*Demographics* - Age - Gender - Body mass index - NYHA class - Ejection fraction <30% - Ischemic etiology of heart failure - Systolic blood Pressure <160 mm Hg - Diuretic dose (mg/kg per day) - Allopurinol use *Laboratory* - Serum sodium - Serum creatinine - Serum cholesterol - WBC count - Hemoglobin (g/dL) - Percentage of lymphocytes - Uric acid (mg/dL) *Medications* - ACE inhibitor use - Beta-blocker use - ARB use - Potassium sparing diuretic - Statin use *Device use* - ICD implantation - Biventricular pacemaker - implantation - VAD implantation	- Well validated in all populations with optimal medical therapy and device therapy	- Not validated in populations in whom isosorbide dinitrate and hydralazine have been beneficial - Developed using clinical trial database - May not be completely relevant to clinical practice

Contd...

Contd...

Table 41: Comparison of heart failure prognostic risk scores

Risk scoring system	Variables included	Advantages	Disadvantages
MUSIC score	<ul><li>Previous atherosclerotic event</li><li>Left atrial enlargement</li><li>LVEF <35%</li><li>Atrial fibrillation</li><li>Left bundle branch block or IVCD</li><li>NSVT or frequent PVCs</li><li>eGFR <60 mL/min/1.73 m$_2$</li><li>Sodium <138 mEq/L</li><li>NT-proBNP <1.0 ng/L</li><li>Positive troponin</li></ul>	<ul><li>Developed in ambulatory heart failure population</li><li>Validated for both causes of mortality-pump failure and sudden cardiac death</li></ul>	<ul><li>Data regarding post-transplant outcomes is not available</li><li>Population was not racially diverse</li></ul>

(Abbreviations: ACE: Angiotensin converting enzymes; ARB: Angiotensin receptor blockers; BP: Blood pressure; eGFR: Estimated glomerular filtration rate; ICD: Implantable cardioverter defibrillator; LVEF: Left ventricular ejection fraction; MUSIC: MUerte Subita en Insuficiencia Cardiaca; NSVT: Nonsustained ventricular tachycardia; NYHA: New York Heart Association; PVCs: Premature ventricular contractions; VAD: Ventricular assist device; WBC: White blood cell)

expensive therapies, such as implantable cardioverter defibrillators and biventricular pacemaker. Another important prognostic indicator, which is not included in the risk scores, is repeated hospitalizations.

It is important to remember when interpreting the risk scores and the individual determinants that these act as a guide to decision making and not the sole criteria in deciding selection of patients for advanced cardiac therapies.

Functional Assessment

New York Heart Association classification of heart failure is the most widely used tool for evaluation of functional status. It has been shown to have prognostic value, and class IV (patients with symptoms at rest) heart failure is associated with mortality of greater than 50% in 1 year. Cardiopulmonary exercise testing not only helps in discerning the cause of poor functional status but also provides valuable prognostic information. The American College of Cardiology/American Heart Association has recommended cardiopulmonary exercise testing as a class I indication for use in transplant patient selection. Use of different variables of cardiopulmonary exercise testing in patient selection is listed in Table 42.

❑ HEART TRANSPLANTATION

Indications and Contraindications

The absolute and relative contraindications are institution specific but most of them follow the broad guidelines set in the International Society of Heart and Lung Transplantation (ISHLT) guidelines for transplant candidate selection (Table 43).

Management of Patients on the Transplant List

Transplantation requires an elaborate set-up of support structure to ensure timely identification and management of donor, expeditious procurement, and

Table 42: Cardiopulmonary stress testing and indications for transplantation

Use of cardiopulmonary stress testing and indications for cardiac transplantation	Class of recommendation (level of evidence)
1. In patients not on or intolerant to beta-blocker, peak VO_2 <14 mL/kg/min	Class I (B)
2. In patients on beta-blockers, peak VO_2 <12 mL/kg/min	Class I (B)
3. In patients younger than 50 years and women, percent of predicted (<50%) peak VO_2 should be used in conjunction with absolute VO_2 max	Class IIa (B)
4. In the presence of a submaximal CPX test (RER <1.05), use of ventilation equivalent of carbon dioxide (VE/VCO2) slope of >35 as a determinant in listing for transplantation	Class IIb (C)
5. In obese (body mass index >30 kg/m^2) patients, lean body mass adjusted peak VO_2 <19 mL/kg/min can be used to guide pretransplant prognosis	Class IIb (B)

(Abbreviations: CPX: Cardiopulmonary exercise; RER: Respiratory exchange ratio; VE/VCO$_2$: Minute ventilation/carbon dioxide elimination; VO$_2$: Oxygen consumption)

Table 43: Commonly accepted absolute and relative contraindications to transplantation

Age
- Greater than 70 years

Malignancy
- Current active malignant conditions
- Preexisting malignancies which have high rates of recurrence

Obesity
- Body mass index >35 kg/m^2
- Insulin-dependent diabetes mellitus
- Uncontrolled diabetes mellitus with hemoglobin A1c >7.5
- Presence of end-organ damage

Vascular disease
- Severe symptomatic peripheral vascular disease not amenable to intervention
- Symptomatic cerebrovascular disease not amenable to revascularization

Substance abuse
- Active tobacco, alcohol and drug use

Psychosocial issues
- No demonstrated ability to comply with medical regimen

transplantation. In the United States, UNOS is a private not-for-profit agency, which manages transplant system. The selection of recipients is based on the UNOS criteria, which are listed in Table 44.

Patients listed for transplantation have to be meticulously managed so that they are well optimized when the donor heart becomes available. The preoperative care of these patients falls into the following categories:
- Optimization of heart failure
- Preventing infections
- Prevention of allosensitization.

Table 44: United Network of Organ Sharing (UNOS) status and criteria

UNOS status	Inclusion criteria	Patients receiving transplantation (%) (UNOS report 2008–2009)

1A	1. Mechanical circulatory support for acute hemodynamic decompensation that includes at least one of the following:
	  a. Left and/or right ventricular assist device implanted (includes patients discharged with total artificial heart)*
	  b. Hospital admitted patients with:
	    • Total artificial heart†
	    • Intra-aortic balloon pump†
	    • Extracorporeal membrane oxygenator†
	2. Mechanical circulatory support with objective medical evidence of significant device-related complications like device infection, thromboembolism, pump failure and/or life-threatening ventricular arrhythmias†
	3. Continuous mechanical ventilation†
	4. Continuous infusion of a single high-dose intravenous inotrope (dobutamine ≥7.5 mcg/kg/min, or milrinone >0.50 mcg/kg/min), or multiple intravenous inotropes, in addition to continuous hemodynamic monitoring of with a pulmonary artery catheter‡
		50

1B	1. Left and/or right ventricular assist device implanted 2. Continuous infusion of intravenous inotropes	41
2	A candidate who does not meet the criteria for status 1A or 1B	9
7	A candidate listed as status 7 is considered temporarily unsuitable to receive a thoracic organ transplant	

*Candidates may be listed for 30 days at any point after being implanted as status 1A once the treating physician determines that they are clinically stable. Admittance to the listing transplant center hospital is not required.
†Status valid for 14 days and must be recertified by an attending physician every 14 days extend the status 1A listing.
‡Status valid for 7 days and may be renewed for an additional 7 days for each occurrence of a status 1A listing under this criterion for the same candidate.

Donor Selection and Perioperative Period

Preoperative management of the heart not only involves meticulous search of contraindications but also the optimization of the organ with preexplant donor management and postexplant organ preservation. Donors have to be screened for various characteristics, which have been commonly agreed upon to have a deleterious effect on post-transplant outcome (Table 45).

Donor Management

Brain death imposes several physiological responses, which can have a deleterious effect on the heart. These include an initial Cushing's response (coronary vasospasm due to release of catecholamines) and Anrep effect (maintenance of coronary circulation despite increased afterload) followed by loss of vasomotor tone and hypotension. These physiological states require appropriate management with vasodilators and vasopressors as required. Myocardial depression in the setting of increased catecholamines may require brief inotropic support. Prolonged high doses of inotropes indicate myocardial injury, which would be a contraindication.

Table 45: Criteria for donor heart selection	
Donor heart screening (Mostly accepted contraindications)	**Class of recommendation (level of evidence)**
Age	Class IIa (B)
• Greater than 55 years	
Donor infection	Class IIa (C)
• HIV, Hepatitis B and Hepatitis C, HTLV-1	
• Bacterial infection	
▪ Donor infection is community acquired and death occurs before 96 hours	
▪ Repeat blood cultures are positive	
▪ Pathogen-specific antibiotic not administered	Class IIa (C)
▪ Endocarditis	
Potential drug use	
• Intravenous cocaine use	Class I (B)
• Chronic alcohol use	
• Carbon monoxide poisoning	
Evaluation of cardiac function	
• LV ejection fraction <40%	
• Discrete wall motion abnormalities	
• Excessive use of inotropes	Class IIa (C)
• Intractable ventricular arrhythmias	
Evaluation of cardiac structure	
• Electrocardiograph evidence of LV hypertrophy or echocardiography evidence of wall thickness >1.4 cm	Class I (C)
• Coronary artery disease involving major coronary artery	Class I (C)
Donor-recipient size matching	
• Donors whose body weight is >30% below that of the recipient	
Projected ischemic time	
• Greater than 4 hours	

(Abbreviations: HIV: Human immunodeficiency virus; HTLV-1: Human T-lymphotropic virus type I; LV: Left ventricular)

Organ Explantation and Preservation

The donor heart explantation procedure begins with decompression of left ventricle and the right ventricle with an incision of the left atrium and inferior vena cava, respectively. Subsequently, the aorta is cross-clamped and the preservation solution is infused along with topical cooling. The superior vena cava and main pulmonary artery are subsequently transected to completely excise the heart. The heart is then bagged with preservation solution and ice. The preservation solution contains ice slush, potassium, magnesium, lactiobionate, raffinose and free radical scavengers.

Donor Heart Implantation

Traditionally, biatrial technique was used for implantation, which involved anastomoses of the donor and recipient atria. Due to increased incidence of atrial tachyarrhythmias, sinus node dysfunction and tricuspid regurgitation, this technique is being abandoned for the bicaval technique. Bicaval technique involves performance of left atrial anastomoses initially followed by inferior vena cava, superior vena cava, and aortic anastomoses.

Immediate Post-transplant Physiology and Management
Hemodynamic Stabilization

Left ventricular (LV) dysfunction in the immediate postoperative period points either to hyperacute/acute rejection or primary graft failure (defined as systolic dysfunction of either LV, right ventricular (RV) or both not due to obvious anatomic or immunologic cause). Diastolic dysfunction is common in the early postoperative period due to ischemic and preservation related injury to the allograft.

Primary graft failure often manifests as RV dysfunction and is related to poor organ preservation, elevated pulmonary venous resistance or injury to right ventricle during implantation. RV failure is recognized by the elevation of right atrial pressure (above 15 mm Hg) in the presence of decreased cardiac output with increased or normal pulmonary artery pressures. Management of primary graft failure broadly falls into following categories:

Afterload reduction: The use of pulmonary vasodilators, such as inhalational nitric oxide, prostanoids, or sildenafil.

Inotropic and vasopressor support: Predominantly isoproterenol, dobutamine and milrinone and vasopressors (epinephrine, norepinephrine or vasopressin), if there is hypotension despite use of inotropes.

Preload reduction: Diuretics are often needed in higher doses especially in patients with preoperative diuretic resistance to unload the right ventricle. Ultrafiltration or continuous venovenous hemofiltration can be used in case of postoperative oliguric renal failure.

Mechanical circulatory support: Intra-aortic balloon pump or temporary assist devices, such as Extracorporeal Membrane Oxygenation (ECMO) or Tandem Heart or Levitronix Centrimag device can be used as a bridge to recovery or retransplantation in case of persistent graft failure with endorgan dysfunction.

Rhythm management: Postoperatively between 14% and 60% of the patients have bradyarrhythmias predominantly due to sinus node dysfunction needing chronotropic support with agents such as isoproterenol and dobutamine or temporary pacing. Need for temporary pacing has decreased from since the widespread adoption of the bicaval technique to 18–27% from about 37% with biatrial technique.

Early Immunosuppressive and Antimicrobial Management

Successful prevention of rejection and infections in the immediate postoperative period is the key to decreasing early morbidity and mortality. Immunosuppressant and regimens with their adverse effects are listed in Table 46. Commonly used antimicrobial regimen is also listed in Table 47. Induction therapy usually begins intraoperatively during the removal of the cross clamp and continues as soon as the patient is moved to the ICU.

Long-term Management of Transplant Patients

This requires meticulous management of their immunosuppression and long-term management of the sequelae of transplantation.

Table 46: Commonly used immunosuppressants with their mechanism of action and common side effects

Immunosuppressant class	Mechanism of action	Indications for use	Major adverse effect
Antilymphocyte preparations			
Polyclonal antilymphocyte preparation (ATGAM or thymoglobulin)	T and B lymphocyte depletion due to complement dependent opsonization	Steroid resistant acute rejection	• Urticaria • Cytokine release syndrome: fever, chills and rash
Monoclonal antilymphocyte antibodies (muromonab or OKT3)	Binds to CD3 molecule of T cell causing depletion due to opsonization	Steroid resistant rejection	• Cytomegalovirus infections • Cytokine release syndrome
Anti-interleukin (IL)-2 receptor antibodies			
Basiliximab and daclizumab	Blocks IL-2 receptor alpha chain and inhibits proliferation of T lymphocytes	Induction therapy	Hypersensitivity
Corticosteroids			
Prednisone, Prednisolone and Methylprednisolone	Increased death, decreased proliferation and function of leukocytes, including T and B lymphocytes, macrophages, and monocytes	Induction and maintenance therapy	• Hypertension • Hyperglycemia, diabetes mellitus and weight gain • Osteoporosis and proximal myopathy • Gastric ulcer
Antiproliferative agents			
Azathioprine	Decreases proliferation of T and B lymphocytes by inhibiting purine synthesis	Maintenance therapy	• Myelosuppression • Pancreatitis and hepatitis
Mycophenolate mofetil	Inhibits lymphocyte proliferation by blocking purine synthesis	Induction and maintenance therapy	Nausea, vomiting, and diarrhea
Calcineurin inhibitors			
Cyclosporine and tacrolimus	Reduces function of T lymphocytes by calcineurin dependent transcription particularly by preventing production of IL-2	Induction and maintenance therapy	• Nephrotoxicity • Hypertension, dyslipidemia, and diabetes mellitus • Neurological toxicity
Mammalian target of rapamycin (mTOR) inhibitors			
Sirolimus	Inhibits growth and proliferation of T and B lymphocytes by inhibiting IL-2 and IL-6	Maintenance therapy in place of CI, in patients with CNI related renal dysfunction	• Dyslipidemia • Pancytopenia • Wound healing impairment

(Abbreviation: CNI: Calcineurin inhibitors)

The sequelae can be broadly divided into:

Graft related: This includes acute rejection and coronary allograft vasculopathy (CAV), which some believe to be primarily a manifestation of chronic rejection. These two problems lead to chronic allograft dysfunction, which can eventually lead to death if retransplantation is not an option.

Detailed discussion of rejection and transplant vasculopathy along with its management is given in Figure 42 and Table 48.

Table 47: Post-transplant infection prophylaxis		
Organisms and common antimicrobial agent	**Indications**	**Adverse effects and interactions**
Pneumocystis jirovecii (carinii)		
Trimethoprim-sulfamethoxazole	• Induction therapy • Acute and chronic rejection • Use of antilymphocyte agents	• Rash • Renal insufficiency • Hyperkalemia • Bone marrow suppression
Aspergillus sp and Candida sp		
Nystatin	Induction therapy	Not significant
Cytomegalovirus		
Ganciclovir or valganciclovir	Induction therapy	Bone marrow suppression

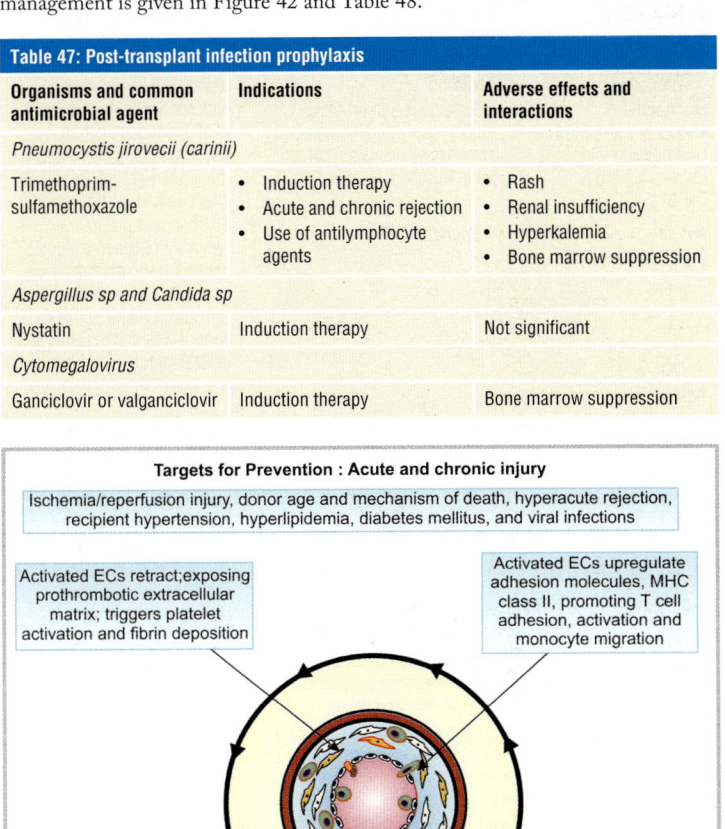

FIGURE 42: Pathogenesis of transplant vasculopathy (Abbreviation: EC: Endothelial cell)

Table 48: Types of rejection

Type of rejection	Pathophysiology and diagnostic modalities	Management medications and principles
Acute cellular rejection		
<ul><li>Classified based on histopathology</li><li>Grade 1R (mild rejection)</li><li>Grade 2R (moderate rejection)</li><li>Grade 3R (severe rejection)</li></ul>	<ul><li>T lymphocyte mediated damage to the myocardium</li><li>Diagnosed by endomyocardial biopsy and staining with hemotoxylin/eosin</li><li>Gene expression profiling (GEP) tests evaluating the lymphocyte activation can be used to screen for rejection</li></ul>	<ul><li>High dose corticosteroids and polyclonal/monoclonal antithymocyte antibody are mainstay of treatment</li><li>All grades of rejection are treated in symptomatic patients and in the presence of allograft dysfunction</li><li>Asymptomatic patients with moderate to severe grades of rejection have to be treated</li><li>Treatment of resistant or recurrent rejection include methotrexate, photopheresis or total body irradiation</li><li>Surveillance with periodic endomyocardial biopsies and/or GEP tests</li></ul>
Antibody mediated rejection		
<ul><li>Hyperacute (occurs within minutes to hours of implantation of the heart)</li><li>Acute (occurs anytime post-transplant)</li></ul>	<ul><li>Complement mediated destruction due to production of recipient antibodies against the allograft</li><li>Hyperacute rejection often involves preformed antibodies to donor HLA or endothelial antigens</li><li>Diagnosed by endomyocardial biopsy with immunofluorescence staining against complement fragments in the tissue</li></ul>	<ul><li>Management of hyperacute rejection includes use of IV immunoglobulin (IVIg), plasmapheresis, high dose steroids and cytolytic therapy</li><li>Management of acute rejection includes high dose IV corticosteroids, plasmapheresis, IVIg and rituximab</li><li>Screening of donor anti-HLA antibodies to prevent antibody mediated rejection</li></ul>

(Abbreviations: HLA: Human leukocyte antigen; IV: Intravenous)

Immunosuppression-related organ dysfunction: Minimizing adverse effects, while maintaining adequate immunosuppression to prevent rejection, are one of the main challenges of long-term post-transplant management. Common problems associated with transplant in the long term are described in Table 49.

Cardiac Retransplantation

Cardiac retransplantation is common in the pediatric and young adult patients who have received their first hearts as children. CAV, early graft failure (within 6 months of first transplantation) and acute rejection are common indications of retransplantation. The survival rates with retransplantation are lower with 1-year survival of about 54% compared to 84% with first transplant. The rates of retransplantation are about 3% and coming years may see an increase in retransplantation rates due to the improvement in survival of patients with heart failure on MCS, making retransplantation less of an ethical issue.

Table 49: Long-term problems associated with heart transplantation

Problems	Post-transplant incidence and prevalence	Pathophysiology and	Management risk factors
Coronary allograft (Transplant) Vasculopathy	Prevalence of 42% at 5 years (moderate-severe CAV of 15%)	Endothelial injury which begins time of procurement with further insults from prolonged ischemic time, acute rejection, immunosuppressants, and post-transplant metabolic syndrome	1. Periodic monitoring with coronary intravascular ultrasonography (IVUS), coronary angiography or CT angiography. 2. Choice of Immunosuppressant: preferred use of sirolimus. 3. Vitamin C and vitamin E supplementation. 4. Choice of statin: pravastatin better than other statins. 5. Choice of antihypertensive: calcium channel blocker or ACE inhibitor better. 6. Percutaneous coronary intervention in patients with obstructive CAV. 7. Retransplantation in patients with established CAV and allograft dysfunction.
Opportunistic infections			
CMV, *Pneumocystis jirovecii*, *Aspergillus* sp, *Candida* sp	Incidence and prevalence vary for different organisms during different post-transplantation periods	• Decreased T lymphocyte function • Main risk factor included induction therapy with cytolytic agents	1. Periodic screening for CMV especially during first year in recipients who were CMV seropositive or received hearts from seropositive donor 2. Antimicrobial prophylaxis 3. Season age appropriate vaccinations
Metabolic syndrome			
Diabetes mellitus	5-year cumulative incidence of 32%	Steroid and calcineurin inhibitor induced	1. Frequent screening with hemoglobin A1c and fasting glucose 2. Early weaning of steroids in diabetes prone individuals
Hypertension	5-year prevalence of 95%	Steroid and calcineurin inhibitor related	1. Use of calcium channel blocker or ACE-I depending on comorbidities 2. Lifestyle modifications
Dyslipidemia	Lifetime prevalence of 60–80%	Immunosuppressants, loop diuretics	1. HMG-CoA inhibitors (pravastatin preferred)
Osteoporosis	1-year incidence of fractures of 21–36%	• Steroid and calcineurin inhibitor induced • Hypogonadism can contribute	1. Early weaning of steroids 2. Limiting calcineurin inhibitors 3. Screening and treating hypogonadism in men

Contd...

Contd...

Table 49: Long-term problems associated with heart transplantation

Problems	Post-transplant incidence and prevalence	Pathophysiology and	Management risk factors
Chronic kidney disease	5-year prevalence of 10.9%	• Calcineurin inhibitor use • Preexisting renal dysfunction, old age and female gender are risk factors	1. Minimizing CNI use. Sirolimus (Rapamycin) can be used instead 2. Management of risk factors, including hypertension and diabetes mellitus 3. Use calcium channel blockers as a preferred antihypertensive agent
Malignancy (in the order of frequency) • Skin (50%) • Lymphomas (10%) or post-transplant lymphoproliferative disorder (PTLD) • Other solid malignancies including lung, breast and prostate (40%)	• 20-year cumulative Incidence 14.4% (all malignancies) • 5-year cumulative prevalence 15.1% • 10-year cumulative prevalence of 31.9%	• Decreased activity of NK lymphocytes due to chronic immunosuppression • Epstein Barr virus (EBV) is implicated in the development of lymphoma or PTLD	1. Decrease use of cytolytic therapy especially if antiviral prophylaxis 2. Use of antiproliferative agents (specifically MMF) 3. Yearly skin screening and risk reduction by modification of patient behavior 4. Age appropriate screening for colon, breast and genitourinary cancers

(Abbreviations: ACE: Angiotensin converting enzyme; CAV: Coronary allograft vasculopathy; CNI: Calcineurin inhibitor; CT: Computed tomography; MMF: Mycophenolate mofetil; NK: Natural killer)

Survival with Cardiac Transplantation

Survival with cardiac transplantation has improved over years and, as per the latest UNOS report, the 1-year survival is about 88% and 10-year survival is about 50%. Median survival of patients who survive up to 1 year is about 13 years. The mortality risk is highest in the first six months after transplant and drops off subsequently to 3–4% per year, which is still high compared to the general population.

Risk factors for 1-year mortality are:
- Long-term circulatory support dependence (RR = 1.3; 1.02-1.7; $p = 0.03$),
- Ischemic cardiomyopathy (RR = 1.2; 1.02-1.3; $p = 0.02$), and
- Congenital cause of heart failure (RR = 2.27; 2.02–3.68; $p < 0.0001$).

Other comorbidities at the time of transplantation, including temporary circulatory support, dialysis dependence, ventilator dependence and infections portend a higher risk as well. Risk factors for mid- to long-term mortality include being female recipient, male recipient receiving female allografts, recipient history of stroke, age at both extremes and lack of treatment with mycophenolate, azathioprine or rapamycin at the end of one year.

❏ MECHANICAL CIRCULATORY SUPPORT

The current generation of devices has rotary pumps with non-physiologic continuous flow but offer durability. Successful results from the Thoratec HeartMate II trial as a bridge to transplantation has led to transition from pulsatile devices (HeartMate XVE) to continuous flow devices as the foremost choice in bridge to transplantation. Currently, about 25–30% of patients undergoing heart transplantation undergo assist device implantation prior to transplantation. The VADs have been classified in several different ways though most common ones are based on indication of use and ventricle being assisted (Table 50).

Unlike guidelines for patient listing for transplantation, consensus guidelines for implantation do not exist. In 2005, INTERMACS has put forth a classification consisting seven categories based on the severity of heart failure to aid in patient selection (Table 51).

Indications and Contraindications for Mechanical Circulatory Support

Evaluation for VAD implantation begins with thorough search for conditions, which would:
- Limit survival
- Prevent therapeutic anticoagulation
- Cause intraoperative mortality
- Impair ability to follow complex medical regimens.

The indications and contraindications (Table 52) are institution specific but most of them follow the broad guidelines set in the CMS approved indications for durable mechanical support (Table 53).

The essential characteristics of such devices include easy implantability and removal, reliable and sufficient cardiac support, and easy transportability. Some of the most common devices used today are summarized in Table 50.

Important consideration in deciding the type of assist device also depends on the right ventricular function. If a patient has severe preoperative RV failure or has a high-risk of developing RV failure postoperatively, he may need biventricular support. In different trials of LVADs, the incidence of RV failure is 10–20%, and 6–17% needed right ventricular assist device (RVAD) implantation.

Table 50: Classification of ventricular assist devices

Classification of VADs	What they mean	Examples
Position		
Extracorporeal	Pumping system outside the patient	Levitronix CentriMag
Paracorporeal	Pumping system on the body of the patient	Thoratec PVAD
Intracorporeal	Pumping system inside the body of the patient	Thoratec HeartMate II
Ventricle supported/replaced		
Left ventricular assist device (LVAD)	Supports the LV	Thoratec HeartMate II
Right ventricular assist device (RVAD)	Supports the RV	Levitronix CentriMag
Biventricular assist device (BiVAD)	Supports both LV and RV	Thoratec PVADS
Orthotopic replacement of heart	Replaces the heart	Total artificial heart
Pumping principle/flow mechanics		
Displacement pumps or pulsatile pumps Rotary pumps or continuous flow pumps (two types): — Axial flow — Centrifugal flow	• Similar to native heart; Work by displacement of blood from a filling chamber • Has an impeller, which spins at high speed to propel blood forward continuously • Inflow and outflow are parallel to the rotational axis • Inflow is parallel but outflow is orthogonal to rotational axis	• Thoratec HeartMate XVE • Thoratec PVAD • Thoratec HeartMate II • HeartWare VAD
Purpose of use		
Bridge to decision • Reversal of end-organ dysfunction • Ascertain transplant candidacy	Temporary mechanical support in patients who present with cardiogenic shock and their transplant candidacy is uncertain	• Levitronix CentriMag • TandemHeart
Bridge to transplantation • Reversal of end-organ (especially renal dysfunction) • Decreasing PVR	Durable mechanical support to help patients survive till transplantation	• Thoratec HeartMate II • HeartWare VAD
Destination Therapy	Durable mechanical support as a palliative support till end of life	Thoratec HeartMate II

(Abbreviations: LV: Left ventricular; NYHA: New York Heart Association; PVAD: Paracorporeal ventricular assist device; PVR: Pulmonary vascular resistance; RV: Right ventricular; VAD: Ventricular assist device)

Table 51: INTERMACS classification of advanced heart failure patients

Class	Description	Time to mechanical circulatory support	National percentage of patients receiving VAD implantation (%)
1	"*Crashing and burning*"; critical cardiogenic shock	Emergent intervention within hours	27
2	"*Sliding on inotropes*"; deteriorating end-organ function on inotropes	Urgent or semi-elective intervention within days	41.4
3	"*Dependent stability*"; stable blood pressure and organ function on inotrope	Elective intervention within days to weeks	15.7
4	"*Resting symptoms*"; daily rest symptoms of volume overload with intensive diuretic dose management	Elective intervention within days to weeks	9.5
5	"*Exertion intolerant*"; comfortable at rest but homebound due to exertional symptoms often needing extensive symptomatic management	Dependent on progression of symptoms and deterioration of organ function	2.3
6	"*Exertion limited/walking wounded*"; comfortable at rest and minor activities. Fatigability and SOB with minor activity	Dependent on progression of symptoms and deterioration of organ function	2.1
7	*NYHA Class III*; living comfortably with activity limited to mild exertion	Advanced cardiac therapies not currently indicated	1.8

(Abbreviations: INTERMACS: Interagency Registry for Mechanically Assisted Circulatory Support; NYHA: New York Heart Association; VAD: Ventricular assist device)

Table 52: Contraindications to ventricular assist device implantation

- Recent stroke or stroke in evolution
- Neurological or psychiatric illness impairing the ability to manage device
- Metastatic cancer deemed incurable
- Advanced cirrhosis
- Dialysis dependent renal failure
- Abdominal aortic aneurysm >5 cm
- Peripheral arterial disease
- Active systemic infection or major chronic risk for infection such as diabetic neuropathy/stasis ulcers
- Severe pulmonary dysfunction (FEV1 <1 liter)
- Inability to tolerate anticoagulation
- Lack of social support and inability to comply with medical instructions

(Abbreviation: FEV1: Forced expiratory volume in 1 second)

Table 53: Center for Medicare services approved indications for ventricular assist device implantation

1. Postcardiotomy cardiogenic shock
2. Bridge to transplantation
   - Listed for transplantation at a Medicare approved transplantation site
3. Destination therapy
   - Severely decreased LVEF (< 25%)
   - NYHA class IV heart failure for at least 90 days
   - Failure to respond to medical management in 60 of 90 days
   - Not a transplant candidate
   - Life expectancy <2 years
   - Peak oxygen consumption <12 ml/kg/min
   - Continuous need for intravenous inotropic support limited by symptomatic hypotension, renal failure or pulmonary congestion

(Abbreviations: LVEF: Left ventricular ejection fraction; NYHA: New York Heart Association)

Postoperative RV failure is associated with decrease postoperative survival and increased length of stay. Inotropic support with pulmonary vasodilators is often needed postoperatively but suboptimal cardiac output with chronically elevated venous pressure can often result in end-organ dysfunction.

There are several preoperative predictors of postoperative RV failure. Predominantly low RV stroke work index (<600 mm Hg mL/m^2), increased bilirubin (>2.0 g/dL), and increased creatinine and increased liver enzymes. Though patients with higher risk of RV failure can undergo LVAD placement, postoperative vigilance is necessary for early detection and prompt management with inotropes and pulmonary vasodilators.

Design of Ventricular Assist Device and Impact on Post-implant Physiology

A VAD consists of a pump to circulate blood which could be external or housed within the body. The pump has an inflow cannula, which drains the chamber of the heart that is being supported into the pump (Figs 43 and 44). The outflow cannula is another conduit, which connects the pump to the outflow tract of the chamber being supported. The power is usually supplied by an external power source through an electrical lead.

In contrast, the pulsatile pumps, especially BiVADs, have the capability of functioning in asynchronous mode with the no dependence on native rhythm for functioning.

Insertion of VAD into the circulatory system establishes two systems, which are parallel and competing for flow. The blood from the left atrium has two conduits that it can go to aortic or the inflow cannula of the pump. So the flow through the VAD is mostly preload dependent. The cardiac output becomes heart rate dependent for a given preload per cardiac cycle. Since both the LV and the pump face the same systemic vascular resistance (SVR), the work done (power consumed) by the pump will increase with increasing SVR. For the most part if the pump is functioning optimally, the LV will act as a passive conduit. Most continuous flow devices work in a synchronous mode with maximum flow through the device occurring during native systole.

Mechanical unloading leads to remodeling of the ventricle, which includes a reduction in LV end-diastolic and end systolic dimension with reduction of size

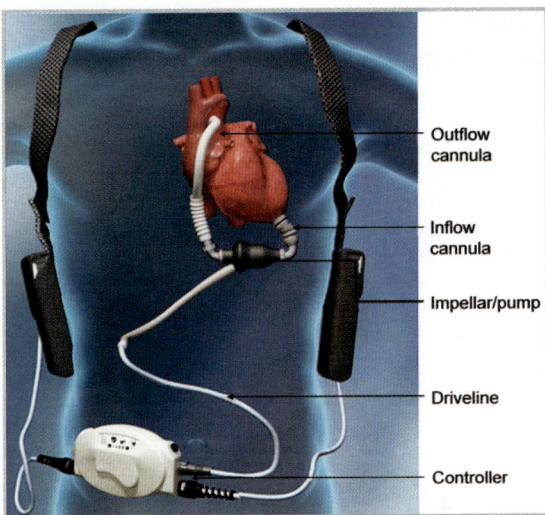

FIGURE 43: Parts of an LVAD (HeartMate II as a prototype)

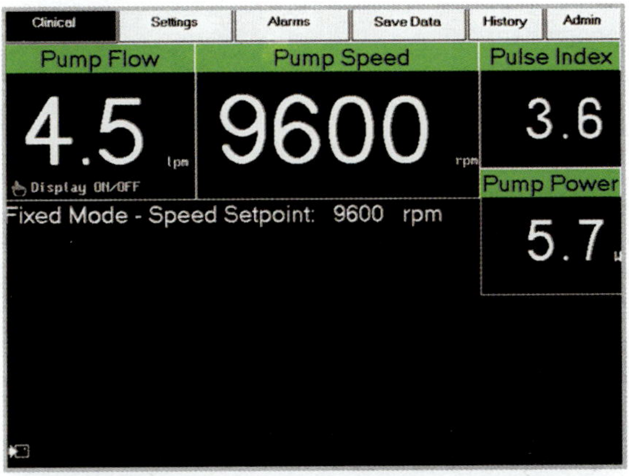

FIGURE 44: Display clinical screen of Thoratec HeartMate II VAD

primarily seen in the radial dimension. In most cases, there is an improvement in LV and RV ejection fraction. The QRS duration and QT duration shortening suggestive of electrical remodeling has been observed as well.

At the molecular level, improvements are seen in myocardial filament structure, metabolic gene expression and function and calcium handling by myocytes.

Optimization of patients prior to surgery primarily involves optimization of end-organ function and improving nutritional status. Certain intraoperative considerations are extremely important in determining optimal functioning of the pump and, in turn, affect the survival and quality of life postimplantation. These include repair of concomitant valvular lesions and appropriate positioning of inflow cannula and percutaneous lead.

Postoperative Patient and Device Management

Hemodynamic Stabilization

Hemodynamic instability in LVAD patients is usually due to RV dysfunction the postoperative period. Preexisting RV dysfunction and perioperative fluid shifts and transfusions can affect this. Often higher pump speed can result in greater return of blood to the right compared to preoperative state resulting in RV failure.

Management of RV failure is similar to that in post-transplant patients and consists of afterload reduction (with inhalational nitric oxide, prostanoids or sildenafil), inotropic support and preload reduction with diuresis or ultrafiltration. Failure to resolve end-organ dysfunction and hypotension with conservative management should be managed with an insertion of an RVAD.

Hemodynamic instability in BiVAD patients often occur due to an increased incidence of postoperative bleeding in these patients. Volume shifts in these patients need to be managed well to prevent decrease in preload.

Anticoagulation

Therapeutic anticoagulation with warfarin and aspirin is required. The international normalized ratio (INR) goal varies depending on the type of VAD being implanted and other patient comorbidities. The goal INR for Thoratec HeartMate II device is between 1.5 and 2.5. This is often achieved by starting warfarin postoperatively without a heparin bridge to prevent bleeding complications.

Pump Management

Monitoring a ventricular assist device: The display modules of VADs show data regarding the electromechanical functioning and flow characteristics (Fig. 45).

Electrical and mechanical data: Continuous flow device modules display the speed of the rotor and the power consumed by the rotor to generate the given flow through the device. Displacement pumps often display the rate of the pump along with the time spent in filling and emptying. Pulsatile pumps often display the pressure being applied to suction and displace the blood.

Flow characteristics: Both pulsatile and continuous flow pumps either display a measured flow (measured by a flow meter) or calculated flow (calculated based on a normogram of power consumption for a given flow).

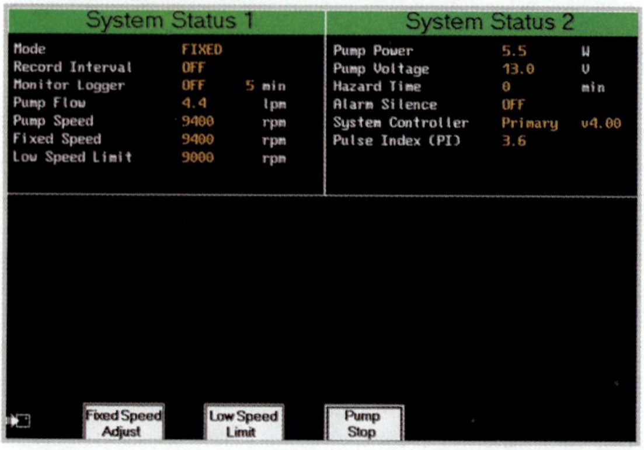

FIGURE 45: Display of setting screen of Thoratec HeartMate II VAD

Pump optimization: Optimal pump management in the postoperative period is geared toward the following two goals:
1. Delivering optimal cardiac output: This can be achieved by anticipating the postoperative fluid shifts and maintaining adequate filling pressures on the right side.
2. Preventing failure of unsupported RV: In patients with BiVAD, matching the flows in RVAD and
LVAD with appropriate speed changes are important. In patients with LVAD, pump speeds can be reduced to prevent the amount of return to the RV, hence, decreasing the chances of postoperative RV failure.

Long-term Management of Ventricular Assist Device Patients

Antiplatelet and thrombosis management: Individualization of INR goals is essential to balance these risks. Optimization of pump speed and preload to avoid suction events also decreases thrombotic risks.

Infection prevention: Stabilization of percutaneous lead to prevent local trauma and sterile cleaning or dressing techniques is the key to preventing percutaneous lead infections.

Heart failure management: Resumption of optimal medical therapy of heart failure is essential to prevent neurohormonal excitation, which exists despite mechanical unloading. Angiotensin converting enzymes inhibitors are usually well tolerated. Beta-blockers may be harder to use in the presence of RV failure but has an additional benefit of suppressing post-VAD implant arrhythmias. Some of the common complications and their prevention strategies are listed in Table 54.

Survival with Mechanical Circulatory Support

Survival data from INTERMACs registry reveals a 1-year survival of 74% for patients undergoing LVAD implantation. Actuarial survival is better in bridge to transplantation (84%) and bridge to candidacy (72%) patients when compared to destination therapy patients (64%; $p < 0.0001$). LVAD patients fared better with 74% 1-year survival compared to BiVAD patients with a 50% 1-years survival ($p < 0.001$). Primary cause of early death being cardiac (30%) and infection is the primary late cause of death (20%).

Small percentages of patients with VAD implantation undergo explantation successfully and have recurrence-free survival with good quality of life. Most of the explant experience comes from a few centers across the world with greatest success reported from Harefield Hospital, London, UK. In two prospective studies, one involving pulsatile device and recently with a continuous flow device, this group has shown up 60% explants rates in carefully selected patients, out of which 80–90% of patients stay successfully explanted. Most of these patients are young and have nonischemic cardiomyopathy for a short duration (<3–4 years).

❏ FUTURE DIRECTIONS

Organ re-engineering with stem cells is an exciting new development in the field of heart transplantation. Three dimensional biologic scaffold is built from decellularization of organs from allogeneic or xenogenic donors. Subsequently, these are populated with progenitor cells. In animal models, this has resulted in formation of organs, which have worked in vivo the short-term (few hours). Vascular regeneration and scar formation during organ growth are some of the challenges,

Table 54: Long-term complications in patients with ventricular assist device support

Complications	Incidence with newer generation LVADs (per 100 patient months)	Pathogenesis and risk factors	Clinical presentation	Management
Hardware-related complications				
• Pump stops • Percutaneous lead fracture • Motor failure	0.82	• Due to device/hardware malfunction or loss of electrical power	• Syncope • Heart failure symptoms • Decrease in arterial blood pressure with increase in pulse pressure	• Pump replacement • Replacement of controller if it is damaged
Device-related infection				
• Driveline site infection • Pump pocket infection	11.8	• Improper stabilization of driveline • Obesity • Improper exit site dressing techniques	• Redness and discharge at the exit site • Abdominal pain and fever with sepsis	• Intravenous antibiotics • Chronic infection may require suppressive oral antibiotics • Pump replacement for resistant and recurrent infections
Right heart failure	2.23	• Pump being run at high speeds • Inadequate diuresis • Preoperative right ventricular dysfunction • Unrepaired severe tricuspid insufficiency	• Heart failure symptoms • Diuretic resistance • Intermittent inflow cannula obstruction	• Pulmonary artery vasodilators • Intravenous inotrope infusions • Exchange LVAD for a BiVAD
Major bleeding				
• Hemorrhagic stroke • Gastrointestinal bleeding, epistaxis	17.41	• Over anticoagulation • Acquired von Willebrand's (VW) disease due to shearing of platelets and loss of VW multimers	• Syncope and hypotension • Other symptoms dependent on type of bleed	• Avoid over anticoagulation • Avoid hypertension (Keep MAP range between 70–90 mm Hg)

Contd...

Contd...

Table 54: Long-term complications in patients with ventricular assist device support

Complications	Incidence with newer generation LVADs (per 100 patient months)	Pathogenesis and risk factors	Clinical presentation	Management
Thromboembolic complications				
• Pump thrombus • Arterial thrombosis • Venous thrombosis	1.84	• Subtherapeutic anticoagulation • Inadequate antiplatelet therapy	• Heart failure symptoms • Hemolysis • Systemic embolization	• CT angiography or echocardiography to confirm presence of thrombus • Thrombolysis can be tried along with heparin • Pump replacement is definitive treatment
Cannula obstruction				
• Inflow cannula • Outflow cannula		• Malpositioning during surgery • Remodeling of LV leading to suctioning of septum/LV lateral wall during part of cardiac cycle	• Heart failure symptoms • Hemolysis	• Chest X-ray, echocardiography or CT angiography to evaluate cannula position • Hydration to improve LV end-diastolic volume • Decreasing pump speed • Surgical repositioning

(Abbreviations: CT: Computed tomography; LV: Left ventricular; LVAD: Left ventricular assist device; MAP: Mean arterial pressure; VAD: Ventricular assist device)

which still have to overcome prior to medium term *in vivo* experiments. MCS has entered its third generation with newer devices having magnetically levitated rotor to prevent friction and decrease energy loss. Development of transcutaneous energy transfer system (TETS) would obviate the need for a percutaneous lead decreasing infection rate. Ideal VAD would be one which could be completely implantable within the thoracic cage powered by TETS with enhanced durability.

❑ SUGGESTED READINGS

1. Center for Medicare Services. Available from http://www.cms.gov/MLNMattersArticles/downloads/MM7220.pdf.
2. John R. Donor management and selection for heart transplantation. Semin Thorac Cardiovasc Surg. 2004;16:364-9.
3. Kalogeropoulos AP, Georgiopoulou VV, Giamouzis G, et al. Utility of the Seattle Heart Failure Model in patients with advanced heart failure. J Am Coll Cardiol. 2009;53:334-42.
4. Kearney MT, Fox KA, Lee AJ, et al. Predicting death due to progressive heart failure in patients with mild-to-moderate chronic heart failure. J Am Coll Cardiol. 2002;40:1801-8.
5. Kirklin JK, Naftel DC, Kormos RL, et al. Second INTERMACS annual report: more than 1,000 primary left ventricular assist device implants. J Heart Lung Transplant. 2010;29:1-10.
6. Lietz K, Miller LW. Patient selection for left-ventricular assist devices. Curr Opin Cardiol. 2009;24:246-51.
7. Lindenfeld J, Miller GG, Shakar SF, et al. Drug therapy in the heart transplant recipient: Part II: immunosuppressive drugs. Circulation. 2004;110:3858-65.
8. Lindenfeld J, Page RL 2nd, Zolty R, et al. Drug therapy in the heart transplant recipient: Part III: common medical problems. Circulation. 2005;111:113-7.
9. Mehra MR, Kobashigawa J, Starling R, et al. Listing criteria for heart transplantation: International Society for Heart and Lung Transplantation guidelines for the care of cardiac transplant candidates—2006. J Heart Lung Transplant. 2006;25:1024-42.
10. Mudge GH Jr, Fang JC, Smith C, et al. The physiologic basis for the management of ventricular assist devices. Clin Cardiol. 2006;29:285-9.
11. Slaughter MS, Rogers JG, Milano CA, et al. Advanced heart failure treated with continuous-flow left ventricular assist device. N Engl J Med. 2009;361:2241-51.
12. Stehlik J, Edwards LB, Kucheryavaya AY, et al. The Registry of the International Society for Heart and Lung Transplantation: twentyseventh official adult heart transplant report—2010. J Heart Lung Transplant. 2010;29:1089-103.
13. United Network of Organ Sharing. Available from http://optn.transplant.hrsa.gov/
14. Vazquez R, Bayes-Genis A, Cygankiewicz I, et al. The MUSIC risk score: a simple method for predicting mortality in ambulatory patients with chronic heart failure. Eur Heart J. 2009;30:1088-96.

Chapter 8

Myocardial and Pericardial Diseases

8.1 Hypertrophic Cardiomyopathy

❏ INTRODUCTION

Hypertrophic cardiomyopathy (HCM) is a clinically heterogenous, autosomal dominant heart muscle disorder due, primarily, to mutations in the genes encoding the cardiac sarcomere myofilament proteins. This culminates in the protein's altered structure and function with myofibrillar disarray, marked ventricular hypertrophy (frequently asymmetric), diastolic dysfunction and, in some patients, sudden cardiac death as its most devastating outcome. Hypertrophic cardiomyopathy is the most prevalent, monogenic heritable cardiovascular disease, affecting approximately 1 in 500 people (0.2% of the population) and is the most common cause of sudden cardiac death in young people, including competitive athletes. The HCM is global and found with equal frequency in males and females as well as across all populations, including non-Hispanic whites, Hispanic whites, blacks and Asians (Chinese included). The HCM is caused by mutations (inherited in an autosomal dominant pattern) in genes that encode sarcomeric proteins. The morphologic and functional changes associated with HCM result in complex and multiple interrelated changes in cardiac physiology, including diastolic dysfunction, left ventricular outflow tract (LVOT) obstruction, mitral regurgitation (MR), myocardial ischemia, arrhythmias and, in a minority of patients over time, overt systolic dysfunction (Table 1).

Table 1: Pathophysiologic hallmarks of hypertrophic cardiomyopathy

Diastolic Dysfunction
Multifunctional etiology:
1. Molecular function (e.g. mutations, calcium economy and sensitivity)
2. Myocardial tissue function (e.g. hypertrophy, fibrosis, and disarray)
3. Global function (e.g. geometry and ischemia)

LVOT Obstruction
Multifunctional etiology:
1. Septal hypertrophy and configuration
2. Systolic anterior motion and SAM-septal contact
3. Elongated, redundant and often anteriorly positioned mitral apparatus
4. Altered ventricular loading conditions
5. Reduced ventricular chamber volume

Midventricular obstruction:
1. Mid-septal hypertrophy
2. Hypertrophic papillary muscles
3. Anomalous papillary muscle insertion

Contd...

Contd...

Table 1: Pathophysiologic hallmarks of hypertrophic cardiomyopathy

Arrhythmogenic Substrate

Tachyarrhythmias:
1. Myocardial disarray
2. Interstitial fibrosis
3. Small-vessel disease:
    a. Structurally abnormal intramural arterioles with thickened media and narrowed lumina
    b. Silent myocardial ischemic with replacement fibrosis/scarring (perivascular fibrosis)
4. Apical pouch
5. Dilated left atrium (diastolic dysfunction ± mitral regurgitation)

Bradyarrhythmias:
1. Conduction system disease
2. Chronotropic incompetence
3. Left bundle branch block; uncommonly, right bundle branch block
4. Spontaneous complete heart block (rare)

Dilated Hypokinetic Phase (burnt-out stage)

(Abbreviations: LVOT: Left ventricular outflow tract; SAM: Systolic anterior motion)

❑ PATHOLOGY

The HCM is characterized by a thick ventricle (symmetrical or asymmetrical) and hypertrophy (increased LV mass) involving particularly substantial portions of the LV wall (Fig. 1, Table 2). Histology (Table 2) remains the cornerstone for the diagnosis of HCM. At the microscopic level, pathological hallmarks of HCM include myocyte hypertrophy (maximal in the subendocardial region) and disarray (with bizarre enlarged nuclei, hyperchromasia, and pleomorphism) together with expansion of the interstitial collagen compartment (Fig. 2).

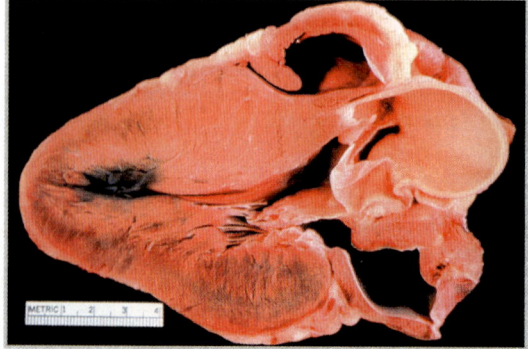

FIGURE 1: Autopsy specimen of the heart of a young patient with hypertrophic cardiomyopathy who had sudden death. Massive asymmetric hypertrophy of the myocardium can be recognized, which dwarfs the cavity size of the left ventricle in comparison. Also observe the grossly visible area of necrosis toward the apical septum. (*Source:* WD Edwards, MD, Rochester, MN)

Table 2: Gross anatomic and microscopic features of HCM

Gross examination:
1. Asymmetrically or symmetrically thick ventricle
2. Basal septal bulge or sigmoid septum
3. Endocardial fibrosis
4. "Septal callus" or subaortic mitral impact friction lesion (plaque on the interventricular septum where mitral–septal contact has repeatedly occurred)#
5. Elongated and/or thickened chordae tendineae
6. Increased anterior leaflet length of the mitral valve
7. Increased number of posterior leaflet scallops
8. Abnormal attachments of mitral valve chordal apparatus to septum
9. Hypertrophied papillary muscles with or without anterior displacement
10. Abnormal attachment of papillary muscle heads directly into the mitral leaflets
11. Dilated atria

Microscopy (characterized by disorganization or "whorling" of muscle fibers):
1. Myocardial disarray characterized by severely hypertrophied myocytes aligned perpendicularly or obliquely to each other around central cores of collagen in a pinwheel configuration or herringbone pattern
2. Fibrosis (pericellular, patchy or extensive)
3. Degenerating muscle fibers
4. Intimal and medial smooth muscle hyperplasia of intramural coronary arteries and capillaries (small-vessel disease)
5. Reduced arteriolar density
6. Microscopic evidence of subacute/acute myocardial necrosis

#This lesion is an exact mirror image of the anterior cusp of the mitral valve and chordae and is characterized by a sharper lower edge, corresponding to the lower border of the valve cusp.

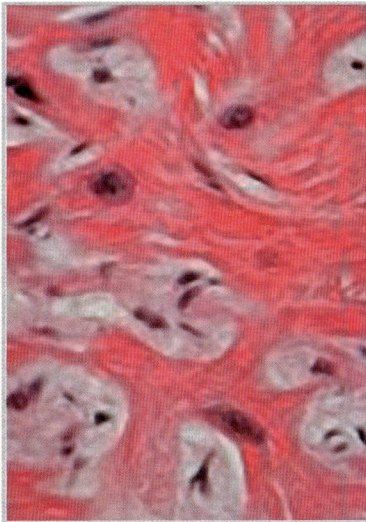

FIGURE 2: Microscopic sections of the myocardium from a young patient with hypertrophic cardiomyopathy who had sudden death. There is myocardial disarray characterized by hypertrophied myocytes aligned perpendicularly to each other around central cores of collagen. Also note the pericellular patchy fibrosis. (*Source:* WD Edwards, MD, Rochester, MN)

❏ CLINICAL PRESENTATION

Symptoms

In HCM, there are at least four interacting pathophysiological mechanisms (Fig. 3) that may be responsible for symptoms: (i) LVH, (ii) diastolic dysfunction, (iii) LVOT obstruction and subsequent MR, and (iv) myocardial ischemia. A characteristic pattern of day-to-day variation in the activity needed to cause symptoms is also unique to HCM.

Dyspnea occurs in the vast majority of patients, either at rest or with exertion, and is primarily due to elevated LV diastolic filling pressures caused by impaired LV filling. Angina pectoris is also a frequent symptom, occurring in the absence of epicardial coronary disease and primarily related to small vessel disease and oxygen supply-demand mismatch. Patients with HCM may also be present with presyncope and syncope due to either a rhythm or hemodynamic alteration. Other, less commonly reported symptoms include palpitations, paroxysmal nocturnal dyspnea, dizziness, and symptoms of heart failure (HF).

Physical Examination

Classic physical examination findings in HCM (Fig. 4) relate to the obstructive variant, with minimal findings (save the presence of an LV lift or a palpable or audible fourth heart sound) in the nonobstructive or apical form. However, variants of HCM may all develop LVOT obstruction at various times, and these physical signs refer to HCM with LVOT obstruction.

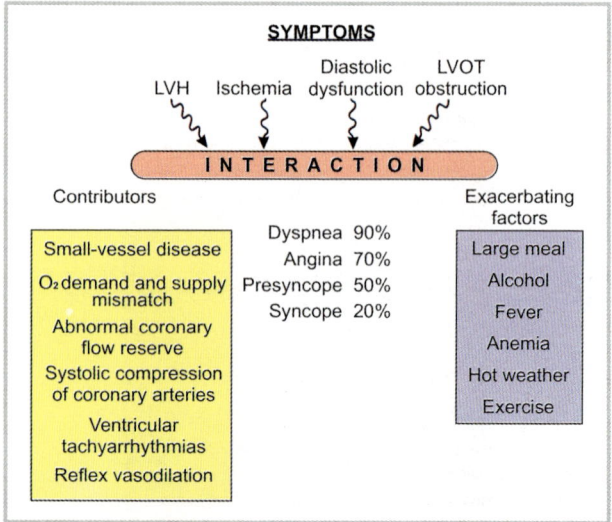

FIGURE 3: The symptoms of hypertrophic cardiomyopathy (HCM) arise from a close interaction of left ventricular outflow tract (LVOT) obstruction, diastolic dysfunction, small-vessel ischemia, and left ventricular hypertrophy (LVH). These symptoms are often exacerbated (purple box) by factors that can increase LVOT obstruction, either by decreasing preload or afterload or increasing left ventricular contractility. Several other factors (yellow box) may also interact to contribute to the symptom complex of HCM

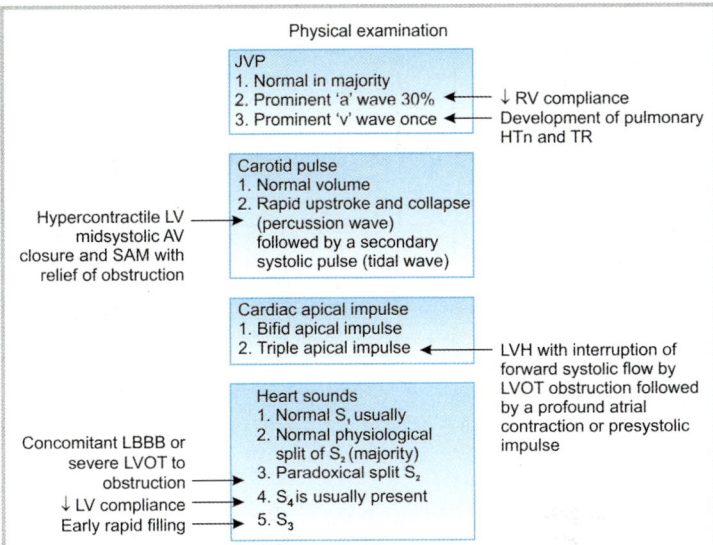

FIGURE 4: Common findings on physical examination in patients with hypertrophic cardiomyopathy. Potential pathophysiological mechanisms are shown by arrows. (Abbreviations: AV: Atrioventricular; JVP: Jugular venous pressure; HTn: Hypertension; LBBB: Left bundle branch block; LV: Left ventricle; LVH: Left ventricular hypertrophy; LVOT: Left ventricular outflow tract; RV: Right ventricle; SAM: Systolic anterior motion; TR: Tricuspid regurgitation)

❏ DIAGNOSIS

Electrocardiogram

The vast majority of patients with HCM have an abnormal ECG manifest either as left-axis deviation, LVH or abnormal Q-waves simulating myocardial infarction (representative of massive septal hypertrophy and/or fibrosis) (Table 3). ST-segment changes with T-wave abnormalities are common (due primarily to LVH) (Fig. 5).

Table 3: Electrocardiographic features of HCM

1. Normal axis 60–70%
2. Left axis 30%
3. LVH 70–80% (tallest QRS complexes in mid-precordial leads)
4. Abnormal Q-waves 25% (pseudoinfarct pattern)
5. Grant diffuse symmetric T-wave inversions (apical HCM)
6. Left anterior hemiblock
7. First-degree atrioventricular block
8. Complete left bundle branch block
9. Left atrial abnormality
10. Prominent delta wave of ventricular preexcitation may also be seen
11. Biventricular hypertrophy when RV involvement (mostly in children)
12. Normal electrocardiogram (5–10%)

(Abbreviations: HCM: Hypertrophy cardiomyopathy; LVH: Left ventricular hypertrophy; RV: Right ventricular)

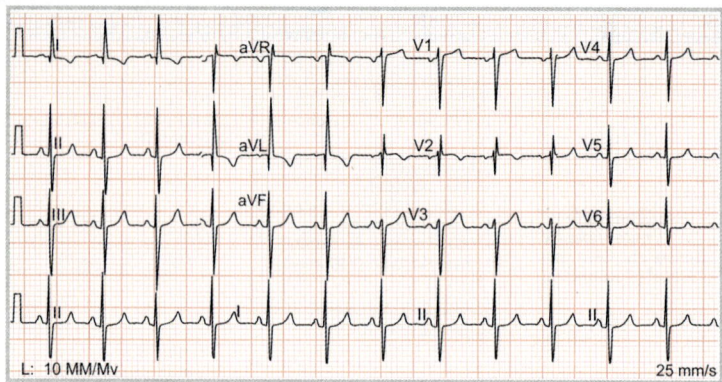

FIGURE 5: A 12-lead surface electrocardiogram from a patient with hypertrophic cardiomyopathy revealing left ventricular hypertrophy (LVH). Note the nonspecific ST-T segment changes and T-wave inversions in the lateral leads, which can be part and parcel of LVH

Holter Monitoring

Holter monitoring demonstrates the basic rhythm in most patients to be normal sinus, but will occasionally demonstrate a high incidence of supraventricular tachycardia (46%), premature ventricular contractions (43%) and nonsustained VT (26%). AF is also commonly seen in patients with HCM, with a reported prevalence of approximately 22% and an annual incidence of up to 2% per year.

Chest X-ray

A normal chest X-ray (CXR) is common in HCM patients, although it may show an enlarged cardiac silhouette. Evidence of elevated LV filling pressures may be evident in the form of increased pulmonary interstitial markings, and left atrial enlargement may also be noted, particularly when accompanied by MR or AF. An important differentiation on the CXR from patients with aortic stenosis may be the absence of aortic root dilation and aortic valve calcification.

Echocardiography

Two-dimensional and Doppler echocardiographies are the essential parts of the evaluation of all patients with suspected HCM and are the current gold standard for diagnosis. Echocardiographic evaluation of HCM involves assessment of (i) presence, magnitude and distribution of LVH, (ii) LVOT obstruction, (iii) MR, (iv) diastolic dysfunction, and (v) identification of HCM variants and screening of all first-degree relatives for occult HCM. Table 4 summarizes the classic echocardiographic features of HCM.

Cardiac Magnetic Resonance Imaging

In contemporary clinical practice, CMR has become a useful complementary imaging tool for the diagnosis of HCM and follow-up of patients after either surgical myectomy or septal ablation therapy. In addition, CMR imaging can help discriminate HCM from closely related morphological cardiomyopathies and cardiac disorders, e.g. amyloidosis, Fabry's disease, athlete's heart and isolated apical hypertrophy. CMR provides high-resolution moving images of the

Table 4: Classic echocardiographic features of HCM

1. Thick LV (≥13 mm)[#]
2. Increase in LV mass (HCM is the leading cause of the heaviest hearts)[§]
3. Small LV end-diastolic volume
4. Increase in left atrial volume index
5. E/A reversal, prolonged DT and prolonged IVRT
6. Restrictive filling dynamics (increased E/A ratio, short DT and short IVRT)
7. Decrease in tissue early diastolic velocity (E') and increased E/E' ratio
8. Pulmonary hypertension as measured by tricuspid regurgitation jet
9. Increase in circumferential strain and strain rate
10. Decrease in longitudinal strain and strain rate
11. Clockwise mid-LV rotation (opposite to normal)
12. Time to peak systolic twist shorter
13. Time from peak to trough twist (untwist) longer (obstructive HCM >nonobstructive HCM)

[#]A septal-to-posterior wall thickness ratio of 1.3:1 is evidence of asymmetric septal hypertrophy. However, pulmonary hypertension with right ventricular hypertrophy and inferior wall infarction in the presence of left ventricular hypertrophy also can cause such septal-to-posterior wall thickness ratio.
[§]LV mass = 1.04 [(LV end-diastolic diameter in diastole + posterior wall thickness in diastole + interventricular septal thickness in diastole)3—LV end-diastolic diameter in diastole3] × 0.8 + 0.6.
(Abbreviations: DT: Deceleration time; HCM: Hypertrophy cardiomyopathy; IVRT: Isovolumetric relaxation time; LV: Left ventricle)

myocardium accurately determining the site (e.g. segmental hypertrophy) and extent of hypertrophy. The strengths of CMR imaging include its ability to identify macroscopic areas of abnormal myocardium with delayed gadolinium-enhanced imaging.

Currently, increasing interest in CMR imaging for HCM has evolved due to delayed hyperenhancement magnetic resonance imaging (DHE-MRI), which makes it possible to accurately detect areas of myocardial fibrosis/scarring in vivo with a high degree of sensitivity. In the past, this was possible only in histopathologic specimens. Areas of DHE on CMR have been shown to correlate with, histologically proven myocardial scar as well as with wall thickness, regional function and ventricular tachyarrhythmias.

Cardiac Catheterization

Because 2D and Doppler echocardiographic assessment with or without CMR usually establishes the diagnosis of HCM in a given clinical situation, cardiac catheterization is seldom necessary in the vast majority of cases. However, in cases of inadequate or difficult echocardiographic imaging (suboptimal), cardiac catheterization may be of benefit in demonstrating the presence and severity of an LVOT obstruction.

Stress Test

Stress testing in HCM for the diagnosis of obstructive coronary artery disease (CAD) is of limited value because the combination of the supply–demand mismatch and the small coronary arteriolar disease can result in findings of myocardial ischemia on ECG and nuclear imaging, even in the absence of obstructive epicardial coronary disease. However, under careful ECG and hemodynamic monitoring, exercise can be used as a physiological provocation maneuver to attempt to detect latent LVOT obstruction. Besides, exercise in a patient with HCM can be used to obtain substantial information on (i) exercise hemodynamics and MR, diastolic dysfunction and pulmonary artery pressures, (ii) blood pressure response, (iii) chronotropic incompetence, (iv) exercise tolerance, and (v) arrhythmic potential.

❏ NATURAL HISTORY

The HCM is a unique disease that may present during any phase of life from infancy to old age with a variable clinical course. Although patients with HCM may remain stable over long periods of time and achieve normal longevity (>75 years), many patients have their natural course punctuated by SD, embolic stroke and development of HF. In general, the natural history of HCM follows one of several profiles (Table 5).

Early literature on HCM described a poor prognosis for patients with this disease, suggesting a high incidence of SD and overall high mortality rates (3–6% per year). This most likely represented a selection bias, since much of the published clinical data emanated from a few select tertiary centers in North America and Europe. Nevertheless, subgroups of patients within the broad HCM spectrum that are clearly at high risk for death (including SD) and in whom annual mortality exceeds 1% do exist (Table 6).

Table 5: Spectrum of natural history of hypertrophic cardiomyopathy

1. Stable benign course with normal longevity
2. Premature sudden death
3. Progressive symptomatic deterioration
   Exertional dyspnea
   Chest pain (either typical of angina or atypical in nature)
   Syncope, near-syncope or presyncope (i.e. dizziness/lightheadedness)
4. Progression to advanced diastolic heart failure or so-called "end-stage phase" or "burnt-out" phase with left ventricular remodeling and systolic dysfunction
5. Complications attributable to atrial fibrillation, including embolic stroke

Table 6: High-risk cohort for sudden death in HCM

1. Prior cardiac arrest or sustained ventricular tachycardia
2. Family history of premature SD due to HCM in a first-degree relative
3. Repetitive nonsustained ventricular tachycardia
4. Massive ventricular hypertrophy (wall thickness >30 mm)
5. Hypotensive response to exercise
6. Unexplained syncope
7. Atrial fibrillation
8. Systemic embolism
9. Vigorous physical activity and/or competitive sports
10. Development of end-stage HCM
11. Marked outflow gradient
12. Abnormal aortic stiffness as measured by increased pulse-wave velocity with VENC-MRI
13. Myocardial fibrosis as demonstrated by late gadolinium enhancement on CMR
14. Genotypic expression
    a. MYH7-R403Q mutation
    b. Multiple sarcomeric defects or "gene-dosage effect" (double, triple or compound hetezygosity)
    c. TNNT2 (troponin T)-HCM genotype

(Abbreviations: CMR: Cardiac magnetic resonance imaging; HCM: Hypertrophy cardiomyopathy; SD: Sudden death; VENC-MRI: Velocity-encoded magnetic resonance imaging)

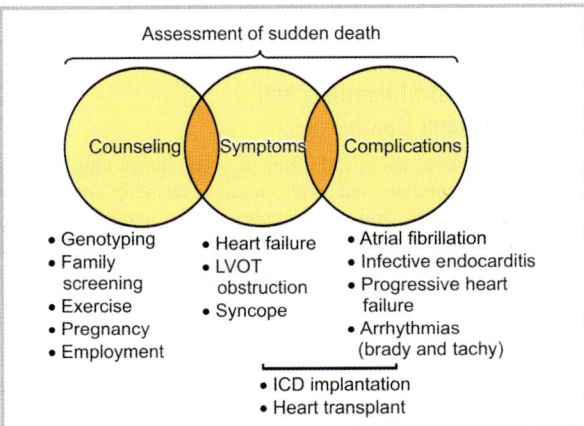

FIGURE 6: Illustrated is the complicated and formidable management plan in a given patient with hypertrophic cardiomyopathy. The physician needs to incorporate multiple facets of patient care, including the medical, social and family aspects of disease management. Not only does the physician have to be vigilant about the symptoms and complications of the disease process (an ongoing management issue) but also manage issues related to family counseling and employment. (Abbreviations: ICD: Implantable cardioverter-defibrillator; LVOT: Left ventricle outflow tract)

❏ MANAGEMENT

The management of HCM is complex and challenging (Fig. 6) and can change over a period of time. It involves not only management of the symptomatic HCM patient with pharmacological interventions, but also considerable personal commitment by the treating physician toward both patient and family counseling as well as due consideration and introduction of life-changing interventions such as exercise restrictions, ICD and/or pacemaker implantation and, sometimes, heart transplant.

Genotyping, Genetic Counseling, and Family Screening

Currently, four US laboratories (Harvard Partners, Correlagen, PGxHealth, and GeneDX) offer testing for the eight most common myofilament-associated HCM genes. As pointed out previously, echocardiography may help guide genetic testing by providing anticipatory guidance and a pretest probability of a positive genetic test result.

In contemporary clinical practice, genetic testing of the index case has the potential of providing the diagnostic gold standard for his/her offspring, siblings, parents and more distant relatives. A positive genetic test enables scrutiny of the index case's relatives to separate "those at risk" from "those not at risk" (positive vs negative test). In other words, the genetic testing of the index case risk stratifies the family, enabling two very different courses to be charted: (i) close surveillance of the genotype-positive, preclinical individual and (ii) standard observation or dismissal of the genotype-negative/phenotype negative relative and his/her future progeny. However, irrespective of genetic testing, once a clinical diagnosis of HCM is made, all first-degree relatives and probably "athletic" second-degree relatives to the index case should be screened by an ECG and echocardiogram. Annual screenings are recommended for adolescents, young adults (age 12–25) and athletes, and every 3–5 years thereafter.

Assessment, Risk Stratification, and Prevention of Sudden Death

Precise risk stratification in HCM remains a challenge due to its clinical heterogeneity of presentation and expression, its relatively low prevalence in general cardiology practice, and the complexity of potential pathophysiologic mechanisms. Nevertheless, it is possible to identify most high-risk patients by noninvasive clinical markers, and only a small minority of those HCM patients who die suddenly (about 3%) are without any of the currently acknowledged risk markers (Fig. 7).

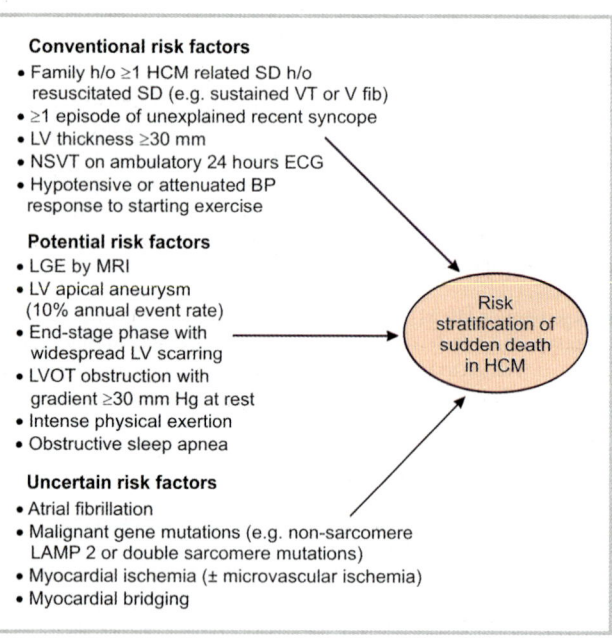

FIGURE 7: Sudden death (SD) risk stratification in hypertrophic cardiomyopathy (HCM). Top arrow identifies a clinical profile currently used to identify those patients at highest risk for SD who are potential candidates for implantable cardioverter-defibrillators (ICD). The middle and bottom arrows identify a number of disease features that can be regarded as arbitrators when the level of risk based on conventional markers is ambiguous. These may be useful in resolving otherwise uncertain ICD decisions on a case-by-case basis. Also note that sustained ventricular tachyarrhythmias have been reported in a significant minority of patients (~10%) over the short-term after alcohol septal ablation. A direct relation exists between magnitude of left ventricular (LV) hypertrophy (maximum wall thickness by echocardiography) and SD risk. Mild hypertrophy conveys generally lower risk; extreme hypertrophy (wall thickness = 30 mm) conveys the highest risk as a marker for SD. (Abbreviations: BP: Blood pressure; ECG: Electrocardiogram; LGE: Late gadolinium enhancement; MRI: Magnetic resonance imaging; NSVT: Nonsustained ventricular tachycardia; V Fib: Ventricular fibrillation, VT: Ventricular tachycardia, LVOT: Left ventricular outflow tract)

The HCM patients (particularly those <60 years old) should undergo comprehensive clinical assessments on an annual basis for risk stratification and evolution of symptoms, including, (i) careful personal and family history, (ii) noninvasive testing with 2D echocardiography (primarily for assessment of magnitude of LVH and outflow obstruction), (iii) a 24- or 48-hour ambulatory (Holter) ECG recording for VT, and (iv) blood pressure response during maximal upright exercise (treadmill or bicycle). Subsequent risk analysis should be performed periodically and when there is a perceived change in clinical status.

Although most clinical markers of SD risk in HCM patients have low positive predictive values (due to low event rates), their negative predictive value is high (at least 90%), suggesting that the absence of these markers and certain other clinical features can be used to profile HCM patients into a low-likelihood cohort for SD or other adverse events. Patients with such features apparently have a favorable prognosis and constitute an important proportion of the overall HCM population.

With the availability of implantable cardioverter-defibrillators ICDs, prevention of SD by administration of drugs such as beta-adrenergic blocking agents (beta blockers), verapamil and type 1A antiarrhythmic agents (i.e. quinidine, procainamide) is of historical interest now. In contemporary clinical practice, ICD is the most effective and reliable treatment option available, harboring the potential for absolute protection and altering the natural history of this disease in some patients. Based on current evidence, there is universal agreement that an ICD is indicated in HCM patients for secondary prevention after cardiac arrest or sustained episodes of VT, including the American College of Cardiology/European Society of Cardiology 2003 consensus HCM panel. However, ICD selection in patients for primary prevention can be a contentious issue based on available clinical evidence (risk stratification) in a particular patient scenario, the level of risk acceptable to the patient and family, and the potential complications largely related to lead systems and inappropriate device discharges.

Athletes with Hypertrophic Cardiomyopathy

To reduce SD risk in athletes with HCM, the generally accepted recommendation of Bethesda Conference 36 is withdrawal from intense training and competition associated with most competitive sports due to the linkage between SD and intense exertion in trained athletes with underlying cardiovascular disease (including HCM) and in athletes with HCM even in the absence of conventional markers. However, stringent lifestyle or employment modifications for other HCM patients (who are not participants in organized athletics) do not seem justified or practical, although intense physical activity involving burst exertion (e.g. sprinting) or systematic isometric exercise (e.g. heavy lifting) should always be discouraged. In genetically affected but phenotypically normal family members, and in the absence of cardiac symptoms, family history of SD or a mutant gene regarded as malignant, activity restrictions are not mandated, although such subjects may undergo periodic (usually annual) noninvasive clinical evaluation directed toward risk assessment. Healthy-appearing competitive athletes may harbor unsuspected cardiovascular disease (e.g. HCM) with the potential to cause SD. This fact raises issues of physician responsibility in pre-participation screening and eligibility disqualification decisions.

Medical Therapy

The accepted standard clinical practice in patients with symptomatic obstructive HCM is to start beta-blockade as the initial therapy and increase the dose to optimal range. Should beta-blocker not be tolerated due to adverse effects, a CCB, usually verapamil should be substituted. In case of severe LVOT obstruction and symptoms, it is advisable to start the CCB under monitored conditions in the hospital. If patients with obstructive HCM tolerate large doses of either a beta-blocker or CCB and continue to have severe symptoms, disopyramide may be added to either. Currently, no existing data support the combination of beta-blocker and CCBs as being better than one drug alone. When patients continue to be symptomatic and medical therapy is ineffective, septal myectomy, septal ablation or dual-chamber pacing are then considered.

Septal Myectomy

The ventricular septal myectomy (SM) operation (also known as the Morrow procedure) is regarded as the gold standard therapeutic option for adults and children with obstructive HCM and drug-refractory symptoms. Transaortic septal myectomy involves the resection of a carefully defined, relatively small amount of myocardium from the proximal septum (about 5–10 g), extending from near the base of the aortic valve to beyond the distal margins of mitral leaflets (about 3–4 cm), thereby enlarging the LV outflow tract. In the vast majority of patients, septal myectomy:
1. Relieves the LVOT gradient,
2. Abolishes any significant mechanical impedance to ejection and mitral valve SAM,
3. Normalizes LV systolic pressures,
4. Abolishes MR and, ultimately,
5. Reduces LV end-diastolic pressures.

Percutaneous Alcohol Septal Ablation

It is estimated that septal ablation (SA) procedures are 15–20 times more common than SM for HCM, and at some centers the frequency of SM has been reduced by more than 90% in favor of performing SA as the definitive treatment strategy. Alcohol septal ablation produces a controlled myocardial infarction of the proximal septum, which produces shrinkage and scarring of the septal wall, resulting in a widening of the LVOT, thereby lessening the SAM of the mitral valve (thereby reducing/eliminating LVOT obstruction) and MR.

While SA represents an option available to HCM patients and a selective alternative to surgery, current guidelines do not recommend SA as the standard and primary therapeutic strategy for all severely symptomatic patients refractory to medical management with marked obstruction to LV outflow. In real-world practice, the choice of SA versus SM for the treatment of HCM is guided by several considerations (Table 7) and, although SM continues to be the gold-standard treatment for refractory HCM, SA has emerged as an attractive alternative.

❑ DUAL-CHAMBER PACEMAKER

Initial observational and uncontrolled studies reported dual-chamber pacing to be associated with a substantial decrease in outflow gradient and amelioration of symptoms in most patients with HCM. Subsequent randomized trials where

Table 7: Considerations to decide choice of procedures for the treatment of HOCM

Feasibility of each approach:
1. Institutional expertise
2. Patient characteristics
3. Anatomy (septum, papillary muscles, septal perforator, mitral valve, midventricular, or apical variants)

Different mechanism:
1. Size and location of septal reduction

Heterogeneous disease:
1. SAM-independent
2. SAM-related
    a. Anterior coaptation
    b. Positive angle between the LVOT and the leaflets
3. Chordal slack

Informed decision after detailed discussion about both therapies

(Abbreviations: HOCM: Hypertrophic obstructive cardiomyopathy; LVOT: Left ventricular outflow tract; SAM: Systolic anterior motion). (Source: Agarwal S, et al. Updated meta-analysis of septal alcohol ablation versus myectomy for hypertrophic cardiomyopathy. J Am Coll Cardiol. 2010;55:823-34, with permission)

patients received 2–3 months of pacing and backup AAI mode (no pacing) as a control did not, however, demonstrate this consistently. Currently, no known parameters exist that can identify the patients who would uniformly benefit from dual-chamber pacing. Thus, the role of dual-chamber pacing is limited in contemporary practice to patients who are at high risk for other therapeutic modalities, e.g. SA and SM. Candidates for dual-chamber pacing may include: (i) patients who have significant bradycardia in which pacing may allow an increased dosage of medication, and (ii) patients who are receiving an ICD for high-risk status and in whom obstruction to LV outflow is also present.

❏ SUGGESTED READINGS

Binder J, Ommen SR, Gersh BJ, et al. Echocardiography-guided genetic testing in hypertrophic cardiomyopathy: septal morphological features predict the presence of myofilament mutations. Mayo Clin Proc. 2006;81:459-67.

Bonow RO, Rosing DR, Bacharach SL, et al. Effects of verapamil on left ventricular systolic function and diastolic filling in patients with hypertrophic cardiomyopathy. Circulation. 1981;64:787-96.

Bos JM, Towbin JA, Ackerman MJ. Diagnostic, prognostic and therapeutic implications of genetic testing for hypertrophic cardiomyopathy. J Am Coll Cardiol 2009;54:201-11.

Epstein AE, DiMarco JP, Ellenbogen KA, et al. ACC/AHA/HRS 2008 guidelines for device-based therapy of cardiac rhythm abnormalities: a report of the American College of Cardiology/American Heart Association Task Force on Practice Guidelines (Writing Committee to Revise the ACC/AHA/NASPE 2002 Guideline Update for Implantation of Cardiac Pacemakers and Antiarrhythmia Devices) developed in collaboration with the American Association for Thoracic Surgery and Society of Thoracic Surgeons. J Am Coll Cardiol. 2008;51:e1-e62.

Frank MJ, Abdulla AM, Canedo MI, et al. Long-term medical management of hypertrophic obstructive cardiomyopathy. Am J Cardiol. 1978;42:993-1001.

Kuhn H, Gietzen F, Leuner C, et al. Induction of subaortic septal ischaemia to reduce obstruction in hypertrophic obstructive cardiomyopathy. Studies to develop a new catheter-based concept of treatment. Eur Heart J. 1997;18:846-51.

Maron BJ, McKenna WJ, Danielson GK, et al. American College of Cardiology/European Society of Cardiology clinical expert consensus document on hypertrophic cardiomyopathy. A report of the American College of Cardiology Foundation Task Force on Clinical Expert

Consensus Documents and the European Society of Cardiology Committee for Practice Guidelines. J Am Coll Cardiol. 2003;42:1687-713.

Maron BJ, Nishimura RA, McKenna WJ, et al. Assessment of permanent dual-chamber pacing as a treatment for drug-refractory symptomatic patients with obstructive hypertrophic cardiomyopathy. A randomized, double-blind, cross-over study (M-PATHY). Circulation. 1999;99:2927-33.

Maron MS, Olivotto I, Zenovich AG, et al. Hypertrophic cardiomyopathy is predominantly a disease of left ventricular outflow tract obstruction. Circulation. 2006;114:2232-9.

Morrow AG, Reitz BA, Epstein SE, et al. Operative treatment in hypertrophic subaortic stenosis. Techniques and the results of pre and postoperative assessments in 83 patients. Circulation. 1975;52:88-102.

Spirito P, Seidman CE, McKenna WJ, et al. The management of hypertrophic cardiomyopathy. N Engl J Med. 1997;336:775-85.

Wigle ED, Rakowski H, Kimball BP, et al. Hypertrophic cardiomyopathy. Clinical spectrum and treatment. Circulation. 1995;92:1680-92.

8.2 Dilated Cardiomyopathy

❑ INTRODUCTION

The determination of the true incidence and prevalence of idiopathic dilated cardiomyopathy (IDC) is hampered by the lack of unified definition, the difficulty in establishing the absence of coronary artery disease and other causes of dilated cardiomyopathy (DCM), and the under recognition of asymptomatic cases. The reported incidence varies between 2.5 and 8.3 cases per 100,000 of the population. The risk of IDC is 2.5 fold higher in African Americans even after adjusting for socioeconomic factors.

❑ DEFINITION

The most recent definition and classification of the cardiomyopathies was proposed in a scientific statement published by the American Heart Association (AHA) (Flowchart 1) in which cardiomyopathies were defined as "a heterogeneous group of diseases of the myocardium associated with mechanical and/or electrical dysfunction that usually (but not invariably) exhibit inappropriate ventricular hypertrophy or dilatation and are due to a variety of causes that frequently are genetic. Cardiomyopathies either are confined to the heart or are part of generalized systemic disorders, often leading to cardiovascular death or progressive heart failure-related disability."

❑ PATHOLOGY

The major morphologic feature of IDC is dilation of both ventricular cavities with the left ventricle typically more severely affected than the right; in addition, both atria are usually dilated. The weight of the heart is always increased (mean 615 gm in men and 551 gm in women) due to massive dilation. The large end systolic ventricular volume coupled with poor contractility contributes to the relative stasis of blood and the formation of intracavitary thrombi. Likewise, dilation of atria along with the poor atrial emptying leads to the formation of thrombi in atrial appendages. Thrombi are found most frequently in the left ventricle followed by the right ventricles, right atrial and left atrial appendages.

FLOWCHART 1: Classification of cardiomyopathies

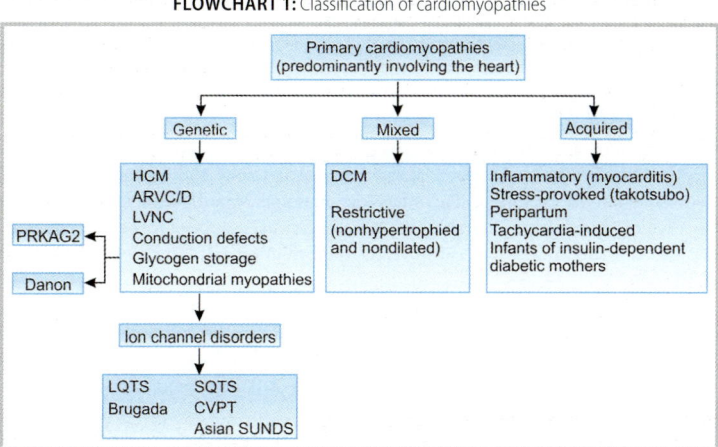

(Abbreviations: HCM: Hypertrophic cardiomyopathy; DCM: Dilated cardiomyopathy; ARVC/D: Arrhythmic right ventricular cardiomyopathy/dysplasia; LVNC: Left ventricular non-compaction; LQTS: Long QT syndrome; SQTS: Short QT syndrome; CVPT: Catecholaminergic polymorphic ventricular tachycardia; SUNDS: Sudden unexpected nocturnal death syndrome)

Microscopic examination reveals marked variation in myocyte size with extensive areas of interstitial and perivascular fibrosis involving mainly the left ventricular (LV) subendocardium.

❏ ETIOLOGY

Ischemic Versus Nonischemic Etiology

A proposed definition of assigning an ischemic etiology to the impairment of ventricular systolic function requires the presence of more than or equal to 75% stenosis of left main or proximal left anterior descending or the presence of more than or equal to 75% stenosis of two or more epicardial vessels. However, coronary microvascular and endothelial dysfunction have been well documented in patients with DCM. It should be noted that the presence or absence of regional wall motion abnormalities alone does not establish the presence or absence of an ischemic etiology.

Cardiac magnetic resonance imaging (CMRI) can help in differentiating ischemic from nonischemic etiology of LV dilatation using two criteria: regional wall motion abnormalities with reduction in wall thickness combined with hyperenhancement extending from the subendocardium up to the epicardium confined to the perfusion territories of the coronary arteries.

Clinical Course

The clinical presentation may be similar in ischemic and nonischemic HF, but symptoms appear at a younger age in patients with DCM. Chest pain, including typical angina, may be present in 40% of patients with DCM and should not be used as a determinant of etiology. One notable difference in the clinical course is the consistent finding of worse prognosis in patients with ischemic etiology of systolic HF that may be secondary to recurrence of ischemic events leading to more impairment in ventricular systolic function and/or potentially more arrhythmic events.

Response to Treatment

Contemporary trials with angiotensin-converting enzyme inhibitors, angiotensin-receptor blockers, beta-blockers, aldosterone antagonists and biventricular pacers demonstrated an overall similar effect on outcome regardless of the etiology of ventricular dysfunction. Notable differences, however, appear to be present with the use of synchronization, cardioverter defibrillation (ICD) and the inodilator milrinone.

The benefits of ICD were clearly established in patients with systolic HF of ischemic etiology. It was also shown that sustained reverse remodeling occurred to a much larger extent in patients with nonischemic etiology. It is interesting to note that the differential effect on remodeling was not associated by any differences on mortality suggesting that the mechanism for survival benefit was not related to improvement in LV function but perhaps to favorable effect on substrates for arrhythmias. Milrinone infusion was associated with an increase in the composite of death or rehospitalization, while the opposite was noted in the nonischemic patients. Thus, a differential effect for milrinone appears to be present based on etiology and the speculated mechanism is acceleration of HF progression in hibernating myocardium.

Myocarditis

There is mounting evidence that supports the contribution of autoimmunity to the development of IDC including a higher prevalence of the major histocompatibility complex class II proteins HLA-DR4 and HLA-DQ_4/6 subtypes that interact with CD4+ T-helper cells leading to the activation of B-lymphocytes. In addition, several autoantibodies have been identified, such as myosin autoantibodies, which have been reported to be present in 23–66% of patients with IDC and were correlated with worsening LV systolic function and increased diastolic stiffness. The B1 adrenoreceptor antibodies have been found in 26–46% of patients with IDC and were associated with increased all cause mortality and sudden death. Interestingly, they have been found to induce a dose-dependent increase in cardiomyocytes apoptosis.

The clinical manifestations of myocarditis are highly variable and range from asymptomatic nonspecific electrocardiographic abnormalities to cardiogenic shock or sudden death. A history of viral prodrome is variable. Giant cell myocarditis should be considered in patients with acute DCM associated with thymoma, autoimmune disorders, ventricular tachycardia, or high-grade heart block.

There are no specific biomarkers or features in the electrocardiogram or echocardiogram that establish the diagnosis of myocarditis. The CMRI has been used to localize biopsy sites or as an alternative noninvasive method for diagnosing myocarditis. Histopathological confirmation is required and myocardial biopsy should be performed in patients with unexplained, new onset HF of less than 2 weeks' duration with hemodynamic compromise and in patients with unexplained, new onset HF of 2 weeks' to 3 months' duration in the presence of dilated left ventricle and new ventricular arrhythmia or advanced atrioventricular (AV) block and in patients with suspected giant cell myocarditis if they do not show a response to usual care within 1–2 weeks.

The treatment of myocarditis is primarily supportive, including the occasional need for ventricular assist devices or heart transplantation. Antiviral therapy is unlikely to be of value considering the difficulty in establishing the diagnosis in the acute viral phase. The role of immunosuppression therapy has been evaluated in several randomized controlled trials and has not been found to be of significant benefit in the acute phase. On the other hand, there appears to be a better response in patients with chronic DCM following the acute phase with significant improvement in LV function with immunosuppression (prednisone and azathioprine) and interferon beta. The data on the benefit of intravenous gamma globulin are insufficient to recommend their routine use for acute myocarditis. For giant cell myocarditis, prolongation of transplant-free survival was clearly documented with a combination of cyclosporine and steroids.

Familial Dilated Cardiomyopathy

Familial dilated cardiomyopathy (FDC) is predominantly a genetic disease and more than 30 genes causing IDC have been identified. The diagnosis of (FDC) is made when IDC is diagnosed in two closely related family members. The current practice guidelines recommends screening, every 3–5 years, beginning in childhood, and every 1–3 years in adults if a mutation is present (Table 8).

The presence of sinus/AV node dysfunction including first, second, and third degree heart block, with or without atrial flutter, fibrillation, tachy-brady syndrome is an indication for genetic testing. Mutations in LMNA gene can cause DCM with conduction disease and portends high risk of sudden death. Genetic testing should be considered for the person most clearly affected in a family to facilitate screening and management, because it increases the likelihood of detecting a relevant mutation.

Tachycardia-induced Cardiomyopathy

This is a reversible form of DC that is caused by any rhythm disturbance associated with rapid ventricular rate and is either completely or partially reversible after the normalization of heart rate. Postulated mechanisms include depletion of myocardial energy stores, abnormal calcium handling, oxidative stress, angiotensin converting enzyme gene polymorphism, and myocardial ischemia. The management is primarily restoration of a normal heart rate by either pharmacological or interventional approach.

Table 8: Clinical screening of disease

It is recommended that clinical screening consists of:
- History (with special attention to heart failure symptoms, arrhythmias, presyncope and syncope)
- Physical examination (with special attention to the cardiac, and skeletal muscle systems)
- Electrocardiogram
- Echocardiogram
- CK-MM (at initial evaluation only)
- Signal-averaged electrocardiogram (SAECG) in ARVD only
- Holter monitoring in HCM, ARVD
- Exercise treadmill testing in HCM
- Magnetic resonance imaging in ARVD

(Level of Evidence = B) (Abbreviations: CK-mm: Creatine kinase, muscle; HCM: Hypertrophic cardiomyopathy; ARVD: Arrhythmic right ventricular dysplasia)

Stress-induced Cardiomyopathy

This is a relatively new entity also called takotsubo cardiomyopathy, transient apical ballooning syndrome and broken heart syndrome. It accounts for 2% of ST-segment elevation infarcts and primarily occurs in postmenopausal women (90% of reported cases) who may present with chest pain (68%) or dyspnea (18%); ST-elevation occurs in 82%, T-wave abnormalities in 64% and Q-waves in 32%. The onset of symptoms may often be preceded by emotional (27%) or physical (38%) stress. Despite a marked impairment of LVEF, all patients experience a dramatic improvement with full recovery of most patients.

Hemodialysis and End-stage Renal Failure

Impairment of LV systolic function has been identified in one third of new dialysis patients. In addition to the traditional risk factors for HF, the uremic milieu itself contributes to the development and progression of HF. Biopsies from patients with dilated left ventricles on dialysis demonstrate more severe hypertrophy and disarray compared to patients with comparable degree of LV systolic dysfunction not on dialysis, and the ultrafiltrate and serum of uremic patients have been shown to have negative inotropic effects.100 Furthermore, renal transplantation results in significant improvement in LV systolic function and HF functional status.

Cirrhosis

In a significant number of cirrhotic patients and up to 50% of those undergoing liver transplantation, there is an evidence of cardiovascular dysfunction that include systolic and diastolic dysfunction, inotropic and chronotropic incompetence, peripheral and splanchnic vasodilation and prolonged QT interval. Although, the recommended management is to follow the standard guidelines, the value of digitalis beta blockers and angiotensin-aldosterone inhibitors in improving clinical picture and outcome has not been proven.

Nutritional Deficiency

Several factors contribute to nutritional deficiency in HF, including loss of appetite, dietary restriction, social isolation, malabsorption and increased metabolic rate. Selective deficiency of several micronutrients has been associated with impaired systolic function and HF; however, knowledge of this subject is very limited. These include selenium deficiency, vitamin D and calcium insufficiency, thiamine deficiency, carnitine deficiency, and accumulation of trace elements like mercury, antimony, and lesser increase in gold, chromium, cobalt, etc.

❏ PROGNOSIS

Despite the recent evidence that the prognosis of HF has been improving, it remains a lethal disease. The one year mortality rate for patients with moderate systolic HF selected in clinical trials has declined from 17 to 7%. Community HF patients, however, due to their older age and comorbidities have higher mortality rates. In mild-to-moderate HF, sudden death is the most common mode of death; while in advanced HF, pump failure becomes the predominant mode of death. Both, the presence as well as the absence of diurnal variation with morning peak, have been described with sudden death in HF. The mortality rate in patients with HF increases with the age, most likely due to the cumulative exposure to comorbidities as well as the higher prevalence of comorbidities. Women have better prognosis than men regardless of etiology and the more favorable outcome may be related to sex hormones. Mortality rates after hospitalization for HF are lower in blacks as compared to whites.

❑ SUGGESTED READINGS

Cooper LT, Berry GJ, Shabetai R. Idiopathic giant-cell myocarditis—natural history and treatment. N Engl J Med. 1997;336:1860-6.

Felker GM, Shaw LK, O'Connor CM, et al. A standardized definition of ischemic cardiomyopathy for use in clinical research. J Am Coll Cardiol. 2002;39;210-8.

Ferrans V. Pathologic anatomy of the dilated cardiomyopathies. Am J Cardiol. 1989;64:9-11C.

Gianni M, Dentali F, Grandi AM, et al. Apical ballooning syndrome or takotsubo cardiomyopathy: a systematic review. Eur Heart J. 2006;27:1523-9.

Harnett JD, Foley RN, Kent GM, et al. Congestive heart failure in dialysis patients: prevalence, incidence, prognosis and risk factors. Kidney Int. 1995;47:884-90.

Hershberger RE, Lindenfeld J, Mestroni L, et al. Genetic evaluation of cardiomyopathy—a Heart Failure Society of America practice guideline. J Card Fail. 2009;15:83-97.

Indolfi C, Piscione F, Perrone-Filardi P, et al. Inotropic stimulation by dobutamine increases left ventricular regional function at the expense of metabolism in hibernating myocardium. Am Heart J. 1996;132:542-9.

Lappe JM, Pelfrey CM, Wilson Tang WH. Recent insights into the role of autoimmunity in idiopathic dilated cardiomyopathy. J Cardiac Fail. 2008;14:521-30.

Maron BJ, Towbin JA, Thiene G, et al. Contemporary definitions and classification of the cardiomyopathies: an American Heart Association scientific statement from the council on clinical cardiology, heart failure and transplantation committee; Quality of care and outcomes research and functional genomics and translational biology interdisciplinary working groups; and council on epidemiology and prevention. Circulation. 2006;113:1807-16.

Metropolol CR/XL randomized intervention trial in congestive heart failure (MERIT-HF) MERIT-HF Study Group. Effect of metoprolol CR/XL in chronic heart failure. Lancet. 1999;353:2001-7.

Moss AJ, Zareba W, Hall WJ, et al. Prophylactic implantation of a defibrillator in patients with myocardial infarction and reduced ejection fraction. N Engl J Med. 2002;346:877-83.

Robinson JL, Hartling L, Crumley E, et al. A systematic review of intravenous gamma globulin for therapy of acute myocarditis. BMC Cardiovasc Disord. 2005;5:12.

Soukoulis V, Dihu JB, Sole M, et al. Micronutrient deficiencies: an unmet need in heart failure. J Am Coll Cardiol. 2009;54:1660-73.

Wikstrom G, Blomström-Lundqvist C, Andren B, et al. The effects of aetiology on outcome in patients treated with cardiac resynchronization therapy in the CARE-HF trial. Eur Heart J. 2009;30:782-8.

Zardi EM, Abbate A, Zardi DM, et al. Cirrhotic cardiomyopathy. J Am Coll Cardiol. 2010;56:539-49.

8.3 Restrictive and Obliterative Cardiomyopathies

❏ INTRODUCTION

Restrictive and obliterative cardiomyopathies are characterized by impaired ventricular filling with normal ventricular wall thickness and systolic function. They are the best examples of the syndrome of 'heart failure with normal ejection fraction' (HFNEF) and can be recognized by near normal ventricular size and ejection fraction with abnormal diastolic function and dilated atrial chambers. Unlike dilated and hypertrophic cardiomyopathies, where the definition is morphological, the definition of restrictive cardiomyopathy is based on the hemodynamic abnormality.

❏ RESTRICTIVE CARDIOMYOPATHIES

Restrictive cardiomyopathies are classified as 'primary' when the heart alone is affected and 'secondary' when it forms part of a systemic disorder or due to a known cause or association. Table 9 shows the recent modification of classification of cardiomyopathies, as applicable to restrictive heart diseases.

Restrictive cardiomyopathies form 5% of the pediatric cardiomyopathies, and there is an increase in its prevalence as the age advances. Children and adults usually present with episodes of breathlessness due to pulmonary venous congestion, which gets mistaken as reactive airway disease. This soon progresses to pulmonary arterial hypertension and congestive cardiac failure. The late stage of the disease is dominated by the development of ventricular systolic dysfunction, complex ventricular arrhythmias and heart blocks leading to sudden cardiac death, which occasionally could be the first manifestation.

Physical examination reveals features of pulmonary hypertension and congestive cardiac failure with mild cardiomegaly or near normal heart size. Third heart sound in gallop rhythm is the most common physical finding followed by accentuated pulmonary component of the second heart sound. Systolic murmurs of atrioventricular valve regurgitation are a common finding. Chest X-ray shows signs of pulmonary venous and arterial hypertension with atrial dilatation. Myocardial calcification is characteristic of EMF. Electrocardiogram may show biatrial enlargement and nonspecific ST-T changes. Two dimensional echocardiography and Doppler recordings help to document the normal ventricular dimensions, systolic function, absence of myocardial hypertrophy and atrial dilatation and features of systemic venous congestion.

Table 9: Restrictive cardiac disorders

- Primary/idiopathic restrictive cardiomyopathy
- Secondary restrictive disorders:
  - Infiltrative disorders: Amyloidosis
  - Endomyocardial: EMF and Loeffler's endocarditis (hypereosinophilic syndromes)
  - Inflammatory: Sarcoidosis, post-irradiation syndromes
  - Storage diseases: Hemochromatosis, Fabry's disease, glycogen storage diseases
  - Neuromuscular diseases
  - Connective tissue diseases and disorders (scleroderma, pseudoxanthoma elasticum)

Myocardial and Pericardial Diseases

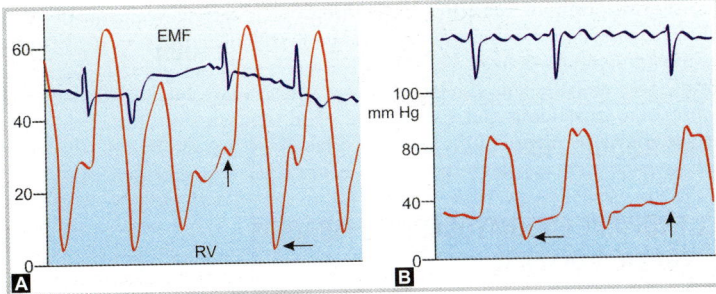

FIGURES 8A AND B: Typical hemodynamic patterns of right and left ventricular pressure tracings in EMF with dip and plateau pattern, elevated dip diastolic pressures (side arrows) and end-diastolic pressures (upward facing arrows). Right ventricular pressure tracing shows absence of post-ectopic potentiation, and the left ventricular pressure tracing shows no 'a' wave impression because of atrial fibrillation

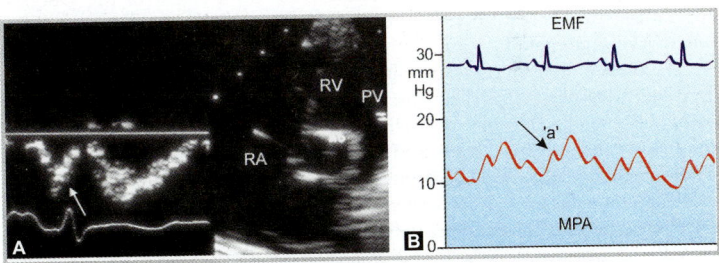

FIGURES 9A AND B: (A) Pulse Doppler across the pulmonary valve and (B) pulmonary artery pressure tracing showing presystolic forward flow because of atrial systole (arrow)

The typical hemodynamic signature of restrictive physiology is the square root sign seen in the ventricular pressure tracings (Figs 8A and B). The rapid short early diastolic filling is followed by the steep elevation of diastolic pressures. An inability to fill further is reflected as the square root sign of the pressure tracing in ventricular diastole. Atrial systole further elevates the end diastolic pressures, at times opening the pulmonary valve during late diastole (Figs 9A and B). Restrictive cardiomyopathies affecting the left side are characterized by elevated pulmonary artery pressures of more than 50 mm of systolic pressure.

The common differential diagnosis of restrictive cardiomyopathy is the pericardial disorder of constriction, where the ventricular function is restricted from outside and the hemodynamic outcome of restricted cardiac output dominates the clinical picture. In restrictive cardiomyopathy, diastolic filling pressures can show variation of more than 5 mm Hg. Mitral flow propagation velocity (color M-mode echocardiography) of more than 100 cm/sec and mitral annular early diastolic velocity of more than 10 cm/sec and normal S waves are characteristic of constrictive pericarditis. Electron beam computed tomography and various modalities of magnetic resonance imaging (MRI) are also useful to differentiate constrictive pericarditis from restrictive cardiomyopathy and to identify the cause for myocardial restriction. But, at times, the extensive involvement of visceral pericardium can result in restrictive features and rarely both disorders can coexist.

The treatment of restrictive cardiomyopathy is largely symptomatic with diuretics and aldosterone antagonists. The rhythm abnormalities are treated on their own merits with pacemakers, rate control measures and adequate anticoagulation. Intractable cardiac failure is an indication for cardiac transplantation. The systemic causes, like amyloidosis and eosinophilia, when adequately treated in the early stages can cause reversal of the restrictive physiology. Significant atrioventricular valve regurgitation requires valve replacement or repair with endocardectomy.

❑ TROPICAL ENDOMYOCARDIAL FIBROSIS (DAVIE'S DISEASE)

Endomyocardial fibrosis (EMF) is an obliterative cardiomyopathy characterized by fibrotic thickening and obliteration of either right ventricular endomyocardial fibrosis (RVEMF), left ventricular endomyocardial fibrosis (LVEMF) or both ventricles endomyocardial fibrosis (BVEMF) with a predilection to selectively involve the ventricular apices and inflow region and sparing the outflow tract. The fibrotic process does not involve the valve leaflets, the atria, or the great vessels, and extracardiac involvement is not known. The involvement of the subvalvar apparatus in the fibrotic process plasters and hinders the leaflet mobility leading to progressive regurgitation.

The disease often starts as an acute febrile illness in young children or middle aged individuals like acute rheumatic carditis. There is pancarditis with peripheral blood eosinophilia in some reported series. Patients develop pericarditis and/or thrombotic endocarditis complicated by cerebral embolism. The sudden and early development of cardiac failure in some, speaks in favor of acute myocarditis as the more predominant form. Mitral regurgitation, often mild, with gallops completes the clinical picture. The endomyocardial biopsy at this phase of the disease shows presence of mild myocarditis. The peripheral blood eosinophilia is associated with degranulated eosinophils and intracytoplasmic vacuolations. This may indicate a causal relationship with myocarditis. Immunosuppressive treatment with prednisolone was effective in lowering the eosinophil count but did not avoid the development of endocardial fibrotic disease.

Three phases of EMF could be identified from history and pathological features. The first phase involves eosinophilic infiltration of the myocardium with necrosis of the subendocardium and a pathologic picture consistent with acute myocarditis. This is reportedly present in the first 5 weeks of the illness. The second stage, typically observed after 10 months, is associated with thrombus formation over the initial lesions, with a decrement in the amount of inflammatory activity present. Ultimately, after several years of disease activity, the fibrotic phase is reached, when the endocardium is replaced by collagenous fibrosis. Fibrosis involves the inflow tract of both ventricles and the outflow tracts are spared. The involvement of the mitral and tricuspid subvalvar apparatus results in varying degrees of valve regurgitation. Calcification in areas of extensive fibrosis marks the late stage of the disease. Echocardiography and angiocardiography are useful in identifying the disorder in asymptomatic subjects.

❑ RIGHT VENTRICULAR ENDOMYOCARDIAL FIBROSIS

Right ventricular endomyocardial fibrosis (RVEMF), the most common form of the disease in many published reports, is readily diagnosed at the bedside in countries where it is commonly seen. Dominant or isolated RVEMF presents in an emaciated adolescent with cachexia, massive pericardial effusion and gross ascites.

The classical clinical triad of RVEMF, viz. distended jugular veins, hepatomegaly and ascites, is present in symptomatic subjects.

The two-dimensional echocardiographic findings are dominated by the aneurysmal right atrium. The RV apex will be filled by a dense fibrous mass, which encroaches on to the inflow tract involving the chordopapillary structures of the tricuspid valve. The RV cavity is shrunken with an apical notch to the right of interventricular groove due to the apical fibrosis, pulling the RV apex inward. The RV endocardial calcification is diagnostic. Fibrosis does not involve the outflow tract, which becomes dilated and hyperdynamic. The late stages of the disease will show a common right atrial and ventricular cavity with low pressure tricuspid regurgitation as in Ebstein's anomaly. An echocardiographic classification was proposed on the basis of involvement of ventricular cavity obliteration and plastering of AV valves.
- Grade 1: RV involvement confined to apex; apical dimpling or minimal apical obliteration
- Grade 2: Obliteration of RV apex up to mid cavity
- Grade 3: RV cavity obliteration, distortion and outflow dilatation.

Degree of cavity obliteration in RV chamber is graded as follows:
- Grade 1: Minimal RV involvement confined to trabecular alterations at apex and along septal border; normal contour of RV
- Grade 2: Obliteration of RV apex and adjacent body up to mid cavity, but sparing tricuspid annulus (saucer shaped RV)
- Grade 3: RV cavity obliteration, including area near annulus, and outflow dilatation
- Grade 4: RV body as well as RV outflow narrowed.

❏ LEFT VENTRICULAR ENDOMYOCARDIAL FIBROSIS

Isolated left ventricular endomyocardial fibrosis (LVEMF) often presents as mitral regurgitation or severe pulmonary hypertension. Moderate cardiomegaly, well felt apex beat, left para-sternal heave, loud pulmonary component of the second heart sound, loud LV third heart sound and varying degrees of mitral regurgitation are the salient clinical features. The onset of the atrial fibrillation heralds profound clinical deterioration. The left atrial P waves and the LV hypertrophy with strain are often seen in the electrocardiogram. Plain X-ray film closely resembles that of patients with rheumatic mitral valve disease. The LV calcification when present is diagnostic. Biventricular EMF can be recognized in an equal subset of patients with EMF but their signs and symptoms overlap and, at times, is dominated by the dominant chamber involvement.

An echocardiographic classification was proposed on the basis of involvement of ventricular cavity obliteration and plastering of AV valves.
- Grade 1: Involvement at apex or only papillary muscles
- Grade 2: Apex blunted, with disease extending to cavity
- Grade 3: Obliteration involving up to mid cavity, transverse diameter more than longitudinal, PML plastering

Angiographic Diagnosis of EMF

Angiography was the most reliable method of confirming EMF, especially the milder forms. The LVEMF can be recognized angiographically as smoothening of the LV cavity due to loss of fine trabeculae (earliest change), irregular outline, filling defects, cervices and out-pouching (Figs 10A and B). Crevices and out-

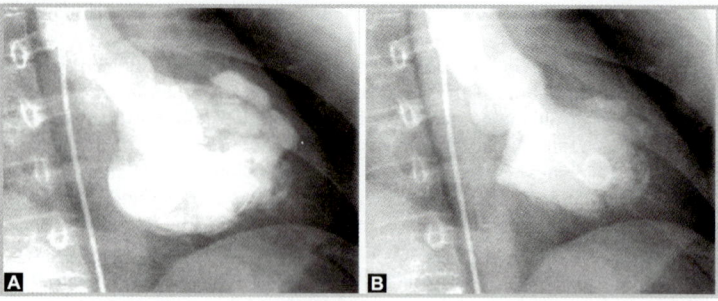

FIGURES 10A AND B: Left ventricle (LV) angiogram from a patient with LVEMF, diastolic frame on the left and systolic frame on the right. Note the obliteration of the left ventricular apex, transverse diameter more than the longitudinal diameter and absence of mitral regurgitation

pouching are filling defects within ventricular chamber extending beyond contrast filled cavity. Varying degree of mitral regurgitation is common. Left atrium is seldom markedly enlarged. Coronary angiography reveals normal vascular pattern, although asymptomatic burned out cases may present with acquired coronary artery disease.

Treatment

Management of cardiac failure is the mainstay in the treatment of EMF. Atrial fibrillation will require use of antiarrhythmic drugs and oral anticoagulants. The patients with RVEMF may require repeated abdominal paracentesis, and rarely pericardiocentesis. For surgical management, a plane of cleavage is easily developed and all of the yellow-white thickened endocardium removed. Other options are LV endocardectomy with mitral valve repair or replacement, exclusion of fibrotic right ventricle in RVEMF by a bidirectional Glenn connection. Surgical treatment has always been contemplated only for NYHA classes III and IV patients. A detailed 2D echo Doppler evaluation can identify the ideal surgical candidates of EMF with a fair amount of certainty.

❏ LOEFFLER'S ENDOCARDITIS

Loeffler, in 1936, described the syndrome of eosinophilia with multiorgan involvement, wherein the cardiac involvement was characterized by congestive heart failure and thromboembolism. The disease is now considered to represent the specific form of endomyocardial involvement in hypereosinophilic syndromes (HESs). It manifests as restrictive cardiomyopathy and resembles EMF in the burnt out phase. Both the disorders are considered to represent different spectrum of damage to the heart by activated eosinophils. Activated eosinophils generate a spectrum of myocardial damage ranging from acute coronary syndrome, intracardiac thrombus formation, thromboembolic phenomena and sudden cardiac death to congestive cardiac failure.

Clinical features are rather diverse from asymptomatic incidental detection to multiorgan dysfunction. The incidence of HES peaks in the fourth decade, and there is a male preponderance of 9:1. Half the patients with HES have cardiac involvement, which adversely affects the prognosis. The signs and symptoms of cardiac involvement could manifest as myocardial ischemia, pericarditis, arrhythmia, cardiac failure and thromboembolic phenomena. Mitral regurgitation is the most common valve lesion but aortic valve lesions are also reported.

One-third of the individuals with Loeffler's endocarditis have electrocardiographic abnormalities, and echocardiogram typically shows the fibrothrombotic obliteration of ventricular apices with atrial dilatation and atrioventricular valve regurgitation. Cardiac MRI is superior to identify layered thrombus and tissue characterization, and is superior to echocardiography for early detection of eosinophilic endocardial disease. Myocardial biopsy is diagnostic but needs to be deferred as thromboembolic complications are anticipated.

Constrictive pericarditis should be considered in the differential diagnosis for all restrictive cardiomyopathies, since the diagnosis gives an option of surgical correction. The treatment option in eosinophilic endomyocardial disease could be symptomatic or specific. The management of cardiac failure, anticoagulation to prevent thromboembolism, antiarrhythmics for the variety of arrhythmias and vasodilators for the atrioventricular valve regurgitation are suggested. Once hypereosinophilia is confirmed, specific treatment with corticosteroids, chemotherapeutic agents and monoclonal antibodies impart a favorable outcome, especially in the early stages. Organized fibrotic lesions can be treated with selective endocardectomy and mitral valve replacement. Cardiac transplant is an option, but the disease can recur in the transplanted heart.

❏ IDIOPATHIC RESTRICTIVE CARDIOMYOPATHY

Idiopathic restrictive cardiomyopathy is a rare disease primarily affecting the heart, and no other systemic disorders are apparent at the time of diagnosis. The majority of the patients are above the age of 40 years with a slight female preponderance. Dyspnea is the most common presenting feature, followed by edema. Ventricular third heart sound, systolic murmurs, jugular venous distension, pulmonary rales, ascites and edema are the common clinical features.

The term idiopathic restrictive cardiomyopathy was coined when no clinically identifiable cause could be ascertained in an individual with primary myocardial disease with restrictive physiology. Linkage associations studied in large multigenerational pedigrees by various laboratories specializing in various loci, and sharing of the DNA data in the last two decades, have revealed more of the genomics of these rare disorders.

The electrocardiographic features are nonspecific with three-fourth patients have atrial fibrillation or nonspecific STT changes. Cardiomegaly is common in chest skiagram and 20% of the subjects presenting with restrictive cardiomyopathy have normal cardiothoracic ratio. The echocardiogram is diagnostic in the majority with atrial dilatation, and ventricles with normal dimensions and wall thickness.

❏ SUGGESTED READINGS

Bozcali E, Aliyev F, Agac MT, et al. Unusual case of aortic valve involvement in patient with Löffler's endomyocarditis: management, follow-up and short review of the literature. J Thromb Thrombolysis. 2007;24:309-13.

Bukhman G, Ziegler J, Parry E. Endomyocardial fibrosis: still a mystery after 60 years. PLoS Negl Trop Dis. 2008;2:e97.

Callis TE, Jensen BC, Weck KE, et al. Evolving molecular diagnostics for familial cardiomyopathies: at the heart of it all. Expert Rev Mol Diagn. 2010;10:329-51.

Kleinfeldt T, Nienaber CA, Kische S, et al. Cardiac manifestation of the hypereosinophilic syndrome: new insights. Clin Res Cardiol. 2010;99:419-27.

Kushwaha SS, Fallon JT, Fuster V. Restrictive cardiomyopathy. N Engl J Med. 1997;336:267-76.

Maurer MS, King DL, El-Khoury Rumbarger L, et al. Left heart failure with a normal ejection fraction: identification of different pathophysiologic mechanisms. J Card Fail. 2005;11:177-87.

Mogensen J, Arbustini E. Restrictive cardiomyopathy. Curr Opin Cardiol. 2009;24:214-20.

Mousseaux E, Hernigou A, Azencot M, et al. Endomyocardial fibrosis: electron-beam CT features. Radiology. 1996;198:755-60.

Sivasankaran S. Restrictive cardiomyopathy in India: the story of a vanishing mystery. Heart. 2009;95:9-14.

Tharakan J, Bohora S. Current perspective on endomyocardial fibrosis. www.ias.ac.in/currsci/aug102009/405.pdf. Available from www.ias.ac.in/currsci/aug102009/405.pdf.

Vijayaraghavan G, Davies J, Sadanandan S, et al. Echocardiographic features of tropical endomyocardial disease in South India. Br Heart J. 1983;50:450-9.

Vijayaraghavan G. Angiographic features of endomyocardial fibrosis in 'endomyocardial fibrosis in India'. In: Sapru RP (Ed). Indian Council of Medical Research, New Delhi, India. 1983. pp. 104-6. Available from http://www.gvr.co.in/publications.

8.4 Specific Cardiomyopathies

AMYLOID HEART DISEASE

❏ INTRODUCTION

The amyloidoses are a large group of hereditary or acquired diseases characterized by the deposition of extracellular proteinaceous material known as amyloid. Amyloid is a homogenous material composed of specific highly insoluble fibrillar proteins that accumulate primarily in the extracellular spaces in certain tissues and organs, leading to architectural disruption and organ dysfunction. Although the histochemical properties and morphology of all amyloid deposits are similar, the underlying amyloid precursor proteins (APP) are highly variable. To date, 27 human and 9 animal amyloidogenic proteins have been identified. Amyloid is an amorphous, homogenous extracellular substance, which stains pink with hematoxylin and eosin and exhibits characteristic apple-green birefringence when viewed under polarized light after Congo red staining. Likewise, when viewed with electron microscopy, all types of amyloid demonstrate rigid, nonbranching fibrils with a consistent diameter of 7.5–10 nm. The propensity for cardiac involvement depends on the specific APP type. Cardiac amyloidosis has a wide spectrum of clinical manifestations but the most frequent presentation is heart failure related to restrictive cardiomyopathy (CMP) due to the deposition of amyloid fibrils within the myocardial interstitium.

❏ OVERVIEW OF CARDIAC AMYLOIDOSIS

Amyloid CMP is a progressive infiltrative disease, typically with distinct features seen on the macroscopic anatomy, histology, echocardiography and cardiac magnetic resonance (CMR) imaging. The heart infiltrated with amyloid appears tan and waxy with a firm, rubbery consistency and increased thickness of all four-chamber walls. In addition, the valves are typically thickened with a shiny, waxy appearance (Fig. 11). The extracellular deposition of amyloid within the myocardium leads to increased ventricular wall stiffness and diastolic dysfunction

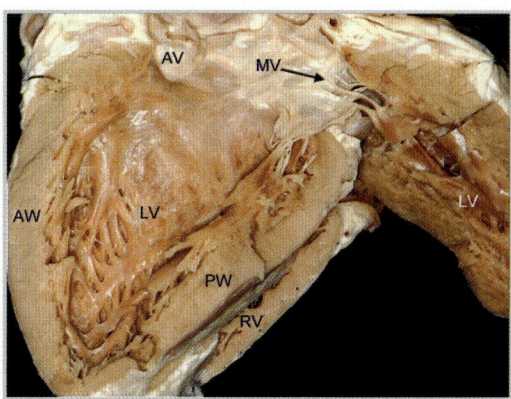

FIGURE 11: Macroscopic view of heart with amyloidosis obtained from a patient who underwent heart transplantation for advanced amyloid cardiomyopathy. Right and left ventricular walls are thick, and the formalin-fixed myocardium is pale and unusually glistening. (Abbreviations: LV: Left ventricle; RV: Right ventricular wall; AW: Anterior wall of the left ventricle; PW: Posterior wall of the left ventricle; MV: Mitral valve; AV: Aortic valve)

of increasing severity as the disease progresses. In its advanced state, amyloidosis classically leads to restrictive physiology. Indeed, according to the two main international classifications of myocardial diseases, amyloid CMP is a restrictive CMP that is characterized by steep rises in ventricular pressure in association with small increases in volume. At a later stage, amyloid CMP may present as a dilated CMP with predominant systolic dysfunction. Very rarely, amyloid deposits have been reported to cause epicardial coronary artery obstruction that is indistinguishable from cholesterol-laden plaques. Amyloid can also infiltrate the pulmonary vasculature, causing pulmonary hypertension, and patients can present with symptoms and signs of cor pulmonale. Pericardial and pleural effusions may be present when heart failure is present, but they may also be due to amyloid deposits in pericardium or pleura, respectively. The most common mode of death in patients with amyloid CMP is cardiac arrest related to electromechanical disassociation (pulseless electrical activity).

❏ CLASSIFICATION OF AMYLOIDOSIS

In the past, the amyloidoses were classified mainly according to the clinical phenotype when the amyloid disease processes were poorly understood. However, the current system classifies amyloid based upon the chemical structure of the major fibrillar APP, which makes for a more logical nomenclature as the understanding of the chemical diversity of amyloid fibril proteins has increased. In the current system of nomenclature, the amyloid fibril type is designated as the capital letter A followed by a suffix that is an abbreviated form of the precursor protein name.

❏ CARDIAC AMYLOIDOSIS

Among the 27 known amyloid fibril proteins in humans, only four proteins have been associated with 5 different cardiac amyloid phenotypes. In decreasing order of frequency, the APP leading to cardiac amyloidosis are: (i) AL amyloid (phenotypically referred to as primary amyloidosis) originates from clonal populations of immunoglobulin light chains, and it is the most common type in developed countries; (ii) ATTR amyloid, phenotypically responsible for both SSA (due to amyloidogenic wild-type transthyretin protein deposition) and familial/hereditary amyloidosis (originates from transthyretin gene mutations); (iii) AA amyloid, also described as secondary amyloidosis, is due to serum amyloid A (SAA) protein deposition in the setting of chronic infections or untreated inflammatory conditions, and (iv) isolated atrial natriuretic factor (AANF) amyloid, which causes isolated atrial amyloidosis (IAA), a common autopsy finding in elderly patients with unclear clinical significance, but it may be associated with atrial fibrillation. The major APP in this case is atrial natriuretic peptide.

History and Physical Examination

Patients often present with dyspnea and symptoms predominantly of right sided heart failure, such as ankle edema and increased abdominal girth. Although the reasons are poorly understood, ascites is often more marked than peripheral edema much like it is with other causes of restrictive CMP and constrictive pericarditis. Occasionally, patients may present with palpitations due to atrial or ventricular arrhythmias. Orthostatic hypotension may occur from volume depletion related to diuretics or due to autonomic neuropathy from amyloid infiltration. Amyloid may also infiltrate multiple different tissues leading to diverse manifestations of the disease such as skin and soft tissue thickening, vocal cord infiltration and hoarseness, adrenal gland or thyroid infiltration with resultant hypoadrenalism or hypothyroidism, lymphadenopathy, pulmonary infiltrates, factor X inhibition with bleeding diathesis and mesenteric infiltration with diarrhea.

Although very specific for the diagnosis, macroglossia and periorbital purpura are seen in less than 20% of patients with AL, and may be easily overlooked. More frequent are recurrent petechial lesions of the eyelids, which may occur after coughing or rubbing the eye area, and result from vascular fragility. The cardiac exam reveals evidence of restrictive filling of the right ventricle with elevated jugular venous pressure, which may paradoxically increase with inspiration (Kussmaul's sign), hepatomegaly and ascites, and peripheral edema. There may also be signs of low cardiac output with cool extremities and delayed nailbed capillary refill. Auscultation often reveals a third heart sound (S3); however, a fourth heart sound (S4) is often absent because amyloid infiltration of the atria markedly impairs atrial contraction. Systolic regurgitant murmurs may be present due to mitral or tricuspid valve insufficiency; however, they are not usually severe. The blood pressure is often normal or reduced with a narrow pulse pressure consistent with low cardiac output state.

Diagnostic Tests

Tissue Diagnosis

The diagnosis of amyloidosis requires tissue confirmation of its presence and identification of the responsible APP. In cases of suspected cardiac amyloidosis based upon the clinical history, examination and/or echocardiographic findings, a tissue biopsy should be obtained, preferably from an easily accessible site. Although the sensitivity of detecting amyloidosis within the heart via endomyocardial biopsy is virtually 100% due to widespread deposition within the myocardium, it is associated with a risk for myocardial perforation and life threatening cardiac tamponade. Less invasive tissue sampling methods are available for diagnosing systemic amyloid disease. Although rectal submucosa was previously the traditional biopsy site, it can be complicated by bleeding or perforation. Abdominal fat aspiration can be easily performed without serious complications and has sensitivity for detecting systemic amyloidosis in 57–88% of cases. Other potential biopsy sites include the gingiva, bone marrow, liver or kidney when clinical suspicion for the respective organ involvement exists.

Radiological Findings

The chest X-ray is often unremarkable, but there may be cardiomegaly, which is usually due to biatrial dilatation. Pulmonary edema and pleural effusions may be present, particularly when heart failure is present.

Electrocardiography

Patients with cardiac amyloidosis frequently have EKG abnormalities (Fig. 5). The presence of low voltage QRS complexes in the limb and/or precordial leads, particularly in the presence of increased left ventricular mass on echocardiography, is highly suggestive amyloid CMP. Atrial dilatation from restrictive CMP or amyloid infiltration may predispose to atrial fibrillation. Bundle branch block or extreme right or left axis deviation in the absence of hypertrophy may also be present. Atrioventricular conduction defects are not uncommon, particularly in familial amyloidosis with polyneuropathy where it is associated with worse prognosis. Prolonged HV interval appears to be frequent in AL amyloidosis and may be missed on the surface EKG with a narrow QRS complex. It appears to be an independent predictor of sudden death.

Echocardiography

Two-dimensional and Doppler echocardiography is extremely helpful in the diagnosis of amyloid CMP. Typical findings include increased right and left ventricular wall thickness with normal or small ventricular chamber size, thickened interatrial septum and biatrial enlargement. Amyloid infiltration characteristically produces a speckled or granular appearance to the myocardium on echocardiography. Although this is a nonspecific finding that can also be seen in patients with ventricular hypertrophy from hypertrophic CMP, hypertensive heart disease or other infiltrative diseases, such as Fabry's disease, this finding should prompt the consideration of amyloidosis in the differential diagnosis. Diffuse valvular leaflet thickening without significant valve dysfunction is also characteristic of the disease. Left ventricular systolic function as determined by the ejection fraction is normal in the early course of the disease. However, as amyloid infiltration within the myocardium progresses, ventricular systolic dysfunction deteriorates, and the ventricle may even dilate in the later stages of disease. Doppler echocardiography is used to evaluate ventricular diastolic function. Varying degrees of left ventricular diastolic dysfunction are often present, depending on the disease stage. A restrictive pattern consistent with advanced left ventricular diastolic dysfunction with an increased E wave velocity, short deceleration time, and low A wave velocity is characteristic of advanced amyloid CMP; however, early in the course of the disease, mild (grade I) left ventricular diastolic dysfunction may be present. A Doppler index combining systolic and diastolic myocardial performance has been shown to be predictive of survival in patients with cardiac amyloidosis.

Laboratory Findings

In patients suspected of having cardiac amyloidosis, the initial investigation should include serum and urine analysis for the presence of a monoclonal immunoglobulin light chains, in addition to standard blood tests, such as blood count, urea, electrolytes, liver function tests, clotting screen, glucose and thyroid function tests. Once the diagnosis of AL amyloid is suspected based on serologic testing and/or clinical presentation, a bone marrow biopsy is necessary to confirm the diagnosis of a plasma cell dyscrasia, exclude coexistent multiple myeloma and evaluate for bone marrow amyloid infiltration. In the past several years, serum cardiac biomarkers have been introduced as adjunctive markers for the presence and severity of cardiac amyloidosis, especially in AL amyloidosis. Elevated levels of cardiac troponin T (cTnT) or cardiac troponin I (cTnI) and/or serum brain-type natriuretic peptide (BNP) or N-terminal pro-brain natriuretic peptide (NT pro-BNP) levels can diagnose the presence of cardiac involvement in AL amyloidosis with greater sensitivity than all other noninvasive diagnostic modalities.

Cardiac Magnetic Resonance Imaging

Cardiac magnetic resonance imaging has been shown to detect cardiac amyloidosis with a high sensitivity. CMR imaging of amyloid CMP shows a characteristic pattern of subendocardial delayed hyper-enhancement (DHE) and rapid clearance of gadolinium from the blood pool leaving it colored black. In addition, other findings supportive of the diagnosis of amyloidosis include diffuse thickening of all cardiac walls and late gadolinium enhancement the walls of the atria. CMR is probably most useful as a noninvasive test to detect amyloidosis when noncardiac tissue stains have been negative for amyloid, but the diagnosis of cardiac amyloid is suspected. CMR may also have prognostic value in patients with AL-CMP.

Cardiac Catheterization Hemodynamics

It is used to perform an endomyocardial biopsy and confirm the diagnosis amyloidosis, assess the hemodynamics for signs of restrictive physiology and evaluate coronary artery anatomy when clinically indicated. In advanced amyloid CMP, right heart catheterization typically reveals restrictive physiology, which is characterized by elevated biventricular filling pressures and a prominent early diastolic dip followed by mid-to-late diastolic plateau. Depending on the extent and severity of amyloid infiltration and restrictive CMP, the cardiac output may be low and varying degrees of passive or mixed precapillary and postcapillary pulmonary hypertension may be present.

Serum Amyloid P Component Scintigraphy

Serum amyloid P (SAP) is a cofactor which presents all of the amyloidoses. SAP scintigraphy imaging with ^{123}I-labeled human SAP is useful for locating and monitoring the extent of systemic amyloidosis, because the P component is present in all types of amyloid. It allows the quantification of amyloid burden in systemic amyloidosis; however, it is not useful for the identification of amyloid in the heart because uptake by the heart may be obscured by the high blood flow and the slow passage of the tracer across myocardial capillary endothelia.

❏ TREATMENT

Heart Failure Medical Management

The medical management of heart failure in patients with amyloid CMP is very challenging, and none of the traditional therapies for heart failure has been shown to improve symptoms or survival with this disease. The mainstay of the medical treatment is the careful titration of diuretics and fluid volume restriction to relieve symptoms of volume overload. Due to the steep pressure–volume relationship that is present in patients with restrictive CMP, it is often challenging to find an optimal fluid balance. Anticoagulation should be considered and appears to be protective in cases of atrial fibrillation or if there is evidence of severe atrial dilatation and mechanical atrial failure. Large, recurrent pleural effusions may require thoracentesis and even pleurodesis if they are diuretic refractory.

Device Therapies

Patients with amyloid CMP often have sinoatrial node dysfunction and/or atrioventricular block that occasionally require permanent pacemaker insertion. Internal cardioverter defibrillator (ICD) placement in AL amyloidosis should be limited to patients with documented malignant arrhythmias with the understanding that it still may not prevent sudden cardiac death.

Treatment of the Underlying Amyloid Disease

No therapy is uniformly effective in the management of AL amyloidosis. Currently, the best outcomes of treatment for AL amyloidosis appear to be achieved with the combination of high dose melphalan (HDM) and stem cell transplantation (SCT) (HDM/SCT), with eligible patients who survive the post-transplant period experiencing a median survival of 57 months (4.75 years), which includes nearly 50% of patients with cardiac involvement. In patients considered to be too high risk for HDM/SCT, melphalan and dexamethasone combination is still considered to be the standard intervention because of its low toxicity profile, its demonstrated ability to produce hematologic responses even in the presence of advanced disease, and the orally available formulations of both agents. For cases of hereditary or familial amyloidosis caused by variant transthyretin (ATTR), fibrinogen (AFib) and apolipoprotein (AApo-AI and AApo-AII), liver transplantation may be an effective treatment because APP is produced in the liver. However, much like with SCT, the presence of cardiac amyloidosis generally excludes patients from being eligible for liver transplantation. The mainstay of treatment for AA amyloidosis is directed at treatment of the underlying inflammatory or infective etiology. An algorithm for the diagnosis and management of suspected cases of cardiac amyloidosis is provided in Flowchart 2.

Heart Transplantation

Patients with AL amyloidosis who present with severe heart failure due to cardiac amyloidosis have an extremely poor prognosis with a median survival of only 4–6 months. Criteria for transplant eligibility is center dependent; however, the acronym DANGER has been used to predict adverse outcomes in patients undergoing evaluation for cardiac transplantation and it can be used to identify patients who are unlikely to be eligible for cardiac transplantation. DANGER stands for diarrhea, involvement of the autonomic nervous system, poor nutritional status, gastrointestinal tract (history of bleeding), elimination problems (i.e. renal

FLOWCHART 2: Diagnostic and management algorithm for suspected cardiac amyloidosis. In suspected cases of cardiac amyloidosis, based on history, physical examination, echocardiographic findings, electrocardiogram and cardiac magnetic resonance imaging, the diagnostic workup should be based on the confirmation of the presence of amyloidosis in tissue and identification of the underlying amyloid precursor protein using immunohistochemical staining. Based upon the specific amyloid fibril type, adjunctive tests to evaluate the status of the underlying disease and other organs involved as discussed earlier in the chapter. Treatment involves management of heart failure with diuretics and anticoagulation in some cases, and also importantly, treatment directed to reducing the production of the amyloid fibril protein as previously discussed

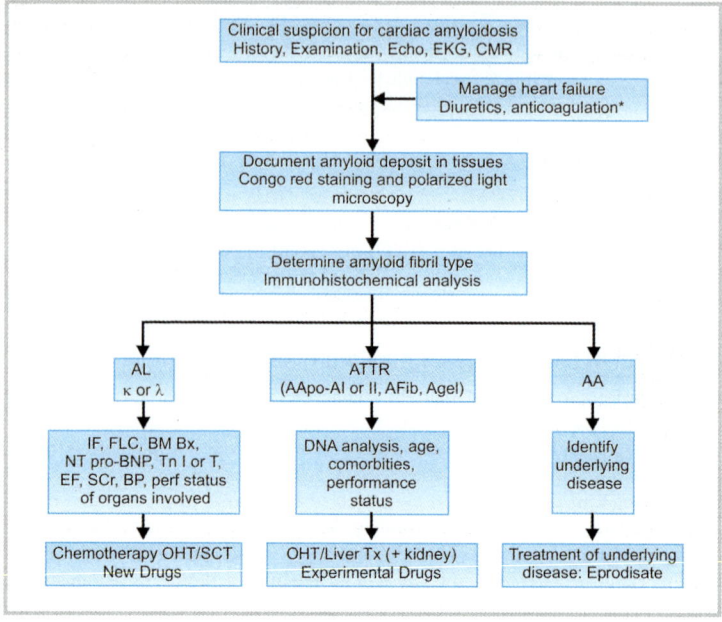

*Recommended in patients at high risk for thromboembolic events, such as history of thromboembolic events, atrial fibrillation, or severe left atrial failure as evidenced by echo-Doppler evaluation
(Abbreviations: BM Bx: Bone marrow biopsy; BP: Blood pressure; CMR: Cardiac magnetic resonance imaging; Echo: Echocardiography; EF: Left ventricular ejection fraction; EKG: Electrocardiogram; FLC: Free light chain assay; IF: Immunofluorescence; OHT: Orthotopic heart transplantation; perf status: Performance status; SCr: Serum creatinine; SCT: Stem cell transplantation; Tn I or T: Troponin I or T levels; Tx: Transplant; AL: Light chain amyloidosis; ATTR: Senile systemic amyloidosis)

impairment or nephritic syndrome) and respiratory dysfunction. Less than 5% of patients with advanced heart failure related to AL amyloidosis have disease isolated to the heart. Therefore, the vast majority of AL amyloid patients are not eligible for OHT, and among eligible patients, 30–50% die on the waitlist from progressive disease. However, for selected patients with advanced amyloid CMP, sequential OHT/SCT can profoundly alter the otherwise grim prognosis. In contrast to cardiac transplantation for AL amyloidosis, patients with amyloid CMP from hereditary ATTR have similar survival rates compared with nonamyloid heart transplant recipients.

PERIPARTUM CARDIOMYOPATHY

❏ INTRODUCTION

The definition of peripartum cadiomyopathy (PPCM) has been recently updated by a working group on PPCM of the European Society of Cardiology to "idiopathic cardiomyopathy presenting with heart failure (HF) secondary to left ventricle (LV) systolic dysfunction toward the end of pregnancy or in the months following delivery where no other cause of HF is found. The LV may not be dilated but the ejection fraction (EF) is nearly always reduced below 45%". The cause of PPCM is still unknown and many potential theories have been proposed and discussed in details in a recent review. Most recent hypothesis is based on experimental work suggesting that unprotected increase in oxidative stress leads to increased expression and proteolytic activity of cardiac cathepsin D, which results in conversion of the nursing hormone prolactin into an antiangiogenic and proapoptotic 16 kDa form with a detrimental effect on coronary microvasculature resulting in a myocardial insult due to hypoxemia and apoptosis.

The incidence of PPCM has been found to be higher in women older than 30 years, in patients with history of hypertension and preeclampsia, multifetal pregnancies and in the United States, in African-American women. In addition, recent studies have demonstrated a high incidence of PPCM in families with dilated cardiomyopahies suggesting that a proportion of patients with PPCM may be due to genetic cause. Many of the signs and symptoms of PPCM are similar to those of HF due to other etiologies.

❏ DIAGNOSIS

B-type natriuretic peptide (BNP) levels remain grossly unchanged during normal pregnancy and are only mildly elevated in women with preeclampsia. Similar to other form of HF, BNP levels rise significantly in symptomatic patients with PPCM. Troponin can be slightly elevated especially in patients with a substantial myocardial insult at the time of diagnosis.

Electrocardiogram usually shows sinus tachycardia, nonspecific ST segment and T wave changes. LV hypertrophy and conduction abnormalities can also be seen. Chest X-ray commonly demonstrates cardiomegaly, pulmonary venous congestion and occasionally pulmonary edema and pleural effusion. Echocardiogram shows a dilated LV size in the majority of the patients but can also be within normal range, dilation of the other cardiac chambers is also commonly found. LV systolic dysfunction is the rule with moderate to severe depression of LVEF and a small pericardial effusion. Doppler evaluation usually shows moderate to severe mitral and tricuspid valve regurgitation, mild to moderate pulmonic regurgitation and pulmonary hypertension.

❏ PROGNOSIS

PCM can be associated with severe complications, including pulmonary edema, cardiogenic shock, arrhythmias, thromboembolic event and mortality. It continues to be an important cause of pregnancy related death in the United States and other countries. Risk of death increases with older age, severe myocardial insult (LVEF <25%), multiparity, African-American ethnicity and when diagnosis is delayed.

Most recent publications have demonstrated improvement of LV function in at least 50% of patients with PPCM, mostly occurring within 6 months after diagnosis and race, ethnicity and environmental differences as well as access to medical care may be responsible for poorer outcome. Rate of unfavorable maternal and fetal outcome was even higher especially in women with persistent LV dysfunction.

❏ TREATMENT

Standard drug therapy for acute and chronic HF includes the potential use of several drugs, including diuretics, angiotensin converting enzyme (ACE) inhibitors or angiotensin receptor blockers (ARB) as well as beta blockers, spironolactone, digoxin, intravenous (IV) and oral vasodilators, and IV inotropes. In general, the treatment of HF in patients with PPCM should follow recent guidelines recommendations, although drug therapy may need to be changed during pregnancy and lactation to prevent side effects to the fetus or the lactating infant.

Since improvement of LV function is common and failure to improve cannot be predicted early after diagnosis, the use of a wearable external defibrillator or an entirely subcutaneous implantable cardioverter-defibrillator rather than implantable cardioverter defibrillators (ICD) should be considered in high risk patients, as a bridge to recovery or to ICD in cases with persistent LV dysfunction in spite of appropriate trial of medical therapy.

Intra-aortic balloon pump, extracorporeal membrane oxygenation and LV assist devices have been used successfully as bridge for recovery or transplantation in patients with PPCM and should be considered in a rapidly deteriorating patient not responding to medical therapy, including vasoactive medications.

This procedure has been performed successfully in patients with PPCM with slightly higher risk of rejections, lower risk of infections and similar rate of vascular cardiac allograft vasculopathy and mortality compared to comparable women undergoing transplantation for reasons other than PPCM.

A successful effect of IV immune globulin was reported in a small number of women with PPCM compared with 11 historical control patients who received conventional therapy alone. The treatment was associated with a significantly larger rate of LV recovery and decreased rate of mortality and symptomatic HF at 6 months compared with a control group of 10 PPCM patients treated with standard therapy alone.

❏ LABOR AND DELIVERY

In a patient who is diagnosed during pregnancy continuation of pregnancy in order to allow fetal maturity may be possible under close monitoring in a woman who can be stabilized with therapy. Termination of pregnancy often results in the improvement of both symptoms and cardiac function and should be considered in a patient with deteriorating symptoms or cardiac function. Mode of delivery in a stable patient with PPCM should be decided jointly by the obstetrician and the cardiologist. In general, vaginal delivery is preferred in the stable patient and cesarean section should be performed for obstetrical reasons or due to maternal instability. In case of vaginal delivery, instrumental delivery is recommended to reduce maternal efforts and shorten labor. Hemodynamic monitoring for labor and delivery is advisable in a patient who is diagnosed during pregnancy for hemodynamic optimization prior to delivery and monitoring during and after the delivery.

CHEMOTHERAPY-INDUCED CARDIOMYOPATHY

❏ INTRODUCTION

Chemotherapy-induced cardiotoxicity remains a major limitation for the use of chemotherapeutic agents. Chemotherapy-induced cardiotoxicities commonly classified into two types: (1) Acute or subacute which occurs anytime up to 2 weeks from the initiation to the termination of the chemotherapy and (2) chronic which manifests after months or years after termination of chemotherapy. The chronic type is further classified into two subtypes: (i) early, which is evident within 1 year and (ii) late, after 1 year of termination of therapy. It should be appreciated that the timing of the onset of the complications of chemotherapy-induced cardiotoxicity and classification based on this timing is arbitrary. The manifestations of acute or subacute cardiotoxicity are usually hypertension, electrocardiographic changes such as prolongation of the QT interval and other repolarization abnormalities, supraventricular and ventricular arrhythmias, chest pain syndromes, myopericarditis and rarely acute heart failure. Most of these cardiotoxicities are reversible. The manifestations of chronic cardiotoxicity are related to the type of chemotherapeutic agents used. The risk factors for anthracycline cardiotoxicity are summarized in Table 10.

❏ PATHOPHYSIOLOGY OF ANTHRACYCLINE-INDUCED CARDIOMYOPATHY

The cardiac morphologic and functional derangements of doxorubicin cardiomyopathy are characterized by reduced contractile and pump functions. The morphologic and functional changes in doxorubicin cardiomyopathy are summarized in Table 11. It is relevant to subclassify the chronic cardiotoxicity on histological basis into type I (e.g. doxorubicin) and type II (e.g. trastuzumab). Type I agents cause cell death and biopsy changes while type II agents cause

Table 10: The risk factors for anthracycline cardiotoxicity

- High total dose
- High peak serum level
- Combination therapy with other cardiotoxic antitumor drugs
- Mediastinal radiation therapy
- Age—very young and very old
- History of cardiac diseases—hypertension, reduced LVEF
- Liver diseases
- Whole-body hyperthermia

Table 11: Chronic doxorubicin cardiotoxicity: cardiac manifestations

- Dilatation of all cardiac chambers
- Mural thrombi
- Diastolic dysfunction
- Systolic dysfunction
- Increased wall stress
- Overt systolic heart failure

Table 12: Doxorubicin cardiomyopathy: Light microscopy findings

Cardiac morphologic changes: Light microscopy
- Multifocal patchy interstitial fibrosis
- Scattered vacuolated cardiomyocytes (Adria cells)
- Frank necrotic cardiomyocytes are rare
- Fibroblast proliferation and histiocyte infiltration

Table 13: Doxorubicin cardiomyopathy: Electron microscopic findings

Cardiac morphologic changes
Cardiomyocytes:
- Partial or total loss of myofibrils
- Vacuolar degeneration
- Distention of SR and T tubules
- Formation of membrane-bound spaces
- Nuclei-chromatin disorganization
- Replacement of chromatin by pale filaments

(Adapted from Takemura G, Fujiwara H, Progr Cardiovasc Dis. 2007;49: 330)

Table 14: Doxorubicin cardiomyopathy: Proposed mechanisms for cardiotoxicity

- Increased levels of ROS and lipid peroxidation
- Decreased levels of antioxidants and sulfhydryl groups
- Inhibition of nucleic acid and protein synthesis
- Release of vasoactive amines
- Altered adrenergic function
- Decreased expression of cardiac-specific genes

cellular dysfunction with no ultrastructural abnormalities. The histopathologic changes are summarized in Tables 12 and 13.

❏ MECHANISM OF CHEMOTHERAPY-INDUCED CARDIAC DYSFUNCTION

Anthracyclines

The proposed principal mechanisms of doxorubicin cardiotoxicity are summarized in Table 14. Increased oxidative stress, as evident from increased levels of ROS and lipid peroxidation is the principal mechanism.

Alkylating Agents

Cyclophosphamide

The pathogenesis of cyclophosphamide-induced cardiotoxicity is poorly understood. The proposed hypothesis is that it causes direct endothelial injury followed by extravasation of plasma proteins, erythrocytes and toxic metabolites which damage the cardiomyocytes. Hemorrhagic myocarditis with fibrin-platelet capillary microemboli and fibrin strands are detected in myocardium. Intracapillary microemboli may cause ischemic myocardial necrosis. The interstitial edema and hemorrhage lead to wall thickening which is associated with decreased left ventricular compliance and restrictive cardiomyopathy.

Ifosfamide

Ifosfamide is a nephrotoxic agent and reduces glomerular filtration rate. It may also produce renal tubular acidosis. Reduced renal function may lead to delayed elimination of its cardiotoxic metabolites.

Antimetabolites

The risks of cardiotoxicity in humans have not been adequately studied. The antimetabolite clofarabine can produce left ventricular dysfunction, which is usually reversible. The animal studies have suggested that it can interfere with mitochondrial function and energy production.

Monoclonal Antibody-based Tyrosine Kinase Inhibitors

The mechanism of heart failure with bevacizumab may be due to uncontrolled hypertension resulting left ventricular hypertrophy. It has also been suggested that there might be a reduction in myocardial capillary density, inducing myocardial ischemia, cardiac fibrosis and contractile dysfunction and heart failure. Also the vascular endothelial growth factor signaling is inhibited which may decrease angiogenesis. The cardiomyocyte HER2 intracellular pathway can also modulate response to oxidative stress. The anthracycline induced myocardial damage leads to transient upregulation in the HER2 in the myocardial cells as a compensatory mechanism. Thus, the incidence of cardiac dysfunction is increased when trastuzumab is used concurrently with anthracyclines.

Small Molecule Tyrosine Kinase Inhibitors

In animal models, imatinib treatment causes impairment of left ventricular contractile function and cellular abnormalities compatible with toxic cardiomyopathy. In addition to inhibition of tyrosine kinases, other mechanisms might be involved in inducing its cardiotoxicity.

❏ DIAGNOSIS

The diagnosis of chemotherapy-induced cardiotoxicity should consist of taking appropriate history to assess the likelihood of the diagnosis. A clinical evaluation of the cardiovascular system should be performed to determine presence of signs of overt heart failure, such as elevated jugular venous pressure and S3 gallop. An electrocardiogram should be obtained which usually demonstrates nonspecific ST-T wave changes and occasionally low voltage QRS complexes. A plain chest X-ray to assess the presence of cardiomegaly and signs of pulmonary venous congestion should be included during clinical evaluation.

Transthoracic echocardiography with Doppler studies is commonly used to detect diastolic and systolic left ventricular dysfunction. Doppler tissue imaging (DTI) has been employed for early detection of doxorubicin cardiomyopathy. The changes in DTI may precede changes in left ventricular ejection fraction. The Tei index, which simultaneously evaluates ventricular systolic and diastolic function, has been used to assess chemotherapy-induced cardiac dysfunction.

Radionuclide ventriculography is also used to assess left ventricular systolic function and may provide a more accurate determination of left ventricular ejection fraction. Increasingly cardiac magnetic resonance (CMR) is being used not only for assessing left ventricular function but also to determine the degree of fibrosis.

The irreversible myocardial damage is detected by late gadolinium enhancement in patients with chemotherapy-induced cardiotoxicity.

Metaiodobenzylguanidine (MIBG) nuclear imaging is employed for determination of cardiac adrenergic denervation. In doxorubicin cardiomyopathy, abnormal glucose and fatty acid metabolism can occur which can be assessed by positron emission tomography (PET) using fluorine-18-F-deoxyglucose.

Antimyosin antibody study with the use of 111-In-labeled monoclonal antimyosin antibody imaging has been employed for the diagnosis of doxorubicin cardiomyopathy. The B-type natriuretic peptide (BNP) and N-terminal pro-BNP plasma levels are elevated in patients with established cardiac dysfunction and the magnitude of increase in the plasma levels of these natriuretic peptides correlates with the severity of congestive heart failure. The abnormal levels of troponin T or I indicate myocardial injury and should be measured in patients with anthracycline cardiomyopathy. The endomyocardial biopsy, which can provide a definitive diagnosis of doxorubicin cardiomyopathy is occasionally employed in clinical practice.

❑ MONITORING

The American Heart Association and the American College of Physicians recommend close monitoring of cardiac function during and after chemotherapy (Table 15). The hemodynamic grading has been proposed before institution of chemotherapy with doxorubicin. Presence or absence and severity of both right and left ventricular failure are considered for grading (Table 16).

Table 15: Doxorubicin cardiomyopathy: Diagnostic and monitoring procedures

- Assessment of left ventricular function:
  - Radionuclide angiography
  - Echocardiography
- Assessment of adrenergic denervation:
  - MIBG
  - Precedes reduction in LVEF, nonspecific
- Assessment of myocardial energy metabolism:
  - F-FDG, I-BMIPP
  - Measurement of humoral factors
  - ANP, BNP, endothelins, troponins
- Detection of cardiomyocyte death:
  - In-labeled monoclonal antimyosin antibody
  - Tc-99m labeled Annexin V imaging
  - (sensitivity—high, specificity—low)

Table 16: Doxorubicin cardiomyopathy: Hemodynamic grading

Hemodynamic grading of patients before therapy:
- Grade 0: no RVF or LVF
- Grade 1: Mild RVF or LVF
- Grade 2: Moderate RVF or LVF
- Grade 3: Severe RVF or LVF

Worse the hemodynamic grade prior therapy, higher the incidence of cardiotoxicity and mortality

Table 17: Anthracycline cardiomyopathy: Prevention—proposed approaches

- Risk factors modification
- To limit the cumulative dose of DOX to less than 450 mg/m^2
- To use anthracycline analogues
- Alternative methods of drug delivery
- Continuous slow infusion

Table 18: Doxorubicin cardiomyopathy: Prevention—pharmacologic

Prevention
- Mercaptopropionyl glycine (MPG)
- Probucol
- Dexrazoxane
- Amlodipine
- Carvedilol
- Angiotensin-converting enzyme inhibitors
- PDE-5 inhibitor (sildenafil)
- Nitric oxide
- Superoxide dismutase
- Endothelin receptor antagonist (bosentan)
- Erythropoetin, thrombopoetin
- Granulocyte colony-stimulating factor

❏ PREVENTIVE STRATEGIES

As currently available treatment of established anthracycline induced cardiomyopathy does not appear to be very effective to improve prognosis, there is a major emphasis on prevention, and many strategies have been proposed (Tables 17 and 18).

❏ TREATMENT

Presently there is no specific treatment available for the management of patients with established cardiotoxicity with or without overt heart failure. Heart failure due to chemotherapeutic agents should be managed similarly to other causes of systolic heart failure and the recommendations of the American College of Cardiology, American Heart Association and the Heart Failure Society of America should be considered.

The treatment strategies for heart failure stages B, C, and D are highly desirable for chemotherapy-induced cardiomyopathy. Complete recovery of function may occur following discontinuation of the chemotherapeutic agent. Early institution of standard therapy with angiotensin and adrenergic inhibition therapy may be associated with full recovery of systolic function.

A modern approach of care of cancer patients, which is based on prevention and early detection of cardiotoxicity is illustrated in Flowchart 3.

FLOWCHART 3: The traditional and the modern approaches for management of cancer patients at risk of developing chemotherapy-induced cardiomyopathy

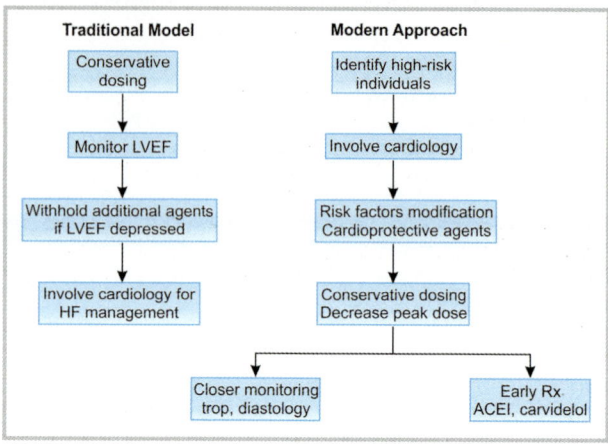

(Abbreviations: LVEF: Left ventricular ejection fraction; HF: Heart failure; Rx: Treatment; ACEI: Angiotensin-converting enzyme inhibitors)

❏ SUGGESTED READINGS

Cardinale D, Colombo A, Lamantia G, et al. Anthracycline-induced cardiomyopathy: clinical relevance and response to pharmacologic therapy. J Am Coll Cardiol. 2010;55:213-20.

Elliott P, Andersson B, Arbustini E, et al. Classification of the cardiomyopathies: a position statement from the European Society of Cardiology Working Group on Myocardial and Pericardial Diseases. Eur Heart J. 2008;29:270-6.

Goland S, Modi K, Bitar F, et al. Clinical profile and predictors of complications in peripartum cardiomyopathy. J Card Fail. 2009;15:645-50.

Hilfiker-Kleiner D, Kaminski K, Podewski E, et al. A cathepsin D-cleaved 16 kDa form of prolactin mediates postpartum cardiomyopathy. Cell. 2007;128:589-600.

Hunt SA, Abraham WT, Chin MH, et al. American College of Cardiology Foundation; American Heart Association. 2009 Focused update incorporated into the ACCF/AHA 2005 Guidelines for the Diagnosis and Management of Heart Failure in Adults. A Report of the American College of Cardiology Foundation/American Heart Association Task Force on Practice Guidelines Developed in Collaboration with the International Society for Heart and Lung Transplantation. J Am Coll Cardiol. 2009;53:e1-90.

Kristen AV, Sack FU, Schonland SO, et al. Staged heart transplantation and chemotherapy as a treatment option in patients with severe cardiac light-chain amyloidosis. Eur J Heart Fail. 2009;11:1014-20.

Libbey CA, Skinner M, Cohen AS. Use of abdominal fat tissue aspirate in the diagnosis of systemic amyloidosis. Arch Intern Med. 1983;143:1549-52.

Skinner M, Sanchorawala V, Seldin DC, et al. High-dose melphalan and autologous stem-cell transplantation in patients with AL amyloidosis: an 8-year study. Ann Intern Med. 2004;140:85-93.

Sliwa K, Hilfiker-Kleiner D, Petrie MC, et al. Current state of knowledge on aetiology, diagnosis, management and therapy of peripartum cardiomyopathy: a position statement from the Heart Failure Association of the European Society of Caridology Working Group on peripartum cardiomypathy. Eur J Heart Fail. 2010;12:767-78.

Westermark P, Benson MD, Buxbaum JN, et al. A primer of amyloid nomenclature. Amyloid. 2007;14:179-83.

Yeh ET, Bickford CL. Cardiovascular complications of cancer therapy: incidence, pathogenesis, diagnosis and management. J Am Coll Cardiol. 2009;53:2231-47.

8.5 Pericardial Disease

❑ INTRODUCTION

The pericardium is a thin covering that separates the heart from the remaining mediastinal structures, consisting of an outer sac (fibrous pericardium) and inner double layer sac (serous pericardium). There are two layers of serous pericardium: (i) the visceral layer (epicardium) covers the heart and great vessels and (ii) the parietal layer is fused to the fibrous pericardium. Diseases of the pericardium may present as inflammation (acute pericarditis), exudation (pericardial effusion or tamponade) or fibrosis (constrictive pericarditis). Although these appear to be three simple pathophysiologic processes, diseases of the pericardium present one of the most misdiagnosed and undertreated cardiac problems today.

❑ ACUTE PERICARDITIS

Inflammation of the pericardium (acute pericarditis) can be a manifestation of an underlying systemic disease, but most commonly presents as an isolated entity. The presentation is usually that of a young otherwise healthy patient who develops sudden pleuritic chest pain accompanied by systemic symptoms of fever, malaise and myalgias. In most patients, the etiology of acute pericarditis thought to be due to a viral etiology. Known secondary causes of acute pericarditis include bacterial or tuberculosis infection, systemic diseases (such as immune mediated diseases), neoplastic invasion of the pericardium, chronic renal disease, prior myocardial infarction or bypass operation, or chest wall trauma.

The typical chest pain of a patient presenting with acute pericarditis is usually sharp in nature and substernal in location, radiating to the neck and arms, exacerbated by either inspiration or position. Patients with acute pericarditis typically assume an upright sitting position, which appears to lessen the pericardial pain.

Examination

If there is a pulsus paradoxus and/or elevation of venous pressure, pericardial tamponade or constriction should be suspected. The classic pericardial friction rub is a "scratchy" three component sound heard mainly at the left sternal border. Auscultation should be performed with the patient in multiple positions, including the left lateral decubitus position, supine and sitting upright, as the pericardial rub may be effervescent and heard only in certain positions.

Diagnosis

The diagnosis of acute pericarditis should include at least two of the following criteria: (i) characteristic pleuritic chest pain; (ii) a pericardial friction rub, and (iii) typical electrocardiographic changes (Flowchart 4). In the acute setting, an upward concave ST segment elevation in two or more locations as well as PR segment depression are commonly present (Figs 12A to D). The evolution of electrocardiographic changes with pericarditis includes normalization of the ST and PR segments with the development of widespread T-wave inversions, some of which may persist indefinitely.

Once the diagnosis is made, further work-up of a patient presenting with acute pericarditis is mainly to rule out other etiologies for the presenting symptoms.

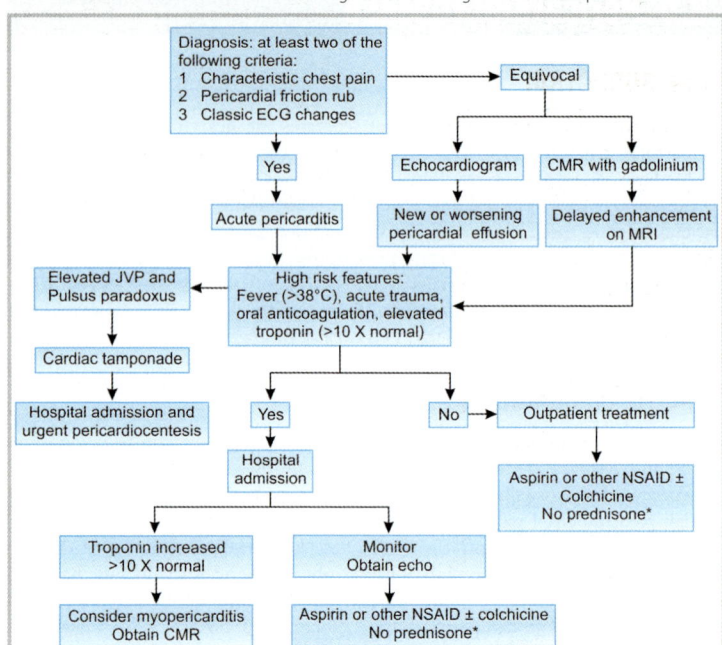

FLOWCHART 4: Overview of the diagnosis and management of acute pericarditis

*Corticosteroids should not be routinely used initially unless rheumatologic etiology or contraindication of NSAIDs and colchicine

Treatment

The high-risk features for hospitalization include a high fever (temperature >38°), and an immunocompromised state, concurrent oral anticoagulation, previous failure of nonsteroidal therapy or a marked elevation of troponin (>10 × upper limit normal).

The treatment of acute pericarditis depends upon the absence or presence of an underlying etiology. For instance, if pericarditis is due to a secondary cause, such as uremia, aggressive dialysis should be performed (i.e. dialysis). In the presence of systemic autoimmune diseases, appropriate treatment for the underlying disease should be implemented. However, for the majority of patients presenting with isolated acute pericarditis, the treatment should be with high dose salicylates or nonsteroidal anti-inflammatory agents. The dosage of salicylates is 900–1200 mg every 4–6 hours while awake for a period of 7–10 days, followed by gradual tapering for an additional 3 weeks. Indomethacin or other nonsteroidal anti-inflammatory agents can also be used, but large dosages are necessary (up to 150–200 mg/day). Nonsteroidal anti-inflammatory agents should not be used in patients who present with a concomitant myocardial infarction or known coronary artery disease. Proton pump inhibitors should be used in all patients on these large dosages of salicylates or nonsteroidals. Colchicine should be used in all patients unless there is a contraindication (Flowchart 4). It is recommended that all patients with acute pericarditis who can tolerate colchicine be treated with 0.6 mg twice a day for 1 week, then taper to 0.6 mg per day for at least 6 months. Colchicine should

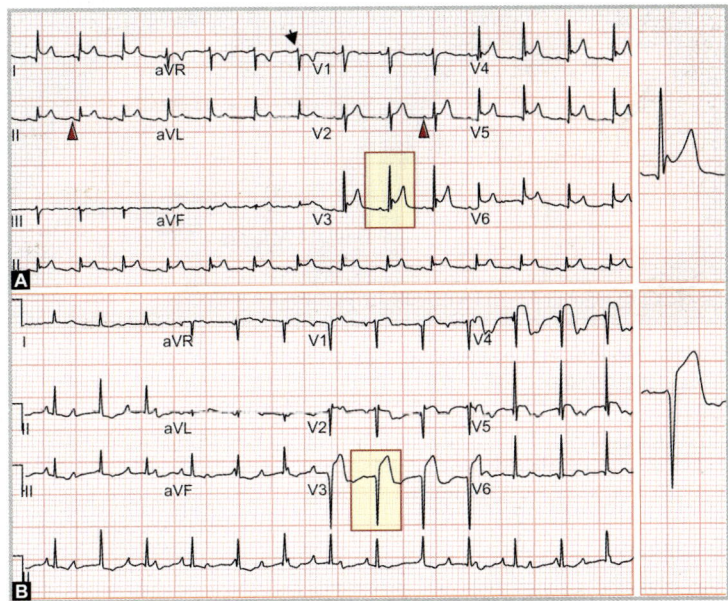

FIGURES 12A TO D: ECG abnormalities in acute pericarditis versus acute myocardial infarction. (A) Acute pericarditis reveals diffuse concave upsloping ST-segment elevation is seen in leads I, II, aVL, aVF and V2 to V6. There is also PR-segment elevation in aVR (arrow) and subtle PR-segment depression in leads II and V_2 (arrowheads). Reciprocal ST-segment depression is seen in aVR; (B) In acute myocardial infarction, the ST-segment elevation is convex upward or "humplike". (C and D) These panels demonstrate the difference in the ST-segment elevation in acute pericarditis (C) and acute myocardial infarction (D)

be avoided in patients with renal insufficiency, hepatobiliary disorders, blood dyscrasias and gastrointestinal motility disorders. Corticosteroids should rarely be used, as the use of steroids to treat acute pericarditis has been shown to result in a higher incidence of relapsing pericarditis.

❏ CHRONIC RELAPSING PERICARDITIS

Chronic relapsing pericarditis is a severe debilitating disease of the pericardium in which patients develop multiple recurrent episodes of pericarditis weeks to months after an initial episode of acute pericarditis. The frequency of chronic relapsing pericarditis following about of acute pericarditis is unknown, due to a paucity of studies with small patient populations; the frequency in many clinical series varies between 8% and 80%. The etiology is unknown but appears to be consistent with an autoimmune reaction activated by the initial episode. The pericardium is often thickened and fibrinous due to chronic inflammatory changes (Figs 13A and B).

This devastating disease entity appears to be particularly frequent in patients who have received prior corticosteroid therapy for acute pericarditis. These relapses may occur weeks to months after the initial event, and frequently corticosteroids are restarted for pain relief. When the steroid dose is dropped below physiologic levels upon weaning, the signs and symptoms of pericarditis will then return. Increasing the steroid dose will result in temporary resolution of the pericarditis,

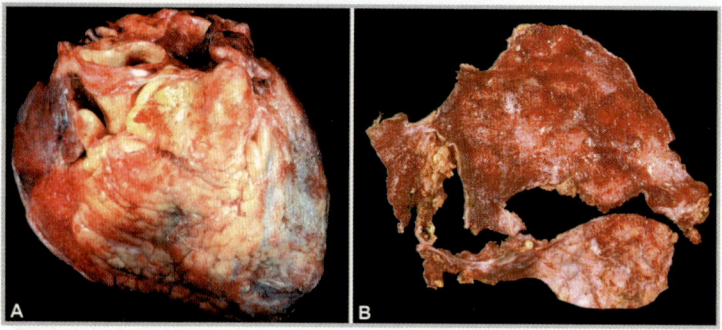

FIGURES 13A AND B: Gross features of relapsing pericarditis. (A) Anterior view of fibrinous pericardium in a patient with recurrent pericarditis; (B) Following surgical pericardiectomy, the thickened fibrinous pericardium is demonstrated. (*Source:* William D Edwards)

but as soon as the steroids are dropped below a certain level (usually 10–15 mg equivalent of prednisone), the relapses will recur.

Diagnosis

The diagnosis of chronic relapsing pericarditis uses the same diagnostic criteria as acute pericarditis for determining the presence of pericardial inflammation. It is helpful to have concomitant findings of either an elevated sedimentation rate or C-reactive protein (CRP) at the time of the relapse. MRI scanning with gadolinium enhancement will show delayed gadolinium enhancement in areas of inflamed pericardium and may be helpful in some patients in whom the diagnosis remains equivocal.

Treatment

An aggressive medical therapy with high dose salicylates or nonsteroidal anti-inflammatory agents should be implemented while the steroid dose is above the level at which relapses occur. Following the relief of all pericardial pain by the combination of prednisone and the salicylates or nonsteroidal anti-inflammatory agents, the steroids should then be very slowly weaned over a long period of time, while maintaining high levels of salicylates or nonsteroidal anti-inflammatory agents. The weaning process should be as slow as 1 mg taper per month, necessitating duration of up to 18–24 months before the patient is completely off the steroids. Following the taper off steroids, the salicylates and nonsteroidal anti-inflammatory agents should be continued for at least months after complete withdrawal of the steroids. Colchicine is effective in preventing recurrent episodes if given after the first episode of acute pericarditis and thus should be administered during this process and continued for at least 1 year after the last episode of pericarditis. A subset of patients who are not be able to respond to this very slow steroid taper and in these patients, complete pericardiectomy may be effective.

❑ PERICARDIAL EFFUSION AND PERICARDIAL TAMPONADE

The development of a pericardial effusion can either be idiopathic or due to a number of underlying etiologies. The effect of the pericardial fluid on cardiac hemodynamics depends more on the rate at which the effusion accumulates rather than the amount of the effusion. In a patient with slow accumulation of pericardial fluid, the pericardium is able to expand, thus accommodating up to several liters of fluid without compromising cardiac hemodynamics. However, when the amount of fluid exceeds the ability of the pericardium to expand, all four cardiac chambers are compressed as a result of increased intrapericardial pressure comprising systemic venous return and cardiac tamponade ensues. Acute pericardial tamponade can occur with rapid accumulation of less than 100 cc of fluid. This is a life-threatening entity if not treated rapidly. Acute tamponade may occur due to a malignancy or left ventricular rupture from a myocardial infarction. It is being seen more frequently as a result of complications from invasive cardiac catheterization and electrophysiologic procedures.

Examination

In a patient with pericardial tamponade, sinus tachycardia is usually present, as the increased heart rate is a physiologic response to the drop in stroke volume to maintain cardiac output. The venous pressure is elevated, with preservation of the "x" descent, but there is blunting of the "y" descent, as the high pericardial pressure prevents early rapid diastolic filling of the right ventricle at the time of tricuspid valve opening. Pulsus paradoxus, is always seen in pericardial tamponade, defined as a drop of systolic pressure greater than 10 mm Hg during inspiration.

Diagnosis

In a patient suspected of having pericardial tamponade, echocardiography is the diagnostic procedure of choice. Typical findings on echocardiography (Figs 14A to C), Doppler and cardiac catheterization are listed in Table 19.

Treatment

The treatment of acute pericardial tamponade is drainage of the high pressure pericardial fluid. Although a rapid infusion of volume and decrease in afterload with nitroprusside can result in a mild transient improvement in hemodynamics, it is essential to remove the pericardial effusion as soon as possible by pericardiocentesis. If possible, pericardiocentesis should always be performed under echocardiographic guidance. Two-dimensional echocardiography is able to identify the optimal site for the pericardiocentesis by visualizing the location and distribution of the pericardial effusion. In the presence of a bloody pericardial effusion associated with malignancy, continued drainage for 48–72 hours is required to prevent recurrence of the effusion.

❑ CONSTRICTIVE PERICARDITIS

Constrictive pericarditis occurs when there is thickening and fibrosis of the pericardium, causing limitation of expansion of the cardiac chambers. Due to the resultant decrease in ventricular filling and an increase in diastolic pressures, constrictive pericarditis results in signs and symptoms of heart failure, similar to that seen with left ventricular systolic dysfunction. Tuberculosis remains a common cause of constrictive pericarditis in the third world countries. However constrictive pericarditis now is most commonly seen following cardiac surgery, radiation therapy for prior malignancies or years after a bout of acute idiopathic pericarditis. There is a subset of patients who present with constrictive pericarditis in whom no obvious etiology is evident.

Table 19: Diagnostic testing in cardiac tamponade

Initial findings	Echocardiography	Cardiac catheterization
Symptoms: • Chest pain • Shoulder discomfort • Abdominal discomfort • Nausea	Two-dimensional: • Late diastolic collapse of RA • Early diastolic collapse of RV • Collapse of LA • Ventricular interdependence • IVC dilatation with <50% inspiratory collapse	*Early:* • Increased RA pressure with loss of "y" descent *Late:* • Decreased aortic systolic pressure • Decreased aortic pulse pressure • Pulsus paradoxus • Prominent decrease in pulse pressure with inspiration • Intracardiac diastolic pressure equilibration

Examination:
• Sinus tachycardia
• Elevated JVP-loss "y" descent
• Pulsus paradoxus
• Friction rub
	Doppler:
	• Blunted initial transmitral E velocity
	• Expiration
	  - Increased mitral E velocity
	  - Increased transmitral pressure gradient
	  - Decreased IVRT \
	  - Hepatic vein diastolic flow reversal
	• Inspiration
	  - Further drop in mitral E velocity	

ECG: • Sinus tachycardia • Low voltage QRS • Widespread concave ST-segment elevation and PR-segment depression • Electrical alternans		

The most common presentation of a patient with constrictive pericarditis is that of progressive fatigue, peripheral edema and abdominal swelling. Patients can present primarily with a low output state, so that the major complaint is decreased exercise tolerance and fatigue. Other patients may present with liver failure and cirrhosis, for the longstanding elevation of RA pressure can cause hepatic congestion and secondary cirrhosis. Recurrent pleural effusions may sometimes be the initial presentation of constrictive pericarditis.

Examination

The physical examination of a typical patient with constrictive pericarditis is that of an emaciated patient with severe ascites and edema. The sine qua non of constrictive pericarditis is a marked elevation of venous pressure with a rapid "x" and "y" descent (Fig. 15). The observation of a rise in jugular venous pressure with inspiration (Kussmaul's sign) is also often present and suggests impaired diastolic filling of the right ventricle due to restriction by an inelastic pericardium. Examination of the lung fields may reveal dullness in both bases consistent with pleural effusions. The heart sounds are usually distant without significant murmur. An early diastolic filling sound may be present, heard best with inspiration at the left sternal border.

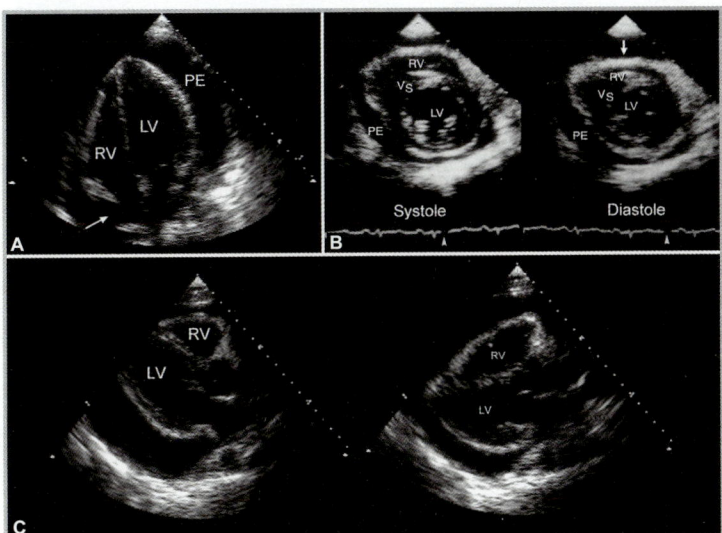

FIGURES 14A TO C: Two-dimensional echocardiographic features of cardiac tamponade. (A) Still frame image of an apical four-chamber view demonstrating late diastolic collapse of the right atrium (arrow). Persistence of right atrial (RA) collapse for more than one-third of the cardiac cycle is highly sensitive and specific for tamponade; (B) Early diastolic collapse (arrow) of the RV is specific for tamponade; (C) Parasternal long-axis views demonstrate the swinging motion of the heart within the pericardial cavity of a large pericardial effusion. The swinging motion is responsible for the electrocardiographic manifestation termed electrical alternans. (*Source:* Oh JK, Seward JB, Tajik AJ. The Echo Manual, 3rd edn. Lippincott, Williams and Wilkins; 2007)

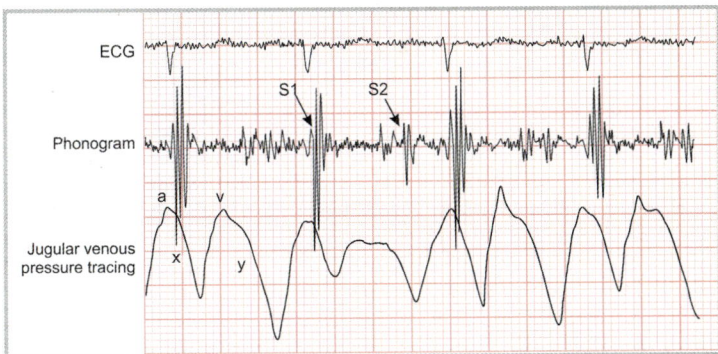

FIGURE 15: Jugular venous pressure tracings in constrictive pericarditis. Simultaneous jugular venous pressure tracings, phonogram and ECG tracings are shown in a patient with constrictive pericarditis. The "a" wave is generated by atrial contraction and occurs just prior to S1. The "v" wave is generated by ventricular contraction. The "x" descent reflects movement of the lower portion of the right atrium toward the right ventricle during ventricular systole. The "y" descent represents the abrupt termination of the downstroke of the "v" wave during early diastole after the tricuspid valve opens and the right ventricle begins to fill passively. In a patient with constrictive pericarditis, the "a" and "v" waves are more pronounced due to contraction against higher ventricular filling pressures resulting in marked JVP elevation. Impaired diastolic filling of the right ventricle combined with enhanced longitudinal motion of the heart in constrictive pericarditis results in unusually rapid "x" and "y" descents

It is usually closer to the second heart sound than a typical third heart sound heard in patients with left ventricular dysfunction, and represents a pericardial knock.

Diagnosis

Constrictive pericarditis should be suspected when a patient presents with severe right heart failure in the absence of a definable etiology such as left ventricular dysfunction, valvular heart disease or pulmonary hypertension. Classic findings of constrictive pericarditis obtained at cardiac catheterization are severe elevation and end equalization of pressures in all four cardiac chambers. There is the presence of early rapid filling seen as a dip and plateau sign on the ventricular pressure traces and the rapid "x" and "y" descent on the atrial pressure traces (Fig. 16).

A comprehensive echocardiogram can many times confirm the clinical suspicion of constrictive pericarditis. It should first rule out other causes of heart failure such as left ventricular systolic dysfunction, valvular disease or pulmonary hypertension. A normal left ventricular systolic function with a dilated IVC should raise the suspicion of constrictive pericarditis. Subtle changes in septal motion are usually present. A septal "bounce" reflects the effect of increased and equalized right ventricular and left ventricular diastolic pressures. Early rapid filling can be seen as a rapid expansion of the left ventricular cavity on M-mode (Fig. 17). A septal "shift" into the left ventricular occurs during inspiration indirectly representing enhanced ventricular interaction. Doppler echocardiography can further delineate the respiratory changes in hemodynamics.

About 25% of patients with constrictive pericarditis will have calcification on chest X-ray. However the absence of calcification does not necessarily rule

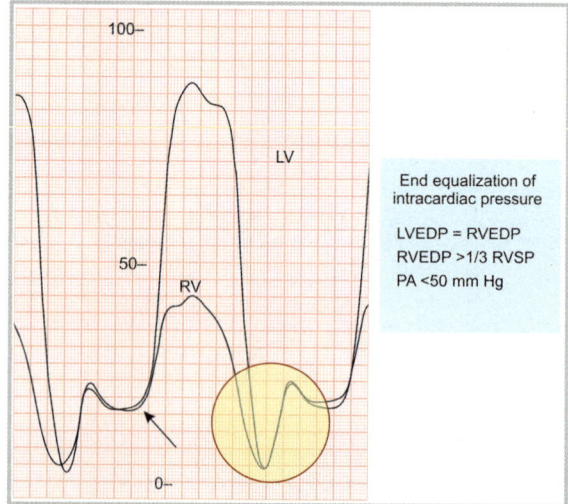

FIGURE 16: Left and right ventricular pressure tracings in constrictive pericarditis. Simultaneous pressure recordings from the left ventricle (LV) and the right ventricle (RV) in a patient with constrictive pericarditis are demonstrated. At end diastole, there is elevation and equalization of the LV and RV pressures (arrow). Other hemodynamic features include an increase in the RV end diastolic pressure (RVEDP) to greater than one-third of the RV systolic pressure (RVSP) and a pulmonary artery pressure of less than 50 mm Hg. In first third of diastole, there is rapid ventricular filling and an abrupt increase in ventricular pressure (circle), called the dip and plateau sign (circle). However, these findings can also be seen in patients with restrictive cardiomyopathy

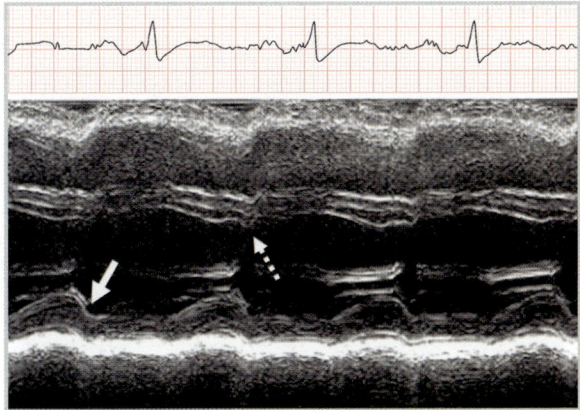

FIGURE 17: M-mode echocardiography demonstrating septal bounce and left ventricular posterior wall flattening in constrictive pericarditis. There are several M-mode signs that are indicative of the diagnosis of constrictive pericarditis. The septal bounce (dashed arrow) represents the result of increased and equalized right and left ventricular diastolic pressure. In early diastole, the left ventricular (LV) posterior wall expands rapidly and posteriorly, followed by an abrupt cessation of ventricular filling in mid to late diastole (solid arrow)

out constriction. MRI and CT scanning are useful in demonstrating increased pericardial thickness and calcification. In addition, myocardial imaging can show the deformed ventricular contours, angulation of the ventricular septum and inferior vena cava dilatation. Failure of pulmonary structures to pulsate during the cardiac cycle in the presence of a thickened pericardium is suggestive of constrictive pericarditis.

Treatment

Patients presenting with constrictive pericarditis should be considered for open heart surgery (Flowchart 5). The surgery is a complete pericardiectomy, resecting the pericardium from phrenic nerve to phrenic nerve. A complete pericardiectomy does pose an increased operative mortality, greater than 5–6% even at experienced centers. The independent adverse predictors of long-term outcome by surgery include: over age, worsening of the heart association class at presentation, renal dysfunction, left ventricular dysfunction and prior radiation. However, a complete pericardiectomy may result in significant improvement of symptoms and possibly prolongation of life.

If there is a history of a more acute onset of symptoms coupled with laboratory findings of inflammation (elevated sedimentation rate, CRP or gadolinium enhancement defects by MRI scan), it is beneficial for a trial of high dose nonsteroidal anti-inflammatory agents, salicylates or even steroids to determine whether or not resolution of the constrictive process might be possible.

Effusive constrictive pericarditis is a unique condition in which there is both a pericardial effusion as well as constrictive pericarditis. In these patients, a decision then needs to be made as to whether more aggressive medical therapy or surgery is required. In those patients in whom active inflammation is present, a trial of anti-inflammatory medications should be considered. In other patients, a surgical pericardiectomy is not necessary.

FLOWCHART 5: Overview of the diagnosis and management of constrictive pericarditis

*Unless aggressive diuresis; **If recent onset of symptoms. Rule out transient constrictive pericarditis. Obtain inflammatory markers +/− CMR (Abbreviations: IVC: Inferior vena cava; RV: Right ventricle; LV: Left ventricle)

❏ SUGGESTED READINGS

Breen JF. Imaging of the pericardium. J Thorac Imaging. 2001;16:47-54.

Brucato A, Brambilla G, Moreo A, et al. Long-term outcomes in difficult-to-treat patients with recurrent pericarditis. Am J Cardiol. 2006;98:267-71

Holmes DR Jr., Nishimura R, Fountain R, et al. Iatrogenic pericardial effusion and tamponade in the percutaneous intracardiac intervention era. JACC Cardiovasc Interv. 2009;2:705-17.

Imazio M, Bobbio M, Cecchi E, et al. Colchicine as first-choice therapy for recurrent pericarditis: results of the CORE (Colchicine for Recurrent pericarditis) trial. Arch Intern Med. 2005;165:1987-91.

Khandaker MH, Espinosa RE, Nishimura RA, et al. Pericardial disease: diagnosis and management. Mayo Clin Proc. 2010;85:572-93.

Maisch B, Seferovic PM, Ristic AD, et al. Guidelines on the diagnosis and management of pericardial diseases executive summary; the task force on the diagnosis and management of pericardial diseases of the European society of cardiology. Eur Heart J. 2004;25:587-610.

Misselt AJ, Harris SR, Glockner J, et al. MR imaging of the pericardium. Magn Reson Imaging Clin N Am. 2008;16:185-99.

Soler-Soler J, Sagrista-Sauleda J, Permanyer-Miralda G. Relapsing pericarditis. Heart. 2004;90:1364-8.

Spodick DH. Acute cardiac tamponade. N Engl J Med. 2003;349:684-90.

Talreja DR, Nishimura RA, Oh JK, et al. Constrictive pericarditis in the modern era: novel criteria for diagnosis in the cardiac catheterization laboratory. J Am Coll Cardiol. 2008;51:315-9.

8.6 Radiation-induced Heart Disease

❏ INTRODUCTION

During therapeutic irradiation of the chest, the heart and other intrathoracic structures are predisposed to radiation injury. Acute radiation injury is usually transient and, in general, benign. However, long-term cardiovascular complications of chest irradiation can be devastating. Typically, there is a long latency period between radiation exposure and clinical manifestations of the cardiovascular complications. Radiation induced cardiotoxicity primarily occurs in patients who received radiation for Hodgkin's lymphoma or breast cancer. However, it can also occur after radiation therapy for lung and esophagogastric cancers, thymomas and peptic ulcer disease. It should be appreciated that brachytherapy, occasionally used for coronary artery stenosis, is not associated with radiation-induced cardiotoxicity.

❏ RADIATION-INDUCED PERICARDIAL DISEASE

Pericardial disease is the most frequent complication of mediastinal radiation therapy. Acute radiation injury often manifests as inflammatory pericarditis with or without pericardial effusion. Acute radiation pericarditis usually manifests a few weeks after radiation treatment. The typical clinical presentation includes fever, tachycardia, chest pain and pericardial friction rub. The pericardial fluid shows variable amount of protein rich exudates. Acute pericarditis is not a contraindication for continuation of radiation therapy; however, a dose adjustment may be necessary.

Approximately 20% of patients who develop acute irradiation-induced inflammatory pericarditis progress to develop chronic constrictive pericarditis. The rate of progression is slow and it usually takes 5–10 years to develop clinically relevant features of constrictive pericarditis. Fibrosis of the parietal and visceral pericardium, with or without calcification, produces the pathophysiologic, clinical and hemodynamic features of constrictive pericarditis. The mechanism of fibrosis in radiation-induced constrictive pericarditis remains unclear. It has been postulated that ischemia resulting from injury to the microvascular network to the pericardium may be contributory.

The clinical presentation of radiation-induced constrictive pericarditis is similar to that of other etiologies of constriction. The physical findings in patients with overt constrictive pericarditis are elevated jugular venous pressure with a positive Kussmaul's sign, a quiet precordium, abdominal swelling, peripheral edema and absence of signs of pulmonary hypertension. The hemodynamic features are characterized by equalization of left and right ventricular diastolic pressures, "square root sign" and exaggerated ventricular interdependence (Fig. 18). For the assessment of pericardial thickening, cardiac tomographic study or cardiac resonance imaging are usually employed.

The treatment of radiation-induced constrictive pericarditis is surgical pericardiectomy. It should be appreciated; however, that pericardiectomy may not always result in significant clinical and hemodynamic improvement due to concomitant presence of restrictive cardiomyopathy. The prognosis of patients with radiation-induced constrictive pericarditis remains poor.

Asymptomatic chronic pericardial effusion is another complication of radiation-induced pericardial disease. The latent period may vary from months to years after mediastinal irradiation. The pericardial fluid may be clear, hemorrhagic or serosanguinous. Most asymptomatic pericardial effusions resolve spontaneously.

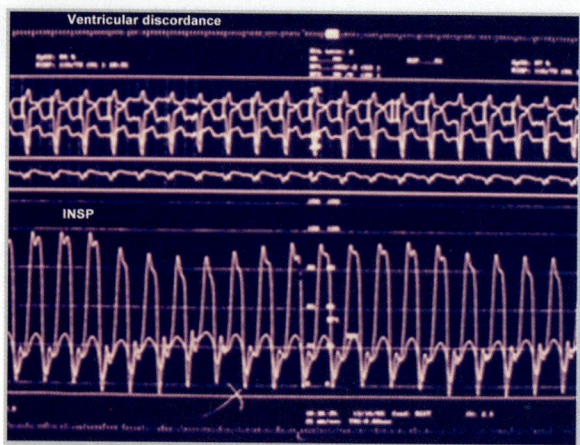

FIGURE 18: The characteristic hemodynamic features of constrictive pericarditis showing equalization of left and right ventricular diastolic pressure and exaggerated ventricular interdependence and exaggerated ventricular interdependence (the systolic pressures generated in the left ventricle and the right ventricular vary in opposite directions in relation to breathing)

Only a minority of patients develop cardiac tamponade. In some patients, the constrictive physiology persists even after pericardiocentesis and in these patients a diagnosis of effusive-constrictive pericarditis should be entertained.

❏ RADIATION-INDUCED MYOCARDIAL DISEASE

Overt clinical cardiomyopathy due to radiotherapy is rare. However, autopsy studies reported that the frequency of asymptomatic myocardial fibrosis is over 60%. Myocardial fibrosis consists of proliferation of bands of collagen separating and/or replacing cardiac myocytes. It occurs in patches, often in the anterior wall of the left ventricle. The mechanisms of radiation-induced cardiomyopathy remain unclear.

The predominant cardiac functional derangement in patients with radiation-induced cardiomyopathy is diastolic dysfunction. Diastolic dysfunction may or may not be associated with clinical heart failure. Older age, hypertension, diabetes and coronary artery disease are the risk factors for diastolic dysfunction. A larger dose of radiation is also associated with an increased risk of developing abnormalities of left ventricular diastolic function. The diagnosis of the radiation-induced restrictive cardiomyopathy should be only made after exclusion of other more common causes.

The symptoms of heart failure resulting from restrictive cardiomyopathy, irrespective of its etiology, are fatigue and dyspnea, which initially occur during exertion but later at rest, with the deterioration of the hemodynamic abnormalities. The physical findings are characterized by elevated jugular venous pressure, positive Kussmaul's sign and evidences of pulmonary hypertension. Ascites and lower extremity edema are common in patients with advanced heart failure.

Transthoracic echocardiography demonstrates, normal left ventricular size, normal or slightly reduced left ventricular ejection fraction (LVEF) and restrictive filling pattern. In addition, impaired exercise tolerance and a decrease in LVEF during exercise have been observed. The hemodynamic studies by cardiac catheterization reveal the dip-and-plateau or square-root contour of the ventricular diastolic pressure, left ventricular end diastolic pressure higher than right ventricular end diastolic pressure and pulmonary arterial hypertension.

There is no specific treatment for radiation-induced restrictive cardiomyopathy. Diuretic therapy is necessary for relief of congestive symptoms. As usually stroke volume is fixed, heart rate should not be decreased excessively, otherwise cardiac output will decrease.

❏ RADIATION-INDUCED CORONARY ARTERY DISEASE

Epicardial coronary artery stenosis is a recognized complication of mediastinal irradiation. The coronary artery lesions have characteristic features and location. The manifestations of coronary artery stenosis usually occur 10–15 years after radiation therapy. Due to the anterior location in the chest, there is a disproportionately higher incidence of ostial lesions and a predilection for the involvement of the right coronary artery, left main coronary artery and proximal left anterior descending coronary artery.

The pathophysiologic mechanisms of epicardial coronary artery stenosis following radiation therapy are similar to those of established mechanisms for the development of atherosclerotic coronary artery disease. Experimental studies have shown that radiation not only can initiate atherosclerosis but also can predispose plaque disruption. The prognosis of patients with radiation-induced coronary artery stenosis appears to be worse than that of patients with nonradiation-induced coronary artery atherosclerosis.

Patients with radiation-induced coronary artery disease are often asymptomatic. The overt clinical manifestations of irradiation-induced coronary artery disease are similar to those of nonradiation-induced coronary artery stenosis. The presentations can be typical effort angina, acute myocardial infarction or sudden cardiac death.

The diagnosis of radiation-induced coronary artery disease can be established by both invasive and noninvasive investigations. Coronary artery angiography by cardiac catheterization, computerized contrast tomographic angiography or cardiac catheterization, or computerized contrast tomographic angiography can be used to assess presence and severity of coronary artery stenosis. Presence or absence of myocardial ischemia can be detected by pharmacologic and nonpharmacologic stress tests.

The treatment of radiation-induced coronary artery disease is similar to that of nonradiation atherosclerotic coronary artery disease. Adequate treatment of dyslipidemia, diabetes, hypertension and obesity should be undertaken. The cessation of smoking should be encouraged. Angiotensin inhibitors, betaadrenergic antagonists and antiplatelet agents should be used. Coronary artery revascularization is recommended in appropriate patients. Both percutaneous coronary artery intervention and coronary artery bypass surgery have been used. Both in patients with stable or unstable coronary artery disease, coronary angioplasty has been successfully performed.

❏ RADIATION-INDUCED VALVULAR HEART DISEASE

The overall incidence of valvular heart disease following radiotherapy is variable and has been reported to be between 6% and 11% after approximately 22–23 years after radiation exposure. Aortic valve disease is the most frequent valvular complication in patients with radiation-induced heart disease (RIHD). The aortic root may also be calcified in these patients. The aortic valves leaflets are fibrotic, markedly thickened and calcified. Valvulitis and rupture of the aortic valve have also been reported. Mitral valve may also be affected following mediastinal irradiation. Mitral valve stenosis has been reported, although mitral regurgitation is more common. Isolated tricuspid valve disease is rare; however, severe tricuspid valve regurgitation following radiation therapy has been reported.

Physical examination, echocardiographic studies and, if required, cardiac catheterization should be performed for establishing the diagnosis of presence and severity of radiation-induced heart valve disease. It is also essential to assess ventricular function. Coronary angiography should also be performed to assess the presence of significant coronary artery disease. The hemodynamic severity, pulmonary artery pressure and pulmonary vascular resistance should also be determined.

The timing of surgical intervention of radiation-induced valve disease is similar to that of patients without radiation-induced valve disease. Asymptomatic patients should be followed and surgery is not recommended. There is no specific therapy for asymptomatic patients. Antibiotic prophylaxis for bacterial endocarditis is not recommended. Surgical intervention should be considered in symptomatic patients or in patients with decreasing LVEF even in the absence of symptoms.

❑ CONDUCTION SYSTEM DISEASE

A variety of cardiac conduction system abnormalities have been observed following mediastinal radiation therapy. Atrioventricular blocks, bundle branch block, sick sinus syndrome and prolonged Q-T intervals have been reported. The mechanisms of radiation-induced conduction system disturbances are not entirely clear. Autonomic dysfunction has been postulated as a potential mechanism. Presyncope and syncope are the presenting symptoms of conduction system disease and the patients usually have complete heart block. Electrocardiographic evaluation is essential to establish the diagnosis. In patients with intermittent symptoms, the use of Holter monitor or event recorder may be necessary. The treatment of symptomatic heart block or sick sinus syndrome is implantation of a permanent pacemaker.

❑ PREVENTION

The reduction of dose of radiation is of paramount importance in reducing the risk of RIHD. The higher fractional dose is also associated with a higher risk of development of RIHD, thus it is desirable to reduce the fractional dose. When a larger volume of heart is irradiated, the higher is the risk of cardiac complications.

Table 20: Risk factors for RIHD	
Patient-related risk factors	• Younger age at exposure • Presence of traditional cardiac risk factors • Presence of tumor next to the heart
Treatment-related risk factors	• Higher total dose • Higher fractionated dose • Increased volume of heart irradiated • Longer time since exposure • Concomitant or previous cardiotoxic chemotherapy • Type of radiation source (cobalt)

Table 21: Strategies for prevention of RIHD

- Decreased total dose
- Decreased fraction size
- Treatment planning to reduce cardiac volume exposed
- Employ the minimum dose of adjunctive chemotherapy
- Screening and aggressive treatment for traditional cardiac risk factors
- Long-term monitoring
- Anti-free radical agents

Thus reduction of cardiac volume exposed to radiation should be attempted. The risk factors for RIHD and the strategies for its prevention are summarized in Tables 20 and 21.

❏ SUGGESTED READINGS

Benoff LJ, Schweitzer P. Radiation therapy-induced cardiac injury. Am Heart J. 1995;129:1193-6.

Bovin JF, Hutchison GB, Lubin JH, et al. Coronary artery disease mortality in patients treated for Hodgkin's disease. Cancer. 1992;69:1241-7.

Caus T, Canavy I, Mesana T, et al. Rescue revascularization for acute coronary occlusion late after radiotherapy. Ann Thorac Surg. 1999;67:236-8.

Daitoku K, Fukui K, Ichinoseki I, et al. Radiotherapy-induced aortic valve disease associated with porcelain aorta. Jpn J Thorac Cardiovasc Surg. 2004;52:349-52.

Darby SC, Cutter DJ, Boerma M, et al. Radiation-related heart disease: current knowledge and future prospects. Int J Radiat Oncol Biol Phys. 2010;76:656-65.

Darby SC, McGale P, Taylor CW, et al. Long-term mortality from heart disease and lung cancer after radiotherapy for early breast cancer: prospective cohort study of about 300,000 women in US SEER cancer registries. Lancet Oncol. 2005;6:557-65.

Fajardo LF, Stewart JR, Cohn KE. Morphology of radiation-induced heart disease. Arch Pathol. 1968;86:512-9.

Hancock SL, Donaldson SS, Hoppe RT. Cardiac disease following treatment of Hodgkin's disease in children and adolescents. J Clin Oncol. 1997;1:1208-15.

Hull MC, Morris CG, Pepine CJ, et al. Valvular dysfunction and carotid, subclavian and coronary artery disease in survivors of Hodgkin's lymphoma treated with radiation therapy. JAMA. 2003;290:2831-7.

Konings AW, Smit Sibinga CT, Aarnoudse MW, et al. Initial events in radiation-induced atheromatosis. II. Damage to intimal cells. Strahlentherapie. 1978;154:795-800.

Lee PJ, Mallik R. Cardiovascular effects of radiation therapy: practical approach to radiation therapy-induced heart disease. Cardiol Rev. 2005;13:80-6.

Chapter 9

Pulmonary Vascular Disease and Adult Congenital Heart Disease

9.1 Pulmonary Arterial Hypertension

❑ DEFINITIONS AND CLASSIFICATIONS

Hemodynamic Classification of Pulmonary Hypertension

Pulmonary hypertension (PH) is defined hemodynamically by invasive right heart catheterization (RHC) as a mean pulmonary artery pressure (mPAP) greater than 25 mm Hg. The exercise criteria has been removed during the 4th World Symposium on PH due to the lack of data regarding its meaning and clinical relevance. Given the diverse array of diseases that can lead to PH, it can be useful to classify PH based on the anatomical location of the "lesion" that results in elevated pulmonary pressures (Fig. 1).

PH from lesions proximal to the pulmonary capillary bed are hemodynamically classified as "precapillary" and are characterized by an mPAP greater than 25 mm Hg, pulmonary arterial wedge pressure (PAWP) or left ventricular end-diastolic pressure (LVEDP) less than or equal to 15 mm Hg and PVR greater than three Wood units (WU)(or >240 dynes sec cm^{-5}). In contrast, "postcapillary" PH is defined as an mPAP greater than 25 mm Hg, PAWP and/or LVEDP greater than 15 mm Hg, and PVR less than three WU. Some patients have "mixed" precapillary and postcapillary PH, which is defined as an mPAP greater than 25 mm Hg, PAWP greater than 15 mm Hg, and PVR greater than 15 mm Hg. Rarely, increased pulmonary blood flow from a high cardiac output (CO) state leads to PH without elevations in PAWP or PVR.

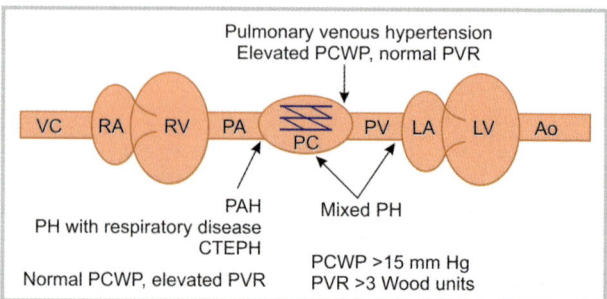

FIGURE 1: Schematic of precapillary and postcapillary pulmonary hypertension.
(Abbreviations: Ao: Aorta; CTEPH: Chronic thromboembolic pulmonary hypertension; LA: Left atrium; LV: Left ventricle; PA: Pulmonary artery; PAH: Pulmonary arterial hypertension; PC: Pulmonary capillary; PCWP: Pulmonary capillary wedge pressure; PH: Pulmonary hypertension; PV: Pulmonary veins; PVR: Pulmonary vascular resistance; RA: Right atrium; VC: Vena cava)

Clinical Classification of Pulmonary Hypertension

The clinical classification system for PH continues to evolve as our understanding of the pathological basis of the various diseases that underlie the syndrome improves. The most current clinical classification was developed in 2008 during the 4th World Symposium on PH in Dana Point, California, which resulted in a revision of the Venice clinical classification of 2003 (Table 1).

Table 1: Clinical classification of pulmonary hypertension (Dana Point, 2008)

1. Pulmonary arterial hypertension (PAH)
    1.1 Idiopathic PAH (IPAH)
    1.2 Heritable
        1.2.1 BMPR2
        1.2.2 ALK, endoglin (with or without hereditary hemorrhagic telangiectasia)
        1.2.3 Unknown
    1.3 Drug and toxin induced
    1.4 Associated with:
        1.4.1 Connective tissue diseases
        1.4.2 HIV infection
        1.4.3 Portal hypertension
        1.4.4 Congenital heart diseases
        1.4.5 Schistosomiasis
        1.4.6 Chronic hemolytic anemia
    1.5 Persistent pulmonary hypertension of the newborn
1. Pulmonary veno-occlusive disease (PVOD) and/or pulmonary capillary hemangiomatosis (PCH)
2. Pulmonary hypertension owing to left heart disease
    2.1 Systolic dysfunction
    2.2 Diastolic dysfunction
    2.3 Valvular disease
3. Pulmonary hypertension owing to lung diseases and/or hypoxemia
    3.1 Chronic obstructive pulmonary disease
    3.2 Interstitial lung disease
    3.3 Other pulmonary diseases with mixed restrictive and obstructive pattern
    3.4 Sleep-disordered breathing
    3.5 Alveolar hypoventilation disorders
    3.6 Chronic exposure to high altitude
    3.7 Developmental abnormalities
4. Chronic thromboembolic pulmonary hypertension (CTEPH)
5. Pulmonary hypertension with unclear multifactorial mechanisms
    5.1 Hematologic disorders: myeloproliferative disorders, splenectomy
    5.2 Systemic disorders: sarcoidosis, pulmonary Langerhans cell histiocytosis: lymphangioleiomyomatosis, neurofibromatosis, vasculitis
    5.3 Metabolic disorders: glycogen storage disease, Gaucher disease, thyroid disorders
    5.4 Other: tumoral obstruction, fibrosing mediastinitis, chronic renal failure on dialysis sarcoidosis, histiocytosis X, lymphangiomatosis, compression of pulmonary vessels (adenopathy, tumor, fibrosing mediastinitis)

(Abbreviations: ALK: Activin receptor-like kinase; BMPR2: Bone morphogenetic protein receptor type 2; HIV: Human immunodeficiency virus)

Pulmonary Arterial Hypertension (WHO Group 1 PH)

With an estimated prevalence of 15 cases per million, PAH affects women more than men, with female to male ratios from 1.5:1 to 4.1:1. Age of onset is typically in the fourth to fifth decade although it appears to be increasing. Causes of PAH include idiopathic and heritable cases, drug and toxins, PAH associated with connective tissue disease (CTD), human immunodeficiency virus (HIV) infection, portal hypertension, congenital heart disease (CHD), schistosomiasis, chronic hemolytic anemia and persistent PH of the newborn. Pulmonary veno-occlusive disease (PVOD) and pulmonary capillary hemangiomatosis (PCH) are classified as PAH; as they differ from other types of PAH with the variable amounts of disease affecting the pulmonary capillaries and pulmonary veins, which leads to differences in their prognosis and variable responses to treatment compared with other WHO Group 1 (PAH) diseases.

Pulmonary Venous Hypertension (WHO Group 2 PH)

Elevated pulmonary artery pressure may also be related to upstream high left atrial pressure as a consequence of left-sided heart disease (WHO Group 2 PH). Any cause of elevated left atrial pressure, including left ventricular (LV) systolic and/or diastolic dysfunction (most common), left-sided valve disease (e.g. mitral or aortic regurgitation or stenosis), pericardial disease, or a congenital membrane within the left atrium (cor triatriatum) can all lead to this type of pulmonary hypertension. In these cases, the PCWP and/or LVEDP is greater than or equal to 15 mm Hg. WHO Group 2 PH has been often described as "pulmonary venous" or "post-capillary" pulmonary hypertension, and most often the PVR is normal. Due to the prevalence of left-sided heart failure, postcapillary PH accounts for the majority of cases of PH.

However, in the setting of chronically elevated left-sided filling pressures, pulmonary vascular remodeling can occur such that the PVR and transpulmonary gradient increase out of proportion to the degree of PCWP and/or LVEDP elevation. In such cases, the transpulmonary gradient (TPG) is greater than the normal 10 mm Hg or less (usually 12–15 mm Hg or greater).

Pulmonary Hypertension Due to Lung Disease and/or Chronic Hypoxemia (WHO Group 3 PH)

Precapillary PH can develop in patients with parenchymal lung disease and/or chronic hypoxia. Examples of this type of PH include chronic obstructive pulmonary disease (COPD), interstitial lung disease (ILD), other pulmonary diseases with mixed restrictive and obstructive lung pattern, sleep-disordered breathing, alveolar hypoventilation disorders, chronic exposure to high altitude, and developmental abnormalities. Of the parenchymal lung diseases, ILD most commonly results in PH through capillary destruction and hypoxic vasoconstriction. Patients with CTD, in particular those with the scleroderma spectrum of CTD, are at increased risk for development of ILD.

Chronic Thromboembolic Pulmonary Hypertension (WHO Group 4 PH)

The defining features of chronic thromboembolic pulmonary hypertension (CTEPH) are pulmonary arterial mural thrombi, webbing, bands and obliteration of the larger pulmonary vessels. In addition, patients with CTEPH may have pathologic changes in nonoccluded pulmonary artery segments that are typically seen in PAH, including medial hypertrophy and intimal hyperplasia. Although acute pulmonary embolism (PE) can lead to PH and RV dysfunction, in the majority of patients it resolves after the acute episode. There is limited evidence that patients treated with thrombolysis due to RV dysfunction following acute PE have decreased incidence of CTEPH. Approximately 2–4% of patients, who suffer from PE, go on to develop CTEPH despite anticoagulation.

Pulmonary Hypertension with Unclear Multifactorial Mechanisms (WHO Group 5 PH)

Group 5 consists of several forms of PH for which the etiology is unclear or multifactorial. For instance, PH may be related to hematologic disorders, such as chronic myeloproliferative disorders including by polycythemia vera, essential thrombocythemia, chronic myeloid leukemia, and postsplenectomy state. In addition, systemic disorders that are associated with an increased risk of developing PH include sarcoidosis, pulmonary Langerhans cell histicytosis and neurofibromatosis type 1 (also known as von Recklinghausen disease). Finally, metabolic disorders, such as type Ia glycogen storage disease (a rare autosomal recessive disorder caused by a deficiency of glucose-6-phosphatase), Gaucher disease, and thyroid disease (both hyper- and hypothyroidism) have been associated with a risk for developing PH. In each of these disorders, the pathophysiology of PH is either unclear or related to multiple potential underlying mechanisms.

❑ PATHOPHYSIOLOGY OF PULMONARY ARTERIAL HYPERTENSION

There is no unifying pathobiologic mechanism to explain the development of PAH in all cases, and multiple independent factors may play a role, such as mutations in bone morphogenetic protein receptor type 2 (BMPR2), high volume systemic to pulmonary shunts and inflammatory changes in CTD that lead to similar disease phenotypes.

The normal pulmonary circulation is a high-flow, low resistance circuit with great capacity to recruit more pulmonary capillaries and reduce PVR when needed without an increase pulmonary artery pressure. Fundamental to the development of PAH is smooth muscle cellular proliferation, decreased apoptosis, vasoconstriction, platelet dysregulation and inflammation. Pathologically, these changes manifest as medial hypertrophy, intimal hyperplasia, adventitial proliferation of the small pulmonary arteries and *in situ* thrombosis (Fig. 1). The hallmark of advanced PAH is the plexiform lesion, which consists of endothelial cell channels lined by myelofibroblasts, smooth muscle cells and connective tissue matrix (Fig. 2).

On a molecular level, multiple pathways have been identified which have served as therapeutic targets. Arachidonic acid metabolism is altered in PAH, which leads to decreased activity of prostacyclin synthase and reduced levels of prostaglandin I_2 (prostacyclin) with a shift toward increased thromboxane A2 production. This imbalance favors cellular proliferation, vasoconstriction and platelet aggregation. PAH is also characterized by a deficit of nitric oxide through decreased endothelial nitric oxide synthase activity. The effects of nitric oxide are mediated through cyclic guanosine monophosphate (cGMP), which is an important modulator of vascular tone and is broken down by cGMP phosphodiesterase type-5A (PDE5A). PDE5A is found in high concentrations in the pulmonary vascular bed, which has made it an attractive target for drug development. Endothelin-1, which leads to smooth muscle cell vasoconstriction and proliferation, is elevated in PAH, and

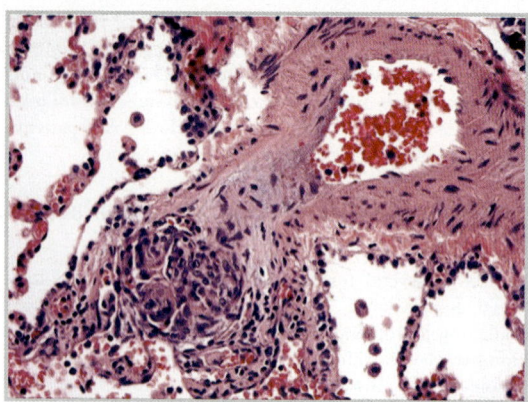

FIGURE 2: Pulmonary arterial hypertension. Plexiform lesion: a tangle of slit-like vascular channels are noted adjacent to a pulmonary arterial branch (Hematoxylin and eosin stain, 400x)

higher levels are associated with worse outcomes. Other mediators that appear to impact the development and progression of PAH include increased activity levels of serotonin, angiopoietin-1 and angiopoietin-2, plasminogen activator inhibitor-1, growth factors, oxidant stress, and inflammation and reduced activity levels of vasoactive intestinal peptide, Kv channels and fibrinolysis. The role of estrogen in the development of PAH, if any, remains unclear; however, altered estrogen levels, signaling and metabolism may play a role in idiopathic PAH (IPAH).

The pathologic outcome of the above physiologic and molecular changes is progressive elevation in PAP and PVR, leading to RV failure, poor LV filling, decreased CO, ventricular dysrhythmias and ultimately death. In PAH, increasing PVR leads to abnormal loading conditions, forcing the RV to undergo pathologic changes and remodel (Flowchart 1).

In the initial stages of the disease, the RV adapts to increased PVR by increasing RV wall thickness, which tends to decrease RV wall stress. During this phase, both CO and right atrial pressure (RAP) are normal. However, progressive increases in PVR lead to RV chamber enlargement, fibrosis and distortion of the normal RV architecture. As the RV begins to fail, right ventricular end-diastolic pressure (RVEDP) and thus RAP begin to rise. Due to decreased ability of the pulmonary vasculature to dilate in response to exercise, the RV is unable to augment CO and exercise tolerance decreases.

As the RV begins to dilate, the typical triangular shape of the RV is distorted, resulting in tricuspid annular dilatation and regurgitation, which further increases RV preload and decreases CO. Because the RV and LV are interdependent and contained within the pericardium, RV morphologic distortion affects LV filling, compliance and shape. As RV pressure continues to increase, the septum flattens during systole. However, once RV volume overload develops, the LV becomes progressively "D" or crescent shaped as the septum flattens in both systole and diastole. In addition to direct compression of the LV, decreased RV CO leads to poor filling of the LV and decreased LV CO. Increased RVEDP leads to increased coronary sinus pressure, which leads to ventricular edema and decreased ventricular compliance. Decreased CO further exacerbates RV ischemia due to decreased coronary perfusion pressure in the setting of low MAP and high RVEDP. Furthermore, in decompensated RV failure, LVEDP can increase as a result of ventricular interdependence and pericardial constraint.

FLOWCHART 1: Pathophysiology of right ventricular failure in pulmonary arterial hypertension

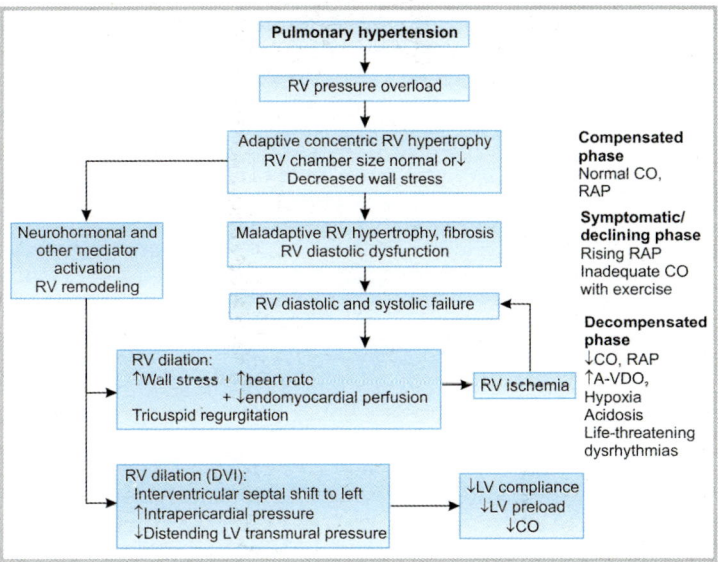

(Abbreviations: A-VDO$_2$: Arterial venous oxygen difference; CO: Cardiac output; LV: Left ventricle; RAP: Right atrial pressure; RV: Right ventricular). (*Source:* DeMarco T, McGlothlin D. Managing right ventricular failure in pulmonary arterial hypertension—An algorithmic approach. Advances in pulmonary hypertension. 2005;4(4):16-26)

❏ DIAGNOSTIC EVALUATION

The steps, necessary to establish the diagnosis of PH and which WHO Group patients belong to, are outlined in the diagnostic algorithm (Flowchart 2), which was published as part of the most recent ACCF/AHA consensus statement guidelines on PH. It should be recognized that definitive diagnosis might require additional specific evaluations not necessarily included in this general guideline.

Physical examination findings in PAH are listed in Table 2. An abnormal chest radiograph (X-ray) is present in 90% of IPAH patients at diagnosis. Typical findings include clear lung fields with enlarged central pulmonary arteries and "pruning" of the peripheral vasculature. In addition, the presence of RV enlargement can be suggested on a lateral chest X-ray by a reduction or obliteration of the normal retrosternal space (Figs 3A and B). Infiltrates on the chest X-ray may suggest the presence of ILD or pulmonary venous hypertension due to left heart abnormalities as the cause of PH. In addition, hilar adenopathy may be suggestive of sarcoidosis. Of note, a normal chest X-ray does not exclude postcapillary PH since many patients with chronic pulmonary venous hypertension may not have pulmonary venous congestion on chest imaging.

The electrocardiogram (ECG) (Fig. 4) may provide evidence of PH by showing RV hypertrophy (R > S in lead V1 and/or V2, right axis deviation, S1Q3T3 pattern); incomplete or complete right bundle branch block; strain pattern (ST depressions and/or T wave inversions in the anterior precordial leads and occasionally in the inferior leads) and right atrial enlargement

FLOWCHART 2: Diagnostic approach to pulmonary arterial hypertension

Pivotal tests	Contingent tests	Contribute to assessment of:
History, Examination, CXR, ECG		• Index of suspicion of PH
Echocardiogram	TEE, Exercise echo	• RVE, RAE, RVSP, RV Function • Left heart disease • VHD, CHD
VQ scan	Pulmonary angiography, Chest CT angiogram, Coagulopathy profile	• Chronic PE
PFTs	ABGs	• Ventilatory function • Gas exchange
Overnight oximetry	Polysomnography	• Sleep disorder
HIV ANA LFTs	Other CTD serologies	• HIV Infection • Scleroderma, SLE, RA • Porto-PH
Functional test (6MWT, CPET)		• Establish baseline • Prognosis
RH cath	Vasodilator test, Exercise RH cath, Volume loading, Left heart cath	• Confirmation of PH • Hemodynamic profile • Vasodilator response

(Abbreviations: 6MWT: Six-minute walk test; ABGs: Arterial blood gases; ANA: Antinuclear antibody serology; Cath: Catheterization; CHD: Congenital heart disease; CPET: Cardiopulmonary exercise test; CT: Computed tomography; CTD: Connective tissue disease; CXR: Chest X-ray; ECG: Electrocardiogram; Exam: Examination; HIV: Human immunodeficiency virus screening; LFT: Liver function test; PE: Pulmonary embolism; PFT: Pulmonary function test; PH: Pulmonary hypertension; RAE: Right atrial enlargement; RA: Rheumatoid arthritis; RH Cath: Right heart catheterization; RVE: Right ventricular enlargement; RVSP: Right ventricular systolic pressure; SLE: Systemic lupus erythematosus; TEE: Transesophageal echocardiography; VHD: Valvular heart disease; VQ Scan: Ventilation-perfusion scintigram)

Table 2: Physical examination findings in pulmonary arterial hypertension

Findings in pulmonary arterial hypertension
- Left parasternal lift
- Increased intensity of P2
- Holosystolic murmur of tricuspid regurgitation
- Diastolic murmur of pulmonary regurgitation
- Right ventricular S3 and S4
- Elevated jugular venous pressure
- Positive hepatojugular reflux
- Hepatomegaly
- Ascites with abdominal distention
- Lower extremity edema

Contd...

Contd...

Table 2: Physical examination findings in pulmonary arterial hypertension

Findings that may suggest causes of associated pulmonary arterial hypertension or pulmonary hypertension
- Pulmonary rales
- Central cyanosis
- Digital clubbing
- Raynaud's phenomenon
- Sclerodactyly, telangiectasias, Raynaud's phenomenon, calcinosis
- Spider angiomata

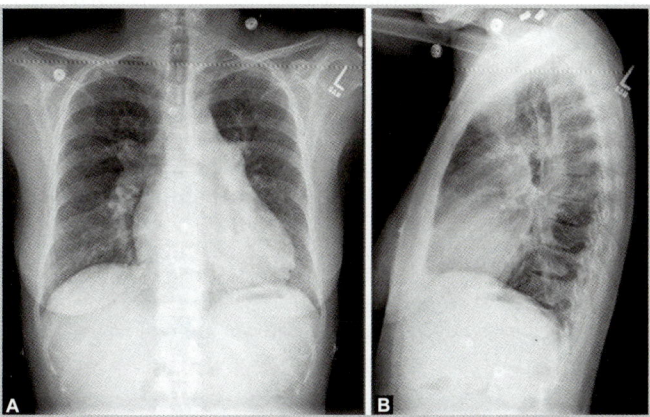

FIGURES 3A AND B: Chest radiograph of a patient with pulmonary arterial hypertension. (A) Posteroanterior chest radiograph showing enlarged pulmonary arteries with pruning of peripheral vasculature. (B) Lateral view demonstrating obliteration of retrosternal space due to right ventricular enlargement

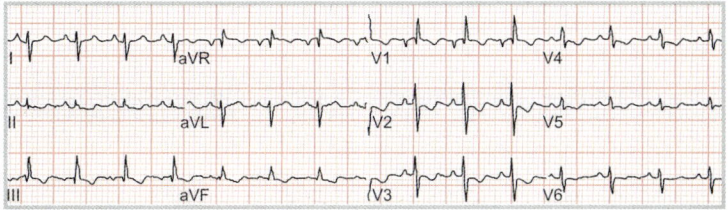

FIGURE 4: Electrocardiogram of 44-year-old woman with right axis deviation, right ventricular hypertrophy with repolarization abnormality and right atrial abnormality

(tall P wave in lead II). RV hypertrophy on the ECG is present in 87% and right axis deviation in 79% of patients with IPAH. It is important to note that the ECG has insufficient sensitivity (55%) and specificity (70%) to be the sole screening tool for detecting significant PAH.

Role of Echocardiography

Transthoracic echocardiography (TTE) with Doppler interrogation is the most useful and readily available noninvasive tool to screen for PH. In most cases of moderate-to-severe PH, the RV is hypertrophied and dilated, often with reduced systolic function. The right atrium is often dilated to various degrees, depending on the degree of RV failure and tricuspid regurgitation, and the left heart chamber volumes are typically reduced, also depending on the degree of RV enlargement and severity of PAH disease (Figures 5 to 7).

Laboratory Studies

Laboratory evaluation for CTD, HIV infection and liver disease should be performed including serologic studies for antinuclear antibody, HIV and liver function tests. A history of stimulant or toxin exposure, in particular anorexigens, methamphetamines and cocaine should be queried and toxicology studies should be performed if indicated. Thyroid function tests should also be evaluated as hyperthyroidism can contribute to PH (WHO Group 5 PH).

Pulmonary Function Testing

DLCO corrected for alveolar volume can be useful in discriminating between SSc related PAH and SSc associated ILD. A disproportionately low DLCO in patients with SSc (Forced vital capacity/DLCO ratio of >1.4) suggests that pulmonary arterial disease may also be present. If PFT testing indicates the presence of a significant obstructive or restrictive ventilatory defect, then high resolution computed tomography (HRCT) should be considered to evaluate for the presence

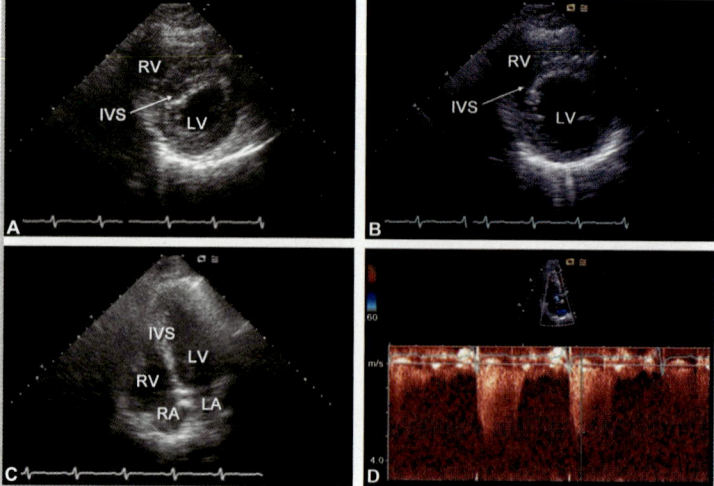

FIGURES 5A TO D: Mild pulmonary arterial hypertension suggested by parasternal short axis views showing flat IVS during (A) systole, but not in (B) diastole indicating RV pressure overload. (C) Apical four-chamber view showing borderline increased RV volume. (D) Continuous wave Doppler image of the TR jet velocity of 2.7 m/sec, equivalent to a PASP of 30 mm Hg plus the RA pressure. (Abbreviations: LA: Left atrium; LV: Left ventricle; RA: Right atrium; RV: Right ventricle; IVS: Interventricular septum; TR: Tricuspid regurgitation; PASP: Pulmonary artery systolic pressure)

Pulmonary Vascular Disease and Adult Congenital Heart Disease

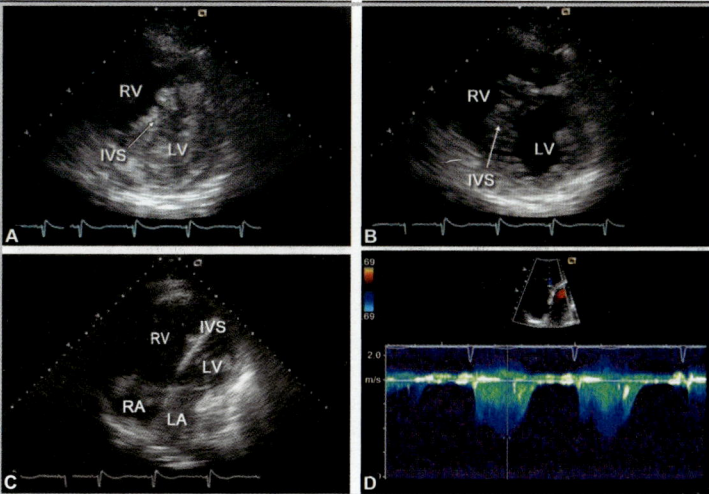

FIGURES 6A TO D: Moderately severe pulmonary arterial hypertension. (A) Parasternal short axis view demonstrates flattening of the IVS during systole, indicating RV pressure overload, (B) but not in diastole. (C) Apical four-chamber view showing moderately to severely enlarged RV. (D) Continuous wave Doppler image of the TR jet velocity of 4.7 m/sec, equivalent to a PASP of 89 mm Hg plus the RA pressure. (Abbreviations: LA: Left atrium; LV: Left ventricle; RA: Right atrium; RV: Right ventricle; IVS: Interventricular septum; TR: Tricuspid regurgitation; PASP: Pulmonary artery systolic pressure)

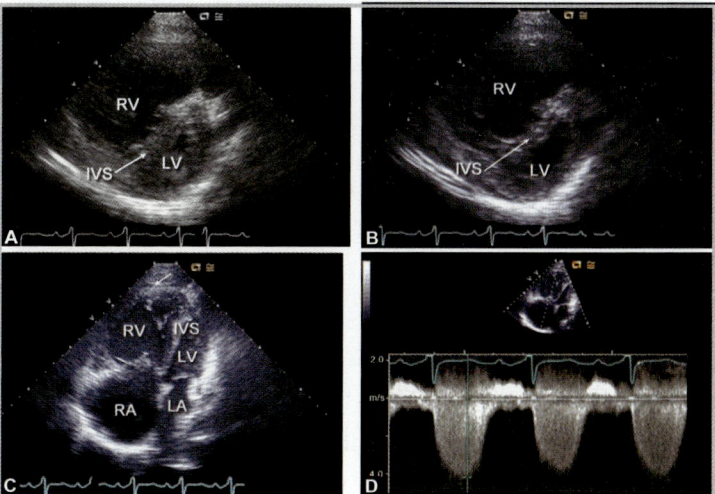

FIGURES 7A TO D: Severe pulmonary arterial hypertension. (A) Parasternal short axis demonstrating flattening of the IVS during both systole and (B) diastole, suggesting both pressure and volume overload. (C) Apical four-chamber view demonstrates severe enlargement and hypertrophy of the RV and severe RA enlargement with small, compressed left heart chambers. (D) The RV/RA pressure gradient in this case is estimated to be 69 mm Hg, so depending on the RA pressure, the PASP may be severely elevated, or it could be relatively lower because of RV failure and inability of the RV to generate a higher PASP. (Abbreviations: arrow: RV hypertrophy; LA: Left atrium; LV: Left ventricle; RA: Right atrium; RV: Right ventricle; IVS: Interventricular septum; TR: Tricuspid regurgitation; PASP: Pulmonary artery systolic pressure)

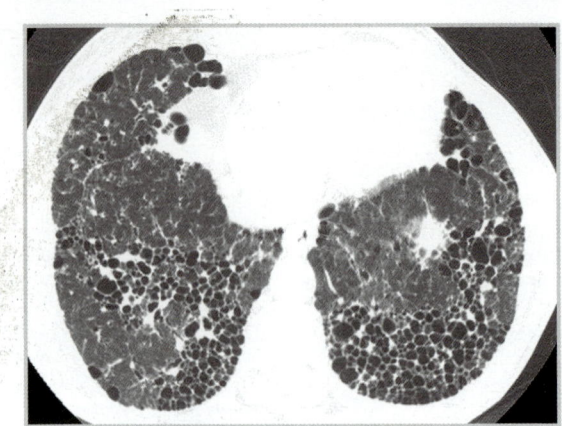

FIGURE 8: High resolution computed tomography of the chest showing severe interstitial lung disease with diffuse honeycombing

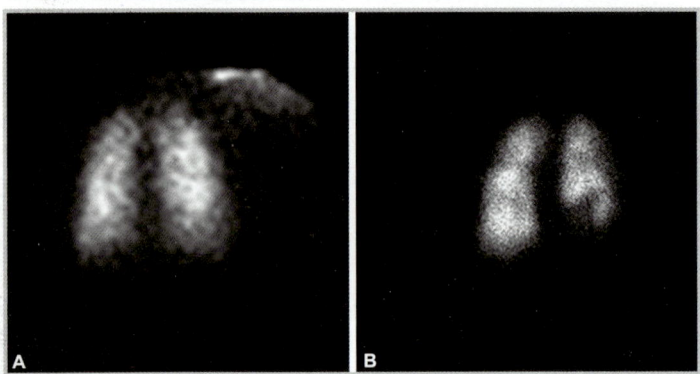

FIGURES 9A AND B: Pulmonary ventilation-perfusion (V/Q) scan. (A) Ventilation image demonstrating homogenous uptake of radioisotope. (B) Perfusion image demonstrating multiple bilateral peripheral subsegmental mismatched defects consistent with chronic thromboembolic disease

of COPD/emphysema or ILDs, such as IPF, usual interstitial pneumonia, nonspecific interstitial pneumonia and hypersensitivity pneumonitis, etc. (Fig. 8).

Screen for Chronic Thromboembolic Pulmonary Hypertension

All patients with PH should be screened for CTEPH, which in selected patients can be surgically treated. Although chest computed tomographic angiography (CTA) has adequate sensitivity for the detection of acute PE, it can miss chronic thromboemboli affecting the more distal, small pulmonary arteries. The ventilation/perfusion (V/Q) scan has greater sensitivity for detecting chronic pulmonary thromboemboli and is, therefore, the preferred initial screening modality for CTEPH (Fig. 9). A patient whose V/Q scan is suggestive of CTEPH should be further evaluated with chest CTA and/or pulmonary angiography to evaluate the extent and location of pulmonary emboli and to exclude other causes of pulmonary arterial obstruction such as endovascular tumors or extrinsic compression from mass lesions.

Right Heart Catheterization

All patients suspected of having PAH by noninvasive studies should have a diagnostic RHC by clinicians trained in its performance and hemodynamic interpretation. In addition to providing confirmation of PH as suggested by echocardiogram and measuring its severity, the RHC provides important prognostic information including RAP, PVR and CO. Determination of the PAWP is of fundamental importance to distinguish between precapillary and postcapillary PH, as the treatment is distinct. If the PAWP is elevated despite multiple attempts and, especially, if blood obtained in the wedge position is not fully saturated, direct measurement of LVEDP should strongly be considered so as not to incorrectly diagnose patients with pulmonary venous hypertension who in fact have PAH. A shunt evaluation with blood oximetry sampling from the superior vena cava and pulmonary artery should be obtained in every case; however, in patients suspected of having CHD, a complete shunt evaluation should always be performed. Coronary angiography is also frequently indicated to exclude coronary artery disease as the potential cause of a patient's symptoms when there are risk factors.

Vasoreactivity Testing

A vasodilator challenge should be performed in all patients with IPAH to identify the small proportion (~12% of IPAH patients) who might respond to calcium channel blocker (CCB) therapy.

Common agents used for acute vasoreactivity testing include inhaled nitric oxide (iNO), intravenous epoprostenol and intravenous adenosine. Other vasodilators, such as nitroprusside or CCBs should not be used in cases of precapillary PH due to the possibility of profound systemic hypotension and hemodynamic collapse. In patients with pulmonary venous hypertension from left-heart disease who are being considered for heart transplantation, vasodilator testing with nitroprusside may be performed. A typical vasoreactivity test protocol for PAH is to administer iNO at 20 ppm for 10 minutes after which hemodynamics are reassessed. The current definition of a positive test is defined as a decrease in the mPAP greater than 10 mm Hg to an mPAP to less than 40 mm Hg with near normal or improved CO. In patients with a positive acute vasoreactivity test, hemodynamic assessment to confirm the response to CCBs should be performed before discharging the patient on this therapy. Patients with severe RV failure (cardiac index <2.2 and/or RAP >15 mm Hg) are not candidates for CCB therapy because of their negative inotropic properties.

❏ THERAPEUTIC OPTIONS FOR THE TREATMENT OF PULMONARY ARTERIAL HYPERTENSION

Conventional therapy with coumadin, diuretics and digoxin, and CCBs are largely based on empiric evidence and retrospective studies. The currently approved disease specific therapies for PAH are directed primarily toward three distinct pathways that are involved in the pathogenesis of PAH, including the endothelin, nitric oxide and prostacyclin pathways. In general, the goals of therapy with these agents are to improve functional capacity, decrease time to clinical worsening and to improve mortality.

Adjuvant/Conventional Therapies

Anticoagulation

The evidence for favorable effects of oral anticoagulant treatment in patients with IPAH, HPAH or PAH associated with anorexigens is based on retrospective analyses from seven studies, of which five were positive and two were negative. The survival of anticoagulated patients selected on the basis of clinical judgment was improved, as compared with a concurrent population that was not treated with oral anticoagulants. Three-year survival improved from 21 to 49% in the series reported by Fuster et al., and the 3- and 5-year survival rates increased from 31 to 47% and from 31 to 62%, respectively, in the series reported by Rich et al.

A goal international normalized ratio (INR) of 1.5–2.5 is currently recommended for patients with PAH. The role of newer oral anticoagulants, such as dabigatran, is uncertain.

Diuretics

Diuretics are frequently required to control congestion in patients with PAH and RV failure. In particular, loop diuretics, such as furosemide, bumetanide, and torsemide, are used in clinical practice. Goals of therapy should be to reduce jugular venous pressure to normal, and eliminate renal venous and hepatic congestion while avoiding hypotension.

Digitalis

Data regarding the use of digoxin in PAH is limited to a single study, which demonstrated that the short term administration of digoxin was associated with increase in CO and reduction in neurohormonal activation. As with all patients treated with digoxin, there is a narrow therapeutic window and the goal serum digoxin concentration should be less than 0.8 ng/mL.

Calcium Channel Blockers

Patients with IPAH who during RHC have a positive vasodilator may benefit from therapy with CCBs, and 5-year survival can be as high as 95% for those who have clinical response. Patients who have not had a vasodilator study should not be started on CCBs. Typical agents include the dihydropyridines amlodipine or nifedipine, or the nondihydropyridine diltiazem. These drugs should be initiated cautiously as hypotension and hemodynamic collapse can occur. Verapamil should not be used due to its potential negative inotropic effects. Patients being treated with CCBs should have invasive hemodynamics monitored at least yearly to ensure a sustained response (mPAP <40 mm Hg with normal or near-normal CO and NYHA/WHO class I or II) since a substantial proportion of patients fail to respond long term and should be considered for PAH specific therapy. Indeed, only approximately 8% of IPAH will continue to respond to CCB therapy over the following year.

Disease-specific Therapies for Pulmonary Arterial Hypertension

Prostacyclin Analogues

Epoprostenol (Flolan® and Veletri®), a prostacyclin analogue, is administered as a continuous intravenous infusion through a central venous catheter. Flolan was the first FDA approved therapy for PAH and remains the only therapy proven to improve survival. Epoprostenol (Flolan®) has to be reconstituted into solution and it is characterized by a short half-life of 3–6 minutes and instability at room temperature that requires it to be maintained on ice in order to prevent degradation. Importantly, because epoprostenol has a short half-life, if the drug infusion is interrupted, patients can develop rebound worsening of PH, which can be life threatening. Likewise, inadvertent bolus administration can lead to life-threatening systemic vasodilation and hypotension.

In the landmark 12-week prospective, randomized, multicenter, open-label trial by Barst et al., 81 patients with IPAH and FPAH were studied in an open-label trial of intravenous epoprostenol versus conventional therapy. At 12 weeks, patients in the epoprostenol group had significant increases in the primary endpoint of 6MWD from 315 to 362 m as compared to a decrease from 270 to 204 m in the control group. The difference in change between the two groups was 60 m. There were significant improvements in mPAP, cardiac index, stroke volume and PVR with epoprostenol therapy. Most importantly, eight patients in the control group and none in the treatment group died during the 12-week study period, the difference of which was highly statistically significant.

It should also be noted that there are limited data regarding the use of epoprostenol in treating other WHO Groups of PH and its use is currently restricted to PAH (WHO Group 1 PH). Moreover, its use can be associated with increased pulmonary shunt flow and hypoxemia in patients with ILD (WHO Group 3 PH) and reduced survival in patients with systolic heart failure (WHO Group 2 PH).

Due to its longer half-life of 4.5 hours and stability at room temperature, treprostinil (Remodulin®) can offer an alternative to epoprostenol. It was originally developed and studied as a subcutaneous infusion but currently can be administered as an intravenous infusion, or as an inhaled formulation.

Simonneau et al. conducted a 12-week, double-blind, placebo-controlled multicenter trial in 470 patients with PAH and NYHA functional classes II–IV symptoms who were randomized to subcutaneous treprostinil versus placebo. 6MWD in the treprostinil group improved at week 12 by 10 m but was unchanged in the placebo group with a difference in mean distance walked between the two groups of 16 m (95% CI, 4.4–27.6 m, P = 0.006). Improvements in 6MWD were dose dependent. In addition, improvements in walk distance were greatest among the sicker patients but were independent of PAH disease etiology.

Inhaled delivery exists for both iloprost (Ventavis®) and treprostinil (Tyvaso™). Iloprost is administered via the handheld portable I-neb Adaptive Aerosol Delivery System every two hours while the patient is awake for a total of six to nine times daily. It is breath activated and tailors the administration to the patient's breathing pattern to precisely deliver the intended amount of drug. The device also contains a computer microchip, which can be analyzed with insight software that provides useful information, such as patient compliance and treatment times. Inhalational treprostinil is administered via an ultrasonic nebulizer and the total dose is administered in less than one minute with 3–9 breaths. Dosing is four times daily (approximately every four hours while awake).

The recently published randomized, double-blind, 12-week placebo-controlled TRIUMPH-1 trial (TReprostinil Sodium Inhalation Used in the Management of Pulmonary Hypertension-1) studied inhaled treprostinil in 235 patients with NYHA function class III–IV symptoms with PAH who remained symptomatic on bosentan or sildenafil. The primary endpoint, or change from baseline to week 12 in 6MWD measured at 10–60 minutes after treprostinil inhalation, was 21.6

m in the treprostinil group and 3.0 m in the placebo group. Between the group median difference was 20 m (95% CI 8.0–32.8 m, p = 0.0004). Although quality of life measures and NT-proBNP improved with therapy, there was no change in the secondary endpoint of time to clinical worsening, perhaps because to overall event rate was lower than expected.

The choice of prostacyclin or prostacyclin analogue and the route of administration are determined by a combination of degree of illness and patient factors, including strong preference of route, social support, manual dexterity and distance of the patient from hospitals with staff trained their management. Common side effects of prostacyclins and prostacyclin analogues include headache, flushing, jaw pain, nausea, diarrhea, hypotension, dizziness, and leg pain. Patients with intravenous catheters are at risk for infection and thrombosis, as well as interruption of therapy. The inhaled agents are commonly associated with a cough.

Endothelin Receptor Antagonists

Endothelin receptor antagonists were the first oral therapy approved by the FDA for treatment of PAH and offered an alternative to the more complex prostacyclin based therapies. Channick et al. initially evaluated the dual ERA bosentan (Tracleer®) as compared to placebo in a 12-week pilot trial

(Study 351) of 32 patients with PPH (IPAH or FPAH) and SSc-PAH, and WHO functional class II–III symptoms. Patients treated with bosentan increased 6MWD at week 12 from 360 to 430 m. In contrast, placebo treated patients decreased from 355 to 349 m. The mean change in 6MWD was 76 m further for treated as compared to placebo patients (95% CI 12–139 m, p = 0.021). In addition, significant benefits were seen in cardiac index, PVR, mPAP, PAWP and mean RAP.

The BREATHE-1 trial corroborated these findings in a pivotal 16-week, double-blind, placebo-controlled randomized trial in 213 patients with WHO functional class III–IV symptoms due to IPAH/FPAH or CTD-PAH. Bosentan resulted in an increase in 6MWD by 36 m whereas patients receiving placebo experienced a decrease in 8 m (mean difference of 44 m) (95% CI 21–67 m, p <0.001). Notably, patients in BREATHE-1 experienced a significantly greater time to clinical worsening as compared to placebo treated patients and 89% of the patients on bosentan were event free after 28 weeks as compared to 63% of the patients treated with placebo (p = 0.0038).

Ambrisentan (Letairis®), which is an endothelin receptor-A selective antagonist, was studied as an alternative to bosentan. The ARIES-1 and -2 studies were concurrent, randomized, double-blind, placebo-controlled studies that compared different doses of ambrisentan versus placebo. The ARIES-1 trial compared 5 mg and 10 mg of ambrisentan, whereas the ARIES-2 trial compared 2.5 mg and 5 mg of bosentan versus placebo. The placebo-corrected 6MWD at 12 weeks was significantly improved with all doses of ambrisentan as compared to placebo. Time to clinical worsening was also significantly delayed in patients taking ambrisentan as compared to placebo in the combined analysis of ARIES-1 and -2, although the difference were not significantly different in the ARIES-1 trial alone.

Side effects of ERAs include peripheral edema, potential for liver toxicity, anemia, reduced hormonal contraceptive efficacy, reduced sperm count and drug-drug interactions with strong inducers or inhibitors of cytochrome P450 enzymes.

Phosphodiesterase Type 5 Inhibitors

Due to the lack of significant difference in 6MWD among the dosing regimens, the FDA only approved sildenafil for PAH at 20 mg three times daily, although the study had shown a trend toward improved walk distances with higher doses.

In contrast to sildenafil, tadalafil (Adcirca®) is longer acting with a half-life of 17.5 hours, and can be dosed once daily. The PHIRST (PAH and Response to Tadalafil) trial evaluated 405 patients with idiopathic or associated PAH in a 16-week randomized, double-blind, dose-ranging double-dummy, placebo-controlled trial. Patients were randomized to 2.5 mg, 10 mg, 20 mg, or 40 mg daily of tadalafil versus placebo. A statistically significant improvement in 6MWD was only seen in the 40 mg dose strata with mean placebo-corrected treatment effect of 33 m (95% CI, 15–50 m, p <0.01). Additionally, tadalafil at 40 mg daily, but not in the other dosing groups, demonstrated increased time to clinical worsening as compared to placebo (P = 0.041). Notably, there were no significant differences in change in WHO functional class or Borg dyspnea score between any of the treatment groups, although improvements in quality of life were seen with 40 mg daily of tadalafil as compared to placebo.

Sildenafil and tadalafil are metabolized by the cytochrome P450 (CYP) 3A4 pathway, although about 20% of sidenafil's metabolism is also by CYP2C9. Simultaneous use with other inhibitors of CYP3A4 or CYP2C9, such as ketoconazole, erythromycin, HIV protease inhibitors and grape fruit juice, should be used with caution. It is an absolute contraindication to use nitrates with any of the PDE5Is as life-threatening hypotension can develop. Clinically relevant side effects of PDE5 inhibitors include headaches, dizziness, nausea, and priapism. Sildenafil, and to a lesser extent, tadalafil, can cause epistaxis, possibly through inhibition of platelet aggregation.

Invasive and Surgical Options

Atrial septostomy (AS) can be a useful strategy to increase CO and unload the right ventricle by creating an interatrial communication to allow right to left shunting in patients with severe RV failure despite vasodilator therapy or intolerance to vasodilator therapy. In addition, in resource poor settings where the cost of vasodilator therapy may be prohibitive, it can be a viable alternative. The procedure should not be performed in patients with severely decompensated right heart failure (RA pressure >20 mm Hg) because the degree of right to left shunting with resultant hypoxemia can be substantial and outcomes are worse.

The eventual need for lung transplantation should be anticipated early in the course of the disease and patients with advanced disease (WHO functional class III–IV) should be referred to centers that specialize in lung transplantation.

❏ TREATMENT ALGORITHM AND EVALUATING RESPONSE TO THERAPY

Therapeutic decisions should be based on assessment of clinical status, risk factors for deterioration or death and response to vasodilator testing. Flowchart 3 shows the algorithm for the management of PAH as outlined in the latest American College of Cardiology Foundation/American College of Chest Physicians guidelines. There is emerging evidence that earlier initiation of therapy when patients are mildly symptomatic improves functional and clinical status.

Theoretically, combination therapy is attractive as targeting the separate pathways (i.e. endothelin, nitric oxide and prostacyclin pathways) may have

FLOWCHART 3: Algorithm for the treatment of PAH

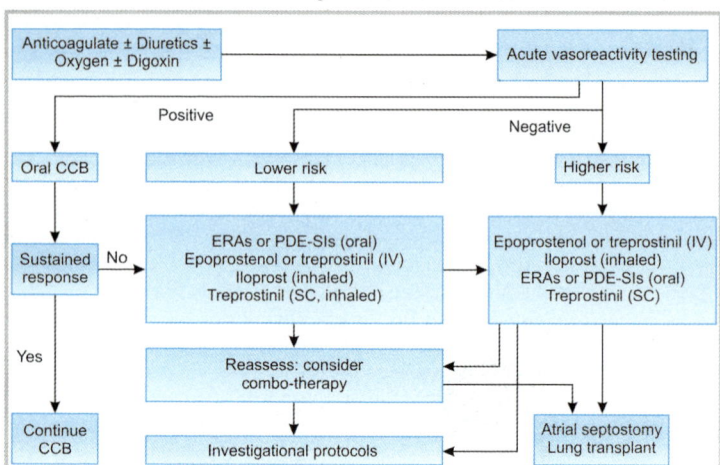

(Abbreviations: CCB: Calcium channel blocker; ERAs: Endothelin receptor antagonists; IV: Intravenous; PDE-5Is: Phosphodiesterase type 5 inhibitors; SC: Subcutaneous)

additive effects. However, there are few studies to guide this approach, and combination therapy is an active area of research. Based on the very poor expected survival and few therapeutic options, as well as the results of the above studies, most PAH specialists will institute combination therapy in higher risk patients, patients who do not improve to functional class I or II, or those patients whose disease progresses while on monotherapy. Patients may experience increased side effects, such as flushing and headaches, with combination therapy and the potential for drug interactions should be closely monitored.

❏ THERAPY OF DECOMPENSATED RIGHT HEART FAILURE IN PULMONARY ARTERIAL HYPERTENSION

Patients presenting with acute or progressive right heart failure with decompensation pose a unique clinical challenge. An algorithm for the management of acutely decompensated RV failure in patients with PAH has been outlined in Flowchart 4. Efforts should be made to distinguish acute decompensation due to progressive right-sided failure as compared to events that can acutely lead to decompensation, such as PE, anemia, thyroid disorders and hypoxia. In patients with a central venous catheter for infusion of a prostacyclin analogue, infection should always be considered. Patients should be monitored in an intensive care unit or transferred to a facility skilled in the management of patients with PAH. A central line can be useful to administer inotropes, measure central venous pressures and to obtain central venous oxygen saturation, which can be used to estimate CO. If central access cannot be obtained, echocardiographic estimates of CO through pulmonary and LV outflow tract velocity time integral can give estimates of CO, which can be helpful to guide therapy.

FLOWCHART 4: Algorithm for management of acutely decompensated right ventricular failure

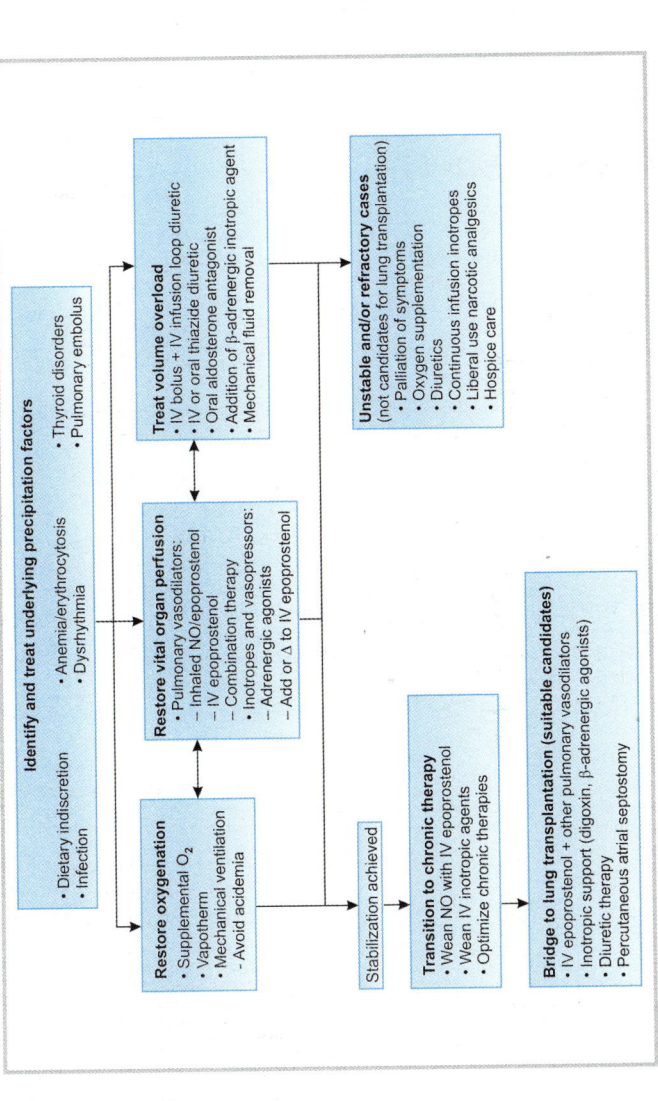

(Abbreviations: IV: Intravenous; NO: Nitric oxide). (*Source*: DeMarco T, McGlothlin D. Managing right ventricular failure in pulmonary arterial hypertension: an algorithmic approach. Advances in pulmonary hypertension. 2005;4(4):16-26)

CONCLUSION

In summary, PAH is a rare disease with poor survival, especially if left undiagnosed and inadequately. There are many disease states that are associated with PAH, each of which has unique prognosis and epidemiology, but all of which result in similar pathologic manifestations. Therapy for PAH has evolved significantly in the modern era, and outcomes have improved with treatment with prostacyclin analogs, ERAs and PDE5Is. Continued research is needed to further improve the prognostication, treatment and outcome of this devastating disease.

SUGGESTED READINGS

Barst RJ, Rubin LJ, Long WA, et al. A comparison of continuous intravenous epoprostenol (prostacyclin) with conventional therapy for primary pulmonary hypertension. The Primary Pulmonary Hypertension Study Group. N Engl J Med. 1996;334:296-302.

Channick RN, Simonneau G, Sitbon O, et al. Effects of the dual endothelin-receptor antagonist bosentan in patients with pulmonary hypertension: a randomised placebo-controlled study. Lancet. 2001;358:1119-23.

Chatterjee K, De Marco T, Alpert JS. Pulmonary hypertension: hemodynamic diagnosis and management. Arch Intern Med. 2002;162:1925-33.

Galie N, Brundage BH, Ghofrani HA, et al. Tadalafil therapy for pulmonary arterial hypertension. Circulation. 2009;119:2894-903.

Hoeper MM, Welte T. Sildenafil citrate therapy for pulmonary arterial hypertension. N Engl J Med. 2006;354:1091-3.

McGoon M, Gutterman D, Steen V, et al. Screening, early detection, and diagnosis of pulmonary arterial hypertension: ACCP evidence based clinical practice guidelines. Chest. 2004;126:14S-34S.

McLaughlin VV, Archer SL, Badesch DB, et al. ACCF/AHA 2009 expert consensus document on pulmonary hypertension a report of the American College of Cardiology Foundation Task Force on Expert Consensus Documents and the American Heart Association developed in collaboration with the American College of Chest Physicians; American Thoracic Society, Inc.; and the Pulmonary Hypertension Association. J Am Coll Cardiol. 2009;53:1573-619.

McLaughlin VV, Benza RL, Rubin LJ, et al. Addition of inhaled treprostinil to oral therapy for pulmonary arterial hypertension: a randomized controlled clinical trial. J Am Coll Cardiol. 2010;55:1915-22.

O'Callaghan DS, Savale L, Jais X, et al. Evidence for the use of combination targeted therapeutic approaches for the management of pulmonary arterial hypertension. Respir Med. 2010;104:S74-80.

Pugh ME, Hemnes AR. Pulmonary hypertension in women. Expert Rev Cardiovasc Ther. 2010;8:1549-58.

Rubin LJ, Badesch DB, Barst RJ, et al. Bosentan therapy for pulmonary arterial hypertension. N Engl J Med. 2002;346:896-903.

Simonneau G, Barst RJ, Galie N, et al. Continuous subcutaneous infusion of treprostinil, a prostacyclin analogue, in patients with pulmonary arterial hypertension: a double-blind, randomized, placebo-controlled trial. Am J Respir Crit Care Med. 2002;165:800-4.

Simonneau G, Robbins IM, Beghetti M, et al. Updated clinical classification of pulmonary hypertension. J Am Coll Cardiol. 2009;54:S43-54.

9.2 Congenital Heart Disease in the Adult Patient

ACYANOTIC HEART DISEASE

Acyanotic heart disease includes the following lesions: left-sided heart obstructive lesions, aortic valve disease, subvalvular and supravalvular aortic stenosis, and coarctation of the aorta.

❑ CONGENITAL VALVAR AORTIC STENOSIS

Congenital aortic stenosis in children and young adults occurs secondary to leaflet dysplasia and/or fusion of one or more leaflets, creating a functionally bicuspid or unicuspid aortic valve. Unicuspid aortic valves can produce severe obstruction are more likely to present in infancy or before 1 year of age. Bicuspid aortic valves (BAVs) occur more frequently than unicuspid valves and can be asymptomatic until middle age (Figs 10A to D). The valve is often dysplastic and, with time, may

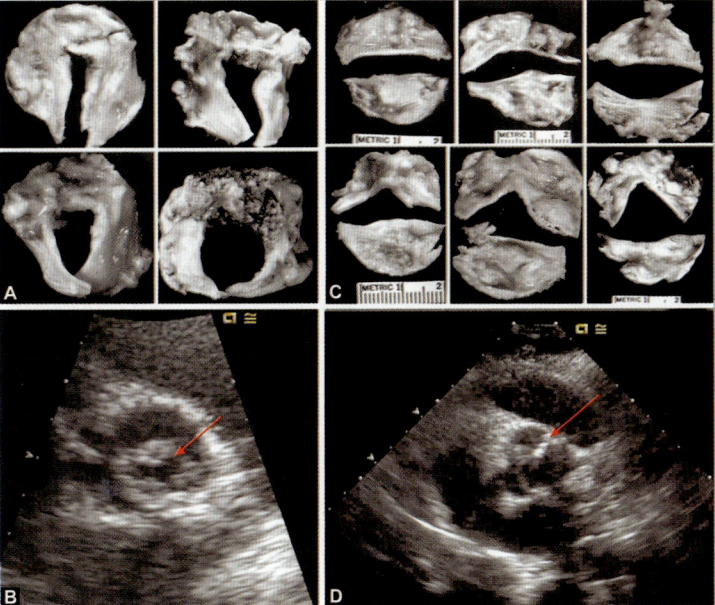

FIGURES 10A TO D: (A) Pathologic specimens from excised valves demonstrating unicommissural morphology. (B) Still frame of parasternal short axis (PSAX) view demonstrating unicommissural valve in end-systolic frame with a "keyhole" appearance (arrow). (C) Excised specimens of bicuspid aortic valves. (D) Still frame of PSAX view at end-systole demonstrating bicuspid valve with fusion of the raphe between the right and left coronary cusps (arrow). (*Source:* Roberts WC, Ko JM. Frequency by decades of unicuspid, bicuspid, and tricuspid aortic valves in adults having isolated aortic valve replacement for aortic stenosis, with or without associated aortic regurgitation. Circulation. 2005;111:920-5, with permission)

become thickened with rolled and calcified leaflets. As a consequence, stenosis and/or regurgitation develop with a left ventricular (LV) to aortic pressure gradient.

The most common fusion is of the right and left coronary cusp, in which case both coronaries arise from the same large anterior sinus. The second most common pathology of fusion is the right and noncoronary cusp, in which case the coronaries arise from two separate cusps. The male-to-female ratio is approximately 2–3:1.

The BAV can be associated with subaortic stenosis, parachute mitral valve, coarctation of the aorta, ventricular septal defect (VSD) and patent ductus arteriosus (PDA). Shone's syndrome is the presence of multiple left-sided heart obstructions, which may include subaortic stenosis, BAV, coarctation, parachute mitral valve or supravalvular mitral valve ring.

A mutation in the NOTCH1 gene has been described in families with an inheritance pattern for BAV. It is autosomal dominant with incomplete penetrance pattern.

Clinical Findings

An individual with congenital BAV is usually asymptomatic unless hemodynamically significant stenosis or regurgitation is present. Dyspnea, chest pain, and exertional syncope are the classic presenting symptoms.

A patient with BAV reveals an early systolic click and a crescendo-decrescendo systolic murmur at the second right intercostal space radiating to the left carotid. With increasing severity of stenosis the murmur will peak later in systole. If complicated by aortic regurgitation there will be an early diastolic murmur over the aortic area. Once stenosis predominates, the carotid upstroke is delayed and diminished, and the systolic click is no longer present. S2 is single.

Diagnostic Studies

Electrocardiogram (ECG) findings depend on the extent of the hemodynamic derangement, which leads to left ventricular hypertrophy (LVH). Left atrial enlargement may also be present.

Chest X-ray findings are also nonspecific.

Echocardiogram is the primary imaging modality for evaluation of aortic stenosis and aortic regurgitation. On M-mode interrogation, the point of BAV closure may be eccentric. Subaortic stenosis may be associated with early closure of the aortic valve. Two-dimensional (2D) imaging allows for structural assessment of the valve and location of the fused leaflets as well as the origin of the coronary arteries in young patients. According to the 2006 ACC/AHA guidelines for the management of patients with valvular heart disease, the severity of aortic stenosis is assessed by jet velocity, mean gradient, valve area by continuity equation and valve area indexed to body surface area (m^2). The primary echocardiographic parameters for the evaluation of aortic regurgitation are color Doppler jet width, vena contracta width, regurgitant volume, regurgitant fraction, regurgitant orifice area, LV size.

Magnetic resonance imaging and computed tomography must be followed routinely for disease progression. Gadolinium-enhanced magnetic resonance angiography imaging provides an accurate and reproducible alternative for follow-up without exposure to radiation. Post-repair patients also require routine surveillance of the aorta and repair site for which magnetic resonance angiography is accepted as standard of care.

Cardiac catheterization for hemodynamic measurement is recommended for the assessment of severity of aortic stenosis in symptomatic patients when noninvasive tests are inconclusive or where there is discrepancy between noninvasive tests and clinical findings regarding severity of aortic stenosis. Coronary angiography should be performed before valve surgery in high-risk individuals.

Treatment

Medical

Current guidelines do not recommend endocarditis prophylaxis for the native valve. Patients with aortopathy associated with BAV could benefit from beta blockers; however, there is no direct evidence to recommend their use except in the setting of hypertension. In patients with moderate to severe aortic regurgitation, aggressive afterload reduction to reduce LV wall tension with nifedipine and angiotensin-converting enzyme (ACE) inhibitors has been studied and conflicting data exists. There is no data that afterload reduction in these patients delays the need for surgery or intervention and current guidelines recommend their use only in hypertensive patients who are otherwise not candidates for surgery.

Surgical

Surgery is indicated in symptomatic patients with severe aortic stenosis and in asymptomatic patients with severe aortic stenosis who require other cardiac surgery or have reduced ejection fraction less than 50%.

The surgical approach to aortic valve disease is, most frequently, aortic valve replacement. Torn leaflets, prolapsed leaflets and perforated leaflets are more amenable to aortic valve repair. Percutaneous valvuloplasty has been successful in children and adolescents with noncalcified aortic valves.

Pregnancy

Women with mild aortic stenosis and normal LV function can be carried through term with conservative medical management throughout pregnancy. Symptomatic women with moderate to severe aortic stenosis should be advised to delay conception until the aortic stenosis has been treated surgically. Valve replacement prior to pregnancy should be considered if there is evidence of LV dysfunction or reduced exercise tolerance. If a woman, who was asymptomatic prior to pregnancy, develops new symptoms balloon valvotomy prior to labor and delivery may be required, which is a high-risk procedure.

❏ COARCTATION OF THE AORTA

Coarctation of the aorta is a stenosis of the proximal descending thoracic aorta (usually adjacent to the origin of the subclavian artery) or the abdominal aorta. The most common location is distal to the origin of the left subclavian artery (postductal); however, an uncommon manifestation of this disease is stenosis proximal to the left subclavian artery (preductal) (Fig. 11). Coarctation of the thoracic aorta is a fairly common defect accounting for 5% of all the congenital heart lesions. It is two to five times more common in males than in females. Natural history of unrepaired coarctation of the aorta shows a mean age of death of 34 years.

Coarctation of the aorta is often associated with an abnormal aortic valve, most commonly a bicuspid valve, which occurs in up to 50% of patients. When more than one level of obstruction is present, this is termed Shone's syndrome.

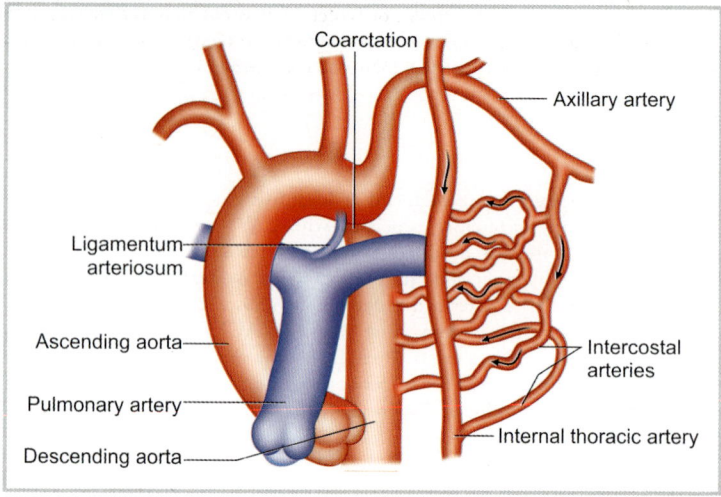

FIGURE 11: Coarctation causes severe obstruction of blood flow in the descending thoracic aorta. Collateral channels from the axillary and internal thoracic arteries through the intercostal arteries (arrows) perfuse the descending aorta and its branches. (*Source:* Brickner ME, Hillis LD, Lange RA. Congenital heart disease in adults. First of two parts. N Engl J Med. 2000;342:256-63, with permission)

Additional associated conditions are VSD, Turner syndrome and berry aneurysms in the circle of Willis occur in 3–5% of the patient with coarctation.

Clinical Findings

Patients with isolated coarctation of the aorta are usually asymptomatic and diagnosis is commonly made on routine physical examination presenting with hypertension. There may be exertional dyspnea, headaches, epistaxis and claudication or leg fatigue.

The systolic blood pressure is elevated in the right arm and usually in the left arm (postductal) with reduced systolic blood pressures in the lower extremities. Diastolic blood pressures are generally unaffected. Delayed arrival of the femoral pulse is noted during simultaneous palpation of the brachial and femoral pulses.

Cardiac examination reveals a nondisplaced but is sustained LV impulse. The first heart sound is normal; the aortic component of the second heart sound may be accentuated. Jugular venous pulse is normal. Carotid upstrokes are brisk. A late systolic murmur, heard best between the scapulae, might be heard as a result of the coarctation. An ejection click and a systolic murmur may be associated with BAV along with a blowing diastolic murmur associated with aortic regurgitation.

Diagnostic Studies

Electrocardiogram is nonspecific with LVH and in later stages left atrial enlargement. *Chest X-ray* shows rib notching which is highly specific for coarctation of the aorta. Another classic radiographic finding is the "3" sign, with the dilated left subclavian forming the upper curvature and the dilated distal aorta forming the lower curvature.

Echocardiogram may miss the region of coarctation if routine suprasternal notch images are not obtained. Doppler evidence of flow acceleration in the descending aorta can be useful even when the 2D images are suboptimal (Figs 12A to C). Localization of the coarctation is possible with multiplanar transesophageal echocardiography (TEE).

Gadolinium-enhanced cardiac magnetic resonance angiography can localize, define and magnify the extent of the coarctation. It provides an estimate of the extent of collateralization, which is helpful in therapeutic decision-making (Fig. 12B).

Computed tomography (CT) angiography provided excellent anatomic definition; however, it does not provide physiologic information.

Catheterization for diagnosis is only necessary when all of the noninvasive imaging methods are inconclusive.

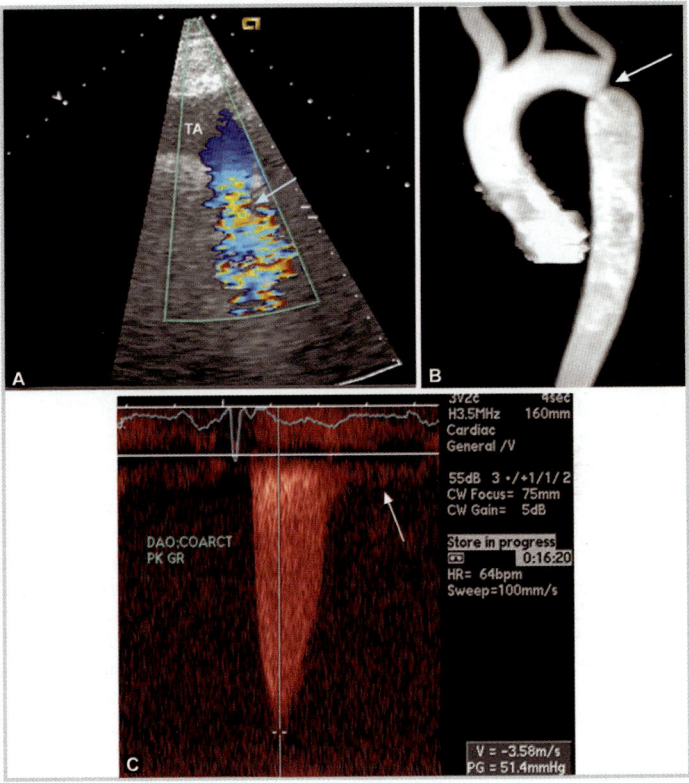

FIGURES 12A TO C: (A) Suprasternal notch view demonstrating flow acceleration by color Doppler through the narrowed region of coarctation (arrow); (B) corresponding image from magnetic resonance angiography of the aorta demonstrating discrete coarctation; (C) continuous wave Doppler peak velocity of 3.5 m/sec through region of coarctation in descending aorta with diastolic runoff (arrow). The gradient, as estimated by the modified Bernoulli's equation, may not correlate with invasively measured gradient, although the presence of diastolic runoff suggests hemodynamically significant coarctation. (Abbreviation: TA: Transverse aorta)

Treatment

Medical

Medical therapy should be geared toward treating hypertension with beta-blockers, ACE inhibitors or angiotensin II receptor blockers as first-line medications. When hypertension persists following either percutaneous or surgical intervention, these medications should be continued.

Surgical and Interventional Correction

The repair strategy often depends upon the age of presentation as well as the anatomy and location of the coarctation. Children often undergo surgical correction. The removal of the abnormal coarctation followed by end-to-end anastomosis is the most desirable procedure. The morphologic variability has precluded the dominance of any one single method. The repair depends on the length of the coarctation and the location of the subclavian artery relative to the coarct.

Surgery for correction in patients, over the age of 15 years, can be challenging because of huge intercostal aneurysms and atheromatous changes in the shelf near the coarctation site. Over the last 10 years, endovascular repair of coarctation has grown in popularity. Compared with surgery, endovascular stents have similar morbidity and mortality but are associated with higher degree of recoarctation, need for repeat interventions, and persistent hypertension. In the light of these differences, there is ongoing controversy about the best treatment.

Treatment of coarctation, either primary or repeat, is indicted if
(a) the peak-to-peak coarctation gradient is greater than or equal to 20 mm Hg, or
(b) peak-to-peak coarctation gradient is less than 20 mm Hg in the presence of significant coarctation with radiological evidence of significant collateral flow.

Pregnancy

It is essential to screen women of childbearing age for postrepair aortic dilatation because of high risk of rupture during pregnancy. The concern is about the integrity of the paracoarctation tissue in these young women. Now, in these patients consideration for removal of the paracoarctation tissue is given.

❏ VALVAR PULMONIC STENOSIS

Congenital pulmonary valve stenosis is characterized by a conical or dome shaped valve formed by the fusion of the valve leaflets. The valve may be tricuspid, bicuspid, unicuspid or dysplastic. Acquired PS is rare but may occur with rheumatic disease and carcinoid heart disease. Valvar PS is the second most common form of CHD and comprises 7% of all congenital heart lesions in adults. The natural history of the isolated mild PS is benign and rarely progresses to severe obstruction.

Congenital PS often coexists with other congenital cardiac abnormalities such as ASD, VSD or PDA. PS may also occur as a part of a more complex congenital heart process such has tetralogy of Fallot (TOF), aortic valve (AV) canal defect, double outlet RV and a univentricular heart.

Clinical Findings

Patients with severe PS usually have exercise intolerance and present with exertional fatigue, dyspnea or chest pain. Exertional syncope or light-headedness may occur if there are systemic or suprasystemic RV pressures, especially in association with dehydration leading to decreased preload.

The physical examination demonstrates a parasternal RV heave and delayed or diminished P2 and a late peaking crescendo-decrescendo murmur. If the valve is pliable, an ejection click may be heard before the murmur. The jugular venous pressure shows a prominent wave as a result of diminished RV compliance. Once RV failure occurs, the jugular venous pressure increases.

Diagnostic Studies

Electrocardiogram demonstrates right ventricular hypertrophy (RVH) with right axis deviation, prominent R waves in the right precordial leads and deep S waves in the left precordial leads.

There may also be evidence of P pulmonale with peaked inferior P waves.

Chest X-ray shows enlarged cardiac silhouette in severe PS especially with right heart failure occurs.

Echocardiography is the method of choice for the diagnosis, assessment of PS. Associated findings, such as RVH, subpulmonic stenosis, septal defects, can also be identified. Color flow Doppler imaging demonstrates high-velocity flow within the PA. Continuous wave (CW) Doppler interrogation demonstrates the high velocity jet and estimates the gradient across the RVOT.

According to the 2006 ACC/AHA guidelines on the management of valvular heart disease, the severity of pulmonary stenosis is defined as follows:
Severe stenosis: A peak jet velocity of 4 m/s (peak gradient 64 mm Hg).
Moderate stenosis: A peak jet velocity of 3–4 m/s (peak gradient 36–64 mm Hg).
Mild stenosis: A peak jet velocity of 3 m/s (peak gradient <36 mm Hg).

Cardiac catheterization is now reserved for patients in whom balloon valvuloplasty is indicated and should be performed in centers capable of this procedure to avoid duplicated procedures.

Treatment

According to current guidelines, patients with untreated or treated pulmonary valve stenosis do not require antibiotics for endocarditis prophylaxis. Most patients, including adults, are treated with balloon valvuloplasty. The long-term results after balloon valvuloplasty are excellent. Surgery is still usually required for the dysplastic valve often seen in Noonan syndrome. Surgical valvotomy via transpulmonary artery incision can be effective with excellent long-term outcomes to avoid prosthetic valve replacement.

Pregnancy

Volume overload combined with a low systemic vascular resistance in pregnancy may precipitate right heart failure in patients with severe PS. Symptomatic patients with severe stenosis during pregnancy may require pulmonary valvotomy during pregnancy, which can be performed safely with uterine shielding especially during the second trimester.

Guidelines

In adults, the treatment for PS according to the "2008 focused update incorporated into the ACC/AHA 2006 guidelines for the management of patients with valvular heart disease" are:
- Patient with mild gradients should be observed

- Symptomatic patients in whom the catheterization peak-to-peak gradient is more than 30 mm Hg (class I)
- Asymptomatic patients, intervention is recommended when gradients across the stenosis is more than 40 mm Hg (class I); however, may be reasonable with gradient 30–39 mm Hg (class IIa)
- Intervention in the absence of pulmonary insufficiency is almost always performed in the catheterization laboratory with balloon valvuloplasty. Some pulmonary regurgitation almost invariably occurs after valvuloplasty, but it is rarely clinically important
- If severe pulmonary insufficiency is present, treatment is surgical, often with a pulmonary valve with a conduit.

❑ ATRIAL SEPTAL DEFECTS

An ASD results in an interatrial communication due to deficient septal tissue causing left-to-right shunting. ASDs make up 7% of CHD in newborns and are relatively commonly encountered in adults.

Classification of ASDs is based on anatomic location (Figs 13A to C):
- Ostium secundum—in the region of the fossa ovalis
- Ostium primum—in the lower portion of the atrial septum
- Sinus venosus defect of the superior vena cava (SVC) results in the SVC overriding both atria
- Coronary sinus defects are rare with an opening of the wall of the coronary sinus communicating to the left atrium allowing left-to-right shunting

As opposed to congenital aortic stenosis, ostium secundum ASD have a 2:1 female preponderance. The ostium primum and sinus venosus ASDs have a 1:1 ratio.

Clinical Findings

The most common presenting symptoms in adults are exercise intolerance and palpitations. Patients with large shunts will have signs and symptoms consistent with right heart failure because of pulmonary hypertension and volume overload. A pathognomonic finding is a fixed split second heart sound. A prominent RV impulse along the left lower sternal border and a palpable PA can be palpated. A systolic ejection murmur is heard secondary to increased flow across the pulmonary valve.

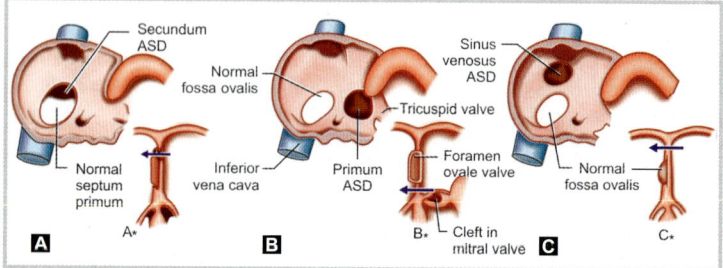

FIGURES 13A TO C: Classification of ASDs based on anatomic location

Diagnostic Studies

Electrocardiogram shows RV conduction delay ["incomplete right bundle branch block (RBBB)"] in 90% of the cases. In ostium secundum ASDs and sinus venosus ASDs, the QRS axis is vertical or rightward. In patients with ostium primum ASDs, the axis is superior and leftward. Abnormal sinus node function in patients with sinus venosus ASD often results in ectopic atrial rhythm with superior P wave axis.

Chest x-ray shows prominent aortic and pulmonary arteries and RV enlargement.

Echocardiogram visualizes most cases of primum and secundum ASDs. However only 70% of sinus venosus defects are visualized by transthoracic imaging and require a high level of clinical suspicion and further imaging with TEE or magnetic resonance. Echocardiographic findings of an ASD include RV enlargement, paradoxical septal motion consistent with volume overload and increased PA flow. Color flow Doppler can identify in the interatrial flow, especially in the four-chamber view.

MRI and CT imaging are especially useful in patients with ASDs to assess anatomy of the pulmonary veins and SVC. Also, phase contrast MRI is another noninvasive way of determining the Q_p/Q_s ratio, with good correlations to invasive measures.

Catheterization is required when equivocal finding are there on noninvasive imaging. Right heart catheterization with repeat blood sampling for oxygenation levels reveals oxygen step-up from the vena cava to the right atrium. A value greater than 90% suggests a large shunt.

Treatment

In adults, hemodynamically insignificant ASDs with Q_p/Q_s less than 1.5 do not require closure unless there is concern for paradoxical emboli. Symptomatic or large ASDs should be closed. In patients with pulmonary hypertension, closure can be considered as long as the pulmonary blood flow is greater than 70% of systemic blood flow.

Endocarditis is rare in patients with ASDs, and prophylaxis is not routinely indicated. Prophylaxis is, however, indicated for the 6 months after surgical and percutaneous ASDs closure.

Pregnancy

Pregnancy in the absence of pulmonary hypertension is generally uncomplicated and well-tolerated. The risk or paradoxical is increased in the peripartum and postpartum period. In women with large shunts detected prior to conception, closure of the ASD is recommended. Pregnancy is contraindicated in Eisenmenger's syndrome.

Guidelines

Class I

- Closure of an ASD either percutaneously or surgically is indicated for right atrial and RV enlargement with or without symptoms. (Level of Evidence: B)
- A sinus venosus, coronary sinus or primum ASD should be repaired surgically rather than by percutaneous closure. (Level of Evidence: B)
- Surgeons with training and expertise in CHD should perform operations for various ASD closures. (Level of Evidence: C)

Class IIa

- Surgical closure of secundum ASD is reasonable when concomitant surgical repair/replacement of a tricuspid valve is considered or when the anatomy of the defect precludes the use of a percutaneous device. (Level of Evidence: C)
- Closure of an ASD, either percutaneously or surgically, is reasonable in the presence of:
  - Paradoxical embolism. (Level of Evidence: C)
  - Documented orthodeoxia-platypnea. (Level of Evidence: B).

Class IIb

- Closure of an ASD, either percutaneously or surgically, may be considered in the presence of net left-to-right shunting, PA pressure less than two-thirds systemic levels, pulmonary vascular resistance (PVR) less than two-thirds systemic vascular resistance, or when responsive to either pulmonary vasodilator therapy or test occlusion of the defect (patients should be treated in conjunction with providers who have expertise in the management of pulmonary hypertensive syndromes). (Level of Evidence: C)
- Concomitant maze procedure may be considered for intermittent or chronic atrial tachyarrhythmias in adults with ASDs. (Level of Evidence: C).

Class III

Patients with severe irreversible pulmonary arterial hypertension (PAH) and no evidence of a left-to-right shunt should not undergo ASD closure. (Level of Evidence: B)

❑ VENTRICULAR SEPTAL DEFECTS

Ventricular septal defect is an abnormal connection between the systemic and pulmonary circulation at a level, which reflects arterial pressures, in contrast to ASDs, and pulmonary venous anomalies, which connect at venous pressure levels. VSD is the most common of all forms of CHD. Twenty percent of all children with CHD have an isolated VSD. This figure is as high as 30% in the newborn population and 10% in the adult congenital population. Acquired VSDs occur secondary to trauma and ischemia.

Most VSDs present in childhood as a murmur or with CHF. Up to 40% close spontaneously so it is uncommon to encounter adults with a previously unrecognized significant VSD. Therefore, most adults present with either small defects of no hemodynamic consequence or large defects associated with Eisenmenger's syndrome.

Classification of VSDs can be based on anatomic location and/or physiology. The anatomic classification includes both the membranous and muscular portions of the ventricular septum (Fig. 14).

Membranous VSDs: This is the most common site for VSDs. The membranous septum lies beneath the aortic valve and behind the tricuspid septal leaflet. Membranous VSDs are subclassified as supracristal (also known as doubly committed subarterial), perimembranous (the inlet portion of the membranous septum) and malalignment (found in TOF with the overriding aorta). These latter defects occur as a result of anterior malalignment of the conal septum; however, the anatomical location is similar to perimembranous VSDs.

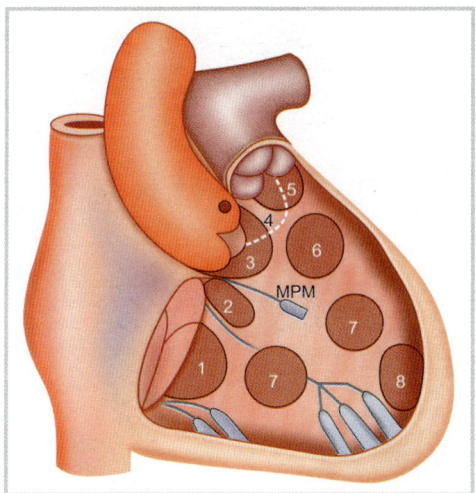

FIGURE 14: Classification of the site of ventricular septal defects as viewed from ventricle. (1–5) subvalvular: 1. Inlet; 2. Subtricuspid; 3. Subaortic; 4. Subarterial doubly committed; 5. Subpulmonary. (6–8) muscular: 6. Outlet; 7. Central; 8. Apical. (Abbreviation: MPM: Medial papillary muscle)

Muscular VSDs: About 10% of the VSDs are muscular defects. They are often multiple and may be located in the inlet or outlet regions or within the trabeculae portion of the septum.

Physiologically they can be divided into two categories:

Restrictive VSDs: A small defect with a large gradient between the ventricles such that the RVSP is less than 50% of the LV systolic pressure.

Non-restrictive VSDs: A large defect with a small gradient between the ventricles such that the RVSP is more than 50% of the LV systolic pressure.

Clinical Findings

Adults with small uncorrected VSDs with normal PA pressures are usually asymptomatic. Rarely, large VSDs without pulmonary hypertension may cause dyspnea, especially if the condition is complicated by aortic regurgitation. Adults with Eisenmenger's syndrome are markedly symptomatic with diminished exercise tolerance, air hunger, headaches, hemoptysis and angina on exertion.

The patient with an uncomplicated VSD is acyanotic. Generally it is held that small VSDs produce the loudest murmurs, but if they are small enough, they may produce little to no acoustic energy and may be soft in intensity. The murmur associated with a VSD is pansystolic and begins during isovolumic contraction before the aortic and pulmonic valve open. It is generally heard at the left sternal border in the fourth or fifth intercostal space, radiating rightward except in the case of a supracristal VSD, where radiation is usually to the left clavicle. The murmur is often associated with a systolic thrill.

When Eisenmenger's physiology develops, the systolic murmur across the VSD diminishes. The patient will have a loud P2 with a wide but physiologically split S2. The murmurs of pulmonic regurgitation and TR may be audible as a result of the pulmonary hypertension.

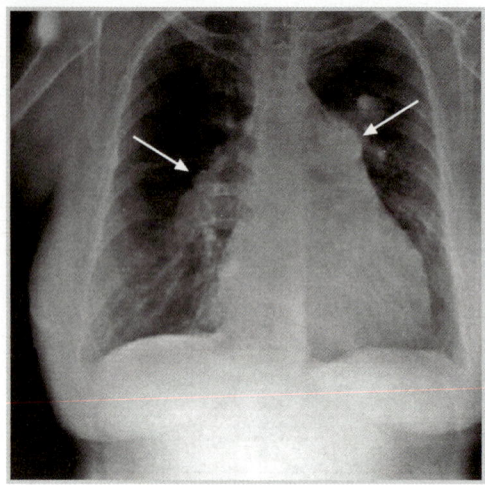

FIGURE 15: Pulmonary arterial view of chest radiograph in a patient with Eisenmenger's syndrome showing severely dilated pulmonary arteries (arrows)

Diagnostic Studies

ECG may be normal. In presence of a large shunt, the ECG is suggestive of LVH or biventricular hypertrophy with biphasic QRS complexes in the precordial leads.

Chest X-ray in a patient with a VSD shows a normal to slightly increased cardiothoracic ratio due to an increase in size of the left atrium and left ventricle. Increase pulmonary vascular markings consistent with large pulmonary blood flow are common. Pulmonary vascular plethora will not be present in adults or in Eisenmenger's syndrome. In stable Eisenmenger's syndrome, the cardiothoracic ratio will be normal, although RV prominence may be noted on the lateral chest X-ray. The main PA will be very prominent and central hilar vessels will be enlarged (Fig. 15).

Echocardiography and color flow Doppler interrogation can define the size and location of the VSD. The basal short axis view allows for assessment of perimembranous and supracristal VSDs. Mid ventricular and apical short axis views can visualize muscular VSDs, which are also well seen in the apical and subcostal views. The presence of left atrial and LV enlargement suggest that the left-to-right shunt is hemodynamically significant.

Cardiac catheterization has a little role to play in the diagnosis of patients with small VSDs. However, the decision to close a VSD requires accurate measurements of shunt fraction and PVR.

Treatment

Surgery prior to the age of 2 years in infants with large VSDs, high pulmonary blood flow and preoperative pulmonary hypertension almost always prevents the development of pulmonary vascular obstructive disease. However, current guidelines do not recommend closure of small VSDs in the absence of a history of endocarditis when the shunt ratio ($Q_p:Q_s$) is less than 1.5.

Closure of a VSD is indicated when the Qp/Qs is greater than 2.0 and is reasonable with the Qp/Qs is greater than 1.5 with a PA pressure less than two-thirds of the systemic pressure and the PVR is less than two-thirds of the systemic vascular closure. Closure of a VSD is indicated when the patient has a history of infective endocarditis. VSD closure is not recommended in patients with severe irreversible PAH. Pulmonary vasodilator therapy should be considered in these patients.

There are two options for closure catheter base device and surgical patch closure. Catheter based device closure of muscular VSDs in a location remote from the tricuspid valve has been gaining attention. Initial results show high success rates and low complication rates. Surgery with patch closure has a low perioperative mortality and high success rate.

Pregnancy

In women with small VSDs and no pulmonary hypertension pregnancy is generally well-tolerated. Women with VSD and severe PAH (Eisenmenger's syndrome) have excessive maternal and fetal mortality and should be counseled strongly against pregnancy with appropriate contraceptive measures.

Guidelines

Class I

- Surgeons with training and expertise in CHD should perform VSD closure operations. (Level of Evidence: C)
- Closure of a VSD is indicated when there is a Qp/Qs (pulmonary-to-systemic blood flow ratio) of 2.0 or more and clinical evidence of LV volume overload. (Level of Evidence: B)
- Closure of a VSD is indicated when the patient has a history of infective endocarditis. (Level of Evidence: C).

Class IIa

- Closure of a VSD is reasonable when net left-to-right shunting is present at a Qp/Qs greater than 1.5 with PA pressure less than two-thirds of systemic pressure and PVR less than two-thirds of systemic vascular resistance. (Level of Evidence: B)
- Closure of a VSD is reasonable when net left-to-right shunting is present at a Qp/Qs greater than 1.5 in the presence of LV systolic or diastolic failure. (Level of Evidence: B).

Class III

VSD closure is not recommended in patients with severe irreversible PAH. (Level of Evidence: B).

❏ PATENT DUCTUS ARTERIOSUS

The PDA is a remnant of the normal fetal circulation, which connects the main PA to the proximal descending aorta (just distal to the left subclavian) to deliver systemic venous return from the right ventricle to the placenta for oxygenation (Fig. 16). The ductus normally closes within the first hours to days of life. If it does not close and a shunt persists then it is considered a PDA.

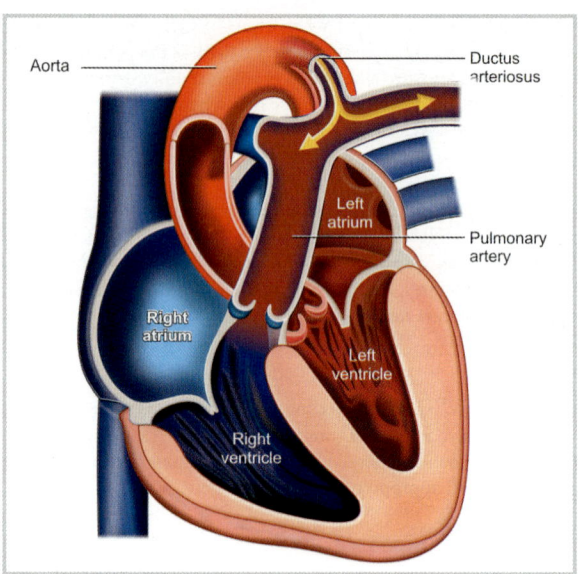

FIGURE 16: Patent ductus arteriosus with resultant left-to-right shunting. Some of the blood from the aorta crosses the ductus arteriosus and flows into the pulmonary artery (arrows). (*Source:* Brickner ME, Hillis LD, Lange RA. Congenital heart disease in adults. First of two parts. N Engl J Med. 2000;342:256-63, with permission)

Clinical Findings

Most small PDAs are asymptomatic in adults. CHF rarely develops in early adulthood. This is largely dependent on the shunt size, if large enough to cause LV volume overload, the patient may experience exertional dyspnea, chest pain, and palpitations. When pulmonary vascular disease has progressed to cause right-to-left shunting, cyanosis and clubbing are predominantly seen in the lower extremities often sparing the upper extremities (the left hand may show clubbing if the left subclavian origin is distal to the PDA).

The LV impulse is hyperdynamic and often laterally displaced. The classic murmur of the uncomplicated PDA is best heard below the left clavicle. The murmur is continuous machinery like. With significant LV volume overload caused by a large shunt, a mitral diastolic rumble and a left-sided S3 may be heard. As the PVR increases and shunt reverses, the murmur changes. Initially there is a decrease in the diastolic component and then a decrease in the systolic component. Finally, the murmur is silent with physical findings consistent with Eisenmenger's syndrome and pulmonary hypertension.

Diagnostic Studies

ECG is normal if the shunt is small. Larger shunts will show findings consistent with LVH. With pulmonary hypertension and shunt reversal the ECG may show P pulmonale, right axis deviation and evidence of RVH.

Chest X-ray is normal in the presence of a small shunt. With a large shunt, LV prominence is evident with an enlarged cardiac silhouette and pulmonary vascular plethora. The ductus may be calcified in the older adults.

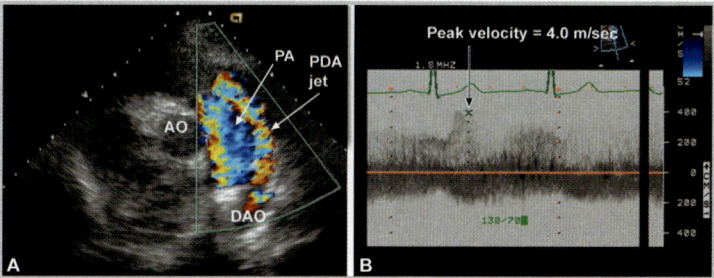

FIGURES 17A AND B: The high velocity jet from the patent ductus arteriosus into the pulmonary artery is visualized (blue arrow). It arises from the descending aorta. The high velocity jet seen on continuous wave peaks at 4.0 m/sec with a gradient of 64 mm Hg between the aorta and the pulmonary artery at point when systolic blood pressure was 130 mm Hg. The estimate pulmonary artery systolic pressure of 65 mm Hg suggested only mildly increased pulmonary vascular resistance on the basis of extremely high pulmonary blood flow due to the large and persistent left-to-right shunt. (Abbreviations: AO: Aorta; DAO: Descending aorta; PDA: Patent ductus arteriosus; PA: Pulmonary artery)

Echocardiogram will show left atrial and ventricular enlargement. The ductus itself can be difficult to visualize; however, it can be detected in the basal short axis and suprasternal notch views by the presence of continuous flow signal into the PA using color Doppler. Spectral Doppler shows a continuous jet with a peak velocity in systole (Figs 17A and B).

Right heart catheterization may be performed to measure the PA pressure, PVR and flow ratio (Qp:Qs). The oxygen step-up is at the level of the PA.

Treatment

Medical

Treatment in premature infants who are not dependent on the PDA flow consists of indomethacin administration to stimulate closure, surgical ligation or percutaneous closure with coils or a device.

Surgical and Interventional

In adults, surgical ligation or percutaneous coil or device occlusion of a PDA can be performed with low morbidity and mortality and is recommended because of high risk of endocarditis in uncorrected cases. Adults with mildly elevated PVR (<4 Wood units) can undergo surgical ligation or percutaneous closure with good results. In patients with elevated PVR (> 10 Wood units), survival is poor and right heart failure may occur if the ductus is closed.

Closure of a PDA, either percutaneously or surgically, is indicated if: (a) left atrial size and/or LV enlargement or if PAH is present as long as there is net left-to-right shunting; (b) prior history of endocarditis.

Pregnancy

Generally, pregnancy is well-tolerated in women with a small PDA. In women with larger shunts, pregnancy may precipitate right heart failure. Closure of these shunts is recommended prior to conception.

Guidelines

Class I

- Closure of a PDA either percutaneously or surgically is indicated for the following:
  - Left atrial and/or LV enlargement or if PAH is present, or in the presence of net left-to-right shunting. (Level of Evidence: C)
  - Prior endarteritis. (Level of Evidence: C)
- Consultation with ACHD interventional cardiologists is recommended before surgical closure is selected as the method of repair for patients with a calcified PDA. (Level of Evidence: C)
- Surgical repair by a surgeon experienced in CHD surgery is recommended when:
  - The PDA is too large for device closure. (Level of Evidence: C)
  - Distorted ductal anatomy precludes device closure (e.g. aneurysm or endarteritis). (Level of Evidence: B).

Class IIa

- It is reasonable to close an asymptomatic small PDA by catheter device. (Level of Evidence: C)
- PDA closure is reasonable for patients with PAH with a net left-to-right shunt. (Level of Evidence: C).

Class III

PDA closure is not indicated for patients with PAH and net right-to-left shunt. (Level of Evidence: C).

OTHER ACYANOTIC LESIONS

❑ EBSTEIN'S ANOMALY

Ebstein's anomaly is a rare congenital heart defect and comprises of less than 1% of all congenital heart lesions. Ebstein's anomaly is characterized by the apical displacement of the attachment of the posterior and/or septal leaflets of the tricuspid valve and adherence to the underlying myocardium.

A variable portion of the inflow of the right ventricle lies above the tricuspid valve creating "atrialization" of the right ventricle. The anterior leaflet is often large and redundant and is often described as "sail-like" and may contain fenestrations, contributing to the TR.

More than 50% of the patients have a shunt at the atrial level with either a secundum ASD or PFO, which results in varying degree of cyanosis. The degree of cyanosis is greater with severe TR and high right atrial pressure.

Clinical Findings

Patients over the age of 10 years often present with electrophysiological rather than hemodynamic manifestations at presentation. Hemodynamic symptoms in adulthood can include dyspnea on exertion, fatigue, palpitations and cyanosis (depending on degree of right-to-left shunting). Cyanosis may be present only during exercise.

Physical examination reveals right parasternal lift, widely split S1, systolic clicks (from delayed tricuspid valve closure) and systolic murmur of the TR. The jugular venous pulse is usually normal. An early diastolic snap from opening of the elongated anterior leaflet may be present. Pulse oximetry at rest and at stress can be useful in the diagnostic evaluation of Ebstein's anomaly in adult patients.

Diagnostic Studies

ECG shows right atrial enlargement and right ventricular conduction defect of the RBBB type. The PR interval may be prolonged, except in the presence of an accessory pathway.

Chest X-ray can be normal in mild cases. In more severe cases, right atrial enlargement with reduced pulmonary vascularity.

Transthoracic echocardiography findings often help in making the diagnosis of Ebstein's anomaly. Classic M-mode description of this anomaly included increased excursion of the anterior tricuspid valve leaflet and delayed tricuspid valve closure (>40 ms) following mitral valve closure. Often, the mitral and tricuspid valves are seen simultaneously on M-mode. It is mandatory to perform a saline contrast examination to reliably exclude a PFO or an ASD. TEE should be used for confirming diagnosis and defining the anatomy of the interatrial communications.

Catheterization is rarely necessary for diagnosis. However, simultaneous recording of a RV ECG and a right atrial pressure tracing are obtained with a specialized catheter in the atrialized portion of the right ventricle.

Treatment

Medical Treatment

Anticoagulation is recommended for patients with Ebstein's anomaly with a history of paradoxical embolus or atrial fibrillation. Supraventricular tachycardias may be resistant to medical therapy.

Catheter-based Intervention

In patients with mild TR, who have cyanosis due to an interatrial shunt or a history of paradoxical embolus, percutaneous closure of the interatrial septal defect may provide symptomatic relief. Many of the supraventricular arrhythmias are now amenable to catheter ablation at experienced centers. Given that, often there is presence of multiple accessory pathways, the overall success rates are lower than those reported in a structurally normal heart.

Surgical Intervention

Surgery for the tricuspid valve is dependent on the degree of anatomic and physiologic abnormalities. Surgery for the mild cases usually involves tricuspid valve repair when feasible or valve replacement. Tricuspid valve annuloplasty and tricuspid valve reconstruction, with creation of a monocuspid valve are often possible in experienced centers. However, valve replacement with a mechanical or heterograft bioprosthesis may be required in some patients. A right reduction atrioplasty is often performed.

Tricuspid valve surgery, with concomitant closure of ASD, for patients with (a) symptoms of deteriorating capacity, (b) cyanosis, (c) paradoxical embolus, (d) progressive cardiomegaly on chest X-ray, and (e) progressive RV dilatation or reduction of RV systolic function.

Pregnancy

Most women can have a successful pregnancy. However, if there is significant right-to-left shunting and cyanosis, there is increased risk of low-birth weight and fetal loss. The risk of CHD in the offspring is approximately 6%. It may be higher in patients with a family history of Ebstein's anomaly. Thromboprophylaxis should be considered in those with interatrial shunts and a modified delivery plan may be needed.

Guidelines

Class I

- Surgeons with training and expertise in CHD should perform tricuspid valve repair or replacement, with concomitant closure of an ASD, when present, for patients with Ebstein's anomaly with the following indications:
    - Symptoms or deteriorating exercise capacity. (Level of Evidence: B)
    - Cyanosis (oxygen saturation <90%). (Level of Evidence: B)
    - Paradoxical embolism. (Level of Evidence: B)
    - Progressive cardiomegaly on chest X-ray. (Level of Evidence: B)
    - Progressive RV dilatation or reduction of RV systolic function. (Level of Evidence: B).
- Surgeons with training and expertise in CHD should perform concomitant arrhythmia surgery in patients with Ebstein's anomaly and the following indications:
    - Appearance/progression of atrial and/or ventricular arrhythmias not amenable to percutaneous treatment. (Level of Evidence: B)
    - Ventricular pre-excitation not successfully treated in the electrophysiology laboratory. (Level of Evidence: B).
- Surgical repair or replacement of the tricuspid valve is recommended in adults with Ebstein's anomaly with the following indications:
    - Symptoms, deteriorating exercise capacity, or New York Heart Association functional class III or IV. (Level of Evidence: B)
    - Severe TR after repair with progressive RV dilatation, reduction of RV systolic function, or appearance/ progression of atrial and/or ventricular arrhythmias. (Level of Evidence: B)
    - Bioprosthetic tricuspid valve dysfunction with significant mixed regurgitation and stenosis. (Level of Evidence: B)
    - Predominant bioprosthetic valve stenosis (mean gradient >12–15 mm Hg). (Level of Evidence: B)
    - Operation can be considered earlier with lesser degrees of bioprosthetic stenosis with symptoms or decreased exercise tolerance. (Level of Evidence: B).

CYANOTIC CONGENITAL HEART DISEASE

All abnormalities resulting in cyanosis require a right-to-left shunt, which may be at the atrial, ventricular or vascular level. Cyanotic heart lesions can be further divided into categories based on the degree of pulmonary blood flow, excessive or deficient, and the pressure in the pulmonary circuit. The status of the PVR, pulmonary blood

FLOWCHART 5: Systematical classification of various cyanotic heart diseases

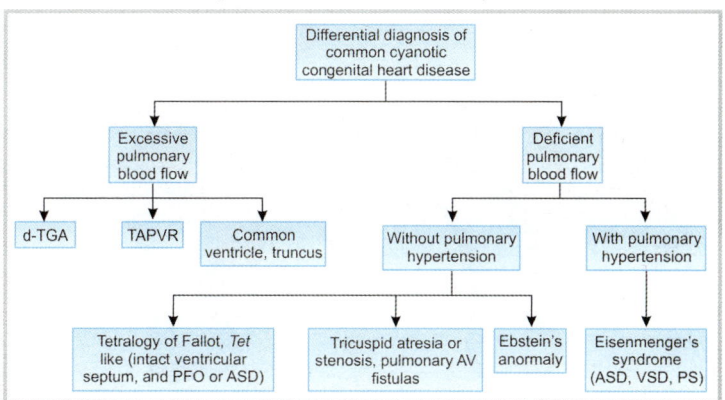

flow and pulmonary vascular anatomy determine survival, functional capacity and operability. The various cyanotic CHDs can be systematically classified based on one of two categories: excessive pulmonary blood flow or deficient pulmonary blood flow (Flowchart 5). This classification is based on the initial presentation in childhood and is altered by the various palliative procedures performed.

❏ PALLIATIVE SHUNTS

Wide spectrums of palliative shunts have been used in patients with cyanotic CHD (Figs 18A to D). They are broadly classified into those that increase pulmonary blood flow through a systemic artery to PA connection or those that divert systemic venous blood flow directly to the PA. The systemic artery to PA shunts includes the Blalock-Taussig shunt, Waterston shunt, Potts anastomosis, and central shunts. The systemic venous to PA shunts include the Glenn anastomosis and the Fontan operations. The Fontan circulation will separate the systemic and PA circulations.

❏ TETRALOGY OF FALLOT

Tetralogy of Fallot is the most common cyanotic congenital heart lesion, accounting for 10% of all CHD. It consists of a malalignment VSD in conjunction with RVOT obstruction, overriding aorta and consequent RVH (Fig. 19). The RVOT obstruction may be subvalvar, valvar or supravalvar. Often it is a combination of infundibular stenosis with valvar stenosis.

Clinical Findings

Most adult patients presenting with TOF have often undergone palliative or restorative surgery. They usually present with symptoms related to long-term complications of surgery.

Physical examination in an adult with TOF depends on the type of repair performed and the residual defect. In the increasingly rare adult patient with a persistent aortopulmonary shunt, such as Blalock-Taussig shunt, Waterston shunt or Potts anastomosis, there should be a continuous murmur, a single S2 and a harsh systolic murmur. In the patient with tetralogy with pulmonary atresia, continuous

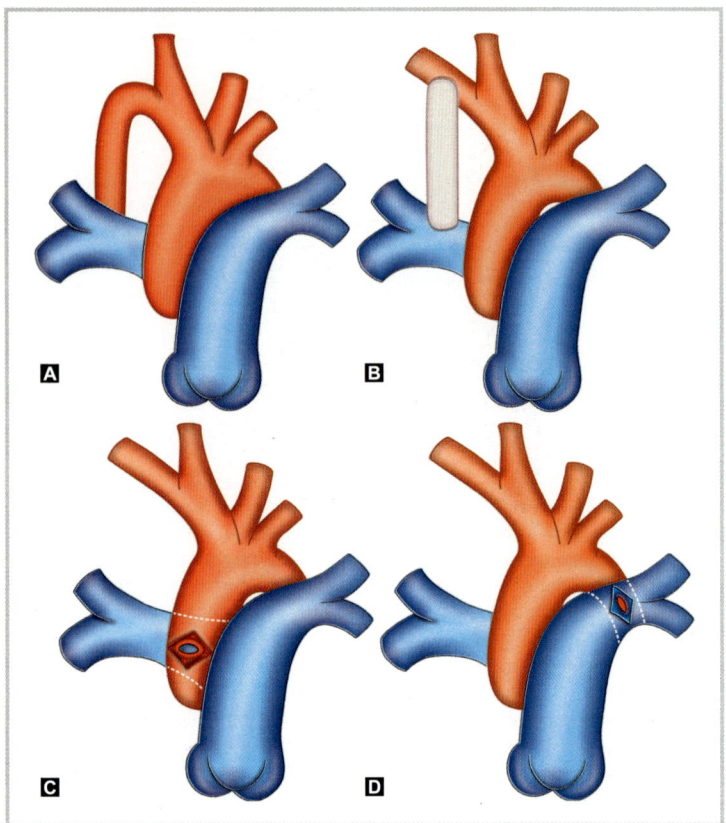

FIGURES 18A TO D: (A) Classic Blalock-Taussig shunt. (B) Modified Blalock-Taussig shunt. (C) Waterston shunt. (D) Potts anastomosis. (*Source:* Khairy P, Poirier N, Mercier LA. Univentricular heart. Circulation. 2007;115:800-12, with permission)

murmurs may be audible over the patient's back due to the aortopulmonary collaterals.

After total repaired of TOF, there is usually a prominent and often sustained right ventricular impulse, a single S2, a systolic ejection murmur with intensity and timing dependent on the severity of residual stenosis and, a low-pitched decrescendo murmur of pulmonary valve insufficiency. A right sided S3 and/or S4 may be present. In the presence of dilated aortic root, a second high-pitched diastolic murmur of aortic valve regurgitation may be present.

Diagnostic Studies

ECG shows right ventricular hypertrophy with right axis deviation in childhood. RBBB with left anterior hemiblock is seen commonly in patients after tetralogy repair surgery. The degree of QRS prolongation should be noted and followed as it has been used as clinical marker for sudden death risk.

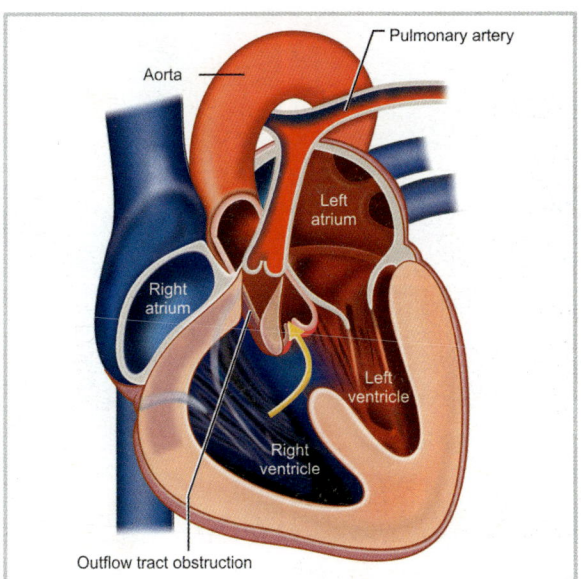

FIGURE 19: Tetralogy of Fallot. (*Source:* Brickner ME, Hillis LD, Lange RA. Congenital heart disease in adults. Second of two parts. N Engl J Med. 2000;342:334-42, with permission)

Chest X-ray in the unrepaired is typically shows the boot shaped heart (Coeur en sabot), which is seen when the PS is severe and a prominent right ventricle. Right-sided aortic arch (25%) is a variant seen with TOF may be seen on chest X-ray.

Echocardiography in the rare adult with unrepaired TOF shows a perimembranous VSD, RVOT obstruction, RVH and an overriding aorta (Figs 20A to D and 21A and B). The large overriding aortic root can be appreciated and attention must be paid to the presence of aortic regurgitation and prolapse of the aortic valve leaflets. The right ventricle is rarely dilated and the tricuspid regurgitant jet velocity reflects the degree of outflow tract obstruction. The level of RVOT obstruction is variable. There may be a small PA with a thickened pulmonary valve. The infundibulum is usually hypertrophied. Color flow Doppler shows right-to-left shunting across the VSD unless the outflow obstruction is mild. The velocity across the VSD by CW Doppler is usually low.

In the adult with repaired TOF, echocardiography should focus on the right ventricular infundibular region, the pulmonary valve and RV size and function. Residual RVOT obstruction with a persistent subvalvular gradient or valvular gradient is less common that severe pulmonary valve regurgitation (Figs 22A to D). When a gradient is detected, the shape of the jet can provide a clue as to the level of obstruction; a late peaking "dagger-shaped" jet suggests dynamic subvalvular obstruction and an early to mid-peaking jet is consistent with valvular obstruction. Residual VSDs due to patch leaks and ASDs should be sought.

Transesophageal echocardiogram can be useful to define the anatomy of the RVOT and the pulmonary valve when precordial imaging is suboptimal.

Magnetic resonance imaging is an important noninvasive modality in assessing patients with repaired TOF, primarily to provide accurate assessment of RV size, ejection fraction, volume, and the pulmonic regurgitant fraction.

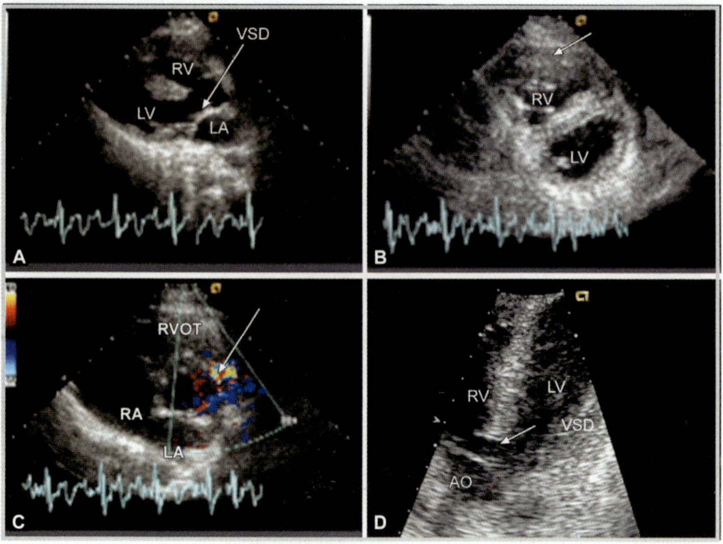

FIGURES 20A TO D: Transthoracic echocardiogram in cyanotic patient with unrepaired tetralogy of Fallot. (A) Parasternal long axis view in a patient with large malalignment ventricular septal defect and overriding aorta (arrow). (B) Parasternal short axis view demonstrating flattened septum consistent with right ventricular pressure overload and severe right ventricular hypertrophy (arrow). (C) Parasternal short axis view showing the narrowed right ventricular outflow tract and high velocity jet at the level of the hypoplastic pulmonary valve (arrow). (D) Magnified apical five-chamber view showing aorta overriding septum with moderate sized ventricular septal defect. (Abbreviations: AO: Aorta; LA: Left atrium; LV: Left ventricle; RV: Right ventricular; RVOT: Right ventricular outflow tract; VSD: Ventricular septal defect)

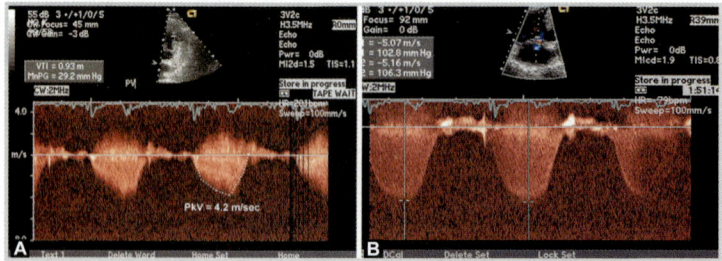

FIGURES 21A AND B: (A) Continuous wave Doppler jet through the right ventricular outflow tract with a peak velocity of 4.2 m/sec consistent with a peak gradient of 70 mm Hg suggestive of severe right ventricular outflow tract obstruction. The late peaking jet suggests a component of dynamic obstruction associated with infundibular hypertrophy. (B) High velocity tricuspid regurgitant jet estimated right ventricular systolic pressure as 110 mm Hg based on a right atrial pressure of 5 mm Hg. Therefore, the pulmonary artery systolic pressure is low enough (110–70 mm Hg = 40 mm Hg) to consider a total repair in this patient

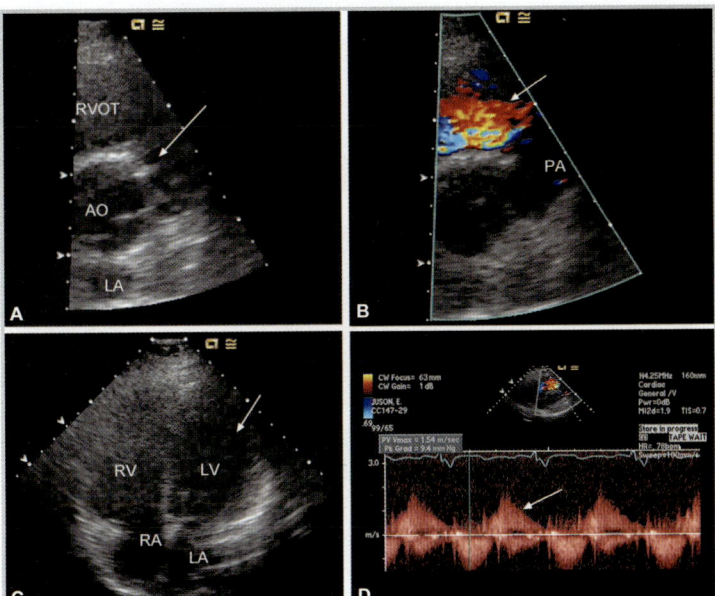

FIGURES 22A TO D: Transthoracic echocardiogram in a patient with repaired tetralogy of Fallot. (A) Parasternal short axis view in a patient with dilated right ventricular outflow tract, remnants of pulmonary valve tissue (arrow). (B) Parasternal short axis view demonstrating broad low velocity jet of pulmonary valve regurgitation (arrow). (C) Four-chamber view showing dilated right ventricle. (D) Continuous wave Doppler jet of low-velocity dense pulmonary valve regurgitant jet with steep slope and short pressure half-time consistent with severe pulmonary valve regurgitation. There was no evidence of residual stenosis. (Abbreviations: AO: Aorta; LA: Left atrium; LV: Left ventricle; PA: Pulmonary artery; RA: Right atrium; RV: Right ventricular; RVOT: Right ventricular outflow tract)

Computed tomography scanning can be used as a secondary alternative to make measurements of the right ventricle and systolic function and is potentially helpful in patients who cannot have an MRI due to a pacemaker or defibrillator.

Catheterization should be performed prior to any surgical intervention in patients with TOF, whether it is for primary surgery or repeat surgery. Additionally, in post-repair patients, catheterization can offer therapeutic interventions to eliminate residual native or palliative systemic to PA shunts, such as ASDs or VSDs, and to address branch pulmonary stenosis. Percutaneous pulmonic stent valves for patients who develop PR, remains investigational; however, this procedure is promising.

Treatment

Many older adults require palliative aortopulmonary shunts prior to total repair, which is often not performed until age 4–5 years. Restorative surgery involves closure of the VSD and relief of the pulmonary or infundibular stenosis (Fig. 23). Closure of the VSD is usually done with a synthetic patch. Late survival after surgery is excellent and 35-year survival nears 85–95%.

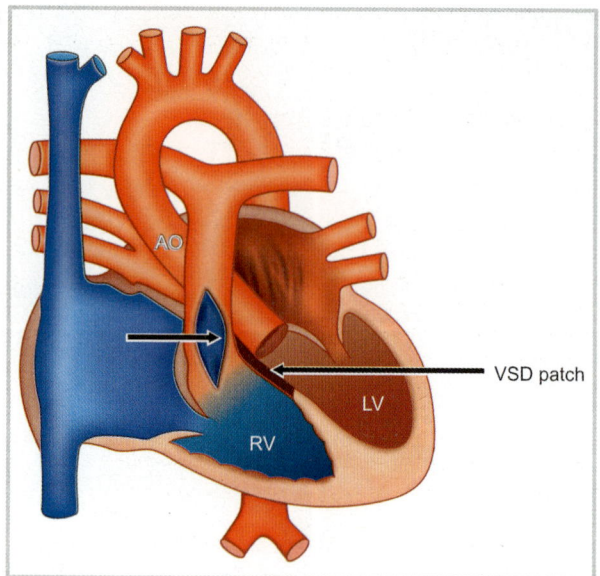

FIGURE 23: Repaired tetralogy of Fallot with ventricular septal defect patch, patch augmentation of the pulmonary artery (small arrow). (Abbreviations: AO: Aorta; LV: Left ventricle; RV: Right ventricular; VSD: Ventricular septal defect). (*Source:* Mayer CD, Mullins CE. Congenital Heart Disease: A Diagrammatic Atlas. New York: Alan R Liss Inc; 1988. p. 5)

Pregnancy

In uncorrected patients, pregnancy poses significant risks to both mother and fetus. The fall in systemic vascular resistance may increase cyanosis due to increase in right-to-left shunting. In corrected patients, the risks depend upon their hemodynamic status. In patients with good hemodynamics and minimal symptoms, pregnancy is fairly low-risk.

However, in women with severe PR, residual RVOT obstruction and RV dysfunction pregnancy may lead to worsening RV failure and arrhythmias. Pregnancy should be managed and delivery should be performed in a center for ACHD.

Guidelines

Evaluation and Follow-up

Class I

- All patients should be seen at least yearly by a cardiologist who has expertise in the management of ACHD. (Level of Evidence: C)
- Echocardiograms and MRIs should be performed by staff with expertise in ACHD. (Level of Evidence: C)
- Screening for heritable causes of their condition (e.g. chromosome 22q11 deletion) should be offered to all patients with TOF. (Level of Evidence: C)
- Before pregnancy or if a genetic syndrome is identified, consultation with a geneticist should be arranged for patients with TOF. (Level of Evidence: B)

- Patients with unrepaired or palliated forms of tetralogy should have a formal evaluation at an ACHD center regarding suitability for repair. (Level of Evidence: B).

Recommendations for Surgery in Patients with Previous Repair of Tetralogy of Fallot

Class I
- Surgeons with training and expertise in CHD should perform operations in adults with previous repair of TOF. (Level of Evidence: C)
- Pulmonary valve replacement is indicated for severe pulmonary regurgitation and symptoms or decreased exercise tolerance. (Level of Evidence: B)
- Coronary artery anatomy, specifically the possibility of an anomalous anterior descending coronary artery across the RVOT, should be ascertained before operative intervention. (Level of Evidence: C).

Class IIa
- Pulmonary valve replacement is reasonable in adults with previous TOF, severe pulmonary regurgitation, and any of the following:
  - Moderate to severe RV dysfunction. (Level of Evidence: B)
  - Moderate to severe RV enlargement. (Level of Evidence: B)
  - Development of symptomatic or sustained atrial and/or ventricular arrhythmias. (Level of Evidence: C)
  - Moderate to severe TR. (Level of Evidence: C).
- Collaboration between ACHD surgeons and ACHD interventional cardiologists, which may include preoperative stenting, intraoperative stenting or intraoperative patch angioplasty, is reasonable to determine the most feasible treatment for PA stenosis. (Level of Evidence: C)
- Surgery is reasonable in adults with prior repair of TOF and residual RVOT obstruction (valvular or subvalvular) and any of the following indications:
  - Residual RVOT obstruction (valvular or subvalvular) with peak instantaneous echocardiography gradient greater than 50 mm Hg. (Level of Evidence: C)
  - Residual RVOT obstruction (valvular or subvalvular) with RV/LV pressure ratio greater than 0.7. (Level of Evidence: C)
  - Residual RVOT obstruction (valvular or subvalvular) with progressive and/or severe dilatation of the right ventricle with dysfunction. (Level of Evidence: C)
  - Residual VSD with a left-to-right shunt greater than 1.5:1. (Level of Evidence: B)
  - Severe AR with associated symptoms or more than mild LV dysfunction. (Level of Evidence: C)
  - A combination of multiple residual lesions (e.g. VSD and RVOT obstruction) leading to RV enlargement. (Level of Evidence: C).

Recommendations for Arrhythmias: Pacemaker/ Electrophysiology Testing

Class I
Annual surveillance with history, ECG, assessment of RV function, and periodic exercise testing is recommended for patients with pacemakers/automatic implantable cardioverter defibrillators. (Level of Evidence: C)

Class IIa

Periodic Holter monitoring can be beneficial as part of routine follow-up. The frequency should be individualized depending on the hemodynamics and clinical suspicion of arrhythmia (Level of Evidence: C).

Class IIb

Electrophysiology testing in an ACHD center may be reasonable to define suspected arrhythmias in adults (Level of Evidence: C).

❏ TRUNCUS ARTERIOSUS

Truncus arteriosus (TA) is a rare lesion, accounting for only 1% of all congenital heart defects. TA is defined as a single arterial trunk arising from both ventricles due to failure of septation of the TA, which gives rise to the systemic, pulmonary and coronary circulation. It is always accompanied by a VSD.

Classifications

Several anatomic classifications based upon the PA anatomy are available (Fig. 24). The variant that was called type IV where there were no main pulmonary arteries, and the flow arose from the descending aorta is now classified as pulmonary atresia with VSD.

Type I truncus—The common PA exits the lateral aspect of the trunk, near the truncus valve. This is the most common type, and lends itself to easier repair.

Type II truncus—There are separate origins of the right and left pulmonary arteries from the posterior aspect of the ascending trunk.

Type III truncus—Each PA arises from the lateral aspect of the truncus.

Clinical Findings

Most infants, if not surgically corrected before one year, die from CHF. As the PVR increases in infancy, there degree of cyanosis and right-to-left shunting increases. Adults presenting with unrepaired TA typically present with Eisenmenger's syndrome.

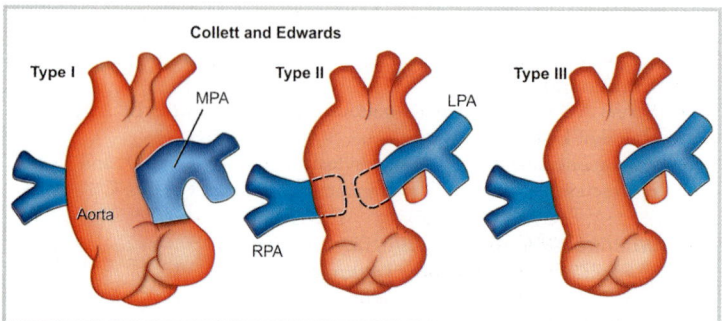

FIGURE 24: Variations of truncus arteriosus (Abbreviations: LPA: Left pulmonary artery; MPA: Main pulmonary artery; RPA: Right pulmonary artery). (*Source:* Bashore TM. Adult congenital heart disease: right ventricular outflow tract lesions. Circulation. 2007;115:1933-47, with permission)

Diagnostic Studies

ECG shows biventricular hypertrophy is common in infants. If pulmonary vascular disease develops, there is RVH. In repaired adults, the ECG findings will depend on the presence of residual lesions. A RBBB may found due to VSD closure.

Chest X-ray shows cardiomegaly with prominent pulmonary arterial markings in infants. In the repaired adult, the appearance depends on the presence of residual lesions. Approximately 30% of patients have a right-sided aortic arch.

Echocardiography helps in the diagnosis. In the absence of repair, there is an overriding common arterial trunk with a common truncal valve, which has a variable number of truncal valve cusps. Truncal valve may associated with stenotic or regurgitant lesions. The origin of the pulmonary arteries is more readily visualized in type I lesions. Also, the VSD size and location should be noted. In the adult with repaired TA, the truncal root may show varying degrees of dilatation with valvular regurgitation. The gradient across the conduit should be evaluated as well as the presence of conduit valve regurgitation.

Treatment

Surgery consists of VSD closure, surgical separation of the pulmonary arteries from the truncus followed by placement of a valved conduit from the RV to the PA. Adults with repaired TA must be followed for progressive RV to PA conduit obstruction, ventricular dysfunction, truncal root dilatation and truncal valve regurgitation.

Repeat surgery in the adult is usually required when there is conduit obstruction due to pseudointimal hyperplasia and regurgitation due to degeneration of the bioprosthetic valve. There is increasing investigational use of implantable percutaneous valves similar to patients with TOF.

Pregnancy

Patient with successful repairs and no residual lesions are able to tolerate pregnancy. Patients with residual lesions/conduit obstructions may require correction prior to considering a safe pregnancy. In uncorrected adults with Eisenmenger's syndrome, pregnancy is contraindicated. Genetic testing with chromosome analysis is recommended prior to conception, and fetal echocardiography is advised.

❏ TOTAL ANOMALOUS PULMONARY VENOUS RETURN

In total anomalous pulmonary venous return (TAPVR), the pulmonary venous flow enters the right atrium either directly or by connecting to the coronary sinus, SVC, IVC, portal vein, hepatic vein and ductus venosus. If pulmonary venous obstructions are present, it is called "obstructed TAPVR". Obstruction can be within the pulmonary venous system or compression from adjacent structures like left bronchus or PA.

Several anatomic variants exist based on the level of the drainage:

1. Supracardiac (49%): The pulmonary vein confluence drains upward through a vertical vein into the left innominate vein and into the SVC (Fig. 25).
2. Cardiac (25%): All pulmonary veins drain directly into the right atrium or into the coronary sinus.
3. Infradiaphragmatic (18%): The pulmonary vein confluence passes down thorough the diaphragm into the portal vein, ductus venosus or hepatic vein and into the IVC (Fig. 26).

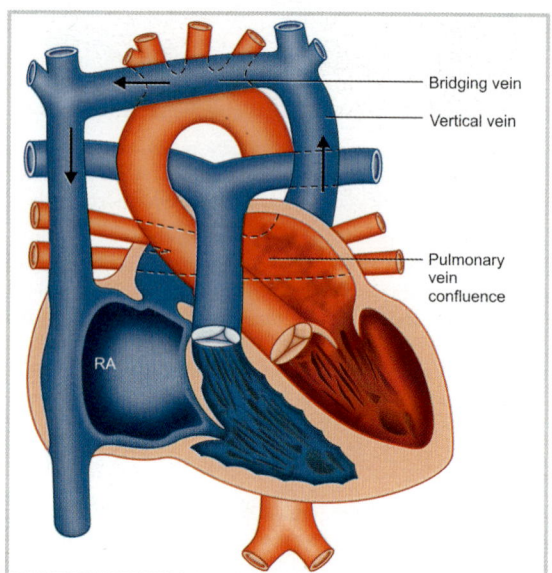

FIGURE 25: Supradiaphragmatic variant of total anomalous pulmonary veins. (Abbreviation: RA: Right atrium). (*Source:* Mayer CD, Mullins CE. Congenital Heart Disease: A Diagrammatic Atlas. New York: Alan R Liss Inc; 1988. p. 5, with permission)

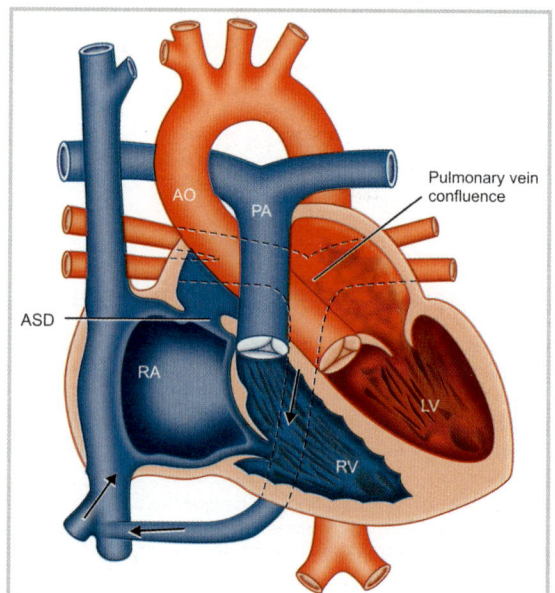

FIGURE 26: Infradiaphragmatic variant of total anomalous pulmonary veins. (Abbreviations: AO: Aorta; ASD: Atrial septal defect; LV: Left ventricle; PA: Pulmonary artery; RA: Right atrium; RV: Right ventricular). (*Source:* Mayer CD, Mullins CE. Congenital Heart Disease: A Diagrammatic Atlas. New York: Alan R Liss Inc; 1988. p. 5)

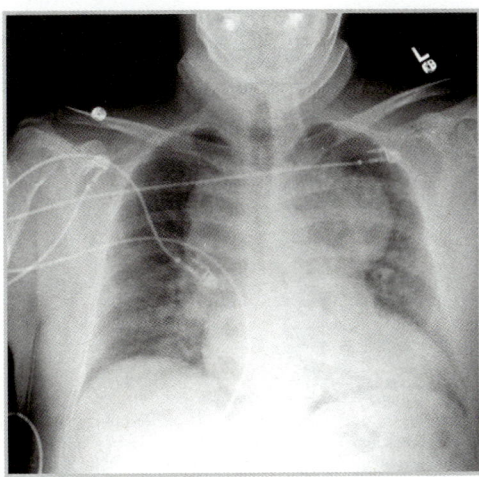

FIGURE 27: Chest radiograph of 45-year-old man with uncorrected total anomalous pulmonary venous drainage demonstrating the "snowman" appearance of the mediastinal structures

There is an atrial communication and the degree of cyanosis depends upon the size of the ASD and the PVR. If the flow is unobstructed the clinical presentation is similar to an ASD. Infants with obstructive TAPVR present more cyanotic. This anomaly often requires emergency surgery in infancy and 80% of patients will die if not treated within the first year of life. In the rare patient who is diagnosed in adulthood, the lesion is most commonly the supradiaphragmatic type. There is usually mild cyanosis and the chest X-ray shows the typical "snowman" pattern (Fig. 27). Surgical repair can usually be done with low morbidity and mortality.

Surgical correction consists of connecting the common pulmonary venous channel to the left atrium. The postoperative course is usually uncomplicated and they can live a normal life span as adults without CHD.

❑ SUGGESTED READINGS

Bonow RO, Carabello BA, Chatterjee K, et al. 2008 Focused update incorporated into the ACC/AHA 2006 guidelines for the management of patients with valvular heart disease: a report of the American College of Cardiology/American Heart Association Task Force on Practice Guidelines (Writing Committee to Revise the 1998 Guidelines for the Management of Patients With Valvular Heart Disease): endorsed by the Society of Cardiovascular Anesthesiologists, Society for Cardiovascular Angiography and Interventions, and Society of Thoracic Surgeons. Circulation. 2008;118:e523-661.

Bonow RO, Carabello BA, Kanu C, et al. ACC/AHA 2006 guidelines for the management of patients with valvular heart disease: a report of the American College of Cardiology/American Heart Association task force on practice guidelines (writing committee to revise the 1998 guidelines for the management of patients with valvular heart disease): developed in collaboration with the Society of Cardiovascular Anesthesiologists: endorsed by the Society for Cardiovascular Angiography and Interventions and the Society of Thoracic Surgeons. Circulation. 2006;114:e84-231.

Campbell M. Natural history of coarctation of the aorta. Br Heart J. 1970;32:633-40.

Frescura C, Angelini A, Daliento L, et al. Morphological aspects of Ebstein's anomaly in adults. Thorac Cardiovasc Surg. 2000;48:203-8.

Gabriel HM, Heger M, Innerhofer P, et al. Long-term outcome of patients with ventricular septal defect considered not to require surgical closure during childhood. J Am Coll Cardiol. 2002;39:1066- 71.

Garg V, Muth AN, Ransom JF, et al. Mutations in NOTCH1 cause aortic valve disease. Nature. 2005;437:270-4.

Klieverik LM, Takkenberg JJ, Bekkers JA, et al. The Ross operation: a Trojan horse? Eur Heart J. 2007;28:1993-2000.

Masura J, Tittel P, Gavora P, et al. Long-term outcome of transcatheter patent ductus arteriosus closure using Amplatzer duct occluders. Am Heart J. 2006;151:755 e7-755. e10.

Michielon G, Di Donato RM, Pasquini L, et al. Total anomalous pulmonary venous connection: long-term appraisal with evolving technical solutions. Eur J Cardiothorac Surg. 2002;22:184-91.

Nistri S, Sorbo MD, Marin M, et al. Aortic root dilatation in young men with normally functioning bicuspid aortic valves. Heart. 1999;82:19-22.

Reller MD, Strickland MJ, Riehle-Colarusso T, et al. Prevalence of congenital heart defects in metropolitan Atlanta, 1998-2005. J Pediatr. 2008;153:807-13.

Williams JM, de Leeuw M, Black MD, et al. Factors associated with outcomes of persistent truncus arteriosus. J Am Coll Cardiol. 1999;34:545-53.

Wilson PD, Correa-Villaseñor A, Loffredo CA, et al. Temporal trends in prevalence of cardiovascular malformations in Maryland and the District of Columbia, 1981-1988. The Baltimore-Washington infant study group. Epidemiology. 1993;4:259-65.

Chapter 10

Secondary Disorders of the Heart

10.1 Alcohol and Arrhythmia

❏ DIRECT EFFECTS OF ETHANOL EXPOSURE ON HEART CELLS AND TISSUES

Alcohol has long been recognized as an important modulator of cell membrane potentials, action potential duration, conduction and contractility in the heart tissues. Action potential amplitudes, transmembrane resting potentials and conduction times were not altered by physiologically relevant concentrations of ethanol or acetaldehyde. Acetate had no effect on action potential configuration or conduction time. Interestingly ethanol, acetaldehyde and acetate at every concentration examined did not increase the rate of spontaneous depolarization of the guinea pig atria. At clinically relevant concentrations, ethanol shortened the action potential duration and reduced L-type Ca^{2+} currents (I_{Ca}), by shifting channel availability curves toward more negative potentials. In contrast, there were no changes in fast Na^+ currents (I_{Na}) in the same experimental system. The group proposed I_{Ca} inhibition as one major contributor to the negative inotropy, action potential shortening and arrhythmia seen in heavy drinkers.

❏ ETHANOL INGESTION AND THE NORMAL CARDIAC CONDUCTION SYSTEM

Heavy drinking is consistently linked to the clinical arrhythmias. However, there is controversy as to whether alcohol-mediated rhythm disorders are primarily triggered by direct effects on cardiac conduction or indirect effects on nutritional status and myocardial viability; although it has been demonstrated that heavy ethanol consumption did not cause cardiac hypertrophy, inflammation, or necrosis.

Randomized controlled studies of humans who drink are rare but suggest the dose-related effects of ethanol on cardiac conduction. More recently, Spaak et al. examined dose-related effects of red wine and ethanol on heart rate variability (HRV). They concluded that moderate alcohol ingestion diminishes time and frequency indices of parasympathetic heart rate modulation in a dose-dependent manner and augments frequency domain indices of sympathetic rate modulation. Spaak's findings are most consistent with centrally mediated sympathoexcitatory and vagolytic actions on HRV, with no differences between intakes of red wine versus other ethanol solutions.

❏ BINGE DRINKING AND TRANSIENT CLINICAL ARRHYTHMIAS— HOLIDAY HEART

Of more immediate interest to the general public and health professionals is the association between heavy drinking and acute cardiac rhythm disorders, better known as "Holiday heart". Ettinger et al. published an important case series that documented experience with patients who drink heavily and habitually with superimposition of especially heavy ingestion prior to the cardiac arrhythmia. Most hospital admissions occurred after weekends and holidays, prompting staff to coin the term "Holiday heart". The most common arrhythmia was atrial fibrillation (AF), followed by atrial flutter (AFL) or isolated ventricular premature beats. Several patients had supraventricular beats, paroxysmal atrial tachycardia (PAT) and junctional tachycardia. The mean heart rate of alcoholics during systolic time interval testing was higher than controls, as was the ratio of pre-ejection period (PEP) to left ventricular ejection time (LVET). Mean PRc, QRS, and QTc intervals were higher in alcoholic patients compared to controls. Mean cardiac index (MCI) was lower in heavy drinkers, and stroke volume index did not increase normally in response to angiotensin infusion, further supporting alcohol-related left ventricular dysfunction. Ettinger concluded that preclinical cardiomyopathy was likely to be present in the majority of cases.

❏ ALCOHOL CONSUMPTION, CHRONIC ATRIAL FIBRILLATION, AND ATRIAL FLUTTER

Recent prospective cohort studies validate the association of heavy ethanol intake with a higher risk of AF. Mukamal et al. tested the association between self-reported alcohol use and incident AF among more than 16,000 women and men enrolled for up to 18 years in the Copenhagen City Heart Study (CCHS). The investigators documented 1,071 cases of AF—68 by study ECG, 891 from the hospitalization records and 112 from both sources. In both age- and multivariable-adjusted analyses, risk of AF was similar between abstainers and those consuming up to 14 drinks per week. The risk of AF increased significantly at a threshold of 35 drinks per week (HR, 1.45; 95% CI, 1.02–2.04), with a relatively flat relationship at lower levels of intake. Blood pressure, incident CHD during follow-up and incident congestive heart failure during follow-up was independently associated with the risk of AF.

Marcus et al. address mechanisms connecting alcohol and atrial arrhythmia in their investigation of 200 patients presenting for ablation or cardioversion of AF or AFL to a university medical center. After multivariate adjustment, patients less than or equal to 60 years of age who drank daily had greater odds of having AFL than nondrinkers. Patients less than or equal to 60 years of age exhibited a significant linear association between increasing amounts of alcohol and greater odds of having AFL. Greater intake was associated with decreased high right atrial atrial effective refractory period (AERP), approximately 50 milliseconds shorter than in nondrinkers. Interestingly, neither proximal nor distal coronary sinus (DCS) ERPs showed a linear association with self-reported alcohol ingestion. Marcus et al. postulated that the lack of association between alcohol and AF may be a consequence of the relatively small patient cohort. However, their observations advance the field by (a) suggesting that the association between alcohol and AFL may be stronger than between alcohol and AF and (b) raising the possibility that AERP shortening may be a key atrial arrhythmia mechanism.

❏ ALCOHOL CONSUMPTION AND SUDDEN CARDIAC DEATH

Beyond holiday heart and chronic atrial arrhythmias looms the specter of alcohol-induced sudden cardiac death. Wannamethee and Shaper found that mortality from IHD actually decreased with greater alcohol intake up to levels of moderate drinking. In contrast, heavy drinkers had a higher rate of sudden death than all other groups combined (relative risk 1.6; 95% confidence interval 1.0–2.6; p = 0.05). Heavy drinkers did not have excess risk of overall death from ischemic heart disease (IHD), but death was more likely to be sudden. Subsequent adjustments for social class and cigarette smoking did not alter the association between heavy alcohol intake and sudden cardiac death. However, adjustment for age showed that heavy drinking was associated with increased risk of sudden death only in the older participants (50–59 years). Moreover, death in the event of a heart attack in heavy drinkers was likely to be sudden and that alcohol intake discriminated between sudden death and nonsudden death, perhaps by triggering ventricular arrhythmias.

Mukamal et al. subsequently evaluated the effects of binge drinking on mortality after acute myocardial infarction (AMI) using data from the Determinants of MI Onset Study. Interestingly, there were similar associations between binge drinking and mortality among light and heavier drinkers, based on usual alcohol intake, and among patients who reported binges up to once per week and more often. Risks associated with binge drinking were similar among patients who reported heavy intake of beer, wine, liquor or multiple beverages. For the majority of binge drinkers, there was a positive relation between binge frequency and mortality. Further adjustments for use of nicotine, caffeine, marijuana, cocaine or heroin did not alter these findings. The investigators postulated that binge alcohol use could be a trigger for lethal ventricular arrhythmias. Heavy intake appears to lower ventricular fibrillation threshold and increase risk in postinfarction patients, who are susceptible to sudden cardiac death.

❏ SUMMARY AND CLINICAL GUIDELINES

- Physiologically relevant concentrations of ethanol cause direct, acute and reversible shortening of action potential duration in isolated heart cell and tissue preparations
- Randomized controlled studies of ethanol consumption by humans and experimental animals demonstrate slowing of cardiac conduction and modulation of HRV that are independent of ethanol-mediated effects on nutritional status and myocardial viability
- Chronic heavy drinkers are more likely to develop "holiday heart", a condition in which transient supraventricular arrhythmias develop after weekend and holiday binge episodes
- Individuals who consume more than 2 drinks every day are more likely to develop sustained atrial arrhythmias, possibly through effects on the AERP
- Heavy consumption is also associated with increased risk of sudden cardiac death, possibly through ethanol-mediated effects on the threshold for ventricular fibrillation
- Binge drinking is a major risk factor for cardiovascular mortality, including sudden death, even among individuals who are usually light-to-moderate consumers of alcoholic beverages.

In response to these important findings, the American College of Cardiology, American Heart Association and European Society of Cardiology recommend: (i) complete abstinence from alcohol when there is a suspected correlation between intake and ventricular arrhythmias and (ii) optimal evidence-based treatment, including an implantable cardioverter defibrillator (ICD), if necessary, for individuals who have an expectation of survival of greater than 1 year.

❑ SUGGESTED READINGS

Ettinger PO, Lyons M, Oldewurtel HA, et al. Cardiac conduction abnormalities produced by chronic alcoholism. Am Heart J. 1976;91:66-78.

Ettinger PO, Wu CF, De La Cruz C, et al. Arrhythmias and the "Holiday Heart": alcohol-associated cardiac rhythm disorders. Am Heart J. 1978;95:555-62.

Habuchi Y, Furukawa T, Tanaka H, et al. Ethanol inhibition of Ca2+ and Na+ currents in the guinea-pig heart. Eur J Pharmacol. 1995;292:143-9.

Majchrowicz E. Metabolic correlates of ethanol, acetaldehyde, acetate, and methanol in humans and animals. Adv Exp Med Biol. 1975;56:111-40.

Marcus GM, Smith LM, Whiteman D, et al. Alcohol intake is significantly associated with atrial flutter in patients under 60 years of age and a shorter right atrial effective refractory period. PACE. 2008;31:266-72.

Mukamal KJ, Maclure M, Muller JE, et al. Binge drinking and mortality after acute myocardial infarction. Circulation. 2005;112: 3839-45.

Mukamal KJ, Tolstrup JS, Friberg J, et al. Alcohol consumption and risk of atrial fibrillation in men and women: the Copenhagen City Heart Study. Circulation. 2005;112:1736-42.

Spaak J, Tomlinson G, McGowan CL, et al. Dose-related effects of red wine and alcohol on heart rate variability. Am J Physiol Heart Circ Physiol. 2010;298:H2226-31.

Wannamethee G, Shaper AG. Alcohol and sudden cardiac death. Br Heart J. 1992;68:443-8.

Zipes DP, Camm AJ, Borggrefe M, et al. ACC/AHA/ESC 2006 Guidelines for management of patients with ventricular arrhythmias and the prevention of sudden cardiac death: a report of the American College of Cardiology/American Heart Association Task Force and the European Society of Cardiology Committee for Practice Guidelines. J. Am Coll Cardiol. 2006;48:e247-346.

10.2 Insulin Resistance and Cardiomyopathy

❑ INTRODUCTION

Insulin resistance, the underlying abnormality responsible for the metabolic syndrome, is associated with the development of hypertension, adiposity, glucose intolerance and the characteristic dyslipidemia that are used to define the metabolic syndrome (Fig. 1). Insulin-resistance is important in the progression of heart failure, while in some patients insulin resistance may also serve a primary role in the development of heart failure. The hereditary and environmental factors that combine to produce insulin resistance provide the nidus for the development of heart failure; both by contributing to the causes of heart failure, and by aggravating the response to myocardial injury or stress which characterizes the progression of cardiomyopathy.

❑ DIASTOLIC HEART FAILURE AND INSULIN RESISTANCE

As it became more apparent that the relationship between insulin resistance and heart failure is not necessarily mediated by CAD, attention turned to the relationship between insulin resistance and diastolic heart failure.

The association between insulin resistance and hypertension is well established. Multiple prospective studies have noted that insulin resistant individuals are more likely to develop hypertension than insulin sensitive individuals. LVH, an important factor closely linked to the development of heart failure in epidemiological studies, is closely related to the presence of hypertension. An interaction between insulin

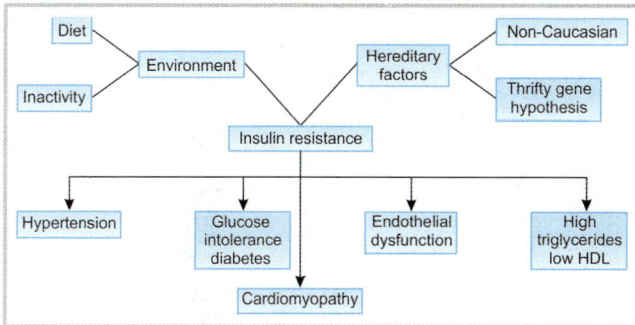

FIGURE 1: Insulin resistance and cardiomyopathy.
(*Source:* Modified from Michael B Fowler)

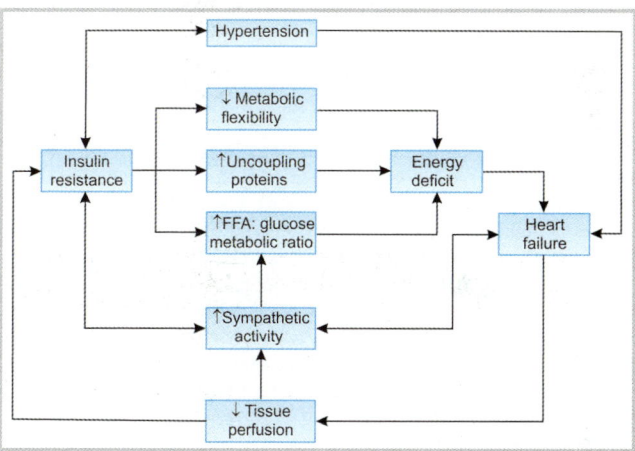

FIGURE 2: Relationships/mechanisms linking insulin resistance to heart failure.
(*Source:* Modified from Witteles and Fowler, JACC. 2008)

resistance and hypertension has been described in the development of LVH. The relationship linking insulin resistance to heart failure is shown in Figure 2. Evidence supports the concept that a superimposed myocardial insult (such as ischemia or pressure overload) and the presence of insulin resistance contributes to the development of a cardiomyopathic state. Importantly, whether insulin resistance initiates myocardial damage or impairs the response to myocardial injury, in both cases, the resultant myocardial performance leads to worsening insulin resistance, compounding myocardial stress and engendering a cycle of ever worsening cardiac function and insulin metabolism (Fig. 3).

❏ MYOCARDIAL ENERGY METABOLISM

To explain the role of insulin resistance in heart failure, an understanding of myocardial energy metabolism is required. The heart turns over its ATP supply in

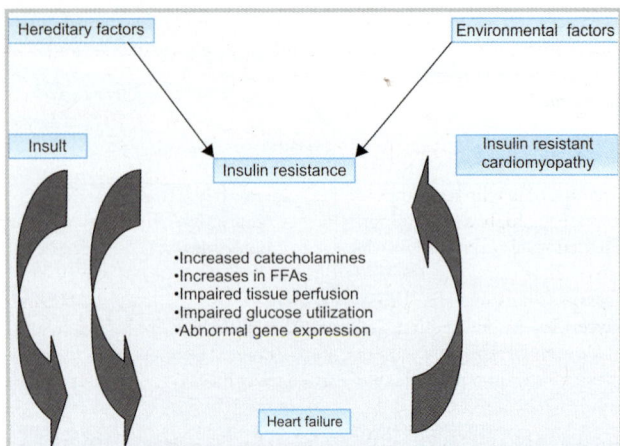

FIGURE 3: Vicious cycle of insulin resistance in HF.
(*Source:* Modified from Michael B Fowler)

4–5 seconds and has a limited capacity for intracellular energy storage. Thus the myocardium needs a steady supply of energy to function optimally and safely. Two major energy sources are available to the heart. Glucose, the more efficient fuel, which yields a higher number of ATP per amount of oxygen consumed, and free fatty acids (FFA), predominant fuel used in normal heart, which in the setting of abundant oxygen yield a greater total amount of ATP.

In the failing heart, a switch is initially made to the more efficient fuel glucose, in an attempt to reduce myocardial oxygen consumption and thus myocardial workload. This switch is accompanied by a reversion of the failing heart to the fetal gene program (the fetal condition itself an energy deprived environment), with increased transcription of genes such as glucose transporters (GLUT-1 and GLUT-4), atrial natriuretic peptide, MHC beta and skeletal actin, and by the repression of metabolic 'adult' genes alpha myosin heavy chain and SERCA. Energy metabolism is closely linked to gene expression: increased myocardial work spurs increased glucose uptake via insulin secretion, which stimulates transcription of genes encoding glucose transporters and inhibits nonesterified fatty acid (NEFA) release, leading to lower NEFA levels.

❏ METABOLIC EFFECTS OF INSULIN RESISTANCE

Energy Metabolism

The switch to the fetal gene program and resultant increase in glucose utilization is an adaptive response to myocardial stress. In the setting of insulin resistance, however, this switch is ineffective, since glucose utilization is impaired, and the heart enters an 'energy starved state'. It should be emphasized here that insulin resistance can both initiate this cycle, by producing the stress that leads to reversion to the fetal gene program, and perpetuate this cycle, by subverting the metabolic efficiency of the fetal gene program by inhibiting glucose utilization. Heart failure can in turn worsen insulin resistance by increasing sympathetic activity, endothelial dysfunction and inflammatory cytokine production. Thus, insulin resistance can initiate a cardiomyopathic state and subsequently exacerbate a cardiomyopathic state. Importantly, heart failure itself engenders insulin resistance, and a cycle of worsening efficiency perpetuates until there is either treatment or correction of the underlying insult.

Dyslipidemia or Lipotoxicity

Characteristic of insulin resistance is a dyslipidemia with an increase in triglycerides and decrease in high density lipoprotein concentration. This is partially due to the increased level of NEFAs in the serum that results from impaired utilization of glucose. These excess fatty acids bind to PPAR alpha and influence gene transcription. The excess of FFA in the heart also leads to an accumulation of triglycerides in myocardial cells, causing mitochondrial dysfunction, lipid peroxidation and myocardial dysfunction, a phenomenon known as lipotoxicity. Among the most deleterious effects of insulin resistance upon the heart is an increase in serum catecholamine levels (norepinephrine) and beta-adrenergic receptor density, leading to augmentation in chronic beta-adrenergic receptor stimulation. Insulin resistance is also an inflammatory state, and as with atherosclerosis, this inflammatory milieu leads to adverse effects upon the vasculature, particularly the endothelium of blood vessels.

In its most extreme form, insulin resistance leads to hyperglycemia when the excess insulin produced by the pancreas is insufficient to maintain normal blood glucose levels. Hyperglycemia replicates and compounds many of the effects of insulin resistance including increased inflammation (IL-6, TNF-alpha and IL-18), increased reactive oxygen species generation (peroxidation of LDL) and impaired microcirculation (nitric oxide derangement). Hyperglycemia also causes increased platelet aggregation, reduced fibrinolysis and the formation of advanced glycosylation end products, which accumulate in many tissues, including the myocardium.

❏ STRUCTURAL EFFECTS OF INSULIN RESISTANCE

Detection of the metabolic effects of insulin resistance requires specialized, often investigational tools. Energy use in the myocardium can be examined through phosphorous magnetic resonance (MR) spectroscopy; the phosphocreatine to ATP ratio is low in heart failure, and a low ratio independently predicts mortality in heart failure. Fluorodeoxyglucose positron emission tomography (FDG PET) cardiac imaging has revealed impaired myocardial glucose uptake in diabetics and shown that this uptake worsens in advanced heart failure.

The metabolic effects of insulin resistance, as they accumulate over time, eventually lead to macroscopic changes in the structure and function of the heart. Both diastolic and systolic dysfunction can arise from long-standing insulin resistance.

Diastolic Dysfunction

The direct hypertrophic effect of insulin resistance upon cardiomyocytes plays a primary role in LVH, and is largely mediated by the Akt-1 pathway in the acute phase as well as by B2 adrenergic receptors in chronic insulin resistant states. Other contributing factors to diastolic dysfunction in the insulin resistant state include myocardial fibrosis (arising from myocardial cell apoptosis and collagen deposition in the gaps left by cellular death), endothelial dysfunction (which can lead to reactive fibrosis and cellular injury) and altered calcium metabolism (decreased sarcoplasmic reticulum calcium protein expression occurs in diabetes, leading to slower myocardial relaxation). Finally, myocardial steatosis, another effect of insulin resistance described above, is increased in insulin resistant individuals compared with controls and is associated with diastolic dysfunction.

Detection of Diastolic Dysfunction

Echocardiography can detect increases in LV mass as well as diastolic dysfunction by measuring transmitral flow and mitral annular velocity. Newer techniques, such as strain imaging, also show promise for earlier detection of diastolic dysfunction, while measures of coronary flow reserve (CFR) via echocardiography or coronary catheterization can also characterize diastolic dysfunction. Multiple studies have demonstrated increased LV mass in individuals with insulin resistance (up to 70%) as measured by echocardiography, and the presence of diastolic dysfunction in diabetic cohorts has been described to be as high as 60%. Cardiac MR spectroscopy also shows promise in the early detection of diastolic dysfunction in insulin resistant cardiomyopathy.

Systolic Dysfunction

Systolic dysfunction in insulin resistant individuals is less well described than diastolic dysfunction. The effects of insulin resistance that contribute to systolic dysfunction of the heart include impairment of the coronary microcirculation, mitochondrial dysfunction and lipotoxicity. The CFR is impaired in diabetic patients; these findings have been extended to nondiabetic individuals, with more severe insulin resistance associated with lower CFR. Diabetes has been shown to reduce mitochondrial oxidative capacity by suppressing genes that produce proteins active in oxidative phosphorylation and through impaired calcium homeostasis; the resultant decline in ATP production can lead to impaired myocardial contractile efficiency.

Detection of Systolic Dysfunction

Echocardiographic studies have noted impairment of systolic function in patients with metabolic syndrome as compared to controls as measured by the Tei index, a combination of systolic and diastolic dysfunction, while subclinical systolic dysfunction has been unmasked in diabetic individuals using dobutamine stress echocardiography: with stress, diabetics had lower measures of systolic function than controls. Others have shown cardiac steatosis detected by cardiac MRI in patients with impaired glucose tolerance when compared to normal controls, which is also associated with systolic dysfunction. Though not specific to insulin resistant cardiomyopathy, late gadolinium enhancement detected by cardiac MRI predicts subsequent cardiovascular outcomes likely due to an association with ventricular tachycardia; the prevalence of this in patients with insulin resistance is not known. Finally, invasive angiography and measurement of CFR had been shown to predict prognosis in both diabetic and nondiabetic patients: patients with abnormal CFR exhibited higher rates of death and myocardial infarction than those with normal CFR.

❏ TREATMENT

As the role of insulin resistance in the development and propagation of cardiomyopathy has only recently been investigated, there are no large scale clinical trials of therapy targeting insulin resistance in individuals with heart failure. Thus,

Table 1: Potential therapeutic options		
Medication	**Mechanism**	**Other/side effects**
Metabolic modulators		
Trimetazidine	↓ FFA metabolism	Not approved in US
Prehexiline	↓ FFA metabolism	Not approved in US, liver/neurotoxicity
Ranolazine	↑ Glu metabolis,	Might not be primary mechanism, ↑ QT interval
L-carnitine	↑ FFA/Glu metabolism	
Diabetic medications		
Insulin	↑ Ins	Hypoglycemia
Sulfonylureas	↑ Ins	Hypoglycemia
Metformin	↑ Ins sensitivity	Lactic acidosis (rare)
TZDs ("glitazones")	↑ Ins sensitivity	Fluid retention/edema
GLP-1	↑ Ins/↑ Ins sensitivity	Very short half-life (1–2 min)
Exenatide	↑ Ins/↑ Ins sensitivity	Nausea/weight loss, subcutaneous injection
DPP-IV inhibitor	↑ Ins/↑ Ins sensitivity	

(Abbreviations: DPP: Dipeptidyl peptidase; FFA: Free fatty acid; GLP: Glucagon-like peptide; Glu: Glucose; Ins: Insulin; TZD: Thiazolidinedione).
(Source: Modified from Witteles and Fowler. JACC. 2008)

much of the evidence supporting treatment modalities for this condition are based upon extrapolation from other clinical populations or from small scale animal and human studies (Table 1).

Antiadrenergic Therapy

Since insulin resistance worsens with heart failure, therapies that lead to significant myocardial remodeling and improved systolic function could conceivably lead to improved insulin resistance.

Thus, the recommended therapies for heart failure, including beta-blockers (BB), angiotensin-converting enzyme inhibitors (ACEI) or angiotensin receptor blockers, and aldosterone antagonists will improve the insulin resistant state in patients with systolic heart failure. Antineurohormonal therapy can also directly modify insulin resistance. ACEIs have been shown to reduce insulin resistance in various patient cohorts, although BB have been shown to adversely affect insulin resistance and increase fasting glucose levels in diabetics.

Insulin Therapy

The benefit of insulin therapy in modifying the progression of cardiovascular disease has become more controversial due to recent data. The large, prospective trials of glycemic control, including UK Prospective Diabetes Study (UKPDS) have shown a decrease in microvascular complications with better glucose control, whether with provision of insulin or insulin secretagogues, such as the sulfonylureas. Macrovascular complications have not been shown to decrease with tight glycemic control in patients with diabetes. This may in part be due to the reduced effect of insulin in patients with heart failure, an insulin resistant state; insulin infusions have been shown to improve systolic function in nondiabetics more than in diabetics.

Insulin Sensitization

While adrenergic antagonists can directly affect insulin resistance, more specific agents that target insulin resistance exist. Among these are the thiazolidinediones, rosiglitazone and pioglitazone. These directly affect insulin resistance by altering DNA expression, binding to the PPAR gamma receptor in cell nuclei. Other ancillary data suggesting improved outcomes with agents that directly improve insulin resistance include a study by Shannon et al. that employed infusions of GLP-1, a peptide that increases insulin sensitivity, which was found to increase glucose uptake and improve LV performance in patients with reduced LV systolic function following acute infarct. Some promising data have arisen from the bariatric surgery field. The striking weight loss from bariatric surgery has been shown to improve insulin resistance and to improve LV mass and diastolic function as measured by cardiac MRI.

Metabolic Modulators

Given the preference for glucose utilization in the failing heart but a paradoxical increase in FFA concentrations, another hypothetical approach to treating insulin resistant cardiomyopathy would be to decrease FFA utilization or production, or increase carbohydrate metabolism. Trimetazidine, etoxomir, and perhexiline are agents that decrease FFA metabolism, the former by inhibiting beta-oxidation of FFAs, and the latter two by inhibiting mitochondrial transport of FFAs. Trimetazidine is one of the more promising agents to be studied in patients with heart failure and has been found to improve LV systolic function while reducing LV dimensions.

❏ SUGGESTED READINGS

Fragasso G, Palloshi A, Puccetti P, et al. A randomized clinical trial of trimetazidine, a partial free fatty acid oxidation inhibitor, in patients with heart failure. J Am Coll Cardiol. 2006;48:992-8.

Haffner SM. Insulin-resistance, inflammation, and the prediabetic state. Am J Cardiol. 2003;92:18J-26J.

Kinoshita M, Nakaya Y, Harada N, et al. Combination therapy of exercise and angiotensin-converting enzyme inhibitor markedly improves insulin sensitivities in hypertensive patients with insulin-resistance. Circ J. 2002;66:655-8.

Neubauer S. The failing heart—an engine out of fuel. N Engl J Med. 2007;356:1140-51.

Nikolaidis LA, Sturzu A, Stolarski C, et al. The development of myocardial insulin-resistance in conscious dogs with advanced dilated cardiomyopathy. Cardiovasc Res. 2004;61:297-306.

Page A, Dumesnil JG, Clavel MA, et al. Metabolic syndrome is associated with more pronounced impairment of left ventricle geometry and function in patients with calcific aortic stenosis: a substudy of the ASTRONOMER (Aortic Stenosis Progression Observation Measuring Effects of Rosuvastatin). J Am Coll Cardiol. 2010;55:1867-74.

Poirier P, Bogaty P, Garneau C, et al. Diastolic dysfunction in normotensive men with well-controlled type 2 diabetes: importance of maneuvers in echocardiographic screening for preclinical diabetic cardiomyopathy. Diabetes Care. 2001;24:5-10.

Reaven GM. Insulin-resistance/compensatory hyperinsulinemia, essential hypertension and cardiovascular disease. J Clin Endocrinol Metab. 2003;88:2399-403.

Rider OJ, Francis JM, Ali MK, et al. Beneficial cardiovascular effects of bariatric surgical and dietary weight loss in obesity. J Am Coll Cardiol. 2009;54:718-26.

Verdecchia P, Reboldi G, Schillaci G, et al. Circulating insulin and insulin growth factor-1 are independent determinants of left ventricular mass and geometry in essential hypertension. Circulation. 1999;100:1802-7.

Witteles RM, Fowler MB. Insulin-resistant cardiomyopathy clinical evidence, mechanisms, and treatment options. J Am Coll Cardiol. 2008;51:93-102.

10.3 Cardiac Complications of Substance Abuse

❑ INTRODUCTION

The use of mood-altering substances occurs quite frequently in modern society and ranges from the social use of alcohol to the intravenous administration of cocaine, heroin, and other illegal substances. Many of these substances produce cardiac complications, particularly if taken in large enough quantities over long enough periods of time. The spectrum of pathology ranges from the acute overdose at one end to the more subtle chronic issues related to long-standing usage patterns at the other. The distinction between these two ends of the spectrum offers some value to the clinician as the clinical presentations are generally quite different.

❑ SUBSTANCES OF ABUSE

Cocaine

Coca leaves, the source of cocaine, have been chewed and ingested for thousands of years, making cocaine one of the oldest known stimulants. Cocaine was second only to marijuana as the most commonly used illicit drug in the United States from 2005 to 2006 and was first in terms of the illicit drug leading to the most emergency department evaluations from 1995 to 2002. Although there appears to be significant movement in terms of decreasing usage patterns, the current numbers still fall near the two million mark and will continue to present the health care community with the various cocaine related issues that have been seen and studied in the past.

Pharmacologically active diluting agents include procaine (with its local anesthetic effect), methamphetamine, and others. The two forms of cocaine that are abused are the water soluble hydrochloride salt and the water insoluble cocaine base (freebase). The water soluble form, the fine white crystalline powder, can be snorted or injected. The insoluble base form results from processing with ammonia or sodium bicarbonate and water, and heating to remove the hydrochloride. The final product can then be smoked. The term "crack" refers to the street name given to freebase cocaine which produces a crackling sound when smoked.

Cardiovascular Complications

The activation of the postsynaptic alpha-adrenergic receptors in the vascular system causes vasoconstriction and hypertension, while activation of the beta-adrenergic receptors of the myocardium causes tachycardia and enhanced contractility. In addition, cocaine increases end-systolic wall stress and reduces left ventricular function. Of interest in this regard is that plasma levels of cocaine are not linearly related to central nervous system effects, and the subjective "high" sought by the user dissipates at a time when plasma levels are still significantly elevated. The practice of repeating cocaine administration to maintain the "high" over a number of hours can lead to progressively more elevated plasma levels (with corresponding cardiac toxicity) without the similarly improved mood sought by the user.

Coronary Artery Vasoconstriction

Small medically indicated doses of intranasal cocaine (10% cocaine hydrochloride, 2 mg/kg) have been shown to cause vasoconstriction of coronary arteries, increased heart rate and BP, and reduction of coronary sinus blood flow in patients with or without atherosclerotic coronary artery disease (CAD). The degree of vasoconstriction may be more prominent in patients with CAD. Cocaine-induced vasoconstriction has been shown to be alpha-adrenergic receptor mediated, more pronounced in stenotic as opposed to nonstenotic coronary segments, and is generally believed to be accentuated by beta-adrenergic-blockade (unopposed alpha-adrenergic effects). Vasoconstriction may also occur via other mechanisms, including cocaine precipitated release of plasma endothelin-1 which causes vasoconstriction and impaired production of nitric oxide, a vasodilator.

Acute Coronary Artery Thrombosis

There are a number of different mechanisms by which the propensity for clot formation and coronary artery thrombosis increases in the presence of circulating cocaine. There is an increase in plasminogen activator inhibitor. There are also a number of changes in the platelets, including an acute increase in the number of platelets, an increased platelet activation, and increased platelet aggregation. Cocaine users have also been found to have increased levels of C-reactive protein, von Willebrand factor and fibrinogen which probably contribute to the coagulopathic issues.

Direct Myocardial Damage

Autopsy studies of patients who used cocaine but died from an unrelated cause (trauma) have demonstrated that cocaine may exert direct toxic effects on the heart, with myocardial inflammation and interstitial fibrosis. Myocardial biopsy specimens in the setting of acute cocaine toxicity have demonstrated focal myocyte necrosis, focal myocarditis, sarcoplasmic vacuolization, and myofibrillar loss. Contraction band necrosis has been reported to occur in the myocardium of patients who died of complications of cocaine abuse. It probably represents this adrenergic stress and may be linked to malignant terminal arrhythmias, such as ventricular fibrillation.

Recent animal studies of neonates born from cocaine-treated hamster mothers demonstrate irreversible focal ischemic damage to the Purkinje cells, as well as endocardial damage, and myocardial cell vacuolization. These findings were felt to be consistent with the pharmacotoxicity of cocaine.

Coronary Artery Atherosclerosis

Accelerated atherosclerosis has been demonstrated at autopsy in young cocaine users and in patients with cocaine related sudden death. Premature coronary atherosclerosis is common in young cocaine abusers.

Cardiac Arrhythmias

Among the rhythms seen, sinus tachycardia is commonplace. In anesthesia, cocaine is associated with a greater incidence of arrhythmias, particularly premature ventricular beats. Cocaine has also been implicated in the production or exacerbation of supraventricular tachycardias, ventricular tachycardia (VT), torsades de pointes, accelerated idioventricular rhythm, sinus bradycardia, asystole and ventricular fibrillation. The conduction system of the heart has a prominent place in these discussions as cocaine disrupts normal electrical activity, causing increased PR, QRS and QT intervals on the electrocardiogram (ECG). These effects are generally attributed to direct effects on the potassium, sodium and calcium channels.

Channelopathies

Cocaine has also been shown to block K^+ channels, increase L-type Ca^{2+} channel current, and inhibit Na^+ influx during depolarization, all possible causes for arrhythmia. Electrocardiogram changes in the setting of cocaine abuse are generally attributed to the direct effects of cocaine on these cardiac ion channels where multiple sites of action have been demonstrated. Cocaine inhibits L-type calcium currents, delays potassium channel currents, and inhibits sodium currents providing influx during repolarization, and these actions are thought to have direct effects in the arena of cocaine induced arrhythmia. The sympathomimetic effects of cocaine may also be related to actions on the cardiac ion channels.

Myocardial Ischemia and Infarction

Several mechanisms may contribute to cocaine related MI. The adrenergic physiology with tachycardia and hypertension may produce ischemia in patients with preexisting atherosclerotic CAD. Decrease or total interruption of coronary blood flow resulting from spasm or thrombosis may also occur, and this likelihood seems higher in patients with normal coronary arteries at cardiac catheterization or autopsy. Thrombosis may also cause AMI in the presence of anatomically normal coronary arteries. Catecholamine mediated direct myocardial injury is another potential mechanism. Angina or silent myocardial ischemia may occur in patients using cocaine and the incidence of episodes of silent ischemia may be as high as 87% in these patients and may be observed during the first weeks of withdrawal. Cocaine and methamphetamine are probably the major risk factors for young people who present with an acute coronary syndrome (ACS). Finally, although approximately a third of patients with cocaine-induced MI develop complications, such as congestive heart failure (CHF) or arrhythmias, the overall mortality in hospitalized patients remains exceedingly low.

ECG Changes

Cocaine can cause prolongation of the PR interval, of the QRS duration, and of the QT interval of the ECG. The interpretation of ECGs in patients with cocaine-associated chest pain can be challenging. Cocaine-induced MI has been documented in patients with normal ECGs as well as with abnormal ECGs. On the other hand, a significant proportion of patients meeting the electrocardiographic criteria for ST-elevation myocardial infarction (STEMI) may not have MI.

Chest Pain

Cocaine chest pain is a frequent presentation in routine emergency medical practice. Many other causes of chest pain occur in the setting of cocaine abuse, and due consideration should be given to them in terms of differential diagnosis. Aortic dissection should always be a consideration in patients with severe chest pain. Acute rupture of the ascending aorta has been reported in cocaine users. Cocaine has also been reported to cause coronary artery aneurysms and ectasia. Barotrauma also occurs in this population. Smoking freebase cocaine may cause lung damage and noncardiac pulmonary edema. Spontaneous pneumomediastinum and pneumopericardium have been reported.

Treatment

Volume adjustment: If some degree of tachycardia arises from a volume down status, poor oral intake or blood loss for example, that should be addressed. Likewise, if the patient has pump problems, ACS or CHF for example, the underlying issues must be identified and the management adjusted accordingly.

Analgesics: This should be treated and the component of the adrenergic physiology removed from the equation. If the pain arises from some source other than cocaine, some secondary orthopedic injury for example, that should be addressed in the appropriate fashion.

Benzodiazepines: They reduce heart rate and systemic arterial pressure, thereby decreasing myocardial demand and directly addressing the agitation and anxiety which occurs so commonly in these patients. The downside of sequential IV benzodiazepine titration in these patients should be minimal unless specific mental status or neurological examination findings mandate inclusion of differential diagnoses such as intracranial hemorrhage, meningitis or traumatic brain injury, all of which may be seen and any of which may dictate a more nuanced approach to the situation.

Nitroglycerin: Nitrates or benzodiazepines are effective when used alone or in combination and can resolve chest pain and improve cardiac performance. The agent of choice may be influenced by CNS symptomatology.

Oxygen, aspirin, heparin, PCI, thrombolytics: Oxygen should be a part of the routine management of cocaine associated chest pain patients, along with venous access, cardiac monitoring, ECG, and laboratory work with troponins. Aspirin administration to inhibit platelet aggregation in patients with cocaine-induced myocardial ischemia is reasonable and should also be done. Heparin and coronary catheterization and thrombolytics should be the next consideration, and these are site specific in terms of availability. A cardiologist should be involved in this decision making process. The American College of Cardiology/American Heart Association guidelines advocate the use of thrombolytic therapy if ST segments remain elevated despite nitroglycerin and calcium antagonists and if coronary arteriography is not possible (class II A indication). The updated ACC/AHA guidelines for STEMI management and for PCI do not offer any additional recommendations regarding cocaine, other than to include the recent use of cocaine as a low likelihood factor in determining whether the patient's signs and symptoms represent an ACS secondary to CAD.

Bicarbonate: The potential use of sodium bicarbonate in cocaine-induced sodium channel blockade arises from the action of bicarbonate in reversing QRS prolongation and stabilizing arrhythmias due to sodium channel blocking drugs, such as tricyclic antidepressants and Class Ic anti-arrhythmic drugs like flecainide. Models of flecainide toxicity, a drug which has similar properties to cocaine, show that sodium bicarbonate partially reversed the QRS prolongation. This effect does not occur in patients with mild QRS prolongation due to therapeutic use of flecainide.

Beta-blockers: There has been a perennial debate regarding the use of beta-blockers to manage the adrenergic physiology of cocaine, particularly with cocaine precipitated ACS. Underlying theoretical support for the use of beta blockade involves the use dependent kinetics of cocaine binding to sodium channels, in which the degree of cocaine binding increases with tachycardia. Reduction of the heart rate in isolation, in this model, could theoretically reduce cocaine binding to sodium channels resulting in normalization of the QRS prolongation. This was tested in animals and found not to be true. In a relatively strong toxicology editorial, on the other hand, it was noted that the majority of patients with cocaine chest pain will continue to use cocaine after discharge, and the usual practice of starting patients on long-term beta blockade may be unwise.

Subacute and Chronic Problems

These include chest pain presentations beyond the period of acute intoxication, an advanced rate of atherosclerosis, the issue of hypercoagulable states with non-cardiac related clot formation, myocarditis, cardiomyopathy and CHF. With regard to long-term therapy and outpatient management, the primary goal should be abstention from cocaine. Many case reports have shown improvement in LVF after stopping cocaine. LVD and heart failure may recur if the patient returns to cocaine use. Patients should be advised that continued cocaine use increases their risk of heart attack, heart failure, stroke and sudden death.

Cocaine Washout

The syndrome of "cocaine washout" (also seen as methamphetamine washout) occurs as a state of deep depression of the level of consciousness following a hyperadrenergic state, particularly one which has gone on for some time. The acuity of the situation often dictates the specific evaluation and workup required, and the clinical question often becomes not just whether cocaine was involved, but whether only cocaine was involved. A perennial concern lies with deciding whether the washout phase may really represent some other underlying pathology requiring an approach other than observation and watchful waiting.

Polysubstance Abuse

The use of cocaine in combination with tobacco causes more tachycardia and more vasoconstriction than does the use of tobacco or cocaine alone. The use of cocaine in combination with tobacco causes more tachycardia and more vasoconstriction than does the use of tobacco or cocaine alone. The metabolism of cocaine with ethanol (transesterification) occurs in the liver and results in the metabolite cocaethylene, which is considered to be more lethal than the parent cocaine. Cocaethylene blocks reuptake of dopamine and may be responsible for the increase in cardiovascular complications observed in this setting.

Methamphetamine

The amphetamines are a group of chemically related drugs, which produce similar effects. Methamphetamine (also referred to as meth, speed, ice, crystal, chalk and glass) may be the most widely circulated compound of this group. Synthetic amphetamine compounds may be synthesized in clandestine laboratories with variable purity and potency. The potential routes of administration may be oral, inhalation or parenteral (intravenous).

Cardiovascular Complications

A number of complications have been connected to methamphetamine use, including the usual adrenergic physiology findings of tachycardia and hypertension. Other cardiovascular complications include myocarditis, necrotizing vasculitis, cardiomyopathy, pulmonary hypertension (cor pulmonale), and cardiac arrhythmias. There have also been reports of acute coronary syndromes (ACS) and sudden death. One recent review mentions accelerated atherosclerosis, hypercoagulable states and epicardial coronary artery spasm similar to those issues with cocaine.

Noncardiac Complications

Among the other complications seen with methamphetamine abuse are aortic dissection, central nervous system pathology, such as ruptured berry aneurysms and cerebral hemorrhage, and rhabdomyolysis. Chronic use of these drugs can produce insomnia, anxiety, confusion, mood and other psychiatric disorders, behavioral disorders, violence as well as severe dental problems. With parenteral use, the usual infectious complications of IVDU also occur. These may include hepatitis, endocarditis and HIV/AIDS.

Phenylpropanolamine

Phenylpropanolamine (PPA) hydrochloride is a sympathomimetic compound, structurally and functionally similar to amphetamine and ephedrine. It is a component of more than one hundred over the counter medications, including nasal decongestants, anorectics and stimulants. The cardiovascular effects of PPA, including vasoconstriction and increased cardiac output, are related to its alpha- and beta-adrenergic activity. This may or may not benefit weight control effort programs or symptoms of the common cold, but the use of PPA in patients with heart disease and hypertension can clearly be hazardous.

The sympathomimetic effects are well recognized and more an effect of the drug than a complication, but the elevated BP can present as a hypertensive emergency. Additional cardiac complications may include atrial and ventricular arrhythmias, myocarditis, myocardial damage, MI, and cardiac arrest. The noncardiac complications relate to the central nervous system with psychosis, headaches, seizures, and fatal CVAs with an area of predilection, hemorrhagic strokes in young women. Another complication related to vasospasm includes ischemic bowel.

❏ MARIJUANA, TETRAHYDROCANNABINOL, HASHISH

Marijuana is the most commonly used illegal drug in the US. It is made up of dried parts of the cannabis sativa hemp plant, and can be smoked or taken orally. Tetrahydrocannabinol (THC) is the main found in the plant. Hashish is a concentrated form of marijuana, which is smoked, the use of which is much more common in Europe. Given the prevalence of the use of this drug, there are surprisingly few complications. Occasional cases of increases in the mean arterial pressure, ventricular fibrillation, and coronary vasospasm have been reported.

❏ CLUB DRUGS: MDMA, GHB, KETAMINE, ROHYPNOL

The term "club drugs" refers to a group of drugs used by young adults often associated with nightclubs and parties, particularly all night dance parties called "raves" that take place in nightclubs and other venues. The US Office of National Drug Control Policy identifies four specific club drugs: (i) methylenedioxymethamphetamine or "ecstasy" (MDMA), (ii) gammahydroxybutyrate (GHB), (iii) ketamine, and (iv) rohypnol (flunitrazepam). A study of club drug usage by medical students encompassed a somewhat larger group of drugs, classifying them as Generation I (cocaine and LSD) and Generation II (MDMA, ketamine, GHB, methamphetamine, rohypnol and dextromethorphan). These categories were based upon "their initial widespread use in club settings". The usage pattern was based upon an anonymous questionnaire.

Methylenedioxymethamphetamine

Methylenedioxymethamphetamine (MDMA) or ecstasy is a synthetic drug with stimulant and psychoactive properties. MDMA affects neurotransmitters, principally in the serotonin system where it acts as a serotonin agonist.

Given that MDMA is structurally related to the amphetamines, there is less by way of cardiac complications than one might expect. MDMA may lead to mild to moderate valvular heart disease and valvular strands. Dilated cardiomyopathy has been reported in conjunction with liver damage attributed to MDMA. MI has also been reported in a single patient.

Gammahydroxybutyrate

Gammahydroxybutyrate (GHB) is structurally related to gamma-aminobutyric acid (GABA) and inhibits dopamine release and activates tyrosine hydroxylase, both of which increase central dopamine levels which may be associated with the clinical effects. Apart from its other systemic effects, cardiovascular complications were not a major issue. Those occurred in less than 10% of the patients, and included only bradycardia, tachycardia and hypertension.

Ketamine

Ketamine distorts perception producing a dissociative state which may be quite useful clinically, in controlled settings and dosages. It is an N-methyl-D-aspartate (NMDA) receptor antagonist. It decreases excitatory amino acid neurotransmission mediated by NMDA receptors through calcium channel blockade, and has been associated with altered perception, memory and cognition. Numerous effects of ketamine have been described and many are directly related to the actions of the drug. There appear to be no specific cardiac complications associated with ketamine, other than issues with the tachycardia and hypertension in patients for whom these issues would be problematic.

Rohypnol

Flunitrazepam (Rohypnol) is a benzodiazepine used as a sedative hypnotic. It acts as a GABA agonist, mediating inhibitory neurotransmission in the brain and spinal cord. Adverse effects include the expected sedation and impaired functioning, along with visual disturbances, confusion, GI disturbances and urinary retention. In terms of cardiovascular complications, hypotension has been noted, but as with any benzodiazepine overdose, the process may include loss of consciousness and respiratory failure if sufficient quantities of the drug have been taken.

❑ BODY IMAGE DRUGS

Anabolic Steroids

Synthetic anabolic androgenic steroids are widely used by professional athletes in many sports, perhaps somewhat less at present given the rigid proscriptions and testing now in place, but for weight lifters and body builders the issue persists. Among the various cardiovascular complications which have been reported are sudden cardiac death, LV hypertrophy, reduced LVF, cardiomyopathy, CHF, arterial thrombosis, pulmonary embolism and AMI. Anabolic steroids also cause a thrombotic state by increasing platelet aggregation. There is also data showing alterations of lipid metabolism, with elevations of low-density lipoprotein (LDL) and decreases of high-density lipoproteins (HDL), which increase the risk of CAD.

Diet Drugs

Fenfluramine, dexfenfluramine and phenteramine (fen fen) have an established role in the development of valvular heart disease; along with other drugs such as MDMA (ecstasy). The FDA received five reports of similar series of patients on these drugs with an overall incidence of 32% having valvular heart disease. The risk was increased for patients taking the drug for more than 6 months. On the basis of these reports, fenfluramine and dexfenfluramine were voluntarily withdrawn from the market.

Anorexia and Bulimia

There continue to be issues among young people (mostly female) with pathologic concerns about weight leading to induced vomiting, abuse of furosemide and other diuretics, and purging with emetics and laxatives. They may present with hypokalemia and ECG abnormalities including low voltage, bradycardia, ST and T wave changes, prolonged QT interval, and U waves due to hypokalemia. The prolonged QT interval in anorexia nervosa has led to ventricular arrhythmias and death. Cardiomyopathy has been seen as well.

❑ NARCOTICS

Heroin

Heroin, the prototype of illicit drugs, is processed from morphine and is highly addictive. It can be used by injection, nasal insufflation, or by smoking and usually causes euphoria, clouded thinking and altered mental states. The researchers have described heroin associated cardiomyopathy in some historical detail along with a number of other cases. The pathophysiology of heroin-induced cardiomyopathy was felt to be uncertain, but one fatal case had microscopic findings at autopsy in the myocardium that resembled those in skeletal muscle with focal myolysis.

Methadone

Methadone appears in the clinical arena as an analgesic for chronic pain patients, particularly cancer-related pain, and as a pharmacologic adjunct to assist in weaning patients from illegal opiates. Cardiac complications with methadone may involve QT interval prolongation, which has been noted to provoke ventricular arrhythmias and particularly torsades de pointes. Sudden cardiac death has also been reported with methadone therapy.

❑ SUGGESTED READINGS

Afonso L, Mohammad T, Thatai D. Crack whips the heart: a review of the cardiovascular toxicity of cocaine. Am J Cardiol. 2007;100:1040-3.

Antman EM, Hand M, Armstrong PW, et al. 2007 Focused Update of the ACC/AHA 2004 Guidelines for the Management of Patients with ST-Elevation Myocardial Infarction: a report of the American College of Cardiology/American Heart Association Task Force on Practice Guidelines: developed in collaboration with the Canadian Cardiovascular Society endorsed by the American Academy of Family Physicians: 2007 Writing Group to Review New Evidence and Update the ACC/AHA 2004 Guidelines for the Management of Patients with ST-Elevation Myocardial Infarction, Writing on Behalf of the 2004 Writing Committee. Circulation. 2008;117:296-329.

Callaham M. Cardiac complications of substance abuse. In: Chatterjee K, Rapaport E, Cheitlin M, Parmley W, Scheinman M (Eds). Cardiology: An Illustrated Text/Reference. Philadelphia, PA: Gower Medical Publishing; 1991. pp. 13. 74-13.81.

Connolly HM, Crary JL, McGoon MD, et al. Valvular heart disease associated with fenfluramine-phentermine. N Engl J Med. 1997;337:581-8.

Ehret GB, Desmeules JA, Broers B. Methadone-associated long QT syndrome: improving pharmacotherapy for dependence on illegal opioids and lessons learned for pharmacology. Expert Opin Drug Saf. 2007;6:289-303.

Foltin RW, Fischman MW, Pedroso JJ, et al. Marijuana and cocaine interactions in humans: cardiovascular consequences. Pharmacol Biochem Behav. 1987;28:459-64.

Gawin FH, Ellinwood EH. Cocaine and other stimulants. Actions, abuse, and treatment. N Engl J Med. 1988;318:1173-82.

Leo PJ, Hollander JE, Shih RD, et al. Phenylpropanolamine and associated myocardial injury. Ann Emerg Med. 1996;28:359-62.

McCord J, Jneid H, Hollander JE, et al. Management of cocaine-associated chest pain and myocardial infarction: a scientific statement from the American Heart Association Acute Cardiac Care Committee of the Council on Clinical Cardiology. Circulation. 2008;117:1897-907.

SAMHSA. Results from the 2008 National Survey on Drug Use and Health: National Findings, NSDUH Series H-36, HHS Publication No. SMA 09-4434. In: Substance Abuse and Mental Health Services Administration OoAS, Division of Population Surveys, SAMSHA ed. Rockville, MD; 2009.

Vanberg P, Atar D. Androgenic anabolic steroid abuse and the cardiovascular system. Handb Exp Pharmacol. 2010:411-57.

Wu LT, Schlenger WE, Galvin DM. Concurrent use of methamphetamine, MDMA, LSD, ketamine, GHB, and flunitrazepam among American youths. Drug Alcohol Depend. 2006;84:102-13.

10.4 HIV/AIDS and Cardiovascular Disease

❑ INTRODUCTION

According to data from the Joint United Nations Programme on HIV/AIDS and the World Health Organization in 2008, an estimated 1.4 million people were living with human immunodeficiency virus (HIV) or acquired immunodeficiency syndrome (AIDS) in North America and there were over 33 million living with HIV or AIDS worldwide. As patients are living longer, chronic health complications, such as cardiovascular disease (CVD), represent an increasing important health issue in this patient population. The mechanism underlying CVD in the setting of HIV is most likely multifactorial and related to inflammation in the setting of HIV infection, side effects from antiretroviral medication and HIV-related immune responses.

❑ HIV AND CORONARY HEART DISEASE

Since the initial reports of myocardial infarction (MI) in HIV-infected patients on antiretroviral treatment in 1998, an increasing number of observational studies have reported higher rates of coronary heart disease (CHD) among HIV-infected individuals. While the data regarding coronary events in HIV disease are conflicting, the majority of studies suggest the concept that antiretroviral therapy is associated with increased CHD risk among individuals with HIV. These studies also suggested that, although long-term treatment with HAART, especially PIs, may lead to detrimental cardiovascular effects, there may be beneficial effects of HAART in the short-term, providing additional evidence that HIV itself is mechanistically associated with increased CHD risk.

Clinical Characteristics of CHD in HIV-infected Individuals

Compared to uninfected controls, HIV patients, who develop acute coronary syndrome, are more than a decade younger, with a mean age of 50 years. They are also more likely to be male, to be current smokers and to have low high density lipoprotein (HDL) cholesterol. As expected, HIV patients tend to have low thrombolysis in myocardial infarction (TIMI) risk scores, and tend to have single, rather than multiple-vessel coronary artery disease. In general, HIV patients hospitalized with acute coronary syndrome have excellent immediate outcomes, with successful percutaneous coronary intervention procedures. However, when compared with noninfected controls, HIV patients tend to develop higher rates of future stent-related complications.

Pathogenesis of Coronary Heart Disease in HIV Infection

Compared to the general population, atherosclerosis in HIV patients may represent a pathologically distinct entity, although autopsy studies have had mixed results. Chronic inflammation and T cell activation are thought to play a central role in the development of atherosclerosis. The underlying mechanism of early atherosclerosis in HIV disease is not well understood, but may be due to direct viral effects, the use of highly active antiretroviral therapy (HAART) and associated metabolic changes or host immune responses. Specifically, the HIV envelope protein gp-120 has been linked to higher endothelin-1 levels. Clinical observations also support the potential role of HIV disease in the pathogenesis of early atherosclerosis, as both CD4+ count and viral load appear to influence cardiovascular risk. The CD4+ count nadir predicts subclinical carotid atherosclerosis, and a low CD4+ count on HAART has been associated with increased risk of CVD. From a mechanistic standpoint, endothelial cells appear to play a central role in the pathogenesis of HIV-associated atherosclerosis, as do procoagulant changes, fibrinolytic effects, and increased activation of platelets. Elevations in levels of endothelial cell derived markers, such as von Willebrand factor antigen, have been reported in HIV disease, particularly in patients with a high viral burden or advanced disease. Circulating levels of the adhesion molecules—intercellular adhesion molecule-1 (ICAM-1) and vascular adhesion molecule-1 (VCAM-1)—have also been shown to be elevated in HIV patients compared with noninfected controls, and were directly related to the degree of inflammation as assessed by soluble receptor type 2 for TNFalpha (sTNFR2). HIV-infected individuals also have higher high sensitivity C-reactive protein (hsCRP) levels and T cell activation compared with uninfected individuals. Lastly, chronic activation of the immune system in HIV infection may also be due to microbial translocation in the gastrointestinal tract, leading to elevated levels of circulating microbial products, such as lipopolysaccharide, which may activate immune and inflammatory pathways.

HIV and Cardiovascular Risk Factors

HIV infection and antiretroviral therapy are also associated with a variety of traditional risk factors, including dyslipidemia, metabolic syndrome, hypertension and cigarette smoking. In the early stages of HIV infection before treatment, the predominant changes appear to be hypertriglyceridemia, low HDL and low LDL levels with predominant small, dense LDL particles when compared with controls. In contrast, after initiation of HAART, LDL and total cholesterol levels appear to increase, while HDL cholesterol appears to remain low, findings that are particularly associated with the use of PIs.

The HIV-associated lipodystrophy is a syndrome characterized by fat accumulation in the neck and dorsocervical region along with subcutaneous and peripheral fat loss, with relative preservation or increase in visceral fat, resulting in relative central adiposity. After starting HAART, these abnormalities are clinically evident in 20–35% of patients. The use of PIs as well as the concomitant use of the two NRTIs, stavudine and didanosine is strongly associated with the development of lipoatrophy. Lipodystrophy in HIV patients is commonly associated with different features of metabolic syndrome, including insulin resistance, impaired fasting glucose tolerance, elevated triglycerides, low HDL cholesterol and hypertension.

Treatment

Although treatment should largely be guided by existing recommendations in uninfected patients, two aspects particular to HIV-infected patients deserve attention: (i) the potential role of HAART with regard to CVD and (ii) the treatment of hyperlipidemia in HIV disease, for which separate recommendations have been devised.

Highly Active Antiretroviral Therapy

While long-term HAART may have adverse effects, it is becoming clearer that uncontrolled HIV replication leads not only to increased cardiovascular risk, but also to other non-AIDS complications. Current recommendations by the International AIDS Society USA Panel guidelines, thus, support HAART initiation for asymptomatic individuals at CD4+ counts less than 350 cells/μL, with 'individualized' therapy at CD4+ count greater than or equal to 350 cells/μL. Whether earlier initiation of HAART at higher CD4+ counts in the course of HIV disease improves cardiovascular risk is not known; however, guidelines do support earlier initiation of HAART in the setting of high cardiovascular risk, in addition to other high risk clinical features (high viral loads >100,000 copies/mL, rapidly declining CD4+ count >100/μL per year, active hepatitis B or C infections or the presence of HIV-associated nephropathy). The initial choice of HAART regimen is primarily targeted at viral suppression; however, metabolic profiles of drugs should be considered in patients at high cardiovascular risk. While traditional HAART may be constrained by HIV resistance and medication tolerability, novel antiretroviral agents, such as integrase inhibitors and viral entry inhibitors may in the future provide better options with regard to cardiovascular side effect profiles.

FLOWCHART 1: Treatment of hyperlipidemia in HIV-infected individuals

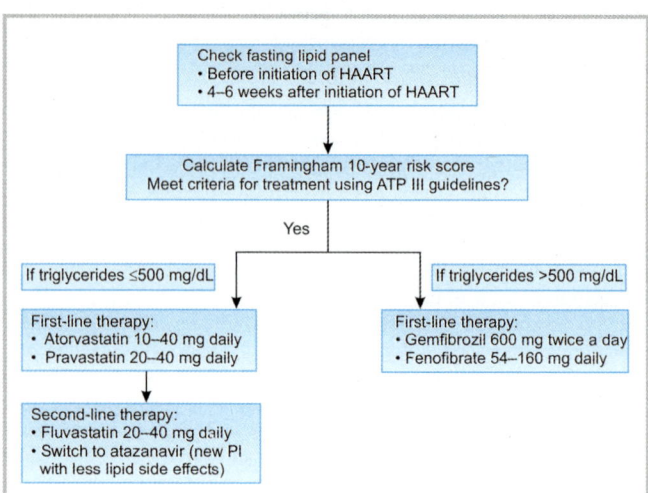

Hyperlipidemia

The Infectious Disease Society of America (IDSA) and Adult AIDS Clinical Trials Group (AACTG) have developed specific guidelines for the evaluation and management of HAART-related hyperlipidemia. These recommendations are largely based on National Cholesterol Education Program Adult Treatment Panel III (NCEP ATP III) guidelines, and advocate adjusting individual cholesterol targets to the underlying cardiovascular risk based on the Framingham predicted 10-year risk. A general algorithm of treatment of hyperlipidemia has been summarized in Flowchart 1.

Modification of Other Risk Factors

Smoking cessation, lifestyle changes in diet and exercise, and the appropriate treatment of hypertension and diabetes mellitus are all measures which should be pursued aggressively in this population. The most widely used screening tool is the Framingham risk score, which appears to underestimate CHD risk in HIV patients who are smokers. The IDSA/HIV Medicine Association (HIVMA) recommendations include checking fasting lipid panels before and within 4–6 weeks after starting HAART, fasting glucose levels before and during HAART, and routine measurements of body weight and changes in body shape.

❏ SURROGATE MEASURES OF ATHEROSCLEROSIS

Carotid Artery Intima-Media Thickness

In HIV-uninfected patients, carotid artery intima-media thickness (IMT) as assessed with B-mode ultrasound has been strongly correlated with coronary atherosclerosis, and is directly associated with increased risk of MI and stroke in older patients without known CVD. In general, the impact of HIV and HAART on subclinical atherosclerosis is still incompletely understood; however, most studies appear to demonstrate premature atherosclerosis in the HIV-infected population. The effect of HAART and PI use in particular on cardiovascular risk is no clearer in carotid IMT studies as it was in observational studies, and studies demonstrating a correlation between carotid IMT and clinical outcomes are lacking in the HIV-infected population. One of the current limitations of carotid IMT measurement is the lack of uniform methodology.

Brachial Artery Flow-mediated Dilation

Endothelial dysfunction is thought to play a central role in the development and progression of atherosclerosis and in non-HIV infected patients has been shown to predict future cardiovascular events. The hallmark of endothelial dysfunction is impaired endothelium-dependent vasodilation, which can be noninvasively assessed using brachial artery FMD. Whereas, carotid IMT is thought to reflect long-term exposure to atherogenic factors, brachial artery FMD is a measure of current vascular function and short-term exposures.

The relative contribution of HAART to endothelial dysfunction in HIV-infected individuals is complex. Data from numerous studies examining endothelial function and the use of HAART, in particular PI-based regimens are conflicting. Initiation of HAART in treatment-naïve patients however resulted in dramatic improvement in endothelial function both at 4 and 24 weeks of therapy, irrespective of whether a PI was used or not.

Coronary Artery Calcium Scoring

The quantification of coronary artery calcium (CAC) by electron beam computed tomography is a noninvasive marker of atherosclerosis that has been shown to predict coronary death and nonfatal MI in the noninfected population. Interestingly, a cross-sectional study of 400 HIV-infected patients showed that over 40% of individuals had evidence of increased vascular age as calculated on the basis of CAC scores published from the MESA study which was associated with current CD4+ T cell count.

❑ HIV-RELATED LEFT VENTRICULAR DYSFUNCTION AND MYOCARDITIS

The incidence of HIV-related dilated cardiomyopathy before HAART was 15.9 per 1,000 person-years, and has decreased significantly after introduction of HAART. The etiology of HIV-related cardiomyopathy is likely multifactorial, and may be due to direct infection of myocardial cells by HIV-1 virions, immune activation or coinfection with other viruses such as coxsackievirus B3 and cytomegalovirus, as well as nutritional deficiencies, autoimmune factors (increased anti-alpha myosin antibodies), and HAART toxicity (AZT). The treatment of HIV-related cardiomyopathy is unclear, and usual treatment for heart failure with afterload reduction appears reasonable. The prognosis of HIV-related cardiomyopathy appears to be worse than other nonischemic cardiomyopathies.

❑ CEREBROVASCULAR DISEASE

Although up to 40% of AIDS patients appeared to have neurologic complications, most of these were related to encephalopathy or infectious causes, although both ischemic stroke and intracranial hemorrhage have been described in HIV patients.

❑ MISCELLANEOUS

Pericardial effusion is the most common cardiac manifestation of HIV infection with prevalence up to 20%. Although most patients are asymptomatic and effusions are generally small, the presence of a pericardial effusion appears to be an independent predictor of mortality and poor prognosis. The risk of bacterial endocarditis in HIV-infected patients is similar to cohorts with similar risk behaviors, and the diagnosis and management is the same as in uninfected patients. Cardiac malignancies are quite rare in HIV patients, and include Kaposi's sarcoma and malignant lymphoma. HIV patients also have been noted to have prolonged QTc intervals, a finding which may be associated with myocarditis, cardiomyopathy and autonomic neuropathy.

❑ SUGGESTED READINGS

Arad Y, Spadaro LA, Goodman K, et al. Prediction of coronary events with electron beam computed tomography. J Am Coll Cardiol.2000;36:1253-60.

Barbaro G. HIV-associated cardiomyopathy etiopathogenesis and clinical aspects. Herz. 2005;30:486-92.

Davignon J, Ganz P. Role of endothelial dysfunction in atherosclerosis. Circulation. 2004;109:III27-32.

Hammer SM, Eron JJ, Reiss P, et al. Antiretroviral treatment of adult HIV infection: 2008 recommendations of the International AIDS Society-USA panel. JAMA. 2008;300:555-70.

Hansson GK. Inflammation, atherosclerosis, and coronary artery disease. N Engl J Med. 2005;352:1685-95.

Hsue PY, Giri K, Erickson S, et al. Clinical features of acute coronary syndromes in patients with human immunodeficiency virus infection. Circulation. 2004;109:316-9.

http://data.unaids.org/pub/EPISlides/2007/071118_epi_revisions_factsheet_en.pdf.

Kaplan RC, Kingsley LA, Sharrett AR, et al. Ten-year predicted coronary heart disease risk in HIV-infected men and women. Clin Infect Dis. 2007;45:1074-81.

Levy RM, Bredesen DE. Central nervous system dysfunction in acquired immunodeficiency syndrome. J Acquir Immune Defic Syndr. 1988;1:41-64.

O'Leary DH, Polak JF, Kronmal RA, et al. Carotid-artery intima and media thickness as a risk factor for myocardial infarction and stroke in older adults. Cardiovascular Health Study Collaborative Research Group. N Engl J Med. 1999;340:14-22.

Torriani FJ, Komarow L, Parker RA, et al. Endothelial function in human immunodeficiency virus-infected antiretroviral-naive subjects before and after starting potent antiretroviral therapy: the ACTG (AIDS Clinical Trials Group) Study 5152s. J Am Coll Cardiol. 2008;52:569-76.

Velasquez EM, Glancy DL. Cardiovascular disease in patients infected with the human immunodeficiency virus. J La State Med Soc. 2003;155:314-24.

10.5 Systemic Autoimmune Diseases and the Heart

❏ RHEUMATOID ARTHRITIS

Rheumatoid arthritis is the prototypical systemic autoimmune disease and patients with rheumatoid arthritis have an increased mortality when compared with the general population, due in part to cardiovascular diseases. The spectrum of cardiovascular involvement in rheumatoid arthritis is protean, and it may involve nearly all cardiovascular tissues, including the pericardium, myocardium, coronary arteries, conducting system, endocardium and valves, in addition to the aorta and peripheral vessels.

Clinical Features

Pericardial Involvement

The pericardium becomes involved in rheumatoid arthritis more often than the myocardium, endocardium or vascular structures of the heart. The clinical diagnosis of rheumatoid pericarditis is established in up to 2% of adults with rheumatoid arthritis; the rate rises to 6% in patients with systemic juvenile inflammatory arthritis (Still's disease) and 10% of hospitalized patients with rheumatoid arthritis. Pathophysiologically, acute fibrinous rheumatoid pericarditis involves the inflammatory interplay of leukocytes and immune complexes. The pericardial fluid contains low levels of glucose and complement factor 3 and elevated levels of lactic dehydrogenase, immunoglobulin, and cholesterol; rheumatoid factor is sometimes also detected. Histologically, there is plasma cell infiltration, immunoglobulin deposition and cytoplasmic inclusion of immune complexes, but rheumatoid granulomata (nodules) are unusual. More commonly, the inflammatory changes are nonspecific and include adhesions and scarring.

Compressive complications of rheumatoid pericarditis, such as acute cardiac tamponade and chronic constrictive pericarditis occur in less than 1% of cases. Most patients have positive tests for rheumatoid factor, and extra-articular features are common. Echocardiography, right heart catheterization, computed tomography, and magnetic resonance imaging are the mainstays of diagnosis. Neither tamponade nor constriction responds well to corticosteroid or cytotoxic medications and invasive approaches are usually required. In case of effusive-constrictive pericarditis in which fluid becomes loculated by pericardial adhesions, making needle aspiration or catheter drainage incompletely effective. In such cases, pericardectomy may be called for.

Myocardial Involvement

Disease of the myocardium associated with rheumatoid arthritis is an unusual, but recognized cause of heart failure. Myocarditis typically occurs in either a granulomatous or nonspecific form. The granulomatous form is considered specific for rheumatoid arthritis with nodules. The myocardial nodules have morphology similar to subcutaneous nodules, but a predilection for the left ventricle. The nonspecific form is characterized by infiltration of lymphocytes, plasma cells and histiocytes.

Most echocardiographic studies have focused on pericardial and endocardial changes. Some have reported lower diastolic closure rates (reduced E to F slope) of the anterior mitral valve leaflet in some patients with rheumatoid arthritis and suggested that abnormal ventricular compliance was responsible. Congestive symptoms were infrequent, however, and hemodynamic measurements have not been provided to corroborate the ultrasound findings. Patients with rheumatoid arthritis have a higher prevalence of heart failure compared with controls often on the basis of diastolic dysfunction. In patients with rheumatoid arthritis and cardiomyopathy, evaluation is directed to excluding reversible factors, such as volume overload, hypertension, pulmonary involvement, ischemia and rhythm disturbances. Management entails conventional modalities for treating heart failure.

Endocardial and Valvular Involvement

Like rheumatoid myocarditis, the histologic pattern of endocardial involvement in rheumatoid arthritis is nonspecific. There is infiltration of lymphocytes, histiocytes, plasma cells and occasionally eosinophils accompanied by collagen deposition, fibrosis, and calcific sclerosis. Valvular involvement is characterized by formation of granulomas that morphologically resemble the rheumatoid nodules encountered in subcutaneous tissue.

The order of frequency of involvement of the cardiac valves (mitral the highest, then aortic, tricuspid and pulmonic) parallels that in rheumatic fever and it is difficult to distinguish valvular disease related to rheumatoid arthritis from rheumatic heart disease following streptococcal infection without histological examination of the involved tissue. As in other forms of rheumatoid heart disease, clinical features occur less frequently than histologic abnormalities. Congestive symptoms are cardinal, but auscultatory clues may be misleading. Coexisting anemia or hypertension may distort cardiac murmurs, and auscultatory findings were commonly absent altogether in patients with granulomatous involvement of valvular tissue at necropsy. The hemodynamic consequences may reflect either valvular regurgitation or stenosis.

Disease of the Conducting System

Although progression to complete heart block seldom occurs, lesser degrees of conduction delay are fairly common. Other than direct involvement of the conducting system with granulomas, pathologic processes producing cardiac conducting system disease include extension of the inflammatory process from the base of the aortic or mitral valve leaflets, amyloidosis or hemorrhage into a rheumatoid nodule. Management of patients with symptomatic bradycardia resulting from involvement of the conducting system generally entails permanent cardiac pacemaker implantation. Therapeutic agents used to treat patients with rheumatoid arthritis may be associated with complete heart block. Other than conduction system disorders, patients with rheumatoid arthritis occasionally display abnormalities of impulse generation in the form of sinoatrial block, wandering atrial pacemaker and atrial fibrillation. A significant correlation has been reported between the severity of inflammation in patients with rheumatoid arthritis, heart rate variability on ambulatory cardiac rhythm monitoring, ventricular arrhythmias, myocardial infarction, and sudden cardiac death.

Coronary Artery Disease

A relationship between inflammation and accelerated atherosclerosis has been recognized, and corticosteroid therapy has also been thought to accelerate the progression of the atherosclerotic process. Inflammatory markers, such as C-reactive protein, are associated with atherosclerotic risk, but the mechanisms of this relationship are incompletely understood. Tumor necrosis factor (TNF)-alpha and interleukin (IL)-6 are associated with coronary atherosclerosis in patients with rheumatoid arthritis, and therapy directed against TNF may decrease cardiovascular morbidity. Inhibition of IL-6 is another potential avenue for decreasing atherosclerosis, but in a double blind trial in patients with rheumatoid arthritis, the anti-IL-6 receptor antibody, tocilizumab, raised blood cholesterol levels. Myocardial revascularization surgery is commonly performed in patients with coronary disease and rheumatoid arthritis, and the clinical course of these patients is not appreciably different from the remainder of the coronary bypass population.

❑ SPONDYLOARTHROPATHIES

This group of diseases is characterized by enthesitis (inflammation at the attachment site of ligaments to bone), sacroiliitis, peripheral arthritis, and dactylitis (fusiform swelling of a digit caused by inflammation in the joint space and along tendon sheaths). The prototype is ankylosing spondylitis, but this group of diseases includes reactive arthritis (formerly called Reiter's syndrome), psoriatic arthritis and enteropathic arthritis (associated with inflammatory bowel disease, celiac disease or Whipple's disease). There is a strong association of the spondyloarthropathies with the histocompatibility antigen, HLA-B27.

Ankylosing Spondylitis

There are four principal cardiac sites of involvement in ankylosing spondylitis: (i) the region around the aortic root, (ii) the conduction system, (iii) the myocardium, and rarely, (iv) the pericardium. The histopathologic features of proximal aortic root and subaortic involvement were described by Bulkley and Roberts and include focal destruction of the muscular and elastic structures of the media, intimal and adventitial thickening, and obliterative vascular disease.

Extension of the inflammatory process into the conduction system has been associated with atrioventricular and fascicular block. Myocardial involvement affects diastolic function before systolic contraction. Left atrial diameter, left ventricular cavity size and wall thickness are typically normal early in the course of the disease. Fibrosis may occasionally involve the endocardium at the base of the anterior mitral leaflet and upper portion of the interventricular septum. Mitral regurgitation as an isolated valvular lesion is unusual in this disease but may develop as a consequence of left ventricular enlargement in patients with severe aortic regurgitation.

Reactive Arthritis

The classic presentation of reactive arthritis (formerly called Reiter's syndrome) involves conjunctivitis, urethritis and arthritis, although all three of these features typically are not present. Atrioventricular block and aortic valve incompetence are the most frequent cardiac manifestations, but other forms of conduction system disease have been described in reactive arthritis as well. The histopathology is similar to that in ankylosing spondylitis.

Scleroderma

Scleroderma, or systemic sclerosis, is characterized by progressive fibrosis of the skin, although much of the morbidity of the disease results from visceral involvement and vasculopathy. The pathophysiology of systemic sclerosis is not well understood, but seems to begin with vascular injury and infiltration of mononuclear cells into perivascular tissues. Tissue factors, including endothelin and platelet-derived growth factor, induce smooth muscle cell differentiation into myofibroblasts, resulting in intimal proliferation and narrowing of the vascular lumen. The most frequent cardiovascular manifestation is cutaneous vasospasm, classically manifesting as episodic attacks of Raynaud's phenomenon characterized by well-demarcated triphasic color change of pallor, cyanosis and rubor. Arteriographic studies of patients with scleroderma most commonly demonstrate occlusions in the digital arteries and ulnar artery. The coronary circulation can be affected early in disease by transient, reversible, cold-induced constriction of distal coronary arteries and arterioles and impaired coronary flow reserve thought to be due to fixed, structural abnormalities of small vessels. Intramyocardial blood flow is abnormal, both at rest and after exercise in the majority of patients with diffuse systemic sclerosis.

While cardiac symptoms may develop as a consequence of renal or pulmonary disease related to scleroderma, primary cardiac involvement and its hallmark, myocardial fibrosis, is increasingly appreciated. Fibrosis is typically patchy and may result from chronic microvascular ischemia. The cardiomyopathy that sometimes develops in patients with scleroderma may be a consequence of both microvascular insufficiency and myocardial fibrosis leading to heart failure and conduction defects.

Clinical Features

Pericardial disease is a frequent histological finding in patients with scleroderma. However, pericarditis becomes clinically apparent in only 5–15% of patients with scleroderma and is sometimes recurrent. Large effusions (>200 mL) are associated with a poor prognosis. In patients with scleroderma-related interstitial lung disease, the presence of pericardial abnormalities is strongly associated with pulmonary hypertension unless cardiac tamponade develops. Management of pericardial disease in scleroderma typically involves administration of nonsteroidal anti-inflammatory medications, although these agents may adversely affect renal hemodynamics and function. Administration of corticosteroid medication has not been systematically evaluated and doses of prednisone greater than 15 mg daily have been associated with an increased risk of renal crisis.

Myocardial disease in scleroderma may produce systolic or diastolic dysfunction, conduction abnormalities, exertional chest pain or sudden death. Exertional dyspnea may result from elevation of left ventricular filling pressure or pulmonary involvement, and pulmonary hypertension may lead to right ventricular failure. Heart failure related to cardiomyopathy may be either insidious or fulminant and cardiac disease appears prior to cutaneous manifestations in one-fourth to one-third of cases of progressive systemic sclerosis. Myocarditis is a rare, but life threatening complication, usually associated with myositis. It typically occurs early in the course of the disease and requires prompt diagnosis and treatment with immunosuppressive medications.

Abnormal coronary perfusion was identified by myocardial perfusion imaging using thallium-201 scintigraphy in patients with systemic sclerosis. Cold-provoked and exercise-induced defects suggesting abnormal coronary vasomotor regulation and more extensive defects are associated with subsequent cardiac disease or death.

Atherosclerotic disease does not appear more pronounced in patients with systemic sclerosis than in the general population. Coronary angiography in patients with scleroderma and exercise-induced perfusion defects may show no evidence of atherosclerotic obstruction, supporting a microvascular mechanism of ischemia. Vascular narrowing, fibrosis, fibrinoid necrosis and concentric intimal hypertrophy have been described more frequently in patients with systemic sclerosis than in controls, and these lesions are similar to those found in the kidneys and other organs.

Management of patients with scleroderma-associated myocardial disease is guided by predominant clinical features. For those with heart failure, standard therapy with digoxin, diuretics, and vasodilator agents is employed. Control of hypertension is essential, and angiotensin converting enzyme (ACE) inhibitors are often effective. ACE inhibitors are crucial components of treatment for scleroderma renal crisis, which usually manifests as acute renal failure, hypertension and active urinary sediment. Cutaneous vasospastic symptoms can be managed both through lifestyle modification (avoiding cold exposure and smoking, and application of moisturizing emollients affected skin to prevent dryness and cracking) and by administration of vasodilator drugs, such as α-adrenergic antagonists, calcium-channel blockers, ACE inhibitors and angiotensin-II receptor antagonists.

Pulmonary hypertension is the leading cause of mortality in patients with systemic sclerosis and when identified is associated with a poor prognosis. Pulmonary function testing and right heart catheterization are recommended in symptomatic patients to guide treatment, the approach to which is similar to that for idiopathic pulmonary hypertension by often less successful.

Conduction disturbances in patients with systemic sclerosis may develop as a consequence of ischemia or fibrosis, and some require electronic pacemaker therapy. Ventricular ectopic arrhythmias should be managed as they would be for patients with coronary atherosclerotic disease. Those patients who develop overt cardiac symptoms typically face a poor prognosis and require aggressive management.

❏ POLYMYOSITIS—DERMATOMYOSITIS

Polymyositis and related disorders of skeletal muscle may occur as isolated diseases or in association with rheumatologic disorders such as systemic lupus erythematosus (SLE), scleroderma or mixed connective tissue disease (MCTD). Characteristic findings in dermatomyositis are predominantly perifascicular vascular inflammation and CD4+ T cell, macrophage and occasional B cell infiltration. The presence of the C5b-9 membrane attack complex in the vessel walls of patients with dermatomyositis suggests that complement activation plays a role in pathogenesis Although the reported prevalence varies, cardiac involvement is often subclinical, and when present may be a predictor of mortality. Cardiac lesions have been identified most frequently in the conducting system with lymphocytic infiltration and fibrosis of the sinoatrial node. Valvular and coronary structures are generally spared. Mononuclear inflammatory cells may infiltrate the myocardial tissue as they do in skeletal muscle, leading to degeneration of cardiac myocytes, clinical myocarditis and fibrosis. While associated malignancy portends the worst outcomes, respiratory muscle and cardiac involvement also have prognostically unfavorable implications.

Cardiovascular symptoms have been reported in 10–15% of cases and include palpitations, chest pain, dyspnea and edema. Serum levels of creatine kinase (CK-MB) may be elevated due to either myocardial damage or skeletal muscle regeneration. Inflammatory myositis without cardiac involvement may be associated with a higher of CK-MB to total CK. Serum troponin-I has the highest specificity for myocardial tissue and is a more reliable marker of myocardial damage in patients with polymyositis or dermatomyositis. Atrioventricular and fascicular conduction block have been reported repeatedly in polymyositis and seems to correlate with the severity of skeletal muscular and myocardial involvement. Pericarditis is relatively rare.

Corticosteroids are the accepted initial treatment for patients with polymyositis or dermatomyositis, typically augmented by immunosuppressive medication therapy. Nonsteroidal anti-inflammatory medication may be useful for the treatment of pericarditis.

❏ SYSTEMIC LUPUS ERYTHEMATOSUS

Systemic lupus erythematosus is characterized by development of autoantibodies, prototypically antinuclear antibody. The pathogenesis seems to involve formation of immune complexes of these antibodies with circulating antigen and complement that are deposited on the microvascular endothelium, producing organ dysfunction. Attention was drawn to the heart in SLE in 1924 when Libman and Sacks described a nonbacterial form of endocarditis characterized by verrucous valvular vegetations. Clinical evidence of cardiac involvement is seldom florid, but astute physicians have identified features of cardiac disease in over 50% of patients.

Clinical Features

Pericarditis

Acute or chronic pericardial inflammation has been described as the most common cardiac lesion associated with the disease. Acute pericarditis may be serous or fibrinous, but the chronic form is most often fibrinous. Pericardial effusions may cause cardiac tamponade, but constrictive pericarditis occurs rarely, and a remitting, episodic course is the rule.

Treatment of pericarditis in patients with SLE includes nonsteroidal anti-inflammatory drugs or corticosteroids in low to intermediate doses. In moderate or severe cases, higher doses of corticosteroids (prednisone 1 mg/kg or high dose intravenous methylprednisolone bolus administration) may be needed. In patients with recurrent or chronic pericarditis, immunosuppressive therapy with methotrexate, azathioprine, mycophenolate or intravenous immunoglobulins (IVIG) have been used. In patients with large pericardial effusions associated with SLE, pericardiocentesis has been suggested to carry a greater risk of hemorrhagic complications than in patients without this disease, and it may be prudent to leave a drainage catheter in place for several hours following the procedure to reduce the need for repeated puncture. Surgical pericardiectomy is seldom required since few cases of chronic constriction have been reported in patients with SLE.

Myocarditis

Signs and symptoms of myocarditis are similar to those in myocarditis due to other causes.

Corticosteroid therapy in high doses is indicated in patients with myocarditis complicating SLE and was associated with clinical improvement in heart failure in nearly 90% of cases in an older report. Immunosuppressive therapy, such as cyclophosphamide, azathioprine or IVIG, may also be beneficial. Patients with SLE who develop heart failure associated with myocarditis should also receive other standard treatment, including diuretic vasodilator and inotropic medications.

Endocarditis

The characteristic of Libman-Sacks form of endocarditis, verrucous lesions, most commonly affect the mitral and aortic valves in two histologic forms: lesions with fibrin clumps, focal necrosis and mononuclear cell infiltrates or vascularized fibrous tissue occasionally accompanied by calcification. An association between antiphospholipid antibodies and valvular lesions is controversial, and an association between valvular abnormalities, clinical cardiovascular disease, hyperhomocysteinemia and hypertriglyceridemia has also been reported.

Antibiotic prophylaxis has been suggested for patients with valvular abnormalities associated with SLE receiving immunosuppressive therapy, but the efficacy of this approach has not been established. Asymptomatic Libman-Sacks endocarditis generally does not require treatment; when actively symptomatic, high dose corticosteroid therapy (e.g. 1 mg/kg per day with prednisone) has been recommended with surveillance for the development of clinical hemodynamic compromise.

Electrophysiological Disturbances

In patients with SLE who develop conducting system disease, coronary atherosclerosis or vasculitis involving the sinoatrial or atrioventricular nodal arteries are more common than active myocarditis, but progressive fibrosis of the conducting system is common in chronic cases. Atrioventricular block and bundle branch blocks are rare in adults. Maternal lupus is also a recognized cause of congenital complete heart block. The risk of congenital heart block complicating subsequent pregnancies is approximately 19% or ninefold greater than the risk in a primigravida with SSA or SSB antibodies. As a consequence, serial fetal echocardiography is recommended weekly between 16 weeks and 26 weeks of gestation and thereafter, alternate weeks until the 34th week for pregnant women with antibodies to SSA and/or SSB. Dexamethasone therapy may ameliorate incomplete heart block, but data are insufficient to support prophylactic therapy during gestation in high-risk mothers.

Coronary Artery Disease

A report from the National Heart, Lung and Blood Institute found the lumens of at least major epicardial coronary artery more than 50% obstructed by atherosclerotic plaque in 42% of patients with SLE treated with long-term corticosteroid medication, despite an average patient age of 35 years. Lipid abnormalities provoked or aggravated by corticosteroid therapy, along with hypertension, physical inactivity and hyperhomocysteinemia have been implicated in the development of atherosclerosis in patients with SLE. Symptomatic myocardial ischemia and myocardial infarction are now commonly encountered in young women with corticosteroid-treated SLE, altering the spectrum of cardiac involvement more than any other aspect of the disease and representing a major cause of premature mortality in this patient population.

❑ SUGGESTED READINGS

Bulkley BH, Roberts WC. Ankylosing spondylitis and aortic regurgitation: description of the characteristic cardiovascular lesion from study of eight necropsy patients. Circulation. 1973;48:1014-27.

Bulkley BH, Roberts WC. The heart in systemic lupus erythematosus and the changes induced in it by corticosteroid therapy: a study of 36 necropsy patients. Am J Med. 1975;58:243-64.

Cosh JA, Barritt DW, Jayson MI. Cardiac lesions of Reiter's syndrome and ankylosing spondylitis. Br Heart J. 1973;35:553.

Das SK, Cassidy JT. Antiheart antibodies in patients with systemic lupus erythematosus. Am J Med Sci.1973;265:275-80.

Dimachkie MM. Idiopathic inflammatory myopathies. J Neuroimmunol. 2011;231:32-42.

Kahn AH, Spodick DH. Rheumatoid heart disease. Semin Arthritis Rheum. 1972;1:327-37.

Lebowitz WB. The heart in rheumatoid arthritis (rheumatoid disease). A clinical and pathological study of 62 cases. Ann Intern Med. 1963;58:102-23.

Seferovic PM, Ristic AD, Maksimovic R, et al. Cardiac arrhythmias and conduction disturbances in autoimmune rheumatic diseases. Rheumatology. 2006;45:iv39-42.

Steen VD, Powell DL, Medsger TA Jr. Clinical correlations and prognosis based on serum autoantibodies in patients with systemic sclerosis. Arthritis Rheum. 1988;31:196-203.

Van Doornum S, McColl G, Wicks IP. Accelerated atherosclerosis: an extra-articular feature of rheumatoid arthritis? Arthritis Rheum. 2002;46:862-73.

10.6 Neurogenic and Stress Cardiomyopathy

❑ INTRODUCTION

The brain is capable of exerting profound influence on the heart through direct effects of innervation and indirect effects of chemical mediators. Due to this relationship, brain injury or psychological stress may result in abnormal autonomic outflow to the heart, causing a diverse spectrum of cardiac injury and dysfunction which may present diagnostic and therapeutic challenges.

❑ NEUROGENIC CARDIOMYOPATHY

Myocardial activity is mediated by multiple sites in the central nervous system (CNS). Through systemic release of catecholamines and direct innervation by the autonomic nervous system (ANS), the heart can meet a broad range of metabolic demands. Not surprisingly, brain injury may have numerous effects on the heart, including contractile dysfunction, arrhythmia and even sudden cardiac death. The syndrome of CNS-mediated cardiac injury has also been referred to as stunned neurogenic myocardium, neurogenic heart disease and neurocardiogenic injury. Cardiac abnormalities are observed in a variety of intracranial disturbances including brain trauma, ischemic stroke, brain hemorrhage, seizure disorders, post-electroconvulsive therapy and in brain dead organ donors.

The mechanism of neurogenic myocardial injury involves complex interactions between specific components of the ANS and the heart (Flowchart 2).

Clinical Features

Conscious patients may report symptoms such as chest discomfort, dyspnea, palpitations and presyncope or syncope. Some cases of sudden cardiac deaths have

FLOWCHART 2: Proposed pathophysiological pathways resulting in neurogenic cardiomyopathy

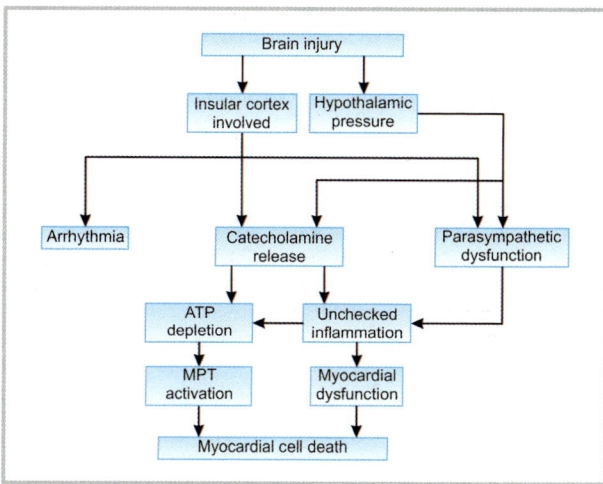

(*Source:* Mashaly HA, Provencio JJ. Inflammation as a link between brain injury and heart damage. Cleve Clin J Med. 2008;75(Suppl 2):S26-30. Copyright 2008 The Cleveland Clinic Foundation. All rights reserved, with permission)

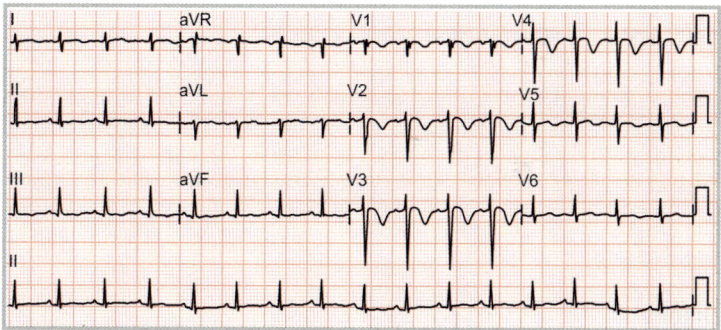

FIGURE 4: QT prolongation and deep anterior T wave inversions in a patient with subarachnoid hemorrhage

been attributed to neurogenic mechanisms. In general, women appear more likely to experience many forms of neurogenic heart disease.

ECG Abnormalities

Prominent U waves, prolonged QT interval and inverted T waves (Fig. 4) are common ECG changes after stroke and other forms of brain injury. The most common ECG abnormality is QT prolongation, which is observed most frequently in SAH but also occurs after intraparenchymal hemorrhage and ischemic stroke. The ECG may also reveal ST changes or new Q waves; the latter are not necessarily indicative of myocardial infarction (MI). ECG evidence of left ventricular hypertrophy (LVH) has been observed in SAH patients, even in the absence of a prior history of hypertension. In this setting, as well as in brain dead organ donors, the ECG LVH pattern may reverse over time and might be due to myocardial edema or another acute process.

Arrhythmias

A variety of cardiac arrhythmias can be seen after brain injury and are quite common in some circumstances, occurring in up to 100% of SAH patients and 20% of patients with ischemic stroke. The observed arrhythmias include bradycardia, supraventricular tachycardias (SVT) including atrial fibrillation, premature ventricular contractions (PVCs), ventricular fibrillation and torsades de pointes. The frequency and severity of arrhythmias are most severe during the first 48 hours after presentation.

Release of Cardiac Biomarkers

Elevation of cardiac biomarkers is common in ischemic and hemorrhagic stroke. Creatine kinase (CK) and CK-MB isoenzyme can be elevated in 10–45% of stroke patients. Unlike MI from coronary atherosclerosis, however, CK-MB is elevated 4 days after stroke, peaks more slowly and plateaus at a lower value. In approximately a quarter of patients with SAH, cardiac troponin I (cTnI) is elevated and is associated with greater SAH severity and female gender. Plasma levels of B-type natriuretic peptide (BNP) are frequently elevated to a modest degree after SAH and are more significantly elevated (>600 pg/mL) in 9% of cases.

Left Ventricular Dysfunction

It is particularly common, however, after SAH, where a reduced left ventricular ejection fraction (LVEF) has been observed in 15–30% of patients. Both global and regional LV systolic dysfunction has been described. Diastolic dysfunction is more common than systolic dysfunction, occurring in 71% of patients after SAH. High grade diastolic dysfunction is strongly associated with pulmonary edema. The presence of LV systolic dysfunction correlates with the severity of neurologic injury and may occasionally escalate to severe congestive heart failure in patients with SAH.

Diagnosis

Diagnosing neurogenic cardiac injury may be challenging. Cardiac enzyme elevation, electrocardiographic changes, echocardiographic changes, including regional wall motion abnormalities can occur in both neurogenic myocardial dysfunction and acute coronary syndrome (ACS). Cardiac enzyme elevation, electrocardiographic changes, echocardiographic changes including regional wall motion abnormalities can occur in both populations. Thus the most important clue in diagnosing neurogenic stunned myocardium is an appropriate clinical setting. A relatively young patient with no previous cardiac history, who suffers an acute brain injury that is not associated with vascular atherosclerosis and has elevated cardiac enzymes and global hypokinesis, should prompt a physician to think about neurologic associated myocardial damage. Similarly, an LV wall motion pattern of basal hypokinesis of the septum is atypical of MI. In general, cardiac catheterization should be preserved for patients with specific features suggestive of ACS, such as chest discomfort, ST elevation on ECG, an echo wall motion pattern that fits a coronary distribution, a troponin level that continues to rise beyond 2–3 days after brain injury and hypotension that could be due to cardiogenic shock.

Treatment

Treatment of neurogenic cardiac injury and dysfunction should focus on treating the underlying cause. Cerebral function and outcomes should be given clinical priority and neurointerventional and neurosurgical interventions should not be withheld due to cardiac concerns. Additionally, SAH patients at the risk of cerebral vasospasm should be treated using "triple-H therapy" (HHH—hypertension, hypervolemia and hemodilution). Nimodipine, a cerebral vasodilator is also useful in prevention of vasospasm. In cases of relative hypotension, vasoactive medications, such as phenylephrine, are commonly used to maintain cerebral perfusion pressure and prevent vasospasm. However in the setting of poor systolic function even a potent peripheral vasoconstrictor may not provide adequate blood pressure support. In such cases, addition of an inotrope to a peripheral vasoconstrictor may assist in providing adequate cerebral perfusion pressure. In severe cases of neurocardiogenic injury, intraaortic balloon counterpulsation can be used to maintain cerebral perfusion pressure until LV systolic function improves.

Since excessive catecholamine release is thought to be a central cause of neurogenic cardiac injury, adrenergic-blocker therapy makes theoretical sense. Due to blood pressure lowering effects, clinicians may believe that beta-blockers are contraindicated in the window of cerebral vasospasm after SAH. In some SAH treatment centers, beta-blockers are used transiently when systolic blood pressure (SBP) is being lowered prior to clipping or coiling.

Pulmonary edema occurs frequently after brain injury and in many cases may be due to LV systolic and/or diastolic dysfunction, or volume overload. However direct pulmonary catecholamine toxicity may occur and results in neurogenic pulmonary edema. Several experimental models have shown that alpha-blockers can prevent pulmonary edema associated with neurologic injury. Similarly, the use of phentolamine may be beneficial in patients with myocardial dysfunction as long as hypotension does not occur and cerebral perfusion is not compromised. No clinical trials currently exist that explore this possibility. Further research is needed to elucidate the benefit of alpha and beta-blockers after neurogenic cardiac injury.

❑ STRESS CARDIOMYOPATHY

Although carrying a different name, stress cardiomyopathy, originally known as takotsubo cardiomyopathy, can be considered a variant of neurogenic cardiac injury. The condition has also been called stress-induced cardiomyopathy, transient apical ballooning syndrome and the broken heart syndrome. The original name stems from the pattern of ventricular systolic dysfunction recognized on left ventriculogram, resembling the shape of a Japanese octopus trap, or takotsubo. The hallmark of the condition is transient LV systolic dysfunction with characteristic LV apical and midventricular regional wall motion abnormalities in the absence of significant coronary artery disease.

No single pathophysiologic process can explain all cases of stress cardiomyopathy. Excessive release of catecholamines is probably an important mechanism, similar to cases of neurogenic cardiac injury. Another possible mechanism is epicardial coronary spasm. Some researchers have suggested myocarditis as an underlying process, although myocardial biopsies taken from stress cardiomyopathy patients did not support this theory. Future studies will need to focus on identification of further risk factors, risk stratification and potential preventive measures.

Clinical Features

Patients with stress cardiomyopathy have typically experienced some sort of acute emotional or physical stress. Emotional triggers may include heated arguments, severe anxiety and the death of a friend or family member. Reported physical stressors have included exacerbations of chronic obstructive pulmonary disease, advanced cancer, severe infection (sepsis), trauma, gastrointestinal bleeding and various surgical procedures. Potential pharmacologic triggers include high doses of beta-agonist bronchodilator drugs. Rare cases without a specific trigger have also been reported.

Postmenopausal women are most commonly affected by stress cardiomyopathy. Classic coronary risk factors, such as hypertension, diabetes mellitus, hyperlipidemia, a positive family history of MI and tobacco use, have been found to have a lower incidence in the patient population presenting with stress cardiomyopathy compared to patients with MI. The most commonly reported symptom is substernal chest pain. In a minority of cases, the presenting symptom has been dyspnea or syncope. Sudden cardiac death and cardiac arrest upon presentation have been reported rarely.

ECG Abnormalities

The 12 lead ECG of stress cardiomyopathy classically demonstrates QT prolongation and deep, symmetric T wave inversions, similar to ECGs observed in patients with SAH. However other ECG abnormalities may also occur, including anterior ST elevation, anterior Q waves, nonspecific ST and T wave abnormalities, left bundle branch block and right bundle branch block.

Arrhythmias

Diverse arrhythmias, including atrial fibrillation, can occur in patients with stress cardiomyopathy. In rare cases, life-threatening ventricular arrhythmias, such as torsades de pointes, have occurred on initial presentation or later during the course. There are also case reports of atrioventricular block occurring in the setting of stress cardiomyopathy.

Release of Cardiac Biomarkers

Serum levels of cardiac troponin are mildly elevated in most cases. A systematic review determined that levels of cardiac troponins or the CK-MB fraction were elevated in 86% and 74% of patients respectively. The severity of presentation is not well correlated with troponin release.

Left Ventricular Dysfunction

The main complication of stress cardiomyopathy is left-sided heart failure. The typical mechanism of heart failure is LV systolic dysfunction and this can be demonstrated with a variety of imaging techniques, including left ventriculography, echocardiography and magnetic resonance imaging of the heart. Most commonly, midventricular and apical akinesis or dyskinesis are described. Right ventricular systolic dysfunction has also been reported in patients with stress cardiomyopathy. In some cases, left heart failure may be caused by LV outflow tract obstruction which is related to hyperdynamic systolic function of the basal LV segments. Mitral regurgitation may accompany this finding secondary to systolic anterior motion of the mitral valve leaflets.

Diagnosis

Prior to making the diagnosis of stress cardiomyopathy, significant underlying coronary artery disease must be excluded. The following diagnostic criteria have been proposed by the Mayo Clinic:
- Transient akinesis or dyskinesis of the LV apical and midventricular segments with regional wall motion abnormalities extending beyond a single epicardial vascular distribution
- Absence of obstructive coronary disease or angiographic evidence of acute plaque rupture
- New electrocardiographic abnormalities (either ST segment elevation or T wave inversion)
- Absence of:
  - recent significant head trauma
  - intracranial bleeding
  - pheochromocytoma
  - obstructive epicardial coronary artery disease
  - myocarditis
  - hypertrophic cardiomyopathy.

In clinical practice, the regional wall motion abnormalities are most often demonstrated by left ventriculography or echocardiography, although cardiac CT or magnetic resonance imaging may also be used for this purpose.

Treatment

Most stress cardiomyopathy patients presenting to an emergency department will initially be suspected of having an ACS, ultimately resulting in coronary angiography. Once a diagnosis of stress cardiomyopathy is made, treatment should focus on relief of chest pain and treatment of LV dysfunction and heart failure symptoms. Appropriate medical therapies may include beta-blockers (such as carvedilol), angiotensin-converting enzyme inhibitors, and diuretics. If transient coronary thrombosis or vasospasms are suspected as possible mechanisms, aspirin, clopidogrel, calcium channel blockers and nitrates may also be considered. If LV systolic function is not improving rapidly (over a few days), anticoagulation with warfarin needs to be considered in order to prevent thrombus formation and cardioembolus. Warfarin can be discontinued when LV apical systolic function has normalized. Long-term treatment with beta-blockers may have a protective effect and should be used in patients with more than one episode.

❑ SUGGESTED READINGS

Bybee KA, Kara T, Prasad A, et al. Systematic review: transient left ventricular apical ballooning: a syndrome that mimics ST segment elevation myocardial infarction. Ann Intern Med. 2004;141:858-65.

Cheung RT, Hachinski V. Cardiac effects of stroke. Curr Treat Options Cardiovasc Med. 2004;6:199-207.

Di Pasquale G, Pinelli G, Andreoli A, et al. Holter detection of cardiac arrhythmias in intracranial subarachnoid hemorrhage. Am J Cardiol. 1987;59:596-600.

Naidech A, Du Y, Kreiter KT, et al. Dobutamine versus milrinone after subarachnoid hemorrhage. Neurosurgery. 2005;56:21-6.

Neil-Dwyer G, Walter P, Cruickshank JM. Beta-blockade benefits patients following a subarachnoid hemorrhage. Eur J Clin Pharmacol. 1985;28:25-9.

Sharkey SW, Lesser JR, Zenovich AG, et al. Acute and reversible cardiomyopathy provoked by stress in women from the United States. Circulation. 2005;111:472-9.

Sommargren CE, Zaroff JG, Banki N, et al. Electrocardiographic repolarization abnormalities in subarachnoid hemorrhage. J Electrocardiol. 2002;35:257-62.

10.7 Kidney and the Heart

❏ INTRODUCTION

Chronic kidney disease (CKD) is defined as the persistence for 3 or more months of structural and/or functional abnormalities of the kidneys. These abnormalities can be any of the following: microalbuminuria (or proteinuria), an abnormal urinalysis or imaging studies or an estimated glomerular filtration rate (eGFR) that is less than 60 ml/min per 1.73 m^2. Among patients with CKD, cardiovascular disease (CVD) is 2–4 times more prevalent and advances at twice the rate, resulting in a 5–10 times greater likelihood of dying from CVD than reaching end-stage renal disease (ESRD). This appears to be a graded association between reduced eGFR and the risk of death and cardiovascular (CV) events. Besides the decreased GFR, albuminuria and proteinuria have emerged as independent risk factor for myocardial infarction, stroke and death.

❏ PATHOPHYSIOLOGY

Patients with CKD have a high prevalence of arteriosclerosis which may occur in the presence or absence of significant atherosclerosis; this is a result of the calcification of the intimal and medial layers of blood vessels. Abnormalities of bone mineral metabolism, including elevations in serum phosphorus, calcium and calcium-phosphorus product, are involved in promoting vascular calcification. These vessels become stiff, leading to an increase in systolic blood pressure (BP), a decrease in diastolic BP, a widened pulse pressure and an increased pulse wave velocity. A higher systolic BP increases left ventricular (LV) afterload and contributes to the development of left ventricular hypertrophy (LVH), while the reduced diastolic pressure compromises coronary artery perfusion leading to myocardial ischemia.

The traditional CV risk factors—advanced age, diabetes mellitus (DM), hypertension (HTN), low high-density lipoprotein (HDL), smoking and LVH—are more prevalent in subjects with CKD. Most patients have more than one of these risk factors, resulting in an even higher risk of adverse outcomes. More unusual is the fact that ESRD patients have a "reverse epidemiology" and a "U-shaped" mortality curve: patients with low cholesterol, not obese and with low BP paradoxically have an increased mortality. To explain this "reverse epidemiology" the so-called nontraditional risk factors (anemia, abnormalities of calcium and phosphate metabolism, inflammation, oxidative stress, prothrombotic factors, hyperhomocysteinemia, hypoalbuminemia and elevated apolipoprotein B) have been invoked; although these factors have been linked to the increased CVD in CKD, a causal relationship has not been proven.

❏ CARDIOVASCULAR RISK FACTORS IN CHRONIC KIDNEY DISEASE

Hypertension

The Seventh Report of the Joint National Committee on Hypertension and American Diabetic Association recommends a therapeutic BP target of 130/80 mm Hg. BP goals are: less than 130/85 mm Hg for individuals with renal parenchymal disease, DM or with less than 1 g/day of proteinuria. Achieving this degree of BP reduction in individuals with CKD typically entails the use of two to three antihypertensive agents including a renin angiotensin aldosterone system (RAAS) blocker and a diuretic. Achieving this degree of BP reduction in individuals with CKD typically entails the use of two to three antihypertensive agents including a renin–angiotensin–aldosterone system (RAAS) blocker and a diuretic. Sympathetic nervous system activity is increased in CKD and contributes to the CV risk. In a post hoc analysis of the Bezafibrate Infarction Prevention (BIP) study, β-blockers were found to reduce cardiac risk in patients with coronary heart disease (CHD) to a similar magnitude as in patients without CKD. Large relative risk reductions in all-cause mortality have been reported for patients who receive β-blockers with ESRD after CAD events. Metoprolol and nebivolol are the two β-blockers that do not accumulate in CKD and have no active metabolites.

Hyperlipidemia

Lipid abnormalities are more prevalent in patients with CKD than in the general population. Patients with CKD have increased serum triglyceride (TG), very low-density lipoprotein (VLDL) and low-density lipoprotein (LDL) with unchanged total cholesterol (TC) and low HDL. HD patients usually have normal TC and LDL levels but higher HDL and serum TG levels. However, in patients with nephrotic syndrome, LDL, TG and TC are markedly elevated whereas HDL decreases.

If statin therapy is administered to dialysis patients, the guidelines recommend: a serum LDL cholesterol of lesser than 100 mg/dL and a non-HDL cholesterol of lesser than 130 mg/dL in patients who have already achieved the target LDL cholesterol level but have TG greater than or equal to 200 mg/dL.

Diabetes Mellitus

The presence of DM in patients with moderate to severe CKD predicts CV deterioration in patients with or without CVD at baseline. Diabetic patients are more prone to CAD, impaired LV function and LVH. Only 11% of diabetic patients had normal echocardiographic dimensions compared with 25% of nondiabetic patients, predominantly due to severe LVH (34% vs 18%). Only limited data are available regarding potential benefits of tight glycemic control.

Left Ventricular Hypertrophy

Left ventricular hypertrophy increases in prevalence with declining renal function and is already evident in 30–45% of patients with moderate CKD90 and in up to 75% of those commencing dialysis. In dialysis patients, LVH is a strong predictor for the subsequent development of congestive heart failure (HF), CAD and SCD.

Anemia

One of the causes of anemia in patients with CKD is a relative deficiency of erythropoietin. Among patients with CHF, for each 1 g/dL decrement in Hb, there is a 13% increase in risk for all-cause mortality. Anemia is an independent risk factor for the development and progression of LVH, CHF, CAD, stroke and increased mortality in patients with CKD. There is an inverse relationship between hemoglobin (Hb) and LV mass index. Randomized trials in CKD showed that correction of anemia to higher Hb targets (>12 g/dL) results in worsened CVD outcomes.

Increased Extracellular Volume

At all stages of CKD, sodium and water retention may cause plasma volume expansion, LV dilatation and LVH. Greater interdialytic weight gain is independently associated with higher BP which is a risk factor for cardiac events.

Miscellaneous

Smoking has been independently associated with de novo HF, peripheral vascular disease and death in CKD patients. However, there are no studies demonstrating that cessation of smoking improves the outcome of CKD. Hyperhomocysteinemia is an adverse prognostic factor for CVD outcomes in dialysis patients. Oxidative stress and inflammation and abnormal divalent ion metabolism vascular calcifications have also been reported as CV risk factors in CKD. Elevated levels of procoagulant factors are observed in CKD and hyperfibrinogenemia has been linked to increased coronary events.

❑ SPECTRUM OF CARDIOVASCULAR DISEASE IN CHRONIC KIDNEY DISEASE

Ischemic Heart Disease

Coronary Heart Disease in Chronic Kidney Disease

Chronic kidney disease and/or albuminuria alone are independent risk factors for the development and progression of CHD. The risk of CHD is lower in young, nonobese and nonsmoking patients. The risk of acute myocardial infarction (AMI) is related to the high prevalence of HTN, inflammation, ECV overload, anemia, hypotension and hypoxia during HD, and increased blood flow through the arteriovenous fistula. Even mild renal disease is considered a major risk for mortality after an acute coronary event and the risk increases with declining GFR. Other contributing factors to the higher mortality are older age, presence of comorbidities and receiving fewer effective therapies (less reperfusion, glycoprotein IIb/IIIa (GPIIb/IIIa) receptor inhibitors, early angiography and less aggressive medical therapies). For all these reasons, the National Kidney Foundation and the American College of Cardiology/American Heart Association to recommend that CKD be considered a CHD risk equivalent.

Coronary Heart Disease as a Risk Factor for Chronic Kidney Disease

The presence of CVD increases the risk of developing ESRD. CKD is prevalent among patients with incident CAD (30%) and is associated with an increased mortality, particularly after an acute coronary syndrome. Patients undergoing coronary angiography, those treated with percutaneous coronary intervention (PCI) and coronary artery bypass grafting (CABG), and those with atherosclerotic disease are at increased risk of CKD.

Medical Therapy

To avoid a significant decrease in BP, the administration of CV medications must be avoided when the preload is low, such as the end of an HD session; these medications may be dosed nocturnally. Thus unfractionated heparin is generally preferred as its clearance is not through renal route. The use of fibrinolytic agents and platelet GPIIb/IIIa inhibitors for acute coronary syndrome is less clear due to the markedly increased risk of bleeding in dialysis patients. Bivalirudin, a direct thrombin inhibitor, when used with PCI in patients with CKD, resulted in lower death rate, lower AMI rate or need for urgent revascularization, as well as lower risk of bleeding compared with heparin. Abciximab and tirofiban (GPIIb/IIIa inhibitors) do not require dose changes in dialysis patients. Regarding the combination of aspirin and clopidogrel, it is known that it is associated with increased bleeding when it was used for the prevention of arteriovenous graft stenosis.

Interventional Therapy

Patients with ESRD and CAD who receive only conservative medical management tend to fare the worst. In view of the propensity for restenosis after PCI, there is a consensus in favor of CABG for left main or extensive three-vessel disease and in favor of PCI for single-vessel disease. In the remaining cases of multivessel disease with culprit lesions, it appears that PCI with stenting had similar clinical outcomes to CABG, but repeated revascularization procedures had to be done. PCI provides excellent angiographic success (90% in most published series), but (with or without stenting) is associated with increased restenosis (over 80% in some series) and the need for revascularization as well as an increased mortality which is proportional with the degree of renal dysfunction. Therefore, provocative stress imaging should be considered to detect clinically silent restenosis 12–16 weeks after a PCI procedure.

Congestive Heart Failure

There is a high incidence of HF in CKD, a high prevalence of HF when starting dialysis (35%), a high incidence of *de novo* HF in HD patients as well as a higher rate of *de novo* symptomatic HF in renal transplant recipients than in the general population. The pathogenesis of heart failure is multifactorial with contributions from LVH, CHD, valvular heart disease, chronic extracellular fluid volume expansion, disturbances in divalent ion metabolism, anemia and the presence of arteriovenous fistulas. Patients may have systolic dysfunction, diastolic dysfunction or both. The K/DOQI guidelines recommend that, at initiation of dialysis, all patients should undergo baseline echocardiography and electrocardiography. Heart failure has not been well studied in CKD patients. Thus studies in the general population are the only basis upon which to guide treatment in CKD.

Pericardial Disease

Pericarditis, uremic or dialysis related is encountered in 5–20% of patients requiring chronic dialysis. Due to hypervolemia from inadequate dialysis, pericardial effusions are frequent but they rarely lead to cardiac tamponade. Pericardial contents are usually sterile. Pericardiocentesis with or without catheter drainage should be reserved for cases of circulatory collapse associated with cardiac tamponade.

Infective Endocarditis

Bacteremia in patients receiving HD is often the result of access site infections, access manipulation and procedures such as dental work. *Staphylococcus aureus* is the causative organism in 60–80% cases of infective endocarditis (IE) in HD patients. Methicillin-resistant *S. aureus* is more common than methicillin-susceptible *S. aureus* (67% vs 33%). In the HD population, the mitral valve is more often infected than the aortic valve, and, together, both are more often affected than the right-sided valves. Treatment guidelines recommend a minimum of 4 weeks of antimicrobial therapy after a diagnosis of IE is made in an HD patient. Surgical indications and contraindications for acute IE in ESRD patients are similar to those for general population.

Valvular Heart Disease

Impaired renal function has been linked to dystrophic calcifications of the valvular annulus and leaflets, particularly the aortic and mitral valves. Age, duration of dialysis, hyperphosphatemia and an elevated calcium phosphate product appear to be important risk factors for the development of aortic stenosis; additional factors include specific involvement of the posterior cusp, left atrial dilatation, duration of dialysis and duration of predialysis systolic HTN.

Arrhythmias

Uremia, LVH, LV dilation, CHF, ischemic and valvular heart disease, calcification of the conduction system from secondary hyperparathyroidism, pericarditis, dialysis-associated hypotension, acid-base and electrolyte disturbances and hypoxemia are all potential causes for the various types of arrhythmias encountered in CKD. Serious arrhythmias are uncommon except in patients with underlying heart disease, those receiving digitalis or those with severe hyperkalemia. Dialysis-associated hypotension seems to be an important factor in precipitating high-grade ventricular arrhythmias, irrespective of the type of dialysis. The finding of high-grade ventricular arrhythmias in the presence of CAD has been associated with an increased risk of cardiac mortality and SCD. CKD and ESRD patients have elevated defibrillation thresholds and a high failure rate of implantable cardioverter defibrillators (ICDs). Many antiarrhythmic medications (digoxin, sotalol and procainamide) require dose adjustments in renal insufficiency. The risk for arrhythmias in dialysis patients receiving digitalis increases sharply during dialysis due to rapid shifts of potassium. Therefore, digitalis should be prescribed with the lowest therapeutic dosage and the potassium concentration in the dialysate can be increased. Considering the high rates of sudden death in patients with ESRD, clinical trials of prophylactic ICDs in this population are under consideration.

❏ DIAGNOSTIC TESTS

Cardiac Markers

Creatine and troponin elevations are frequently observed in asymptomatic ESRD patients (more often with troponin T than with troponin I). For this reason, obtaining serial levels of troponin I is a good approach for diagnosing acute ischemic events. Cardiac troponin T is a predictor of asymptomatic multiple vessel coronary artery stenoses and all-cause mortality. B-type natriuretic peptide (BNP) and N-terminal proBNP (NT-proBNP) increase by 20.6% and 37.7%, respectively for every 10 mL/min per 1.73 m² reduction in eGFR. In euvolemic CKD patients, plasma BNP concentration was predicted by LV mass index and β-blocker usage. The NT-proBNP levels were associated with the same parameters and also GFR and Hb.

Electrocardiography

Hemodialysis induces or changes in serum electrolytes and volume status. These, coupled with the presence of LVH and the effect of medications contribute to the changes seen in the resting electrocardiogram. There are changes in the ST-T segment morphology (in the absence of ischemia) as well as an increase in: QT interval and dispersion, P wave duration, amplitude of the QRS complex (especially with LVH). Ectopy and tachyarrhythmias are more common in patients with advanced renal disease, transplant recipients and in patients with uremic cardiomyopathy, explaining the higher risk of sudden death.

Echocardiography

LV disease is common in dialysis patients and manifests as LVH, dilated cardiomyopathy and systolic dysfunction. Although echocardiography overestimates LV mass in HD patients, the echocardiogram is most accurate when performed at the patient's "dry weight" and there is a true increase in LV mass in patients on HD compared with predialysis patients.

Stress Tests

In patients with CKD and stable CAD, an increased prevalence of exercise-induced ischemia was noted. Exercise ECG and thallium scintigraphy stress tests are of limited utility in renal failure because patients are unable to attain their target heart rate (poor exercise tolerance, autonomic neuropathy, use of medications that impair the chronotropic response to exercise) and because of abnormalities of the resting ECG. The National Kidney Foundation recommends noninvasive stress testing in the following dialysis patients:
- Kidney transplant waitlist patients who have diabetes, have a high Framingham risk score, have known CHD (but not revascularized) or, prior to 1 year ago, underwent angioplasty or stent placement
- Selected dialysis patients with a high risk of an adverse CV event and that are not kidney transplant candidates
- History of complete coronary revascularization with coronary artery bypass surgery that occurred at least 3 years ago
- History of incomplete coronary revascularization with coronary artery bypass surgery that occurred at least 1 year ago
- LV systolic ejection fraction less than 40%
- Change in symptoms related to ischemic heart disease or change in clinical status.

Coronary Angiography

This is the "gold standard" test. In predialysis patients, the procedure may worsen renal function by causing contrast nephropathy or cholesterol embolization. The K/DOQI guidelines suggest that a limited amount of iso-osmolar radiocontrast media should be administered to patients with residual renal function who have been treated with prophylactic N-acetylcysteine, to help decrease the risk of contrast nephropathy and volume overload.

❏ PRINCIPLES OF TREATMENT OF CARDIOVASCULAR DISEASE

The CV medications are less frequently used in patients with renal dysfunction and this is associated with significantly increased risk for subsequent mortality. It is likely that underutilization of effective therapies occurs in patients with CKD and that optimal targets for treatment are not achieved. However there is enough data to support the idea that patients with concurrent CKD and CVD likely benefit from many of the interventions implemented in individuals with CVD alone (or at the highest risk for development of CVD), incuding the same secondary prevention measures employed in the general population; observational studies indicate that heart failure patients may derive a mortality benefit from ACEIs and β-blockers.

Peritoneal dialysis is less efficient at removing drugs than HD and is most effective for smaller molecular weight drugs that are not extensively bound to serum proteins. Drug clearance in dialysis patient is affected by their water solubility, protein binding, distribution volume and diffusion across the dialysis membrane. In patients with ESRD but without preexisting CVD, different renal replacement modalities lead to similar CV outcomes. Exercise training during HD significantly improves both interdialytic and treatment-related BP. There is evidence that tight glycemic control in DM, reduction of BP to below 130/80 mm Hg, with either ACEIs or ARBs, weight loss in obese patients and dietary protein restriction to the recommended daily allowance of 0.8 g/kg per day reduce the risk of progressive kidney disease and risk of CVD. Close follow-up is required for potentially dangerous complications that may be more common in CKD, such as hyperkalemia with the use of ACEIs, ARBs or aldosterone antagonists. Correction of anemia to a target of 10–12 g/dL is currently recommended.

❏ KIDNEY TRANSPLANT RECIPIENTS

After renal transplantation, systolic dysfunction, LV dilatation, LVH and risk of hospitalization for HF improve despite levels of BP that are similar with those found prior to grafting. It is not clear yet what is it about transplantation (and improved renal function) that provides protection against CVD despite the fact that immunosuppression can exaggerate known CVD risk factors such as hyperlipidemia, HTN, anemia and DM. Despite these positive results, there is significant progression of CAC and atherosclerotic CVD is one of the most frequent causes of morbidity and mortality after transplantation.

Pretransplant CVD is a major risk factor for developing post-transplant CVD. Other risk factors associated with CV complications are: male gender, age, HTN before transplantation, smoking, high CRP, abnormal Hb, cytomegalovirus seropositivity, longer pre-transplantation dialysis, post-transplantation diabetes, increased pulse pressure after transplantation, use of corticosteroids, lower serum albumin, higher serum TG levels after transplantation and metabolic syndrome. Attention has been focused in recent years on so-called nontraditional risk factors, including inflammation and oxidative stress, which are prevalent in patients with CKD and are not effectively controlled by dialysis. CAD progression is most likely to occur in white patients and is associated with clinical factors such as BP, body mass index, renal function and baseline CAC score.

The vasoconstrictive effects of calcineurin inhibitors in particular worsen HTN after transplantation. Calcium channel blockers are widely used because they are well tolerated and due to their effects in counter-acting calcineurin-mediated vasoconstriction. In transplant patients, levels of TC, LDL and TG are usually higher than in the general population but HDL is usually normal. Clinical practice guidelines for managing dyslipidemia in transplant patients suggest that changes in the immunosuppressive protocol (reduction in prednisone dose, reduction in cyclosporine dose or switching from cyclosporine to tacrolimus, and discontinuation or replacement of sirolimus) be considered when LDL levels remain elevated (>100 mg/dL) despite optimal medical management. The risk of CVD, cerebrovascular disease and death is increased with smoking. DM has also been found to be an independent risk factor for ischemic heart disease and for cardiac failure in renal transplant recipients. Hypoalbuminemia, anemia, and presence of LVH during the first year are also independent predictors for the development of heart failure and death.

❏ SUGGESTED READINGS

American Diabetes Association. Clinical Practice Recommendations 2005. Diabetes Care. 2005;28:S1-79.

Antman EM, Anbe DT, Armstrong PW, et al. ACC/AHA guidelines for the management of patients with ST-elevation myocardial infarction—executive summary. A report of the American College of Cardiology/American Heart Association Task Force on Practice Guidelines (Writing Committee to revise the 1999 guidelines for the management of patients with acute myocardial infarction). J Am Coll Cardiol. 2004;44:671-719.

Chonchol M, Benderly M, Goldbourt U. Beta-blockers for coronary heart disease in chronic kidney disease. Nephrol Dial Transplant. 2008;23:2274-9.

K/DOQI Workgroup. K/DOQI clinical practice guidelines for cardiovascular disease in dialysis patients. Am J Kidney Dis. 2005;45:S1-153.

Kasiske BL, Guijarro C, Massy ZA, et al. Cardiovascular disease after renal transplantation. J Am Soc Nephrol. 1996;7:158-65.

Kidney Disease Outcomes Quality Initiative (K/DOQI) Group. K/DOQI clinical practice guidelines for management of dyslipidemias in patients with kidney disease. Am J Kidney Dis. 2003;41:I-IV, S1-91.

Lenfant C, Chobanian AV, Jones DW, et al. Seventh report of the Joint National Committee on the prevention, detection, evaluation, and treatment of high blood pressure (JNC 7): resetting the hypertension sails. Hypertension. 2003;41:1178-9.

McCullough PA, Lepor NE. The deadly triangle of anemia, renal insufficiency, and cardiovascular disease: implications for prognosis and treatment. Rev Cardiovasc Med. 2005;6:1-10.

National Kidney Foundation. K/DOQI clinical practice guidelines for chronic kidney disease: evaluation, classification and stratification. Am J Kidney Dis. 2002;39:S1-266.

Schwenger V, Zeier M, Ritz E. Hypertension after renal transplantation. Ann Transplant. 2001;6:25-30.

Tadros GM, Herzog CA. Percutaneous coronary intervention in chronic kidney disease patients. J Nephrol. 2004;17:364-8.

Tonelli M, Bohm C, Pandeya S, et al. Cardiac risk factors and the use of cardioprotective medications in patients with chronic renal insufficiency. Am J Kidney Dis. 2001;37:484-9.

10.8 Endocrine Heart Disease

❑ INTRODUCTION

Endocrine disorders, which include diabetes mellitus commonly affect the heart. This section reviews the cardiovascular manifestations of a number of endocrine disorders and the impact of treatment on ameliorating the cardiovascular manifestations.

❑ DIABETES MELLITUS

People with diabetes mellitus are at increased risk for angina, myocardial infarction (MI), congestive heart failure (CHF) and sudden death.

Coronary Artery Disease

There are a number of explanations for this increased risk for heart disease with diabetes. The majority of people with diabetes have type 2 diabetes (~ 95% of the 25.8 million people with diabetes in the United States); and type 2 patients in addition to hyperglycemia typically also have additional risk factors for heart disease including hypertension, dyslipidemia, hypercoagulability and hyperuricemia. These various risk factors act in concert on the vascular wall to increase the risk for atherosclerosis (Fig. 5).

Experimental and epidemiological evidence suggests that the increased blood pressure affects both the arterial media and the endothelium. In the media the elevated pressure increases the total smooth muscle mass and connective tissue content. Endothelial changes include an increase in number and change in shape of endothelial cells; increased endothelial permeability to macromolecules (including lipoproteins); impaired nitric oxide (NO) induced relaxation and increased cell surface adhesion molecules such as the selectins and vascular adhesion molecule 1 (VCAM 1). These molecules in turn mediate recruitment of inflammatory cells such as monocytes and T cells. When there are other atherogenic factors, such as dyslipidemia, these hypertensive changes promote the development of atherosclerosis. The lipid abnormalities that are typically present in type 2 diabetes patients—increased triglycerides, low HDL cholesterol levels, and increased

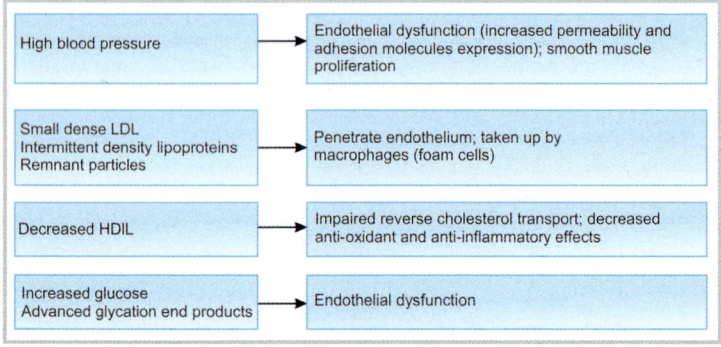

FIGURE 5: Principal mechanisms by which hypertension, dyslipidemia, and hyperglycemia in type 2 diabetes promote atherosclerosis

small dense LDL particles—are also those that in experimental systems promote atherosclerosis. The increased adipose tissue that is present in many patients with type 2 diabetes, especially visceral fat, is a source of a number of factors including free fatty acids, plasminogen activator inhibitor-1 (PAI-1), tumor necrosis alpha (TNF-α) that negatively affect endothelial function.

The role of hyperglycemia as an independent risk factor for cardiovascular disease remains a controversial issue. Only a proportion of people with diabetes develop significant microvascular complications; and microvascular disease, particularly nephropathy predicts cardiovascular disease. The link between microvascular and macrovascular disease in some instances may therefore reflect the susceptibility of the individual to both conditions, and, in other instances, the macrovascular disease may be secondary to the microvascular condition. Hypertension and acquired lipid abnormalities in diabetic nephropathy may play an important pathological role in the development of atherosclerosis.

Type 2 diabetes is also associated with changes in homeostatic mechanisms in the direction promoting atherosclerosis. Type 2 diabetes has been associated with increased levels of PAI-1 which suppresses fibrinolysis. PAI-1 is a risk factor for coronary events in patients with angina and for reinfarction post-MI. Elevations of factor VII coagulant activity (FVII:c); von Willebrand factor, fibrinogen, and activated factor XII (XIIa) have been inconsistently reported in patients with diabetes. Many studies, but not all, have also reported that platelets from patients with type 2 diabetes aggregate more readily than in healthy subjects. Gout is more common in patients with type 2 diabetes, and hyperuricemia is associated with increased risk of cardiovascular disease. It is unclear, however, if it is an independent risk factor for heart disease.

Metabolic Syndrome

The conditions of central obesity, dyslipidemia (elevated triglycerides and/or low HDL cholesterol), glucose intolerance and hypertension co-occur in individuals more often than might be expected by chance. The term "metabolic syndrome", "syndrome X" or the "insulin resistance syndrome" has been used to describe this cluster, and individuals who have this cluster of abnormalities are at higher risk of cardiovascular disease. There is considerable debate as to whether "metabolic syndrome" meets these criteria. First, since not all the risk factors have to be present to have the diagnosis of metabolic syndrome, patients can be categorized into 16 distinct groups using the National Cholesterol Education Program Treatment Panel III (ATP III) definition and 11 different groups using the International Diabetes Federation definition. As a result the risk for cardiovascular disease is not equivalent across the different risk factor combinations. Second, the risk for cardiovascular disease in those with the syndrome does not appear to be greater than that conferred by constituent components. Third, the treatment of the syndrome as a whole is no different from that of each of its components. Fourth, since type 2 diabetes identifies individuals who have central obesity, dyslipidemia and hypertension, including glucose intolerance in the definition of metabolic syndrome is questionable. Fifth, the hypothesis that insulin resistance is the mechanism that underlies the metabolic abnormalities remains controversial. Sixth, the definition does not include other important risk factors for cardiovascular disease, such as age, sex, family history, smoking history, previous cardiovascular events and LDL cholesterol. There are other risk prediction algorithms for cardiovascular disease including the Framingham risk score and the Heart score that outperform the metabolic syndrome in predicting cardiovascular events.

Congestive Heart Failure

Diabetes is a well-established risk factor for CHF. Much of the excess risk for heart failure is thought to be due to ischemic heart disease and its complications. A number of etiologic mechanisms have been implicated. Hyperglycemia may increase glycation of interstitial proteins such as collagen resulting in myocardial stiffness and impaired contractility. Hyperglycemia may also increase intracellular generation of superoxide leading to cellular injury. In experimental systems, strategies that enhance mitochondrial reactive oxygen species (ROS) scavenging systems have been shown to reverse diabetes-induced cardiac dysfunction. Lipid accumulation within the cardiac myocytes may also be important.

Sudden Death

Sudden cardiac death in people with diabetes is most often due to atherosclerotic heart disease. The risk for sudden death may be increased if cardiac autonomic neuropathy is present—the hypothesized mechanisms include silent myocardial ischemia and infarction, impaired central control of respiration and predisposition to cardiac arrhythmias because of alterations in the QTc intervals. QTc prolongation and cardiac rate or rhythm disturbances to episodes of nocturnal hypoglycemia in ambulant patients with type 1 diabetes have been documented. As might be expected, multifactorial interventions targeting hyperglycemia, blood pressure and dyslipidemia can substantially reduce risk for cardiovascular events in people with diabetes.

❏ THYROID DISEASE

Hyperthyroidism

The common cardiac physiologic manifestations of hyperthyroidism include increases in resting heart rate, left ventricular contractility and blood volume and decreased systemic vascular resistance. Cardiac output may be increased by about 50–300%, and the increased oxygen demand and reduced cardiac reserve leads to decreased exercise tolerance. With appropriate treatment of hyperthyroidism, these physiologic changes completely reverse and match euthyroid controls. Hyperthyroidism is also associated with several pathophysiologic cardiac complications, including atrial fibrillation (AF), cardiomyopathy and pulmonary hypertension.

Atrial fibrillation is usually persistent rather than paroxysmal and develops in about 9–22% of patients with hyperthyroidism. The risk factors for fibrillation in hyperthyroid patients include being male, older, having a history of ischemic heart disease, valvular disease and CHF. Subclinical hyperthyroidism (a suppressed or below normal thyroid-stimulating hormone (TSH) with normal T4 and T3 levels) is also associated with increased risk of AF. These patients with hyperthyroidism and AF are at high risk for thromboembolic events but not higher than AF from other causes.

Treatment of AF initially includes beta blockade to control the ventricular rate but successful conversion to sinus rhythm depends upon return to a euthyroid state. Predictors for successful reversion to sinus rhythm were lower blood pressure measurements at baseline, age, absence of underlying heart disease and a hypothyroid state induced by therapy. Electrical or pharmacologic cardioversion, with anticoagulant treatment for at least 3 weeks before and continued for at least 4 weeks after cardioversion, should be considered for patients who have persistent

AF for 4 months or more after returning to a euthyroid state. Hyperthyroid patients need lower doses of warfarin as they have increased clearance of clotting factors and reduced binding proteins.

Rate related cardiomyopathy can occur in hyperthyroidism due to persistent tachycardia, and rate control improves left ventricular dysfunction even before the euthyroid state is restored. Pulmonary hypertension is quite frequent in patients with hyperthyroidism. Usually the patients are asymptomatic and the pulmonary pressures normalize on return to a euthyroid state.

Hypothyroidism

The common cardiac physiologic manifestations of hypothyroidism include bradycardia, decreased myocardial contractility and increased peripheral vascular resistance. Usually patients have elevated blood pressure and treatment reverses these physiological changes. Severe hypothyroidism can cause a prolongation of QTc interval predisposing the patient to ventricular irritability. Rarely, torsade de pointes may result. Cardiac enlargement most often due to pericardial effusion can occur but cardiac tamponade however is unusual. Hypothyroidism is also associated with increased risk for coronary atherosclerosis. An increase in LDL cholesterol and diastolic hypertension are two factors that may contribute to this increased risk. Levothyroxine replacement should be performed cautiously in elderly patients with longstanding and severe hypothyroidism because too rapid replacement can precipitate or worsen myocardial ischemia.

Amiodarone-induced Thyroid Disease

Amiodarone, a benzofuran derivative, structurally resembles thyroid hormone and it inhibits deiodinase activity. Amiodarone therapy causes thyroid dysfunction in about 15–20% of patients. The drug affects thyroid function in two ways—first, by its inherent effects on the thyroid follicles and on deiodinase activity, and second, by its high iodine content. A 200 mg maintenance dose releases 7 mg of iodide into the circulation. This is 70-fold in excess of the daily iodine requirements of 100–150 μg. This excess iodine can cause both hypothyroidism and hyperthyroidism–which condition develops depends on the sufficiency of iodine intake of the population and the underlying thyroid disorder. The presence of a positive thyroid peroxidase antibody increases the likelihood of hypothyroidism by sevenfold to eightfold. The hypothyroidism is permanent in the majority of patients with positive antibodies but may resolve in patients who appear to have a normal gland and negative antibodies within 2–4 months of discontinuing the amiodarone.

In patients with autonomously functioning nodular goiters (or those patients with latent Graves' disease), the increased iodine availability leads to excessive synthesis and release of thyroid hormone (type 1 amiodarone induced thyrotoxicosis). The thyrotoxicosis can occur early after initiation of amiodarone therapy and may be heralded by worsening of the underlying cardiac disorder and heart failure. Treatment includes methimazole therapy or surgery. Potassium perchlorate depletes intrathyroidal iodine stores and can be used in conjunction with methimazole therapy. Amiodarone withdrawal usually results in slow remission because the drug is highly lipid soluble and has a long elimination half-life (~40–60 days). The decision to withdraw depends on the availability of other therapeutic options to treat the cardiac arrhythmia.

Both amiodarone and the excess iodine can occasionally cause an acute, sometimes painful, destructive inflammatory thyroiditis. Glucocorticoids (prednisone 30–40 mg daily) tapered over 2–3 months can be used for treatment.

Finally, dronedarone, also a benzofuran derivative, does not contain iodine, and may be an option for patients who are at risk for amiodarone induced thyroid dysfunction. The drug, however, has been reported to cause severe liver injury.

❏ PITUITARY DISORDERS

Growth Hormone Excess

Cardiomegaly is a prominent feature of acromegaly with reported ranges of between 70% and 90% in autopsy studies. The enlargement of heart is generally proportionate to that of other visceral organs and so is unlikely to be only due to the hypertension. A direct effect of growth hormone and IgF-1 is likely. Growth hormone and IgF-1 receptors are present on cardiac myocytes, and in cultured rat cardiomyocytes, IgF-1 induces hypertrophy. Growth hormone also stimulates matrix metalloproteinases which may be involved in the remodelling process of the extracellular matrix that occurs with cardiac hypertrophy. Hypertension, however, is important in exacerbating the hypertrophy—in a multistep regression analysis, diastolic blood pressure was the best predictor of cardiac hypertrophy.

Echocardiography in patients with acromegaly confirms biventricular involvement with increase in left ventricular mass index and right free wall thickness. The chambers are not dilated. Impairment in left and right ventricular diastolic filling is present but the overall ejection phase indices are normal. The ejection fraction, however, is impaired with exercise. About 10% of patients with acromegaly develop heart failure.

The presence of myocardial interstitial fibrosis may affect the conduction system leading to cardiac arrhythmias. Valvular heart disease is also seen in patients with acromegaly. There is an increase in prevalence of risk factors for CAD (hypertension, diabetes, insulin resistance and dyslipidemia) in patients with acromegaly.

Normalization of serum IgF-1 and growth hormone levels (<1 µg/L) by surgery or using somatostatin analogs reduces overall mortality to normal. Successful treatment also improves cardiovascular parameters with reduction in cardiac mass and improvement in diastolic filling. Patients with shorter duration of disease were more likely to have reversal of cardiomyopathy. Treatment with the growth hormone antagonist—pegvisomant—has been shown to significantly improve blood pressure and fasting blood glucose levels in those patients who normalized their IgF-1 levels.

Hypopituitarism

Hypopituitarism, a deficiency of one or more hormones of the anterior or posterior pituitary gland, is associated with an increase in all cause mortality. Hypopituitary patients have a reduction in lean mass and increase in central obesity and are significantly insulin resistant compared to normal matched controls. Increases in triglycerides and PAI-1 levels and decrease in Low HDL cholesterol have also been reported. Growth hormone deficiency may play a role in the development of these abnormalities. Indeed growth hormone replacement reverses the body composition abnormalities and improves the lipid profile. Sustained improvement in carotid intimal media thickening has also been reported. Growth hormone replacement however does not uniformly improve cardiovascular risk factors; it increases plasma glucose and also lipoprotein (a)—an independent risk factor for cardiovascular disease.

Traditionally, the daily hydrocortisone dose for adrenal insufficiency was 30 mg daily (normal cortisol production is ~10 mg/day). It is possible that the subtle increased glucocorticoid exposure with the traditional 30 mg dose might contribute to the increased morbidity and mortality. Similarly, the adequacy of thyroid hormone replacement in central hypothyroidism is difficult to assess because TSH levels cannot be used to titrate the T4 dose. Both over-replacement and under-replacement with T4 could have negative cardiovascular effects. There is little information on the role of estrogen and testosterone replacement on morbidity and mortality in hypopituitarism. The increased cerebrovascular risk in hypopituitary patient may be a reflection of treatment rather than any particular hormone deficiency. Stereotactic radiosurgery is a relatively new therapy and most of the mortality data in hypopituitary patients dates from the era of conventional radiotherapy.

❏ ADRENAL DISORDERS

Pheochromocytoma and Paraganglioma

Pheochromocytomas arise from the adrenal medulla and paragangliomas arise from the non-adrenal chromaffin tissue. Most of these tumors secrete catecholamines in excess—sometimes as much as 27 times the usual amount. The increased levels of epinephrine and norepinephrine lead to activation of alpha 1 and beta 1 adrenergic receptors with resulting increases in heart rate, contractility and vasoconstriction. Pheochromocytomas can also secrete other peptide hormones that have vascular effects such as neuropeptide Y, a very potent noradrenergic vasoconstrictor. The clinical picture is of hypertension, left ventricular hypertrophy, dilated cardiomyopathy and arrhythmias.

Electrocardiographic abnormalities include left ventricular hypertrophy and T wave inversion. Patients can also present with electrocardiographic evidence of ischemia due to coronary artery vasoconstriction and increased oxygen demand. Sinus tachycardia, paroxysmal supraventricular tachycardia and supraventricular ectopic activity occur from direct chronotropic effects of the catecholamines. Marked prolongation of QT interval and widened deep T waves may predispose to ventricular arrhythmias.

Surgical resection of the pheochromocytoma or paraganglioma usually reverses the abnormalities although in some patients with longer duration of disease, cardiovascular remodeling and organ damage can lead to persistence of complications especially hypertension. Those patients with hypertension without recurrence of tumor should be managed as if they have essential hypertension.

Primary Aldosteronism

Aldosterone increases the number of open epithelial sodium channels in the renal cortical collecting tubule, increasing sodium and water absorption and potassium excretion. The hypertension may be a consequence of volume expansion or possibly due to direct actions of sodium itself. The etiology of the primary aldosteronism may modulate the severity of hypertension—patients with adrenal adenomas have been reported to have higher pressures (181/112 mm Hg) compared to patients with adrenal hyperplasia (161/105 mm Hg).

The hypertension may explain some of the cardiovascular morbidity and mortality but it appears that aldosteronism per se has additional cardiovascular and renal sequelae. The mineralocorticoid receptor is expressed on cardiomyocytes, endothelial cells, vascular smooth muscles and on renal cells other than the collecting tubules and in experimental systems aldosterone induces inflammation, oxidative stress, endothelial dysfunction and fibrosis. Patients with primary aldosteronism have greater left ventricular wall thickness (posterior and septal wall), concentric remodeling and impaired diastolic filling when compared to controls matched for age, sex, body mass index, blood pressure and duration of blood pressure. Primary aldosteronism is also associated with increased risk of AF, MI, heart failure and stroke.

Surgery is the preferred treatment for primary aldosteronism due to adenoma (30–60% of cases) and the occasional patient with unilateral hyperplasia (~3% of cases). Medical therapy with mineralocorticoid receptor antagonists is used for nonsurgical candidates or those with bilateral hyperplasia. Salt restriction can also lower blood pressure since sodium retention is the primary mechanism for hypertension.

Cushing's Syndrome

The greatly increased risk of cardiovascular disease in Cushing's syndrome is due to the presence of multiple risk factors for atherosclerosis including hypertension, dyslipidemia, hyperglycemia and coagulopathy. Active Cushing's patients have been documented to have premature development of carotid atherosclerotic plaques; even in subclinical Cushing's, the prevalence of these risk factors is substantially increased. Glucocorticoid excess is associated with increased visceral fat deposition.

The mechanisms underlying this effect are not fully elucidated, but it has been reported that glucocorticoids have a tissue specific effect on AMP-activated protein kinase (AMPK)—inhibiting its activity in the heart and visceral adipose cells and stimulating it in the liver and hypothalamus resulting in hypertension. Additional factors thought to contribute the development of hypertension in hypercortisolemia include vascular hyper-reactivity to adrenergic agonists, inhibition of peripheral catabolism of catecholamines, inhibition of the vasodilatory system (including NO synthase, prostacyclin and kinin-kallikrein) and increased activity of the renin-angiotensin system. An increase in plasma clotting factors, especially Factor VIII and von Willebrand factor complex, as well as impaired fibrinolysis due to elevated PAI-1 levels also occur and may contribute to the increased risk of thromboembolic events in this population.

Cushing's patients have normal left ventricular dimension but increased left ventricular hypertrophy and impaired left ventricle diastolic function when compared to controls matched for age, sex, body surface area, blood pressure, and left ventricular ejection fraction. With biochemical normalization of cortisol levels, these changes in cardiac structure and function appear to reverse independent of changes in blood pressure.

Surgical cure of the Cushing's syndrome significantly reduces cardiovascular risk but some risk factors may persist. There is only limited long-term mortality data in patients with Cushing's disease who have persistent disease or are in remission.

Adrenal Insufficiency

Arterial hypotension is the most common cardiovascular finding in patients with adrenal insufficiency. In adrenal crisis, recumbent hypotension or shock is almost always present. Rarely, cardiomyopathy and heart failure have been reported as the presenting manifestation of adrenal insufficiency. The cardiomyopathy reverses with glucocorticoid replacement. The mechanisms resulting in the cardiomyopathy are not well understood. Excess catecholamine effect without the protective effect of glucocorticoids may be important. Glucocorticoid deficiency could also affect membrane calcium transport function and impair excitation contraction coupling.

❑ PARATHYROID DISORDERS

Primary Hyperparathyroidism

Both mild and severe primary hyperparathyroidism is associated with increased mortality mostly from cardiovascular events. There are parathyroid hormone (PTH) receptors on the vascular endothelium and on vascular smooth muscle cells, and hyperparathyroid patients have evidence for endothelial dysfunction compared to controls. Hypertension is nearly twice more common in patients with primary hyperparathyroidism than in the general population. Acute administration of PTH in normal subjects induces vasodilatation and lowers blood pressure but chronic continuous infusions on the other hand caused persistent hypercalcemia and hypertension.

Primary hyperparathyroidism is associated with hypertension, left ventricular hypertrophy, and valvular, myocardial and coronary calcification.

In earlier studies, surgery reduced but did not eliminate the excess mortality associated with primary hyperparathyroidism. More recent studies have not reported persistence of excess mortality after surgical treatment. Surgery partly reverses the changes in cardiac structure—a reduction in mean left ventricular mass index in the 6 months following surgery has reported. The regression seems to occur in normotensive and not hypertensive patients. Cardiac calcification persists but does not appear to progress post-surgery.

Hypoparathyroidism

The hypocalcemia of hypoparathyroidism can occasionally result in cardiac complications. Hypocalcemia characteristically causes lengthening of the QTc interval, and this can result in early after depolarizations and trigger dysrhythmias including supraventricular tachycardia, ventricular fibrillation and torsades de pointes. In neonates hypocalcemia has been reported to induce atrioventricular block.

Long-standing poorly controlled hypoparathyroidism has been associated with dilated cardiomyopathy and CHF. The patients tend to have a long history of hypocalcemia and insidious development of signs and symptoms of CHF that are improved with vitamin D and calcium replacement.

❑ CARCINOID SYNDROME

Carcinoid tumors secrete a number of vasoactive amino acids and peptides. 5-hydroxytryptamine (5-HT) is the most prominent secretory product. Other molecules include 5-hydroxytryptophan, bradykinin, histamine, substance P, prostaglandins and calcitonin gene related peptides. Carcinoid heart disease occurs in about 70% of patients. The typical findings are white plaques or diffuse pearl gray endocardial thickening on the right side of the heart affecting the tricuspid and pulmonary valves. The tricuspid valve leaflets and the pulmonary cusps are thickened and retracted by the fibrotic process. Papillary muscles and chordae tendineae of the tricuspid valves are shortened impairing the mobility of the valves. Patients develop symptoms and signs of tricuspid and pulmonary valve regurgitation. Pulmonary outflow obstruction due to pulmonary annular constriction can also occur. Left sided carcinoid syndrome can occur if the liver tumor burden is very high or if there is a patent foramen ovale.

Treatment is directed at removing tumor by surgery, chemoembolization, radiofrequency ablation. Octreotide can be used to control symptoms. Valvular disease is a major cause of morbidity and mortality and valve replacement even in the presence of significant tumor burden improves outcomes.

❏ SUGGESTED READINGS

- Alberti KG, Eckel RH, Grundy SM, et al. Harmonizing the metabolic syndrome: a joint interim statement of the International Diabetes Federation Task Force on Epidemiology and Prevention; National Heart, Lung, and Blood Institute; American Heart Association; World Heart Federation; International Atherosclerosis Society; and International Association for the Study of Obesity. Circulation. 2009;20:1640-5.
- De Leo M, Pivonello R, Auriemma RS, et al. Cardiovascular disease in Cushing's syndrome: heart versus vasculature. Neuroendocrinology. 2010;92:50-4.
- Eskes SA, Wiersinga WM. Amiodarone and thyroid. Best Pract Res Clin Endocrinol Metab. 2009;23:735-51.
- Galetta F, Franzoni F, Bernini G, et al. Cardiovascular complications in patients with pheochromocytoma: a mini-review. Biomed Pharmacother. 2010;64:505-9.
- Giles TD, Iteld BJ, Rives KL. The cardiomyopathy of hypoparathyroidism. Another reversible form of heart muscle disease. Chest. 1981;79:225-9.
- Hedbäck G, Odén A. Increased risk of death from primary hyperparathyroidism—an update. Eur J Clin Invest. 1998;28:271-6.
- Johansson JO, Fowelin J, Landin K, et al. Growth hormone-deficient adults are insulin-resistant. Metabolism. 1995;44:1126-9.
- Klein I, Danzi S. Thyroid disease and the heart. Circulation. 2007;116:1725-35.
- Kulke MH. Clinical presentation and management of carcinoid tumors. Hematol Oncol Clin North Am. 2007;21:433-55; vii-viii.
- Lehto S, Ronemma T, Haffner SM, et al. Dyslipidemia and hyperglycemia predict coronary heart disease events in middle-aged patients with NIDDM. Diabetes. 1997;46:1354-9.
- Melmed S, Colao S, Barkan A, et al. Guidelines for acromegaly management: an update. J Clin Endocrinol Metab. 2009;94:1509-17.
- N J, Francis J. Atrial fibrillation and hyperthyroidism. Indian Pacing Electrophysiol J. 2005;5:305-11.
- Takeda R, Matsubra T, Miyamori I, et al. Vascular complications in patients with aldosterone producing adenoma in Japan: comparative study with essential hypertension. The Research Committee of Disorders of Adrenal Hormones in Japan. J Endocrinol Invest. 1995;18:370-3.
- Tanenberg RJ, Newton CA, Drake AJ. Confirmation of hypoglycaemia in the "dead-in-bed" syndrome, as captured by a retrospective continuous glucose monitoring system. Endocr Pract. 2010;16:244-8.
- Tomlinson JW, Holden H, Hills RK, et al. Association between premature mortality and hypopituitarism. West Midlands Prospective Hypopituitary Study Group. Lancet. 2001;357:425-31.
- Whiteley L, Padmanabhan S, Hole D, et al. Should diabetes be considered a coronary heart disease risk equivalent?: results from 25 years of follow-up in the Renfrew and Paisley survey. Diabetes Care. 2005;28:1588-93.

10.9 Venous Thromboembolism and Cor Pulmonale

❑ VENOUS THROMBOEMBOLISM

Venous thromboembolism (VTE), most commonly originating from deep venous thrombosis (DVT) of the legs, ranges from asymptomatic pulmonary emboli, incidentally discovered emboli to massive embolism causing immediate death. Acute pulmonary embolism (PE) may occur rapidly and unpredictably and may be difficult to diagnose. Treatment can reduce the risk of death, and appropriate primary prophylaxis is usually effective. The interaction of an extensive pulmonary artery obstruction and the presence of cardiopulmonary comorbidity may lead to right ventricular dysfunction. The result is hemodynamic instability and, in severe cases, death.

In 1856, Virchow defined a triad of primary risk factors for thromboembolism: (i) local trauma to the vessel wall, (ii) hypercoagulability, and (iii) venous stasis. VTE is a multifactorial disease with genetic and genetic-environmental interaction. The risk factors responsible are summarized in Table 2. The majority of

Table 2: Risk factors for venous thromboembolism	
Hereditary factors	
Antithrombin deficiency	Protein C deficiency
Congenital dysfibrinogenemia	Factor V Leiden (G1691A mutation)
Thrombomodulin	Plasminogen deficiency
Hyperhomocysteinemia	Dysplasminogenemia
Anticardiolipin antibodies	Protein S deficiency
Excessive plasminogen activator inhibitor	Factor XII deficiency
Prothrombin G20210A mutation	Homozygous C677T mutation
Acquired factors	
Trauma/fractures	Surgery
Stroke	Immobilization
Advanced age	Malignancy (chemotherapy)
Central venous catheters	Obesity
Chronic venous insufficiency	Heart failure
Smoking	Long distance travel
Pregnancy/puerperium	Oral contraceptives or hormone replacement therapy
Crohn's disease	Antiphospholipid syndrome
Nephrotic syndrome	Prosthetic surfaces
Hyperviscosity (polycythemia, Waldenstrom's macroglobulinemia)	Acute medical illness
Platelet abnormalities	Spinal cord injury

cases of secondary thrombosis have more than one underlying condition, with the combination of surgery and malignancy occurring with highest frequency. The role of combined risk factors in thromboembolic disease hints at a probable multi-hit pathophysiology underlying VTE.

Pathophysiology

Acute PE causes major pulmonary physiologic derangements. Pulmonary embolism acutely increases peripheral vascular resistance (PVR) with mean pulmonary artery pressures increasing in proportion to the degree of vascular obstruction in patients without preexistent pulmonary vascular disease. In contrast to the muscular left ventricle (LV), the thin-walled right ventricle (RV) is poorly suited to compensate for acute increases in afterload produced by PE. The impact of VTE on the pulmonary outflow tract precipitates an increase in right ventricular impedance, increasing the pressure load on the RV producing stroke volume reduction, which will later depress cardiac output resulting in right ventricular dilatation. As a consequence, left ventricular preload will decrease along with an additional leftward shift of the interventricular septum related to right ventricular dilation that will further impair left-sided function. The additional decrease of left ventricular flow results in systemic hypotension, which associated with increasing right ventricular end-diastolic pressure and increased oxygen demands, will precipitate right ventricular ischemia, which may lead to right ventricular failure.

Vasoactive mediators may also contribute to an increase in right ventricular impedance. Decreased arterial partial pressure of oxygen (hypoxemia) and an increase in alveolar-arterial oxygen tension gradient are the most common gas exchange abnormalities. Although PE impairs efficient pulmonary elimination of CO_2 as a result of increased dead space, hypercapnia, and respiratory acidosis rarely accompany PE. This is the result of compensatory hyperventilation.

The lungs have a certain capacity to dispose of thromboemboli by endogenous thrombolysis making pathological investigation difficult. Large emboli obstructing the pulmonary trunk or main pulmonary arteries can be detected during autopsy, but lobar and segmental pulmonary arteries are not regularly evaluated. As a result, thrombosis in those vessels may escape detection. Large thrombi present in major elastic pulmonary arteries are thought to be embolic in nature in the absence of underlying disease of the vascular wall. A fresh thrombus is particularly susceptible to fragmentation in transit; however, older organized thrombus is more likely to pass intact into the pulmonary circulation and to lodge on bifurcations. If a patient survives the initial PE, the thrombus undergoes endogenous thrombolysis. The remaining thrombus then undergoes organization into vascularized connective tissue. The final step is recanalization. Residual thrombosis, however, is common after anticoagulation. Complete resolution of thrombus is not achieved in more than 50% of patients at 6 months after diagnosis. Pulmonary infarction is the death of lung tissue distal to embolic obstruction and is usually associated with an obstruction of a medium-sized pulmonary artery.

Outcomes

The short-term prognosis of PE depends on hemodynamic status and underlying disease. The hemodynamic status and underlying disease states, mainly malignancy, were the main prognostic factors for major adverse events at 30 days. There are other factors associated with poor outcomes, for example, right ventricular dysfunction assessed by echocardiography or spiral CT as well as increased levels of brain natriuretic peptide (BNP), pro-BNP and troponin T. Patients with acute symptomatic PE and concomitant DVT have a higher short-term risk for all-cause mortality, PE-related death and recurrent VTE than patients solely diagnosed with VTE over a 3-month follow-up.

Clinical Manifestations

Deep venous thrombosis usually starts in the calf veins; it may extend to the proximal veins, and subsequently break free to cause PE. Each of these stages of thromboembolism may or may not be associated with symptoms. The development of symptoms depends on the extent of thrombosis, the adequacy of collateral vessels and the severity of associated vascular occlusion and inflammation. An additional factor is the capacity of the patient to tolerate thrombosis. Clinical syndromes in patients with PE have been described as the syndrome of hemoptysis or pleuritic pain, uncomplicated dyspnea syndrome and the circulatory collapse syndrome.

New dyspnea at rest or with exertion was the most frequent symptom. Orthopnea was associated with dyspnea in 38% of patients. Pleuritic chest pain was more frequently reported than hemoptysis. Description of hemoptysis varied from pinkish to blood streaked to grossly bloody sputum. Commonly reported symptoms in patients with suspected DVT, including leg pain and swelling are neither sensitive nor specific for this condition.

Signs

Tachypnea and tachycardia are present in a large number of cases. Abnormal cardiac examination with increased P2, right ventricular lift or jugular venous distention is seen. Crackles and decreased breath sounds were reported frequently, while ronchi and wheezes were uncommon. Hepatomegaly is infrequently seen and may herald right ventricular compromise. Signs of suspected DVT include pitting edema, warmth, dilated superficial veins and erythema. Homans sign, pain in the calf or popliteal region on forceful and abrupt dorsiflexion of the ankle with the knee in flexed position, may be demonstrated in these patients.

Arterial blood gas analysis commonly demonstrates hypoxia and hypocapnia; however, a PaO_2 higher than 80 mm Hg is not uncommon in patients with the hemoptysis or pleuritic pain syndrome. A normal A-a gradient did not distinguish patients with acute PE from patients with no PE.

Chest radiographs are nonspecific in PE. Electrocardiography is also nonspecific and may show a normal pattern, sinus tachycardia, T wave inversion in V1 to V3 leads, the S1Q3/S1Q3T3 pattern (Fig. 6) or a right bundle branch block.

Diagnostic Testing

Plasma D-dimer is a marker of endogenous fibrinolysis and should therefore is detectable in patients with thromboembolic disease. The D-dimer assay has a high negative predictive value, and it is a sensitive but nonspecific marker of thromboembolism. Contrast venography is the diagnostic gold standard for patients with suspected lower extremity DVT. Noninvasive testing with compression ultrasonography has largely replaced venography to diagnose proximal DVT. It should be emphasized that compression ultrasonography needs to be repeated over the course of a week, since 6% of the cases of DVT were detected during serial testing.

Ventilation/perfusion scan or V/Q scan is frequently used to investigate potential PE; however, its use has been plagued by a nondiagnostic rate as high as 30%, particularly if PE is limited to subsegmental pulmonary arteries. Diagnostic

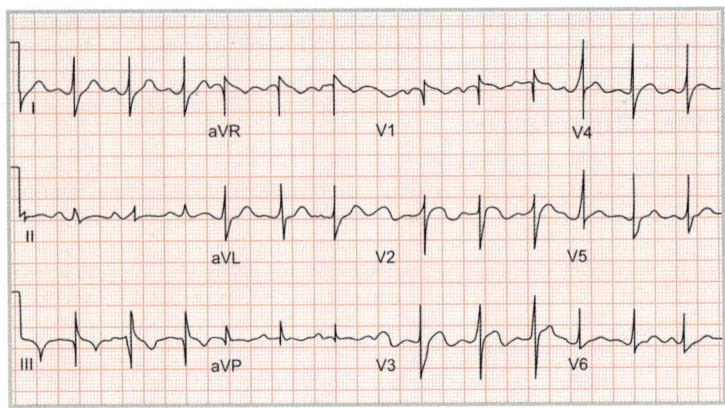

FIGURE 6: The S1Q3T3 pattern. (*Source:* Reprinted with permission from Stein PD, Woodard PK, Weg JG, et al. Diagnostic pathways in acute pulmonary embolism: recommendations of the PIOPED II investigators. Am J Med. © 2008 with permission from Elsevier)

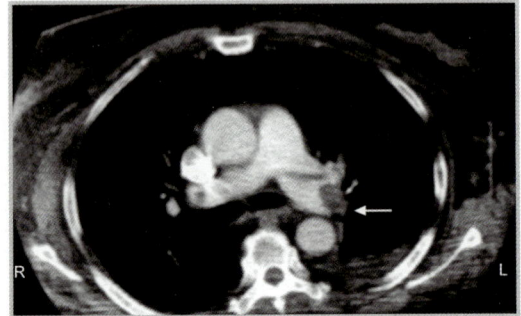

FIGURE 7: Spiral computerized tomographic pulmonary arteriography. (*Source:* Reprinted with permission from Stein PD, Woodard PK, Weg JG, et al. Diagnostic pathways in acute pulmonary embolism: recommendations of the PIOPED II investigators. Am J Med. © 2008 with permission from Elsevier)

uncertainty occurs whenever scans are either low or intermediate probability. Computed tomographic pulmonary angiography (Fig. 7) is an alternative that provides a clear result (either positive or negative) and may detect alternative nonthrombotic causes of symptoms. Pulmonary angiography is thought to be the most definitive of the techniques used for the diagnosis of PE; however, it is not ideal because it is invasive, expensive, and has a 6% risk of morbidity and 0.5% risk of mortality. Pulmonary angiography is generally reserved for patients in whom the clinical suspicion of PE remains high despite negative computed tomographic pulmonary angiography and bilateral lower extremity venous evaluations (by computed tomographic venography or ultrasonography), or for those with contraindications to computed tomographic pulmonary angiography and an indeterminate V/Q scan.

Magnetic resonance imagings (MRI) of pulmonary and deep venous system remain as second-line diagnostic tools due to higher costs, technical limitations, limited availability and logistical constraints. Magnetic resonance direct thrombus imaging (MRDTI) is a technique that has demonstrated accuracy and reproducibility for DVT diagnosis in limited studies. It detects the presence of methemoglobin in clots, allowing visualization of thrombus without using intravenous contrast and making it useful for detection of subacute thrombosis. The potential major advantages of MRDTI over conventional modalities include: (i) early data suggesting that it is highly accurate for the detection of both DVT and PE, providing a single imaging modality for the detection of VTE, (ii) direct visualization of thrombus, avoiding the pitfalls of conventional techniques that have either identified thrombus as a filling defect or in terms of surrogates, and (iii) simultaneous imaging of the legs and chest, allowing a comprehensive assessment of thrombus load, minimizing the importance of overlooked subsegmental PE and potentially facilitating more titrated treatment.

Echocardiography is a convenient and safe imaging technique that may provide critical insight into the pathophysiologic effect of VTE on right ventricular function.

Diagnostic Approach

The choice of diagnostic tests depends on the clinical probability of PE, condition of the patient, availability of diagnostic tests, risks of ionizing radiation exposure and cost; thus a clinical assessment should be made before imaging and by an objective method. In order for a test, or combination of test, to be considered accurate enough to diagnose the presence of PE, it should have a positive predictive value of 85%. To exclude the presence of VTE, such a test should have a negative predictive value of 95%. The most frequently used clinical prediction rule, the Wells score, uses both a three-category scheme (low, moderate or high clinical probability) and a two-category scheme (PE likely or PE unlikely); however, the interobserver reproducibility is variable. The revised Geneva rule is also widely used; it comprises four variables not included in the Wells score: (i) age, (ii) unilateral lower limb pain; (iii) heart rate, and (iv) signs of DVT; this rule has also been extensively validated (Table 3). The pulmonary embolism rule-out criteria (PERC) is an eight-factor decision rule designed to support the decision not to order a diagnostic test for VTE in patients with low clinical suspicion for disease. The use of assessment of probability allows patients to be classified into three groups on the basis of the approximate prevalence of PE: (i) low clinical probability (a prevalence of 10% or less; Flowchart 3), (ii) intermediate clinical probability (a prevalence of approximately 30%; Flowchart 4), and (iii) high clinical probability (a prevalence of 70% or higher; Flowchart 5).

Acute Management

The acute management of VTE begins during workup. Patients judged to be moderate or high clinical probability for PE should be started on anticoagulation therapy as arrangements are being made for confirmatory testing. The morbidity and mortality of undiagnosed PE outweighs the risk inherent in anticoagulation.

In parallel with the assessment of clinical probability, the patient should be assessed for mortality risk. Two clinical findings identify patients at high risk of mortality associated with PE: the presence of shock or hypotension defined by systemic systolic blood pressure less than 90 mm Hg, or a drop from baseline of greater than or equal to 40 mm Hg for greater than 15 minutes with no other identifiable cause. Table 4 provides a scheme for stratification of patients on the basis of mortality risk.

Table 3: The revised Geneva rule is compared with the Wells score

Revised Geneva score		Wells score	
Variable	Points	Variable	Points
Predisposing factors		*Predisposing factors*	
Age > 65 years	+1		
Previous DVT or PE	+3	Previous DVT or PE	+15
Surgery of fracture within 1 month	+2	Recent surgery or immobilization	+1.5
Active malignancy	+2	Cancer	+1
Symptoms		*Symptoms*	
Unilateral lower limb pain	+3		
Hemoptysis	+2	Hemoptysis	+1
Clinical signs		*Clinical signs*	
Heart rate		Heart rate	
75–94 beats/min	+3	>100 beats/min	+1.5
> 95 beats/min	+5	Clinical signs of DVT	+3
Pain on lower limb deep vein at palpitation and unilateral edema	+4		
		Clinical judgment Alternative diagnosis less likely than PE	+3
Clinical probability	Total	*Clinical probability (3 levels)*	Total
Low	0–3	Low	0–1
Intermediate	4–10	Intermediate	2–6
High	> 11	High	≥7
		Clinical probability (2 levels)	
		PE unlikely	0–4
		PE likely	>4

(Source: Torbicki A, Perrier A, Konstantinides SU, et al. Guidelines on diagnosis and management of acute pulmonary embolism. Task Force for the Diagnosis and Management of Acute Pulmonary Embolism of the European Society of Cardiology (ESC). Eur Heart J. 2008;29:2276-315)

Management of Patients at High Risk of Death

Shock or hypotension in a patient with PE is a medical emergency and rapid therapy should be initiated to prevent death. Fluid resuscitation is the cornerstone of therapy in many forms of shock. Although no prospective clinical trials have been performed, vasopressors and inotropes may provide temporary benefit though they do not address or correct the cause of shock in this clinical scenario. Mechanical ventilation may be required in extreme cases but should be initiated with caution given the unstable nature of these patients.

FLOWCHART 3: Pathway for diagnosis with CT angiography or CT angiography/CT venography following testing with D-dimer in combination with low probability clinical assessment

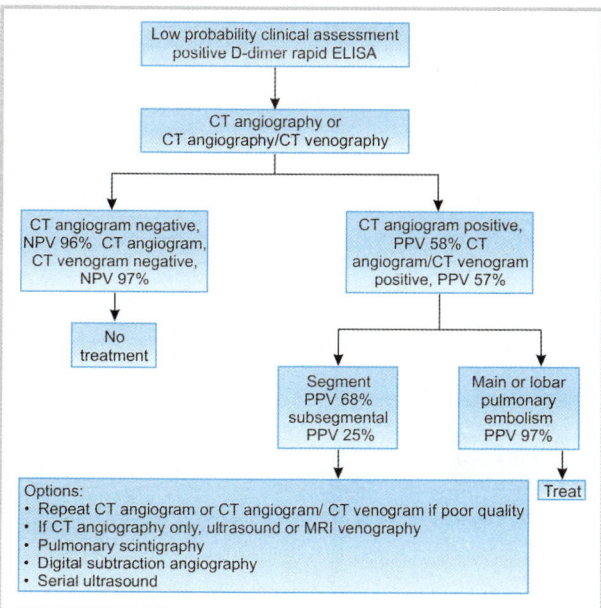

(Abbreviations: CT angiography: Contrast-enhanced multidetector computed tomographic pulmonary angiography; CT venography: Contrast-enhanced multidetector computed tomographic venous phase imaging of the veins of the lower extremities; NPV: Negative predictive value; PPV: Positive predictive value). (*Source:* Stein PD, Woodard PK, Weg JG, et al. Diagnostic pathways in acute pulmonary embolism: recommendations of the PIOPED II investigators. Am J Med. ©2008 p. 1052 with permission from Elsevier)

Thrombolysis

Current guidelines support treating patients presenting with shock or hypotension associated with PE with thrombolytic therapy. Resolution of obstruction and prevention of end-organ damage associated with shock are postulated as possible benefits. Catheter delivery of thrombolytic agents directly into the pulmonary artery did not show improved efficacy over systemic therapy, and was associated with bleeding at the introducer site. Contraindications to thrombolytic therapy include recent major trauma or surgery, intracranial disease and uncontrolled hypertension at presentation.

Surgical and Catheter-based Thrombectomy

In patients judged to have high-mortality risk due to shock or hypotension who have contraindications to thrombolytic therapy, surgical thrombectomy may be a good choice, and is the preferred choice. Surgery may also be necessary in patients who fail a trial of systemic thrombolysis. Catheter thrombectomy is another alternative, although more data is needed before it can be recommended.

FLOWCHART 4: Pathway for diagnosis with CT angiography or CT angiography/CT venography following testing with D-dimer in combination with moderate probability clinical assessment

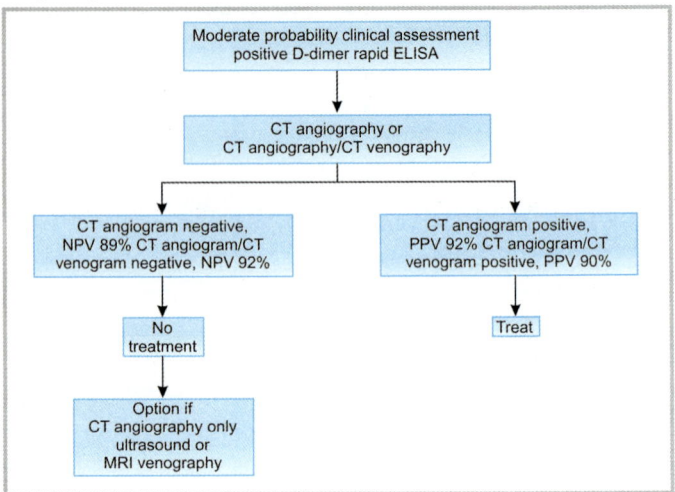

(Abbreviations: CT angiography: Contrast-enhanced multidetector computed tomographic pulmonary angiography; CT venography: Contrast-enhanced multidetector computed tomographic venous phase imaging of the veins of the lower extremities; NPV: Negative predictive value; PPV: Positive predictive value). (*Source:* Reprinted with permission from Stein PD, Woodard PK, Weg JG, et al. Diagnostic pathways in acute pulmonary embolism: recommendations of the PIOPED II investigators. Am J Med. © 2008 with permission from Elsevier)

Intermediate Risk Populations

Several markers of poor outcome have been identified. Broadly, they include markers of right ventricular dysfunction and markers of myocardial injury (Table 4). Use of markers of right ventricular strain and myocardial injury assist in the identification of patients who, although they may not demonstrate hemodynamic instability, may be at increased (intermediate) risk for mortality. The current American College of Chest Physicians guidelines recommend a case by case assessment of these intermediate risk patients in order to identify those who may benefit from thrombolysis despite absence of shock or hypotension. Regardless, this population represents a group of patients that warrant close attention.

Low Risk Populations

These patients may be candidates for early discharge or possibly even home therapy as long as appropriate anticoagulation strategies are employed.

Anticoagulation Therapy

The main aim of VTE therapy is to prevent extension of thrombosis and embolization to the lungs. Other long-term goals include reduction in the incidence of recurrent VTE, prevention of post-thrombotic syndrome and avoidance of pulmonary hypertension. Anticoagulants remain the mainstay of VTE therapy.

Therapy for Acute Decompensation

As the only vasodilator shown to have benefit in patients with cor pulmonale, oxygen is the cornerstone of therapy for acute decompensation. Maintenance of oxygen saturation at 90% promotes pulmonary vasodilation, reducing right ventricular afterload, thus improving cardiac output and inducing a diuretic effect. Care must be taken to monitor for worsening of coexisting hypercapnia. If elevated PCO_2 is detected, ventilatory support may be indicated. Diuretic therapy should be utilized with care and close monitoring of fluid and electrolyte status. Treatment of bronchospasm with beta 2 agonists and anticholinergics in combination with noninvasive ventilation may help alleviate airflow obstruction. Antimicrobial therapy should also be considered in patients in acute exacerbation of COPD with cor pulmonale. Additionally, corticosteroid therapy is recommended for this patient population.

Long-term Therapy

Continuous oxygen therapy treats the persistent alveolar hypoxia that is thought to be the triggering mechanism in cor pulmonale. Therapy may reduce chronic elevation of pulmonary pressures despite progression of airflow limitation resulting in improvement in right ventricular function, quality of life and mortality.

❑ SUGGESTED READINGS

Budev MM, Arroliga AC, Wiedemann HP, et al. Cor pulmonale: an overview. Semin Respir Crit Care Med. 2003;24:233-43.

Hirsh J, Bauer KA, Donati MB, et al. Parenteral anticoagulants: American College of Chest Physicians Evidence-Based Clinical Practice Guidelines (8th edition). Chest. 2008;133:141S-59S.

Hirsh J, Fuster V, Ansell J, et al. American Heart Association/American College of Cardiology Foundation guide to warfarin therapy. J Am Coll Cardiol. 2003;41:1633-52.

Kearon C, Kahn SR, Agnelli G, et al. Antithrombotic therapy for venous thromboembolic disease: the eight ACCP conference on antithrombotic and thrombolytic therapy. Chest. 2008;133:454S-545S.

Kruip MJ, Slob MJ, Schijen JH, et al. Use of a clinical decision rule in combination with D-dimer concentration in diagnostic workup of patients with suspected pulmonary embolism: a prospective management study. Arch Intern Med. 2002;162:1631-5.

Libby P, Zipes DP, Mann DL, et al. Braunwald's heart disease. A Textbook of Cardiovascular Medicine, 8th edition. pp. 1863-79.

Mason RJ, Murray JF, Nadel JA, et al. Murray and Nadel's Textbook of Respiratory Medicine, 5th edition. pp. 1186-223.

Musset D, Parent F, Meyer G, et al. Diagnostic strategy for patients with suspected pulmonary embolism: a prospective multicentre outcome study. Lancet. 2002;360:1914-20.

Pauwels RA, Buist AS, Calverley PM, et al. Global strategy for the diagnosis, management and prevention of chronic obstructive pulmonary disease. Am J Respir Crit Care Med. 2001;163:1256-76.

Stein PD, Terrin MC, Hales CA, et al. Clinical, laboratory, roentgenographic, and electrocardiographic findings in patients with acute pulmonary embolism and pre-existing cardiac or pulmonary disease. Chest. 1991;100:598-603.

Tapson VF. Acute pulmonary embolism. N Engl J Med. 2008;358:1037-52.

Torbicki A, Perrier A, Konstantinides S, et al. Guidelines on diagnosis and management of acute pulmonary embolism. Task force on pulmonary embolism. European Society of Cardiology. Eur Heart J. 2008;29:2276-315.

to lung disease and/or hypoxia. Disease entities included in this group include such diverse states as chronic obstructive pulmonary disease (COPD), interstitial lung disease, sleep disordered breathing and diseases of alveolar hypoventilation.

The increased load on the RV is driven by hypoxic vasoconstriction, acidemia, hypercarbia, structural changes to the vascular bed including scarring and destruction, elevated cardiac output and elevated blood viscosity. Prolonged hypoxia also mediates vascular remodeling by interacting with the nitric oxide and endothelin pathways. The PVR rises and the RV, which is a low pressure pump, develops pressure overload.

The initial symptom of cor pulmonale is dyspnea. If untreated the process progresses to overt right heart failure resulting in bilateral lower extremity edema, chest pain, presyncope and syncope. Advanced COPD has been associated with edema in the absence of right heart failure, so further investigation should be considered in the clinically stable COPD patient with leg swelling.

Diagnosis

Multiple classic electrocardiographic findings have been described, including a rightward p wave axis, the S1S2S3 pattern, the S1Q3 pattern, right bundle branch block and evidence of RV hypertrophy. These findings are helpful when present, but are often absent.

The chest film in cor pulmonale will demonstrate large central pulmonary arteries, obliteration of the retrosternal air space and right-sided chamber enlargement. Another important feature is the absence of evidence of left-sided heart failure, including diffuse vascular congestion, cephalization, Kerley B lines, significant pleural effusions and left ventricular enlargement.

It has been demonstrated that as many as 40% of patients with COPD who have an forced expiratory volume in one second (FEV1) of less than 1 liter have evidence of cor pulmonale. Conversely, patients suspected of having cor pulmonale secondary to obstructive or restrictive disease that have normal pulmonary function testing should be assessed for other causes of their pulmonary hypertension.

The combination of echocardiographic evidence of right ventricular hypertrophy or dysfunction and severe COPD or interstitial lung disease is consistent with cor pulmonale. The echo can also be used to estimate the right ventricular systolic pressure and thus the severity of the pulmonary hypertension.

Therapy

Direct pulmonary vasodilator therapy includes the prostacyclin analogs epoprostenol, iloprost and treprostinil; the endothelin receptor antagonists bosentan and ambrisentan and the phosphodiesterase-5 inhibitors sildenafil and tadalafil. Their efficacy in the treatment of pulmonary arterial hypertension has been proven by well-designed clinical trials and they have been approved by the FDA for use in patients with Group 1 pulmonary hypertension. They have not, however, been approved for patients with Group 3 PH. Multiple clinical trialsare under way in this patient population. Unfortunately, preliminary data are contradictory at best.

Oxygen is the only therapy that has been proven to treat cor pulmonale in patients suffering from COPD. The nocturnal oxygen therapy trial (NOTT) and the British Medical Council long-term domicillary oxygen treatment trial actually demonstrated hemodynamic benefit of therapy.

however, it can be used for prophylaxis similar to enoxaparin. Tinzaparin is only indicated for therapy in patients with VTE.

Enoxaparin is used most often in the hospital setting, and dosing is listed below. For specific dosing on dalteparin and tinzaparin, please refer to their package insert. Treatment dosing for enoxaparin is 1 mg/kg twice daily or 1.5 mg/kg daily. In patients with creatinine clearance (CrCl) of less than or equal to 30 mL/min, dosing is decreased to 1 mg/kg daily. Prophylactic dosing for surgeries is normally 40 mg daily or 30 mg twice daily. In renal dysfunction, the dose is decreased to 30 mg daily. Fondaparinux was as effective and safe as UFH for the treatment of PE, and as effective and safe as enoxaparin for the treatment of DVT. The drug is also used for prophylaxis of VTE and is contraindicated in patients with CrCl less than 30 mL/min, hemorrhage, bacterial endocarditis, thrombocytopenia, allergy to the drug itself and for prophylaxis in patients weighing less than 50 kg. Fondaparinux is dosed based on body weight for treatment and at a fixed dose for prophylaxis. As with LMWHs, Fondaparinux is customarily not monitored.

Direct thrombin inhibitors also have the advantages of predictable dose response and reduced incidence of thrombocytopenia. However they do not have an antidote for cases of severe bleeding. Argatroban and lepirudin are two intravenous direct thrombin inhibitors that are FDA approved for the prevention and/or treatment of VTE in patients with HIT.

Oral Agents—Vitamin K Antagonists-warfarin

While there are many ongoing studies to find a new anticoagulant medication, warfarin remains the only oral anticoagulant available on the market in the United States. Indications for warfarin include VTE, atrial fibrillation, mechanical and bioprosthetic heart valve replacement, MI and hypercoagulable conditions. Warfarin dosing is highly individualized and must take into account comorbid disease states. The recommended initiation dose for warfarin is 5 mg, which was shown to achieve therapeutic international normalized ratio (INR) as fast as the 10 mg loading dose. In patients at high risk for developing another event and in need of immediate anticoagulation, heparin/LMWH is used alongside warfarin for at least 4–5 days and pending two therapeutic INR levels. The therapeutic INR range for most indications continues to be 2–3 (target 2.5).

Inferior Vena Cava Filters

Inferior vena cava filters are indicated for patients for whom anticoagulation is contraindicated, those who experience recurrent PE despite adequate anticoagulation, and possibly those with patients with PE who have poor cardiopulmonary reserve. However there has been only one randomized clinical trial evaluating the efficacy of IVC filters to prevent recurrent VTE. Patients in the IVC filter group had significantly fewer total PE after 12 days and fewer symptomatic pulmonary emboli at 8 years. Retrievable IVC filters are approved as an alternative for patients with temporary contraindication to anticoagulation, but data for these are limited.

❑ COR PULMONALE

Cor pulmonale or "pulmonary heart disease" is characterized by right heart dysfunction secondary to underlying lung disease. All forms of cor pulmonale share the unifying feature of pulmonary hypertension and are classified in group 3 of the revised classification of pulmonary hypertension— pulmonary hypertension owing

FLOWCHART 5: Pathway for diagnosis with CT angiography or CT angiography/CT venography following testing with D-dimer in combination with high probability clinical assessment

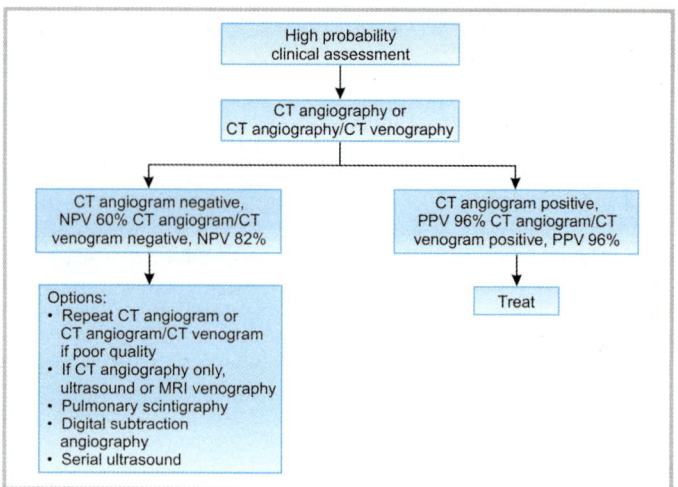

(Abbreviations: CT angiography: Contrast-enhanced multidetector computed tomographic pulmonary angiography; CT venography: Contrast-enhanced multidetector computed tomographic venous phase imaging of the veins of the lower extremities; NPV: Negative predictive value; PPV: Positive predictive value). (*Source:* Reprinted with permission from Stein PD, Woodard PK, Weg JG, et al. Diagnostic pathways in acute pulmonary embolism: recommendations of the PIOPED II investigators. Am J Med. © 2008 with permission from Elsevier)

Table 4: Risk stratification—expected pulmonary embolism-related mortality				
PE-related early mortality risk	**Clinical (shock/hypotension)**	**RV dysfunction**	**Myocardial injury**	**Treatment implications**
High >15%	+	Na	Na	Thrombolysis (consider embolectomy)
Intermediate (3–15%)	–	+	+	Hospital admission
		+	–	
		–	+	
Low	–	–	–	Early discharge

(*Source:* Torbicki A, Perrier A, Konstantinides SV, et al. Guidelines on the diagnosis and management of acute pulmonary embolism: the Task Force for the Diagnosis and Management of Acute Pulmonary Embolism of the European Society of Cardiology (ESC). Eur Heart J. 2008;29:2276-315)

Parenteral Anticoagulants

Enoxaparin is indicated in the prophylaxis of VTE, as well as in the treatment of VTE and ST segment elevation MI. The medication is also used in patients with unstable angina and non-ST elevation MI for prevention of ischemic embolisms during treatment of these disease states. Dalteparin is not indicated in the treatment of VTE unless the patient has cancer and a history of blood clots;

Chapter 11

Relevant Issues in Clinical Cardiology

11.1 Noncardiac Surgery in Cardiac Patients

❏ INTRODUCTION

Patients with cardiovascular disease or major risk factors incur a significant risk of adverse cardiac events during major noncardiac surgery. Since the prevalence of cardiovascular disease, especially coronary heart disease (CHD), increases with age, the development of perioperative cardiac complications may also increase substantially. Adverse perioperative cardiac events, mainly nonfatal myocardial infarction (MI) and cardiac death, usually occur in patients with known or occult CHD, left ventricular (LV) dysfunction or severe valvular heart disease (VHD) who are undergoing surgical procedures that produce prolonged hemodynamic aberrations and cardiac stress response. Perioperative cardiac complications have implications not only for the immediate postoperative period but also influence long-term patient outcomes.

❏ PREOPERATIVE CARDIAC RISK ASSESSMENT

The key element of perioperative management of patients with cardiac disease undergoing noncardiac surgery is a thorough preoperative assessment of the risk of cardiac events. This process involves two equally important elements: (i) factors related to the patient and (ii) factors related to the specific surgery being performed.

Although patient related factors are an important tool in assessing risk, it is important to remember that emergency surgery should not be delayed for preoperative risk stratification. Once it is clear that surgery can be delayed, the patient should be examined closely to evaluate the perioperative risk, beginning with a thorough history and physical examination.

General Risk Stratification

For the practitioner who is asked to see a patient prior to surgery, the ACC/AHA guidelines provide a useful framework. By following a simple, stepwise approach to the patient based mainly on history and physical examination, one can quickly assess the risk of adverse cardiac events during the perioperative period (Flowchart 1).

Initial risk stratification prior to noncardiac surgery should be based upon the stepwise integration of all elements mentioned above: urgency and type of surgery; presence or absence of an active cardiac condition; the patient's functional status and the number of the patient's clinical risk predictors.

762 Manual of Cardiology

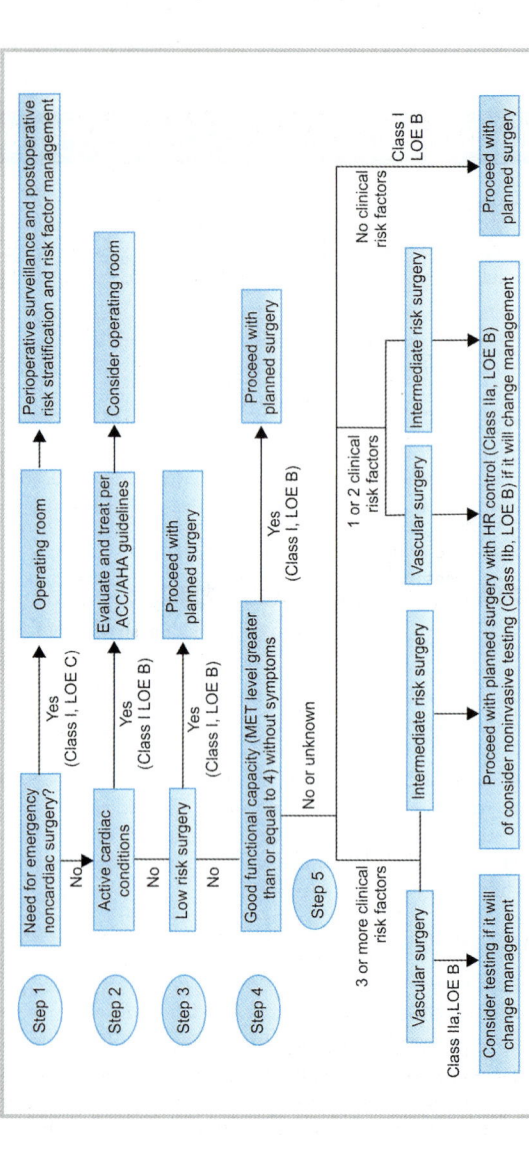

FLOWCHART 1: Cardiac evaluation and care algorithm for noncardiac surgery-based on active clinical conditions (high-risk predictors), known cardiovascular disease, or cardiac risk factors for patients aged more than or equal to 50 years

(Abbreviations: HR: Heart rate; LOE: Level of evidence; MET: Metabolic equivalent. (Source: Fleisher LA, Beckman JA, Brown KA, et al. 2009 ACCF/AHA Focused Update on Perioperative Beta Blockade Incorporated into the ACC/AHA 2007 Guidelines on Perioperative Cardiovascular Evaluation and Care for Noncardiac Surgery, J Am Coll Cardiol. 2009;54:e13-118; originally published online Nov 2, 2009. With permission from the American College of Cardiology)

Ischemic Heart Disease

Patients with known ischemic heart disease are at considerable risk for developing an adverse cardiac event in the perioperative period. Evaluation of these patients should include an assessment of symptoms, the patient's ischemic threshold, amount of myocardium at jeopardy (if known), LV function and whether the patient is on optimal medical therapy. Estimation of functional status is especially important in patients with CHD because if their functional capacity is limited to less than four METs, either due to angina, dyspnea or noncardiac limitation of activity, consideration should be given to further testing.

Hypertension

There is some controversy regarding whether isolated hypertension is an independent risk factor of perioperative complications. Hypertension increases the risk of ischemic disease (both CHD and stroke). Additionally, it can worsen the ischemic burden in the setting of stress situations such as surgery. Patients with stage III hypertension (SBP >180) and those who have evidence of end-organ damage have an increased risk of intraoperative blood pressure lability and possibly of perioperative complications. If a new diagnosis of hypertension is made during preoperative assessment evaluation for secondary causes of hypertension and standard treatment guidelines should be applied.

Heart Failure

Clinical evidence of heart failure (HF) has been identified as a predictor of poor clinical outcomes in the surgical setting in every analysis that has examined the question. Decompensated HF is considered an "active cardiac condition" that requires treatment prior to surgery. Due to the clear link between HF and surgical risk, a careful history and physical examination should be undertaken prior to surgery in any patient for whom HF is a potential diagnosis. Decreased exercise tolerance due to shortness of breath, paroxysmal nocturnal dyspnea or new orthopnea, elevation of the jugular venous pressure (JVP), peripheral edema, or the presence of an S3 should prompt further evaluation prior to surgery to either confirm or rule out a diagnosis of HF.

Valvular Heart Disease

Valvular disease includes a broad and varied set of pathologies, and each disease process affects surgical risk in different ways. Murmurs and valve-related symptoms must be identified during the initial patient assessment. TIn general, severe valvular obstructive lesions carry the highest risk of perioperative cardiac complications whereas regurgitant lesions are better tolerated.

Congenital Heart Disease

In patients with congenital heart disease, it is the physiology of the underlying defect and the consequences of the repair that drive risk. Consequently, the risk of a particular patient with a congenital cardiac defect is difficult to generalize. However, there is general consensus that patients with pulmonary hypertension including those with Eisenmenger's physiology, those with cyanotic congenital defects those in New York Heart Association Functional Class III or IV and those with severe left sided obstructive lesions (aortic stenosis, coarctation of the aorta) or severe systemic ventricular dysfunction (EF < 35%) are at highest risk. Patients with Eisenmenger's physiology are at significantly higher risk of complications during and after surgery. The right to left shunt can increase due to increased intrathoracic pressure from ventilation during surgery and from the systemic vasodilatation induced by anesthesia. In one small study, the perioperative mortality of such patients was approximately 10% and was not altered by the type of anesthesia.

Arrhythmias

Many cardiac dysrhythmias discovered preoperatively are benign, especially if they are asymptomatic and incidentally found on ECG monitoring. Occasional premature atrial or ventricular beats and even short runs of nonsustained ventricular tachycardia (VT) in the preoperative setting have not been associated with increased perioperative cardiac events.

Sustained atrial arrythmias, such as atrial fibrillation, found during preoperative evaluation frequently indicate the presence of underlying structural heart disease and have been identified as independent risk factors for perioperative cardiac complications. Sustained VT found in the preoperative setting significantly increases the risk of intraoperative arrhythmias and is suggestive of serious structural or ischemic heart disease.

❏ PREOPERATIVE DIAGNOSTIC TESTING

Supplemental tests are frequently used to help risk stratify patients prior to noncardiac surgery and arrive at a decision whether a preoperative intervention is warranted.

12-Lead Resting Electrocardiography

A resting 12-lead electrocardiogram (ECG) is performed commonly as part of preoperative cardiovascular risk-assessment in patients with established CHD undergoing noncardiac surgery. The preoperative ECG contains important prognostic information and is predictive of long-term morbidity and mortality independent of clinical findings and the presence of perioperative myocardial ischemia. AHA guidelines recommend preoperative electrocardiography for patients with known atherosclerotic vascular disease or at least one clinical risk factor who are to undergo vascular or intermediate-risk surgery.

Ambulatory Electrocardiography

Several studies have evaluated the positive and negative predictive value of ambulatory electrocardiography for perioperative cardiac complications. The frequency of ST-segment abnormalities consistent with silent myocardial ischemia has ranged from 9 to 39% and the positive predictive value for perioperative MI and cardiac death from 4 to 15%, whereas the negative predictive value ranged from 3 to 16%.

Heart Rate Variability

Decreased heart rate variability (HRV) is a more powerful predictor for cardiovascular mortality, including sudden cardiac death than other established clinical predictors. Decreased HRV in the preoperative period is also thought to be an independent predictor for postoperative cardiac death or MI after major surgery or trauma. However, no guideline recommendations regarding preoperative HRV determination have been published.

Assessment of Left Ventricular Function

Studies that have evaluated the role of left ventricular (LV) function in relation to perioperative risk have generally concluded that LV dysfunction has poor sensitivity and a low positive predictive value for perioperative cardiac events. The current ACC/AHA guidelines suggest that such assessment might be useful only for patients with dyspnea of unknown origin and for patients with HF and worsening symptoms.

Noninvasive Studies for Myocardial Ischemia

Several noninvasive diagnostic tests have been proposed to assess the presence and extent of CHD before noncardiac surgery. Exercise electrocardiography has traditionally been used to evaluate individuals for the presence of CHD and myocardial ischemia. However, a substantial number of high-risk patients are either unable to exercise or have contraindications to exercise. Therefore, pharmacologic stress testing with imaging has been employed commonly as a preoperative test in patients undergoing high risk and especially vascular surgery. A large body of knowledge has accumulated showing that the presence of a distribution defect on dipyridamole perfusion scintigraphy (DPS) or extensive wall motion abnormalities on a dobutamine stress echocardiographic (DSE) study predict perioperative adverse cardiac events with high sensitivity, but overall low positive predictive value. Current ACC/AHA guidelines recommending such testing only if it will change patient management.

Coronary Angiography

Invasive coronary angiography is a well-established diagnostic technique, which is infrequently indicated preoperatively to assess the risk of noncardiac surgery since randomized clinical trials have not demonstrated much benefit in perioperative risk assessment, and there is little information derived from such trials on its usefulness in this setting. The advent of noninvasive CT angiography may introduce changes in current practice. However, the role of CT coronary angiography for preoperative risk assessment has not been rigorously studied so far.

Cardiac Biomarkers

Cardiac biomarkers have been found to have major prognostic significance in the nonoperative setting and also provide important prognostic information in cardiac patients about to undergo noncardiac surgery. Cardiac troponin T and I (cTnT and cTnI) have superior sensitivity and tissue specificity for myocardial injury compared to other markers. Evidence suggests that even small increases in cTnT in the perioperative period reflect clinically important myocardial injury and poor cardiac prognosis and outcomes.

Brain natriuretic peptide (BNP) and N-terminal pro-BNP (NT pro-BNP) are produced by cardiac myocytes in response to increased myocardial wall stress independent of the presence or absence of myocardial ischemia and have emerged as important prognostic indicators in patients with HF in nonsurgical settings. Inflammatory markers, such as C-reactive protein (CRP), are thought to be associated with unstable coronary artery disease in population studies. However routine assessment of cardiac biomarkers is not recommended because of lack of data from prospective controlled trials.

❏ PREOPERATIVE RISK MITIGATION STRATEGIES

Pharmacologic Interventions

Beta-adrenergic Blockade

Beta-blocking agents are the mainstay of anti-ischemic therapy in many clinical settings. Beta-blocking agents are used perioperatively to decrease myocardial oxygen consumption by reducing heart rate and decreasing myocardial contractility. Additional cardioprotective benefits may include redistribution of coronary blood flow to the subendocardium, increased threshold of ventricular fibrillation and possibly plaque stabilization.

Careful preoperative administration of beta blockers with gradual dose titration to achieve tight heart rate control is beneficial for high-risk patients who are undergoing noncardiac surgery. The ACC/AHA focused update of the perioperative guidelines dealing specifically with beta-blockade recommends that beta blockers be continued in patients undergoing surgery if they are receiving these agents for the treatment of preexisting conditions and that it is reasonable to administer beta blockers titrated to appropriate heart rate and blood pressure to high-risk patients undergoing vascular surgery

Statin Therapy

In addition to their lipid lowering effects, statins (3-hydroxy-3- methylglutaryl coenzyme A reductase inhibitors) improve endothelial function, stabilize atherosclerotic plaques, and reduce vascular inflammation. By these mechanisms statins may reduce perioperative cardiac events.

Recent guidelines recommend the initiation of statin therapy in high-risk surgery patients starting ideally between 30 days and one week before surgery and continuation of statin therapy perioperatively for patients taking these agents chronically.

Calcium Channel Blockers

The pharmacologic effects of calcium channel blockers on myocardial oxygen supply/demand balance make them theoretically useful for perioperative risk reduction. However, this applies primarily to calcium channel blockers that lower heart rate such as diltiazem and verapamil, and not to dihydropyridines. The ACC/AHA perioperative guidelines offer no recommendations regarding the perioperative use of calcium channel blockers.

Alpha-2 Adrenergic Receptor Agonists

The role of alpha-2 receptor agonists in the perioperative period is still evolving. These agents reduce postganglionic norepinephrine output and theoretically may reduce the catecholamine surge that develops during anesthesia and surgery. Current ACC/AHA guidelines provide a weak class IIb recommendation stating that these agents may be considered for perioperative control of hypertension in patients with known CHD or with at least one clinical risk factor who are undergoing surgery.

Nitrates

Nitrates, especially nitroglycerine, have been used for many years to effect coronary vasodilatation and reverse myocardial ischemia in patients with chronic stable angina. Nitroglycerin administration during surgery has been proposed as a way to ensure good coronary flow and maintain myocardial oxygenation in the setting of surgical stress. Countering this theoretical beneficial effects are its complex hemodynamic effects of arterial and venous dilatation. This makes the use of nitroglycerin in the perioperative setting highly debatable. Both the ACC/AHA and the ESC guidelines offer only a weak class IIb recommendation for the use of nitroglycerin during noncardiac surgery.

Antiarrhythmic Agents

In contrast to a large body of literature covering the use of antiarrhythmic agents to prevent perioperative arrhythmias in patients undergoing cardiac surgery, there is limited evidence available regarding their prophylactic use in noncardiac surgery; most of the evidence available is derived primarily from studies of patients undergoing pulmonary resection.

Both the ACC/AHA and the ESC guidelines do not provide specific recommendations regarding the prophylactic use of antiarrhythmic agents for cardiac patients undergoing noncardiac surgery. However, it is explicitly stated in the discussion of betablockers that these agents reduce the incidence of new-onset perioperative atrial fibrillation along with their overall beneficial effects. We must therefore conlude that, with the exception of beta-blockade, the strictly prophylactic use of antiarrhythmic drugs to prevent the dvelopment of perioperative arrhythmias is not warranted.

Aspirin

Aspirin is widely prescribed to patients with CHD both prior to and after coronary revascularization, whether by surgery or percutaneous intervention. However, evidence of beneficial actions of aspirin in the noncardiac perioperative setting is limited.

There is a consensus that aspirin should be continued perioperatively and should be discontinued only if the bleeding risk outweighs the potential cardiac benefits. The ESC guidelines recommend that aspirin discontinuation in patients previously treated with this agent should be considered only in those in whom hemostasis is difficult to control during noncardiac surgery. The ACC/AHA perioperative guidelines do not provide a general recommendation regarding aspirin therapy in this setting.

Nonpharmacologic and Other Interventions

Coronary Revascularization

Preoperative myocardial revascularization has been advocated as means of preventing perioperative fatal and nonfatal MIs. However, it has become abundantly clear that whereas revascularization is quite effective in treating high-grade coronary stenosis and relieving stress-induced myocardial ischemia, it does not prevent coronary thrombosis due to disruption of a vulnerable plaque during the stress of surgery. Since approximately one half of perioperative infarcts are due to plaque disruption and coronary thrombosis the efficacy of coronary revascularization in preventing a perioperative MI has been called to question.

The role of prophylactic preoperative coronary revascularization in reducing perioperative cardiac complications is limited to two general categories of patients with CHD:

- Patients who are found to have prognostically high-risk coronary anatomy and in whom long-term outcomes would likely be improved by coronary revascularization under all circumstances (e.g. stable angina with significant left main coronary artery disease, or stable angina and 3-vessel disease with depressed LV ejection fraction)
- Patients with unstable coronary syndromes, such as acute ST-segment elevation MI, high-risk unstable angina or non-ST-segment elevation MI.

Arrhythmias and Conduction Abnormalities

The presence of sustained ventricular or supraventricular arrhythmias in the preoperative period requires thorough evaluation for underlying structural heart disease and institution of appropriate therapy according to relevant guidelines. Nonsustained ventricular arrhythmias, including complex ventricular ectopy and nonsustained VT do not usually require specific therapy unless they are associated with hemodynamic compromise, myocardial ischemia or severe LV dysfunction. Several studies have reported that beta-blockers reduce the incidence of arrhythmias during the perioperative period and provide better control of heart rate in chronic atrial fibrillation than nondihydropyridine calcium channel blockers or digoxin. Digoxin may be used as a first line drug for rate control only in patients with HF since it cannot effectively block atrioventricular conduction in high adrenergic tone situations such as surgery. Rate control therapy in patients with chronic AF should be continued with minimal interruptions perioperatively.

❏ INTRAOPERATIVE MANAGEMENT

Intraoperative management of a cardiac patient undergoing noncardiac surgery involves both an understanding of the physiologic implications of anesthesia for a particular patient and an integration of all aspects of patient status and the type of surgery. This is the role of the anesthesiologist and beyond the scope of the consulting cardiologist. The choice of anesthesia should be made by the anesthetist. The consultant cardiologist can be helpful by providing some general principles as they apply to a particular patient.

❏ MANAGEMENT OF PATIENTS WITH IMPLANTED ELECTRONIC DEVICES

When a patient with an existing device is scheduled for noncardiac surgery, the consulting cardiologist will frequently be asked to assist in intraoperative management of the device. It is imperative that the device type (ICD or pacemaker) and mode of operation are clearly identified. Pacemaker dependence—the percentage of time the patient is pacer dependent—should be assessed. Intraoperatively, the two main elements of management are to create redundant systems and reduce the risk of electromagnetic interference (EMI).

Intraoperatively, the two main elements of management are to create redundant systems and reduce the risk of electromagnetic interference (EMI).

❏ POSTOPERATIVE MANAGEMENT

The postoperative period is a particularly risky period for cardiac events after noncardiac surgery, especially in the first 48 hours for patients that are at increased risk for cardiac events. Although the routine use of serial ECGs or PA catheters is not indicated, specific patients may benefit from their use.

In selected patients, such as those with clinical signs of HF prior to surgery, intraoperative fluid shifts may significantly worsen loading conditions and create severe hypervolemia. In this case, using a PA catheter to appropriately titrate inotropic therapy, diuresis and management of systemic vascular resistance can restore euvolemia and cardiopulmonary hemodynamics to a compensated state quickly and safely.

Cardiac biomarker assays in the absence of symptoms are unlikely to be helpful in diagnosing perioperative ischemia. ECG abnormalities on surveillance tracings may be more helpful in predicting postoperative infarction and can be considered in patients at elevated risk.

Benign arrhythmias are very common in the postoperative setting. Isolated PACs and PVCs are often the result of electrolyte imbalance, pain, volume shifts or a response to increased adrenergic tone after surgery. These rhythms should be monitored and treated by addressing the underlying cause of the arrhythmia. In most cases, these rhythms disappear when the underlying stimuli are removed.

Aggressive pain control in the perioperative setting is important for patient comfort, increased early mobilization and decreased length of hospitalization. It has the additional effect of blunting the stress response and reduces the metabolic demands on myocardium in the postoperative setting.

❑ SUGGESTED READINGS

Detsky AS, Abrams HB, McLaughlin JR, et al. Predicting cardiac complications in patients undergoing noncardiac surgery. J Gen Intern Med. 1986;1:211-9.

Eagle KA, Guyton RA, Davidoff R, et al. ACC/AHA 2004 guideline update for coronary artery bypass graft surgery: summary article: a report of the American College of Cardiology/American Heart Association Task Force on Practice Guidelines. Circulation. 2004;110:1168-76.

Fleischmann KE, Beckman JA, Buller CE, et al. 2009 ACC/AHA focused update on perioperative beta blockade: a report of the American College of Cardiology Foundation/American Heart Association Task Force on Practice Guidelines. J Am Coll Cardiol. 2009;54:2102-28.

Fleisher LA, Beckman JA, Brown KA, et al. 2009 ACCF/AHA Focused Update on Perioperative Beta Blockade Incorporated Into the ACC/AHA 2007 Guidelines on Perioperative Cardiovascular Evaluation and Care for Noncardiac Surgery. J Am Coll Cardiol. 2009;54:e13-118; originally published online Nov 2, 2009.

Froehlich JB, Karavite D, Russman PL, et al. American College of Cardiology/American Heart Association preoperative assessment guidelines reduce resource utilization before aortic surgery. J Vasc Surg. 2002;36:758-63.

Gibbons RJ, Abrams J, Chatterjee K, et al. ACC/AHA 2002 guideline update for the management of patients with chronic stable angina—summary article. J Am Coll Cardiol. 2003;41:159-68.

Jeger RV, Probst C, Arsenio R, et al. Long-term prognostic value of the preoperative 12-lead electrocardiogram before major noncardiac surgery in coronary artery disease. Am Heart J. 2006;151:508-13.

11.2 Gender and Cardiovascular Disease

❏ INTRODUCTION

Cardiovascular disease (CVD), including ischemic heart disease (IHD), stroke, and other heart diseases, such as hypertension (HTN), and heart failure is the leading cause of mortality and disability for women in the United States. The incidence and severity of CVD among premenopausal women is lower than among men of comparable age, even after correction for various risk factors. The causes of these differences are unclear. Cardiovascular factors strongly associated with sex include vascular function (endothelium-dependent flow-mediated dilation and aortic compliance are greater in females) and a left ventricular (LV) mass index that is greater in males.

❏ PREVALENCE OF IHD IN WOMEN

Most cardiovascular events in women are caused by IHD. IHD, which includes coronary atherosclerotic disease, myocardial infarction, acute coronary syndromes and angina, is the largest subset of CVD mortality, with more than 240,000 women dying annually from the disease. Given the aging population and epidemics of obesity and diabetes, the total number of women dying of IHD is projected to continue to rise.

❏ IDENTIFICATION OF IHD RISK FACTORS IN WOMEN

The incidence of IHD is very low among premenopausal women. Stroke incidence is higher than myocardial infarction, whereas more than 80% of midlife women have one or more traditional cardiac risk factors. Clustering of multiple risk factors is common after menopause, notably with the development of obesity, HTN and dyslipidemia, which is potentially related to hormonally mediated metabolic disturbances. Specifically, women have, on average, greater blood cholesterol levels than men after their 5th decade of life, and reveal mild decreases in high density lipoprotein (HDL) cholesterol after menopause. Low blood levels of HDL appear to be a stronger predictor of heart disease death in women than in men in the over-65 age group; hypertriglyceridemia is a more potent independent risk factor for women than men. Obesity is present in one-third of women, including 7% with BMI greater than or equal to 40 kg/m^2 with associated increased mortality. Diabetic women have significantly increased IHD mortality rate compared with diabetic men. Most notably, 30-year trends reveal marked CVD mortality reduction for diabetic men but not for diabetic women.

In addition to the traditional risk factors, it has been recognized that novel risk factors, such as hormonal disturbances and inflammation due to autoimmune diseases may play prominent roles for IHD sex differences. Disruption of ovulatory cycling indicated by estrogen deficiency and hypothalamic dysfunction or irregular menstrual cycling in premenopausal women is associated with an increased risk of coronary atherosclerosis and adverse CVD events. Polycystic ovary syndrome is prevalent in 10–13% of women and is linked with a clustering of risk factors and adverse IHD events postmenopausally.

Tobacco use is the leading preventable cause of IHD in women, especially in those who have 50 years of age or younger. In numerous population-based studies, diabetic women have a threefold to severe fold increase in IHD death when compared to a twofold to threefold increase in death for diabetic men.

A key to effective blood glucose control is the maintenance of a diet low in saturated fats and cholesterol along with optimal weight control.

HTN is a major risk factor for IHD. A higher percentage of men than women have HTN until age 45. From ages 45–54, the percentage of women is slightly higher. After that a much higher percentage of women have HTN than men do. In addition to traditional risk factors such as dyslipidemia, obesity and diabetes, other factors, such as autonomic mechanisms as well as hemodynamic and metabolic influences, are also implicated in the high prevalence of HTN and CVD in older women.

❏ ASSESSMENT OF SYMPTOMS AND MYOCARDIAL ISCHEMIA IN WOMEN SYMPTOM ASSESSMENT

There are substantial differences between women and men in the type, frequency and quality of symptoms noted during chest pain presentations. A careful medical history and physical examination can provide the key elements to determine IHD likelihood. The likelihood of significant obstructive coronary disease is variable by the type of chest pain symptoms, including noncardiac chest pain, atypical angina or typical angina.

The symptoms, that women experience, often differ from the "classic" symptoms (substernal crushing chest pain radiating to the left arm) typically perceived by men. In women, the pain may be: (i) centred in the chest with or without radiation down one or both arms, (ii) located in the ear, jaw or neck region, or (iii) located in the back or shoulder region. Other reported symptoms are diaphoresis, light-headedness, shortness of breath, nausea and vomiting; these symptoms may or may not accompany chest pain or discomfort. As women present later in life and are more often functionally impaired, their frequency of nonexertional symptoms is higher than that of their male counterparts. Additionally, for elderly women, shortness of breath is more often the initial presenting symptoms for acute MI.

Accumulating evidence over the years also supports the crucial role endothelium plays in vascular homeostasis. Almost all known cardiovascular risk factors, including hypercholesterolemia, HTN, hyperglycemia, smoking and aging, are associated with endothelial dysfunction. The relative importance of endothelial and microvascular dysfunction has only recently been recognized. An integrated understanding of mechanisms and manifestations of ischemia impacting IHD risks in women has been summarized in Figure 1. It is hypothesize that coronary microvascular dysfunction is more prevalent in women than in man as the result of risk factor clustering, vascular inflammation and remodeling, and hormonal alterations and is etiologic for the observed paradoxical frequent yet atypical symptoms, evidence of ischemia, and adverse outcomes.

Approaches for Diagnosing IHD in Women

Recommendations for the workup of women presenting with stable angina are summarized in Flowchart 2. For woman presenting with symptoms of chest pain and suspected IHD, the preferred management approach is to perform a noninvasive stress testing to assess the severity of the residual ischemia. Although specific exceptions were allowed, the guidelines recommended that standard exercise testing be used in the initial female evaluation. Interpretation of the exercise test includes symptomatic response, exercise capacity, hemodynamic response as well as ECG response. Abnormalities in exercise capacity, SBP response to exercise, heart rate response to exercise and occurrence of ischemic chest pain during exercise are

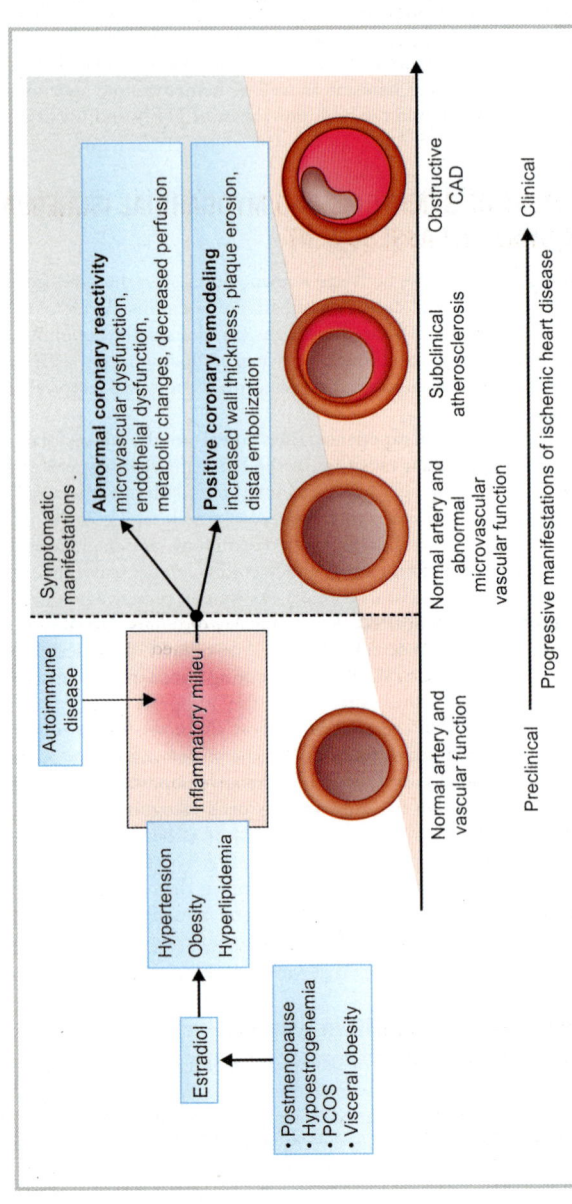

FIGURE 1: Overarching working model of ischemic heart disease pathophysiology in women (Abbreviations: CAD: Coronary artery disease; PCOS: Polycystic ovary syndrome)

Relevant Issues in Clinical Cardiology

FLOWCHART 2: A revision of consensus statement from the American Society of Nuclear Cardiology (ASNC) workup algorithm for noninvasive testing in women

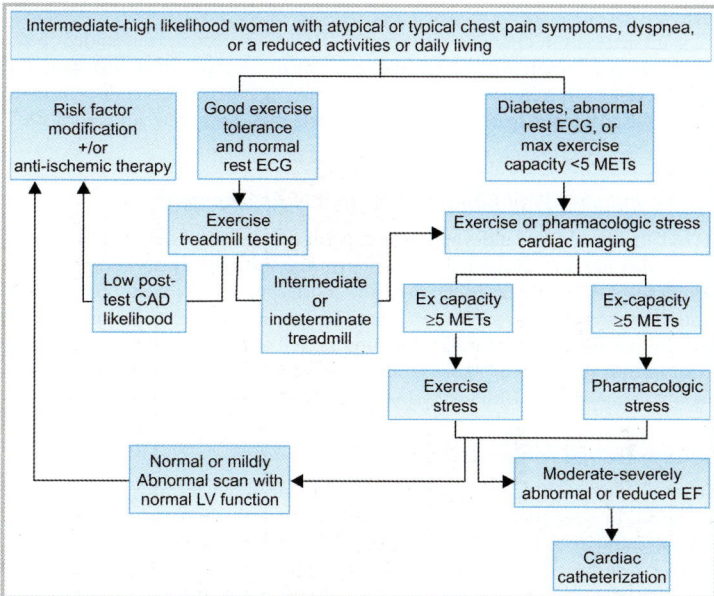

all important findings that carry diagnostic as well as prognostic significance above and beyond ECG interpretations. Therefore, exercise-based test is the preferred diagnostic modality of choice over pharmacological test in those patients who are able to exercise.

For woman presenting with symptoms of chest pain and suspected IHD, the preferred management approach is to perform a noninvasive stress testing to assess the severity of the residual ischemia. Guidelines recommended that standard exercise testing be used in the initial female evaluation. Exercise-based test is the preferred diagnostic modality of choice over pharmacological test in those patients who are able to exercise.

Exercise Electrocardiographic Evaluation

The exercise ECG is the most frequently performed diagnostic test. Using a threshold for abnormality of greater than or equal to 1.0 mm of ST-segment depression, it has a lower diagnostic accuracy (sensitivity and specificity for significant coronary artery obstruction at approximately 60–70%). Multiple factors contribute to the decreased diagnostic accuracy of exercise ECG in women, such as lower CAD prevalence as well as greater comorbidity and functional impairment that preclude women from achieving maximal levels of exercise. A digoxin-like effect of endogenous estrogen can possibly promote false-positive rates in premenopausal women.

Stress-induced Perfusion Abnormality Assessment

Myocardial perfusion single-photon emission computed tomography (SPECT) is a nuclear-based technique that is most commonly used in the evaluation of women presenting with chest pain symptoms. Generally, the literature supports SPECT imaging as a highly sensitive test for the detection of CAD in both women and men.

Cardiac positron emission tomography (PET) has over time ascended to the "gold standard" status for noninvasive assessment of myocardial perfusion and viability, due to its inherently quantitative nature, its superior detection sensitivity, and its advantageous spatial and temporal resolution over conventional SPECT techniques.

Stress-induced Wall Motion Abnormality Assessment

As wall motion abnormalities appear after perfusion abnormalities, identification of this marker has been associated with a higher diagnostic specificity and prognostic significance. Stress echocardiography, the most commonly applied test for wall motion assessment, has advantages due to its low cost, absent radiation exposure and ability to image both cardiac structures as well as ventricular function. Despite these advantages, stress echocardiography can become a suboptimal option due to obesity or lung disease with poor acoustic windows and reducing exercise tolerance.

Cardiovascular MR Assessment

Stress CMR imaging uniquely allows the measurement of subendocardial perfusion. In a report of 19 symptomatic women with abnormal stress tests and normal coronary angiograms, subendocardial ischemia frequently was observed. Further investigation into the prognostic implications of CMR subendocardial ischemia in women with regard to IHD events and its association with future angina burden is needed.

Coronary Computed Tomographic Angiography

Coronary computed tomographic angiography (CCTA) is a noninvasive anatomic technique with a reported high diagnostic accuracy for obstructive CAD. it is important to recognize that women with angina and confirmatory ischemia have an elevated IHD mortality. Abnormalities in functional capacity and noninvasive imaging are valuable IHD risk predictors in symptomatic women.

Coronary Angiography

Coronary angiography use as a diagnostic tool may be indicated if a patient's risk factors, medical history and clinical presentation are consistent with an intermediate-to-high IHD probability. For high-risk women, with either a high coronary disease probability or with unstable symptoms (e.g. increasing chest pain frequency in the proceeding 6 weeks of evaluation, rest angina, etc.), the decision to perform diagnostic angiography is supported by an abundance of evidence. However, angiography may not be an option for women who are not good candidates for revascularization, especially elderly women.

❏ MANAGEMENT OF IHD IN WOMEN

Acute Ischemic Syndromes: Differences in Presentation and Treatment in Women

Women with ACS often present for evaluation with symptom patterns that differ from their male counterparts and are more likely than men to report differences in chest pain quality and frequency. Women who are offered percutaneous coronary revascularization procedures as a therapeutic modality often have clinical characteristics that are associated with an increased risk of major adverse events. For this reason, women are also more likely to be considered suboptimal candidates for surgical revascularization.

Advances in surgical techniques and myocardial protection have increased the availability of surgical revascularization procedures for women with ACS found to have coronary anatomy that warrants surgical intervention. In spite of these advances, in-hospital mortality rates for women are often two to three times higher than for men.

Treatment Strategies for Women with Stable Coronary Artery Disease

While revascularization by PCI or CABG has been shown by many studies to be superior to medical management alone in outcomes in ACS and severely symptomatic patients with complex CAD, in chronic stable angina of mild or moderate severity and in patients with silent ischemia only, there is ongoing debate as to which treatment strategy should be offered to patients: optimized intense medical drug therapy combined with revascularization if medical therapy fails, or direct coronary angiography, both combined with strict risk factor control and secondary prevention.

Medical Therapy and Risk Factor Management for Stable CAD

Optimized medical therapy is the cornerstone of each treatment strategy in patients with chronic CAD, even in patients undergoing revascularization. It includes aggressive risk factor modification with diet, exercise training, treatment of diabetes, HTN and hyperlipidemia as well as smoking cessation and overweight reduction. Current medical therapy and risk factor modification strategies should conform to updated ACC/AHA treatment guidelines as summarized in Tables 1 and 2.

Table 1: Drugs used to treat patients with chronic stable CAD			
Medication	**Indicated in all patients**	**Symptomatically useful**	**Prognostically useful**
Antithrombotic drugs (e.g. aspirin)	Yes	No	Yes
Lipid lowering drugs (e.g. statins)	Yes	No	Yes
Beta-blocking agents	Yes	Yes	Yes (chronic stable CAD?)
Calcium channel blockers	No	Yes	No
Nitrates	No	Yes	No
ACE inhibitors	No	No	Yes (chronic stable CAD?)
Nicorandil	No	Yes	Yes
Ivabradine	No	Yes	No
Chronic stable CAD ® limitations see text			

Table 2: Goals for risk factor management in symptomatic women

Risk factor	Goal	
Smoking	Cessation	
Total dietary fat	<30% calories	
Saturated fat	<7% calories	
Dietary cholesterol	<200 mg/day	
LDL cholesterol (primary goal)	60–85 mg/dL (1.56–2.21 mmol/L)	
HDL cholesterol (secondary goal)	≥40 mg/dL (1.04 mmol/L)	
Triglycerides (TG) (secondary goal)	<150 mg/dL (1.69 mmol/L)	
Physical activity	30–45 minutes of moderate intensity activity 5 times/week supplemented by an increase in daily lifestyle activities	
Body weight by body mass index (BMI)	Initial BMI	Weight loss goal
Desirable <25	25–27.5	BMI <25
Overweight 25.0–29.9	27.5	10% relative weight loss
Obese >30.0	27.5	10% relative weight loss
Blood pressure	<130/85 mm Hg	
Diabetes	HbA1c <7.0%	

All patients with coronary disease and chest pain syndromes should receive antithrombotic therapy with aspirin.. The available evidence supports daily use of aspirin in the range of 75–100 mg for long-term prevention of vascular events. Clopidogrel 75 mg/day may serve as an alternative in the case of aspirin allergy or intolerance. In addition, it may be added to aspirin in patients after stent implantation or after MI. Lipid-lowering drugs and particularly statins improve survival in patients with acute as well as chronic CAD. Current guidelines recommend a goal LDL-C of less than 100 mg/dL in patients with stable CAD. A more stringent goal of less than 70 mg/dL is left to the discretion of treating clinicians. Beta-blockers have powerful anti-ischemic, antihypertensive, and antiarrhythmic properties. In patients with chronic CAD, their main indication is treatment of (exercise-induced) angina. They are the treatment of choice in patients with concomitant HTN or suffering from arrhythmias. Calcium antagonists have anti-ischemic, antihypertensive and in part antiarrhythmic effects similar to beta-blocking agents. They may be added to beta-blockers to enhance therapy with the exception that calcium antagonists with heart rate lowering properties (verapamil or diltiazem) may cause excess heart rate slowing or high-grade AV block in some patients when used in combination with beta blockers. Nitrates provide effective and rapid symptom relief during attacks of angina. However, nitrates have no prognostic benefits in patients with chronic CAD.

For patients with refractory angina symptoms despite optimal medical therapy and revascularization, other newer antiischemic drugs may provide additional symptomatic relief. Ranolazine is a drug with a novel mechanism of action that has been shown in several large trials to be an efficacious adjunctive agent in reducing symptoms of chronic stable angina.

Coronary Angiography and Revascularization for Stable CAD

Revascularization has been shown to reduce angina severity more effectively and more rapidly than medical therapy. PCI is recommended for a proximal coronary artery stenosis that jeopardizes a large myocardium area, which may result in severe inducible ischemia and also angina refractory to medical therapy. Drug-eluting stents and maturation of other catheter-based techniques have improved the procedural success rate and further reduced restenosis rate.

CABG surgery is considered the treatment of choice for patients with significant obstruction of the left-main coronary artery, as well as for those with triple-vessel CAD and LV systolic dysfunction. Women who undergo CABG generally have less symptomatic relief than men. Despite differences in near-term outcomes, female sex is not associated with late morbidity and mortality post CABG.

❏ HEART FAILURE IN WOMEN

Heart failure affects 5 million Americans, and nearly 50% of these are women. Compelling sex differences have been noted regarding the underlying etiology, prognosis, response to treatment and how the disease impacts the quality of life. Hypertension and valvular disease are more likely the culprits for heart failure in women. For both sexes, heart failure contributes to significant morbidity and mortality, but age-adjusted data reveal that women have a better survival. The reasons why survival is better for women remain unclear, but it may be due to differences in the underlying disease.

Medical management recommendations are the same for women and men, because prospective sex-specific clinical trials have not been performed. However, concerns exist that women might respond differently to therapy. Some of the available medications may not be as effective in women, while other therapies, for example beta blockers, aldosterone antagonists and pacemakers, may be very beneficial.

The advent of device therapy including implantable cardioverter-defibrillators (ICDs) and cardiac resynchronization therapy for heart failure further highlights the sex-specific response to novel heart failure management strategies. Implantation of ICDs has expanded to include primary prevention for sudden cardiac death following the publication of randomized clinical trials establishing their efficacy.

CRT has become a significant part of the management of patients with advanced CHF. Several large-scale studies demonstrated the significant improvement in multiple endpoints, including survival in patients with advanced CHF. Studies have shown that women have received significantly fewer CRT devices, despite the facts that more women have left bundle branch block at baseline and the prevalence of heart failure with preserved systolic function is only slightly higher in women. For advanced heart failure patients, Thoratec HeartMate II (Thoratec Corporation, Pleasanton, California) is a ventricular assist device that is recently approved.

❏ GENDER AND CARDIAC ARRHYTHMIAS

Reports have noted differences in the incidence of certain clinical arrhythmias according to the gender of those studied. Some of these differences are related to known variations in the frequency of underlying organic heart disease, such as CAD and associated ventricular arrhythmias. It is long recognized that women have a longer corrected QT interval compared with that of men, and the difference becomes more pronounced at lower heart rate. Indeed, the high incidence of torsade de pointes (TdP) in women has been described in connection with both congenital and acquired long QT syndromes. Female sex and advanced age are both among the risk factors for developing TdP in hospitalized patients.

Atrial fibrillation is the most common supraventricular tachycardia and the incidence increases dramatically with age; the development of AF is associated not only with increased morbidity rates but also with an approximate doubling of all-cause mortality. Men are at greater risk of AF than are women in all age groups. However, because there are almost twice as many women as men who are older than 75 years in the general population, the absolute number of women with AF in older age groups exceeds that of men. Significant sex-related differences in the origins of ventricular tachycardia and sudden cardiac death/arrest (SCD/SCA) were also noted in the Framingham study.

❏ CONCLUSION

In summary, there are clear sex-related differences in the incidence and prevalence of certain cardiac arrhythmias. The exact mechanisms responsible for these differences are as yet unknown. The scant evidence available suggests two general mechanisms: (i) sex steroid hormone effects on ion channels and (ii) modulation of autonomic tone. Better understanding of the basic mechanisms of these differences will facilitate the development of more effective sex-specific methods of diagnosis and treatment.

❏ SUGGESTED READINGS

Arant CB, Wessel TR, Ridker PM, et al. Multimarker approach predicts adverse cardiovascular events in women evaluated for suspected ischemia: results from the national heart, lung, and blood institute-sponsored women's ischemia syndrome evaluation. Clin Cardiol. 2009;32:244-50.

Fraker TD, Fihn SD, Gibbons RJ, et al. 2007 chronic angina focused update of the ACC/AHA 2002 guidelines for the management of patients with chronic stable angina: a report of the American College of Cardiology/American Heart Association Task Force on Practice Guidelines Writing Group to develop the focused update of the 2002 guidelines for the management of patients with chronic stable angina. J Am Coll Cardiol. 2007;50:2264-74.

Gibbons RJ, Abrams J, Chatterjee K, et al. ACC/AHA 2002 guideline update for the management of patients with chronic stable angina summary article: a report of the American College of Cardiology/ American Heart Association Task Force on practice guidelines (Committee on the Management of Patients With Chronic Stable Angina). J Am Coll Cardiol. 2003;41:159-68.

Gibbons RJ, Chatterjee K, Daley J, et al. ACC/AHA/ACP-ASIM guidelines for the management of patients with chronic stable angina: executive summary and recommendations. A Report of the American College of Cardiology/American Heart Association Task Force on Practice Guidelines (Committee on Management of Patients with Chronic Stable Angina). Circulation. 1999;99:2829-48.

Hunt SA, Abraham WT, Chin MH, et al. 2009 focused update incorporated into the ACC/AHA 2005 Guidelines for the Diagnosis and Management of Heart Failure in Adults: a report of the American College of Cardiology Foundation/American Heart Association Task Force on Practice Guidelines: developed in collaboration with the International Society for Heart and Lung Transplantation. Circulation. 2009;119:e391-479.

Mieres JH, Shaw LJ, Arai A, et al. Role of noninvasive testing in the clinical evaluation of women with suspected coronary artery disease: consensus statement from the Cardiac Imaging Committee, Council on Clinical Cardiology, and the Cardiovascular Imaging and Intervention Committee, Council on Cardiovascular Radiology and Intervention, American Heart Association. Circulation. 2005;111:682-96.

Mosca L, Grundy SM, Judelson D, et al. Guide to preventive cardiology for women. AHA/ACC scientific statement consensus panel statement. Circulation. 1999;99:2480-4.

Shaw LJ, Bairey Merz CN, Azziz R, et al. Postmenopausal women with a history of irregular menses and elevated androgen measurements at high risk for worsening cardiovascular event-free survival: results from the National Institutes of Health—National Heart, Lung, and Blood Institute sponsored Women's Ischemia Syndrome Evaluation. J Clin Endocrinol Metab. 2008;93:1276-84.

Shaw LJ, Bugiardini R, Merz CNB. Women and ischemic heart disease: evolving knowledge. J Am Coll Cardiol. 2009;54:1561-75.

11.3 Overview of the Athlete's Heart

❑ INTRODUCTION

The association between cardiac "abnormalities" and participation in athletic activity has been appreciated for more than a century. Initial descriptions of cardiac enlargement in healthy trained athletes, later characterized as global chamber dilation and myocardial hypertrophy, lead to the concept of the athlete's heart. Our understanding of how repetitive exercise affects heart structure and function has advanced considerably since the initial descriptions in the 1890s.

❑ EXERCISE PHYSIOLOGY AND THE ATHLETE'S HEART: OVERVIEW

Successful performance of physical exercise relies on coordinated activity of the lungs and pulmonary vasculature (oxygen uptake), the heart and systemic vasculature (oxygen transport) and the skeletal muscle (oxygen utilization and force generation). Only key aspects relevant to exercise-induced cardiac remodeling (EICR) will be reviewed here. There is a direct relationship between exercise intensity (external work) and the body's demand for oxygen. This oxygen demand is met by increasing pulmonary oxygen uptake (VO_2). The cardiovascular system is responsible for transporting oxygen rich blood from the lungs to the skeletal muscles, a process quantified as cardiac output (L/min). The Fick equation (Cardiac output = VO_2 × arterial-venous O_2 D) can be used to quantify the relationship between cardiac output and VO_2. In the healthy human, there is a direct and inviolate relationship between VO_2 and cardiac output. Cardiac output, the product of stroke volume and heart rate, may increase 5–6-fold during a maximal exercise effort.

Heart rate in the athlete may range from less than 40 beats per minute at rest to greater than 200 beats per minute in young maximally exercising athletes. Importantly, maximal heart rate does not increase with exercise training. In contrast, stroke volume both at rest and during exercise characteristically increases significantly with prolonged exercise training. Cardiac chamber enlargement and the accompanying ability to generate a large stroke volume is a direct result of EICR and is one of the cardiovascular hallmarks of the endurance-trained athlete.

Hemodynamic conditions, specifically changes in cardiac output and peripheral vascular resistance, vary widely across sporting disciplines. Although some overlap exists, exercise activity can be segregated into two forms with defining hemodynamic differences. (1) Isotonic exercise, also referred to as endurance exercise, involves sustained elevations in cardiac output with normal or reduced peripheral vascular resistance. Such activity represents primarily a volume challenge for the heart, which affects all four chambers. This form of exercise underlies activities including long distance running, cycling, rowing, and swimming. (2) Isometric exercise, in contrast, also referred to as strength training, involves activity characterized by increased peripheral vascular resistance and normal or only slightly elevated cardiac output. This increase in peripheral vascular resistance causes transient, but potentially marked systolic hypertension and LV afterload. Strength training is the dominant form of exercise in activities such as weightlifting, track and field throwing events.

❏ ISSUES RELEVANT TO THE CARDIOVASCULAR CARE OF ATHLETES

Overview of the Clinical Approach to the Trained Athlete

The trained athlete is typically regarded as the paradigm of excellent health and there are copious data showing that regular vigorous exercise reduces the incidence of atherosclerotic cardiovascular disease. Nevertheless, trained athletes are frequently referred to general practitioners, internists and cardiovascular disease specialists. Athletic patients may be directed to medical attention due to abnormal findings during pre-participation screening or they may seek medical attention due to symptoms related to their sport participation.

Certain aspects of the medical history may prove particularly valuable in the assessment of the athletic patient. First, a detailed athletic training and participation history must be elicited. This should include characterization of prior athletic achievements (useful for determining the competitive caliber of the athlete), current fitness level, recent training endeavors and future goals. An exercise training history is extremely important in evaluating an athlete. In the symptomatic athlete, it is imperative to determine if changes in training technique, volume or intensity correlate with the onset of symptoms. Second, a detailed family history is important as many conditions that predispose athletic patients to sport-related sudden death are heritable. Finally, athletes of all ages should be questioned about the use of illicit substances.

Etiology of Left Ventricular Hypertrophy

The phenotypic overlap between EICR and pathologic structural heart disease is widely appreciated. The extreme cases of exercise-induced LV hypertrophy and RV dilation may be difficult to differentiate from mild forms of hypertrophic cardiomyopathy and arrhythmogenic right ventricular cardiomyopathy respectively. The overlap between features of the athlete's heart and characteristics of common cardiomyopathic conditions that affect young athletes has been coined "Maron's gray zone".

At the present time, there is no single diagnostic test with adequate accuracy for differentiating adaptive remodeling from pathologic cardiomyopathy. Consequently, clinician's faced with this diagnostic dilemma are encouraged to begin the assessment with an integrated consideration of personal and family medical history, 12-lead electrocardiography and echocardiography. Advanced imaging techniques including tissue Doppler echocardiography, speckled tracking echocardiography, magnetic resonance imaging, cardiopulmonary exercise testing and disease specific genetic testing may be considered on th basis of history and findings. The presence of a previously identified genetic abnormality associated with structural cardiac disease can increase the conviction that a borderline cardiac abnormality in an athlete represents early disease and not exercise-induced adaptation.

Arrhythmia

Arrhythmia and conduction alterations are common in the trained athlete. Bradyarrhythmias including sinus bradycardia, junctional bradycardia, first-degree AV block and Mobitz type I AV block are commonly observed. Athletic patients with these bradyarrhythmias are almost always asymptomatic and profound bradycardia in the context of rest or sleep does not appear to portend a poor prognosis. It has been suggested that heightened parasympathetic tone, specifically increased efferent vagus nerve activity, is responsible for these bradyarrhythmias. More advanced forms of heart block including Mobitz type II second-degree and third-degree heart block. Premature beats (both atrial and ventricular) and nonsustained burst of ventricular tachycardia may be observed in trained athletes. Tachyarrhythmias, specifically atrial fibrillation may also particularly be problematic in the trained athlete.

Syncope

Syncope, defined as a transient loss of consciousness accompanied by loss of postural tone, is common in trained athletes. The vast majority of athletes have syncopal episodes that are attributable to neurocardiogenic mechanisms. Typically, neurocardiogenic syncope in the athlete occurs immediately after exercise and is due to transient cerebral hypoperfusion produced by residual peripheral arterial vasodilatation and a sudden reduction in venous return produced by the cessation of skeletal muscle contraction. The approach to the athletic patient with syncope begins with a detailed history, physical examination and 12-lead electrocardiogram. Exercise testing is frequently normal in individuals with coronary artery anomalies; however, so coronary imaging may be required in athletes with syncope and this clinical possibility. Ambulatory monitoring with a loop or an event recorder may prove useful in patients with symptoms that are not reproduced during a laboratory-based exercise assessment.

Steroids and Sport Performance Supplements

Advances in the science of human performance coupled with increasing societal and financial pressure for athletes to perform has led to increasing the use of PEAs. The most widely known forms of PEAs are androgenic anabolic steroids. Nonsteroidal muscle mass growth stimulators including injectable insulin, human growth hormone and creatine are also popular drugs of abuse in athletes. Finally, erythropoietic stimulants including human recombinant erythropoietin are reportedly widespread use among endurance athletes. Potential complications of erythropoietic stimulant use are related to increased red cell mass and including microvascular sludging and infarction.

Sudden Death and Preparticipation Disease Screening

Sudden death in young athletic individuals is a rare but tragic event. Studies examining sudden death in athletes report a wide range of prevalence. Most cases of sudden, sport-related death in young athletes are attributable to underlying cardiovascular pathology (Table 3). Both the American Heart Association and the American College of Cardiology (AHA/ACC) and European Society of Cardiology (ESC)99 have established sport eligibility criteria for individuals diagnosed with these conditions. Guidelines endorsed by these two groups are largely similar aside from a few notable situations including the management of athletes with asymptomatic Wolff-Parkinson-White syndrome and the approach to athletes with genotype positive/phenotype negative myocardial or electrical heart disease.

The tragic nature of sudden death in young, previously asymptomatic athletes has led to considerable efforts at prevention. The AHA/ACC and the ESC101,102 have published consensus committee-based recommendations for preparticipation athlete screening (Table 4).

Table 3: Common cardiovascular conditions associated with sudden death in athletes

Disorders of the myocardium:
- Hypertrophic cardiomyopathy
- Arrhythmogenic right ventricular cardiomyopathy
- Familiar/idiopathic dilated cardiomyopathy
- Acute and subacute myocarditis

Disorders of myocardial electrical activity and conduction:
- Congenital and acquired long QT syndrome
- Short QT syndrome
- Wolff–Parkinson–White syndrome
- Brugada syndrome
- Catecholaminergic polymorphic ventricular tachycardia
- Commotio cordis

Disorders of the coronary circulation:
- Congenital anomalies of coronary arterial origin and course
- Acquired atherosclerotic disease

Disorders of the heart valves:
- Bicuspid aortic valve disease associated with any of the following:
  - Significant aortic root dilation
  - Marfan syndrome
  - ≥ Moderate stenosis of regurgitation
- Mitral valve prolapse
- Pulmonic stenosis

Table 4: Criteria for abnormality during preparticipation medical history and physical examination screening*

Medical history

Personal history:
1. Exertional chest pain/discomfort
2. Unexplained syncope/near-syncope not clearly attributable to neurocardiogenic/vasovagal mechanism
3. Excessive and unexplained dyspnea/fatigue, associated with exercise
4. Prior recognition of a heart murmur
5. Elevated systemic blood pressure

Family history:
6. Premature death (sudden and unexpected) before age 50 years in >1 relative
7. Disability from heart disease in a close relative ≤ 50 years of age
8. Knowledge of hypertrophic or dilated cardiomyopathy, long-QT syndrome, Marfan syndrome or clinically important arrhythmias in any family member

Physical examination
9. Heart murmur
10. Diminished or asymmetric femoral pulses (to exclude aortic coarctation)
11. Physical stigmata of Marfan syndrome
12. Asymmetric or elevated (>140/90 mm Hg) brachial artery blood pressure

*Criteria adopted from current recommendations from the American Heart Association regarding preparticipation screening of competitive athletes. Circulation. 2007;115:1643-55

CONCLUSION

Our understanding of the athlete's heart has progressed considerably. Today, the findings of global chamber enlargement coupled to normal or enhanced cardiac function are well-established markers of the athlete's heart. As participation in organized sport and individualized vigorous physical exercise continue to grow, the practicing clinician will likely see an increase in the number of patients with possible exercise-induced cardiac adaptations. A basic understanding of the athlete's heart and a familiarity with clinical issues common in athletic patients are essential for effective management of this specific patient population.

SUGGESTED READINGS

Corrado D, Pelliccia A, Bjornstad HH, et al. Cardiovascular preparticipation screening of young competitive athletes for prevention of sudden death: proposal for a common European protocol. Consensus statement of the Study Group of Sport Cardiology of the Working Group of Cardiac Rehabilitation and Exercise Physiology and the Working Group of Myocardial and Pericardial Diseases of the European Society of Cardiology. Eur Heart J. 2005;26:516-24.

Darling EA. The effects of training: a study of the Harvard University crews. Boston Med Surg J. 1899;161:229-33.

Maron BJ, Thompson PD, Ackerman MJ, et al. Recommendations and considerations related to preparticipation screening for cardiovascular abnormalities in competitive athletes: 2007 update: a scientific statement from the American Heart Association Council on Nutrition, Physical Activity, and Metabolism: endorsed by the American College of Cardiology Foundation. Circulation. 2007;115(12):1643-55.

Pelliccia A, Fagard R, Bjornstad HH, et al. Recommendations for competitive sports participation in athletes with cardiovascular disease: a consensus document from the Study Group of Sports Cardiology of the Working Group of Cardiac Rehabilitation and Exercise Physiology and the Working Group of Myocardial and Pericardial Diseases of the European Society of Cardiology. Eur Heart J. 2005;26:1422-45.

Perseghin G, De Cobelli F, Esposito A, et al. Effect of the sporting discipline on the right and left ventricular morphology and function of elite male track runners: a magnetic resonance imaging and phosphorus 31 spectroscopy study. Am Heart J. 2007;154:937-42.

Reindell H, Roskamm H, Steim H. The heart and blood circulation in athletes. Med Welt. 1960;31:1557-63.

Roskamm H, Reindell H, Musshoff K, et al. Relations between heart size and physical efficiency in male and female athletes in comparison with normal male and female subjects. Arch Kreislaufforsch. 1961;35:67-102.

11.4 Cardiovascular Aging

INTRODUCTION

The world population has been aging over the past century, a trend which is expected to continue into the foreseeable future, especially among the oldest-old. Although definitions vary, the term "older adults" in the developed world generally refers to people older than 65 years of age, and within this group the population can be subdivided into the young old (65–74 years), old old (75–84 years), and oldest old (>85 years).

While the burden of CVD in older adults is substantial, an increasing number of interventions have significantly decreased the morbidity and the mortality associated with certain conditions. Procedure-related mortality in older adults appears to be declining as well, with a reduction in mortality attributed to urgent or elective PCI seen in patients older than 80 years since the year 2001. Older adult patients, especially the oldest old, pose many diagnostic as well as therapeutic challenges. Symptoms, such as fatigue and dyspnea, which may be attributable to a single organ system in younger individuals, are more likely to be multifactorial with advancing age. The majority of patients older than or equal to 65 years have two or more chronic medical conditions, and nearly one-third older than or equal to 85 years have four or more chronic conditions. This increasing number of comorbidities makes the application of standard evidence-based therapies that have been proven in younger patients difficult, and balancing the potential cardiovascular benefits against competing risks challenging.

❏ AGE-RELATED CHANGES

Aging results in numerous changes in the cardiovascular system that is caused by various cellular mechanisms resulting in an altered phenotype in properties of the heart and vasculature.

Cellular Aging

The cellular mechanisms underlying cardiovascular aging are numerous and complex. A comprehensive review is beyond the scope of this section.

Telomeres undergo attrition with each division of somatic cells in culture and are hypothesized to contribute to cellular aging by inducing genomic instability, replicative senescence and apoptosis. Several alterations in telomere length have been delineated in the cardiovascular system with aging. In the vascular smooth muscle cells of the distal abdominal aorta, telomere length demonstrates a strong inverse correlation with age, and in patients with severe coronary artery disease the lengths of telomeres are significantly shorter than those of controls. Protein misfolding has been implicated in aging-related diseases as diverse as Alzheimer's disease, type 2 diabetes, in the cardiovascular system and systemic amyloidosis. Inflammation plays a central role in the cellular pathogenesis of atherosclerosis, and advancing age has been described as a "proinflammatory" state. The concentration of inflammatory cytokines increases with age and likely represents a combination of chronic antigenic stress and immune dysregulation, combined with lifestyle factors and comorbid disease.

Vascular Changes

Endothelial cells, which line the luminal surface of the vasculature, regulate diverse functions including angiogenesis and maintenance of vessel tone, undergo a number of changes with aging. Endothelium-dependent vasodilation is impaired in older adults both with and without hypertension. The number of circulating endothelial progenitor cells (EPCs) in patients with coronary artery disease decreases with advancing age, and EPC mobilization after coronary artery bypass grafting (CABG) is impaired in older patients compared to their younger counterparts.

Average systolic blood pressure rises steadily with increasing age in both men and women. However, diastolic blood pressure tends to rise until about age 50 and declines in older adults. This trend is thought to be predominantly due to increased large artery stiffness with aging, a phenomenon which is present in persons with or without clinical CVD.

Myocardial Changes

Several studies have described an increase in left ventricular (LV) mass with aging independent of clinical disease. The rate of early LV diastolic filling progressively decreases after age of 20, even in individuals without clinical CVD. In contrast, LV systolic function as measured by ejection fraction (EF) is usually preserved at rest in healthy older adults, although the ability to augment EF with vigorous exercise is reduced.

Electrophysiologic Changes

The maximum heart rate (MHR) during exhaustive exercise decreases with advancing age, with an accelerated rate of decline in the oldest old. As the MHR decreases, an increasing reliance on stroke volume is necessary to maintain the adequate cardiac output during physical exertion. In addition to MHR, heart rate (HR) variability, or the beat-to-beat fluctuation of HR, declines steadily with age and may be associated with an age-related reduction in parasympathetic function with a concomitant increase in sympathetic activity.

Exercise-related Changes

The maximum oxygen consumption rate (peak VO_2), a measure of aerobic fitness, declines in older adults. The rate of decline, rather than being linear, appears to accelerate with advancing age. Variables influencing peak VO_2 include muscle mass, cardiac output, hemoglobin level, pulmonary reserve and vascular distribution. In normal aging, muscle loss (sarcopenia) accounts for the greatest percentage decline in peak VO_2, since most O_2 consumption during maximal aerobic activity occurs in exercising muscle.

Attenuating Age-related Changes

The interrelation of the various cellular and structural changes in older adults with lifestyle is illustrated in two interventions which may reduce accelerated cardiovascular aging: exercise and caloric restriction. Habitual aerobic exercise is associated with a decreased risk of CVD in older adults, which may be mediated by reductions in large-artery stiffness and improvements in vascular endothelial function. Caloric restriction has long been established as a method of prolonging the lifespan of experimental animals ranging from invertebrates to nonhuman primates, when started in early or middle age. There is emerging evidence that caloric restriction may have similar effects in humans, including an improved cardiovascular risk profile, although studies are small and data remain observational. The cellular mechanisms underlying extended longevity with caloric restriction are still being elucidated, but are likely to include reduction in free radical production and oxidative stress, increased autophagy and modulation of growth factor signaling.

❏ CLINICAL SYNDROMES

Clinical syndromes that disproportionately affect patients older than or equal to 65 years, and particularly patients older than or equal to 80 years of age include HF (especially with a normal or preserved EF), SCA, isolated systolic hypertension, ischemic heart disease (IHD), AF and valve disease [particularly senile calcific aortic stenosis (AS)]. As this segment of the population grows, these disorders will become increasingly prevalent and clinicians will be continued to be challenged by their management.

Heart Failure

Over 80% of patients with HF are aged 65 years or older, and HF represents the most common reason for hospitalization among medicare beneficiaries. Among older adults, the prevalence of HF continues to increase with advancing age. Heart failure with preserved ejection fraction (HFPEF) represents a particular challenge in older adults, both in diagnosis and therapy. The disorder is heterogeneous with a diverse set of related underlying clinical comorbidities that can mimic symptoms of HF and cause or contribute to the pathogenesis of this syndrome.

Therapy

For SCA, treatments have typically been limited to symptomatic management of HF and pacemaker therapy when indicated, although new therapies are emerging which are targeted at preventing the protein misfolding and aggregation that occur when normal TTR tetramers dissociate into monomers. For example, two nonsteroidal anti-inflammatory drugs (NSAIDs), diflunisal and flufenamic acid, have been found to stabilize TTR tetramers in vitro via binding to the T4 binding sites.

For the broader population with hypertensive HFPEF, all major trials of therapy to date have demonstrated no significant reduction in mortality. Interpretation of studies in patients with HFPEF is limited due to heterogeneous enrollment criteria (with differing cutoffs for a "normal" EF) and varied clinical endpoints. Generally, there is no universally accepted therapy for HFPEF, and management strategies remain limited to symptom control as well as modification of coexisting cardiac risk factors such as hypertension.

Vascular Disease—Isolated Systolic Hypertension

Hypertension increases in prevalence with advancing age, and affects over 50% of individuals aged 65–74 and 60% of individuals aged 75 and older. Isolated systolic hypertension is overwhelmingly the most common form of hypertension seen in the oldest-old.

Management

The benefit of treating isolated systolic hypertension in older adults has been well-established by several large trials (Table 5).

Trial	NR	Age range (years)	Relative risk reduction (%)		
			Heart failure	Stroke	MI
SHEP	4,736	≥60	55%*	36%*	33%*
STOP-Hypertension	1,627	70–84	51%*	47%*	13%
STONE	1,632	60–79	68%	57%*	6%
Syst-Eur	4,695	≥60	36%	42%*	30%
HYVET	3,645	≥80	64%*	30%†	28%

Table 5: Effect of antihypertensive therapy on cardiovascular events in older adults

*Achieved statistical significance, p <0.05 NR = Not reported, †Reduction in fatal stroke (39%) statistically significant, p = 0.046

Ischemic Heart Disease

Ischemic heart disease (IHD) is the leading cause of death in older adults, and the prevalence and complications of IHD continue to increase with advancing age. Older adults with MI are more likely to present with atypical symptoms (including nausea, vomiting, syncope and confusion) or to be asymptomaic. In addition, MI is more likely to occur in the setting of acute illness, such as pneumonia, exacerbation of chronic obstructive pulmonary disease, or a fall.

Management

A significant body of research demonstrated that older adults with ACSs were less likely to receive evidence-based treatments, including antiplatelet therapy, beta-blockers and invasive evaluation, despite their greater potential to benefit. However, this paradigm appears to have shifted in recent years and older adults are now receiving more standard medical treatments as well as invasive procedures for ACS. Several issues remain important to address in the management of older adults with ACS. This population has altered pharmacokinetics and is vulnerable to medications with the potential to cause hypotension (beta-blockers, nitrates) as well as bleeding (aspirin, thienopyridines, heparin).

Anticoagulant therapy carries a higher bleeding risk in older patients, especially the oldest old. Observational data have shown an increased risk of bleeding from aspirin and thienopyridine therapy in older adults as well, including gastrointestinal, genitourinary and intracerebral hemorrhage requiring hospitalization. The risk of dual antiplatelet therapy (aspirin plus thienopyridine), which may be indicated in the setting of ACS, stent placement, or a neurologic event such as stroke, appears to be additive; in several observational and randomized studies, bleeding complications with this strategy were as high as twice that with aspirin alone.

Conduction Disease

Cardiac rhythm disturbances are common in older adults and result in substantial morbidity and mortality. One of the most prevalent and important standpoint from a public health is AF. Atrial fibrillation (AF) is a common condition in older adults and increases in prevalence with advancing age. Data from the original Framingham cohort estimated that AF increased the risk of stroke in all participants approximately fivefold, and over onethird of strokes in patients older than or equal to 80 years were associated with AF (which was significantly higher compared to younger subjects).

Management

Anticoagulant therapy with warfarin has been demonstrated to reduce the risk of stroke by approximately two-thirds in several well-designed randomized trials, and this treatment remains a mainstay of stroke prevention in at-risk patients. It has been estimated that the oldest-old stands to benefit the most from anticoagulant therapy, although there is evidence that they are prescribed anticoagulant therapy less often than their younger counterparts for both primary prevention and after admission for ischemic stroke.

Observational studies have found an increased incidence of major bleeding in older adults treated with anticoagulant therapy, although this has not been demonstrated reliably in randomized trials. Bleeding risk appears highest in the oldest old. The decision to proceed with anticoagulation therapy in very advanced ages (>85 years of age), still remains very much an individualized one, based on clinicians' assessment of risk and potential benefit.

Valvular Disease

Arguably, the most relevant valvular disease in older adults is calcific AS, which occurs infrequently in younger patients except in the setting of a bicuspid aortic valve. Aortic stenosis is characterized by restricted excursion of the aortic valve leaflets, leading to LV outflow obstruction and a compensatory increase in LV systolic pressure.

Management

Once AS becomes symptomatic, the only definitive therapy is replacement of the aortic valve. Medical therapy has not been shown to slow disease progression; notably, trials of statin therapy, with the goal of inhibiting the inflammatory process in the valve leaflets, have been negative to date. Balloon valvulotomy, in which one or more balloons have been inserted percutaneously and inflated across a stenotic aortic valve, has not been shown to have any effect on long-term survival despite an immediate post-procedural reduction in the transvalvular gradient. A role may remain as a bridge to surgery in hemodynamically unstable patients, as well as for palliation in severely symptomatic patients who are not operative candidates.

Given the above findings, for nearly all symptomatic patients who are operative candidates, referral for aortic valve replacement (AVR) should be considered.

❏ SPECIAL ISSUES

Prevention

Numerous primary and secondary prevention trials have shown benefits to treating hypertension and hyperlipidemia to delay the onset, or slow progression, of CVD. Treatment with antihypertensive therapy has been associated with an approximately 25% reduction in cardiovascular events (MI, HF, stroke) in a pooled analysis of randomized trials in patients of all ages. However, most hypertension trials, while incorporating older adults, did not enrol substantial numbers of the oldest old (>80 years).

Treatment for hyperlipidemia, particularly statin therapy, has been studied extensively, and in a meta-analysis of over 30,000 patients was found to reduce the rate of major coronary events by 31% and all-cause mortality by 21%. Data on statin therapy for secondary prevention in older adults have generally shown benefit.

End-of-life Care

The majority of serious and chronic illnesses in developed countries occur in older adults, especially the oldest old, and many are accompanied by a long period of functional decline, disability, and loss of independence. While the field of cardiology has enabled older adults with CVD to live longer with an improved quality of life, conditions may progress to the point of being terminal. The final common pathway for pathologies, such as coronary artery disease, AS, hypertension and AF, is often HF, and most of the research to date has been with this condition. Current guidelines recommend end-of-life care (hospice) to be considered in HF patients who, despite maximal therapy, have one of the following:
- Frequent hospitalizations (three or more per year),
- Chronic poor quality of life and inability to perform activities of daily living (ADLs),
- Need for intravenous support inotropic therapy or
- Consideration for destination therapy (ventricular assist device).

The principal goal of palliation for patients with HF is relief of symptoms including pain, fatigue and dyspnea. Standard HF therapies are continued when possible, and diuretics may be titrated to maintain fluid balance. Opioids may be utilized as well, and may relieve dyspnea as well as pain. Psychological and spiritual needs should be screened for and addressed. For terminal HF patients with ICDs, the option of deactivation should be discussed. Multiple ICD shocks near the end of life can be painful, anxiety-provoking, and may not prolong life at a reasonable quality.

CONCLUSION

Cardiovascular disease can be considered a disease of older adults, and changing demographics make it imperative to further understand the aging-related mechanisms underlying various pathologic conditions. Many treatments to date have reduced morbidity and mortality in older patients with heart disease, but the field will continue to be challenged by increasing numbers of patients with very advanced age and multiple medical comorbidities. A multidisciplinary approach in this setting, incorporating the disciplines of cardiology, primary care, geriatrics and palliative care, may be necessary to optimize patients' health outcomes and quality of life.

SUGGESTED READINGS

2006 WRITING COMMITTEE MEMBERS, Bonow RO, Carabello BA, et al. 2008 focused update incorporated into the ACC/AHA 2006 guidelines for the management of patients with valvular heart disease: a report of the American College of Cardiology/American Heart Association task force on practice guidelines (writing committee to revise the 1998 guidelines for the management of patients with valvular heart disease): endorsed by the society of cardiovascular anesthesiologists, society for cardiovascular angiography and interventions, and society of thoracic surgeons. Circulation. 2008;118:e523-661.

Ahmed A, Allman RM, Aronow WS, et al. Diagnosis of heart failure in older adults: predictive value of dyspnea at rest. Arch Gerontol Geriatr. 2004;38:297-307.

Alexander KP, Newby LK, Cannon CP, et al. Acute coronary care in the elderly, part I: non-ST-segment-elevation acute coronary syndromes: a scientific statement for healthcare professionals from the American Heart Association Council on Clinical Cardiology: in collaboration with the society of geriatric cardiology. Circulation. 2007;115:2549-69.

Atrial Fibrillation Investigators: Atrial Fibrillation, Aspirin, Anticoagulation Study, Boston Area Anticoagulation Trial for Atrial Fibrillation Study, Canadian Atrial Fibrillation Anticoagulation Study, Stroke Prevention in Atrial Fibrillation Study, Veterans Affairs Stroke Prevention in Nonrheumatic Atrial Fibrillation Study. Risk factors for stroke and efficacy of antithrombotic therapy in atrial fibrillation: analysis of pooled data from five randomized controlled trials. Arch Intern Med. 1994;154:1449-57.

Fuster V, Ryden LE, Cannom DS, et al. ACC/AHA/ESC 2006 guidelines for the management of patients with atrial fibrillation: a report of the American College of Cardiology/American Heart Association task force on practice guidelines and the European Society of Cardiology Committee for practice guidelines (writing committee to revise the 2001 guidelines for the management of patients with atrial fibrillation): developed in collaboration with the European heart rhythm association and the heart rhythm society. Circulation. 2006;114:e257-354.

Paulus WJ, Tschöpe C, Sanderson JE, et al. How to diagnose diastolic heart failure: a consensus statement on the diagnosis of heart failure with normal left ventricular ejection fraction by the heart failure and echocardiography associations of the European Society of Cardiology. Eur Heart J. 2007;28:2539-50.

Taddei S, Virdis A, Mattei P, et al. Hypertension causes premature aging of endothelial function in humans. Hypertension. 1997;29:736-43.

WRITING GROUP MEMBERS, Lloyd-Jones D, Adams RJ, et al. Heart disease and stroke statistics—2010 update: a report from the American Heart Association. Circulation. 2010;121:e46-215.

Chapter 12

Preventive Strategies for Other Cardiovascular Diseases

12.1 Prevention of Heart Failure

❑ INTRODUCTION

Heart failure is a clinical syndrome due to heterogeneous systemic and cardiac insults resulting in hemodynamic disturbances, neurohormonal dysregulation, leading to subsequent decreased cardiac function and multiorgan dysfunction. Like detecting cancers only at their metastatic stages, the majority of "heart failure" cases present at the late stages of cardiac disease as a result of longstanding hypertension, coronary heart disease, valve disease, diabetes mellitus or primary cardiomyopathies. The prevention of heart failure encompasses primary prevention of cardiovascular disease with risk factor reduction, early recognition of at-risk patients with better understanding of how to protect them from developing heart failure, as well as the detection and management of asymptomatic structural heart diseases.

❑ STAGING OF HEART FAILURE

Over the past decade, the American College of Cardiology (ACC) and the American Heart Association (AHA) have promoted a staging concept of heart failure by identifying four stages with the main objective to emphasize the disease as a continuum in both the development and progression of the disease (Table 1). The "at-risk" stages describe patients who have a structural normal heart and are at high risk due to comorbidities and cardiotoxic exposures that predispose the development of heart failure (stage A), or who have structural abnormalities such as left ventricular hypertrophy or impaired left ventricular function (stage B). The latter two stages describe patients with current or past symptoms of heart failure (stage C) or patients with refractory heart failure symptoms requiring advanced "salvage" therapies or end-of-life care.

Stage A Heart Failure

Screening for and early detection of any disease is quite problematic in that one must define the population most at risk. Established and hypothesized risk factors of heart failure are included in Table 2.

To date, there is limited data to suggest that age, race and gender should influence treatment or preventive strategies in heart failure. While routine comprehensive genetic screening is still controversial, a detailed family history is recommended as part of clinical evaluation for those at risk of developing heart failure.

Elevated systolic (>140 mm Hg), diastolic (>80 mm Hg) and pulse pressure (>60 mm Hg) have been associated with increased risk of heart failure. There is also abundant data to suggest that therapeutic lifestyle changes can prevent the development of hypertension, including aerobic exercise and diet modification.

Table 1: Stages of heart failure

Classification of heart failure by stages

Stage	Description	NYHA class
A	Patients at high risk for developing heart failure • Hypertension, atherosclerotic disease, diabetes, obesity, metabolic syndrome, smoking • Exposure to cardiotoxins • Family history of cardiomyopathy	Not applicable

B	Development of structural heart disease without symptoms
	• Previous myocardial infarction
	• Left ventricular remodeling
	  ▪ Left ventricular hypertrophy
	  ▪ Impaired left ventricular function
	• Asymptomatic valvular disease
		I

C	Symptomatic heart failure • Known structural heart disease with symptoms of heart failure	II–III
D	Refractory end-stage heart failure • Severe symptoms despite maximal medical therapy	IV

Table 2: Established and hypothesized risk factors of heart failure

Major nonmodifiable risk factors	Minor clinical risk factors
• Age, race, sex • Family history	• Smoking • Dyslipidema • Sleep disorders
Major clinical risk factors • Hypertension, left ventricular • hypertrophy • Coronary artery disease, • myocardial infarction • Diabetes mellitus	• Chronic kidney disease • Albuminuria • Homocysteine • Immune activation • Natriuretic peptides • Anemia • Dietary risk factors • Increased heart rate • Sedentary lifestyle • Low socioeconomic status • Psychological stress
Toxin risk precipitants • Chemotherapy • Cocaine • NSAIDs • Thiazolidinediones • Doxazosin • Alcohol	*Genetic/molecular risk predictors* • SNP (a2cDel322-325, b1Arg389) • Cytoskeleton proteins • Sarcomeric proteins • Intermediate filaments *Morphological risk predictors* • Increased left ventricular internal dimension, mass • Asymptomatic left ventricular dysfunction • Left ventricular diastolic dysfunction

Low-dose diuretics are likely the most effective first-line treatment in preventing heart failure, although by default they are also reducing the opportunity of congestion due to their mechanisms of action. However, the paradigm still remains that agents should be chosen based on the patients concomitant comorbidities such as the use of angiotensin converting enzyme (ACE) inhibitors or angiotensin II receptor blockers (ARBs) for patients with diabetes, coronary artery disease or left ventricular dysfunction.

Weight loss, proper diet and increased physical activity have been associated with cardiovascular risk factors such as hypertension, hyperlipidemia, and diabetes type II. The preventative heart failure strategy in patients with diabetes is optimal blood pressure with ACE inhibition or beta blockade as well as optimal management of blood glucose levels. Moreover, aggressive treatment with lipid-lowering medications for hyperlipidemia or dyslipidemia is a reasonable strategy in the prevention of heart failure. Accounting for up to 70% of systolic heart failure, coronary artery disease is a major risk factor for the development of heart failure and a key target for heart failure prevention. In patients with coronary artery disease, many treatments, such as ACE inhibitors, beta blockers, antiplatelet agents, and statins, have been proven to be cardioprotective and prevent the progression to symptomatic heart failure.

Tobacco abusers have a 47% higher risk of incident heart failure compared to prior and nonsmokers. Patients who are current tobacco abusers should be referred for cessation programs and offered pharmacological therapies to best their chances of cessation. An unfortunate and frequent complication of many chemotherapeutic agents is cardiotoxicity. Anthracyclines, alkylating agents, antimetabolites, antimicrotubule agents, tyrosine kinase inhibitors, and proteasome inhibitors have been associated with left ventricular dysfunction, ischemia, hypertension and heart failure. Currently, there are no guidelines for long-term monitoring. Cardiac imaging is the gold standard for detection of chemotherapy-induced cardiotoxicity.

Treatment for Stage A Heart Failure

Current emphasis on the treatment of stage A heart failure remains to be aggressive risk factor modification for those at risk, and avoidance of cardiotoxic exposures. Much work is needed to better identify those at risk of disease progression to more advanced stages of heart failure, which may including genetic and proteomic evaluation as well as electrocardiography and advanced imaging techniques for at risk individuals so that appropriate patient identification for treatment is feasible.

Stage B Heart Failure

"Stage B heart failure" is defined as the presence of structural heart disease without overt clinical presentation of signs and symptoms. Patients may have significant scar territory following a prior or silent myocardial infarction, progressive but preclinical valvular dysfunction, or asymptomatic left ventricular systolic dysfunction. An ill-defined combination of genetic, inflammation and autoimmune responses, and/or pathogen exposure can trigger progressive adaptive and subsequent maladaptive responses leading to development of symptoms (Flowchart 1).

Asymptomatic Left Ventricular Systolic Dysfunction

In asymptomatic patients, the left ventricle enlarges to compensate for impaired contractility in maintaining an adequate stroke volume. Hence, significant cardiac

FLOWCHART 1: Pathophysiology of disease progression of at-risk patients (Stage A) from asymptomatic (Stage B) to symptomatic (Stages C and D) heart failure

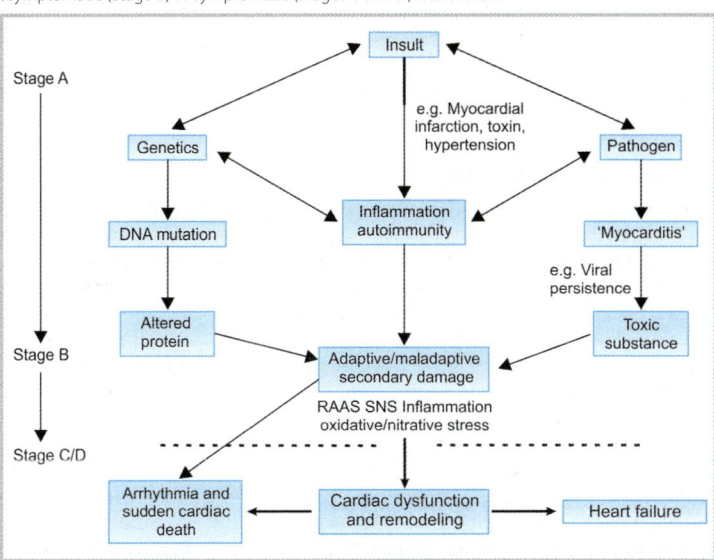

Table 3: Heart Failure Society of America, Guideline recommendations for management of Stage B heart failure with left ventricular systolic dysfunction		
	Recommendation	**Strength of evidence**
5.1	Regular exercise, optimize weight, blood pressure, diabetes control	C
5.2	Smoking cessation	B
5.3	Alcohol abstinence	C
5.4	Optimal blood pressure control	B
5.5	ACE inhibitors for LV systolic dysfunction (LVEF ≤40%)	A
5.6	Angiotensin receptor blockers for ACE inhibitor-intolerant patients (not combined)	C
5.7	Beta-blockers in post-MI	B
	Beta-blockers in non-post-MI	C

pathology ensues, and a negative impact of left ventricular systolic dysfunction even in the absence of overt symptoms has been demonstrated in several large-scale studies. Current guidelines recommended the use of ACE inhibition and to a lower level of evidence antiadrenergic therapy to impede maladaptive left ventricular remodeling and, in hopes, to improve mortality and morbidity (Table 3). Many screening modalities for asymptomatic left ventricular systolic dysfunction have been evaluated in the literature: clinical scores, electrocardiograms, biochemical markers and imaging markers. However, several problems have been encountered: the poor specificity in an asymptomatic population, selecting the correct population and developing cost-effective screening strategies.

Electrocardiogram and Biomarker Evaluation

Plasma B-type natriuretic peptide (BNP) and amino-terminal pro-B-type natriuretic peptide (NT-proBNP) have demonstrated diagnostic usefulness in only certain clinical settings. However, it lacks the specificity and positive predictive value in asymptomatic patients. Electrocardiogram has a high sensitivity but a relatively poor specificity for detecting left ventricular systolic dysfunction.

Cardiac Imaging for Screening

Echocardiography is highly specific in detecting and characterizing structural abnormalities such as left ventricular systolic dysfunction. Screening high-risk patients with limited echocardiography has been demonstrated to be feasible and have substantial yield. Hand-carried cardiac ultrasound offers a promising alternative to the traditional echocardiogram, as it is portable and, perhaps, more cost effective if utilized in a similar manner as a stethoscope. Portable echocardiography has been demonstrated to increase diagnostic accuracy with coupled with a physical examination and has recently gained attention as a possible screening tool in the community. The sensitivity and specificity from these studies approach 90% with experienced operators.

Treatment for Stage B Heart Failure

In the only large, prospective, randomized control trial specifically focused on patients with asymptomatic left ventricular systolic dysfunction, the SOLVD-Prevention study, the use of enalapril was associated with significantly reduced the incidence of heart failure and the rate of heart failure related hospitalizations by 20% when compared to placebo. There was also a trend towards decreased mortality due to cardiovascular related deaths in the enalapril arm compared to placebo. Long-term follow-up data at 12 years in the X-SOLVD study clearly demonstrated mortality benefits with enalapril. Data with beta-blockers are less convincing.

Preventative strategies with the use of statins to retard the progression of coronary artery disease in postinfarction patients have shown significant reduction in incident heart failure cases, most likely due to the prevention of subsequent myocardial infarctions. Adequate blood pressure control remains an important treatment goal to prevent disease progression, since hypertension remains one of the most common causes of heart failure and coronary artery disease. Lowering blood pressure over a 3–5 years period was effective in preventing left ventricular hypertrophy and heart failure regardless of the type of antihypertensive agent. ACE inhibitors and ARBs are the preferred antihypertensive agents for patients with increased left ventricular mass.

❑ FUTURE PERSPECTIVES

Early detection, aggressive treatment and risk factor modification remain the key to advances in the prevention of heart failure. The science in understanding what triggers early development and progression of heart failure and cardiomyopathy in humans continued to evolve. With advances in technologies, handheld imaging modalities, multiple biomarker and genetic profiles, and refined clinical predictors may someday provide the necessary screening and intervention strategies.

❑ SUGGESTED READINGS

Atherton JJ. Screening for left ventricular systolic dysfunction: is imaging a solution? JACC Cardiovasc Imaging. 2009;3:421-8.

Greenberg B, Quinones MA, Koilpillai C, et al. Effects of long-term enalapril therapy on cardiac structure and function in patients with left ventricular dysfunction. Results of the SOLVD echocardiography substudy. Circulation. 1995;91:2573-81.

Hunt SA, Abraham WT, Chin MH, et al. 2009 focused update incorporated into the ACC/AHA 2005 Guidelines for the Diagnosis and Management of Heart Failure in Adults: a report of the American College of Cardiology Foundation/American Heart Association Task Force on Practice Guidelines: developed in collaboration with the International Society for Heart and Lung Transplantation. Circulation. 2009;119:e391-479.

Schocken DD, Benjamin EJ, Fonarow GC, et al. Prevention of heart failure: a scientific statement from the American Heart Association Councils on Epidemiology and Prevention, Clinical Cardiology, Cardiovascular Nursing, and High Blood Pressure Research; Quality of Care and Outcomes Research Interdisciplinary Working Group; and Functional Genomics and Translational Biology Interdisciplinary Working Group. Circulation. 2008;117:2544-65.

The SOLVD Investigators. Effect of enalapril on mortality and the development of heart failure in asymptomatic patients with reduced left ventricular ejection fractions. The SOLVD Investigattors. N Engl J Med. 1992;327:685-91.

Yeh ET, Bickford CL. Cardiovascular complications of cancer therapy: incidence, pathogenesis, diagnosis, and management. J Am Coll Cardiol. 2009;53:2231-47.

12.2 Stroke: Prevention and Treatment

❑ INTRODUCTION

Stroke also is a leading cause of long-term disability and institutionalized care; in many ways stroke is more feared for its potential to lead to dependency than it is for its likelihood to lead to premature mortality. Besides being a leading cause of human suffering, it also has huge economic consequences. The healthcare costs for prevention, acute care and rehabilitation are considerable but even more so are the direct or indirect costs of lost productivity. Thus, the issues related to the prevention and treatment of stroke likely will increase in importance during the 21st century.

❑ DEFINITIONS

The term stroke encompasses a broad spectrum of vascular diseases that affect the central nervous system. Approximately 80% of strokes involve ischemia and the remainder represent bleeding within or adjacent to the brain or spinal cord. Traumatic hemorrhages are not included in the category of hemorrhagic stroke. Vascular events of the spinal cord, while not rare, constitute a small minority of strokes.

Ischemic stroke usually is due to thromboembolism including, *de novo* thrombosis of an artery perfusing the brain (cerebral thrombosis) or a clot that has arisen elsewhere and that has migrated to the brain (embolism). Hemorrhages usually are due to arterial rupture with the primary anatomic site of the bleeding used to describe the pattern of the event: subarachnoid hemorrhage (SAH)—bleeding primarily in the subarachnoid space, intraventricular hemorrhage (IVH)—bleeding in the ventricles, and intracerebral hemorrhage (ICH)—bleeding within the parenchyma of the brain.

Table 4: ABCD₂ score: prediction of TIA and risk of stroke	
Factors	
Age:	
≥ 60	1 point
Blood pressure:	
Systolic >140 mm Hg or diastolic >90 mm Hg	1 point
Clinical features:	
Unilateral weakness	2 points
Speech disturbance without weakness	1 point
Duration of symptoms:	
<10 minutes	0 point
10–59 minutes	1 point
≥60 minutes	2 points
Diabetes mellitus:	
Present	1 point
(Risk of stroke strongly increased if the score is greater than 3 points)	

The time course is also used to describe the type of vascular event. A transient ischemic attack (TIA) in effect is not a risk factor for stroke but rather a relatively mild form of the disease; the patient has had a stroke that spontaneously and completely resolved. While the past definition of TIA included the clearance of symptoms within 24 hours, that time period is excessively long. In general, these events last under 10–20 minutes. Often, brain imaging, in particular magnetic resonance imaging (MRI), will demonstrate an ischemic lesion in the brain in a patient with a TIA, especially if the symptoms have persisted longer than 1 hour. Now a TIA is defined as an event that does not cause changes on brain imaging. The ABCD$_2$ (age, blood pressure, clinical features, symptom, duration, and diabetes mellitus) score is used to predict the risk of stroke among persons with TIA (Table 4).

Because much of the acute treatment of stroke is time-linked, the term acute ischemic stroke (brain attack) often is used to describe those events that are treated within the first few hours of onset; while the time limit for this term may evolve, it probably will remain with the maximal time period of 8–12 hours. The term stroke-in-evolution is used to describe the situation in which a patient's signs are rapidly worsening. A cerebral infarction (completed stroke) describes an event associated with persistent neurological impairments. Multiple strokes may lead to cognitive impairments that directly lead to dementia (vascular dementia) or exacerbate the effects of degenerative brain diseases.

❑ STROKE AS A SYMPTOM

While stroke is a life-threatening or life-changing disease, it also is due to an underlying vascular disease. The cause of stroke greatly affects decisions about prevention, acute treatment, and long-term care. Thus, stroke should be considered to be a symptom and evaluation for the most likely etiology of the vascular event is a crucial component of management.

Preventive Strategies for Other Cardiovascular Diseases

The most obvious division in stroke is between hemorrhages and infarctions (Table 5). Among patients with intracranial hemorrhages, the primary site of bleeding often reflects the most likely diagnosis (Fig. 1). The differential diagnosis for the cause of ischemic stroke is extensive and it is partially influenced by the age of the patient. While atherosclerotic disease and acquired cardiac diseases are important etiologies for stroke in middle-aged adults and the elderly, these conditions are much less common in children and young adults. On the other hand, the relative frequency of inherited hematological disorders and nonatherosclerotic vasculopathies is considerably higher in younger populations.

Table 5: Subtypes and causes of stroke

- Hemorrhagic stroke
  - Hypertension
    - Acute hypertension
    - Sustained hypertension
  - Aneurysms
    - Saccular (berry) aneurysms
    - Other aneurysms
  - Vascular malformations
    - Arteriovenous malformations
    - Other vascular malformations
  - Amyloid angiopathy
  - Hemorrhagic transformation of infarction
  - Bleeding diathesis
    - Congenital/inherited
    - Acquired including medications
  - Drug abuse
  - Tumors
  - Primary brain tumor
    - Metastatic brain tumor
  - Vasculitis
- Ischemic stroke
  - Large artery atherosclerosis
    - Extracranial
    - Intracranial
  - Small artery occlusive disease (lacunes)
  - Cardioembolism
    - Higher risk
      Atrial fibrillation with structural heart disease
      Rheumatic mitral stenosis
      Prosthetic heart valves
      Acute myocardial infarction (anterior wall)
      Dilated cardiomyopathy
      Infective endocarditis
      Nonbacterial thrombotic endocarditis
      Libman-Sacks endocarditis
    - Undetermined or lower risk
      Patent foramen ovale
      Atrial septal aneurysm
      Mitral valve prolapse

Contd...

Contd...

Table 5: Subtypes and causes of stroke
<ul><li>Nonatherosclerotic vasculopathies</li><li>Infectious vasculitis</li><li>Noninflammatory inflammatory vasculitis</li><li>Noninflammatory arteriopathies</li></ul><ul><li>Arterial dissection<ul><li>Fibromuscular dysplasia</li><li>Moyamoya</li><li>Hypercoagulable disorders<ul><li>Genetic</li><li>Acquired</li></ul></li><li>Undetermined cause</li></ul></li><li>Venous thrombosis</li><li>Pituitary apoplexy</li></ul>

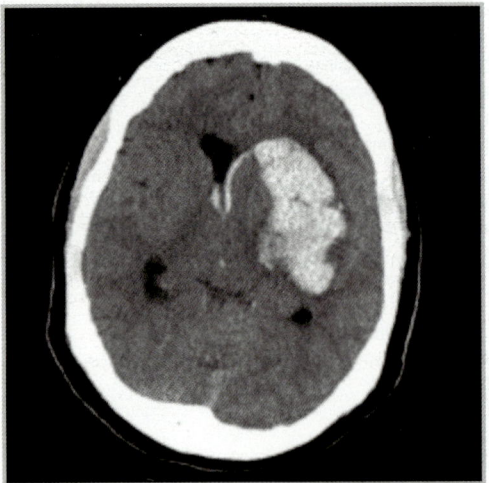

FIGURE 1: Axial CT of the brain demonstrates a hyperdensity in the left hemisphere. The abnormality is consistent with the diagnosis of hypertensive hemorrhage in the basal ganglia (putaminal hemorrhage)

Atherosclerotic disease affecting large intracranial or extracranial arteries, which leads to severe narrowing or occlusion of the vessels, is a leading cause of cerebral infarction. Both the carotid and the vertebrobasilar circulations may be affected. As with coronary artery disease, instability of an atherosclerotic plaque with fracture and secondary thromboembolism may also result. Atrial fibrillation complicating structural heart disease is a leading cause of embolism to the brain. It is the most common etiology of ischemic stroke among women older than 75. While lone atrial fibrillation is not associated with a high risk of embolic infarction, there are factors that are included in the $CHADS_2$ (congestive heart failure, hypertension, age, diabetes mellitus, prior stroke or TIA) score that can predict risk (Table 6).

Preventive Strategies for Other Cardiovascular Diseases

Table 6: CHADS$_2$ score: risk of stroke among persons with atrial fibrillation	
Factors	Score
Congestive heart failure	1 point
Hypertension	1 point
Age > 75 years	1 point
Diabetes mellitus	1 point
Stroke (previous stroke or TIA)	2 points

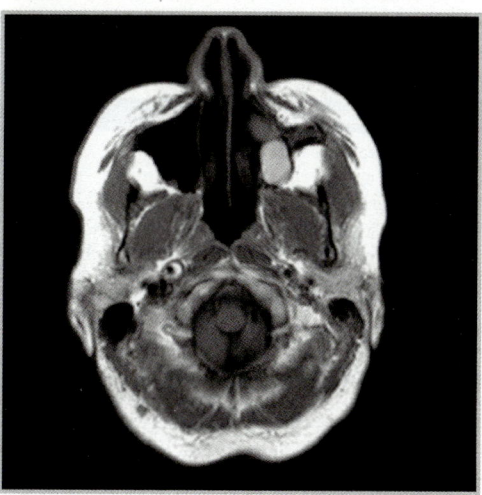

FIGURE 2: An axial view of a T1-weighted magnetic resonance imaging study of the base of the skull and brain shows a "crescent sign" in the right internal carotid artery. The finding is highly suggestive of a dissection of the artery

A large number of nonatherosclerotic vasculopathies that affect intracranial or extracranial arteries may lead to stroke. While each of these conditions is relatively uncommon, they remain important diagnostic considerations particularly among children and young adults. The most common is an arterial dissection, which may occur spontaneously or may complicate trauma (Fig. 2). Genetic or acquired prothrombotic disorders may also lead to ischemic stroke. While these diseases account for a small minority of ischemic strokes, they should be considered if a patient has a personal or family history of venous or arterial thromboembolic events.

Clinical Presentations

As the term stroke implies, vascular events of the brain are of sudden onset. While some patients may have waxing and waning of the symptoms or a slow evolution of the impairments, the deficits usually are of maximal severity shortly after the time of onset. The sudden onset of an unusually severe headache (thunderclap headache) often is the cardinal symptom of aneurysmal SAH. A headache is also a prominent symptom among patients with other intracranial hemorrhages.

While global symptoms, such as lightheadedness or nonspecific dizziness, occasionally occur with a stroke, patients generally have focal neurological symptoms and signs that reflect injury to one part of the brain. The patterns of impairments generally are stereotyped and reflect injury to the dominant or nondominant cerebral hemisphere, deep or more superficial locations of the cerebral hemispheres, the cerebellum or brainstem (Table 7). The patterns of ischemic stroke also fit the vascular territories of the internal carotid artery or vertebrobasilar circulation. The clinical features of a TIA are similar to those of an ischemic stroke but are transient (Table 8). While the presentation of an ICH may mimic an infarction, affected patients generally are sicker and more commonly have altered consciousness, severe headache, nausea and vomiting (Table 9).

While the clinical presentations of stroke and TIA are relatively straightforward, errors in diagnosis occur; both over- and underdiagnosis happen. In particular

Table 7: Clinical features of ischemic stroke

- Sudden onset of focal neurological findings
- Often of maximal severity at onset
- May have stepwise worsening or waxing/waning
- Types of neurological findings
    - Cortical hemisphere involvement—cognitive impairments (aphasia, neglect, etc.), contralateral homonymous hemianopia, contralateral hemiparesis, contralateral hemianesthesia, dysarthria
    - Deep hemisphere involvement—contralateral hemiparesis, dysarthria or contralateral hemianesthesia
    - Brainstem and/or cerebellar involvement—dysarthria, dysphagia, diplopia/abnormal ocular movements, vertigo/nystagmus, hearing loss, unilateral or bilateral weakness, contralateral hemianesthesia, truncal and gait ataxia, ipsilateral limb ataxia
- Headache in approximately 20% of cases
- Nausea and vomiting—brainstem and/or cerebellar involvement
- Loss of consciousness in uncommon
- Coma with large brainstem lesion
- Seizures are uncommon

Table 8: Clinical features of transient ischemic attack

- Usually of sudden onset with gradual resolution
- Usual duration is 5–20 minutes
- Loss of function
- Carotid circulation:
    - Ipsilateral monocular visual loss (amaurosis fugax)
    - Contralateral weakness, numbness, clumsiness arm, hand, side of face, half of body
    - Dysarthria or aphasia
    - Contralateral visual field loss
- Vertebrobasilar circulation:
    - Binocular visual loss
    - Vertigo
    - Diplopia
    - Imbalance or ataxia
    - Dysarthria
    - Unilateral or bilateral weakness, numbness, clumsiness
    - Rarely loss of consciousness
    - Rarely a drop attack

the diagnosis of SAH may be missed if the patient has only a severe headache (Table 10). The occurrence of transient neurological symptoms may or may not be secondary to a TIA. Alternative diagnoses include seizures, migraine, syncope, and metabolic disturbances, such as hypoglycemia (Table 11). In general, the neurological findings, which represent a loss of function, are of sudden onset with TIA; an evolution of symptoms or positive findings (such as involuntary movement or positive visual phenomena) is atypical for a vascular event. The differential diagnosis of ischemic stroke is relatively limited. The most important alternative diagnosis is hemorrhagic stroke (and vice versa) (Table 12).

Table 9: Clinical features of intracranial hemorrhage

- Headache
- Nausea and vomiting
- Photophobia and phonophobia
- Alteration in alertness
- Marked arterial hypertension
- Unstable vital signs
- Signs of meningeal irritation
- Focal neurological signs
  - Hemiparesis
  - Hemisensory loss
  - Homonymous hemianopia
  - Dysarthria
  - Aphasia
  - Ataxia

Table 10: Differential diagnosis of subarachnoid hemorrhage

- Migraine
- Thunderclap headache
- Viral meningitis
- Sinusitis
- Herniated cervical disk
- Drug or alcohol overdose
- Cerebral infarction
- Cerebral hemorrhage
- Myocardial infarction

Table 11: Differential diagnosis of transient ischemic attack

- Migraine
- Syncope
- Seizure
- Metabolic disturbance
  - Hypoglycemia
- Intracranial mass lesion
  - Tumor
  - Subdural hematoma

Table 12: Differential diagnosis of hemorrhagic or ischemic stroke

- Hemorrhagic (ischemic) stroke
- Occult trauma
- Central nervous system infection
  - Encephalitis
- Migraine with residual findings
- Seizures with postictal signs
- Metabolic disorder
  - Hypoglycemia
- Intracranial mass
  - Brain tumor
  - Subdural hematoma

Diagnostic Evaluation

The goals of the diagnostic evaluation are (i) to determine if a hemorrhagic or ischemic stroke is the most likely explanation for the patient's neurological symptoms, (ii) to establish the most likely cause for the patient's stroke, (iii) to screen for risk factors that would predispose to accelerated atherosclerosis and stroke, and (iv) to seek medical or neurological complications of the stroke or severe comorbid diseases. The results of the evaluation affect prognosis and decisions about both acute and longer term treatment. The selection of the diagnostic studies is made on a case-by-case basis; the evaluation may be done in a cost-effective manner through careful selection of studies to order.

Brain imaging remains the cornerstone in the evaluation of patients with suspected stroke. Computed tomography (CT) of the brain revolutionized the diagnosis of stroke (Figs 3 and 4). It has a very high yield in detecting intracranial

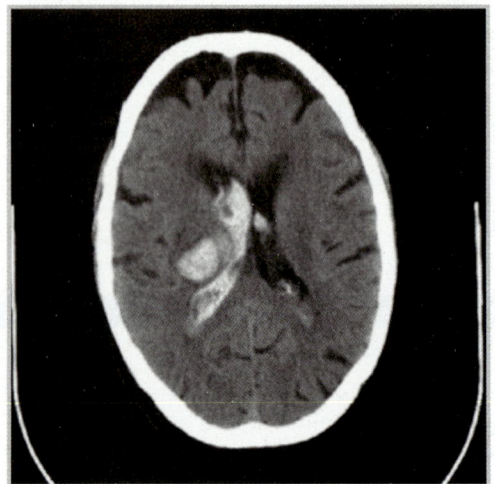

FIGURE 3: Axial CT of the brain shows a hyperdensity in the right thalamus with extension into the right lateral ventricle. The results are consistent with the diagnosis of thalamic hemorrhage with intraventricular extension of bleeding

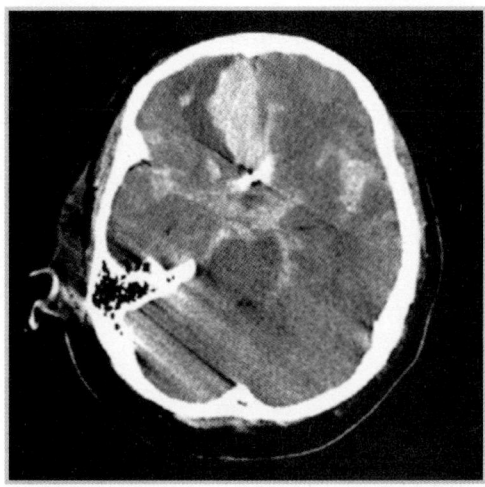

FIGURE 4: Axial CT of the brain reveals hyperdensity in multiple locations at the base of the brain and a focal area of increased signal in the interhemispheric fissure. The findings are those of aneurysmal subarachnoid hemorrhage with the most likely location of the aneurysm being on the anterior communicating artery

hemorrhage and within a few hours of onset, CT usually will detect the changes of cerebral infarction. CT also is useful in identifying neurological complications of stroke, including hydrocephalus, brain edema and hemorrhagic transformation of an infarction. Contrast enhancement may be used to detect early changes of hypoperfusion. Several sequences of MRI are used to assess patients with suspected stroke. Gradient echo studies are particularly useful in defining hemorrhages and diffusion-weighted imaging (DWI) usually detects the changes of cerebral infarction within minutes of the onset of the vascular event.

Patients with decreased consciousness or suspected seizures may be evaluated with an EEG. Examination of the CSF has a limited role in patients with stroke. It may be performed in those patients whose history is highly suggestive of SAH and in whom a CT does not demonstrate bleeding.

Both computed tomographic angiography (CTA) and magnetic resonance angiography (MRA) are used to assess the extracranial and intracranial vasculature. The yields of these tests are relatively high. Magnetic resonance venography (MRV) has become a valuable method to screen for thrombosis of intracranial venous structures. Other noninvasive vascular imaging studies include carotid duplex examination and transcranial Doppler ultrasonography. Arteriography remains the most definitive method to examine the intracranial and extracranial vasculature (Fig. 5). It is invasive and associated with a risk of embolic cerebral infarction.

Because of the strong association between stroke and heart disease, a cardiac evaluation is indicated in most patients with cerebrovascular disease. The usual studies include an ECG and echocardiography. Blood tests include measures of hemoglobin, hematocrit, platelet count, and white blood cell count (complete blood count/CBC). Screening for severe comorbid diseases or risk factors for accelerated atherosclerosis include blood glucose level, hemoglobin A1C level, lipid profile, renal and liver function tests and cardiac enzymes. Screening for an inflammatory

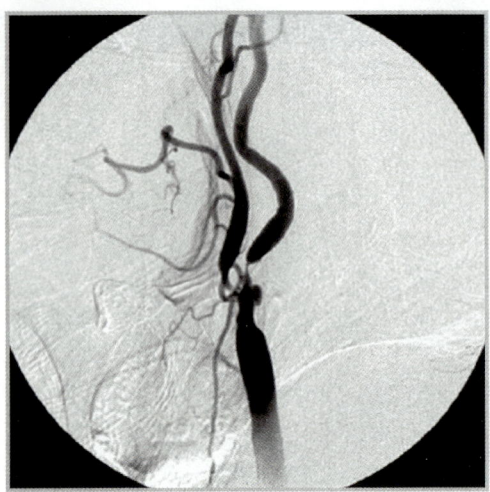

FIGURE 5: A lateral subtraction view of a left carotid arteriogram shows a high-grade stenosis with ulceration of the proximal segment of the internal carotid artery

process would include erythrocyte sedimentation rate and C-reactive protein; elevations may point to an illness such as a multisystem vasculitis. Additional hematological studies to look for acquired or genetic causes of a hypercoagulable disorder or bleeding disorders may be ordered in exceptional cases. The role of genetic testing for specific inherited disorders leading to stroke, such as autosomal dominant polycystic kidney disease or cerebral autosomal dominant arteriopathy with subcortical infarcts and leukoencephalopathy (CADASIL), may also be done. Pharmacogenetic testing may be needed to help guide treatment decisions, such as the use of clopidogrel in prophylaxis.

❏ PREVENTION

The components of management to prevent stroke (Table 13) can be aggregated into three groups: (i) interventions to control or treat those risk factors that promote the course of atherosclerosis and increase the risk of brain ischemia, (ii) antithrombotic medications, and (iii) surgical or endovascular interventions. The selections for treatment are made on a case-by-case basis. Several factors influence decisions about treatment, including (i) the presumed etiology of the patient's ischemic symptoms, (ii) the most likely vascular territory, (iii) responses to prior treatment, (iv) specific contraindications to treatment (for example, allergy to aspirin), and (v) the preferences of the patient.

❏ GENERAL ACUTE TREATMENT

Acute stroke is a medical emergency. Acute treatment includes institution of interventions to limit the neurological injury and use of therapies to prevent or control general medical or neurological complications. Besides a clinical evaluation and ordering diagnostic studies, urgent attention is paid to acute potentially life-threatening complications (Table 14).

Table 13: Prevention of ischemic stroke

- Management of risk factors
- Hypertension (goal systolic blood pressure 120–130 mm Hg and diastolic blood pressure < 80 mm Hg)
  - Lifestyle changes (weight loss, diet, increase exercise)
  - Antihypertensive medications
- Diabetes mellitus (goal of Hgb A1C <7%):
  - Lifestyle changes
  - Insulin or oral medications
- Hyperlipidemia:
  - Lifestyle changes
  - Statins or other lipid-lowering medications
- Smoking:
  - Abstinence
  - Nicotine replacement or other medications
- Antithrombotic agents:
  - Oral anticoagulants
    - Warfarin
  - Thrombin inhibitors
    - Dabigatran
  - Antiplatelet agents
    - Aspirin
    - Aspirin/extended release dipyridamole
    - Clopidogrel
    - Aspirin and clopidogrel
    - Ticlopidine
- Surgical interventions:
  - Carotid endarterectomy
  - Extracranial–intracranial arterial bypass
  - Other operations
  - Angioplasty and stenting

Table 14: General emergency management: acute stroke

- ABCs of life support
  - Protect the airway (intubation)
  - Ventilatory assistance
  - Cardiac monitoring
  - Treat serious cardiac arrhythmias
- Management hypertension
  - Treatment with rt-PA (systolic <185 mm Hg/diastolic <10 mm Hg)
  - Parenteral administration of short acting medications
- Treat fever
- Treat seizures
- Treat hyperglycemia

❑ TREATMENT OF ACUTE ISCHEMIC STROKE

Interventions to restore perfusion to an area of ischemic brain are the engine that drives treatment of acute ischemic stroke. Intravenous thrombolysis has revolutionized emergency management; rt-PA (dosage 0.9 mg/kg—maximum of 90 mg) has been approved for the treatment of carefully selected patients with acute ischemic stroke; 10% of the dose is given as a bolus and the remainder is infused over 1 hour. The original maximum time window was 3 hours, but the results of a European trial permitted expansion of the time period for treatment to 4.5 hours. Guidelines provide recommendations for the administration of rt-PA; the criteria for eligibility for treatment differ for the time periods of less than 3 hours and 3–4.5 hours (Table 15).

Table 15: Treatment of acute ischemic stroke

- Intravenous thrombolysis
- Interval from onset of stroke:
  - <3 hours for persons aged 81 or greater
  - <4.5 hours for younger persons
- Absence of medical contraindications (increased risk of bleeding):
  - History of recent prior stroke
  - History of recent myocardial infarction
  - History of recent major trauma
  - History of recent major operation
  - History of recent serious bleeding
- Absence of other comorbid diseases that may mimic stroke:
  - Blood glucose values are not hypoglycemic
  - Seizures that occur with stroke do not contraindicate treatment
  - A history of diabetes and prior stroke contraindicates treatment in 3–4.5 hours time period
- Survey of medications that the patient is taking:
  - Warfarin may be treated <3 hours if INR is <1.8
  - Any warfarin use precludes treatment in 3–4.5 hours time period
  - Antiplatelet agents are not a contraindication
  - Treatment of stroke with heparin is a contraindication
  - Angiotensin converting enzyme inhibitors appear to increase the risk of angioedema after treatment—not a contraindication
- Findings on general medical examination:
  - Blood pressure: <185 mm Hg systolic and <110 mm Hg diastolic
  - If there is time, blood pressure may be lowered to allow treatment
  - No evidence of acute bleeding
- Findings on neurological examination:
  - Demonstrable focal neurological impairments
  - May be treated even some improvement
  - Patients with severe stroke have higher risk of bleeding
  - Patients with NIH stroke scale score >25 cannot be treated in 3–4.5 hours time period
- Coagulation studies are normal:
  - Platelet count, prothrombin time, aPTT
- Brain imaging findings:
  - Absence of brain hemorrhage
  - Absence of other brain pathology
  - A "normal" CT in a patient with acute symptoms is assumed to be compatible with acute ischemic stroke
  - Detection of ischemic stroke (more likely with DWI sequence on MRI)
- Patient and/or family aware of the risks and potential benefits
  - Overall risk of symptomatic intracranial bleeding is approximately 6% but is higher in severely affected patients

Contd...

Contd...

Table 15: Treatment of acute ischemic stroke

- Administration of rt-PA:
  - Cannot substitute another thrombolytic agent
  - Dosage is 0.9 mg/kg—maximum of 90 mg
  - 10% of dose as intravenous bolus
  - Remainder infused over 1 hour
- Ancillary treatment:
  - Close observation for changes in status
  - Aggressive lowering of increased blood pressure
  - Delay placement of devices (indwelling bladder catheter, etc.) in order to avoid bleeding
  - Do follow-up CT scan of brain to look for hemorrhagic transformation at approximately 24 hours after treatment
  - Delay starting antiplatelet agents or anticoagulants until 24 hours after treatment and CT does not show bleeding

Emergency administration of anticoagulants to persons with acute ischemic stroke was used for several years. At present, there is no strong indication for early administration of anticoagulants to patients with stroke. To date, no neuroprotective agent has been established as safe and effective in treatment of patients with acute ischemic stroke.

❏ TREATMENT OF ACUTE HEMORRHAGIC STROKE

At present, there is not an equivalent to the intravenous administration of rt-PA for treatment of patients with acute intracranial hemorrhage. Current guidelines emphasize general emergency supportive care and treatment of arterial hypertension. The latter component of management is aimed at limiting the extension of the hematoma. Neurosurgical evacuation of the hematoma is recommended for the treatment of mass-producing cerebellar hemorrhages. In addition, neurosurgical management may include placement of intraventricular catheters to remove CSF and to treat increased intracranial pressure.

Other acute treatment depends upon the presumed cause of the hemorrhage. Patients with bleeding secondary to oral anticoagulants are treated with fresh frozen plasma, clotting factors or vitamin K. Protamine sulfate is administered to patients who have bleeding secondary to heparin. Persons with an inherited bleeding disorder, such as hemophilia, are also treated with clotting factors. Transfusions of platelets are given to those patients with intracranial bleeding secondary to thrombocytopenia.

Patients with aneurysmal SAH are at high risk for early recurrent aneurysmal rupture. Due to the markedly increased risk of morbidity and mortality with rebleeding, a focus of early management is aimed at treatment of the aneurysm. A surgical intervention is preferred and the options include direct surgical clipping of the aneurysmal neck or obliteration of the aneurysm through the endovascular placement of coils. The early risk of recurrent hemorrhage is relatively low among patients with bleeding secondary to a ruptured vascular malformation. In general, these patients are allowed to recover from their acute event. Subsequent treatment options include direct surgical resection, endovascular obliteration of feeding vessels, and focused high-intensity radiation to lead to scarring and occlusion of the vascular components of the malformation.

GENERAL IN-HOSPITAL CARE AND REHABILITATION

Patients with recent stroke are seriously ill and are at high risk for major neurological and medical complications that may lead to morbidity and mortality. The complications are similar whether the patient has had a hemorrhagic or ischemic stroke. In addition, patients often have other serious comorbid diseases that need to be treated. As a result, patients with acute stroke are admitted to the hospital for monitoring, evaluation, and treatment. The patient is observed for the development of neurological worsening or other events. Treatment involves both prophylactic measures and interventions aimed at the lessening the consequences of the stroke (Table 16).

Table 16: General management of patients hospitalized with stroke

- Monitoring of neurological status, blood pressure and vital signs:
  - Frequently during first 24 hours and then intervals are expanded
  - Cardiac monitoring for arrhythmias
- Intravenous access to be maintained to ease administration of medications
- Levels of activities:
  - Initially bed rest (usually first 24 hours)
  - Frequent turning in order to avoid pressure sores
  - Then increase level of activity as tolerated
  - Mobilization done with care because of risk for falls
- Diet:
  - Intravenous fluids to maintain hydration
  - No food, liquids or medications by mouth until swallowing is assessed and risk of aspiration is deemed to be low
  - Consistency of oral intake adjusted to ease swallowing
  - Diet modified to meet comorbid diseases and risk factors
  - Nasogastric feedings to maintain nutrition and hydration for patients who cannot swallow
  - If prolonged need for tube feedings, PEG may be needed
  - Laxatives or suppositories as needed to treat constipation
- Bladder treatment:
  - Avoid indwelling bladder catheters if possible
  - Acidification of the urine to help reduce risk of infection
- Prevention of deep vein thrombosis:
  - Subcutaneous administration of heparin or low molecular weight heparin
  - Alternating pressure devices and support hoses for those patients who cannot receive anticoagulants
- Passive range of motion of joints
- Prevention of recurrent stroke depends upon type of stroke and etiology:
  - Antiplatelet agents
  - Anticoagulants
- Consultation to rehabilitation services for assessment and treatment:
  - Physical therapy
  - Occupational therapy
  - Speech pathology
  - Social services and discharge planning
- Symptomatic treatment on a case-by-case basis:
  - Analgesics
  - Stomach protective medication

Contd...

Contd...

Table 16: General management of patients hospitalized with stroke

- Sedatives
- Antidepressants
- Treatment of comorbid diseases and risk factors:
  - Diabetes mellitus
  - Hypertension
  - Heart disease
  - Lung disease
  - Renal disease

Assessment of the individual patient's needs for rehabilitation is done as soon as the patient is medically stable. Physical therapy, occupational therapy and speech therapy form the core efforts in rehabilitation. Physical therapy is focused on improving general mobility and major motor function. Occupational therapy aims at improving fine motor function (especially the hand) and often uses assistive devices. Speech therapy is aimed at improving swallowing, articulation and recovery of language function. Other potential interventions include cognitive rehabilitation, vocational counseling, recreational therapy, music therapy, etc. The setting of the rehabilitation depends upon the severity and types of impairments and the ability of the patient to collaborate in the rehabilitation program. Possible venues include inpatient rehabilitation (in an independent or hospital-based unit); outpatient therapy in which the patient comes to the facility, inhome treatment with professionals, or at-home therapy provided by the patient and family.

❏ SUGGESTED READINGS

Adams H Jr, del Zoppo G, Alberts MJ, et al. Guidelines for the early management of adults with ischemic stroke: a guideline from the American Heart Association/American Stroke Association Stroke Council, Clinical Cardiology Council, Cardiovascular Radiology and Intervention Council, and the Atherosclerotic Peripheral Vascular Disease and Quality of Care Outcomes in Research Interdisciplinary Working Groups: The American Academy of Neurology affirms the value of this guideline as an educational tool for neurologists. Circulation. 2007;115:e478-534.

Adams RJ, Albers G, Alberts MJ, et al. Update to the AHA/ASA Recommendations for the Prevention of Stroke in Patients with Stroke and Transient Ischemic Attack. Stroke. 2008;39:1647-52.

Bederson JB, Connolly ES Jr, Batjer HH, et al. Guidelines for the management of aneurysmal subarachnoid hemorrhage: a statement for healthcare professionals from a special writing group of the Stroke Council, American Heart Association. Stroke. 2009;40:994-1025.

Broderick J, Connolly S, Feldmann E, et al. Guidelines for the Management of Spontaneous Intracerebral Hemorrhage in Adults: 2007 Update: A Guideline From the American Heart Association/American Stroke Association Stroke Council, High Blood Pressure Research Council, and the Quality of Care and Outcomes in Research Interdisciplinary Working Group: The American Academy of Neurology affirms the value of this guideline as an educational tool for neurologists. Stroke. 2007;38:2001-23.

Easton JD, Saver JL, Albers GW, et al. Definition and Evaluation of Transient Ischemic Attack: A Scientific Statement for Healthcare Professionals From the American Heart Association/American Stroke Association Stroke Council; Council on Cardiovascular Surgery and Anesthesia; Council on Cardiovascular Radiology and Intervention; Council on Cardiovascular Nursing; and the Interdisciplinary Council on Peripheral Vascular Disease: The American Academy of Neurology affirms the value of this statement as an educational tool for neurologists. Stroke. 2009;40:2276-93.

Gage BF, van Walraven C, Pearce L, et al. Selecting patients with atrial fibrillation for anticoagulation: stroke risk stratification in patients taking aspirin. Circulation. 2004;110:2287-92.

Josephson SA, Sidney S, Pham TN, et al. Higher ABCD2 score predicts patients most likely to have true transient ischemic attack. Stroke. 2008;39:3096-8.

Sacco RL, Adams R, Albers G, et al. Guidelines for Prevention of Stroke in Patients with Ischemic Stroke or Transient Ischemic Attack: A Statement for Healthcare Professionals From the American Heart Association/American Stroke Association Council on Stroke: Co-Sponsored by the Council on Cardiovascular Radiology and Intervention: The American Academy of Neurology affirms the value of this guideline. Circulation. 2006;113:e409-49.

12.3 Rheumatic Fever

❏ INTRODUCTION

Rheumatic fever (RF) is generally classified as a connective tissue disease or collagen vascular disease. Its anatomical hallmark is damage to collagen fibrils and to the ground substance of connective tissue. The clinical manifestations of RF follow a group A streptococcal infection of the throat after a latent period of approximately 3 weeks.

❏ PATHOGENESIS

For the development of RF, three things are required: (i) streptococcal infection by the group A beta hemolytic group, (ii) susceptible host, and (iii) immune response (Fig. 6).

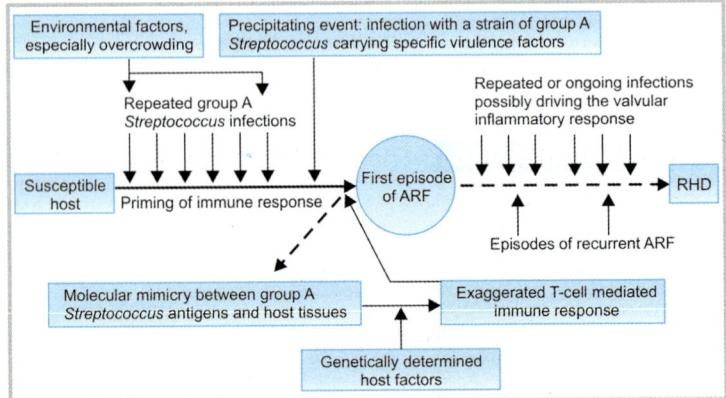

FIGURE 6: Pathogenesis of acute rheumatic fever and rheumatic heart disease.
(Source: Modified from Lancet. 2005;366:155-68)

When a susceptible host develops a group A beta haemolytic streptococci (GABHS) infection, an immune response occurs. There is a molecular mimicry between the epitopes of the strep and many components of the cardiac cell, which leads on to the tissue damage. For example, antibodies formed against the N-acetylglucosamine of the streptococcal carbohydrate cross reacts with the cardiac valve tissue.

Aschoff's body is pathognomonic of RF. This was described in the year 1904. It is made up of perivascular infiltrate of large cells with polymorphous nuclei and basophilic cytoplasm arranged in a rosette around anavascular center of fibrinoid. Some of the cells may be multinucleated or may have an owl eyed nucleus with an eccentric dot and fibrillae radiating to the nuclear membrane or caterpillar nucleus. These cells are called as Antischkow myocyte. Aschoff's bodies are present in the myocardium; these are most marked in the interventricular septum and left atrial appendage. It is not present in areas such as brain or joints. They are found more frequently in younger subjects with mitral stenosis than in those with pure mitral regurgitation.

❏ DIAGNOSIS OF RHEUMATIC FEVER

For the diagnosis of acute rheumatic fever, we have been following the Jone's criteria since 1944. However, there are many patients who do not fulfil the criteria of the Jone's criteria and, presently, a new dimension has been added with the advent of echocardiography. The current guideline was put forward in the year 1992 as an update. These criteria are to be used only for the initial attacks of rheumatic fever. This does not apply for patients with past history of RF or rheumatic heart disease. For the diagnosis of RF, the criteria have been divided into major, minor and supporting evidence. To diagnose RF, patient should have one major plus two minor or two major with evidence of preceding strep infection (Table 17).

Exceptions to Jone's criteria:
- Chorea
- Indolent carditis
- Recurrent rheumatic fever
- Post streptococcal arthritis

With the above four conditions, Jone's criteria do not apply.

Since recurrences are the main reason for worsening of the cardiac damage and due to the fact that recurrences cause only subtle manifestations, WHO has put forward criteria that are given in Table 18.

Table 17: For the diagnosis of initial attacks of rheumatic fever (1992 updated)	
Major	<ul><li>Arthritis</li><li>Carditis</li><li>Chorea</li><li>Erythema marginatum</li><li>Subcutaneous nodules</li></ul>
Minor	<ul><li>Fever</li><li>Arthralgia</li><li>Elevated ESR or CRP</li><li>Prolonged PR interval in ECG</li></ul>
Supporting evidence of preceding strep infection within the last 45 days	Elevated or rising ASO or other strep antibody test or positive throat culture or rapid antigen test

Table 18: WHO criteria (2002–2003) for the diagnosis of rheumatic fever (RHD)	
First episode	Two major or one major and two minor (similar to Jone's criteria)
Recurrent without RHD	Two major or one major + two minor
Recurrent with RHD	Two minor with preceding *Streptococcus* infection
Rheumatic chorea	Preceding *Streptococcus* infection criteria not required

❏ CLINICAL FEATURES

The most common age at which RF occurs is between 5 and 15 years. Recurrences can occur at any age but the rate falls steadily beyond adolescence. Both genders are affected equally for the acute RF, but chorea is more common in women.

Arthritis

- Occurs in 70% of cases
- Asymmetrical and migratory in nature
- Large joint arthritis (knees, ankles, elbows and wrist are involved)
- Pain, swelling, heat and redness are noted
- Lasts for 2–3 weeks
- Rapid response to salicylates within 48 hours
- No residual deformity.

Jaccoud's arthritis is a permanent deformity of small joints, secondary to rheumatic fever, which is very rare. Poststreptococcal reactive arthritis (PSRA) seen early after an episode of streptococcal infection (10 days vs 14–21 days for RF). It also involves small joints, lasts longer and does not respond to salicylates as easily as RF. Experts believe that these patients be treated with secondary prophylaxis for up to one year at least after the onset of symptoms. But in endemic areas of RF, it may be wise to give prophylaxis for 5 years.

Carditis

The cardiac involvement in RF is pancarditis and occurs in 50% of patients with acute rheumatic fever. Since carditis includes some or one of the following, the features are given in increasing order of severity.

- Tachycardia (out of proportion to the degree of fever) is common; its absence makes the diagnosis of myocarditis unlikely
- A heart murmur of valvulitis [caused by mitral regurgitation (MR) and/or aortic regurgitation (AR)] is almost always present; without the murmurs of MR and/or AR, carditis should not be diagnosed
- Pericarditis (friction rub, pericardial effusion, chest pain and ECG changes) may be present
- Cardiomegaly on chest X-ray is indicative of pericarditis or congestive heart failure (CHF)
- Signs of CHF (gallop rhythm, distant heart sounds, cardiomegaly) are indications of severe carditis.

Valve involvement in acute rheumatic fever:
Mitral: 70–75%.
Mitral and aortic: 20–25%.
Aortic: Isolated 5%.

Echo Doppler is extremely useful in the diagnosis of carditis by identifying valvular disease even in patients without clinical evidence of carditis. Echo can

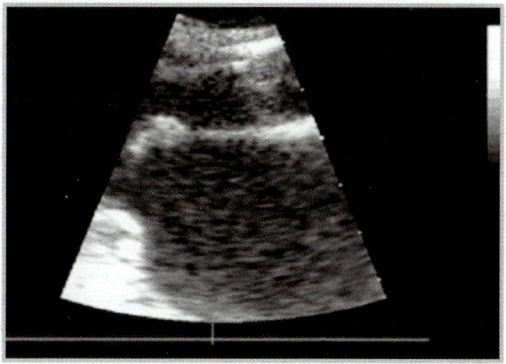

FIGURE 7: Echo showing rheumatic vegetations on the anterior mitral leaflet

also identify the presence of pericardial effusion and in some cases identify the fine rheumatic valvular vegetations. However, echo should not be used as sole criteria for the diagnosis of carditis (Fig. 7).

Chorea

Also called as Sydenham's chorea, or St. Vitus dance is the third most common major manifestation. The period of latency between the GABHS infection and the onset of chorea is around three months.

Chorea can occur in two circumstances:

1. As an isolated manifestation of RF and frequently recurs following a new bout of streptococcal pharyngitis. This is called as pure chorea.
2. It may occur as a part of otherwise active RF with manifestations, such as joint pains, etc.

After puberty, chorea is almost entirely seen only in women. It may last for a few weeks to few months. It seems to be due to immune mediated reaction to auto antibodies of the basal ganglia. Severe chorea responds to treatment with intravenous IgG. The signs are:

- Hyperextension of the fingers, spooning when the arms are extended
- Pronation of hands when arms are raised vertically
- Milkmaid's grip—irregular contraction of the hand muscles when the patient presses the hand of the examiner
- Wormian tongue—gross fasciculations of the tongue when extended
- Clumsiness in fine movements, such as buttoning of the shirt.

Studies suggest that many patients with chorea may eventually have obsessive–compulsive behavior. No residual neurological deficit is seen in most patients. When chorea is associated with other signs of RF, the incidence of valve damage is comparable to that caused by other patients without chorea. When chorea is an isolated event—pure chorea, the valve damage is less frequent, and mitral stenosis is the late manifestation.

Erythema Marginatum

This is the least frequent manifestation of RF and is seen as pink macules with a clear center with serpiginous edge. The usual location is in the trunk and sometimes in the limbs but never seen in the face.

Subcutaneous Nodules

Nowadays, the incidence of the same is only around 5%. They are discrete, nontender, measuring 5–20 mm and are located over the extensor surfaces of elbows, knees, ankles, spinous process of vertebra. They occur in crops, appear late in the course of the disease, often 3 weeks or so. They disappear in 2 weeks' time. Since, it appears late into the disease, it is not useful in the early diagnosis.

Preceding Group A *Streptococcus* Infection

Throat culture is the gold standard for identification of a preceding infection. At the time of diagnosis of acute RF, only about 11% of patients have positive throat culture. Hence, throat culture is less reliable than streptococcal antibody tests.

- RADT: Rapid antigen tests: The specificity is very good but sensitivity is very low
- Antistreptolysin O (ASO) titer is the one that is used routinely. It is elevated in 80% of patients with acute RF and in 20% of normal individuals. ASO titer of at least 333 Todd units in children and 250 Todd units in adults are considered as elevated. If the clinical suspicion is high but the ASO titer is low, this does not exclude the diagnosis of acute rheumatic fever. Then you must do one more test such as antideoxyribonuclease B test (ADNB) or repeat the ASO titer after a week. A rising titer of ASO can be taken as evidence for acute rheumatic fever. Both ASO and ADNB levels rise at 1 week, peak at 3–6 weeks and persist for several months
- Streptozyme test is relatively simple agglutination test but it is less standardized and less reproducible than the other antibody test.

Tests for Active Inflammation (ESR/CRP)

Erythrocyte sedimentation rate: ESR is almost always elevated in patients with acute RF. A normal ESR is uncommon. However, ESR is likely to be normal in patients with chorea or isolated erythema marginatum or severe cardiac failure. CRP reflects rheumatic activity more closely than the ESR, since it is not affected by factors, such as anemia, changes in serum proteins. It is useful in identifying rebounds during withdrawal of suppressive anti-inflammatory drugs.

❑ TREATMENT

The treatment algorithm for RF is given in Flowchart 2.

Eradication of Streptococci: AHA Statement

Of the several regimens given below, intramuscular benzathine penicillin and oral penicillin V are the recommended antimicrobial drugs for the treatment of GABHS except in individuals with penicillin allergy (Table 19). In the 2009 recommendations of AHA, the treatment of choice is oral or intramuscular penicillin. The main changes are following:

- Once-a-day amoxicillin is a suitable alternative for young children who cannot take pills and who can instead take amoxicillin suspension, which also has the advantage of being more palatable than penicillin
- With allergic to penicillin, not type-1, can be given cephalosporin or clindamycin. The macrolides, such as azithromycin are de-emphasized because there is increasing resistance of GAS to this group of antibiotics and they are not as well tolerated, often provoking gastrointestinal symptoms

FLOWCHART 2: Algorithm for rheumatic fever

Table 19: Treatment of strep tonsillopharyngitis			
Drug	**Dose**	**Mode**	**Duration**
Benzathine penicillin	600,000 if weight ≤27 kg 120,000 if weight >27 kg	Intramuscular	Once
Penicillin V	250 mg 3 times daily <27 kg 500 mg 3 times daily >27 kg	Oral	10 days
Amoxicillin	50 mg/kg once daily	Oral	10 days
Cephalexin/Cefadroxil	Variable dose	Oral	10 days
Clindamycin	20 mg/kg divided in 3 doses Maximum 1.8 g/day	Oral	10 days
Azithromycin	12 mg/kg once daily, maximum 500 mg/day	Oral	5 days
Clarithromycin	15 mg/kg divided into 2 doses	Oral	10 days

- For those with severe type-1 allergies to penicillin, clindamycin should be the first choice, because there is a 10% crossover (for allergy) with narrow-spectrum cephalosporins.

Anti-inflammatory Drugs: Salicylates or Steroids

They must not be started until a definitive diagnosis is made. Early therapy with these drugs may interfere with definitive diagnosis of acute rheumatic fever (see the treatment algorithm given below) (Table 20).

Recommended Bed Rest of Varying Duration

The duration depends on the severity of the clinical manifestation. ESR is a helpful guide to the rheumatic activity and, therefore, the duration of restriction of activities. Table 21 will give a general guideline for bed rest/restricted ambulation period.

Table 20: Duration of anti-inflammatory agents

Clinical manifestation	Prednisolone	Aspirin
Arthritis alone	—	1–2 weeks
Mild carditis	—	3–4 weeks
Moderate carditis	—	6–8 weeks
Severe carditis	2–6 weeks*	6 weeks–4 months

*For severe carditis, prednisolone should be tapered and aspirin be started during the final week and the total duration of anti-inflammatory therapy can be between 6 weeks and 4 months, depending on the need.

Table 21: General guidelines of restricted activities in acute rheumatic fever

Clinical feature	Duration of bed rest/limited ambulation
Arthritis alone	Only 2 weeks
Mild carditis	3–4 weeks
Moderate carditis (definite but mild cardiomegaly)	4–6 weeks
Severe carditis (marked cardiomegaly, cardiac failure, pericardial effusion)	Bed rest as long as patient has heart failure and indoor ambulation for a period of 2–3 months

Table 22: Drugs used in secondary prophylaxis

	Drug	Dose	Route
1.	Benzathine penicillin G	1.2 million units every 3–4 weeks	IM
2.	Penicillin V	250 mg twice daily	Oral
3.	Sulfadiazine	0.5 gm once daily for patients ≤27 kg or 1.0 gm once daily for patients >27 kg	Oral
4.	Allergic to penicillin and sulfadiazine: Erythromycin	Erythromycin 250 mg twice daily	Oral

Secondary Prevention of Rheumatic Fever

Tri-weekly regimen of benzathine penicillin is justified and recommended for countries, like India, where the incidence of RF is high. The drugs used for secondary prophylaxis is given in Table 22. The duration of prophylaxis by AHA is given in Table 23 and by WHO is given in Table 24. These two guidelines differ in the duration and age cutoff as given below.

The overall prevention of RF/RHD can be listed as primordial, primary, secondary and tertiary as shown in Flowchart 3.

Management of Chorea

Anti-inflammatory drugs, such as salicylates or steroids, do not alter the course of chorea and are not indicated unless there is clear indication for concomitant carditis. One of the following drugs may be used:
1. Phenobarbital—15–30 mg every 6th hourly.
2. Haloperidol—2 mg every 8th hourly or as needed.
3. Valproate—20 mg/kg/day.

Preventive Strategies for Other Cardiovascular Diseases

Table 23: Duration of secondary prophylaxis—AHA 2009

	Category	Duration
1.	RF with carditis and residual valvular disease	At least 10 years after last episode and at least until age 40 years. Sometimes life-long prophylaxis
2.	RF with carditis but no residual valvular disease	10 years or up to 21 years of age whichever is longer
3.	RF without carditis	5 years or up to 21 years of age, whichever is longer

Table 24: Duration of secondary prophylaxis as per WHO (WHO Tech report 923). The WHO's secondary prophylaxis duration gives a different cut-off age limits in comparison to the ACC/AHA one. The AHA uses a uniform cutoff age of 21 years

Category	Duration
RF with Carditis with severe valvular disease or After Valvular Surgery	Lifelong
RF with carditis (healed or mild mitral regurgitation)	10 years after the last attack or 25 years of age whichever is longer
RF without carditis	5 years or age of 18 years whichever is longer

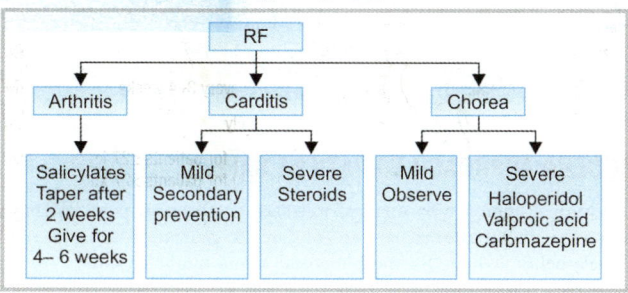

FLOWCHART 3: Types of prevention with RF/RHD

(Source: Modified from NEJM. 2007;357(2):439-41)

❑ SUGGESTED READINGS

Bryant PA, Brown RR, Carapetis JR, et al. Some of the people, some of the time. Circulation. 2009;119:742-53.

Dajani AS, Ayoub EM, Bierman FZ, et al. Guidelines for the diagnosis of rheumatic fever: Jones Criteria. JAMA. 1992;268:2069-73.

Gerber et al. AHA scientific statement. Circulation. 2009;119:1541-51.

Chapter 13

Evolving Concepts

13.1 Preventing Errors in Cardiovascular Medicine

❏ INTRODUCTION

Although medical mistakes have long bedevilled physicians and patients, the patient safety movement is a relatively recent phenomenon. In 2000, the Institute of Medicine published *To Err is Human: Building a Safer Health System*. This seminal report, which estimated that 44,000–98,000 people in the United States die each year from medical errors (the equivalent of a jumbo jet crashing each day), created a revolution in our approach to patient safety. Because patients can be harmed even when receiving pristine care, it is important to separate errors from adverse events. An error is usually defined as "an act or omission that leads to an unanticipated, undesirable outcome or to substantial potential for such an outcome". Adverse events, on the other hand, are injuries due to medical management rather than the patient's underlying illness. Although patients experiencing errors and adverse events may be injured equally, the distinction makes a large difference because the approaches to the two types of problems may be quite different.

❏ MODERN APPROACH TO PATIENT SAFETY

Our traditional approach to medical mistakes has been to point fingers at the provider who was at the "sharp end" of care. A generation ago, the notion of individuals being at fault for most medical errors might well have made some sense. Indeed, in the past decade we have learned that most medical mistakes are committed by hard working, well-trained caregivers. Given this, trying to get people to be more careful, or shaming or suing them is unlikely to be very helpful. Rather, the modern approach to medical errors, drawn largely from safer industries such as commercial aviation and nuclear power, emphasizes "systems thinking", which holds that human error is inevitable, and that the only way to productively deal with the problem is to try to build reliable systems that anticipate errors and either prevent or block them before they cause harm to patients. This model, well known in other industries and among safety scientists, was first introduced to medicine in the mid-1990s and did not become widely accepted until the past decade.

The best accepted mental model for systems thinking is the "Swiss cheese model" of "organizational accidents", articulated by English psychologist James Reason (Fig. 1). It highlights that it is important for us to not immediately focus on the smoking gun—the individual at the "sharp end" whose error began the cascade of events that led to harm—but rather to try to shrink the holes in the cheese and create multiple overlapping layers of protection to decrease the probability that the holes will ever align and let an error slip through to harm a patient.

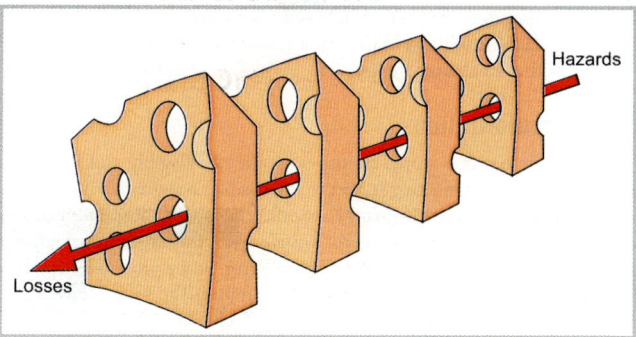

FIGURE 1: The Swiss cheese model for medical mistakes

Even when a physician understands the Swiss cheese model and instinctively tries to shore up the holes in the Swiss cheese rather than assigning blame, improving complex systems is a difficult thing to do. As one example, envision a system with so many robust double and triple checks that no patient with an ST-segment elevation myocardial infarction ever receives the wrong medication in the Emergency Department. That's great, but if the fix was too time-consuming and cumbersome, one of two problematic things would happen: either some patients would have unacceptably long door-to-needle times while their caregivers were performing their triple checks (and some would be harmed by this delay), or the providers would begin bypassing steps in order to give the patient the care he needed (workarounds). These two scenarios do not mean that creating new layers of defense (e.g. a checklist or a new double check) is wrong (it is often the right thing to do), but rather that systems need to be modified thoughtfully, with a lot of attention paid to how providers actually do their work. Some solutions that seem perfectly sensible when they are thought up in a committee meeting turn out to be unfeasible, and even unsafe, when they are implemented in a real-practice setting.

❑ HOW TO IMPROVE PATIENT SAFETY?

Redundancies, Standardization, and Forcing Functions

In keeping with the Swiss cheese model, the modern approach to patient safety focuses on the need to create robust, resilient systems that catch errors before they happen or prevent them from leading to patient harm. For example, errors in routine behaviors (slips) can best be prevented by building in redundancies and cross checks, in the form of checklists, read-backs (Let me read your order back to you) and other standardized safety procedures (e.g. counting the sponges and needles in the operating room to be sure that none have been left inside the patient, signing a surgical site prior to an operation to be sure to operate on the correct limb, asking patients their name before giving them a medication or drawing their blood).

Another important concept in safety is known as the "forcing function". The concept here is that increasing numbers of errors in health care occur as a result of people interacting with complex machinery and technologies. A forcing function is an engineering solution that decreases the probability of human error. In other words, in an error-prone interaction between people and machines, it is best to try to change the machine to prevent the error. This is virtually always easier and more reliable than trying to change the person.

Role of Computerization

Most information today is stored on paper, frequently illegibly and not entered or stored as structured data, making it next to impossible to aggregate it and analyze it for patterns. As patients move from office to office, hospital to hospital, even a clinical laboratory in a town back to their doctor's office down the street, information rarely flows seamlessly. The result is an extraordinarily error-prone process in which crucial data rarely accompanies patients as they move around. The Joint Commission has promoted the value of "medication reconciliation" (checking the medication list for consistency and accuracy at every visit and transition, such as when the patient leaves the ICU and goes to the floor) as a way to try to improve safety.

Luckily, health care is finally on the path to computerization, partly driven by the pressures to improve quality and safety (accompanied by increasingly aggressive requirements to report on clinical care and act on the results. Many hospitals and doctors' offices are implementing computer systems including computerized provider order entry (CPOE), electronic health records and a several other information technology solutions (bar-coding for medication administration, "smart" intravenous pumps). Healthcare information technology systems will become even more useful when they build "decision support", prompting a doctor to use a preferred antibiotic for a given infection, for example, or reminding her to check the creatinine after beginning an angiotensin-converting enzyme inhibitor. And newer decision support engines are emerging that will provide even more sophisticated decision-support, prompting the physician to consider a variety of diagnoses after he enters the patient's history, physical examination and laboratory results.

Ultimately, CPOE systems, when combined with electronic health records that are interoperable (meaning that even different computer systems can "talk to each other", in the same way that you can withdraw money from an ATM of a bank you do not generally use), are likely to provide new levels of safety. Modern systems are improving, becoming more user-friendly and intuitive and building in critical functions sought by caregivers. And patients are becoming key participants, as some modern systems allow them to schedule visits, review their laboratory data and read the literature about their medical problems. While this level of patient engagement will present new challenges (particularly since patients may be misinformed by some of the things they read on the internet), the potential to improve quality and safety is great.

❏ COMMUNICATION AND CULTURE

In the Joint Commission's (the main accreditor of US hospitals) database, communication failures underlie the majority of serious errors. Analysis of these errors has taught us that many are caused by dysfunctional relationships between doctors and nurses, between trainees and supervisors or between patients and providers. We have learned that medicine tends to have "steep hierarchies" in which individuals lower on the totem pole are reluctant to question the opinion of a superior. This problem is also known as an "authority gradient".

The early evidence that healthcare communication or crew resource management (CRM) as in aviation industry will improve patient safety is encouraging but somewhat mixed, partly because changing the culture of a busy med-surg floor or cardiac intensive care unit is substantially more difficult than doing so in a sealed cockpit.

The term "culture of safety" is used as shorthand for an environment in which teamwork, clear communication and openness about errors (both to other health care professionals and to patients) is at work. While this term has, in the past, implied a completely blameless culture, a more mature model has emerged in recent years, often described as a "Just Culture". The Just Culture model recognizes that most errors are, in fact, blameless—committed by good people trying to get it right—and that blaming and finger pointing are counterproductive in these circumstances. On the other hand, willful disregard of safety rules, disruptive behavior or nonremediable incompetence are not blameless, they are blameworthy. The patient safety field is presently grappling with how to get this balance between "no blame" and accountability right.

❑ LEARNING FROM MISTAKES

Another key safety principle is to learn from one's mistakes. Over the past several years, there has been an increasing emphasis on this area, since it is difficult for caregivers and systems to improve if they do not learn from their prior errors. While traditional mortality and morbidity (M&M) conferences often involved only physicians, there is a modern emphasis on interdisciplinary communication (involving the appropriate disciplines, including doctors, nurses and hospital administrators), identifying errors and emphasizing systems thinking and solutions. Moreover, many organizations have embraced a technique drawn from engineering called Root Cause Analysis—a blame-free forum that brings together experts and leaders as well as the involved providers. The goal of these sessions is to analyze major errors in detail, to discover all of the system weaknesses that need to be improved and to create action plans with strong follow-up.

❑ CREATING A SAFE WORKFORCE

While systems are critical to patient safety, there is no substitute for a well-trained, well-staffed and well-rested workforce in delivering safe care. There is now strong evidence linking low nurse-to-patient ratios, long resident work hours and lack of physician board certification to poor patient outcomes. A variety of interventions have been implemented in response to this evidence. Although the impact of these regulations on patient safety is still debated, the new focus on the workforce is overdue and welcome. It seems only a matter of time before some similar work hour restrictions are placed on the work of practicing physicians, mirroring limits on commercial airline pilots and truck drivers.

❑ PREVENTING DIAGNOSTIC ERRORS

Autopsy studies have shown high rates of missed diagnoses, rates that have not gone down appreciably over recent years despite new imaging technologies, such as CAT and MRI scanners, and laboratory studies, such as troponins and BNPs. Part of the reason for the relative inattention to diagnostic errors is that they seem, at first glance, to represent simple human failings and bad thinking. But recent research has demonstrated that some, perhaps many, diagnostic errors can be prevented. As described earlier, some of the improvements will come from modern computerized decision-support systems, which are beginning to develop the capacity to automatically suggest possible diagnoses and point users to helpful resources and articles.

How can the errors caused by faulty thinking be prevented? As always, the answer will come through a systems approach, but here this means the creation of better systems to train physicians to avoid common diagnostic mistakes. The most hopeful approach is known as "metacognition", in which physicians are trained to think about their own thinking, and be aware of risk factors for diagnostic errors. This is often best done by asking hypothetical questions like, "what is the worst thing this could be?" or "if this patient dies tonight and I had missed the diagnosis, what would that diagnosis have been?"

❏ WHAT CAN PATIENTS DO TO KEEP THEMSELVES SAFE?

Without doubt, some errors can be prevented by engaged patients or family members who remain vigilant and are willing to ask questions when they notice something amiss, whether it is a medication that seems wrong or a doctor who has failed to wash his hands before touching them. However, patient engagement has only limited value as a safety strategy.

❏ CHANGING POLICY CONTEXT FOR PATIENT SAFETY

Most American hospitals are accredited by the Joint Commission, which has issued dozens of safety standards in the past several years, and now engages in unannounced surveys at regular intervals. The majority of US states now require reporting of any of these events, reports that can trigger state inspections and fines. Finally, Medicare, the dominant payer for US health care, will now no longer reimburse hospitals for the cost of caring for some of these "never events". Obviously, these policy initiatives, combined with other quality-oriented initiatives that emphasize public reporting of key outcome and process data, create an environment in which hospitals and physicians now must focus on certain quality and safety hazards.

❏ SUGGESTED READINGS

Gawande AA. The Checklist Manifesto: How to Get Things Right. New York: Metropolitan Books; 2010.

Kohn L, Corrigan J, Donaldson M. To Err is Human: Building a Safer Health System. Washington DC Committee on Quality of Health Care in America, Institute of Medicine. National Academy Press; 2000.

Nasca TJ, Day SH, Amis ES Jr. ACGME Duty Hour Task Force. The new recommendations on duty hours from the ACGME Task Force. N Engl J Med. 2010;363:e3.

Pronovost PJ, Faden RR. Setting priorities for patient safety: ethics, accountability and public engagement. JAMA. 2009;302:890-1.

Salas E, Wilson KA, Burke CS, et al. Does crew resource management training work? An update, an extension and some critical needs. Hum Factors. 2006;48:392-412.

Schnipper JL, Hamann C, Ndumele CD, et al. Effect of an electronic medication reconciliation application and process redesign on potential adverse drug events: a cluster-randomized trial. Arch Intern Med. 2009;169:771-80.

Wachter RM, Foster NE, Dudley RA. Medicare's decision to withhold payment for hospital errors: the devil is in the details. Jt Comm J Qual Patient Saf. 2008;34:116-23.

13.2 Integrative Cardiology: The Use of Complementary Therapies and Beyond

❑ NONCONVENTIONAL THERAPIES AND CARDIOLOGY

The use of nonconventional medical therapies is tremendously popular and growing in the United States with 38% of adults using some form of complementary and alternative medicine (CAM) according to the 2007 National Health Interview Survey. Cardiovascular patients are no exception. Select surveys suggest half or more of cardiovascular patients are using CAM. Yet one report reveals that cardiologists have little knowledge about CAM and harbor negative attitudes toward it. This situation begs the question: is it possible to use CAM in cardiology in a way that is evidence-based and integrates CAM therapies with the many effective and powerful conventional cardiovascular therapies? The answer is addressed by the field of integrative cardiology.

❑ WHAT IS INTEGRATIVE MEDICINE?

Integrative medicine is the integration of CAM and conventional medicine, but also much more. Integrative medicine is evidence-based and patient-centered. It recognizes the importance of the relationship with the patient, seeing it as the central therapeutic element. It is holistic in its approach, assessing the mind, body, spirit, social, community and environmental dimensions of health. According to the useful system of categorization proposed by the National Institutes of Health (NIH) [through the National Center for Complementary and Alternative Medicine (NCCAM)], CAM can be divided into the following five categories:
1. Biologically based therapies (e.g. use of natural products such as fish oil, probiotics, botanical medicines, etc.).
2. Mind-body medicine (e.g. biofeedback, meditation, hypnosis, guided imagery).
3. Manual medicine (e.g. osteopathy, chiropractic, massage therapy).
4. Energy medicine (e.g. reiki, therapeutic touch).
5. Whole systems (e.g. traditional Chinese medicine, ayurveda, homeopathy).

❑ WHAT IS INTEGRATIVE CARDIOLOGY?

Integrative cardiology is the application of integrative medicine principles to the field of cardiology. The Lifestyle Heart Trial is an instructional example. This was a rigorous randomized controlled trial with 5-year follow-up. The original trial, published in Lancet in 1990, demonstrated that reversal of coronary atherosclerosis can be achieved with comprehensive lifestyle changes and usual cardiologic care (excluding, importantly, lipid-lowering medications). Five-year follow-up of these patients showed extension of these findings, i.e. the experimental group showed further regression of disease and the control group showed further progression.

There are many other integrative therapies that have evidence of efficacy for cardiovascular conditions. This chapter reviews some of the integrative therapies for the most common cardiovascular conditions.

❑ DYSLIPIDEMIA

Diet

With respect to whole diets controversy continues over which are the most successful whole dietary changes for dyslipidemia. The diet that may be most consistent with integrative medicine is the portfolio diet. This approach begins with a baseline healthy diet for dyslipidemia (e.g. primarily plant-based ATP step III diet) and integrates additional specific foods that have been shown to improve dyslipidemia (soluble fiber, soy, almonds and plant sterols). Outcomes from the portfolio approach have been excellent and comparable to low-dose statin therapy. In addition to whole diets there are several specific foods that have been shown to effectively treat dyslipidemia: plant sterols, soy, nuts, barley, oats, alcohol [increases high density lipoprotein (HDL)], fish (reduces triglycerides, berries (increases HDL), kale juice (increases HDL), olive oil, and cocoa.

Exercise

Studies consistently show that aerobic exercise reduces serum triglycerides and increases HDL cholesterol. This effect is independent of weight loss, although with weight loss the effect is potentiated. There is also a dose-response relationship between exercise and improvement in triglycerides and HDL cholesterol, with greater amount of exercise or more intense exercise resulting in greater lipid benefits. Aerobic exercise can also benefit total and low-density lipoprotein (LDL) cholesterol levels in some patients although results of these studies are not as universally positive.

Botanical Medicines and Supplements

Fish oil: Health benefits from fish oil come from its content of the essential omega-3 fatty acids eicosapentaenoic acid (EPA) and docosahexaenoic acid (DHA). DHA and EPA can be acquired by consuming cold water fatty fish such as herring, sardine, anchovy, kipper, menhaden, salmon and trout. The most potent lipid-related effect that fish oil has is to lower triglycerides. There are multiple mechanisms by which fish oils are thought to lower triglycerides, most notably by decreasing synthesis and secretion of very low-density lipoproteins (VLDLs) and by increasing VLDL apolipoprotein B secretion. There are dozens of clinical trials that have proven the effectiveness of fish oil for reducing serum triglycerides. The magnitude of benefit can be comparable to pharmaceutical treatment. Additional clinical trials examining the combination of a statin with fish oil have shown added benefit on lipid profiles. The American Heart Association recommends that people with hypertriglyceridemia consume 2–4 gm of omega-3 fatty acids per day and there is a proprietary formulation of fish oil that is FDA-approved for use in patients with hypertriglyceridemia. Fish oil supplements should be dosed based on their content of EPA and DHA.

Red rice yeast: Red rice yeast (often called "red yeast rice") is the product of rice fermented with *Monascus purpureus* yeast and has been used in China since at least 800 AD as part of Chinese medicine to enhance circulation and for other indications. Red rice yeast contains a family of naturally occurring substances called monacolins that have 3-hydroxy-3-methyl-glutaryl (HMG)-CoA reductase inhibitor activity. One of these compounds is lovastatin. These compounds constitute about 0.4% of red rice yeast. A typical dose delivers the equivalent of approximately 4 mg of lovastatin daily. The fact that so little lovastatin is present, and that red rice yeast also contains beta-sitosterol, isoflavones and monounsaturated fatty acids, suggests this medicine works to lower cholesterol through multiple mechanisms. The Food and Drug Administration (FDA), however, considers these products to be unapproved drugs when they contain statins.

Plant stanols and sterols: Plant stanols and sterols occur naturally in various plants, and as such they are available through diet. They can be ingested as supplements in the form of enhanced margarine, or other enhanced food products, and as tablets. They inhibit cholesterol absorption from the GI tract by displacing cholesterol from mixed micelles. Beta-sitosterol may also lower cholesterol by increasing bile acid secretion. There are many high-quality studies, including thousands of patients, show plant stanols lower total and LDL cholesterol. There are also good studies showing this is an effective adjunctive therapy to statins. There are no studies, however, that adequately assess clinical endpoints, such as reduced incidence of CAD.

Psyllium: Psyllium is the common name of plants in the genus *Plantago*. Husks of the seeds of *Plantago ovata* are widely used medicinally for constipation, hyperlipidemia and other indications. Psyllium decreases serum cholesterol levels by binding dietary fats in the GI tract and decreasing systemic absorption. Bile acid excretion of cholesterol in the feces is also increased and enterohepatic recirculation is decreased. Furthermore in response the liver uses more cholesterol to make bile acid. Dozens of RCTs and at least three meta-analyses prove the efficacy of psyllium to reduce total and LDL cholesterol levels, both in the 5–10% range. Benefit is additive with statin medications.

Beta-glucan: Beta-glucan is a soluble fiber from the cell walls of plants and microscopic organisms. It is found especially in whole grains such as oats and barley. Most supplements are yeast-derived (*Saccharomyces cerevisiae*). Beta-glucan lowers cholesterol by blocking cholesterol absorption at the luminal surface of the intestinal mucosa, forming a physical barrier. Like psyllium, beta-glucan may also work by binding bile acids in the intestinal lumen. Although not as extensively studied in clinical trials, beta-glucan supplementation does appear to modestly reduce total and LDL cholesterol levels, usually in the 2–8% range.

Artichoke leaf extract: Artichoke is one of the oldest medicinal plants. Artichoke leaf extract stimulate bile flow. Additional mechanisms of action which may account for lipid-lowering effect are inhibition of cholesterol synthesis and inhibition of HMG-CoA reductase by luteolin. Six randomized trials of artichoke leaf extract for the treatment of hypercholesterolemia have been published. A 2009 Cochrane review concluded that the lipid-lowering effects of artichoke extract are supported by *in vitro* and animal studies, but more trials with larger sample sizes are needed to recommend its use for lipid-lowering in humans.

Garlic: Garlic is one of the most popular medicinal herbs in Europe and the United States. It has been used since antiquity for the treatment of cardiovascular and infectious diseases. The German Federal Health Agency Commission E and the European Scientific Cooperative on Phytotherapy have approved its use for the treatment of hyperlipidemia and atherosclerosis. The primary mechanism of action of garlic is theorized to be HMGCoA reductase inhibition. Another proposed mechanism is increased excretion of bile salts. Despite the publication of many dozens of trials over many years, evidence of the effect of garlic on serum lipids is inconclusive.

Cocoa: The blood-pressure lowering effect of cocoa is better understood and better proven than its lipid-lowering effect, but proposed mechanisms for lipid-lowering are: (i) delayed LDL oxidation thereby reducing LDL concentration, and (ii) reduced intestinal absorption of cholesterol and bile acids by decreasing solubility of micellar cholesterol. Although there is good evidence of benefit for reduction of blood pressure and vascular endothelium reactivity, there is only early clinical evidence of cocoa's effect on lipids.

Coenzyme Q10: Although coenzyme Q10 (CoQ10) appears to be effective for some cardiovascular conditions (reducing blood pressure and treating HF—see below) it does not have a lipid-lowering effect. Nevertheless, it merits consideration in the treatment of dyslipidemia because of its possible utility in patients taking statin drugs. Statins block the synthesis of CoQ10, dramatically reduce CoQ10 levels in plasma and skeletal muscle. It has been widely theorized therefore that some of the statin-related side effects, such as myalgia, myositis and rhabdomyolysis, may be mediated through CoQ10 depletion. There have only been two small RCTs to examine whether CoQ10 supplementation can prevent statin-induced myalgias. One reported the positive effect of CoQ10 and the other reported no effect. Further study is needed.

❑ HYPERTENSION

Diet

A variety of dietary modifications are beneficial in the prevention and treatment of hypertension, including the DASH diet (from the Dietary Approaches to Stop Hypertension trial), increased fruit and vegetable consumption, reduction of sodium intake, moderation of alcohol, vegetarian diet and possibly increasing potassium and calcium intake. There are also specific foods that help to lower blood pressure such as cocoa, soy, fish and fiber. Increased fruit and vegetable intake has also been independently shown to reduce blood pressure in hypertensives, as have salt reduction and alcohol reduction. Vegetarian diet also appears to reduce blood pressure, as does a diet with increased fiber. As an individual food, cocoa has also been shown in multiple well-designed studies to be effective at lowering blood pressure. Adding soy or fish to the diet likely also lowers blood pressure.

Exercise

It is well-established that in patients with essential hypertension regular aerobic exercise can lower blood pressure. Resistance training also lowers blood pressure although typically to a lesser degree. Tai Chi, a Chinese martial art that today is practiced more commonly for its health benefits, also appears to lower blood pressure. Yoga similarly can lower blood pressure according to a few studies; however, it has been recommended that patients with cardiovascular risk factors or known cerebrovascular disease should avoid inverted postures (e.g. shoulderstand, headstand) due to risk of acute elevation of intracerebral pressure. Data from the Framingham heart study and elsewhere show that weight loss can reduce blood pressure.

Sleep

Nighttime blood pressure in particular importantly affects cardiovascular health. The common sleep disorder obstructive sleep apnea has a strong correlation with hypertension and cardiovascular mortality. Perhaps more importantly in terms of overall number of people affected, studies have also shown a link between both insomnia and sleep deprivation and the incidence of hypertension.

Mental Health

Although the relationship between depression and cardiovascular morbidity and mortality has been known for some time, the more recent research on positive emotions raises the corollary possibility that cultivating positive emotions may lower blood pressure and improve cardiovascular health. Again, an integrative evaluation and treatment of hypertension would include addressing mental health.

Mind-body Medicine

Biofeedback and meditation are two mind-body medicine modalities, which have been researched for their effects on hypertension. Biofeedback is a behavioral therapy method that teaches a patient to gain greater awareness and control of autonomic nervous function that is not normally under conscious control. This is achieved by using technology that presents to the patient in visual or auditory form the level of activity of a physiologic parameter, such as muscle tension, skin temperature, sweat gland activity, respiratory muscle activity, PCO_2, heart rate variability (HRV) or brain wave pattern. According to the many studies on this topic thermal (i.e. skin temperature) and electrodermal (i.e. galvanic skin response) biofeedback methods most consistently help patients lower their blood pressure more than other types of biofeedback.

The two forms of meditation that have been most thoroughly examined for medical indications are mindfulness meditation and transcendental meditation (TM). With respect to cardiology TM has been more studied. Transcendental meditation is a mantra-based meditation method derived from the ancient Vedic practices of India. Research on the basic science and physiology of TM began in the early 1970s and, although the precise mechanism of action is unknown, extensive studies have been conducted showing reduced respiratory rate, decreased total peripheral resistance, decreased beta-receptor sensitivity, reduced epinephrine and norepinephrine levels, increased alpha wave activity on EEG and reduced skin conductance (a surrogate marker for decreased sympathetic tone).

Botanical Medicines and Supplements

Garlic: The proposed mechanism for the effect of garlic on blood pressure is increased nitric oxide production and endothelium-dependent dilation.

Fish oil: The mechanism by which fish oil lowers blood pressure is increased production of prostacyclin, a prostaglandin which causes vasodilation, and reduces platelet aggregation. Fish oil also appears to improve arterial compliance.

Coenzyme Q10: CoQ10 appears to lower blood pressure by increasing endothelial production of prostacyclin and thereby enhancing endothelium-independent arterial relaxation and endothelium-dependent vasodilation.

Hibiscus (Hibiscus sabdariffa): This red-flowered plant is well-known around the world as an ornamental and as a type of herbal tea. Extracts of hibiscus contain significant amounts of vitamin C, anthocyanins, and polyphenols but the mechanism by which it lowers blood pressure is unknown. *In vitro* and animal studies suggest the possible mechanisms of action which include calcium channel antagonism, diuresis and inhibition of angiotensin-converting enzyme.

Pycnogenol: Pycnogenol® is the brand name for an extract of the bark of the French Maritime Pine tree (Pinus pinaster). Like most botanical products it contains a large number of bioactive compounds. The high concentration of flavonoids, particularly oligomeric proanthocyanidins (OPCs), is particularly noteworthy because of their strong antioxidant activity. Mechanisms by which pycnogenol may reduce blood pressure are increased nitric oxide production, decreased thromboxane B2 levels (a vasoconstrictor) and angiotension-converting enzyme inhibition.

Pomegranate (Punica granatum): Pomegranate juice increases nitric oxide synthetase activity in blood vessel endothelium, thereby increasing nitric oxide levels leading to vasodilation. The juice also reduces angiotensin-converting enzyme (ACE) activity. The polyphenol content of pomegranate juice is very high. Conclusions about the clinical efficacy of pomegranate juice for hypertension have not been drawn yet.

Potassium: Dozens of trials show that potassium supplementation modestly lowers the blood pressure in hypertensive patients. The effect is small (2–4 mm Hg systolic, 0–3 mm Hg diastolic) but significant. Nevertheless, a 2006 Cochrane review concluded that additional high quality trials are needed before a conclusion can be made.

L-arginine: Arginine is an amino acid found in many foods, including dairy products, meat, poultry and fish. Arginine increases nitric oxide levels which causes vasodilation and reduction of blood pressure. Although there are several studies on the use of L-arginine for other cardiovascular conditions (e.g. coronary heart disease, chronic HF, peripheral vascular disease) there are only three trials totaling 66 patients looking at its effect on hypertension. They all show benefit. Interestingly, there is some evidence in humans that arginine supplementation may potentiate the effect of ACE inhibitors.

❏ CORONARY ARTERY DISEASE

Diet

With respect to diet there are whole diets and specific foods that are associated with prevention of CAD. The whole diets are: (i) the Mediterranean diet, (ii) a fruit and vegetable-rich diet, (iii) the Ornish diet, (iv) a low glycemic index diet, (v) a diet that replaces saturated fat and trans fat with monounsaturated or polyunsaturated fat and (6) a high-fiber diet. Specific foods that prevent or improve coronary heart disease are fish, alcohol, red wine and nuts. The Mediterranean diet has been defined as a diet high in fruits and vegetables, whole grains and legumes, with low-to-moderate amounts of fish, poultry and dairy products (mostly as cheese and yogurt), 0–4 eggs per week, and olive oil as the principal fat. The diet is very low in meat and a low-to-moderate amount of wine is consumed. The Ornish diet is a very low-fat vegetarian diet comprised mostly of beans, fruits, vegetables and whole grains.

Exercise

Sedentary lifestyle is a confirmed risk factor for the development of CAD and exercise is proven to beneficially impact CAD risk factors.

Sleep

In prospective observational studies, an inverse relationship is found between all markers of poor sleep quality (i.e. reduced sleep duration, difficulty falling asleep, frequent awakenings and unrefreshing sleep) and risk of CAD. Another prospective study found that difficulty falling asleep correlated with CAD mortality.

Mental Health

The effect that the mind has on cardiovascular health manifests in many ways. The relationship of stress to cardiovascular disease has been a challenging topic for research. At the physiological level stress causes endothelial dysfunction and increases cardiovascular work demand. In humans there is an association between chronic stress and increased CAD. Stress can cause angina and stressful life events are associated with an increase in cardiovascular events. Personality factors that appear to predispose to CAD are hostility and social competitiveness. It should be noted also that there is a correlation between acute anger and myocardial infarction.

Depression has been very strongly correlated with incidence of CHD as well as worsening of CHD outcomes. Although it has been shown that both behavioral and pharmaceutical methods can successfully treat depression in patients with CHD, the research on whether treatment of depression can improve CHD outcomes is less clear. Most observational studies of religious affiliation and participation consistently have shown an inverse correlation with cardiovascular mortality.

Mind-body Medicine Therapies

Biofeedback is a modality that has proven capacity to favorably affect HRV, including in patients with heart disease. Poor HRV in post-MI patients is strongly predictive of short-term and long-term mortality. Guided imagery appears to be effective in reducing pain and anxiety perioperatively in cardiac surgical patients. Transcendental meditation studies have shown benefit from this modality for several CAD risk factors as well as HRV, but there are no randomized, controlled trials with hard clinical CAD outcomes.

Enhanced External Counterpulsation

Enhanced external counterpulsation (EECP) is a nonpharmacologic, noninvasive therapy that uses three sets of pneumatic stockings on each lower extremity (calves, lower thighs and upper thighs/buttocks) whose inflation and deflation are timed to the patient's electrocardiogram. The hemodynamic effect of EECP is similar to the intra-aortic balloon pump in that it increases diastolic coronary blood flow (diastolic augmentation), decreases afterload and increases venous return and preload. EECP may also favorably affect endothelial function and the development of collateral coronary circulation. Comparable rates of survival/Coronary artery bypass grafting/Percutaneous coronary intervention have been found in patients with CAD who received EECP compared to patients who underwent PCI even though EECP patients had more severe disease at baseline. Follow-up studies show benefits are maintained for one, two and 3 years post-EECP.

Botanical Medicines and Supplements

Fish oil: It is likely that multiple mechanisms explain the beneficial effects of omega-3 fatty acids for both primary and secondary prevention of cardiac disease.

These include reductions in dysrhythmias, inflammation, blood pressure, blood clotting, atherosclerotic plaque formation, triglyceride levels and improvements in arterial and endothelial function. The American Heart Association recommends 1 gm/day of omega-3 fatty acids for those with CAD and 500 mg/day for those without CAD.

Garlic: The antiatherosclerotic mechanisms of garlic are thought to be reduction of oxidative stress to endothelial cells, possibly by preventing glutathione depletion in these cells, and inhibition of LDL oxidation.

Carnitine: The precise mechanism by which carnitine may work in CAD is not known. Tissue carnitine levels have been shown to decrease in people with angina and myocardial ischemia, so the known essential role of carnitine in the generation of cellular energy may explain its effect in angina. Carnitine may also have a vasodilatory effect that is prostaglandin-dependent and not nitric oxide-dependent.

Ribose: There is animal evidence that in hypoxic myocardial tissue ribose supplementation helps restore ATP levels. And there is a single human RCT of 20 patients with CAD concluding that ribose significantly prolongs the time to ST-segment depression and angina during exercise treadmill testing.

❏ HEART FAILURE

Diet

High sodium intake has been associated with HF exacerbations. Low sodium intake and fluid restriction are recommended for people with HF, including by the American College of Cardiology. And although there are favorable clinical outcomes documented for patients with hypertension who restrict sodium intake, there is surprisingly little research on HF outcomes.

Exercise

A much better evidence base exists for the benefits of aerobic exercise in HF. Several RCTs have shown outcomes of enhanced exercise capacity, reduced hospitalization, increase survival and improved quality of life. Resistance training has been less extensively studied in HF and some studies that have looked at adding resistance training to aerobic exercise have shown benefit. A specific kind of strength training, inspiratory muscle training (IMT), has been shown in several studies to be effective for reducing symptoms, increasing exercise tolerance and improving quality of life. Neuromuscular electrical stimulation (NMES) that uses electricity to stimulate lower extremity muscles to simulate strength training, Tai Chi, yoga and yogic breathing in HF have all shown benefits, including improved exercise tolerance, dyspnea, endurance and strength.

Mental Health

Depression has an important bidirectional relationship with HF. HF is associated with much higher rates of depression than exists in the general population (or even the chronic disease population) and conversely depression is associated with higher mortality and hospital readmission rate in HF. Although pharmacologic therapy was no more effective than placebo in ameliorating depression or improving cardiovascular status, a combination of exercise plus cognitive behavioral therapy (CBT) versus exercise alone versus CBT alone versus usual care and found that the combined treatment reduced depression and improved 6-minute walk distance at 24 weeks.

Mind-body Therapies

Biofeedback and meditation have been examined for their effect in treating HF. In a controlled pilot study of elders with HF, a 10-week training in HRV-based biofeedback significantly improved psychological parameters and increased 6-minute walk distance. Surprisingly HRV did not change. Studies on meditation and HF showed fewer self-reported symptoms and improved clinical scores compared to controls, reduced norepinephrine levels, improved ventilatory efficiency and improved quality of life.

Enhanced External Counterpulsation

Enhanced external counterpulsation (EECP) increases diastolic filling, reduces afterload and appears to be effective for the treatment of angina. Subsets of patients with HF in angina studies appear to have benefitted from EECP. A RCT of EECP in HF showed significantly improved exercise tolerance, change in NYHA functional class and quality of life.

Botanical Medicines and Supplements

Hawthorn (*Crataegus monogyna*): The plant's content of flavonoids and oligomeric proanthocyanidins are thought to be responsible for most of its physiologic effects. Hawthorn has many mechanisms by which it may affect HF. It increases cardiomyocyte membrane permeability to calcium and inhibits phosphodiesterase (thus increasing intracellular cAMP). At the physiological level hawthorn has been shown to increase cardiac output, increase inotropy, increase coronary blood flow, decrease blood pressure and decrease total peripheral resistance, all of which may be favorable hemodynamic changes for congestive HF. Since hawthorn prolongs the refractory period of cardiomyocytes, it is less arrhythmogenic than other inotropic agents.

Coenzyme Q10 (Ubiquinone): The main proposed mechanism of action of CoQ10 in HF is the replenishment of CoQ10 levels leading to improved myocardial ATP production. Indeed it has been shown that CoQ10 preserves myocardial sodium-potassium ATPase activity, increases in vitro myocardial tolerance to hypoxia-reoxygenation stress and improves diastolic function in patients taking statins. Other mechanisms may include lowering of blood pressure and prevention of oxidative damage.

Fish oil: The main mechanism by which omega-3 fatty acids in fish oils provide clinical benefit in HF appears to be a reduction of dysrhythmias through a membrane stabilizing effect involving sodium, potassium and calcium channels. Other possible mechanisms include vasodilation, improved arterial compliance, reduction of heart rate, anti-inflammatory effect, reduction of BNP and maintenance of favorable renal hemodynamics. Fish oil should not be used in patients with implantable cardiac defibrillators due to conflicting results from clinical trials and the possibility, shown in one study, that fish oil could be pro-dysrhythmic in these patients.

Taurine: The mechanism by which it may affect HF is unknown, but there is evidence that it may reduce catecholamine levels and sympathetic tone as well as increase LV function by modulating intracellular calcium influx.

Carnitine: Carnitine supplementation may enhance myocardial energy production and is the likely mechanism for any effect in HF. Studies have showed benefits, including reduced mortality, reduced symptoms, improved exercise capacity, oxygen consumption and echocardiographic parameters including ejection fraction.

Arginine: Arginine's mechanism of action in HF is likely the same as in hypertension: increased production of nitric oxide and consequent vasodilation. Arginine may also have ACE inhibiting activity. It also seems to potentiate pharmaceutical ACE inhibitors.

Creatine: Creatine as phosphocreatine forms a pool of energy-containing phosphate bonds from which muscle (both skeletal and myocardial) cells can draw when replenishing their ATP levels. The ratio of phosphocreatine to ATP in the myocardium of patients with HF is lower than the ratio found in people without HF and the ratio correlates inversely with the severity of HF. Since creatine is metabolized by the kidneys concern has been raised over potential nephrotoxicity. Creatine supplementation can cause an increase in measured serum creatinine. This usually does not reflect impaired renal function but in such cases further clinical investigation would of course be warranted.

Magnesium (Mg^{++}): Magnesium regulates key ion channels in myocardial cells and helps to maintain the critical transmembrane gradients of sodium and potassium. The purported mechanisms of action of magnesium supplementation in HF are antiarrhythmic effect, decreased coronary vascular resistance, increased coronary artery blood flow and decreased systemic vascular resistance. Hypomagnesemia is one of the most common electrolyte abnormalities in HF patients. Diuretic therapy likely is a common cause as are poor dietary habits. Although hypomagnesemia is associated with increased ventricular ectopic activity in HF, the clinical significance of this is unknown.

Thiamine: It is a water-soluble B vitamin, important as a cofactor in carbohydrate metabolism and production of ATP. Thiamine deficiency can cause a syndrome that includes HF (wet beriberi). Loop diuretics increase urinary thiamine excretion and can cause thiamine deficiency. This may be a common phenomenon.

❑ SUGGESTED READINGS

Anderson JW, Allgood LD, Lawrence A, et al. Cholesterol-lowering effects of psyllium intake adjunctive to diet therapy in men and women with hypercholesterolemia: meta-analysis of 8 controlled trials. Am J Clin Nutr. 2000;71:472-9.

Anderson JW, Liu C, Kryscio RJ. Blood pressure response to transcendental meditation: a meta-analysis. Am J Hypertens. 2008; 21:310-6.

Appel LJ, Moore TJ, Obarzanek E, et al. DASH Collaborative Research Group. N Engl J Med. 1997;336:1117-24.

Arena R, Pinkstaff S, Wheeler E, et al. Neuromuscular electrical stimulation and inspiratory muscle training as potential adjunctive rehabilitation options for patients with heart failure. J Cardiopulm Rehabil Prev. 2010;30:209-23.

Balk EM, Lichtenstein AH, Chung M, et al. Effects of omega-3 fatty acids on serum markers of cardiovascular disease risk: a systematic review. Atherosclerosis. 2006;189:19-30.

Barnes PM, Bloom B, Nahin RL. Complementary and alternative medicine use among adults and children: United States, 2007. Natl Health Stat Report; 2008. pp. 1-23.

Berkman LF, Blumenthal J, Burg M, et al. Effects of treating depression and low perceived social support on clinical events after myocardial infarction: the Enhancing Recovery in Coronary Heart Disease Patients (ENRICHD) Randomized Trial. JAMA. 2003;289:3106-16.

Ceremuzyński L, Gebalska J, Wolk R, et al. Hypomagnesemia in heart failure with ventricular arrhythmias. Beneficial effects of magnesium supplementation. J Intern Med. 2000;247: 78-86.

Hewson MG, Copeland HL, Mascha E, et al. Integrative medicine: implementation and evaluation of a professional development program using experiential learning and conceptual change teaching approaches. Patient Educ Couns. 2006;62:5-12.

Moore CS, Bryant SP, Mishra GD, et al. Oily fish reduces plasma triacylglycerols: a primary prevention study in overweight men and women. Nutrition. 2006;22:1012-24.

Patel C, North WS. Randomised controlled trial of yoga and biofeedback in management of hypertension. Lancet. 1975;2:93-5.

Phillips B, Mannino DM. Do insomnia complaints cause hypertension or cardiovascular disease? J Clin Sleep Med. 2007;3:489-94.

Willett WC, Sacks F, Trichopoulou A, et al. Mediterranean diet pyramid: a cultural model for healthy eating. Am J Clin Nutr. 1995;61:1402S-6S.

Yeh GY, Wang C, Wayne PM, et al. The effect of tai-chi exercise on blood pressure: a systematic review. Prev Cardiol. 2008;11:82-9.

Index

Page numbers followed by *f* refer to figure and *t* refer to table

A

Abciximab 68
Abdominojugular reflux 79
ACE inhibitors 775
Acebutolol 465
Acetazolamide 1, 5, 6
Acetylsalicylic acid 64
Acidosis 315
Acids eicosapentaenoic acid 824
Acquired immunodeficiency syndrome 713
Active ischemia 278
Acute
  aortic
    dissection 73*t*, 164, 483
    regurgitation 195
  care 266
  chest pain syndromes 168
  coronary
    artery thrombosis 706
    syndromes 70, 116, 333, 354, 360, 518, 554, 707, 728
  exacerbation of COPD 760
  heart failure syndromes 545, 555*f*, 556
    management 548
  ischemic syndromes 774
  limb ischemia 472
  management 753
  mitral regurgitation 390*t*
    causes of 389*t*
  myocardial infarction 97*f*, 344, 633*f*, 697, 734
  pericardial tamponade 635
  pericarditis 73*t*, 113*f*, 631, 633*f*, 641
  pulmonary embolism 70, 73*t*, 749
  renal failure 191
  rheumatic fever 816*t*
  right ventricular infarction 364
  severe
    AR 379
    mitral regurgitation 86
  stroke 805*t*
  type B dissection 488
Acyanotic heart disease 665
Adenosine 239, 266, 267, 349
  dinucleotide phosphate 338
    receptor antagonists 338
  monophosphate 33*f*
  triphosphate 33*f*
Adherens junctions 285
Adhesion molecules 188
Adrenal
  disorders 745
  insufficiency 746
Adrenergic
  inhibitors 467
  receptor agonists 32
Adult congenital heart disease 646
Airway management 313, 313
Alagille syndrome 409
Alcohol 695, 791
  abstinence 793
  abuse 462
  consumption 696
Aldosterone 26, 522
  receptor antagonists 3
Aliskiren 467
Alkylating agents 792
Alpha-adrenergic effects 706
Alpha-linolenic acid 53
Alzheimer's disease 784
Ambulatory electrocardiography 764
American
  College of Cardiology 259*f*, 402*t*
  Heart Association 169, 259*f*, 402*t*
  Society of
    Echocardiography 156
    Nuclear Cardiology 550
Amiloride 1, 2, 7, 464
Amiodarone 235, 237, 240, 241, 242, 267, 316
  induced thyroid disease 743
  skin toxicity benign 76
Amlodipine 20, 25, 49
Amoxicillin 431, 814, 815
AMP-activated protein kinase 746
AMPK *See* AMP-activated protein kinase
Amyloid 616
  heart disease 616
  precursor proteins 616
Amyloidosis, classification of 617
Anabolic steroids 712
Anemia 734, 738, 739
Angioedema 351
Angiograms 407*f*
Angiosarcoma 148

Angiotensin
  converting enzyme 479, 522, 667, 723, 792
    inhibitors 19, 22, 351, 357, 393, 466, 521*f*, 555*f*, 703, 820
  receptor
    blockers 24, 393, 555*f*, 624
    blocking agents 531
Ankle brachial index 474
Ankylosing spondylitis 77, 374, 721
Annuloplasty techniques 402
Annulus disorders 389
Anomalous
  coronary arteries 176
  left coronary artery 213
  origin of coronary artery 213
Anorexia 712
Anterior
  axillary line's intersection 103
  mitral leaflet 382*f*
  wall of left ventricle 617*f*
Anterolateral commissure 382*f*
Antero-posterior mitral annulus 413
Anthracycline 626, 792
  cardiomyopathy 629*t*
Antiadrenergic therapy 703
Antianginal drug 356*t*
  therapy 354
Antiarrhythmic
  agents 40
  drug 234
    in lactation 241, 241*t*
    in pregnancy 241, 241*t*
    selection in atrial fibrillation 239
  versus implantable defibrillators 242
Anticardiolipin antibodies 749
Anticoagulation 348, 430, 586, 658
  therapy 756
Antideoxyribonuclease B test 814
Antihypertensive
  agents, classes of 462*t*
  therapy 462
Anti-inflammatory drugs 815
Antimicrotubule agents 792
Antiphospholipid antibody syndrome 58
Antiplatelet
  agents 54, 63, 338, 348
  management 587
  response of clopidogrel 338
  therapy 221
Antischkow myocyte 811
Antithrombin 340
  deficiency 749
Antithrombotic
  agents 54, 55, 339
  drugs 775
  therapy 340, 441, 476
Aorta 159*f*, 163*f*, 164*f*, 180*f*, 404, 404*f*, 679*f*, 686*f*, 687*f*, 692
  coarctation of 667
  descending 679*f*
Aortic
  aneurysm 489
  compliance 770
  component of second heart sound 87*f*, 502*f*
  dissection 70, 164*f*, 165*f*, 483, 483*f*, 484*t*
    classification of 484*f*
  ejection sound 85*f*
  first heart sound 404, 404*f*
  hemodynamic tracings 194*f*
  impedance, components of 19*t*
  insufficiency 84, 99
  intramural hematoma 165
  left ventricular systolic gradient in aortic stenosis 194*f*
  pressure 123
  regurgitation 87, 145, 193, 374
    cause of 374
    characterization of 193
    on aortic angiography 194*f*
  second heart sound 404, 404*f*
  sinus of Valsalva 276
  stenosis 98, 99*f*, 145, 163*f*, 193, 369
    induced left ventricular pressure overload 370
  valve 157*f*, 158*f*, 163*f*, 166*f*, 617
    calcification 99*f*, 370
    closure sound 82*f*, 85*f*
    disease 369
    endocarditis with paravalvular abscess 424*f*
    leaflet mobility 163*f*
    replacement 373, 788
    stenosis 85*f*
  valvuloplasty in special circumstances 415
Aortography 487
Apixaban 60
APLAS *See* Antiphospholipid antibody syndrome
Apoptosis 188
APTT *See* Activated partial thromboplastin time
Arachidonic acid 338
Argatroban 62
Arginine 832
  vasopressin in heart failure 516*t*
Arrhythmia 217, 289, 547, 554, 695, 728, 730, 736, 764, 768, 780
  initiation 226
  mechanisms 226, 234
Arrhythmic right ventricular dysplasia 275*f*
Arrhythmogenic
  right ventricular dysplasia 274, 398
  substrate 592

Arterial
  dissection 798
  nomenclature 211
  oxygen content, determinants of 124
  pressure 80f
  pulse 79
Arteriohepatic dysplasia 409
Arteriolar vasodilators 19
Arterioles arteriovenous 458
Arteriovenous oxygen difference 121, 123
Arthritis 812
Artichoke leaf extract 825
Ascending aorta 424f
ASDS, classification of 672
Aspergillus 421
Aspiration 156
Aspirin 64, 767
  plus thienopyridine 787
Asymptomatic
  diabetic patients 131
  left ventricular systolic dysfunction 792
Atenolol 465
Atherosclerosis 186
Atherosclerotic renal artery stenosis 479, 479t
Athletes with hypertrophic cardiomyopathy 601
ATP-dependent sodium-potassium pump 10
Atrial
  based AV nodal independent SVT 262
  effective refractory period 696
  fibrillation 160, 253, 255t, 390, 442f, 555f, 742, 778, 787
  flutter 262, 696
  ischemia 255
  natriuretic factor 618
  pressure 192
  septal defect 672, 692f
  tachycardia 263
Atrioventricular
  block 105
  nodal reentrant tachycardia 264
  reciprocating tachycardia 262
  reentrant tachycardia 105, 264
Atropine 153
Auscultation 81
Austin flint murmur 84, 87, 87f, 88, 89
Automatic implantable cardioverter defibrillator 314
Autonomic
  nervous system 493, 726
  regulation of cardiovascular system 493
  testing 495
  tone, changes in 255
Autosomal
  dominant disease 287
  recessive disease 287

AV nodal dependent 261
  SVT 264
AV nodal independent 261
  SVT 268
AV node disease 282
AVNRT *See* Atrioventricular nodal reentry tachycardia
Ayurveda 823
Azathioprine 576, 724, 725
Azithromycin 431, 815
Azole antifungals 60
Azygous vein 100

B

Bacteremia, cause of 385
Bacterial endocarditis, antimicrobial therapy of 426t
B-adrenergic
  blocking 29
    drugs 31
  receptors downregulate 29
Balloon
  across mitral valve 411f
  mitral valvotomy 384f
  positioning 165
  valvotomy 407f, 408
    in pulmonic stenosis 416
Baroreflex 494f
  sensitivity 496
Bartonella hensalae 421
Basic
  catechol-phenylethylamine molecule 35
  life support 312
  sense represents 101
Benazepril 25
Benign arrhythmias 769
Benzathine penicillin 815
Benzodiazepines 708
Beta-adrenergic
  blockade 766
  receptor 33f
    blockers 464, 465t
Beta-adrenoceptor blockers 238
Beta-agonist bronchodilator drugs 730
Beta-blockers 242, 708
Beta-blocking agents 775
Beta-glucan 825
Beta-hemolytic streptococci infection 811
Biatrial enlargement 610
Bicarbonate 708
Bicycle ergometry 384
Bilateral hyperplasia 746
Bile acid sequestrants 50
Bioprosthetic valves 434, 454
Bisoprolol 25
Bivalirudin 61, 222, 340
Biventricular diastolic dysfunction 197
Bjork-Shiley tilting disk valve 435f

Blalock-Taussig shunt 683
Blockade of parasympathetic control with atropine 124
Blood
culture 422, 423
exiting pulmonary valve 100
flow, adjacent 184
pressure 125, 470, 496, 547, 600*f*, 729
for adults, classification of 459*t*
tests 245
urea nitrogen 24
Blotchy cyanosis carcinoid heart disease 77
Bluish discoloration of skin 76
BNP *See* Brain natriuretic peptide
Body
demand for oxygen 779
image drugs 712
mass index 330*t*
weight 547
Boot-shaped heart 93
Brachial artery
approach 211
flow-mediated dilation 717
Bradyarrhythmias 366, 592, 781
Bradycardia 280
causes of 280
diseases 280
syndromes 280
Bradykinin 747
Brain
hemorrhage 726
natriuretic peptide 29, 532, 750, 765
Brainstem *See also* Cerebellum
Breast cancer 641
Bronze discoloration 76
Brugada syndrome 278, 294, 320
B-type natriuretic peptide 74, 501, 510, 528, 623, 628, 737
Buerger test 471
Bulimia 712
Bumetanide 1, 6, 536, 658
Bundle
branch
block 284
reentry 273
of HIS *See also* Common bundle
Bypass angioplasty revascularization investigators 212

C

CABG *See* Coronary artery bypass grafting
Calcific aortic stenosis 369
Calcineurin inhibitors 576
Calcitonin gene 747
Calcium
antagonists 466
channel
antagonists 239
blocker 337, 354, 355, 658, 766, 775
blocking agents 40
scoring 373
sensitizers 39
Canadian Cardiovascular Society 72, 208
Functional Classification 73*t*
Candesartan 25
Candida 422
antigenemia 425
Capillary refill test 471
Captopril 25
Carbon dioxide production 561
Carbonic anhydrase inhibitors 3, 5
Carcinoid syndrome 747
Cardiac
amyloidosis 617, 619
anatomy on chest radiographs 91
arrest 311
arrhythmias 232, 706, 710
biomarkers 765
biopsy 201
calcifications 98
catheterization 190, 191*t*, 208*t*, 247, 379, 399, 406, 597, 676
complications of 216
hemodynamics 620
causes of
cardiogenic shock 361
chest discomfort 71*t*
dyspnea 74, 74*t*
heart failure 255*t*
chamber enlargement 92
chest pain 70*t*
computed tomography 173
cycle pressure waveforms 192
dysfunction 135
dyspnea 500
dysrhythmias 764
enzymes 803
imaging for screening 794
injury biomarkers 509
life support, advanced 315
magnetic resonance imaging 379, 512*f*, 531, 596, 605, 620
masses 183
medications 280
morphologic changes 626
light microscopy 626
myocardium 287
myocytes 744
output 123
positron emission tomography 774
rehabilitation 352
resynchronization therapy 149, 296, 297*t*, 396, 555
retransplantation 578
rupture 362
silhouette 100
sympathetic imaging 497

Index

tamponade 199, 270, 487, 637f
thrombi 183
tomography 506
toxicity 705
transplantation 281
veins 177
Cardiogenic
   pulmonary edema 5
   shock 360t, 361, 542, 729
      cause of 360
Cardiomyocyte 285, 626
   sarcolemma 39
Cardiomyopathy 140, 709, 710
   classification of 605
Cardiopulmonary 463
   arrest 311
   exercise testing 560
   hemodynamics 769
   resuscitation 311, 313
      complications of 315
   stress testing 572t
   unit 561f
Cardioregulatory systems 247
Cardiorenal syndrome 534, 535, 535t, 544
   definition of 534
Cardiospecific phosphodiesterase
   inhibitors 524
Cardiothoracic ratio 91
Cardiotoxic
   agents 140
   exposures 790
Cardiotoxins 513
Cardiotropic virus detection 204
Cardiovagal activity 496
Cardiovascular
   aging 783
   complications 705, 710
   disease 11, 27f, 324t, 326, 601, 713,
      725, 741, 744, 770, 790
   disorders 77t
   events 788
   magnetic resonance 178
      assessment 774
      coronary angiography 180
      guided therapy 182
      imaging 392
   pharmacology 1
   system 115
Cardioverter defibrillation 601, 606
Carditis 812
Carnitine 832
Carotid
   artery
      disease 477
      intima-media thickness 716
   endarterectomy 478
   pulse 85f
   sinus massage 245
   stenting 479

Carpentier-Edwards perimount bovine
   pericardial valve 435f
Carvallo's sign 86, 88
Carvedilol 25, 465, 731
Catecholamine 463, 467
   blood measurement 497
   polymorphic ventricular
      tachycardia 278, 320
Catheter
   ablation 260, 269
      for SVT, complications of 270t
   based therapies for aortic stenosis 414
   based treatment of
      mitral valve disease 410
      pulmonary valve disease 413
   for coronary angiography 211
CCB therapy *See* Calcium channel blocker
   therapy
Cefadroxil 815
Cefazolin 431
Ceftriaxone 431
Celiac disease 721
Cellular
   aging 784
   hypertrophy 181
Central
   cyanosis 76
   nervous system 726
   venous pressure 201
Cephalexin 431, 815
Cerebellum 800
Cerebral
   autosomal dominant arteriopathy 804
   edema 1
Cerebrovascular
   accident 54, 207, 217
   disease 718
Cessation of resuscitation 318
CHD in HIV-infected individuals 714
Chemoembolization 748
Chemoreflex influence on heart rate and
   blood pressure 495
Chemotherapy 791
   induced
      cardiomyopathy 625
      cardiotoxicity 627
Chest
   cavity 90
   compressions 313
   film technique 90
   pain 70, 168, 180f, 707, 812
      in acute coronary syndromes 72t
   radiograph 399, 505
   roentgenogram 405, 461
   X-ray 390, 485, 596, 676
Chlamydophila psittaci 421
Chlorothiazide 6, 8
Chlorthalidone 1, 6
Cholesterol 733

Chorea 813
Chronic
　aortic regurgitation 145, 195
　atrial fibrillation 158f, 696
　beta-adrenergic receptor
　　stimulation 701
　digoxin therapy 40
　doxorubicin cardiotoxicity 625t
　heart failure 26
　hemodynamically 87
　hypoxemia 648
　kidney disease 12, 351, 352, 732, 733,
　　734
　mesenteric ischemia 481
　mitral regurgitation 390t
　myeloid leukemia 649
　obstructive pulmonary disease 256,
　　648, 759
　orthostatic intolerance 498
　relapsing pericarditis 633
　resynchronization therapy 149, 555f
　severe
　　aortic regurgitation 87f
　　mitral regurgitation 391f
　thromboembolic pulmonary
　　hypertension 647, 648, 656
　type B dissection 489
Cilostazol 67, 476
Cineangiographic equipment 215f
Cirrhosis 14, 608
Clarithromycin 431, 815
Classic
　Blalock-Taussig shunt 684f
　cardiac silhouette of left atrial
　　dilatation 95f
　waterfall cascade 55f
Clavicular heads of sternocleidomastoid
　muscle 202f
Clindamycin 431, 815
Clopidogrel 65, 338
Closed mitral commissurotomy 386f
Clubbing of fingers and toes 77
Cocaine 705, 709, 791
Coenzyme Q10 826, 827, 831
Cognitive behavioral therapy 830
Colchicine 634
Combination therapy 357
Common bundle 101
Comorbidities 790
Complete blood count 803
Computed
　tomographic angiography 803
　tomography, basic principles of 173
Conducting exercise test 564
Conduction
　disease 787
　disturbances 723
　system disease 644

Congenital
　anomalies of coronary circulation 213
　dysfibrinogenemia 749
　heart disease 255, 263, 276, 321, 648,
　　763
　long QT interval syndrome 276
　pulmonic stenosis 403
　valvar aortic stenosis 665
Congestion, assessment of 547t
Congestive
　heart
　　disease 74
　　failure 14, 96, 97f, 125, 500t, 733,
　　　735, 740, 742, 799
Connective tissue disease 648
Constrictive pericarditis 198, 198t, 631,
　635, 637f, 638f, 642f
Continuous wave Doppler demonstrating
　severe mitral stenosis 147f
Contrast
　CT and coronary angiography 175
　echocardiography 149
　enhanced echocardiography 134
　induced nephropathy 215
Conventional
　angiogram 478
　therapies 658
COPD See Chronic obstructive pulmonary
　disease
Cor pulmonale 710, 758
Coronary
　angiography 36, 191t, 207, 208t, 349,
　　384, 391, 487, 737, 765, 774, 777
　anomalies 213
　artery 187, 212f, 365f
　　absent left main 213
　　atherosclerosis 706
　　bypass grafting 478, 396, 555f, 735,
　　　784
　　calcium 332, 717
　　disease 70, 150, 173, 207, 322, 513,
　　　555f, 597, 720, 725, 740, 772f,
　　　828
　　stenoses 178, 181
　　surgery study 212
　　vasoconstriction 706
　atherosclerosis 725
　computed tomographic
　　angiography 774
　disease 170t
　flow reserve 200, 702
　heart disease 74, 324, 328t, 477, 714,
　　733, 734, 761
　hemodynamics 200
　intervention 223
　perfusion, abnormal 722
　revascularization 767
　sinus 296
　stent 175, 223

Index

Corrected transposition of great arteries 389
Corrigan's pulse 378
Corticosteroid 576, 724
   therapy 725
   treated SLE 725
Corynebacterium 420
Cough 75, 351
Coxiella burnetii 421
Cranial nerve 494*f*
Crataegus monogyna 831
C-reactive protein 634, 765
Creatine 832
   kinase 350, 728
Creatinine
   clearance 758
   kinase 334
Crescendo-decrescendo murmurs 84
Critical limb ischemia 472
Crohn's disease 749
CRT *See* Cardiac resynchronization therapy
CT angiogram 486
Culture-negative endocarditis 419
Cushing's
   disease 746
   syndrome 746
Cutaneous
   lentiginosis 77
   vasospastic symptoms 723
Cyanosis 76, 680
Cyanotic
   congenital heart disease 682
   heart diseases 683
Cyclic
   adenosine monophosphate 33*f*
   guanosine monophosphate 649
Cyclooxygenase 64
Cyclophosphamide 626, 725
Cyclosporine 576

D

Dabigatran 62
Davie's disease 612
Defibrillation 316
Degenerative
   mitral valve disease 392*f*
   valvular disease 453
Dermatomyositis 723
Desmosomal dysfunction 286
Desmosome 285
   function 285
   structure 285
Destructive inflammatory thyroiditis 743
Develop cardiac tamponade 642
Device therapies 621
Diabetes 324, 351, 513
   mellitus 331, 352, 466, 733, 740, 796, 799

Diabetic medications 703
Diagnostic scores 126
Diastolic
   dysfunction 591, 642, 702
      detection of 702
   function 136, 143
   heart failure 527*t*, 528*t*, 530*t*, 533*t*, 698
      definition of 526
   murmurs 84, 87
   regurgitant jet 145
Dietary cholesterol 776
Digital subtraction angiography 475
Digitalis 39
Digoxin 25, 39, 242, 267, 768
Dihydropyridines 466
Dihydroxyphenylacetic acid 497
Dihydroxyphenylglycol 497
Dilatation of ascending thoracic aorta 99*f*
Dilated
   cardiomyopathy 181, 604
   hypokinetic phase 592
Diltiazem 267
Dipyridamole 349
   perfusion scintigraphy 765
   stress protocol 154
Direct
   myocardial damage 706
   thrombin inhibitors 60, 340
Disease
   extent of 211
   of conducting system 720
Disopyramide 235-238, 241
Disorders of
   coronary circulation 782
   heart valves 782
   myocardial electrical activity and conduction 782
   myocardium 782
Distal coronary sinus 696
Distort cardiac murmurs 720
Diuretic
   compounds 1
   induced hypokalemia 15
   optimization strategies evaluation 538
   resistance 542
   sites of action in nephron 2*f*
   tolerance 4
   use in
      edematous disorders 12
      hypertension 11
Dobutamine 35, 153, 349, 363, 524, 573
   infusion 155
   protocol 154
   stress echocardiogram 512*f*
Docohexanoic acid 53
Dofetilide 235, 237, 240-242
Donor heart
   implantation 574
   selection 574*t*

Dopamine 36, 363, 524
Doppler
　echocardiography 505, 619
　parameters of prosthetic aortic and mitral valve stenosis 446t
　tissue imaging 627
　ultrasonography 803
Dorsal motor nucleus of vagus 494f
Doses of corticosteroids 724
Double
　orifice mitral valve surgical repair 395f
　statin dose 50
Down syndrome 77
Doxazosin 468, 791
Doxorubicin cardiomyopathy 625, 626t, 628t, 629t
Dressler's syndrome 351
Dronedarone 235, 237, 241
Dual-chamber pacemaker 602
Duchane's and Baker's, limb girdle 302
Duration of secondary prophylaxis 817t
Duroziez's sign 378
Dysfunction in systolic heart failure 519
Dyslipidemia 701, 740, 824
Dyspnea 72, 180f, 541
　cardiac cause of 74t
　pulmonary cause of 74t
Dysregulation of volume homeostasis 13
Dysrhythmia 156, 350

E

Early
　diastolic
　　motion of mitral annulus 137f
　　murmur 87f, 88
　　transmitral flow 137f
　medical therapy 336, 347
　prosthetic valve endocarditis 421
Ebstein's anomaly 680, 681
ECG
　exercise testing 115
　monitoring, continuous 246
Echocardiography 246, 399, 400t, 406, 422
Edema 75, 547
Edwards Sapien transcatheter pericardial aortic valve 435f
Ehler-Danlos syndrome 77, 374
Eicosopentanoic acid 53
Einthoven's triangle 102
Eisenmenger's
　physiology 763
　syndrome 75, 676f, 677
Ejection
　fraction 179, 377f
　　component of 133
　systolic murmur 85f
Electrocardiogram 101, 246, 256, 334, 343, 399, 405, 503, 595, 794
　component parts of 102

Electrocardiography, basis of 101
Electromagnetic interference 768
Electron beam computed tomography 506
Electrophysiology studies 247, 265
Elevated systolic 790
Embolic protection devices 479
Emergency
　medical services 312
　room evaluation 343
Empiric antimicrobial therapy 425
Enalapril 25
End
　diastolic
　　pressure 190f, 193f
　　volume 132, 134, 377f
　stage renal disease 732
　systolic
　　dimension 584
　　volume 123, 132, 133, 377f
Endocardial fibrotic disease, development of 612
Endocarditis 160, 423, 423t, 430t, 456, 725
Endocrine
　disorders 255
　heart disease 740
Endoleak, absence of 491
Endomyocardial
　biopsy 288, 612
　fibrosis 398, 612
Endotension 491
Endothelial
　cell 577f
　function 331
　progenitor cells 784
Endothelin receptor antagonists 660
Endothelium dependent
　flow-mediated dilation 770
　vasodilation 717
Endovascular
　repair 488
　valve edge-to-edge repair study 413
Energy medicine 823
Enhanced external counterpulsation 829, 831
Enoxaparin 222
Epicardial coronary artery stenosis 178
Epinephrine 38, 316
Episode of Torsades de pointes 272f
Episodic ischemia 213
Epithelial cells 5
Eplerenone 1, 7, 25, 26
Eprosartan 25
Eptifibatide 68
Eradication of streptococci 814
Erythema marginatum 813
Esmolol 267
Estimated glomerular filtration rate 732
Estimation of jugular venous pressure 78

Index

Ethacrynic acid 7
Etoxomir 704
European
 risk scores 325
 Society of Cardiology 259f
Evaluation of
 dyspnea 565
 left ventricular filling pressures 138
 patient with hypertension 458
Examination of
 jugular venous pulse 78
 lung fields 636
 musculoskeletal system 76
 precordial pulsation 81
 skin 76
Excessive plasminogen activator
 inhibitor 749
Exercise
 electrocardiographic evaluation 773
 induced arrhythmias 127
 physiology and athlete's heart 779
 response in heart failure 559
 stress echo 150
 test
  and six-minute walk test 510
  modalities 118
 testing 246
 therapy 476
 training in heart failure 566
Exertional dyspnea 74, 500, 722
External jugular vein 78f
 courses of 78f
Extracorporeal membrane oxygenation 575
Ezetimibe 51

F

Fabry's disease 619
Facilitated percutaneous coronary
 intervention 345
Familial dilated cardiomyopathy 607
Fasicular ventricular tachycardia 232
Fat pad sign 100
Femoral artery
 access site 210f
 approach 209
Fenfluramine, dexfenfluramine and
 phenteramine 712
Fibrates 52
Fibromuscular dysplasia 469, 479t
Fibrous pericardium 631
Flecainide 236, 241, 242
Flufenamic acid 786
Flunitrazepam 711
Fluorodeoxyglucose 187
 positron emission tomography 701
Fluoroscopic imaging system 214
Focal
 ectopic atrial tachycardia 105f

 myocarditis 706
 myocyte necrosis 706
Fondaparinux 57, 340
Fontaine's stages 473
Fontan
 operations 683
 procedure 263
Food and Drug Administration 28, 356
Fosinopril 25
Fractional flow reserve 200
Framingham risk score 325
Frank hypotension, development of 334
Free fatty acids 700
Friction rub 812
Functional tricuspid
 regurgitation 398f
 valve disease 398
Fungal endocarditis, cause of 421
Furosemide 6, 536, 658

G

Galvanic skin response 827
Gamma aminobutyric acid 711
Gammahydroxybutyrate 711
Gastrointestinal symptoms 499
Gated myocardial perfusion
 imaging 167
Gender and
 cardiac arrhythmias 777
 cardiovascular disease 770
Genotype specific therapy 293
Giant cell myocarditis 204
Gingival hyperplasia 466
Global left ventricular 364
Glomerular filtration 540f
Glucocorticoid deficiency 747
Glucose
 6-phosphatase, deficiency of 649
 transporters 700
Goal of blood pressure 351
Growth hormone excess 744

H

HDL cholesterol 776
Healthcare associated
 endocarditis 417
 infections 419
Heart
 block 280
 disease 74, 253, 257
 failure 24, 116, 140, 350, 500, 501t,
  503t, 505, 509t, 525t, 763, 534,
  558, 623, 763, 777, 786, 830
  diagnosis of 505
  management 587
  medical management 621
  Society of America 793t
  survival score 569, 570

valvular heart disease 59
   with preserved ejection fraction 545, 786
murmurs, auscultation of 84
rate 123, 125
   control 495
   recovery 496
   variability 496, 695, 764
stops 75
transplantation 571, 579t, 621, 657
Hematoma 216
Hemiblock 283
Hemodialysis and end-stage renal failure 608
Hemodynamic
   classification of pulmonary hypertension 646
   complications 217
   compromise, clinical 725
   concepts 463
   consequences 530
   disturbances 790
   hallmark of hypertensive disease 463
   impairment 541
   in cardiomyopathy 197
   in pericardial disease 198
   in valvular heart disease 193
   stabilization 586
   symptoms 680
Hemolysis 450
Hemoptysis 75
Hemorrhage 720
Hemorrhagic stroke 797
   category of 795
Heparin 222, 339
   and indirect XA inhibitors 55
Hepatojugular reflux 79
Hibernation 548
Hibiscus sabdariffa 827
High
   ceiling diuretics 5
   density lipoprotein 714, 824
   dose salicylates 632, 634
   grade coronary stenosis 767
   resolution computed tomography 654
Highly active antiretroviral therapy 714, 715
Hirudin 61
Hirudo medicinalis 61
His bundle electrogram 274f
Histamine 747
History of
   blood clots 757
   frothy pink 75
   magnetic resonance imaging 178
HIV
   and cardiovascular risk factors 715
   and coronary heart disease 714

   cardiovascular disease 713
   related left ventricular dysfunction and myocarditis 717
Hodgkin's lymphoma 641
Holter monitoring 305, 596
Holt-Oram syndrome 77
Homans sign 751
Hormonal studies 461
Human immunodeficiency virus 713
Hydralazine 19, 555f
   isosorbide dinitrate 25
Hydrochlorothiazide 1, 6, 9
Hydrogen ion 315
Hyperaldosteronism 463
Hyperbilirubinemia 76
Hypercalcemia 464
Hyperdynamic systolic function 731
Hypereosinophilic syndromes 614
Hyperfibrinogenemia 734
Hyperglycemia replicates 701
Hyperhomocysteinemia 725, 734, 749
Hyperlipidemia 324, 331, 520, 716, 733, 738
Hypertension 253, 324, 331, 513, 729, 733, 740, 763, 799, 826
   causes of 763
Hypertensive
   heart disease, classification of 459t
   hemorrhage 798f
Hyperthyroidism 742
Hypertriglyceridemia 725
Hypertrophic
   cardiomyopathy 140, 181, 245, 591, 594f, 598t, 600f
   obstructive cardiomyopathy 85, 197, 603
Hypertrophied myocytes 593f
Hyperuricemia 740
Hyperviscosity 749
Hypoalbuminemia 739
Hypomagnesemia 464
Hypoparathyroidism 747
Hypopituitarism 744
Hyporesponders 338
Hypotension 156, 366
Hypotensive acute heart failure syndromes 551
Hypovolemia 315, 542
Hypoxemia 156
Hypoxia 243

I

Iatrogenic cause of
   bradycardia 280t
   heart block 280t
Ibutilide 242
ICD therapy 293
Ideal radial artery access site 210f

Identification of
  atrial activity 103
  left-ventricle end diastolic
    pressure 193f
Idiopathic
  left ventricle VT 276
  restrictive cardiomyopathy 615
  VF 279
Idioventricular rhythm 107, 107f
Idrabiotaparinux 58
Ifosfamide 627
IHD, complications of 787
Imaging
  myocardial viability 169
  perfusion 171
Immunosuppression-related organ
    dysfunction 578
Impaired relaxation of left ventricle 136
Implantable
  cardiac defibrillator 555f
  cardioverter defibrillator 294, 600f, 624,
    697, 736, 777
  loop recorders 246, 306, 308
Indapamide 1, 6
Index of microcirculatory
    resistance 200
Indications for
  antiarrhythmic drug therapy 234
  coronary angiography 207
  exercise testing 115
Infarct related artery 341
Infectious Disease Society of America 716
Infective endocarditis 148, 389, 417, 419,
    456, 736
  prophylaxis 393
Inferior vena cava filters 758
Infiltration of mononuclear cells 722
Infiltrative atrial disease 255
Inflammatory
  bowel disease 721
  cytokine 517
    production 700
Infradiaphragmatic variant of total
    anomalous pulmonary veins 692f
Inhibition of tyrosine kinases 627
Inhibitors of platelet
  activation 64
  adhesion 64
  aggregation 68
Inotropes 540
Inotropy 136
Inoue
  balloon mitral valvotomy in mitral
    stenosis 387f
  technique 411, 411f
Inspiratory muscle training 830
Insulin 703
  resistance 513
  and cardiomyopathy 698, 699f
  sensitization 704
  therapy 703
Interatrial septal aneurysm 160f
Intermediate pretest probability 115
Internal jugular vein 78f, 202f, 501f
  courses of 78f
International normalized ratio 758
Interstitial edema 97f
Interventricular septum 141f, 654f, 655f
Intra-aortic balloon
  counterpulsation 36, 729
  pump 348
Intra-atrial reentrant tachycardia 263
Intracardiac
  masses 148
  shunt 183
Intracellular cyclic guanosine
    monophosphate 337
Intracerebral hemorrhage 795
Intracranial hemorrhage 797, 801t
Intracytoplasmic vacuolations 612
Intramural hematoma 483f, 487
Intramuscular benzathine penicillin 814
Intraoperative transesophageal
    echocardiography 165, 403
Intravenous
  immunoglobulins 724
  nitroglycerin 21f, 29
  urography 461
  vasodilators 28
Intraventricular hemorrhage 795
Intrinsic renal disease 542
Ionizing radiation, biological effects of 172
Irbesartan 25
Ischemic
  cardiomyopathy 70
  heart disease 354, 697, 734, 763, 770,
    785, 787
  myocardium 511f
  stroke 797, 800t, 802t
Isolated
  infundibular stenosis 408
  systolic hypertension 786
Isoproterenol 37
Isosorbide dinitrate 555f
Isotope renography and renal scans 461
Isovolumetric ventricular
    contraction 192f
Ivabradine 356, 775

J

Jaundice 76
Jugular venous
  pressure 547, 595f, 763
    tracings 637f
  pulsations 79
  pulse 78, 555f
J-wave syndromes 279

K

Kale juice 824
Kerley lines represent thickening 96
Ketamine 711
Kussmaul's sign 641

L

Labetalol 465
Lactic acid dehydrogenase 460
Large arteries 186
L-arginine 828
Laryngospasm 156
Late
  gadolinium enhancement 600*f*
  occurring complications of endovascular aneurysm repair 491
  precordial transition 112
  prosthetic valve endocarditis 421
Laxative abuse 460
L-carnitine 703
LDL cholesterol 776
Left anterior
  descending coronary artery 180*f*
  fascicle 274*f*
  hemiblock 109
  oblique 91
Left atrial
  enlargement 94, 95*f*
  pressure waveform 192*f*
Left atrium 404
Left bundle branch 282
  block 109*f*, 273, 284, 288, 595*f*
Left cardiac sympathetic
  denervation 293
  techniques 293
Left circumflex coronary artery 180*f*
Left heart disease 397
Left main coronary artery 180*f*
  cannulation 214
Left parasternal lift 502
Left posterior
  fascicle 274*f*
  hemiblock 109
Left pulmonary artery 690*f*
Left ventricle 133, 404
  ejection fraction 81
  end-diastolic pressure 192
  pressure 193*f*
    waveform 190*f*
Left ventricular
  assist devices 363
  diastolic dysfunction 505, 619
  dysfunction 539, 638, 728, 730, 761
  ejection fraction 132, 133, 141, 167, 273, 296, 642, 728
    assessment of 348
  ejection time 696
  end diastolic pressure 377*f*, 646
  endomyocardial fibrosis 612, 613
  enlargement 92, 93*f*
  function, assessment of 765
  hypertrophy 74, 112*f*, 594*f*, 595*f*, 596*f*, 666, 728, 732, 733, 780
  mass 135
  myocardium 167
  noncompaction 181
  outflow tract 591, 594*f*, 595*f*, 600*f*, 603
  outward murmur 87*f*
  pressure and diastolic volume 125
  systolic function 518, 619
  volume overload 390
Legionella 421
Leopard syndrome 77
Lesion of aortic stenosis 369
Leukoencephalopathy 804
Levels of
  cardiac troponins 730
  cyclic adenosine monophosphate 67
Levosimendan 39
Libman-Sacks
  characteristic of 725
  endocarditis 725
Lidocaine 237, 242, 316
Lipid
  lowering
    drugs 775
    therapy 357
  management 352
Lipotoxicity 701
Lisinopril 25
Listeria 420
Loeffler's endocarditis 614, 615
Loeys-Dietz syndrome 483
Long-QT interval syndrome 320
Loop
  diuretics 5, 464
  of Henle 5, 11
Losartan 25
Low
  density lipoprotein 712, 824
  glycemic index diet 828
  high-density lipoprotein 732
  molecular weight heparins 54, 57, 340, 441
Lower extremity edema 519
LQT syndrome 291
L-type calcium channels 337
LV
  diastolic dysfunction 136
  systolic
    dysfunction and heart failure 352
    function 351
LVOT obstruction 591
Lymphocytic myocarditis 204

M

Macrolide antibiotics 60
Macroreentrant tachycardia 264
Macrovascular complications 703
Magnesium 832
Magnetic resonance
  imaging 176, 486, 600f
  venography 803
Main pulmonary artery 404, 404f, 406f, 690f
Maintenance of sinus rhythm 258
Major acute coronary events 357
Malar flush of face 76
Malignant cardiac neoplasm 177
Mammalian target of rapamycin inhibitors 576
Management of
  acute
    CHF 29
    pericarditis 632
  cardiorenal syndrome 542t
  chorea 816
  constrictive pericarditis 640
  IHD in women 774
  pregnancy 456
  pulmonary hypertension 659
  regular SVT in acute setting 268f
Manifestation of heart failure 500
Marfan's syndrome 77, 321, 374
Matrix
  metalloproteinases 528
  remodeling markers 509
Maximum
  heart rate 785
  oxygen consumption rate 785
Mean mitral valve gradient 196f
Measurement of
  arterial pressure 78
  left ventricular end-diastolic dimensions 141f
Mechanical
  circulatory support 575
  devices for cardiopulmonary resuscitation 313
  relief of obstruction 385
  valves 434, 454
Mechanism of
  chemotherapy-induced cardiac dysfunction 626
  secondary mitral regurgitation 388f
Medial papillary muscle 675f
Medical
  disease 280
  management 363, 480
  therapy 373, 379, 425
  treatment 385, 393, 401
Medicine
  alternative 823
  complementary 823

Medtronic Freestyle porcine valve 435f
Medtronic
  Hall tilting disk valve 435f
  Hancock II porcine valve 435f
Mental health 827, 829, 830
Mesenteric
  angiography 481
  ischemia 481
Metabolic
  equivalents 129
  modulators 704
  syndrome 741
Metaiodobenzylguanidine 628
Metformin 703
Methadone 712
Methamphetamine 709
Methemoglobinemia 76
Methicillin-resistant *Staphylococcus aureus* endocarditis 430f
Methodology of exercise testing 117
Methylenedioxymethamphetamine 711
Metolazone 1, 6, 544
Metoprolol 267, 465
  succinate 25
Mexiletine 235-237, 241
Microalbuminuria 732
Mid-diastolic murmur 88
Midodrine 499
Midsystolic murmurs 84
Migration 491
Mild pulmonary arterial hypertension 654f
Milrinone 37, 38
  infusion 606
Mind-body medicine 823, 827
  therapies 829, 831
Mineralocorticoid 10
  receptor blockers 26
Mitraclip device 395f
Mitral
  annular motion during atrial systole 137f
  regurgitation 84, 86, 99, 146, 195, 362, 388, 388f, 389, 389t, 390t, 392f
  stenosis 84, 88, 99, 146, 195, 196f, 381, 383t, 411f
    cause of 381, 382t
    severity, classification of 146t
  valve 382f, 386f, 389, 617f
    anterior leaflet of 440f
    apparatus 381f
    closure sound 82f
    disease 380
    endocarditis 430f
    prolapse 389, 394f, 453
  valvuloplasty in pregnancy 412
Mixed connective tissue disease 723
Mobile cardiac outpatient telemetry 305, 306
Moderate-to-severe claudication 473

Modified Blalock-Taussig shunt 684f
Moexipril 25
Molecular
	CT imaging 187
	genetic analysis 289
	imaging
		modalities 184
		of vascular disease 184, 186
Monascus purpureus yeast 824
Monoclonal antibody-based tyrosine kinase inhibitors 627
Monomorphic ventricular tachycardia 272
Morphine 337, 348
Multifocal atrial tachycardia 262, 264
Multiple system atrophy 498
Murmurs, continuous 89
Muscle
	afferents 124
	loss 785
Mycophenolate 724
	mofetil 576
Myocardial
	and pericardial diseases 591
	capillary endothelia 620
	cells 229
	disease 722
	energy metabolism 699
	fibrosis 512f
		consists of proliferation 642
	hypertrophy 278
	infarction 117, 140, 217, 351-352, 364, 519f, 521f
	involvement 719
	ischemia 511, 768
		and infarction 707
	perfusion imaging 167, 168, 179
	scar 272f
	tissue 230f
	VT in association with
		fibrosis/scar 272
		structural heart disease 272
Myocarditis 606, 709, 710, 719, 724
Myofibrillar loss 706
Myxoma 160f

N

N-acetylcysteine administration 209
Nadolol 465
National Center for Complementary and Alternative Medicine 823
Native valve disease 139
NBTE *See* Nonbacterial thrombotic endocarditis
Nebivolol 25
Neck dilatation 491
Necrotizing vasculitis 710
Nephrons 523
Nephrotic syndrome 15, 749

Nesiritide 29, 37
Neurocardiogenic
	injury 726, 729
	mechanisms 781
Neurogenic
	and stress cardiomyopathy 726
	cardiac injury 729
	cardiomyopathy 726
	heart disease 726
Neurohormonal dysregulation 790
Neurohormones 509
	activation of 546
Neurologic tests 247
Neuromuscular
	diseases 610
	electrical stimulation 830
New York Heart Association
	Classification 503
	Functional Classification 503t
Newer
	antianginal drugs 356
	antiplatelet agents 339
New-onset atrial fibrillation 257
Niacin 51
Nicorandil 775
Nifedipine, alternatives 49
Nitric oxide 661, 740
	derangement 701
Nitroglycerin 708
Nitroprusside 28
Nocturnal oxygen therapy trial 759
Non-adrenal chromaffin tissue 745
Nonbacterial thrombotic endocarditis, development of 418
Noncardiac
	cause of AF 254
	chest pain 71t
	medications 280
	surgery 443, 765
	symptoms 256
Noncommunicating disease 487
Noncontrast CT and coronary calcifications 175
Nonconventional therapies and cardiology 823
Noncoronary artery disease 70
Nonesterified fatty acid 700
Noninvasive
	and hemodynamic evaluation 367
	studies for myocardial ischemia 765
	testing 478
Nonischemic
	cardiomyopathy 322
	systolic heart failure 523
Nonparoxysmal junctional ectopic tachycardia 262
Nonpharmacologic
	therapy 499
	treatments 524

Nonsteroidal
  anti-inflammatory
    agents 523, 632, 634
    drug 52, 786
    medication 724
  muscle mass 781
Nonsustained ventricular tachycardia 600f
Nonvolume dependent forms of
    hypertension 463
Noradrenergic vasoconstrictor 745
Norepinephrine 38, 497
Normal
  carotid upstroke 372f
  PA chest film 92f
Nucleus
  ambiguous 494f
  tractus solitarii 493
Nutritional deficiency 608

O

Obesity 324, 329
  classification of 330
Olmesartan 25
Omega-3 fatty acids 53
Open mitral commissurotomy 386f
Opening of
  mitral valve 502f
  tricuspid valve 192
Oral nitrates 21
Organizational accidents 818
Origins of ventricular tachycardia and
    sudden cardiac death/arrest 778
Orthopnea 74, 500, 541
  test 547
Orthostatic hypotension 247, 495, 498
  development of 498
Osmotic diuretics 10
Ostium
  primum 672
  secundum 672
Oxidative stress 188
  markers 509
Oxygen
  consumption 121
  pulse 563
  uptake 561, 779

P

Pacing device evaluation 140
Palliative shunts 683
Palpable precordial impulses 81
Palpation of pulses 471
Palpitation 74
Papillary muscle 389
Paracoarctation tissue 670
Paraganglioma 745
Parathyroid disorders 747

Paravalvular
  abscess 424f
  regurgitation 450
Parenteral anticoagulant therapy 222
Paroxysmal
  atrial tachycardia 696
  AV block 283
  nocturnal dyspnea 390
  supraventricular tachycardia 104
Paroxysms of cough 75
Partial
  pressure of oxygen 750
  thromboplastin time 55, 222, 339
Parts of LVAD 585f
Parvus et tardus 372f
Patent ductus arteriosus 84, 677, 678f, 679f
Pathogenesis of
  acute rheumatic fever and rheumatic
      heart disease 810f
  coronary heart disease in HIV
      infection 714
  transplant vasculopathy 577f
Pathology of mitral stenosis 382f
Pathophysiology of
  anthracycline-induced
      cardiomyopathy 625
  pulmonary arterial hypertension 649
  right ventricular failure in pulmonary
      arterial hypertension 651f
Patients with valvular heart disease 131
Peak
  aortic systolic pressure 194f
  left ventricular systolic pressure 194f
Pediatric
  cardiomyopathies 610
  population 76
Penetrating aortic ulcer 483f
Pentoxifylline 476
Percutaneous
  alcohol septal ablation 602
  aortic
    balloon valvuloplasty 414
    valve implantation 415
  balloon
    mitral valvuloplasty 410
    valvotomy 411
  catheterization of femoral artery 210f
  coronary intervention 212, 217, 343,
      345
  mitral
    annuloplasty 413
    balloon valvotomy 416
    leaflet repair 413
  pulmonary valve implantation 413
  pulmonic balloon valvuloplasty 413
  revascularization 357
  therapies for mitral regurgitation 412
  transluminal coronary angioplasty 61,
      222

Perhexiline 704
Pericardial
    disease 144, 177, 184, 631, 641, 735
    disorders 100
    effusion 100, 100f, 812
    inflammation
        acute 724
        chronic 724
Pericarditis 724
Pericardium 177, 631
Perindopril 25
Peripartum cardiomyopathy 623
Peripheral
    arterial disease 66, 470
        classification of 473t
    vascular
        disease 469
        resistance 750
    venous blood 461
Periprocedural fluoroscopic time 176
Perivascular tissues 722
Peroxidation of LDL 701
Persistence of perigraft perfusion 490
Persistent fever 430
PET and SPECT technology 169
Pharmacokinetics of thiazides 9
Pharmacologic
    stress echo 152
        protocols 154
    therapy 499
Pharmacotherapy for PCI 221
Pharmacotoxicity of cocaine 706
Phenylephrine 38
Phenylpropanolamine 710
Pheochromocytoma 745
Phosphodiesterase 33f
    antagonism of 540
    inhibitors 38, 67
    type 5 inhibitors 28, 661
Phrenic nerve 639
Pindolol 465
Pituitary
    apoplexy 798
    disorders 744
Plant stanols and sterols 825
Plantago ovata 825
Plasma
    membrane 286f
    renin activity 461
Plasminogen activator inhibitor 706
Platelet abnormalities 749
Platypnea 74
Plavix 65
Pneumocystis jirovecii 577
Polycystic ovary syndrome 772f
Polycythemia 749
Polymerase chain reaction 203
Polymyositis 723
Polysubstance abuse 709

Positron emission tomography 169, 511f
Postballoon mitral valvotomy 387f
Post-electroconvulsive therapy 726
Posterior
    mitral leaflet 382f
    wall of left ventricle 617f
Posteromedial commissure 382f
Postganglionic neuronal depletors 467
Postmyocardial infarction care 348
Postresuscitation care 318
Postsynaptic alpha-receptor
        antagonists 468
Post-transplant infection prophylaxis 577t
Postural orthostatic tachycardia
        syndrome 244, 498
Potassium sparing 3
    agents 464
    diuretics 10, 40
Potential
    duration, action of 235, 292
    of ventricular myocardial cell
        depolarizations 102
Potts anastomosis 683, 684f
PPCM, cause of 623
Prasugrel 66, 339
Prazosin 468
Precapillary and postcapillary pulmonary
        hypertension 646f
Predischarge submaximal test 117
Pre-ejection period 696
Pre-excitation syndromes 108, 265
Prehexiline 703
Premature ventricular contractions 127,
        728
Pretransplant CVD 738
Prevalence of large-vessel peripheral arterial
        disease 470f
Prevention of
    cardiovascular disease 65
    endocarditis 431
    heart failure 790
    ischemic stroke 805t
    RF/RHD 816
    thromboembolism 260
Primary
    aldosteronism 463
    bronchopulmonary disease 75
    chronic autonomic failure 497
    coronary intervention 347
    hyperparathyroidism 747
    tricuspid valve disease 397
    tumors 148
Principles of treatment of cardiovascular
        disease 738
Proarrhythmic
    substrates 232
    triggers 233
Procainamide 236, 237, 241, 242, 316
Prognosis of infective endocarditis 417

Prognostic
  scores 569
  utilization of exercise testing 127
Progression of heart failure 517
Propafenone 235, 236, 241
Prophylactic antithrombic
    therapy 452
Propranolol 465
Prostacyclin 649
  pathways 661
Prosthetic
  heart valves 433, 435*f*
  valve 140,454
    endocarditis 449*t*
    thrombosis 447
Proteinuria 732
Pseudoaneurysm 216
Pseudonormal filling 137
Pseudosepsis syndrome 542
Pseudoxanthoma elasticum 610
Pteridine derivatives 3
Pulmonary
  angiography 752
  arterial
    branch 650*f*
    hypertension 646, 648, 650*f*, 652, 652*t*, 653*f*, 658, 662
    wedge pressure 191, 196*f*, 646
  artery 81, 166*f*, 390, 678*f*, 679*f*, 687*f*, 692*f*
    hypertension 183
    pressure 646
    systolic pressure 198, 654*f*, 655*f*
  capillary
    hemangiomatosis 648
    wedge pressure 21*f*
  congestion 461
  disease 253
  edema 97*f*, 619
  embolism 649
    rule-out criteria 753
  function testing 654
  hypertension 144, 390, 646-649, 710, 723
    classification of 647*t*
  insufficiency 84
  outflow obstruction 85
  oxygen uptake 779
  valve 406*f*
    closure sound 82*f*, 85*f*
    insufficiency 100
    stenosis 100
  vascular
    disease 646
    resistance 674
  vein 162*f*, 176
  veno-occlusive disease 647, 648
  venous hypertension 648
  ventilation-perfusion scan 656*f*
Pulmonic
  component of second heart sound 87*f*, 88, 502*f*
  regurgitant fraction 685
  regurgitation 88, 148, 196
  second heart sound 404, 404*f*
  stenosis 147, 196, 404*f*
  valve stenosis 408
Pulse Doppler across pulmonary valve 611*f*
Pulsus alternans, absence of 81
Punica granatum 828
Purkinje
  cells 101
  fibers 101
Putaminal hemorrhage 798
PVT
  in association with
    long QT interval 276
    short QT syndrome 279
  with normal QT prolongation 278

Q

QRS complex 101
  characterization of 108
QT
  interval 113
  syndrome 230
    acquired long 277
Quantify mitral regurgitation 195
Quinapril 25
Quincke's pulse 378
Quinidine 236-238, 241, 242

R

Radiation induced
  coronary artery disease 643
  heart disease 641, 643
  myocardial disease 642
  pericardial disease 641
  valvular heart disease 643
Radiofrequency ablation 748
Ramipril 25
Randomized aldosterone evaluation
    study 26
Ranolazine 356, 703
Rate of perceived exertion 566
Reactive
  arthritis 721
  oxygen species 226, 742
Recent intracerebral bleed 456
Recurrent chest discomfort 350
Reduced sleep duration 829
Refinement of endomyocardial biopsy 201
Regulation of blood pressure 493
Regurgitant murmurs 84
Relative thrombogenicity of prosthetic
    valves 452*t*

Renal
  arterography 461
  artery stenosis 479
  blood 466
    flow 538
  insufficiency 13
  transplantation 738
Renin
  angiotensin aldosterone 463
    system 22, 23, 536, 733
  inhibitors 467
Renovascular hypertension 458
Reperfusion 345
Respiratory
  exchange ratio 563
  symptoms 541
  variation in mean right atrial pressure 198
Resting heart rate 496
Restoration of sinus rhythm 258
Restricted aortic valve leaflet mobility 163f
Restrictive
  cardiac disorders 610t
  cardiomyopathies 181, 197, 610, 638f
Resuscitation 311
Retrograde technique of balloon aortic valvuloplasty 414f
Return of spontaneous circulation 311
Revascularization 341, 363, 477, 480
Reversible causes of cardiac arrest 315t
Rheumatic
  disease 370
  fever 381, 810, 811, 812t, 815
  heart disease 380, 381
  mitral stenosis 162f
  valvular heart disease 453
Rheumatoid arthritis 77, 719, 720
Rhythm
  disorders and reflexes associated with RVI 366
  management 575
Right anterior oblique 212
Right atrial
  enlargement 143, 95, 95f
  pressure 147
    waveform 192f
Right atrium 92, 404
Right bundle branch block 273, 283, 284, 294, 673
Right coronary artery 180f, 213
  cannulation 214
Right heart
  catheterization 191, 646, 657, 679
  failure 367t
Right internal jugular vein puncture 202f
Right pulmonary artery 690
Right ventricle 404
Right ventricular
  assist device implantation 581
  endomyocardial fibrosis 612
  enlargement 93, 94f
  failure 79, 390
  hypertrophy 671
  infarction 350, 361
  outflow tract 180f, 413, 686f, 687f
  systolic
    and EDP 198
    dysfunction 730
    pressure 405f
Rigler's rule 93
Risk of valve replacement 433
Rivaroxaban 60
Rohypnol 711
Role of
  bystanders 312
  computerization 820
  decreased cardiac output 534
  digoxin 385
  dyssynchrony imaging 300
  echocardiography 654
  elevated central venous pressure 535
  endomyocardial biopsy 205t
  hyperglycemia 741
  left ventricular function 765
  myocardial revascularization 357
Root cause analysis 821
Roth's spots 423
Rutherford's categories 473t
RVOT stenosis 413
Ryanodine 321

S

S. aureus 422, 431, 448
  endocarditis 430
  strains 426
S. gallolyticus 422
Saccharomyces cerevisiae 825
Sarcoplasmic vacuolization 706
Saturated fat 776
Scleroderma 610, 722
Seattle heart failure model 569, 570
Second degree AV block 282
Secondary
  and congenital autonomic failure 498
  disorders of heart 695
  prevention of
    coronary heart disease 352
    rheumatic fever 816
Secundum atrial septal defect 166f
Seizure disorders 726
Selective
  angiography 399
  serotonin reuptake inhibitors 280
Senile calcific aortic stenosis 785
Sensitivity of transesophageal echocardiogram 384

Septal
  lateral dimension of mitral annulus 413
  myectomy 602
Sequela of rheumatic fever 99
Serious comorbid diseases 808
Serotonin 467
Serous pericardium 631
Serum
  albumin 8
  electrolytes 460
  glutamic pyruvic transaminase 460
  levels of creatine kinase 724
Severe
  aortic regurgitation
    acute 88t
    chronic 88t
  aortic stenosis 155
  cardiac failure 814
  congestive heart failure 97f
  heart failure 28
  hemodynamic compromise 366
  LV dysfunction 768
  mitral regurgitation 162f, 392f, 412
  pulmonary arterial hypertension 655f
  symptomatic electrolyte
      imbalance 191
  tricuspid regurgitation 399t, 400t
  valvar pulmonic stenosis 407f
  valvular heart disease 761
Severity of
  aortic
    regurgitation in adults, classification
        of 378t
    stenosis in adults, classification
        of 373t
  prosthetic
    aortic valve regurgitation 444t
    mitral valve regurgitation 446t
  stenosis murmur 666
Shock, absence of 756
Short QT syndrome 320
Shy-Drager syndrome 498
Sick sinus syndrome 282
Signs
  and symptoms of myocarditis 724
  of congestive heart failure 168
Sildenafil 28
  treatment 532
Simultaneous jugular venous pressure
    tracings 637f
Single photon emission computed
    tomography 167, 169, 773
Sinoatrial
  nodal cells 231f
  node 227, 230
  reentry tachycardia 263
Sinus
  arrhythmia 103
  node disease 282
  tachycardia 262
  venosus 672
Sirolimus 576
Sistrurus miliarius barbouri 68
Skeletal muscle changes in heart
    failure 560t
Skin
  abnormalities and cardiovascular
      disorders 76t
  temperature 827
Small
  molecule tyrosine kinase
      inhibitors 627
  vessel ischemia 594f
Smallest measurable orifice 146
Smooth muscle vasodilators 468
Snowman appearance of mediastinal
    structures 693f
Sodium
  bicarbonate 2f
  calcium exchanger 292
  channel
    blockers 237
    gene 293
Sotalol 235, 237, 241, 242
Specific activity scale 73t
Spectrum of cardiovascular disease in
    chronic kidney disease 734
Spiral computerized tomographic
    pulmonary arteriography 752f
Spironolactone 1, 7, 25, 26
Spondyloarthropathies 721
SQT syndrome 293
Stable
  angina 70, 72t, 336
  coronary artery disease 775
Stages of heart failure 791t
Staphylococcus aureus 736
  causing acute endocarditis 417
Starr-Edwards caged-ball
    valve 435f
Statin therapy 766
ST-elevation myocardial infarction 347t,
    707
Stem cell transplantation 621
Stereotactic radiosurgery 745
Sterile vegetation 418
Sternocleidomastoid muscle 78f
Straight back syndrome 77
Strain
  derived indices 135
  pattern 110
Streptococcus and *Streptococcus bovis* 449
Stress
  cardiomyopathy 729, 730
  echo and myocardial viability 154
  echocardiography 150
  induced
    cardiomyopathy 608, 729

perfusion abnormality
  assessment 773
 wall motion abnormality
  assessment 774
 test 597, 737
Stroke 795
 volume 123, 179
Structural
 disease 255
 heart disease 254
 valve
  assessment 161
  deterioration 448
ST-segment elevation myocardial
 infarction 360
Subarachnoid hemorrhage 727f, 795, 801t
Subclavian artery stenosis 480
 cause of 480
Subclinical atherosclerosis 332
Subcortical infarcts 804
Subcutaneous nodules 814
Subsegmental pulmonary arteries 751
Substances of abuse 572, 705
Subvalvular aortic stenosis 85
Sudden cardiac death 179, 293, 696
Sulfonylureas 703
Superior vena cava 92
Supraceliac aorta 489
Supradiaphragmatic variant of total
 anomalous pulmonary veins 692f
Supravalvar stenosis 409
Supraventricular
 beats 696
 tachycardia 104, 261, 262f, 267t, 728
  classification of 261t
Surrogate measures of atherosclerosis 716
Survival with
 cardiac transplantation 581
 mechanical circulatory support 587
Suture techniques 402
Swiss cheese model for medical
 mistakes 819f
Sympathetic nervous system 22
Symptom of heart failure 500
Symptomatic
 peripheral arterial disease 472f
 systolic heart failure 521
Symptoms
 and myocardial ischemia, assessment
  of 771
 of heart failure 594
 of pericarditis 633
Syncope 75, 243, 781
 causes of 244
 classification of 244
Syndrome of
 heart failure with normal ejection
  fraction 610
 organ hypoperfusion 360

Systemic
 hypotension 539
 inflammatory response syndrome 360
 lupus erythematosus 389, 723, 724
 release of catecholamines 726
 tumor dissemination 149
 vascular resistance 18, 584
Systolic
 anterior motion 595f, 603
 blood pressure 729, 732
 dysfunction 702
  detection of 702
 function in nondiabetics 703
 heart failure 19, 26, 502, 502f, 508t,
  514, 515t, 520, 520t, 523
  management 520t
  remodeling 515t
 murmur 84, 404, 404f
 time ratio 91

T

Tachyarrhythmias 592, 781
Tachycardia induced cardiomyopathy 607
Tacrolimus 576
Tadalafil 28
Takotsubo cardiomyopathy 729
Taurine 831
Telmisartan 25
Tendon xanthoma 77
Tenecteplase 345
Terazosin 468
Tetrahydrocannabinol 710
Tetralogy of Fallot 321, 683, 685f-688f,
 689
Thiamine 832
Thiazide 6, 8, 11, 463, 544
 diuretic 8, 523
Thiazolidinediones 791
Thienopyridines 221
Third-degree AV block 283
Thoracic aortic aneurysms and
 dissections 483
Three-dimensional echocardiography
 preballoon mitral valvotomy 387f
Thrombin receptor antagonists 67
Thromboembolic and bleeding
 complications 444
Thrombolysis 345, 755
 in myocardial infarction 336, 343, 714
Thrombomodulin 749
Thrombosis 189
 management 587
Thrombotic valve complications 455
Thyroid
 disease 742
 stimulating hormone 742
Ticagrelor 339
TIMI risk score 336t

Index

Timolol 465
Tirofiban 68
Tissue inhibitors of metalloproteinases 528
Toe-brachial index 474
Torsade de pointes 777
Torsemide 1, 7, 536, 658
Total anomalous pulmonary venous return 691
Trace tricuspid regurgitation 197
Traditional
    CHD risk factors 328
    Chinese medicine 823
Trandolapril 25
Transaortic
    jet velocity 376f
    septal myectomy 602
Transcutaneous
    aortic valve implantation 373, 375f
    energy transfer system, development of 590
Transesophageal echocardiography 148, 156, 158, 158f, 159f, 160, 162f-164f, 183, 399
    image of tricuspid valve 400f
Transient
    ischemic attack 453, 800t, 801t
    throat pain 156
Transmitral flow during atrial systole 137f
Transpulmonary gradient 648
Transthoracic echocardiography 139, 144, 156
Transverse aorta 669f
Treadmill stress testing 384
Treatment of
    acute
        hemorrhagic stroke 807
        ischemic stroke 805, 806t
    cardiorenal syndrome 541
    comorbid diseases 809
    end-stage heart failure 568
    heart failure 522t
    hyperlipidemia in HIV-infected individuals 716f
    hypertension 827
    orthostatic hypotension/intolerance 499
    pulmonary arterial hypertension 657, 662
    secondary mitral regurgitation 396
    strep tonsillopharyngitis 815t
    symptomatic orthostatic hypotension 499
    underlying amyloid disease 621
Trendelenburg position 266
Triamterene 1, 2, 7, 464
Tricuspid
    insufficiency 100
    regurgitation 84, 86, 147, 164f, 197, 398f, 401, 595f, 654f, 655f
    stenosis 84, 88, 89t, 147, 197, 401
    valve 82f, 398f
        closure sound 82f
        disease 397
        obstruction 79
        repair versus replacement 402t
        replacement 401
Triglyceride lowering therapy 52
Trimetazidine 703, 704
Trimethoprim sulfamethoxazole 577
Tropheryma whippelei 422
Tropical endomyocardial fibrosis 612
Troponin 333, 335
Truncus arteriosus 690, 690f
Turner's syndrome 77
Types of
    diastolic dysfunction 136
    prevention with RF/RHD 817
    prosthetic valves 434
    rejection 578t
    stents 223
    transmitral flow 137f
Tyrosine kinase inhibitors 792

U

Ulceration of proximal segment of internal carotid artery 804f
Ultrasmall superparamagnetic iron oxide 186
Uncontrolled hypertension 554
Unfractionated heparin 55, 222, 339, 441
Unstable angina 168, 333
Uremia 736
Urosemide 1
Use of
    amlodipine 523
    automatic external defibrillators 314

V

Vagal tone 281
Vagus nerve 498
Valsalva maneuver 159, 266, 495
Valsartan 25
Valvar pulmonic stenosis 403, 408, 670
Valve
    replacement 402
    thrombosis 455
Valvular
    disease 177, 788
    heart disease 98, 145, 182, 369, 402t, 452t, 736, 763
Valvuloplasty and valve repair 455
Vancomycin plus gentamicin 426
Vascular
    complications 217
    disease 458, 572, 786
    endothelial growth factor 188
    pedicle 98f
        assessment of 98f

Vasodilator drugs and low blood pressure 19
Vasopressin 316, 463
Vasoreactivity testing 657
Vaughan-Williams classification 235
 of antiarrhythmic drugs 235t
VCO_2 *See* Carbon dioxide production
Velocity
 encoding 182
 time integral 134
Venous
 oxygen content, determinants of 124
 stasis 749
 thromboembolism 54, 749
 thrombosis 798
Ventricles endomyocardial fibrosis 612
Ventricular
 arrhythmias 366
 assist devices, classification of 582t
 fibrillation 319, 350, 600f
 myocardial cells 102
 premature beat 390
 pressures 192
 remodeling 514, 526
 septa 84
 septal defect 666, 674, 686f
  classification of site of 675f
 septal
  myectomy 602
  rupture 361, 362
 tachycardia 234, 271t, 319, 600, 764
Ventrolateral medulla 494f
Verapamil 242, 267
Verrucous lesions 725
Very low-density lipoproteins 824

Viridans group streptococci 420
Visual qualitative indicators of systolic dysfunction 135
Vitamin K
 antagonists 58
 epoxide reductase 59f
Volume oxygen consumption 121
Vomiting 460
Von Recklinghausen disease 649
Von Willebrand factor 706, 741
 factor complex 746
Vorapaxar 67
VSDS, classification of 674

W

Waldenstrom's macroglobulinemia 749
Water bottle configuration 100, 100f
Waterston shunt 683, 684f
Wellen's syndrome 334, 335f
Wenckebach second degree AV block 106
Whipple's disease 422, 721
Wilkins valve score 411
Williams-Beuren syndrome 409
Wolff-Parkinson-White
 anomaly 108
 syndrome 116, 126, 265, 321, 781
Worsening renal function 534

X

Xanthomatosis 77

Z

Zofenopril 25